New Therapeutic Agents in Thrombosis and Thrombolysis

FUNDAMENTAL AND CLINICAL CARDIOLOGY

Editor-in-Chief

Samuel Z. Goldhaber, M.D.

*Harvard Medical School
and Brigham and Women's Hospital
Boston, Massachusetts*

Associate Editor, Europe

Henri Bounameaux, M.D.

*University Hospital of Geneva
Geneva, Switzerland*

1. *Drug Treatment of Hyperlipidemia*, edited by Basil M. Rifkind
2. *Cardiotonic Drugs: A Clinical Review, Second Edition, Revised and Expanded,* edited by Carl V. Leier
3. *Complications of Coronary Angioplasty*, edited by Alexander J. R. Black, H. Vernon Anderson, and Stephen G. Ellis
4. *Unstable Angina*, edited by John D. Rutherford
5. *Beta-Blockers and Cardiac Arrhythmias*, edited by Prakash C. Deedwania
6. *Exercise and the Heart in Health and Disease*, edited by Roy J. Shephard and Henry S. Miller, Jr.
7. *Cardiopulmonary Physiology in Critical Care*, edited by Steven M. Scharf
8. *Atherosclerotic Cardiovascular Disease, Hemostasis, and Endothelial Function*, edited by Robert Boyer Francis, Jr.
9. *Coronary Heart Disease Prevention*, edited by Frank G. Yanowitz
10. *Thrombolysis and Adjunctive Therapy for Acute Myocardial Infarction*, edited by Eric R. Bates
11. *Stunned Myocardium: Properties, Mechanisms, and Clinical Manifestations*, edited by Robert A. Kloner and Karin Przyklenk
12. *Prevention of Venous Thromboembolism*, edited by Samuel Z. Goldhaber
13. *Silent Myocardial Ischemia and Infarction: Third Edition*, Peter F. Cohn
14. *Congestive Cardiac Failure: Pathophysiology and Treatment*, edited by David B. Barnett, Hubert Pouleur, and Gary S. Francis
15. *Heart Failure: Basic Science and Clinical Aspects*, edited by Judith K. Gwathmey, G. Maurice Briggs, and Paul D. Allen
16. *Coronary Thrombolysis in Perspective: Principles Underlying Conjunctive and Adjunctive Therapy*, edited by Burton E. Sobel and Désiré Collen
17. *Cardiovascular Disease in the Elderly Patient*, edited by Donald D. Tresch and Wilbert S. Aronow
18. *Systemic Cardiac Embolism*, edited by Michael D. Ezekowitz
19. *Low-Molecular-Weight Heparins in Prophylaxis and Therapy of Thromboembolic Diseases*, edited by Henri Bounameaux
20. *Valvular Heart Diseases*, edited by Muayed Al Zaibag and Carlos M. G. Duran
21. *Implantable Cardioverter-Defibrillators: A Comprehensive Textbook*, edited by N. A. Mark Estes III, Antonis S. Manolis, and Paul J. Wang
22. *Individualized Therapy of Hypertension*, edited by Norman M. Kaplan and C. Venkata S. Ram

ADDITIONAL VOLUMES IN PREPARATION

New Therapeutic Agents in Thrombosis and Thrombolysis

Second Edition, Revised and Expanded

edited by

Arthur A. Sasahara

Brigham and Women's Hospital and
Harvard Medical School
Boston, Massachusetts, U.S.A.

Joseph Loscalzo

Boston University Medical Center,
Whitaker Cardiovascular Institute, and
Boston University School of Medicine
Boston, Massachusetts, U.S.A.

MARCEL DEKKER, INC.   NEW YORK · BASEL

ISBN: 0-8247-0795-8

This book is printed on acid-free paper.

Headquarters
Marcel Dekker, Inc.
270 Madison Avenue, New York, NY 10016
tel: 212-696-9000; fax: 212-685-4540

Eastern Hemisphere Distribution
Marcel Dekker AG
Hutgasse 4, Postfach 812, CH-4001 Basel, Switzerland
tel: 41-61-260-6300; fax: 41-61-260-6333

World Wide Web
http://www.dekker.com

The publisher offers discounts on this book when ordered in bulk quantities. For more information, write to
Special Sales/Professional Marketing at the headquarters address above.

Current printing (last digit):
10 9 8 7 6 5 4 3 2 1

PRINTED IN THE UNITED STATES OF AMERICA

Series Introduction

Marcel Dekker, Inc., has focused on the development of various series of beautifully produced books in different branches of medicine. These series have facilitated the integration of rapidly advancing information for both the clinical specialist and the researcher.

My goal as editor-in-chief of the Fundamental and Clinical Cardiology series is to assemble the talents of world-renowned authorities to discuss virtually every area of cardiovascular medicine. In this second edition of *New Therapeutic Agents in Thrombosis and Thrombolysis*, Arthur A. Sasahara and Joseph Loscalzo have edited a much-needed and timely book. Future contributions to this series will include books on molecular biology, interventional cardiology, and clinical management of such problems as coronary artery disease and ventricular arrhythmias.

Samuel Z. Goldhaber

Preface

Since the publication of the first edition of *New Therapeutic Agents in Thrombosis and Thrombolysis* book five years ago, our understanding of the determinants of the hemostatic cascade has evolved considerably. We continue to learn more about the intricacies of the primary and secondary hemostatic and fibrinolytic pathways, and to be surprised at or disappointed with the results of the clinical applications of different agents targeted to these pathways. Recently, there has been a flurry of activity in developing new pharmaceutical agents that target both conventional and newly characterized pathways of hemostasis. These agents, which generally impair coagulation, include low-molecular-weight heparins, direct thrombin inhibitors, tissue factor pathway inhibitors, and an oral form of unfractionated heparin. New agents have been produced to minimize the prothrombotic activity of activated platelets, such as thienopyridines and the glycoprotein IIb/IIIa receptor antagonists. New thrombolytic agents are also being developed and tested to achieve greater efficacy of thrombolysis and to do so with fewer bleeding complications, especially intracranial hemorrhage.

The book is divided into four parts. The first begins with an overview of new developments in hemostasis and thrombolysis, followed by two other useful overviews. The "Design Issues in Clinical Trials" overview reflects the current thinking of the FDA on the development of these new agents. Parts II and III focus on new heparins, thrombin inhibitors, and other new agents. Chapters on low-molecular-weight heparins have been updated based on newer clinical studies, for example, on hirudin, bivalirudin, and protein C. Notably, new chapters have been added on pentasaccharide, TFP1, and soluble thrombomodulin.

In the last part, on thrombolytic agents, additional clinical studies have been included on variants of t-PA, as well as on staphylokinase and prourokinase. Alfimeprase is a new and novel thrombolytic agent that is not a plasminogen activator. The last chapter discusses recent work on thrombolysis enhancement with ultrasound.

We are grateful to our distinguished section editors who remained with us from the first edition: Jeffrey Weitz, Jack Hirsh, James Willerson, and Marc Verstraete. We are also grateful to our new section editors: Robert Giugliano, Shaker Mousa, and Samuel Goldhaber. We also wish to thank Stephanie Tribuna, editorial assistant to Dr. Loscalzo. Special thanks to Sandra Beberman, Vice President, Marcel Dekker, Inc., who convinced us to undertake this second edition, and to Richard Johnson, Production Editor, who gave us continued support throughout the process.

Arthur A. Sasahara
Joseph Loscalzo

Contents

Contents

PART III.   New Antiplatelet Agents

PART IV.   New Thrombolytic Agents

Contributors

Walter Ageno, M.D.   Assistant Professor of Medicine, Ospedale di Circolo, University of Insubria, Varese, Italy

Sarfraz Ahmad, Ph.D.   Assistant Professor, Department of Thoracic and Cardiovascular Surgery, Loyola University Medical Center, Maywood, Illinois, U.S.A.

Manuela Albisetti, M.D.   University Children's Hospital, Zurich, Switzerland

Maureen Andrew, M.D.[†]   Director, Thrombosis Service, The Hospital for Sick Children, Toronto, Ontario, Canada

Elliott M. Antman, M.D.   Associate Professor of Medicine, Cardiovascular Division, Brigham and Women's Hospital, Boston, Massachusetts, U.S.A.

Deepak L. Bhatt, M.D.   Director, Interventional Cardiology, Department of Cardiovascular Medicine, Cleveland Clinic Foundation, Cleveland, Ohio, U.S.A.

Christoph Bode, M.D.   Professor and Chairman of Medicine, Department of Cardiology and Angiology, University of Freiburg, Freiburg, Germany

Sandra E. Burke, Ph.D.   Research and Development, Hospital Products Division, Abbott Laboratories, Abbott Park, Illinois, U.S.A.

[†] Deceased.

Robert M. Califf, M.D. Donald F. Fortin Professor, Department of Cardiology; Associate Vice Chancellor for Clinical Research; and Director, Duke Clinical Research Institute, Duke University Medical Center, Durham, North Carolina, U.S.A.

Wee Shian Chan, M.D. Assistant Professor, Department of Medicine, University of Toronto, Toronto, Ontario, Canada

Richard Y. Chin, M.D. Associate Director, Department of Biotherapeutics, Genentech, Inc., South San Francisco, and Clinical Instructor, Department of Internal Medicine, Stanford University Medical School, Palo Alto, California, U.S.A.

Désiré Collen, M.D., Ph.D. Professor of Medicine and Director, Center for Molecular and Vascular Biology, Catholic University of Leuven, Leuven, Belgium

R. Bruce Credo, Ph.D. Cancer Research, Global Pharmaceutical Research and Development, Abbott Laboratories, Abbott Park, Illinois, U.S.A.

Mark A. Crowther, M.D. Associate Professor, Department of Medicine, McMaster University, Hamilton, Ontario, Canada

Peter Donner, Ph.D. Head, Protein Chemistry Department, Institute of Cellular and Molecular Biology, Schering AG, Berlin, Germany

John W. Eikelboom, M.B.B.S., M.Sc., F.R.A.C.P., F.R.C.P.A. Department of Medicine, University of Western Australia, Perth, Australia

Charles T. Esmon, Ph.D. Head, Cardiovascular Research Program, Oklahoma Medical Research Foundation, and Investigator, Howard Hughes Medical Institute, Oklahoma City, Oklahoma, U.S.A.

Jawed Fareed, Ph.D. Professor of Pathology and Pharmacology, Loyola University Medical Center, Maywood, Illinois, U.S.A.

Charles W. Francis, M.D. Professor of Medicine, Department of Pathology and Laboratory Medicine, University of Rochester Medical Center, Rochester, New York, U.S.A.

John K. French, B.Med.Sci., M.B., Ch.B., M.Sc. Deputy Director of Coronary Care and Cardiovascular Research, Department of Cardiology, Green Lane Hospital, Auckland, New Zealand

William H. Geerts, M.D. Associate Professor of Medicine, University of Toronto, Toronto, Ontario, Canada

Jeffrey S. Ginsberg, M.D. Professor, Department of Medicine, McMaster University, Hamilton, Ontario, Canada

Robert P. Giugliano, M.D. Assistant Professor of Medicine, Harvard Medical School, and Cardiovascular Division, Brigham and Women's Hospital, Boston, Massachusetts, U.S.A.

Samuel Z. Goldhaber, M.D.   Associate Professor, Department of Medicine, Harvard Medical School and Chief, Thromboembolism and Anticoagulation Services, Cardiovascular Division, Brigham and Women's Hospital, Boston, Massachusetts, U.S.A.

Victor Gurewich, M.D.   Professor of Medicine, Harvard Medical School and Director, Vascular Research Laboratory, Beth Israel Deaconess Medical Center, Boston, Massachusetts, U.S.A.

Robert A. Harrington, M.D.   Associate Professor of Medicine, Duke Clinical Research Institute, Duke University Medical Center, Durham, North Carolina, U.S.A.

Kohki Hayamizu, M.S.   Ethical Products Marketing Department, Sales and Marketing Division, Yamanouchi Pharmaceutical Company, Ltd., Ibaraki, Japan

Jack Henkin, Ph.D.   Cancer Research, Global Pharmaceutical Research and Development, Abbott Laboratories, Abbott Park, Illinois, U.S.A.

Jack Hirsh, M.D.   Professor of Medicine, Emeritus, McMaster University, and Director, Henderson Research Center, Hamilton, Ontario, Canada

Debra A. Hoppensteadt, Ph.D.   Assistant Professor, Department of Pathology, Loyola University Medical Center, Maywood, Illinois, U.S.A.

Russell D. Hull, M.B.B.S., M.Sc.   Professor, Department of Medicine, University of Calgary, Calgary, Alberta, Canada

Omer Iqbal, M.D.   Assistant Professor, Department of Pathology, Loyola University Medical Center, Maywood, Illinois, U.S.A.

Richard M. Jay, M.D.   Assistant Professor of Medicine, University of Toronto, Toronto, Ontario, Canada

Walter P. Jeske, Ph.D.   Assistant Professor of Thoracic and Cardiovascular Surgery and Pathology, Loyola University Medical Center, Maywood, Illinois, U.S.A.

Brigitte Kaiser, M.D.   Associate Professor, Center for Vascular Biology and Medicine, Friedrich Schiller University of Jena, Erfurt, Germany

Ajay K. Kakkar, M.B.B.S., B.Sc., Ph.D.   Consultant Surgeon and Senior Lecturer, Hammersmith Hospital, Imperial College, London, England

Masao Katoh, Ph.D.   Molecular Medicine Laboratories, Institute for Drug Discovery Research, Yamanouchi Pharmaceutical Company, Ltd., Ibaraki, Japan

Chuichi Kawai, M.D.   Professor Emeritus, Kyoto University, and Director, Takeda General Hospital, Kyoto, Japan

Tomihisa Kawasaki, Ph.D.   Pharmacology Laboratories, Institute for Drug Discovery Research, Yamanouchi Pharmaceutical Company, Ltd., Ibaraki, Japan

Konstantinos Konstantopoulos, Ph.D.   Department of Chemical Engineering, Johns Hopkins University, Baltimore, Maryland, U.S.A.

Bruce E. Lewis, M.D.   Associate Professor of Medicine, Loyola University Medical Center, Maywood, Illinois, U.S.A.

H. Roger Lijnen, Ph.D.   Professor and Adjunct-Director, Center for Molecular and Vascular Biology, Catholic University of Leuven, Leuven, Belgium

A. Michael Lincoff, M.D.   Associate Professor of Medicine, Department of Cardiovascular Medicine, Cleveland Clinic Foundation, Cleveland, Ohio, U.S.A.

Jian-ning Liu, Ph.D.   Professor, Institute of Molecular Medicine, Nanjing University, Nanjing, China

Joseph Loscalzo, M.D., Ph.D.   Wade Professor and Chairman, Department of Medicine; Professor of Biochemistry; and Director, Whitaker Cardiovascular Institute, Boston University School of Medicine, Boston, Massachusetts, U.S.A.

Steven Mack, Pharm.D.   Senior Specialist, Department of Medical Information, Centocor, Inc., Malvern, Pennsylvania, U.S.A.

John M. Maraganore, Ph.D.   Senior Vice-President, Strategic Product Development, Millennium Pharmaceuticals, Cambridge, Massachusetts, U.S.A.

Victor J. Marder, M.D.   Professor of Medicine, David Geffen School of Medicine at UCLA, and Director, Vascular Medicine, Los Angeles Orthopedic Hospital, Los Angeles, California, U.S.A.

Ulrich Martin, M.D.   Chief Executive Officer, Scil Biomedicals GmbH, Martinsried, Germany

Edward R. McCluskey, M.D., Ph.D.   Senior Clinical Scientist, Department of Medical Affairs, Genentech, Inc., South San Francisco, California, U.S.A.

Shamir R. Mehta, M.D.   Assistant Professor, Department of Medicine, and Director, Coronary Care, McMaster University, Hamilton, Ontario, Canada

Harry L. Messmore, M.D.   Professor of Medicine, Emeritus, Loyola University Medical Center, Maywood, Illinois, U.S.A.

Paul A. Minella, Pharm.D.   Assistant Professor of Pharmacy, University of Florida College of Pharmacy, Gainesville, Florida, and Manager, Medical Information, Centocor, Inc., Malvern, Pennsylvania, U.S.A.

Joel L. Moake, M.D.   Professor, Hematology-Oncology Section, Department of Medicine, Baylor College of Medicine, and Associate Director, Biomedical Engineering Laboratory, Rice University, Houston, Texas, U.S.A.

Mitsunobu Mohri, Ph.D. Institute for Life Science Research, Asahi Kasei Corporation, Oh-hito, Tagata, Japan

David A. Morrow, M.D. Cardiovascular Division, Brigham and Women's Hospital, Boston, Massachusetts, U.S.A.

Shaker A. Mousa, Ph.D., M.B.A. Professor of Pharmacology, Albany College of Pharmacy, Albany, New York, U.S.A.

J. Conor O'Shea, M.D. Department of Cardiology, Duke Clinical Research Institute, Duke University Medical Center, Durham, North Carolina, U.S.A.

Karlheinz Peter, M.D. Associate Professor of Medicine, Department of Cardiology and Angiology, University of Freiburg, Freiburg, Germany

Gloria Petralia, M.D. Clinical Research Fellow, Hammersmith Hospital, Imperial College, London, England

Graham F. Pineo, M.D. Professor, Departments of Medicine and Oncology, University of Calgary, Calgary, Alberta, Canada

Victor F. C. Raczkowski, M.D., M.S. Acting Deputy Director, Division of Clinical Trial Design and Analysis, U.S. Food and Drug Administration, Rockville, Maryland, U.S.A.

Canio J. Refino, B.S. Department of Physiology, Genentech, Inc., South San Francisco, California, U.S.A.

Dwaine Rieves, M.D. Medical Officer, Division of Clinical Trial Design and Analysis, U.S. Food and Drug Administration, Rockville, Maryland, U.S.A.

M. Michel Samama, M.D. Professor, Laboratoire Central d'Hematologie, Hôtel-Dieu Hospital, Paris, France

Arthur A. Sasahara, M.D. Professor of Medicine, Emeritus, Harvard Medical School, and Senior Physician, Cardiovascular Division, Brigham and Women's Hospital, Boston, Massachusetts, U.S.A.

Andrew I. Schafer, M.D. Department of Medicine, Baylor College of Medicine, and Department of Internal Medicine, The Methodist Hospital, Houston, Texas, U.S.A.

Wolf-Dieter Schleuning, M.D.* Scientific Director, Preclinical Drug Research, Schering AG, Berlin, Germany.

Debra A. Schuerr, M.Tech Vascular Medicine Team, Hospital Products Division, Abbott Laboratories, Abbott Park, Illinois, U.S.A.

---

* *Current affiliation*: Professor, PAION GmbH Research Center, Berlin, Germany.

Gregory A. Schulz, M.S.   Vascular Medicine Team, Hospital Products Division, Abbott Laboratories, Abbott Park, Illinois, U.S.A.

Peter J. Sharis, M.D.   Division of Cardiology, Department of Medicine, Beth Israel Deaconess Medical Center, Boston, Massachusetts, U.S.A.

Jay P. Siegel, M.D.   Director, Office of Therapeutics Research and Review, Center for Biologics Evaluation and Research, U.S. Food and Drug Administration, Rockville, Maryland, U.S.A.

Peter Sinnaeve, M.D.   Staff Scientist, Center for Molecular and Vascular Biology, Catholic University of Leuven, Leuven, Belgium

Jean Marie Stassen, Ph.D.   Thromb-X, N.V., Leuven, Belgium

Dina S. Stolman, M.D., M.S.P.H.   Associate Director, Department of Medical Affairs, GloboMax LLC, Hanover, Maryland

Valentina Suchkova, M.D., Ph.D.   Assistant Professor, Department of Medicine, University of Rochester Medical Center, Rochester, New York, U.S.A.

Masanori Suzuki, Ph.D.   Pharmacology Laboratories, Institute for Drug Discovery Research, Yamanouchi Pharmaceutical Company, Ltd., Ibaraki, Japan

Suguru Suzuki, Ph.D.   Senior Scientist, Tsukuba Research Laboratories, Eisai Company, Ltd., Tsukuba, Japan

James E. Tcheng, M.D.   Associate Professor of Medicine, Department of Cardiology, Duke Clinical Research Institute, Duke University Medical Center, Durham, North Carolina, U.S.A.

Christopher F. Toombs, Ph.D.   Product Development, Amgen, Inc., Thousand Oaks, California, U.S.A.

Alexander G. G. Turpie, M.D.   Professor, Department of Medicine, McMaster University and Hamilton Health Sciences Corporation, Hamilton, Ontario, Canada

Marc Verstraete, M.D., Ph.D.   Professor of Medicine, Center for Molecular and Vascular Biology, University of Leuven, Leuven, Belgium

Jeanine M. Walenga, Ph.D.   Professor, Thoracic and Cardiovascular Surgery and Pathology, Loyola University Medical Center, Maywood, Illinois, U.S.A.

Michael Waller, M.D.   Senior Director, Department of Clinical Research, Centocor, Inc., Malvern, Pennsylvania, U.S.A.

Bruce A. Wallin, M.D.   Head, Vascular Medicine Team, Hospital Products Division, Abbott Laboratories, Abbott Park, Illinois, U.S.A.

Marc K. Walton, M.D., Ph.D. Chief, General Medicine Branch, U.S. Food and Drug Administration, Rockville, Maryland, U.S.A.

Jeffrey I. Weitz, M.D. Professor of Medicine, McMaster University, and Director, of Experimental Thrombosis and Atherosclerosis Group, Henderson Research Center, Hamilton, Ontario, Canada

Harvey D. White, D.Sc. Director, Coronary Care and Cardiovascular Research, Department of Cardiology, Green Lane Hospital, Auckland, New Zealand

James T. Willerson, M.D. President, University of Texas Health Science Center at Houston, and Medical Director, Texas Heart Institute, Houston, Texas, U.S.A.

Salim Yusuf, M.B.B.S., D.Phil. Professor, Division of Cardiology, Department of Medicine, McMaster University, Hamilton, Ontario, Canada

Thomas F. Zioncheck, Ph.D. Director, Department of Clinical and Experimental Pharmacology, Genentech, Inc., South San Francisco, California, U.S.A.

New Therapeutic Agents
in Thrombosis
and Thrombolysis

Overview of Hemostasis and Fibrinolysis

Joseph Loscalzo
Whitaker Cardiovascular Institute, Boston University School of Medicine, Boston, Massachusetts, U.S.A.

Andrew I. Schafer
Baylor College of Medicine and The Methodist Hospital, Houston, Texas, U.S.A.

SUMMARY

Hemostasis and fibrinolysis represent the principal mechanisms for arresting the flow of blood at sites of injury and restoring vascular patency during wound healing, respectively. Under normal circumstances, primary hemostasis (platelet–vessel wall interactions), secondary hemostasis (fibrin formation), and fibrinolysis act in concert to orchestrate these responses. Both during normal hemostasis and (pathological) thrombosis, all three mechanisms become activated simultaneously. The complex regulatory mechanisms that govern the activity of thrombin and of plasmin within the evolving clot or thrombus dictate the net result of the process. The finely tuned interactions among these complex processes have evolved to optimize maintenance of blood fluidity under normal circumstances and rapid cessation of blood flow when vascular integrity has been violated. The equally complex regulatory mechanisms provided both by the endothelial cell and by the plasma milieu limit the extent of these reactions to focus protective hemostasis to the narrowly defined vascular domain in which it is required, without compromising blood flow elsewhere in the vasculature. It is important to recognize that the fine balance between hemostasis and thrombosis and between fibrinolysis and hemorrhage can be readily perturbed, despite the multiple redundancies built into the system. Thus, all antithrombotic or fibrinolytic therapies must be developed, fully cognizant of their potential risks in this important attribute. In the following chapters, specific antithrombotic targets and therapies will be described, and their efficacy and safety profiles considered in detail.

I. INTRODUCTION

Mammalian vascular systems are confronted with two opposing requirements to ensure the viability of the organism: tissue perfusion must be maintained at all times, and hemorrhage must be quickly arrested at sites of vessel injury. Endothelial cells, which line the intimal surface of the entire cardiovascular system, play a central role in maintaining blood fluidity under normal circumstances. At the same time, platelets and the coagulation system are poised to respond quickly to a loss of vascular integrity by promoting the rapid formation of a protective hemostatic plug at sites of injury. Following clot stabilization, local reparative processes restore normal vascular architecture, and the fibrinolytic system reestablishes patency of the vascular lumen. In the setting of endothelial dysfunction or frank vascular disease, the normal subtle balance between endothelial determinants of perfusion and hematological determinants of hemostasis can be perturbed, leading to thrombosis or inappropriate hemostasis. In this overview, we will discuss normal mechanisms of hemostasis and fibrinolysis as a background for the subsequent discussions of selected antithrombotic and fibrinolytic pharmacotherapies for thrombotic disorders.

II. PRIMARY HEMOSTASIS

Platelets respond to vascular injury by first adhering to the subendothelial matrix as a monolayer of cells. The adhesion of platelets to the matrix is mediated by von Willebrand factor, a polymeric plasma glycoprotein that links platelets through their surface glycoprotein Ib/IX receptors to matrix collagen, and by direct association with matrix collagen through their surface glycoprotein Ia/IIa receptors (Fig. 1). Following adhesion, platelets release the contents of their granules and synthesize thromboxane A_2 from arachidonic acid. Released granule contents,

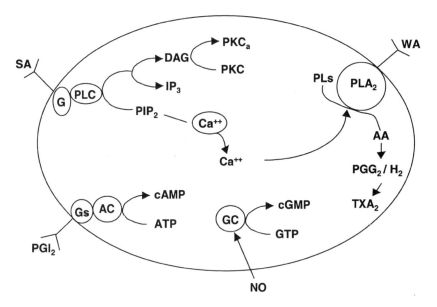

Figure 1 Pathways of platelet activation and inhibition; abbreviations: SA, strong agonist; WA, weak agonist; G, G protein; Gs, adenylate cyclase stimulatory G protein; PIP_2, phosphatidylinositol biphosphate; DAG, diacylglycerol; IP_3, inositol triphosphate; PKC, protein kinase C; PKC_a, activated protein kinase C; PLA_2, phospholipase A_2; AA, arachidonic acid; PGG_2, prostaglandin G_2; PGH_2, prostaglandin H_2; PLs, membrane phospholipids; TXA_2, thromboxane A_2; PLC, phospholipase C; AC, adenylyl cyclase; GC, guanylyl cyclase; NO, nitric oxide; ATP, adenosine triphosphate; GTP, guanosine trisphosphate; cAMP, cyclic adenosine monophosphate; cGMP, cyclic guanosine monophosphate; PGI_2; prostaglandin I_2.

including adenosine diphosphate and serotonin, act in conjunction with thromboxane A_2, to recruit additional platelets to the site of vascular injury. Platelet–platelet interactions within the growing hemostatic plug are mediated by the binding of bivalent fibrinogen to the platelet surface integrin heterodimer glycoprotein IIb/IIIa. The glycoprotein IIb/IIIa complex as a functional fibrinogen receptor is expressed only on the surfaces of activated platelets. Importantly, under conditions of increased shear stress (e.g., diseased coronary arteries), von Willebrand factor preferentially binds to glycoprotein IIb/IIIa in place of fibrinogen.

Throughout its lifetime in the circulation, the platelet is exposed to a variety of external signals that regulate its state of activation [1–3]. Most of these signals mediate their effects on the platelet by binding to surface receptors and initiating a complex series of amplifying mechanisms that transduce these external signals into cellular responses. Many ligand–receptor interactions first transmit information by activating a family of G proteins, which are themselves activated by guanosine triphosphate (GTP). The G proteins, in turn, activate other amplifying enzymes associated with the inner aspect of the platelet surface's membrane bilayer that convert precursor molecules into intracellular second messengers.

Many agonists that activate platelets evoke their responses by a signal–transduction mechanism that involves activation of phospholipase C. This enzyme converts phosphatidy-linositol biphosphate (PIP_2) into diacylglycerol, which activates protein kinase C, and inositol triphosphate (IP_3), which translocates calcium ions from intracellular organelles to the cytosol. An increase in cytosolic free calcium ions initiates actomyosin ATPase activity, resulting in platelet shape change. Increased cytosolic free calcium also activates phospholipase A_2, which cleaves arachidonic acid from the second backbone carbon of membrane phospholipids. Platelet cyclooxygenase, in turn, converts arachidonic acid to cyclic endoperoxides (prostaglandin G_2 and prostaglandin H_2); thromboxane synthase then converts these endoperoxides into thromboxane A_2. Two isoforms of cyclooxygenase, COX-1 and COX-2, are encoded by separate genes. Inducible COX-2 is involved in inflammation, cellular differentiation, and mitogenesis. COX-1 is the constitutive isoform that is present in platelets and serves the "housekeeping" functions of vascular homeostasis and hemostasis. The COX-1 platelet products, prostaglandin G_2, prostaglandin H_2, and thromboxane A_2, are potent vasoconstrictors and platelet activators. By binding to their specific platelet surface receptors, they activate platelet G proteins coupled to phospholipase C, thereby completing a positive feedback loop in the activation process. So-called strong platelet agonists, such as thrombin, activate phospholipase C directly, while weak agonists, such as epinephrine, activate phospholipase A_2 and thereby activate phospholipase C only indirectly through the generation of endogenous thromboxane A_2. Adenosine diphosphate (ADP), another weak agonist, is released from platelet granules and binds to specific ADP receptors on platelet surfaces. In addition to these humoral or biochemical stimuli, fluid shear stress also induces platelet activation directly, possibly through other signal transduction pathways.

A separate class of platelet inhibitors exerts effects through inhibitory signal transduction pathways. These platelet inhibitors are generally elaborated by intact endothelial cells, contributing to the thromboresistant properties of normal vascular intima. Two of these intracellular-signaling molecules predominate: cyclic adenosine monophosphate (cAMP) and cyclic guanosine monophosphate (cGMP). Increases in these cyclic nucleotides impair or reverse platelet activation by inhibiting PIP_2 hydrolysis, calcium mobilization from internal storage granules, arachidonic acid release from membrane phospholipid pools, and the platelets' shape change and secretion.

The primary extracellular molecule that increases platelet cAMP is prostaglandin I_2 [4]. Prostaglandin I_2, a normal product of the endothelial metabolism of arachidonic acid, binds to specific platelet surface receptors associated with G proteins (G_s) that activate adenylyl cyclase, which converts ATP to cAMP. Importantly, many platelet agonists are coupled to G proteins (G_i) that inhibit adenylyl cyclase activation and cAMP formation.

The major molecule that increases cGMP is nitric oxide (NO) [5]. Synthesized by the normal endothelial cell, nitric oxide (endothelium–derived-relaxing factor) exerts its platelet inhibitory effects not by interacting with a specific surface receptor, but by freely diffusing into the platelet cytosol where it binds to the heme activator site of soluble guanylyl cyclase, thereby activating the enzyme. In addition, nitric oxide inhibits nonspecific cation channels limiting calcium ion entry into the cytosol and inhibits phosphoinositide-3-kinase [6] promoting fibrinogen dissociation from glycoprotein IIb/IIIa and platelet disaggregation. The platelet is itself a source of nitric oxide, and this pool of platelet-derived nitric oxide limits recruitment of platelets to the growing platelet plug or thrombus [7]. An important distinction between prostaglandin I_2 and nitric oxide is that although both inhibit platelet activation, aggregation, and secretion, only the latter can prevent platelet adhesion.

Other physiological platelet-inhibitory molecules are elaborated by endothelial cells under normal circumstances to maintain blood fluidity. For example, ADPase (CD39) is an ectonucleotidase that hydrolyzes and inactivates platelet-stimulatory ADP on the endothelial surface [8].

III. COAGULATION

The term secondary *hemostasis*, or coagulation (Fig. 2), refers to the conversion of soluble fibrinogen into insoluble fibrin. This process occurs by way of an amplifying series of enzymatic

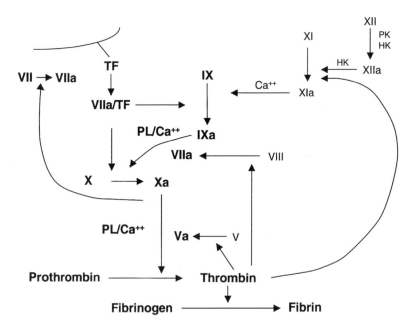

Figure 2 Coagulation pathways; abbreviations used: TF, tissue factor; roman numerals denote specific coagulation factors which, when followed by an "a," indicate their active forms; PK, prekallikrein; HK, high-molecular-weight kininogen; PL, membrane (acidic) phospholipids; Ca^{++}, free ionized calcium. The dominant pathways of coagulation activation are depicted in larger, bolder type; the other reactions are considered to serve more of an amplification role.

reactions in which the product of each reaction converts an inactive plasma protein zymogenic precursor into an active (serine) protease product [9]. Each zymogen is converted to its active form by hydrolysis of one or two peptide bonds. These linked reactions provide dramatic amplification of small initiating stimuli that culminate in rapid and exuberant fibrin formation at sites of vascular injury.

The serine proteases of the coagulation cascade contain a catalytic triad at their active sites, consisting of serine, histidine, and aspartic acid residues, while the peptide bonds required for zymogen activation are located at the carboxyterminal portion of the molecules proximal to the catalytic domains. The conventional view of the coagulation pathway holds that there are two independent pathways converging on the activation of factor X. The intrinsic pathway (factors XII, XI, and IX) is initiated by contact activation, and the extrinsic pathway is activated by tissue factor. Once factor X is activated by either of these two pathways, a common pathway is initiated that leads to thrombin generation and fibrin formation.

This conventional view of coagulation has recently been supplanted by a more complex, but tenable, paradigm in which important interactions between intrinsic and extrinsic pathways are emphasized and by which in vivo correlates are readily explained. Tissue factor, an integral membrane protein of many cell types, is the principal determinant of coagulation in vivo [10]. Although it is not exposed to blood elements under normal circumstances, tissue factor is expressed following injury by activated endothelial cells and leukocytes and is also found constitutively on the surface of subendothelial vascular cells (i.e., smooth-muscle cells and fibroblasts) to which blood is exposed after intimal injury. Tissue factor binds factor VIIa, which exists through low-level endogenous activation in circulating blood, and this interaction leads to a rapid, autocatalytic conversion of factor VII to factor VIIa. The factor VIIa–tissue factor complex can activate factor X, factor IX, or both; factor IXa in conjunction with its cofactor, factor VIIIa, in turn, activates factor X. Importantly, factor Xa can activate additional factor VII, further amplifying the pathway's response.

In the intrinsic pathway, factor XII is converted to XIIa through autoactivation of the protein on negatively charged surfaces; for optimal activation, prekallikrein and high-molecular-weight kininogen are required. Factor XIIa converts factor XI to factor XIa, which, in turn, activates factor IX in a calcium-dependent manner. Analogously, factor IX can be activated by factor XIa or the factor VIIIa–tissue factor complex, and factor X can be activated by factor IXa or the factor VIIa–tissue factor complex.

The sequential activation of coagulation proteins requires their coordinated spatial and temporal assembly, which occurs most efficiently on cell membrane surfaces rather than in fluid-phase plasma. Membrane phospholipids, especially acidic phospholipids, link coagulation proteins through their calcium-binding sites (vitamin K-dependent γ-carboxyglutamic acid residues) to the membrane [11]. Importantly, quiescent cell membranes expose insufficient acidic phospholipids on their surfaces to promote coagulation; following endothelial cell or platelet activation; however, critical surface concentrations of these surface-binding sites are exposed to blood, and assembly of the tenase (Xase) and prothrombinase complexes is facilitated. Factor Xa, generated by membrane-associated tenase complex (factors IXa, VIIIa, and X), diffuses from the complex along the membrane surface to form the prothrombinase complex (factors Va, Xa, and II), which converts prothrombin to thrombin.

Thrombin serves as the central serine protease of the coagulation cascade [12]. Diffusion of thrombin from the membrane site of its generation into blood both converts fibrinogen into fibrin monomer and activates platelets. The activated platelet then provides a membrane surface to activate further the coagulation cascade, generate more thrombin, and thereby amplify and localize the formation of a hemostatic plug. In addition, thrombin sustains the coagulation cascade by feedback activation of other coagulation factors. Once formed, fibrin monomers assemble noncovalently in an end-to-end and side-to-side staggered fashion into fibrin polymers, which form the fibrin clot. Through its activation of factor XIII, thrombin stabilizes the fibrin clot by catalyzing the covalent crosslinking of fibrin polymers through transamidination.

Under normal circumstances, in the absence of vascular injury, activation of the coagulation cascade is suppressed by several physiological antithrombotic (anticoagulant) systems. As with the physiological inhibitors of platelets, these molecules largely depend on the integrity of endothelium. Antithrombin III, a member of the serine protease inhibitor (serpin) class of molecules, inhibits factors XIIa, XIa, IXa, Xa, and thrombin by forming one-to-one complexes with these activated coagulation factors in a reaction catalyzed by glycosaminoglycans, especially heparan sulfate glycosaminoglycans, surface products of the endothelial cell. Heparin cofactor II, another serpin, inhibits thrombin exclusively by a similarly catalyzed mechanism. Tissue factor pathway inhibitor (TFPI) is a lipoprotein-associated coagulation inhibitor that exerts its anticoagulant action by binding to the factor VIIa–tissue factor complex through formation of a quaternary complex with factor Xa. Lastly, activated protein C, in conjunction with its cofactor protein S, retards coagulation by inactivating factors Va and VIIIa. Protein C itself is activated by the action of thrombin when the latter is bound to endothelial cell-surface thrombomodulin.

IV.   FIBRINOLYSIS

The fibrinolytic system (Fig. 3) represents another important endothelium-dependent mechanism for limiting fibrin accumulation [13]. The central molecule of fibrinolysis is plasmin, which is formed from the plasma zymogen plasminogen by the action of endothelial–cell-derived plasminogen activators. Two naturally occurring plasminogen activators exist: tissue-type plasminogen activator (t-PA) and urokinase-type plasminogen activator (u-PA). These enzymes themselves exist in relatively inactive zymogen precursor forms, t-PA as a single-chain species and u-PA as prourokinase. Following the conversion of single-chain t-PA to a two-chain form or of prourokinase to a high-molecular-weight or low-molecular-weight two-chain form, these enzymes convert plasminogen to plasmin by a single peptide bond cleavage. Importantly, t-PA is relatively fibrin selective in that its catalytic efficiency is enhanced several hundredfold after binding to fibrin. Specific cell-surface membrane receptors also facilitate plasminogen activation

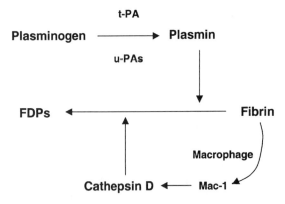

Figure 3 Fibrinolytic pathways; abbreviations: t-PA, tissue-type plasminogen activator; u-PAs, urokinase-type plasminogen activators; FDPs, fibrin(ogen) degradation products; Mac-1, macrophage integrin receptor, CD11b/CD18.

by t-PA and u-PA, and in this way promote degradation of the fibrin clot from the microenvironment of the endothelial cell, macrophage, or platelet surface.

Plasmin, once formed, degrades fibrin into smaller-sized, soluble degradation fragments (FDPs). FDPs themselves have antithrombotic activity owing to their ability to compete with fibrin monomer for fibrin polymer-binding sites and with fibrinogen for platelet-surface glycoprotein IIb/IIIa-binding sites.

Plasminogen activation and plasmin activity are regulated by other members of the serpin class of molecules. α_2-Antiplasmin and plasminogen activator inhibitor (types I and II) inhibit plasmin and plasminogen activators, respectively, by forming one-to-one stoichiometric complexes with the active enzymes.

Another, more recently described pathway for fibrin degradation involves the macrophage [14]. In a series of reactions that first requires the binding of fibrin (monomer) to the pluripotent macrophage integrin Mac-1 (CD 11b/CD) [18], the fibrin(ogen)–Mac-1 complex is next internalized. Once within the macrophage, fibrin is degraded by the action of cathepsin D, a relatively nonselective protease active in the phagolysosome that cleaves fibrin into small, soluble fragments. In contrast to fibrinolysis by plasmin, macrophage-mediated fibrinolysis likely occurs as a later process following fibrin formation during the course of recanalization of the vessel.

REFERENCES

1. Kroll MH, Schafer AI. Biochemical mechanisms of platelet activation. Blood 1989; 74:1181–1195.
2. Andrews RK, Shen Y, Gardiner EE, Dong JF, Lopez JA, Berndt MC. The glycoprotein Ib–IX–V complex in platelet adhesion and signaling. Thromb Haemost 1999; 82:357–364.
3. Shattil SJ. Signaling through platelet integrin alpha IIb beta 3: inside-out, outside-in, and sideways. Thromb Haemost 1999; 82:318–325.
4. Vane JR, Angaard EE, Botting RM. Regulatory functions of the vascular endothelium. N Engl J Med 1990; 323:27–34.
5. Loscalzo J, Welch G. Nitric oxide and the cardiovascular system. Prog Cardiovasc Dis 1995; 38:87–104.
6. Pigazzi A, Heydrick S, Folli F, Benoit S, Michelson A, Loscalzo J. Nitric oxide inhibits thrombin-receptor-activating peptide-induced phosphoinositide 3-kinase activity in human platelets. J Biol Chem 1999; 274:14368–14375.
7. Freedman JE, Sauter R, Battinelli EM, Ault K, Knowles C, Huang PL, Loscalzo J. Deficient platelet-derived nitric oxide and enhanced hemostasis in mice lacking the NOS III gene. Circ Res 1999; 84:1416–1421.
8. Schafer AI. Vascular endothelium: in defense of blood fluidity. J Clin Invest 1997; 99:1143–1144.
9. Furie B, Furie BC. Molecular and cellular biology of blood coagulation. N Engl J Med 1992; 326:800–806.
10. Taubman MB, Giesen PL, Schecter AD, Nemerson Y. Regulation of the procoagulant response to arterial injury. Thromb Haemost 1999; 82:801–805.
11. Zwaal RF, Comfurius P, Bevers EM. Lipid–protein interactions in blood coagulation. Biochim Biophys Acta 1998; 1376:433–453.
12. Coughlin SR. How the protease thrombin talks to cells. Proc Natl Acad Sci USA 1999; 96:11023–11027.
13. Collen D, Lijnen HR. Basic and clinical aspects of fibrinolysis and thrombosis. Blood 1991; 78:3114–3124.
14. Simon DI, Ezratty AM, Francis SA, Rennke H, Loscalzo J. Fibrin(ogen) is internalized and degraded by activated human monocytoid cells via Mac-1 (DC11b/CD18): a non-plasmin fibrinolytic pathway. Blood 1993; 82:2414–2422.

2

A Survey of Animal Models to Develop Novel Antithrombotic Agents

Walter P. Jeske, Omer Iqbal, and Jawed Fareed
Loyola University Medical Center, Maywood, Illinois, U.S.A.

Brigitte Kaiser
Friedrich Schiller University of Jena, Erfurt, Germany

SUMMARY

The development of antithrombotic agents requires preclinical assessment of the biochemical and pharmacological effects of these drugs. It is important to note that the second- and third-generation antithrombotic drugs are devoid of in vitro anticoagulant effects, yet in vivo, by virtue of endogenous interactions, these drugs produce potent antithrombotic actions. The initial belief that an antithrombotic drug must exhibit in vitro anticoagulant activity is no longer valid. This important scientific observation has been possible only because of the availability of animal models.

Several animal models, using species such as rats, rabbits, dogs, pigs, and monkeys, have been made available for routine use. Other animal species, such as the hamster, mouse, cat, and guinea pig, have also been employed. Species variations are an important consideration in selecting a model and interpreting the results, as these variations can result in different antithrombotic effects. Rats and rabbits are the most commonly used species in which both arterial and venous thrombosis have been investigated. Both pharmacological and mechanical means have been used to produce a thrombogenic effect in these models.

Both rat and rabbit models for studying bleeding effects of drugs have also been developed. The rabbit ear blood-loss model is most commonly used to test the hemorrhagic effect of drugs. The rat tail-bleeding models have also been used for the study of several antithrombotic drugs.

These animal models have been well established and can be used for the development of antithrombotic drugs. It is also possible to use the standardized bleeding and thrombosis models to predict the safety and efficacy of drugs. Thus, in addition to the evaluation of in vitro potency, the endogenous effect of antithrombotic drugs can also be investigated. Such standardized methods can be recommended for inclusion in pharmacopeial-screening procedures. Numerous models have now been developed to mimic a variety of clinical conditions for which antiplatelet and antithrombotic drugs are used, including myocardial infarction, stroke, cardiopulmonary bypass, trauma, peripheral vascular diseases, and restenosis.

Whereas dog and primate models are relatively expensive, they have also provided useful information on the pharmacokinetics and pharmacodynamics of antithrombotic drugs. The primate models, in particular, have been extremely useful, as the hemostatic pathways in these species are comparable with those in humans. The development of such agents as the specific glycoprotein IIb/IIIa inhibitor antibodies relies largely on these models. These models are, however, of pivotal value in the development of antithrombotic drugs and provide extremely useful data on the safety and efficacy of new drugs developed for human use.

I. INTRODUCTION

Animal models have played a crucial role in the development of new antithrombotic drugs during the past few decades. Through the use of these animal models, the differentiation between the anticoagulant and antithrombotic effects was first recognized. Drugs that were not able to produce a prolongation of blood clotting time were found to produce antithrombotic effects in animal models, and a recognition that endogenous effects in the intact animal resulting from the metabolic transformation of the drug or release of antithrombotic substances was appreciated. Without the use of intact animal models such an observation would not have been possible.

Antithrombotic and anticoagulant drugs are effective in the control of thrombogenesis at various levels. These drugs are also capable of producing hemorrhagic effects. These effects are not predictable using in vitro testing methods. The bleeding effects of a drug may be direct or indirect; thus, the use of animal models adds to the pharmacodynamic profiling of drugs to project safety/efficacy ratios.

Repeated administration of drugs can result in a cumulative response that may alter the pharmacokinetic and pharmacodynamic indices of a given agent. It is only through the use of animal models that such information can be generated. Furthermore, as antithrombotic drugs represent a diverse class of agents, their interactions with physiologically active endogenous proteins can be studied only by using animal models.

Species variation plays an important role in thrombotic, hemostatic, and hemorrhagic responses. Although there is no set formula to determine the relevance of the results obtained with animal models to humans, the use of animal models can provide valuable information on the relative potency of drugs, their bioavailability after various routes of administration and their pharmacokinetic behavior. Specific studies have provided data on the species relevance of the responses in different animal models to the projected human responses. Thus, the use of animal models in the evaluation of different drugs can provide useful data to compare different drugs within a class. Caution must be exercised in extrapolating such results to the human clinical condition.

The selection of animal models for the evaluation of antithrombotic effects depends on several factors. The interaction of a given drug with the blood and vascular components and its metabolic transformation are important considerations. Thus, ex vivo analysis of blood, along with the other endpoints, can provide useful information on the effects of different drugs. Unlike the screening of other drugs such as the antibiotics, antithrombotic drugs require multiparametric endpoint analysis. Thus, animal models are most useful in the evaluation of the effects of these drugs.

Finally, it should be stressed that the pharmacopeial and in vitro potency evaluations of antithrombotic drugs do not necessarily reflect the in vivo safety–efficacy profile. Endogenous modulation, such as the release of tissue factor pathway inhibitor (TFPI) by heparins, plays a very important role in the overall therapeutic index of many drugs. Such data can be obtained only by using animal models. Therefore, it is important to design experiments in which several data points can be obtained. This information is of crucial value in the assessment of antithrombotic drugs and cannot be substituted by other in vitro or tissue culture-based methods.

II. ANIMAL MODELS OF THROMBOSIS

In most animal models of thrombosis, healthy animals are challenged with thrombogenic (pathophysiological) stimuli, physical stimuli, or both to produce thrombotic or occlusive conditions. These models are useful for the screening of antithrombotic drugs.

A. Stasis Thrombosis Model

Since its introduction by Wessler [1], the rabbit model of jugular stasis thrombosis has been extensively used for the pharmacological screening of antithrombotic agents. This model has also been adapted for use in rats [2]. In the *stasis thrombosis model*, a hypercoagulable state is mimicked by administration of several thrombogenic challenges including human serum [3–7], thromboplastin [8–11], activated prothrombin complex concentrates [10,12], factor Xa [10,13] and recombinant relipidated tissue factor [14]. This administration serves to produce a hypercoagulable state. Diminution of blood flow achieved by ligating the ends of the vessel segments serves to augment the prothrombotic environment. The thrombogenic environment produced in this model simulates venous thrombosis in which both blood flow and the activation of coagulation play a role in the development of a thrombus.

The procedure for the modified stasis thrombosis model of Fareed [15] is outlined here. Male white New Zealand rabbits are anesthetized. A 2-cm segment of each jugular vein, including the bifurcation, is carefully isolated from the facia. The right carotid artery is cannulated to obtain blood samples. The test agent can be administered either subcutaneously in the abdominal region, intravenously through the marginal ear vein, or orally using a nasogastric feeding tube: 7.5 U/kg factor eight inhibitor bypass activator (FEIBA), administered through the marginal ear vein as a thrombogenic stimulus, is allowed to circulate for exactly 20 s before the jugular vein segments are ligated to induce stasis. After 10 min of stasis time, the left vein segment is excised, opened, and the clot graded on a scale from 0 to +4. The right jugular segment is removed after 20 min of stasis time, and the clots are graded using the foregoing scale. Controls are run by administration of the vehicle in place of the antithrombotic agent.

Other more quantitative means of measuring clot formation have also been reported with this model. These include administering radiolabeled fibrinogen or platelets to the test animal before the experiment, thereby allowing clot size to be quantitated by measuring the incorporation of ^{125}I-fibrinogen or ^{111}In-labeled platelets into the thrombus. Even though these techniques can remove the subjectiveness associated with visually grading the clot size, they make the model technically more complex owing to the requirement for using radiolabeled material and to the need to incorporate a means of detecting the radioactivity. Measuring the wet weight of the clot formed has also been used with this model. With either of these clot measurement techniques, careful surgical isolation of the jugular vein is required, for excessive mechanical manipulation of the exposed vessels often results in vasoconstriction. The vessel segments used in such experiments need to be of a consistent size to obtain valid results.

The formation of a thrombus in the jugular vein of rabbits also lends itself to studying the modulation of the fibrinolytic system. Models have been described in which clots formed, as in the stasis thrombosis model, are lysed by administration of a lytic agent by intravenous (iv) bolus or by constant iv infusion [16]. After a set time, any remaining clot can be graded as in the stasis thrombosis model.

Criticisms of this model often revolve around the complete lack of blood flow during the thrombogenic period. The degree to which this model mimics the pathological state is debated. During many pathological conditions in which a thrombus is formed, a certain degree of blood flow remains through the affected site. This model does, however, offer the advantage of allowing the coagulation system to be activated at several distinct points. The activation of the coagulation system in vivo is multivariate relative to various clinical disease states [15]. This model, therefore, can be used to determine the potency of a given agent against a variety of potential thrombogenic triggers.

In addition to differences in the thrombogenic triggers, various other factors can affect thrombus formation in this model [15]. These include the effect of preparatory agents such as anesthetics on various hemostatic parameters, variations in the circulation time of the thrombogenic challenge, and the duration of stasis. Xylazine (Rompun) and ketamine have no known effects of the hemostatic system. When an antithrombotic agent is administered subcutaneously or orally, pharmacokinetic and bioavailability considerations become important in assessing the observed antithrombotic activity. Plasma drug levels are influenced by the extent of drug absorption as well as the time needed for the absorption to occur. During long periods of absorption, drug absorption and drug metabolism may occur simultaneously. It is, therefore, necessary to determine antithrombotic activity at the proper time to assure that maximal plasma drug concentrations have been achieved, particularly if agents with different absorption or metabolism profiles are to be compared.

Figure 1 illustrates the effect of intravenously administered heparin and low-molecular-weight (LMW) heparin on thrombus formation in this model using an activated prothrombin complex concentrate as the thrombogenic trigger. Both agents were tested 5 min following administration. By using this route of administration and short circulation time, little clearance or metabolism of any of the agents is likely to have occurred. In this system, each agent produced a dose-dependent reduction in thrombus formation.

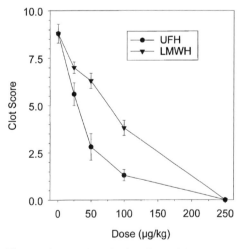

Figure 1 Antithrombotic effect of heparin and LMW heparin in the rabbit stasis thrombosis model following intravenous administration. A stasis time of 10 min was used. The results represent the mean ±standard error of the mean (SEM) of five rabbits per treatment group.

B. Models Based on Vessel Wall Damage

The formation of a thrombus is not solely induced by a plasmatic hypercoagulable state. In the normal vasculature, the intact endothelium provides a nonthrombogenic surface over which the blood flows. The nonthrombogenic properties of the endothelium are partly due to release of such agents as prostacyclin that prevents platelet aggregation, the presence of TFPI, heparin-like glycosaminoglycans, and the synthesis of fibrinolytic activators. Disruption of the endothelium not only limits the beneficial effects just enumerated, but also exposes subendothelial tissue factor and collagen that serve to activate the coagulation and platelet aggregation processes, respectively. *Endothelial damage* can be induced experimentally by physical means (clamping, catheter), chemical means (fluoroscein, rose bengal, ferrous chloride), thermal injury, or electrolytic injury.

1. Rat Jugular Vein-Clamping Model of Thrombosis

The process of thrombus formation following endothelial damage has been modeled in rats [17]. Repeated clamping of the vessel wall with a hemostat produces damage to the endothelium, which has been histologically demonstrated [17,18].

   In this model, male Sprague–Dawley rats are anesthetized, the skin on the neck is shaved, and an incision is made centrally above the trachea. The right jugular vein is isolated and covered with ultrasound transmission gel. A bidirectional Doppler probe is used to measure blood flow through the vessel. Because the carotid artery is located below the jugular vein, it is important to use a bidirectional Doppler probe so that only venous flow is measured. After recording the baseline blood flow, the jugular vein is clamped for 1 min using a mosquito forceps. Following removal of the forceps, blood flow is measured for 5 min by Doppler probe. If measurable flow exists at the 5-min time point, clamping is again initiated. This process is repeated until no flow can be measured 5 min after clamping. The effectiveness of a given antithrombotic agent is determined by the number of clampings required to cause vascular occlusion.

   When high doses of an effective antithrombotic agent is used in this model, the maximal number of vessel clampings needs to be artificially limited. Beyond a certain point, excessive mechanical damage to the vessel leads to bleeding from the clamping site, thereby preventing an accurate determination of the time needed for thrombus formation. As a maximal antithrombotic effect may not be determined, conventional potency designations such as the 50% effective dose (ED_{50}) cannot be used with this model. In setting up this model, one needs to exercise caution in isolating the jugular vein, because excessive physical manipulation or the use of cautery results in a constriction of the vessel. Once constricted, blood flow through the jugular vein cannot be accurately measured by Doppler flow.

   Unfractionated heparin, low-molecular-weight heparin, the synthetic polyanion aprosulate, and several thrombin inhibitors have all dose-dependently increased the number of clampings required for vessel occlusion [18,19].

2. Catheter-Induced Thrombosis Models

Models that use a catheter to induce vessel wall damage of both arteries and veins have been reported [20–23]. Such models in the arterial system mimic potential injuries induced by angioplasty. In these models, the endothelium is damaged either by rubbing the catheter across the luminal surface of the vessel or by air desiccation. Inflation of the balloon and the induction of partial stasis in the area of damage produce additional injury. This procedure exposes vessel wall collagen, elastic tissues, and tissue thromboplastin to the circulating blood. Such models are typically carried out in rabbits or larger animals owing to size considerations for both the vessel and the catheter.

In these models, the formation of thrombi has been detected in various ways. Measurement of flow by a distally placed flowmeter or thermistor has been reported [21]. A decrease in vessel temperature measured distally to the site of injury is reflective of a decrease in blood flow through the segment and the formation of a thrombus. Deposition of radiolabeled platelets at the site of injury and measurement of thrombus wet weight have also been used.

Figure 2 illustrates a typical flow measurement tracing obtained during and after induction of venous thrombus formation in the rabbit jugular vein. In this experiment, recombinant *tissue factor pathway inhibitor* (rTFPI) was administered at doses of either 10 or 20 μg/kg as an intravenous bolus. As observed in the figure, baseline blood flow was measured at approximately 15 mL/min. Following vessel damage by repeated balloon inflation and gentle rubbing of the endothelium, a vessel clamp was placed to reduce blood flow to nearly 90% of baseline. At this time the test agent (TFPI) was administered. A period of partial stasis was carried out for 60 min. Following removal of the vessel clamp, blood flow was observed to immediately increase. Flow was monitored for 3 h after removal of the clamp. At the lower dose of TFPI, full occlusion of the vessel was observed by 120-min postdamage, whereas at the higher dose of TFPI, flow was maintained for at least 240 min.

Platelets appear to play an important role in the formation of thrombi at sites where the endothelium is damaged [24]. Platelets may also play a key role in the initiation of the restenotic process following angioplasty [25]. These models, therefore, provide the opportunity to assess the pharmacological effects of agents that are capable of modulating either immediate platelet function or the coagulation system, which may be useful as adjunctive treatments in angioplasty. It has been demonstrated that both platelets and the clotting system are activated by arterial

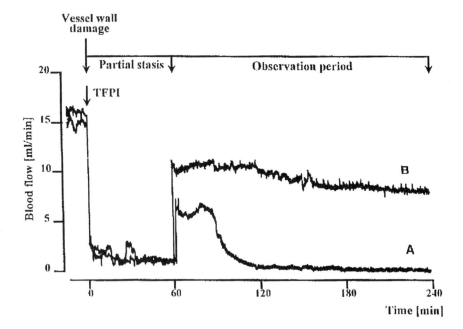

Figure 2 Typical blood flow tracings in the jugular vein of rabbits before, during, and after the induction of venous thrombus formation. The effect of an i.v. bolus injection of tissue factor pathway inhibitor (TFPI) on vascular patency is shown. Rabbits were administered either (A) 10 or (B) 20 μg/kg TFPI.

intervention [25,26] and, with this model, heparin and hirudin are both capable of inhibiting initial thrombosis. In addition, these models have also been used to assess the inhibition of rethrombosis following lysis of the initial clot [21].

3. Chemically Induced Thrombosis Models

The administration of a variety of chemicals, either systemically or locally, can result in damage to the endothelium with subsequent generation of thrombus. Such compounds include *ferric (ferrous) chloride*, fluorescein-labeled dextran, and *rose bengal*.

In models employing ferric (ferrous) chloride [27], the carotid artery of rats is isolated. A flow probe is placed proximal to the intended site of lesion and a 3-mm disk of filter paper that has been soaked in ferric (ferrous) chloride (35–50%) is placed on the artery. The application of ferric (ferrous) chloride results in a transmural vascular injury, leading to the formation of occlusive thrombi. This injury is believed to be a result of lipid peroxidation catalyzed by the ferric (ferrous) chloride. Thrombus formation, measured as a decrease in blood flow through the vessel, typically occurs within 30 min. Microscopic analysis of the thrombi has shown them to be predominantly platelet-rich clots. This model has been used to study the antithrombotic effects of direct thrombin inhibitors [28–30] and heparins.

Endothelial damage can also be induced by fluorescein- or fluorescein isothiocyanate (FITC)-conjugated compounds. A model has been described in which FITC–dextran is administered intravenously to mice. Thrombus formation is induced on exposure of the microvessels of the ear to light of a mercury lamp (excitation wavelength of 450–490 nm) [31]. The endothelial damage induced in this model is believed to be a result of the generation of singlet molecular oxygen produced by energy transfer from the excited dye [32]. Thrombus formation is measured using intravital fluorescence microscopy. This detection technique permits several endpoints to be quantitated, including changes in luminal diameter by thrombus formation, blood flow measurements, and extravasation of the FITC–dextran. This model offers the advantages of not requiring surgical manipulations that can cause hemodynamic or inflammatory changes, which allows repeated analysis of the same vessel segments over time and is applicable to the study of both arteriolar and venular thrombosis. The administration of rose bengal has been used similarly [33].

4. Laser-Induced Thrombosis Model

The physiological responses to injury in the arterial and venous systems vary partly because of differences in blood flow conditions, leading to different clot compositions. This model of arterial thrombosis is based on the development of a platelet-rich thrombus following a laser-mediated thermal injury to the vascular wall. This model was first described by Weichert et al. [34]. In this model, an intestinal loop of an anesthetized rat is exposed through a hypogastric incision and spread on a microscope stage while being continuously irrigated with sterile physiological saline. Vascular lesions are induced on small mesenteric arterioles with an argon laser beam (50 mW at microscope, 150 ms duration) directed through the optical path of the microscope. Exposure of the laser beam is controlled by a camera shutter. Laser shots are made every minute. Antithrombotic potency is evaluated in real-time by microscopic evaluation of vascular occlusion. The number of laser injuries to induce a thrombus with a length of at least 1.5 times the inner diameter of the vessel is taken as an endpoint.

The antithrombotic activity of several thrombin inhibitors has been compared with that of unfractionated heparin by using the *laser-induced thrombosis model*. Each inhibitor was administered intravenously through one of the tail veins and allowed to circulate for 5 min before the initiation of the laser-induced lesions. Saline-treated control rats required an average

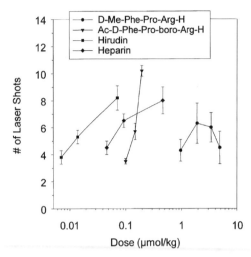

Figure 3. Comparison of the antithrombotic effects of various thrombin inhibitors in the rat laser-induced thrombosis model. Each thrombin inhibitor was administered through the tail vein and allowed to circulate for 5 min before to initiation of the laser injuries. (-●-)D-MePhe-Pro-Arg-H; (-▼-)Ac-D-MePhe-Pro-Arg-boro-OH; (-■-) hirudin, (-◆-) heparin. *Denotes statistical significance compared with saline-treated controls.

of three laser shots to reach an endpoint. Each thrombin inhibitor produced a dose-dependent antithrombotic effect in this model (Fig. 3). In comparing the dose of each agent required to extend the endpoint to six laser shots, heparin was observed to be the most potent antithrombotic agent (0.08 μmol/kg), followed by Ac-(D)-Phe-Pro-boroArg-OH (0.154 μmol/kg) and then by hirudin (0.28 μmol/kg). Consistent with the results obtained with these agents in the rabbit jugular vein stasis thrombosis model, D-Me-Phe-Pro-Arg-H exhibited the weakest effects in the laser-induced thrombosis model (2 μmol/kg).

5.   Folts Coronary Thrombosis Model of Cyclic Flow Variations

The two most commonly used models involving vessel damage as a trigger for thrombosis are the Folts model of *cyclic flow variations* and the Lucchesi model of *coronary thrombosis*. In the Folts model, intimal damage of the coronary artery followed by arterial stenosis leads to acute platelet thrombosis and cyclic flow reductions [35–38]. This model has been successfully used in dog and pig coronary arteries and in monkey and rabbit carotid arteries. After placement of flow probe distal to the site of injury, the circumflex or left anterior descending coronary artery is clamped to produce damage to the endothelium and possibly to the media of the vessel. A plastic cylinder is placed around the damaged vessel to produce a stenosis. This stenosis typically results in a 60–70% decrease in vessel diameter. At such a stenosis, flow is not reduced relative to that through the unstenosed vessel and a hyperemic response to a 20-s complete occlusion of the artery does not occur [39,40]. A combination of vascular damage and vessel lumen stenosis leads to the formation of acute platelet thrombi that eventually occlude the entire lumen. At this point, no blood flows through the artery. When the thrombi embolize, blood flow returns to baseline levels. The size and frequency of these cyclic flow reductions is related to the level of platelet activity [41]. When other factors are controlled, the amount of vascular damage and the degree of stenosis determine the size and frequency of the cyclic flow reductions.

Antiplatelet agents are particularly effective in limiting the formation of cyclic flow reductions. Aspirin, ibuprofen, glycoprotein (GP) IIb/IIIa antagonists such as c7E3 abciximab, serotonin antagonists, and thromboxane synthesis inhibitors effectively inhibited cyclic flow reductions [42–47]. It is suggested that this model is useful for studying the mechanism of arterial thrombosis and agents that can be used for its treatment.

6.   Lucchesi Model of Coronary Thrombosis

In 1961 it was shown that applying anodal electric current to the intravascular lumen by a lumenally placed electrode could induce coronary artery thrombosis [48]. This model was modified [49] such that low-amperage current over a longer duration was used to produce a gradual vessel injury. In this model, following thoracotomy, an electrode is placed into the circumflex artery and a flow probe is placed proximal to the point of insertion of the electrode. Following closure of the chest, electrocardiographic leads are placed subcutaneously and the dog is allowed to recover from surgery. The effect of acute trauma on the experimental results is thereby minimized. In addition, the tests are performed in conscious animals, precluding the effect of anesthetics on platelet function.

C.   Vena-Caval Ligation Model

Vena caval ligation models in rats have been used to study the antithrombotic activities of heparin, thrombin inhibitors, and antiplatelet agents [50–52]. One variation on this model is similar to the stasis–thrombosis model in rabbits in that dilute thromboplastin is administered to the rats before complete ligation of the vessel segment. After a defined time, the vessel segment is opened and the size of the resulting thrombus is determined by weight or protein content. Similar models have been reported in which copper or stainless steel coils are placed in the vena cava, providing a thrombogenic surface on which a thrombus can form.

D.   Disease Models

1.   Microvascular Thrombosis in Trauma Models

Successful replantation of amputated extremities is largely dependent on maintaining the microcirculation. Several models have been developed in which blood vessels are subjected to crush injury, with or without vascular avulsion and subsequent anastomosis [53–55].

In Stockmans' model [55], both femoral veins are dissected from the surrounding tissue. A trauma clamp, which has been adjusted to produce a pressure of $1500\,g/mm^2$, is positioned parallel to the long axis of the vein. The anterior wall of the vessel is grasped between the walls of the trauma clamp and the two endothelial surfaces are rubbed together for 30 s as the clamp is rotated. Formation and dissolution of platelet-rich mural thrombi are monitored over a period of 35 min by transillumination of the vessel. By using both femoral veins, the effect of drug therapy can be compared with control in the same animal, minimizing intra-animal variations.

The models of Korompilias [54] and Fu [53] examine the formation of arterial thrombosis in rats and rabbits, respectively. In these models, either the rat femoral artery or the rabbit central ear artery is subjected to a standardized crush injury. The vessels are subsequently divided at the midpoint of the crushed area and then anastomosed. Vessel patency is evaluated by milking the vessel at various time points postanastomosis. These models have been used to demonstrate the effectiveness of topical administration of LMWH in preventing thrombotic occlusion of the vessels. Such models, while effectively mimicking the clinical situation, are limited by the necessity of a high degree of surgical skill to effectively anastomose the crushed arteries.

2. Cardiopulmonary Bypass Models

Cardiopulmonary bypass (CPB) models have been described in baboons [56], swine [57,58], and dogs [59,60]. In each model, the variables that can affect the hemostatic system such as anesthesia, shear stresses caused by the CPB pumps and the exposure of plasma components and blood cells to foreign surfaces (catheters, oxygenators and such) are comparable with that observed with human patients. With these models, it is possible to examine the potential usefulness of novel anticoagulants in preventing thrombosis under relatively harsh conditions when both coagulation and platelet function are altered. The effectiveness of direct thrombin inhibitors [56,59], LMWHs [61], and heparinoids [60] has been compared with standard heparin. Endpoints have included the measurement of plasmatic anticoagulant levels, the histological determination of microthrombi deposition in various organs, the formation of blood clots in the components of the extracorporeal circuit and the deposition of radiolabeled platelets in various organs and on the components of the extracorporeal circuit. These models, therefore, can be used to assess the antithrombotic potential of new agents for use in CPB surgery and also to assess the biocompatability of components used to maintain extracorporeal circulation.

3. Models of Restenosis

Restenosis develops in about 30–50% of the patients after successful percutaneous transluminal coronary angioplasty (PTCA). Because most animals do not naturally develop atherosclerotic disease and, therefore, do not develop restenosis, experimental changes in the coronary or peripheral arteries must be artificially produced, making it impossible to completely mimic human restenosis [62,63]. The applicability of experimental models of restenosis is limited by a number of factors, including species differences in vessel anatomy, the type and severity of damage induced; and incorporation of a mural thrombus into the experimental lesion [64]. Nevertheless, models such as the balloon catheter-induced denudation of the endothelium are useful to study specific pathophysiological processes involved in the development of restenosis [65,66].

Several experimental restenosis models exist in both small and large animals, although no ideal model for atherosclerosis and restenosis is available [67,68]. Large-animal models such as the porcine coronary model have the advantage of their larger size that permits the use of human interventional devices. In addition, the coronary artery anatomy, the proliferative response after deep coronary artery injury and the susceptibility to atherosclerosis is similar in pigs and humans [69]. The initial injury to the porcine coronary artery is usually caused by balloon oversizing or metallic stent placement. The injury response includes substantial thrombus formation and a resulting neointimal thickening [63].

An advantage of models using nonhuman primates is that the response to angioplasty appears to closely resemble that in humans [70]. In primates there may be a genetic predisposition to neointimal formation and arterial remodeling following vascular injury [71]. Nevertheless, the currently available data indicate that, although large-animal models have been more successful than small-animal models to assess the efficacy of various interventions to reduce restenosis, the results are not always predictive for restenosis inhibition in humans [69].

Small animals, such as rats, guinea pigs, and rabbits, have been used extensively in the field of restenosis research because of the low costs, their ready availability, and the small amounts of experimental agents required for in vivo screening. The value of the data obtained from small animal studies is limited and not very predictive for a successful intervention in human arterial restenosis (69). Nevertheless, small-animal models are still valuable tools for screening purposes as well as to study mechanisms of the formation of intimal hyperplasia, including cellular and molecular processes. The use of transgenic and gene knockout small animals can give additional insights into the mechanisms of atherosclerosis and restenosis.

Balloon catheter-induced denudation of the endothelium and injury of the media is commonly used to study atherosclerosis and restenosis [72,73]. After cannulation of a distal artery, a balloon catheter is brought into the area to be injured. Injuries can range from gentle endothelial denudation to tearing of the internal elastic lamina and damage to the media. Alternative approaches include external injury to the artery using a forceps to crush the artery or internal injury using air or electrical stimulation [62]. Such approaches have been employed in rats, rabbits, transgenic mice, dogs, pigs, and nonhuman primates. They are used to develop intimal hyperplasia that is characterized by the migration and proliferation of smooth-muscle cells into the intima.

The most commonly used experimental model of restenosis involves balloon injury to the rat common carotid artery. This model produces a relatively consistent smooth-muscle cell proliferation response, thereby providing a means to assess the pharmacological mechanism of some antiproliferative therapies. There is little thrombotic component to the injury response in the rat model. An alternative to the injury of normal vessels is the use of double-injury models in which a second injury is performed several weeks after an initial injury. Double injury is associated with a larger thrombotic response than that seen after single injury [62]. Some models include the use of a high-fat–high-cholesterol diet in various species such as rabbits, pigs, or nonhuman primates. In a rabbit restenosis model initial iliofemoral arterial trauma from balloon injury or desiccation is followed by hypercholesterol feeding. The resulting atheromatous lesion is then dilated, producing a reinjury model of restenosis that also includes a thrombotic component. This model is expected to be closer in etiology to the human restenotic lesion [63].

The induction and measurement of vascular smooth-muscle cell proliferation in the rat carotid artery following intraluminal or external vessel wall injury is a rapid and reproducible model to study neointimal formation as well as antiproliferative actions of various agents. In rats, damage of the common carotid artery by external vessel clamps induces proliferation of smooth-muscle cells and formation of a neointima within 2 weeks after vessel wall injury [74]. This can be clearly seen in light micrographs from control and damaged carotid arteries stained with hematoxylin–eosin (Fig. 4). Whereas nondamaged arteries show a regular histological picture with endothelium, media, and adventitia, in damaged arteries a strong neointimal formation is seen. The vascular smooth-muscle cell (VSMC) proliferation can also be demonstrated by the incorporation of precursor molecules such as [^{3}H]thymidine or bromodeoxyuridine (BrdU). Injury of the vessel wall causes a strong increase of [^{3}H]thymidine incorporation, representing the DNA synthesis, and of the protein content of the artery, representing the mass of the vessels (Fig. 5a). In damaged arteries of saline-treated control animals, the incorporation of [^{3}H]thymidine per microgram of protein is increased five- to six fold when compared with nondamaged vessels. Furthermore, morphological and histochemical analyses show that the total number of cells determined by staining with hematoxylin–eosin (see Fig. 5b) as well as the proliferation index measured after labeling the proliferating cells with BrdU (Fig. 5c) in both the media and intima are also significantly enhanced. This model has shown that a direct inactivation of either factor Xa or thrombin by specific inhibitors reduces, but does not completely prevent VSMC proliferation in vivo. The combination of factor Xa and thrombin inhibitors does not lead to a further reduction of the proliferation of VSMCs in the rat carotid artery after external damage of the vessel wall. The inhibition of the known mitogenic activity of factor Xa by specific inhibitors such as DX-9065a or the synthetic pentasaccharide was also demonstrated in other in vitro and in vivo studies [75,76]. The recombinant forms of two naturally occurring factor Xa inhibitors (antistasin and tick anticoagulant peptide) also exert strong antiproliferative actions in a model of atherosclerotic femoral arteries in rabbits [77], in a porcine coronary balloon angioplasty model

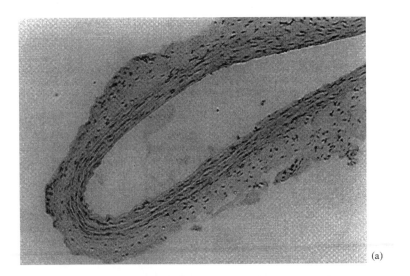

(a)

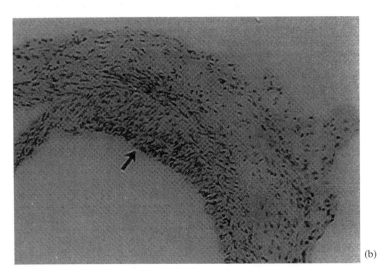

(b)

Figure 4 (a) Light micrograph of a normal, nondamaged carotid artery, 14 days after a sham operation showing a regular vessel wall consisting of intima, media and adventitia without formation of a neointima. The cells were stained with hematoxylin–eosin (magnification 400-fold). (b) Light micrograph of a damaged carotid artery 14 days after vessel wall injury showing the strong formation of a neointima toward the center of the vessel (arrow). The cells were stained with hematoxylin–eosin (magnification 400-fold).

[78] and in hypercholesterolemic minipigs after repetitive balloon hyperinflations [79]. A comparative study on the inhibition of neointimal formation by the thrombin inhibitor hirudin was carried out in several animal models using balloon-induced injury of the carotid artery of rats, rabbits, and hypercholesterolemic minipigs, as well as a double-injury model in rabbits [80]. Short-term application of hirudin reduced neointimal growth in rabbits, but not in rats or minipigs, showing that there are considerable species differences and that the results obtained in a specific model must not be generalized.

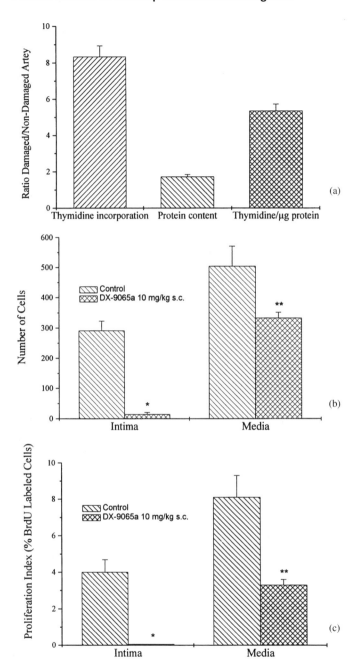

(a)

(b)

(c)

Figure 5 (a) VSMC proliferation in the common carotid artery of rats after injury of the vessel wall by external vessel clamps measured by the uptake of [^{3}H]thymidine and the protein content in the damaged vessel in relation to that in the contralateral, nondamaged artery of the same animal (means + SEM, $n = 22$). (b) Proliferation of VSMCs in the media and intima of injured rat carotid arteries treated by either saline or DX-9065a 10 mg/kg s.c. The total number of cells was determined after staining with hematoxylin–eosin by counting the cells in different parts of damaged vessels (means + SEM, $n = 7$) *$p < 0.001$ to control; ** $p < 0.05$ to control. (c) BrdU-labeling index (percentage of positive nuclei stained by BrdU to total nuclei stained by hematoxylin–eosin) determined in the media and intima of damaged rat carotid arteries after single s.c. injection of either saline or DX-9065a, 10 mg/kg s.c. (mean + SEM, $n = 7$) * $p < 0.001$ to control; ** $p < 0.01$ to control.

III. HEMORRHAGIC MODELS

Hemorrhage is an important side effect of antithrombotic and thrombolytic therapies. Several models have been developed to mimic bleeding observed in clinical situations. Unlike the animal models of thrombosis, the models for studying bleeding in animals are rather limited. Two models have been used extensively to examine the bleeding tendency of antithrombotic agents, the rabbit ear-bleeding model and the rat tail-transection model. Several newer models of hemorrhage have recently been described, including measurements of cuticle and lingual bleeding in rabbits as well as gastrointestinal hemorrhage in mice.

A. Template Bleeding Models

In the rabbit ear-bleeding model, anesthetized rabbits are administered ^{51}Cr-labeled erythrocytes; 10 min later, five standardized incisions are made in the nonvascular portion of the ear. Immediately following the transection, the ear is placed in a bath of isotonic saline for 10 min. Blood loss is quantitated by measuring the radioactivity present in the saline bath [81–83]. This model has also been modified to allow quantitation of the lost red cells with a hemocytometer. This model has been used to determine the hemorrhagic tendencies of heparin (UFH), low-molecular-weight heparins (LMWH), thrombin inhibitors, and thrombolytic agents [12,81,84,85]. Although differences between LMWH and UFH can be demonstrated using this model, the relevance of the results to the human response has not been firmly established. Thus, the results on the bleeding effects of different drugs should be interpreted with caution. Regardless of its limitations, this model offers a unique opportunity to compare the hemorrhagic effects of different agents.

To study the effect of thrombolytic agents on bleeding, a model has been developed in which standardized incisions are made in the rabbit ear and allowed to heal for up to 24 h before administration of the test agent [86,87]. Rebleeding from hemostatically stable wound sites was observed following the administration of streptokinase or recombinant tissue plasminogen activator (t-PA), but not following heparin or hirudin administration. Additionally, in this model with increasing time from injury, there was a decreased susceptibility to rebleeding. Here, the hemorrhagic tendencies of thrombolytic agents can be quantitated by measuring the number of sites that rebleed as well as the time from administration of thrombolytic therapy to the initiation of bleeding.

A similar model has been described in which standardized incisions are made on the tongue of a rabbit [88]. Although this model has demonstrated the effectiveness of topically administered chitosan to reverse a heparin-induced prolongation of bleeding time, its routine use may be limited by a somewhat more involved setup. This model is more complex than the rabbit ear–template-bleeding time model in that the mouth must be held open to expose the tongue and the soft tissues of the tongue must be stabilized to guarantee consistency in the incisions.

Animal models of hemorrhage can be used to predict not only the potential of a hemostatic agent to cause bleeding, but can also be used to study the modulation of such a bleeding effect. Although protamine is effective in neutralizing heparin-like drugs, the anticoagulant effects of direct thrombin inhibitors are not easily reversed. The rabbit ear-bleeding model has been used to study the neutralization of the bleeding time prolongation induced by high levels of argatroban. The increase in bleeding time induced by an intravenous bolus of argatroban could rapidly be reduced by administration of factor VIIa, factor VIII, and various prothrombin complex concentrates (Fig. 6). Such models may also be valuable to assess the potential usefulness of physical and mechanical approaches, such as high-flux membrane dialysis, hemosorption and plasmapheresis for neutralizing antithrombin agents. Figure 7 depicts the results of such a study

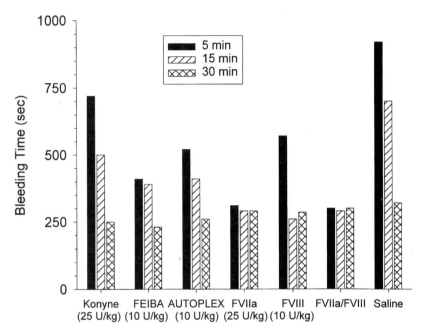

Figure 6 Pharmacological antagonism of the hemorrhagic effects of intravenously administered argatroban in the rabbit ear-bleeding model.

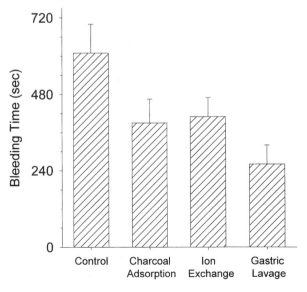

Figure 7 Physical antagonism of the hemorrhagic effects of an orally administered direct thrombin inhibitor in the rabbit ear-bleeding model.

in which charcoal adsorption, ion exchange, and gastric lavage were used to reverse the bleeding time prolongation induced by oral administration of a direct thrombin inhibitor.

B. Rat Tail-Transection and Template-Bleeding Models

Rat tail-transection and rat tail template-bleeding times have been used extensively in the assessment of the bleeding effects of different drugs. Dejana et al. [89] have reviewed the effect of experimental conditions on these models. The methodological considerations play a very important role in the experimental outcome of these methods.

In the rat tail-transection model, the tip of the tail of an anesthetized rat is removed using a scalpel. The bleeding time is used as an index of hemorrhagic potential. This model has been susceptible to several variables, including position of the tail, whether or not the tail is placed in saline, the temperature, and the type of anesthesia. Position of the tail affects the hydrostatic pressure on the capillaries, which can affect clot formation. In this study, bleeding time was observed to be significantly shorter at 37° than at 23°C. When the tail is placed in a saline bath, blood from the injured vessels freely diffuses into the fluid. If the tail is kept out of the bath, filter paper, which can have an effect on the formation of the hemostatic plug, is used to detect bleeding. Transection of the extreme tip of the tail has been reported to be sensitive to coagulation as well as platelet disorders. On the other hand, the template-bleeding time is sensitive only to the effects of platelet function and number. Thus, the selection of the method is dependent on the type of drug to be tested.

C. Gastrointestinal-Bleeding Model in Mice

Internal bleeding can be more hazardous than bleeding associated with a surgical incision or a skin wound because compression is not useful for limiting blood loss, and the time to recognition of a bleeding problem can be significantly longer. A model of gastrointestinal bleeding in mice has been reported [90]. In this model, a blood sample is collected before the test agent is administered for the evaluation of hemoglobin and hematocrit levels. The mice are fasted for 24 h before test agent administration. Following administration of the test agent, the mice receive an oral administration of 0.1 N HCl in 90% ethanol. Twenty-four hours later, a second blood sample is collected, and the animals are sacrificed to determine macroscopically the site of bleeding. The severity of bleeding was defined loosely based on thrombolysis in myocardial infarction (TIMI) criteria, as major, minor, or absent. With this model, dose-dependent hemorrhagic effects have been demonstrated for a variety of antiplatelet agents including aspirin, ticlopidine, and GP IIb/IIIa receptor antagonists.

IV. PRIMATE MODELS OF THROMBOSIS AND RELATED DISORDERS

Primates offer a unique opportunity to investigate the pharmacological effects of antithrombotic drugs in physiological relevant test systems. The results obtained in primates may provide data that is closer to human responses. Furthermore, endogenous interactions of heparin and related drugs exhibit a similar behavior in primates and humans.

Different species of primates have been used for the investigation of various antithrombotic drugs. Although the primate models have been comparable with the human responses, model-dependent variations have been noted between different species of nonhuman primates. The following two models have been used extensively.

The hemostatic parameters and the responses to the anticoagulant action of heparin and its fractions in a primate model (*Macaca mulatta*) are similar to those obtained in humans.

Functional properties of antithrombin III and platelet factor 4 are identical with those of humans in amidolytic and coagulant assays. Infusion of activated prothrombin complex concentrates or homologous primate serum resulted in a prothrombotic state as measured by an increase in fibrinopeptide (FPA) and thromboxane levels. Hemorrhagic tendencies of heparin and heparin fractions have been examined using a modified Simplate bleeding time in the primates. The platelet activation profile of *M. mulatta* is also similar to that in humans, thus allowing this nonhuman primate species to be used in the study of antiplatelet drugs. These studies suggest that plasma and platelet markers, such as the platelet release proteins, products of thrombin activation, surface receptors, and prostaglandin metabolites may provide useful indices for the monitoring of the antithrombotic actions of antithrombotic drugs. Studies have suggested that the pathophysiological responses after a thrombogenic trigger in the primate model and in humans are similar. Studies of drug modulation of such a trigger can provide relevant clinical information.

V. ANIMAL CARE ISSUES

When performing any of the models outlined in the foregoing, it is important to recognize that the welfare of the laboratory animal should be of primary concern for the investigator. All individuals involved in the care and use of laboratory animals in research, teaching, or education must be held responsible for the well-being of the animals (91–94).

An important consideration in the use of laboratory animals is to recognize and implement their humane care when used in biomedical research and for educational and pharmaceutical purposes. Such policies have been clearly defined in various publications. The basic principles that should be followed in designing animal experiments stipulate the following: First, experiments should be designed and performed on the basis of improving health, advancing knowledge, or for the overall benefit of society. Second, the use of the appropriate species, endpoints, and number of animals needs to be considered. Third, the use of alternatives to animal experimentation should be given proper attention. Fourth, efforts should be made to avoid or minimize pain and distress through the appropriate use of sedation, analgesia, or anesthesia. Lastly, only qualified, experienced individuals should conduct animal experimentation.

Committees such as an Institutional Animal Care and Use Committee (IACUC) oversee the proper use of animals in biomedical research and provide guidelines on investigator responsibilities [95,96]. Various independent organizations are actively involved in ensuring proper animal care and use. These include the American Association for Accreditation of Laboratory Animal Care (AAALAC; www.aaalac.org), American Association for Laboratory Animal Science (AALAS; www.aalas.org), American College of Laboratory Animal Medicine (ACLAM), and the Universities Federation for Animal Welfare (UFAW), among others.

Government agencies, such as the United States Department of Agriculture (USDA; www.usda.gov) Animal and Plant Health Inspection Service, Regulatory Enforcement of Animal Care (REAC), and the United States Public Health Service provide guidelines to establish acceptable standards of humane care and monitor compliance with these guidelines. Copies of the guidelines can be obtained from REAC on request.

VI. DISCUSSION

A large variety of animal models have been developed to mimic thrombotic, vascular, bleeding, and cardiovascular disorders. These animal models have provided not only useful information of the pathogenesis of hemostatic and thrombotic disorders, they have also served as crucial models to test the safety and efficacy of newer antithrombotic drugs. The information obtained from animal models remains indispensable and has helped in the designing of human clinical trials. The animal models have played a key role in the development of such newer drugs as the low-molecular-weight heparins, glycoprotein IIb/IIIa antagonists, and hirudin.

It is not possible to survey all of the animal models used in the investigation of antithrombotic drugs in a single manuscript. In this chapter, only the most commonly used animal models have been included. Since rats, rabbits, and monkeys have been used extensively and are available for the investigation of the pathogenesis of thrombosis and pharmacokinetic–pharmacodynamic-modeling studies, these models have been included in this manuscript. Other animal models based on the use of such animals as the mouse, guinea pig, and hamster are not discussed. However, these and other species are used by various investigators.

The original model of jugular vein thrombosis described by Wessler remains the most practical and widely used model for testing antithrombotic drugs. Since its introduction, several modifications have been proposed, including the use of different thrombogenic challenges such as tissue factor, prothrombin complexes, and purified clotting enzymes. The nature of the thrombogenic challenge is the primary determinant of the outcome and has provided a basis for simulating multiple thrombogenic conditions. This model simulates both the decrease in blood flow and the activation of the coagulation system observed in deep venous thrombosis. The use of this model to investigate antiplatelet drugs is rather limited. The jugular vein stasis thrombosis model can be extended to other species as well. In particular, rats have been commonly used with this model. However, significant attenuation of the antithrombotic efficacy for various drugs has been noted in rats in comparison with the effects observed in rabbits.

In both rabbit and rat models, mechanical and physical damage of blood vessels has also been used to trigger thrombogenesis. These lesions eventually lead to occlusive processes and simulate human pathological responses. Stasis and other induced impediments to flow have also been used in conjunction with these models. In both rats and rabbits, ligation has been used to simulate venous thrombosis. The laser-induced thrombosis model has also been developed to test the effects of drugs on the microcirculation of the arterial and venous systems. This model mimics the dynamic condition and allows the direct effect of a test agent to be readily assessed. The thrombogenic trigger in this model involves both the vascular and platelet components. Several other models in dogs have also been developed. These models are very helpful for the study of antithrombotic drugs for cardiovascular indications.

The choice of relevant models to test new antithrombotic drugs depends on several factors such as the intended indication, sites of drug action, route of drug administration, and the nature of the data required. Thus, before choosing an animal model for scientific studies, a careful analysis of the study objectives should be carried out.

The nonhuman primates provide one of the most useful models for studying antithrombotic drugs in simulated conditions mimicking human diseases. The results obtained from the primates closely approximate human responses and the data provide relevant information for developing new antithrombotic drugs in human trials. These primates exhibit significant phylogenetic similarities to the human and the humoral and cellular sites mimic the human receptors. Some of the antibodies engineered for human antigens can be used to investigate the responses in primates. A classic example of this is the development of GP IIb/IIIa antagonists. The platelets from other species, such as the dog, rat, rabbit, guinea pig, and hamster exhibit varying degrees of very low affinity to GP IIb/IIIa, whereas platelets from both the Cynomolgus and *M. mulatta* primates exhibit comparable responses to humans and can be used to investigate the antiplatelet effects of these inhibitors. Similarly, several occlusive disorders such as thrombotic and ischemic stroke can be studied in baboons, where the pathophysiology of tissue damage mimics the human response. Primates have been used extensively for various studies. Because of the cost, many of these studies are not terminal. Primates will be extremely useful in the study of human receptor-specific drugs because of their similarity to humans.

Bleeding is the most common side effect of anticoagulant and antithrombotic drugs. Bleeding models are difficult to develop for methodological reasons. However, several animal models of bleeding have been used to profile the safety of antithrombotic drugs. The rabbit ear-bleeding model reported by Cade remains the most practical and widely used model. In addition, the rat tail-transection and template-bleeding models have also been used. The pathophysiology of the bleeding models is usually based on mechanical damage to the blood vessels. A model based on the endogenous modulation of the hemostatic system is not available at this time.

Microvascular hemorrhagic responses can be mimicked by inducing mechanical damage to rabbit mesenteric arteries. This method, however, is difficult to standardize. Primates also provide a useful model for simulating the bleeding response. Gum bleeding- and ear-bleeding responses have been used to determine the bleeding effects of various agents. Standardization of the bleeding response has been a major problem and a large number of primates are needed to obtain standardized, valid data. Regardless of the limitations of the bleeding models, it is important to profile the pharmacological effects of the antithrombotic drugs using these models.

Despite limitations, the animal models of bleeding and thrombosis have provided invaluable tools for investigating the anticoagulant and antithrombotic drugs. These models provide crucial data on both direct and indirect (endogenous) effects of drugs. Furthermore, the endogenous modulation of drugs can be studied only in intact animals. Species variation, sex, age, and other physiological parameters contribute to the variability of the data obtained and should be assessed with caution in animal studies.

ACKNOWLEDGMENTS

The authors are grateful to Dr. Lee Cera and the staff of the Animal Research Facility of Loyola University Medical Center for their advice and critical input in the development of various animal models. We are also thankful to Drs. Fu and Yang for their expert assistance in carrying out some of the experimental work reported in this manuscript. The expert advice of Dr. Walenga in setting up the stasis thrombosis model is acknowledged. We are also thankful to Professor Breddin of the International Institute for Blood and Vascular Disorders for his assistance in setting up the laser-induced thrombosis model.

REFERENCES

1. Wessler S, Reimer SM, Sheps MC. Biologic assay of a thrombosis-inducing activity in human serum. J Appl Physiol 1959; 14:943–946 .
2. Meuleman DG, Hobbelen PM, Van Dinther TG, Vogel GM, Van Boeckel CA, Moelker HC. Antifactor Xa activity and antithrombotic activity in rats of structural analogues of the minimum antithrombin III binding sequence: discovery of compounds with a longer duration of action than the natural pentasaccharide. Semin Thromb Hemost 1991; 17(suppl 1):112–117.
3. Carrie D, Caranobe C, Saivin S, Houin G, Petitou M, Lormeau JC, Van Boeckel C, Meuleman D, Boneu B. Pharmacokinetic and antithrombotic properties of two pentasaccharides with high affinity to antithrombin III in the rabbit: comparison with CY 216. Blood 1994; 84:2571–2577.
4. Bara L, Bloch MF, Samama MM. A comparative study of recombinant hirudin and standard heparin in the Wessler model. Thromb Res 1992; 68:167–174.

5. Saivin S, Petitou M, Lormeau JC, Dupouy D, Sie P, Caranobe C, Houin G, Boneu B. Pharmacological properties of a low molecular weight butyryl heparin derivative (C4-CY 216) with long lasting effects. Thromb Haemost 1992; 67:346–351.
6. Thomas DP, Gray E, Merton RE. Potentiation of the antithrombotic action of dermatan sulfate by small amounts of heparin. Thromb Haemost 1990; 64:290–293.
7. Walenga JM, Fareed J, Petitou M, Samama M, Lormeau JC, Choay J. Intravenous antithrombotic activity of a synthetic heparin pentasaccharide in a human serum induced stasis thrombosis model. Thromb Res 1986; 43:243–248.
8. Peyrou V, Lormeau JC, Caranobe C, Gabaig AM, Crepon B, Saivin S, Houin G, Sie P, Boneu B. Pharmacologic properties of CY 216 and of its ACLM and BCLM components in the rabbit. Thromb Haemost 1994; 72:268–274.
9. Saivin S, Caranobe C, Petitou M, Lormeau JC, Level M, Crepon B, Houin G, Boneu B. Antithrombotic activity, bleeding effect and pharmacodynamics of a succinyl derivative of dermatan sulfate in rabbits. Br J Haematol 1992; 80:509–513.
10. Walenga JM, Petitou M, Lormeau JC, Samama M, Fareed J, Choay J. Antithrombotic activity of a synthetic heparin pentasaccharide in a rabbit stasis thrombosis model using different thrombogenic challenges. Thromb Res 1987; 46:187–198.
11. Vlasuk GP, Ramjit D, Fujita T, Dunwiddie CT, Nutt EM, Smith DE, Shebuski RJ. Comparison of the in vivo anticoagulant properties of standard heparin and the highly selective factor Xa inhibitors antistasin and tick anticoagulant peptide (TAP) in a rabbit model of venous thrombosis. Thromb Haemost 1991; 65:257–262.
12. Bacher P, Walenga JM, Iqbal O, Bajusz S, Breddin K, Fareed J. The antithrombotic and anticoagulant effects of a synthetic tripeptide and recombinant hirudin in various animal models. Thromb Res 1993; 71:251–263.
13. Millet J, Theveniaux J, Brown NL. The venous antithrombotic profile of naroparcil in the rabbit. Thromb Haemost 1994; 72:874–879.
14. Callas DD, Bacher P, Fareed J. Studies on the thrombogenic effects of recombinant tissue factor. In vivo versus ex vivo findings. Semin Thromb Hemost 1995; 21:166–176.
15. Fareed J, Walenga JM, Kumar A, Rock A. A modified stasis thrombosis model to study the antithrombotic actions of heparin and its fractions. Semin Thromb Hemost 1985; 11:155–175.
16. Bacher P, Welzel D, Iqbal O, Hoppensteadt D, Callas, D, Walenga JM, Fareed J. The thrombolytic potency of LMW-heparin compared to urokinase in a rabbit jugular vein clot lysis model. Thromb Res 1992; 66:151–158.
17. Raake W, Elling H. Rat jugular vein hemostasis—a new model for testing antithrombotic agents. Thromb Res 1989; 53:73–77.
18. Raake W, Klauser RJ, Meinetsberger E, Zeiller P, Elling H. Pharmacologic profile of the antithrombotic and bleeding actions of sulfated lactobionic acid amides. Semin Thromb Hemost 1991; 17(suppl 1):129–135.
19. Hayes JM, Jeske W, Callas D, Iqbal O, Fareed J. Comparative intravenous antithrombotic actions of heparin and site directed thrombin inhibitors in a jugular vein clamping model. Thromb Res 1996; 82:187–191.
20. Kaiser B. Effect of tissue factor pathway inhibitor (TFPI) on venous thrombus formation and rethrombosis after lysis in the jugular veins of rabbits. Thromb Haemost 1995; 73:944.
21. Kaiser B, Simon A, Markwardt F. Antithrombotic effects of recombinant hirudin in experimental angioplasty and intravascular thrombolysis. Thromb Haemost 1990; 63:44–47.
22. Lyle EM, Fujita T, Conner MW, Connolly TM, Vlasuk GP, Lynch JL. Effect of inhibitors of factor Xa or platelet adhesion, heparin, and aspirin on platelet deposition in an atherosclerotic rabbit model of angioplasty injury. J Pharm Toxicol Methods 1995; 33:53–61.
23. Katsuragawa M, Fujiwara H, Kawamura A, Htay T, Yoshikuni Y, Mori K, Sasayama S. An animal model of coronary thrombosis and thrombolysis—comparisons of vascular damage and thrombus formation in the coronary and femoral arteries after balloon angioplasty. Jpn Circ J 1993; 57:1000–1006.
24. Kaiser B, Markwardt F. Experimental studies on the antithrombotic action of a highly effective synthetic thrombin inhibitor. Thromb Haemost 1986; 55:194–196.

25. Heras M, Chesebro JH, Penny WJ, Bailey KR, Lam JYT, Holmes DR, Reeder GS, Badimon L, Fuster V. Importance of adequate heparin dosage in arterial angioplasty in a porcine model. Circulation 1988; 78:654–660.

26. Harker LA. Role of platelets and thrombosis in mechanisms of acute occlusion and restenosis after angioplasty. Am J Cardiol 1987; 60:20B–28B.

27. Kurz KD, Main BW, Sandusky GI. Rat model of arterial thrombosis induced by ferric chloride. Thromb Res 1990; 60:269–280.

28. Schumacher WA, Heran CL, Steinbacher TE, Youssef S, Ogletree ML. Superior activity of a thromboxane receptor antagonist as compared with aspirin in rat models of arterial and venous thrombosis. J Cardiovasc Pharm 1993; 22:526–533.

29. Elg M, Gustafsson D, Carlsson S. Antithrombotic effects and bleeding time of thrombin inhibitors and warfarin in the rat. Thromb Res 1999; 94:187–197.

30. Deschenes I, Finkle CD, Winocour PD. Effective use of BCH-2763, a new potent injectable direct thrombin inhibitor, in combination with tissue plasminogen activator (tPA) in a rat arterial thrombolysis model. Thromb Haemost 1998; 80:186–191.

31. Roesken F, Ruecker M, Vollmar B, Boeckel N, Morgenstern E, Menger MD. A new model for quantitative in vivo microscopic analysis of thrombus formation and vascular recanalisation: the ear of the hairless (hr/hr) mouse. Thromb Haemost 1997; 78:1408–1414.

32. Sanaibadi AR, Umemura K, Matsimoto N, Sakuma S, Nakashima M. Vessel wall injury and arterial thrombosis induced by a photochemical reaction. Thromb Haemost 1995; 73:868–872.

33. Hokamura K, Umemura K, Makamura N, Watanabe M, Takashima T, Nakashima M. Effect of lipo-pro-protaglandin EI, AS-013, on rat inner ear microcirculatory thrombosis. Prost Leukot Essen Fatty Acids 1998; 59:203–207.

34. Weichert W, Breddin HK. Effect of low-molecular-weight heparin on laser-induced thrombus formation in rat mesenteric vessels. Haemostasis 1988; 18S3:55–63.

35. Folts JD, Rowe GG. Cyclical reductions in coronary blood flow in coronary arteries with fixed partial obstruction and their inhibition with aspirin. Fed Proc 1974; 33:413.

36. Folts JD, Crowell EB, Rowe GG. Platelet aggregation in partially obstructed coronary arteries and their inhibition with aspirin. Clin Res 1975; 22:595A.

37. Folts JD, Lalich JJ, Crowell EB, Rowe GG. Platelet aggregation produced by stenosis in dog coronary arteries. Clin Res 1975; 23:183A.

38. Uchida Y, Yoshimoto N, Murao S. Cyclic fluctuations in coronary blood pressure and flow induced by coronary artery constriction. Jpn Heart J 1975; 16:454–464.

39. Elzinga WF, Skinner DB. Hemodynamic characteristics of critical stenosis in canine coronary arteries. J Thorac Cardiovasc Surg 1975; 69:217–222.

40. Gallagher KP, Folts JD, Rowe GG. Comparison of coronary arteriograms with direct measurements of stenosed coronary arteries in dogs. Am Heart J 1978; 95:338–347.

41. Folts J. An in vivo model of experimental arterial stenosis, intimal damage, and periodic thrombosis. Circulation 1991; 83:IV3–IV14.

42. Folts JD. Experimental arterial platelet thrombosis, platelet inhibitors, and their possible clinical relevance: an update. Cardiovasc Res 1990; 6:10–26.

43. Aiken JW, Shebuski RJ, Miller OV, Gorman RR. Endogenous prostacyclin contributes to the efficacy of a thromboxane synthetase inhibitor for preventing coronary artery thrombosis. J Pharm Exp Ther 1981; 219:299–308.

44. Coller BS, Folts JD, Scudder LE, Smith SR. Antithrombotic effect of a monoclonal antibody to the platelet glycoprotein IIb/IIIa receptor in an experimental animal model. Blood 1986; 68:783–786.

45. Folts JD. Inhibition of acute in vivo platelet thrombus formation with U-63557A, a thromboxane A_2 synthase inhibitor, but with renewal of thrombus formation with IV epinephrine. Circulation 1986; 74(suppl II):II-355.

46. Ashton JH, Golino P, McNatt JM, Buja LM, Willerson JT. Serotonin S_2 and thromboxane A_2-prostaglandin H_2 receptor blockades provide protection against epinephrine-induced cyclic flow variations in severely narrowed canine coronary arteries. J Am Coll Cardiol 1989; 13:755–763.

47. Torr S, Noble MIM, Folts JD. Inhibition of acute platelet thrombosis in stenosed canine coronary arteries by the specific serotonin S_2 receptor antagonist retanserin. Cardiovasc Res 1990; 26:465–470.

48. Salazar AE. Experimental myocardial infarction, induction of coronary thrombosis in the intact closed-chest dog. Circ Res 1961; 9:1351–1356.

49. Romson JL, Bush LR, Haack DW, Lucchesi BR. The beneficial effects of oral ibuprofen on coronary artery thrombosis and myocardial ischemia in the conscious dog. J Pharm Exp Ther 1980; 215:271–278.

50. Herbert JM, Bernat A, Maffrand JP. Importance of platelets in experimental venous thrombosis in rats. Blood 1992; 80:2281–2286.

51. Berry CN, Girard D, Lochot S, Lecoffre C. Antithrombotic actions of argatroban in rat models of venous, "mixed" and arterial thrombosis, and its effects on the tail transection bleeding time. Br J Pharm 1994; 113:1209–1214.

52. Seth P, Kumari R, Dikshit M, Srimal RC. Effect of platelet activating factor antagonists in different models of thrombosis. Thromb Res 1994; 76:503–512.

53. Fu K, Izquierdo R, Vandevender D, Warpeha RL, Wolf H, Fareed J. Topical application of low molecular weight heparin in a rabbit traumatic anastomosis model. Thromb Res 1997; 86:355–361.

54. Korompilias AV, Chen LE, Seaber AV, Urbaniak JR. Antithrombotic potencies of enoxaparin in microvascular surgery: influence of dose and administration methods on patency rate or crushed arterial anastomoses. J Hand Surg 1997; 22:540–546.

55. Stockmans F, Stassen JM, Vermylen J, Hoylaerts MF, Nystrom A. A technique to investigate mural thrombus formation in arteries and veins: II. Effects of aspirin, heparin, r-hirudin, and G-4120. Ann Plastic Surg 1997; 38:63–68.

56. Van Wyk V, Neethling WML, Badenhorst PN, Kotze HF. r-Hirudin inhibits platelet-dependent thrombosis during cardiopulmonary bypass in baboons. J Cardiovasc Surg 1998; 39:633–639.

57. Dewanjee MK, Wu SM, Hsu LC. Effect of heparin reversal and fresh platelet transfusion on platelet emboli post-cardiopulmonary bypass surgery in a pig model. ASAIO J 2000; 46:313–318.

58. Dewanjee MK, Wu S, Kapadvanjwala M, et al. Reduction of platelet thrombi and emboli by L-arginine infusion during cardiopulmonary bypass in a pig model. J Thromb Thrombolysis 1996; 3:339–356.

59. Walenga JM, Bakhos M, Messmore HL, Fareed J, Pifarre R. Potential use of recombinant hirudin as an anticoagulant in a cardiopulmonary bypass model. Ann Thorac Surg 1991; 51:271–277.

60. Henny ChP, TenCate H, TenCate JW, Moulijn AC, Sie TH, Warren P, Buller HR. A randomized blind study comparing standard heparin and a new low molecular weight heparinoid in cardiopulmonary bypass surgery in dogs. J Clin Lab Med 1985; 106:187–196.

61. Murray WG. A preliminary study of low molecular weight heparin in aortocoronary bypass surgery. Low molecular weight heparin in surgical practice. (Dissertation) London: University of London, 1985:266.

62. Lieb ME, Taubman MB. General techniques in molecular cardiology. In: EJ Topol, ed., Textbook of Cardiovascular Medicine. Philadelphia: 1998:2353–2369.

63. Moliterno DJ, Topol EJ. Restenosis: epidemiology and treatment. In: EJ Topol, ed. Textbook of Cardiovascular Medicine. Philadelphia: Lippincott-Raven 1998; 2065–2084.

64. De Meyer GR, Bult H. Mechanisms of neointima formation—lessons from experimental models. Vasc Med 1997; 2:179–189.

65. Bauters C, Meurice T, Hamon M, McFadden E, Lablanche JM, Bertrand ME. Mechanisms and prevention of restenosis: from experimental models to clinical practice. Cardiovasc Res 1996; 31:835–846.

66. Bauters C, Isner JM. The biology of restenosis. Prog Cardiovasc Dis 1997; 40:107–116.

67. Narayanaswamy M, Wright KC, Kandarpa K. Animal models for atherosclerosis, restenosis, and endovascular graft research. J Vasc Interv Radiol 2000; 11:5–17.

68. Schwartz RS. Neointima and arterial injury: dogs, rats, pigs, and more. Lab Invest 1994; 71:789–791.

69. Johnson GJ, Griggs TR, Badimon L. The utility of animal models in the preclinical study of interventions to prevent human coronary artery restenosis: analysis and recommendations. Thromb Haemost 1999; 81:835–843.

70. Geary RL, Williams JK, Golden D, Brown DG, Benjamin ME, Adams MR. Time course of cellular proliferation, intimal hyperplasia, and remodeling following angioplasty in monkeys with established

atherosclerosis. A nonhuman primate model of restenosis. Arterioscler Thromb Vasc Biol 1996; 16: 34–43.

71. Coats WD Jr, Currier JW, Faxon DP. Remodelling and restenosis: insights from animal studies. Semin Interv Cardiol 1997; 2:153–158.

72. Clowes AW, Reidy MA, Clowes MM. Mechanisms of stenosis after arterial injury. Lab Invest 1983; 49:208–215.

73. Clowes AW, Reidy MA, Clowes MM. Kinetics of cellular proliferation after arterial injury. I. Smooth muscle growth in the absence of endothelium. Lab Invest 1983; 49:327–333.

74. Kaiser B, Paintz M, Scholz O, Kunitada S, Fareed J. A synthetic inhibitor of factor Xa, DX-9065a, reduces proliferation of vascular smooth muscle cells in vivo in rats. Thromb Res 2000; 98:175–185.

75. Herault JP, Bono F, Avril C, Schaeffer P, Herbert JM. Activation of human vascular endothelial cells by factor Xa: effect of specific inhibitors. Biochem Pharmacol 1999; 57:603–610.

76. Herbert JM, Bono F, Hérault JP, Avril C, Dol F, Mares AM, Schaeffer P. Effector protease receptor 1 mediates the mitogenic activity of factor Xa for vascular smooth muscle cells in vitro and in vivo. J Clin Invest 1998; 101:993–1000.

77. Ragosta M, Gimple LW, Gertz SD, Dunwiddie CT, Vlasuk GP, Haber HL, Powers ER, Roberts WC, Sarembock IJ. Specific factor Xa inhibition reduces restenosis after balloon angioplasty of athero-sclerotic femoral arteries in rabbits. Circulation 1994; 89:1262–1271.

78. Schwartz RS, Holder DJ, Holmes DR, Veinot JP, Camrud AR, Jorgenson MA, Johnson RG. Neointimal thickening after severe coronary artery injury is limited by short-term administration of a factor Xa inhibitor. Results in a porcine model. Circulation 1996; 93: 1542–1548.

79. Abendschein DR, Recchia D, Meng YY, Oltrona L, Wickline SA, Eisenberg PR. Inhibition of thrombin attenuates stenosis after arterial injury in minipigs. J Am Coll Cardiol 1996; 28:1849–1855.

80. Gerdes C, Faber-Steinfeld V, Yalkinoglu O, Wohlfeil S. Comparison of the effects of the thrombin inhibitor r-hirudin in four animal models of neointima formation after arterial injury. Arterioscl Thromb Vasc Biol 1996; 16:1306–1311.

81. Cade JF, Buchanan MR, Boneu B, Ockelford P, Carter CJ, Cerskus AL, Hirsh J. A comparison of the antithrombotic and hemorrhagic effects of low molecular weight heparin fractions: the influence of the method of preparation. Thromb Res 1984; 35:613–625.

82. Carter CJ, Kelton JG, Hirsh J, Cerskus A, Santos AV, Gent M. The relationship between the hemorrhagic and antithrombotic properties of low molecular weight heparin in rabbits. Blood 1982; 59:1239–1245.

83. Carter CJ, Kelton JG, Hirsh J, Gent M. Relationship between the antithrombotic and anticoagulant effects of low molecular weight heparin. Thromb Res 1981; 21:169–174.

84. Racanelli A, Fareed J. Ex vivo activity of heparin is not predictive of blood loss after neutralization by protamine. Thromb Res 1992; 67:263–273.

85. Agnelli G, Pascucci C, Nenci GG, Mele A, Burgi R, Heim J. Thrombolytic and haemorrhagic effects of bolus doses of tissue-type plasminogen activator and a hybrid plasminogen activator with prolonged plasma half-life (K2tu-PA: CGP 42935). Thromb Haemost 1993; 70:294–300.

86. Marder VJ, Sortell CK, Fitzpatrick PG, Kim C, Oxley D. An animal model of fibrinolytic bleeding based on a rebleed phenomenon: application to a study of vulnerability of hemostatic plugs of different age. Thromb Res 1992; 67:31–40.

87. Wikstrom K, Mattsson C, Pohl G. A bleeding model in rabbits demonstrates fresh clot selectivity for a genetically engineered variant of tissue-type plasminogen activator and for streptokinase. Thromb Res 1993; 70:217–224.

88. Klokkevold PR, Fukayama H, Sung EC, Bertolami CN. The effect of chitosan (poly-*N*-acetyl glucosamine) on lingual hemostasis in heparinized rabbits. J Oral Max Surg 1999; 57:49–52.

89. Dejana E, Villa S, de Gaetano G. Bleeding time in rats: a comparison of different experimental conditions. Thromb Haemost 1982; 48:108–111.

90. Horisawa S, Kaneko M, Sakurama T. SM-20302, a non-peptide GPIIb/IIIa receptor antagonist, exhibits a wide therapeutic window in a newly developed hemorrhagic model in mice. Thromb Haemost 1999; 82:1743–1748.

91. National Research Council Guide for the Care and Use of Laboratory Animals. Washington, DC: National Academy Press: 1996.
92. U.S. Government Principles for Utilization and Care of Vertebrate Animals Used in Testing, Research, and Training. Federal Register, May 20, 1985. Washington, DC: Office of Science and Technology Policy.
93. The Future of Animals, Cells, Models, and Systems in Research, Development, Education and Testing. Proceedings of a Symposium of the Institute of Laboratory Animal Resources. Washington, DC: National Academy of Sciences, 1977.
94. Public Health Service Policy on Humane Care and Use of Laboratory Animals. Washington, DC: U.S. Department of Health and Human Services, 1996.
95. Institutional Animal Care and Use Committee Guidebook. NIH/OPPR, 1992. NIH Publication 92–3415.
96. Reference Materials for Members of Animal Care and Use Committees. Berry, DJ, Beltsville, MD: U.S. Department of Agriculture, National Agricultural Library, 1991.

3

Design Issues in Clinical Trials of Thrombolytic and Antithrombotic Agents

Dina S. Stolman
GloboMax LLC, Hanover, Maryland, U.S.A.

Marc K. Walton, Dwaine Rieves, Victor F. C. Raczkowski, and Jay P. Siegel
U.S. Food and Drug Administration, Rockville, Maryland, U.S.A.

Summary

Thrombolytic and antithrombotic agents have been studied in a variety of clinical indications. Issues arise in each clinical setting that are unique to trial design and the interpretation of results, yet certain common principles should govern the design of clinical trials in all settings. This chapter initially reviews general considerations that are common and pertinent to all clinical trials with these agents. A discussion follows of some of the major design issues illustrated by recent trial experiences in selected settings, including acute myocardial infarction, coronary artery disease, acute ischemic stroke, and peripheral arterial occlusion.

I. GENERAL CONSIDERATIONS

A. Specifying Objectives and Hypotheses

Proper protocol design requires a meaningful statement of the objectives of the trial. To define the objectives of a trial, one must first answer the following sets of questions.

1. What is the potential use of the agent under study? Will it be for prophylaxis or for treatment of established disease? Will it be indicated as primary therapy or as an adjunct to other treatment?
2. What are the standard treatments? What treatments are generally accepted as reasonably safe and effective for the selected indication? There may be multiple options for treatment, and the preferred therapy may vary depending on certain patient characteristics or the clinical setting. For example, angina pectoris may be treated with medication alone, with interventional therapy, or with both. The design of the clinical

33

trial should address the therapeutic options and provide a rationale for the therapies being tested.

3.   What are the characteristics of the disease or condition being studied? Is it acute or chronic, and is it nonserious, serious, or life-threatening? What are the incidence and prevalence of the disease? Is the natural history of the process stable over time, fluctuating, or progressive?

4.   Which parameters are to be the focus of the trial? Is it intended to examine the pharmacokinetics and pharmacodynamics of the study agent, or are those data already in hand? Is safety the primary concern, or is clinical efficacy primarily to be examined? Is optimal dosing of study drug to be determined?

5.   What is the hypothesis to be tested in the clinical trial? The hypothesis should be stated clearly, along with the plan for statistical analysis.

B.   Trial Design

Clinical studies in the testing of therapeutic agents may be broadly divided into three phases, based on the major focus of the study [1]. In general, the focus of phase I studies is to establish an initial safety, bioactivity, and pharmacokinetics database. Commonly, the purposes of phase II studies are to determine the appropriate dosage for subsequent studies, to accumulate additional safety data, and to examine clinical activity in one or more indications. Phase III studies are generally considered the definitive trial of a new agent's clinical efficacy [2]. Randomized, controlled trials with parallel treatment arms are most informative for phase 3 clinical trials. In a parallel-arm design, patients are assigned to one of two or more treatment options and tested in separate trial arms. The use of parallel treatment arms eliminates any temporal factors comparing treatment effects among the clinical trial arms.

Crossover trials may be useful in selected settings, in that they may offer the advantage of decreased intrapatient variability. Crossover studies may be accomplished with a relatively small number of subjects. However, the crossover design requires that the disease state be relatively stable over time and that drug effects during one study period do not affect outcomes during a later period. The second condition may sometimes hold true for prophylactic antithrombotic agents, but is not commonly true for thrombolytic agents. An adequate washout period must be established to ensure that there are no residual treatment effects from the prior treatments. Caution should be exercised in the selection of crossover designs for phase III studies when there are uncertainties about the baseline disease stability or residual treatment effects.

Factorial designs may be useful in assessing multiple dosing regimens, optimal regimens for combinations of various modalities of therapy, or when looking for possible interactions among concomitant therapies. Factorial designs offer an efficient means of evaluating multiple therapies that do not interact. When interactions affecting efficacy or safety are anticipated (e.g., when thrombolytics are combined with heparin or aspirin), factorial designs require an adequate number of patients in each cell to assess outcomes of each regimen and to analyze for potential interactions.

C.   Controls

Controls in clinical studies may include the use of a placebo agent, an active agent, or "external" controls (most commonly, historic controls). Inclusion of a placebo control arm enhances the ability to characterize the nature and extent of study treatment effects. However, when a therapy has been effective in prevention of irreversible morbidity or mortality, as have throbolytic agents in the treatment of acute myocardial infarction, active control trials may be necessary. Active control trials to evaluate the superiority of one therapy over another are simpler to design and interpret than trials designed to establish equivalence. In equivalence trials, problems in study design features, study conduct, poor compliance, or the use of marginally active agents can lead to erroneous conclusions [3].

The comparison is more complex between treatments of unestablished efficacy. Direct comparison may be of little value if no significant differences are shown. However, superior efficacy of one therapy over another may be taken as evidence of efficacy of the former if there is reasonable certainty that the latter therapy does not have adverse effects on efficacy parameters.

The use of historic controls is generally not advisable in clinical settings in which the evolution of therapeutic options is rapid, as has been the recent experience with cardiovascular therapies. The use of a control group external to the clinical trial frequently leads to difficulties in interpretation of outcomes. Problems commonly arise in determining whether observed outcome differences are attributable to the study agent or to patient characteristics, ancillary care, adjunctive therapy, or other unidentifiable factors. Historical controls are most likely to be of value when (1) the control group is prospectively defined and well characterized; (2) the disease process has a consistent and predictable outcome; (3) important prognostic variables and covariates have been well studied; and (4) outcomes with the study agent differ markedly from the natural course of the disease.

Dose or concentration controls, a subset of active controls, may be useful in evaluating the dose–response relationship when the use of untreated controls is not feasible. When the dose–response curve is expected to be monotonic (i.e., to show increasing efficacy with increasing doses over a broad range), comparing high and low doses may be of value in establishing efficacy.

D. Endpoints

In efficacy studies, endpoints should be chosen that reflect clinically meaningful consequences of the disease process and the intended clinical benefit of the product or treatment. Generally, for disease processes associated with a substantial case fatality rate, mortality is of greatest interest. Primary endpoints may also reflect the prevention of significant morbidity, such as disability. Clinical endpoints indicating the amelioration of symptoms or an improved functional status are more direct indicators of efficacy than surrogate laboratory or radiologic outcomes.

Surrogate endpoints (e.g., arterial patency rates) may be of value as primary endpoints in exploratory studies or as secondary endpoints in phase III clinical trials. Use of surrogates as primary efficacy endpoints should be limited to settings in which it has been validated that the surrogate predicts clinical benefit. Vascular patency is an important measure of pharmacodynamic activity for a variety of uses of thrombolytics, and reflects the expected mechanism of clinical benefit. The degree of validation of patency as a surrogate for clinical efficacy varies among the clinical settings in which it has been used. In no clinical setting has a change in the frequency and extent of patency at a specific time point been shown to predict quantitatively different outcomes.

Composite endpoints, such as the combination of mortality with myocardial infarction (MI) and stroke rates, may be used to increase the statistical power of a clinical study. A composite endpoint is useful when a single endpoint, such as mortality, is rare, or when there are several endpoints of special clinical interest. Components of a composite endpoint should not span an extremely broad range of clinical importance. A discussion of the effects of an agent on a composite endpoint must always be accompanied by a detailed analysis of its effects on the individual components This analysis should ensure that effects on common, but less clinically significant components (e.g., urgent intervention) do not mask opposite effects of more critical components (e.g., mortality). Such an outcome could lead to misinterpretation of overall benefit based on the composite measure.

E. Patient Selection

The characteristics of the tested population may affect the applicability of clinical trial results to the general population at risk for the disease or condition [2]. Certain covariantes may substantially influence treatment effects. It may be desirable to increase the statistical power of a study by enrichment to include a larger number of patients at higher risk for acute events, for example. A favorable risk–benefit balance in this selected population may not, however, extend to a lower-risk group. Conclusions from the trial may not be generalizable to the larger population in this situation. Phase III trials should include adequate numbers of patients with all covariates of interest, so that the trial results can give guidance for use of the agent.

F. Randomization and Blinding

Randomization of patients to treatment arms ensures that importance covariates are distributed randomly throughout the arms of a study, and is key to avoiding bias. The process of random treatment assignment should generally be simple and expeditious, particularly in trials of acute myocardial infarction (AMI) and stroke, for which the time from the onset of symptoms to initiation of therapy may be an important factor in the therapeutic outcome.

Blinding (masking) is a technique intended to minimize bias in the conduct and analysis of a clinical trial. Confidence in study results may be greatly strengthened by blinding the study treatment assignment. Blinding of treatments to patients and investigators reduces the potential for bias and should be used whenever possible. Certain logistical and technical considerations (dose administration requirements, time constraints, on blinding drug effects) may limit or preclude the use of blinding in a controlled clinical trial. However, the effort incorporated into designing blinded trial will facilitate interpretation of the results and may strongly influence the effect of the conclusions.

Blinding may necessitate the use of a placebo infusion or injection. In addition to matching the appearance of active and control treatments, the manner of administration must be identical for all patients. A nonblinded, separate dose-adjustment investigator may be required to maintain blinding for therapies that must be adjusted during administration by reference to a laboratory parameter. This approach was used in the EPIC and ELILOG trials of abciximab (ReoPro) in PTCA for coronary artery disease and in the Ancrod Stroke Study [4–6] (see Secs. III and IV).

When blinding of treatments is not feasible, it is crucial that guidelines for patient management and criteria for outcome assessments be stated explicitly in the clinical protocol and that adherence to the protocol be monitored. A blinded central clinical endpoint committee may be useful in confirming the determination of MI or stroke or the requirement for a revascularization procedure. There is less potential for bias in the assessment of relatively objective endpoints such as mortality. Relatively objective endpoints should be relied on in nonblinded trials when possible.

G. Dose Optimization

Establishment of the optimal dose range is critical to the development of new agents. The optimal dose range is the dosing regimen that maximizes clinical benefits over the potential risks of treatment. The importance of early dose-finding work cannot be overemphasized. Dose assessment data should initially be collected in phases I and II studies. Surrogate endpoints, such as angiographic patency, and rates of adverse events, such as hemorrhage, may be used to identify a dose range for evaluating clinical efficacy and safety in subsequent trials. Parallel-dose comparisons in phase III trials can also provide dose–response information about both efficacy and safety outcomes. Rates of infrequent, but very serious, adverse events, such as intracranial hemorrhage, may be assessed inadequately powered phase III trials.

H. Concomitant Treatments

Trials of investigational thrombolytic or antithrombotic agents are commonly performed with concomitant treatments, such as heparin or aspirin. Combination therapies may significantly affect both the safety and efficacy of an investigational agent. Such considerations are especially important in the study of agents that affect coagulation, because the risk for hemorrhage may be substantially increased by the use of concomitant medications or invasive therapies. It is also possible that efficacy may be affected by concomitant treatment with anticoagulant or antithrombotic therapies. More work is needed to define the optimal dose ranges and regimens for use of these agents in combination with new therapies. Strategies should be developed for addressing the issues of concomitant treatment and investigational agent interactions as the evaluation of new investigational agents proceeds.

I. Power and Sample Size

Determination of the sample size for a study depends on the expected outcomes in the control arm, the magnitude of the expected treatment effects, and the desired statistical power. Sizing adequately to determine the incidence of serious or life-threatening complications of treatment, such as intracerebral hemorrhage should be given close consideration.

Trials with broad inclusion criteria will allow for easier generalizability of results to the at-risk population. A larger number of subjects may be required to demonstrate treatment effects with a more heterogeneous sample, particularly if subgroup analyses will be performed. The sample size calculation should take this into account.

J. Protocol Adherence

All essential elements of clinical study design should be clearly stated in the protocol. Protocol violations and clinical inconsistencies increase the background variability in outcomes. These findings make it difficult to discern true treatment differences between the investigational agent and the control. An assessment of adherence to the protocol is crucial to validating the quality of clinical study data and conclusions. This is particularly true for eligibility criteria and compliance with dosing regimens and follow-up evaluations. Specification of the statistical analytic plan in the clinical protocol, including the format for interim analyses, is crucial. Once the clinical study is underway, any changes in the prespecified analytic plan should be made in advance of unblinding or knowledge of interim or final outcome data. The clinical protocol should be formally amended to reflect any such changes.

II. ACUTE MYOCARDIAL INFARCTION

A. Background

In 1980, DeWood reported that most patients with acute transmural myocardial infarctions had a thrombus occluding coronary arterial flow [7]. Subsequent clinical investigations clarified the role of thrombus formation in the pathogenesis of an acute myocardial infarction.

B. Clinical Trial Experience

Streptokinase and urokinase were licensed by the U.S. Food and Drug Administration (FDA) in 1982 for intracoronary use in patients with AMI. Licensure of streprokinase was based on the results from a nonrandomized, open-label registry of patients that detailed patency rates and 30-day mortality rates [8]. The utility of a clinical registry, rather than a prospectively designed clinical trial, was questioned in the published literature [9]. Subsequently, the peformance of clinical trials became the standard for assessment of the safety and efficacy of thrombolytic agents.

Large clinical studies examining the use of intravenous thrombolytic agents in the treatment of AMI were conducted in the 1980s [10]. Several of these studies compared thrombolytic agents with placebo using mortality as the primary endpoint. These studies firmly established that the intravenous administration of some thrombolytic agents decreases the early mortality associated with an acute myocardial infarction by approximately 20% [11].

Several clinical trials have examined the role of thrombolytic agents in establishing patency in the infarct-related coronary artery. The Thrombolysis in Myocardial Infarction (TIMI-1) study was initiated in 1984 to compare intravenous alterplase (tissue plasiminogen activator, Activase), with streptokinase (Streptase, Kabikinase) [12]. The primary endpoint of this trial was coronary artery patency. The TIMI-1 trial was terminated early because of a striking advantage of alteplase over streptokinase in reperfusion through the infarct-related artery. Since the TIMI-1 study documented patency and reperfusion effects of alteplase superior to those of streptokinase, it was argued that alteplase implicitly offered a greater mortality benefit. Two studies comparing the effect of streptokinase to alteplase (GISSI-2 [13] and ISIS-3 [14]) did not detect a difference between the agents in mortality, despite the enrolment of approximately 40,000 patients. These findings suggested that coronary artery patency was an incomplete surrogate for clinical benefit and that other factors (perhaps, for example, reocclusion rates, patency at other time points, time to treatment, ancillary therapies) were operative in failure of the cardiac reperfusion advantage seen in the TIMI-1 trial to be translated into a mortality benefit.

Both patency through the infarct-related coronary artery and mortality were studied in the GUSTO-I trial. The GUSTO-I trial compared streptokinase with a new accelerated dose regimen for alteplase [15]. The 90-min coronary artery patency and survival each appeared significantly better for patients treated with alteplase than for those treated with streptokinase. The GUSTO-I trial did not include the alteplase regimen used in other trials. While the GUSTO-I trial demonstrated a significant mortality difference and GISSI-2 and ISIS-3 did not, the confidence intervals around the mortality differences for the trials overlap. It is not possible to determine whether the different mortality findings can be attributed to the alteplase regimen used, to other clinical trial design factors, or to statistical variation. The GUSTO-I experience adds evidence to support the value of patency in assessment of benefit in thrombolytic trials, yet questions remain concerning which circumstances and to what extent differences in coronary artery patency will predict differences in mortality.

C. Issues in Clinical Trial Design

Clinical trials have established the mortality benefit of thrombolytic agents compared with placebo controls. Consequently, placebo-controlled trials are no longer appropriate in evaluating thrombolytic agents in AMI. Most newer thrombolytic agents and regimens will thus be compared with available thrombolytic agents. The design of such trials must make allowances for the integration of newer ancillary therapies, including the use of antithrombotic therapies and invasive procedures. Appropriate endpoint selection and the use of concurrent controls, randomization, and blinding remain the crucial components in the design of these trials.

1. Endpoints

The demonstration of clinical benefit continues to be the most useful outcome measure in therapeutic trials of thrombolytic agents involving patients with AMI. All-cause mortality at 1 month is now considered the most important primary endpoint for efficacy trials. To detect or exclude small but meaningful differences in mortality, it has been necessary to enrol a large number of patients. Large enrollments are also dictated by the need to obtain accurate estimates of the incidence of intracerebral hemorrhage and stroke.

Other clinical endpoints, such as ventricular function, the incidence of congestive heart failure, and 6-month outcomes may also provide important clinical information. Patency is particularly valuable as an endpoint for dose-ranging studies performed in the initial phases of development. Among the recommendations from a Cardiovascular and Renal Drug Advisory Panel to the FDA in 1992 was the suggestion that studies of new thrombolytic agents include an assessment of patency of the infarct-related artery as a function of the dose of the agent administered. The accumulation of data from future clinical trials on the relation to mortality of patency, left ventricular function, and other outcome measures, may increase their value in assessing the efficacy of thrombolytic agents.

2. Design of Active–Controlled Trials

A new thrombolytic agent that produces patency rates largely comparable with those of an existing agent may not be likely to produce a greater mortality benefit than an existing agent. However, the newer thrombolytic agent may offer other benefits, such as ease of administration or a lower incidence of side effects. In a phase III trial comparing such an agent with an existing agent, it would be important to demonstrate that these benefits are not associated with an increased mortality.

Active–controlled clinical trials of a thrombolytic may be used to establish superiority of a study therapy over control or to establish comparability on the primary outcome variable. In either case, the study will determine an observed outcome difference between the therapies and a statistical confidence interval around this observed difference. This is similar to finding a significant p value. To support an inference that a study drug is superior to the control, the confidence interval should not include zero. To support an inference of comparability, the confidence interval may include zero, but should exclude a predetermined degree of inferiority of the study drug.

Comparable outcomes in an active–controlled trial can be taken as evidence of efficacy of the test therapy only if the trial is performed in a setting in which the control therapy has a consistent, predictable effect. Several large, placebo-controlled trials have indicated consistent effects of certain well-studied thrombolytic regimens for AMI. Meta-analysis of these trials has allowed estimates of mortality effects overall and for various subgroups. In the recently completed INJECT trial evaluating the efficacy of reteplase (Retavase), a recombinant tissue plasminogen activator, in the treatment of AMI, streptokinase served as the active control arm [16]. The hypothesis of comparability required that the confidence interval around the observed mortality difference exclude the possibility that retaplase provided less than half the mortality benefit of streptokinase, as estimated by metaanalysis.

In designing an active–controlled trial, knowledge of the expected degree of inferiority of placebo to the active–control agent is critical in determining the degree of inferiority of the new agent to be excluded and, thus, in determining sample size. In trials to establish comparability, it is also crucial that the enrollment criteria select patients likely to benefit from the therapy. The demonstration of comparability in a patient population that is unlikely to benefit from thrombolytic therapy is of little value. The performance of active–control comparability trials mandates strict adherence to the clinical protocol and flawless conduct of the clinical trial. Protocol deviations, missing data, and flaws in trial conduct may obscure true differences in thrombolytic agents.

3. Patient Selection

Clinical trials have suggested that certain key covariates may identify patients with AMI who are more likely than others to benefit or to experience complications from administration of thrombolytic agents (e.g., location of infarction, age, and time to treatment). Characterization of the patient groups most likely to benefit, and the patients most vulnerable to complications, are important considerations in selecting enrollment criteria. Recognition of these factors is critical when comparing therapies, the relative effects of which may differ among subgroups. Depending on the utility of a newer agent, clinical trials may need to be designed to select for certain target patient groups.

4. Blinding

The impact of bias in nonblinded clinical trials in patients with AMI may be reflected in the primary efficacy outcomes, in adverse event assessments, in secondary endpoints, and in the utilization of ancillary therapies such as revascularization. For example, the occurrence of hypotension following the administration of streptokinase in an open-label trial comparing streptokinase with another thrombolytic agent may be more readily assessed as a potential allergic reaction by an investigator aware of the treatment assignment. Bias in open-label clinical trials is more likely also to influence subjectively determined outcome measures, such as the incidence of congestive heart failure. When such endpoints are used in open-label trials, careful protocol definitions of how these endpoints will be assessed and determined may reduce bias, as might the use of endpoint assessment by blinded clinical evaluation. More objective outcomes, such as mortality or coronary arteriographic patency assessments, are less prone to influence by bias related to absent or incomplete blinding.

Nonblinded trials may also be affected by bias in the use of ancillary therapies such as revascularization procedures. Bias might be diminished by providing strict guidelines in the protocol for use of such procedures. However, blinding is the best protection against such bias.

5. Dose Selection

The clinical experience now suggests that certain thrombolytic agents may possess a relatively narrow dose range in which the balance of clinical benefit to potential toxicity is optimized. During the clinical investigation of alteplase, a dose of 150 mg was associated with an excessive incidence of intracranial hemorrhage. Reduction of the recommended dose to a weight-adjusted dose with a maximum of 100 mg was associated with a lower incidence of intracranial hemorrhage, while the coronary thrombolytic effect was retained [17]. The most likely successful method for achieving a targeted effect level in patients of varying sizes is to utilize size-adjusted dosing. While fixed-dose regimens of thrombolytic agents may offer advantages in convenience and cost, the decision to use such a regimen for a newer thrombolytic agent should be based on clinical data demonstrating that the mortality and stroke outcomes do not vary strongly over a range of weight-adjusted–dosing options.

6. Safety Assessment

Prior clinical trials have shown that hemorrhagic complications account for the vast majority of serious adverse events following administration of currently available thrombolytic agents. The experience with hemorrhagic stroke is especially notable. The incidence of nonhemorrhagic stroke has declined since the development of thrombolytic therapy, but the incidence of hemorrhagic stroke was increased. In the prethrombolytic era, the incidence of stroke following a myocardial infarction was approximately 2.5%, with the vase majority of these reported as thromboembolic, nonhemorrhagic strokes [18]. Although the overall incidence of stroke among patients receiving thrombolytic therapy has declined, ranging from 0.5% to approximately 1.5%, almost half of these are associated with intracranial hemorrhage. Stroke rates with thrombolytic agents will vary depending on patient population factors (e.g., age). Comparisons between agents are best based on large randomized trials.

7. Concomitant Therapy

Clinical trials have established that the use of aspirin decreases the 1-month mortality rate in patients with AMI. The combination of aspirin with streptokinase has been superior to streptokinase alone [19]. The beneficial effect of aspirin in these trials has led to the relatively routine use of aspirin as adjunctive therapy in trials of thrombolytic agents. It has been proposed that the thrombolysis of intracoronary clots is followed by a somewhat paradoxical local thrombogenic state and that this phenomenon may be more pronounced with the use of alteplase. Alteration of this thrombogenic rebound phenomenon provides a theoretical basis for the adjunctive use of heparin with t-PA. However, the clinical effects of the use of heparin with thrombolytics have not been fully evaluated in clinical trials. The overall value and optimal dose regimens of such combinations have not been assessed. The use of heparin, aspirin, or other antithrombotic or antiplatelet therapies may not only affect efficacy, but may also increase the hemorrhagic complications associated with thrombolysis. Given the implications for both safety and efficacy outcomes, it is important that the clinical effects of adjunctive therapies be addressed.

III. CORONARY ARTERY DISEASE: DRUGS AS ADJUNCTIVE THERAPIES WITH ANGIOPLASTY

A. History of Adjunctive Drug Therapy

The technique of percutaneous transluminal angioplasty (PTA) developed over several decades. In 1964, Dotter and Judkins performed transluminal angioplasty to treat atherosclerotic obstructions of the femoral artery [20]. In the mid-1970s, after developing a double-lumen dilation catheter with a nonelastic balloon, Grüntzig began dilating obstructions of the iliac and femoropopliteal arteries [21]. He performed the first percutaneous transluminal coronary angioplasty (PTCA) in a patient in 1977 after further modifying this catheter [22]. PTCA is presently used to treat patients with stable angina, acute myocardial infarction, and symptomatic or objective evidence of ischemia after thrombolytic therapy [23].

Adjunctive drug therapy with PTCA has included antithrombotics, antiplatelet agents, anticoagulants, and vasorelaxants. Adjunctive uses of these medications with PTCA began empirically—without prior evidence from clinical trials of the safety or efficacy of these uses, and without prior dose optimization to maximize benefit over risk. For example, Grüntzig and colleagues initially performed PTCA in 50 patients over 18 months, and described the drug treatment used during the procedure as follows:

> The patient is given Aspirin (1.0 g per day) for three days, starting the day before the procedure. Heparin and low-molecular-weight dextran are administered during dilation; warfarin is started after the procedure and is continued until the follow-up study six to nine months later. To prevent coronary spasms, nitroglycerin and nifedipine are given before and during the procedure [24].

In the intervening years only a few studies have been performed to evalute some of the adjunctive therapies. Few prospective randomized clinical trials have been conducted. Certain agents are administered routinely, however. To decrease the likelihood of abrupt vessel closure, low-dose aspirin is typically administered before and after the coronary artery is dilated [25,26]. To prevent thrombosis of the coronary artery, intravenous heparin is commonly given during the procedure [27,28]. Patients are often treated with nitroglycerin and calcium–channel-blocking agents to inhibit coronary artery vasoconstriction after the procedure [29]. The use of any specific drug regimen varies from institution to institution. None of these agents is labeled for use with PTCA in the United States.

Despite adjunctive medical therapy, both acute and long-term complications occur in a substantial proportion of patients undergoing PTCA. Acutely, the treated vessel closes abruptly in up to 8% of cases, usually within 24 h of the dilation [30–34]. Over the longer term, the treated vessel can undergo restenosis in up to 60% of patients [35–40].

In contrast to this empiric evolution, one biological drug has been evaluated systematically in prospective clinical trials, and is the only one pharmacological agent licensed for use in the United States as an adjunctive therapy with PTCA. This agent, abciximab (ReoPro), is a chimeric monoclonal antibody Fab fragment (c7E3 Fab), which is directed against the platelet glycoprotein IIb/IIIa receptor. The remainder of this section focuses on this agent.

B.   Development of Abciximab (ReoPro)

1.   Preclinical Evaluation

Before extensive clinical evaluation of a new agent, preclinical studies should provide an adequate scientific rationale on which to base clinical development. Preclinical pharmacodynamic assessments and evaluations of activity in preclinical models may play a key role in selecting doses and regimens for initial study in humans. Preclinical studies of abciximab showed that the antibody blocks glycoprotein IIb/IIIa receptors in a concentration-dependent manner. The murine $F(ab')_2$ antibody fragment inhibited platelet function in animal studies [41], and the murine Fab fragment inhibited platelet aggregation in early clinical studies [42]. The antibody was also active in animal models of arterial thrombosis.

2.   Clinical Study Design: the EPIC Trial

The principal clinical study supporting licensure of abciximab was the EPIC (Evaluation of C7E3 for the Prevention of Ischemic Complications) trial [4,43]. A critical review of aspects of this trial provides an opportunity to explore issues relating to the designs and interpretation of drug trials in the setting of PTCA.

The EPIC trial was a randomized, double-blind, placebo-controlled multicenter study of abciximab in 2099 patients undergoing PTCA who were felt to be at high risk of abrupt closure of the treated coronary vessel. Three treatment arms were included, comparing an abciximab bolus and infusion, an abciximab bolus and placebo infusion, and a placebo bolus and infusion. Patients were included with (1) unstable angina or a non–Q-wave myocardial infarction ($n = 489$); (2) an acute Q-wave myocardial infarction within 12 h of the onset of symptoms ($n = 66$); or (3) high-risk clinical or morphological characteristics (as adapted from the classification of the American Heart Association and American College of Cardiology) [44] ($n = 1544$). All patients received intravenous heparin during PTCA and for 12 h afterwards. Aspirin was administered orally before the planned procedure and then daily.

The primary efficacy endpoint was a composite of the occurrence of any of the following events within 30 days of PTCA: (1) death from any cause; (2) a myocardial infarction; or (3) an unplanned urgent procedure for recurrent ischemia.

3. Efficacy and Safety Results

Administration of an abciximab bolus and infusion resulted in a decrease in the frequency of the composite primary endpoint events assessed at 30 days as compared with placebo treatment (8.3 vs 12.8%, $p = 0.008$). The effect of abciximab on this composite primary endpoint appeared to be sustained through 6 months. The effects of abciximab on each component of the primary endpoint were also evaluated. Mortality was uncommon, and similar rates (1.3–1.7%) were observed in the three treatment arms. AMI rates were significantly lower in both groups treated with abciximab compared with the group treated with placebo. Most (80%) of the endpoint myocardial infarctions were non–Q-wave infarcations. Urgent intervention rates were also lower in both groups treated with abciximab compared with the group treated with placebo, largely because of lower rates of emergency PTCA and emergency CABG surgery.

Abciximab treatment resulted in significant increases in major and minor bleeding episodes and in the need for transfusions. Bleeding was classified as major or minor by adapting the criteria of the Thrombolysis in Myocardial Infarction (TIMI) study group [45,46]. Treatment with the abciximab bolus and infusion resulted in a 7.4% absolute increase in major bleeding events compared with treatment with placebo (14.0 vs 6.6%, $p < 0.001$).

C. Issues in Clinical Trial Design

1. Patient Selection

Increasing the representation of various groups in clinical trials improves the generalizability of the results and facilitates accrual. Diversity in demographics, baseline disease characteristics, and concomitant therapies and illnesses is an important consideration in trial design. Patients may undergo PTCA for a variety of reasons, and many factors may affect their response to PTCA or adjunctive therapy.

A heterogeneous group of patients were enrolled in the EPIC study, including patients with unstable angina, non–Q-wave MI, Q-wave MI, or high-risk clinical/morphological character-istics. Although the use of a heterogeneous mix of patients could increase the applicability of trial results, it is also potentially problematic. The reduction in the proportion of patients experiencing a primary endpoint event in those treated with abciximab as compared with placebo was statistically significant in those with unstable angina ($n = 489$) or an acute myocardial infarction ($n = 66$). This comprised only one-fourth of the patients evaluated in the trial. In the remaining patients with high-risk clinical and morphological characteristics ($n = 1544$), the beneficial effects were smaller and were not statistically demonstrable.

It is a common finding in clinical trials that there may be insufficient numbers of patients in specific subgroups to establish clinical efficacy directly. The applicability of the overall findings to specific subgroups is based both on the presumption that efficacy would not differ substantially among subgroups and on the absence of data establishing such a differential effect. When either clinical data or other information make it likely that an agent may have different efficacy in different groups, a trial should be sufficiently powered to assess this possibility. It remains to be determined whether variations in clinical characteristics among patients undergoing PTCA will substantially alter responses to adjunctive therapies.

2. Endpoints

When a composite endpoint includes outcomes of varying clinical effects such as death, MI, and urgent intervention, it is important to examine each component, as noted in the General Considerations section. In the EPIC trial, mortality within 30 days occurred infrequently, and was not significantly different among treatment arms. The primary contributions to the treatment effect were seen in myocardial infarctions (80% of which were non–Q-wave MIs) and a lower incidence of urgent interventions. In the setting of adjunctive therapy for PTCA, inclusion of urgent intervention with death and MI may be an appropriate endpoint to demonstrate the influence on a physiological process (e.g., abrupt vessel closure). However, when the objective is to establish net clinical benefit, particularly if the test drug has substantial toxicity, restricting the composite efficacy endpoint to outcomes of higher clinical result (e.g., death and Q-wave MI) should be considered.

3. Blinding and Bias

Determination of whether a revascularization procedure was urgently required, and indeed whether an AMI has occurred, can be significantly subjective. To protect against bias, treatments were double-blinded in the EPIC trial; however, as often occurs, blinding may have been compromised in some patients by drug effects. To further diminish bias and to increase consistency in endpoint assessment, primary efficacy and major safety endpoints in the EPIC trial were reviewed by an independent Clinical Endpoint Committee, which made its determinations blinded to treatment group. Blinded assessments can increase the objectivity of more subjectively determined endpoints, such as procedure rates, and are useful in many trial situations. In addition, each site had a "heparin study coordinator" to prevent revealing the effects of heparin dosage. The coordinator monitored activated partial thromboplastin times and adjusted the heparin infusions accordingly. All other investigators were blinded to this information. Care should be taken in evaluation of newer agents to establish procedures for blinding and to minimize opportunities for bias.

4. Dose Selection

The choice of an appropriate dosage regimen for drug administration must consider both the beneficial and detrimental effects of the drug. Only after the shapes of the dose–effect curves for both beneficial *and* detrimental effects are known can one achieve the goal of selecting a dosage regimen that maximizes benefit over risk. The goal of a drug development program is not merely to maximize benefit; the goal is to maximize benefit compared with risk. The phase III testing program concentrated only on dosage regimens that produced near-maximal (i.e., >80%) blockade of the glycoprotein IIb/IIIa receptors; these dosage regimens were thought to be associated with maximal antithrombotic efficacy. However, the bleeding complications associated with this agent can be serious. It is possible that lower doses might have further reduced this risk. When it is feasible, clinical development should explore a broad range of doses and various dosage regimens to optimize the balance of benefit and risk.

Although the bolus of abciximab in the EPIC trial was adjusted for body weight, the 12-h infusion was not. Similarly, heparin doses were not weight-adjusted. Retrospective analysis of the EPIC trial results found that patients of lower body weight were at greater risk of bleeding and were less likely to benefit from therapy. This suggested the possibility that weight-adjusted dosing might have led to more consistent effects. A fixed-dose regimen of a new drug should ideally be based on clinical data that show that the benefits and risks of the drug are independent of, or only negligibly related to, body size.

5. Concomitant Therapy

Interactions with other medications may alter a drug's safety, efficacy, or both. A drug development program should evaluate drug interactions that may be of clinical significance. The development and study of a new agent should include evaluation of potential influences of concomitant therapies such as heparin and aspirin. In the EPILOG trial (as compared with the EPIC trial), the effects of lower, weight-adjusted doses of heparin were investigated when administered in conjunction with abciximab. Other factors were altered in EPILOG, including the timing of removal of the arterial sheath, management of the arterial access site, and the duration of the heparin infusion. An initial report of the trial results indicates that markedly lower bleeding rates were observed in all treatment arms and suggests that efficacy was preserved [5]. Any or all of the stated factors may have contributed to the decreased rates of bleeding. These findings highlight the importance of optimizing ancillary treatment in combination with new therapeutic agents.

IV. ISCHEMIC STROKE

A. Background

Stroke affects approximately 500,000 individuals in the United States each year. Approximately 85% of these are ischemic strokes. Following the success of antithrombotic and thrombolytic agents for the treatment of prevention of myocardial infarction, there have been efforts to utilize the knowledge gained to develop safe and effective therapies for stroke.

The opportunities for therapeutic intervention can be broadly divided into three categories based on the clinical goal:

1. Prophylactic therapies for patients deemed to be at increased risk for future stroke: These are prolonged treatments, administered for months to years. Oral agents are the most practical. The antiplatelet agents aspirin and ticlopidine (Ticlid) have established roles in this setting.

2. "Stroke in progress" or "threatened stroke": These patients require prompt therapy to interrupt the ischemic process. These therapies are given for briefer periods, over hours to days, and may serve as a temporizing measure until a mechanical intervention (such as endarterectomy or PTCA) can be performed. Antithrombotic agents have been of primary interest, particularly heparin, which is a widely used agent in this setting. There has not been rigorous demonstration of the efficacy of any pharmacological regimen in this circumstance, however.

3. Acute ischemic stroke: Here, it is presumed that the inciting ischemic event has occurred, but the full extent of irreversible damage has not. It is thought that prompt restoration of perfusion to the ischemic penumbra may rescue the hypoxic regions. This hypothesis was explored during investigations of thrombolytic administration in the 1960s and 1970s. These early studies reported a high incidence of hemorrhagic transformation of ischemic strokes. By the late 1980s, pilot studies of thrombolytic and antithrombotic agents were conducted, with some optimistic results [47–50]. The remainder of this section will focus on clinical trials for this indication.

B. Recent Clinical Trial Experience

Several randomized, controlled clinical trials of thrombolytic agents administered intravenously in acute ischemic stroke have recently reported results. The Multicentre Acute Stroke Trial— Europe (MAST-E) of streptokinase versus placebo had enrolled 270 patients when the safety committee recommended halting the trial because of the significantly increased rate of symptomatic intracranial hemorrhage (ICH) and a related increase in mortality in the strepto- kinase group [51,52]. In the Australian Streptokinase Trial (ASK), an interim safety analysis of the first 300 patients showed increased mortality in the patients treated between 3 and 4 h after stroke onset [53]. The trial was halted following the safety committee's recommendation to halt enrolment of patients presenting more than 3 h after the stroke. The Multicentre Acute Stroke Trial—Italy (MAST-I) of streptokinase, or aspirin or both (factorial design) also demonstrated an increased rate of ICH with streptokinase at an interim analysis, and was halted due to this risk and its attendant consequence [54].

The European Cooperative Acute Stroke Study (ECASS) was the first of two major studies with alteplase in acute ischemic stroke to be reported [55]. This study enrolled 620 patients up to 6 h following the onset of a hemispheric stroke. While there was an increase in the number of patients with the most favorable outcome ("minimal or no disability") associated with the alteplase treatment, there was also a notable increase in ICH and mortality. As a result, the median functional outcome assessment was not significantly different between the two treatment arms.

The National Institute of Neurological Disorders and Stroke t-PA Stroke Study (NINDS Study) compared alteplase to placebo and enrolled patients for treatment within 3 h from the onset of a stroke [56]. Two immediately consecutive studies were conducted. Patients treated with alteplase had a higher rate of minimal or no disability at 3 months. In these studies, there was a modest increase in ICH, but there was no increase in either mortality or severe disability. These studies provided the basis for marketing approval of activase for the treatment of patients with acute ischemic stroke. While not without risk, this regimen, in properly selected patients, demonstrated an acceptable benefit–risk balance.

There were many differences among these trials of thrombolytic agents; no single element can be identified as the critical factor determining the success or failure of the interventions studied. These trials have provided experience relevant to the design of future trials in acute ischemic stroke.

C. Issues in Clinical Trial Design

1. Patient Selection

a. Time Window for Enrollment.   One of the prime considerations in patient selection for trials in acute ischemic stroke is the duration of opportunity for benefit from reperfusion after onset of the ischemic event. It is generally considered plausible that this opportunity persists for a limited time. However, there is no strong evidence defining the window of opportunity. Furthermore, there may be an increased risk of ICH with thrombolytics as the time from ischemia onset increases. Thus, each trial should utilize an eligibility criterion that limits enrolment to patients within a specific time frame following the onset of stroke symptoms. If the time window is relatively wide, analyses should be planned and powered to assess differences in therapeutic effects based on the time from onset.

Trials with a short time limit on duration from the onset of symptoms to the initiation of treatment may include only a minority of stroke patients actually screened. This occurred in several of the recently reported trials. The Early Stroke Trial of monosialoganglioside (5-h–time limit) enrolled 9.5% of screened patients, the MAST-I trial (6-h time limit) enrolled only 5% of all patients screened, and the NINDS Studies (3-h–time limit) enrolled only 3.5% of screened patients [57,58]. Presentation to medical care too long after onset was the single most frequent reason for exclusion. However, simply broadening the acceptable time window to accommodate the presentation pattern may add patients who have inadequate salvageable tissue or an increased risk for ICH. This can result in a trial in which there is no observed benefit for an otherwise promising intervention.

b. Comparison to Screened Population. As the enrolled population may be a small minority of screened patients, questions of the generalizability of the results may arise. It is advisable to maintain a screening log of all stroke patients evaluated at treatment sites. This should include demographic information and the reason for exclusion from the trial. This may provide the ability to compare the characteristics of the excluded population with the enrolled population, and assess the applicability of the trial results with the larger stroke population.

c. CT Scan Eligibility Criteria. Administering a thrombolytic or antithrombotic agent in the setting of a small, clinically asymptomatic ICH may risk conversion to a large, life-threatening intracranial hematoma. A sensitive evaluation for hemorrhage is important in the screening evaluation. The most reliable and widely available mechanism for the detection of ICH is currently a cranial computed tomography (CT) scan. Performing and evaluating a CT scan before treatment may delay the administration of study agents, but is felt to be of critical importance.

Certain criteria, if appropriately selected and adequately employed, may enable exclusion of a subpopulation of patients without ICH at presentation, but with excessive risk of developing ICH on therapy. In ECASS, patients with early major infarct signs on the screening CT were felt to be at higher risk for ICH and were to be excluded from the trial. A retrospective review of the screening CT scans determined that some patients were enrolled with such exclusionary findings. The rate of ICH among these patients was relatively high. To be effective in screening out high-risk patients, clear definition of the CT criteria should be included in the protocol. There may need to be training examples for the site investigators to improve diagnostic accuracy.

2. Selection of the Therapeutic Regimen

a. Method of Administration. There are several potential methods of administering thrombolytic agents. The intravenous route is the simplest, and the most quickly initiated. Many investigators have considered the possibility that the restoration of perfusion may be more effective or safer if the thrombolytic agent is delivered directly into or near the thrombus [59]. This necessitates cranial intra-arterial microcatheter placement by an interventional neuroradiologist. If this is the selected method of administration, several complexities must be addressed in advance. The procedure will delay the initiation of the study treatment, and this conflicts with the goal of minimizing the duration between stroke onset and treatment initiation. This may also make enrollment into the trial difficult due to the more limited number of patients presenting early enough to have all procedures performed. Blinding will be possible only if arterial catheterization is performed in the control arm as well.

The intra-arterial procedure necessitates an angiogram to localize the thrombus. This may be performed before or after randomization. In some patients there will be no thrombus visualized. When the angiogram is performed before randomization, the protocol must explicitly address the disposition of the patients without thrombus. If these patients are excluded from the trial, they should be followed for potential adverse events that could be related to the catheterization and angiogram. These procedures are not part of standard care for acute stroke, but are performed as part of the evaluation for study therapy. Any adverse outcomes must thus be incorporated into the eventual comparison of risk and benefit. All randomized patients should be included in the analysis of efficacy to ensure comparability of the groups. When randomization is carried out before the angiogram, patients should not be excluded from analysis of efficacy based on the angiographic findings.

b. Dose Optimization.   The importance of thorough, early dose-finding studies is highlighted by recent trial experiences. In the streptokinase trials, stroke patients were treated with the same dose of streptokinase as that used in treatment of acute MI. Large definitive trials were initiated with little or no examination of the activity of safety of this dose in stroke. All three studies showed excessive rates of ICH, and all were prematurely halted. The two alteplase studies used alteplase from different manufacturers and doses that were modestly different, approximately 22% higher in ECASS than in the NINDS studies. It is possible that the difference in study agent doses may have been an important factor in the different outcomes of the studies. This would suggest a narrow therapeutic window for thrombolytics in acute stroke. Well-conducted dose-ranging studies may help identify doses with a reasonable likelihood of being both safe and effective.

In studies of combinations of thrombolytic agents with other therapies, it is imperative that development include thorough dose optimization. In part owing to concern of inducing excessive rate of ICH, some of the more recent studies have not used any concomitant antithrombotic therapies. This concern may be justified in light of the increased rate of ICH in the streptokinase-with-aspirin group seen in the MAST-I trial. However, preclinical evidence suggests that the thrombolytic activity of some agents is enhanced by the addition of adjunctive antithrombotic agents. In such combination therapies, the dose and schedule of both agents should be addressed in phase II studies. Dose optimization studies may be particularly benefited by judicious use of brain-imaging methods for safety and activity assessments.

c. Dynamically Adjusted Dose Regimens.   Dosing of some therapeutic agents requires ongoing adjustment of the infusion amount, based on a laboratory parameter. Protocols that provide a clear flow of decision-making and guidance for the dosing adjustment are important in these cases. Testing such dosing guidelines under actual trial circumstances is important to ensure that the desired physiological effect is achieved. In the Ancrod Stroke Study, the ancrod dose was adjusted according to plasma fibrinogen levels. Dose adjustment achieved target fibrinogen levels in less than one-fourth of the patients. Drawing conclusions on the safety or efficacy of the intended therapy is difficult in such cases [6].

3.   Efficacy Endpoints and Analyses

Although most patients do not die of an acute ischemic stroke, most will suffer residual impairments. Thus both mortality and functional status outcomes must be evaluated and analyzed. There is no assurance that both outcomes will be directly correlated, or that improvement in one will not be associated with worse outcome on the other. At the present time, patient status at 90 days after the stroke is considered to be the most informative time to assess patient outcome.

Evaluation of a patient who survives the stroke with a residual deficit is a complex assessment. Several types of outcome scales have been utilized to grade the amount of residual deficit.

1. The neurological impairment scales (e.g., the NIH Stroke Scale, Toronto Stroke Scale, and the Scandinavian Stroke Scale) are composites derived from the neurological examination. Interpretation can be complex, as any particular score may derive from patients with very different sets of impairments. This nonequivalence is more marked for comparisons of change in score from baseline. The meaning of any particular point change in score may be quite different for patients with different baseline severity of stroke and constellation of deficits.
2. The multi-item functional scales (e.g., the Barthel Index) can more directly address clinical meaningfulness, but have some of the same difficulties as the neurological impairment scales.
3. The global single-assessment scales (e.g., the Modified Rankin Scale and the Glasgow Outcome Score) use a single, subjective assessment to score the outcome. These suffer from the subjectiveness of the assessment and the coarseness of grading, which may decrease sensitivity to lesser differences.

A deficit in some of the scales is that death is not included as an outcome status. Mortality should be included in the accounting if the scale is to provide a solid basis for forming a conclusion about therapy. Some investigators have modified these ordinal scales by including death, either by assigning the worst possible score to patients who die (often used with the neurological impairment scales and the Barthel Index), or by creating a new category for death, ordered below the category for severely disabled. This modification improves the endpoint by conveying a more complete comparison of the treatment groups on rank analysis. Study conclusions may be questioned, however, if the observed effect between treatment arms is largely dependent on shifting the distribution of patients between the severely disabled and death categories. Such a scale modification implicitly assumes that death is a worse outcome than severely disabled, a subjective judgment that may vary with the individual [60].

Some studies, notably the NINDS study, have utilized these scales in a dichotomized form, comparing the proportion of patients achieving an outcome of minimal or no disability. Some treatments may cause an increase in both the proportion of patients with the most favorable outcome (owing to reperfusion) and the proportion with death or severe disability (owing to ICH). Analysis based on a dichotomized scale may give only a partial representation of the treatment effects. When dichotomized outcomes are used, it is critical to assess whether a shift in outcome distribution from moderate disability toward worse outcome occurs as well.

Results showing treatment effects in the same direction on two or three different scales can further strengthen the conclusions from a study. A single global statistic, incorporating the dichotomized form of four stroke scales, served as the primary endpoint in the NINDS Stroke Study. This method provides a single statistic to determine if the outcomes in the two treatment arms are statistically significantly different. However, this method is unable to assess the clinical meaningfulness of any difference seen. The clinical significance of changes on functional scales is more readily apparent than are changes in a global statistic. When a global stastistic is used, investigators will need to examine each of the outcome scales individually, when judgments about treatment effects can be formed. Any inconsistencies in results between the scales will raise uncertainties about the meaning of the observed treatment effect.

Any of the well-established scales can serve as a good clinical endpoint. The scale should be employed in the same manner as it has been extensively used in the medical community.

4. Concomitant Therapy

Concomitant therapies may have very important effects in treatment of an acute stroke. Study protocols should clearly delineate guidelines for use of ancillary agents to ensure consistency across treatment sites and investigators. Concomitant use of antithrombotic agents with thrombolytic agents may have the potential to markedly increase rates of ICH or other major bleeding complications. The MAST-I trial used a factorial design to evaluate streptokinase, aspirin, and the combination in acute stroke. The rate of ICH was increased with streptokinase alone, but was more markedly increased in the streptokinase-plus-aspirin–treated group, indicating a synergistic effect of the combination on the propensity for ICH. The difference in usage of antithrombotic agents may also have contributed to the difference in results obtained in the ECASS and NINDS studies.

Management of hypertension is another area of concern. Marked systolic hypertension may contribute to the occurrence of ICH, so careful blood pressure control is thought to be desirable. Some recent studies raise the concern that calcium channel blockers may convey a pro-hemorrhagic potential. Consistently applied guidelines for management of hypertension will contribute to the likelihood of meaningful trial results.

5. Randomization

The process of randomization will need to be adapted to allow rapid initiation of treatment. Some studies have chosen to have tentative study medication prepared and brought to the patient's location while the screening is still in progress. Thus, there is no delay from the end of screening to the initiation of treatment. Because a patient may still be deemed ineligible and not enrolled even after vials of medication are opened and prepared, strict binding and accounting for all treatment kits are important to minimize the potential for bias.

It is important to have balance between treatment arms in factors that may be independent predictors of outcome or modifiers of the treatment effect. Considerations include the baseline severity of stroke, patient age, clinical site, and factors that may indicate a propensity to develop an ICH. Stratification in the randomization process may assist in ensuring balance of baseline patient characteristics. There must remain sufficient numbers of patients in each stratum to achieve balance and avoid problems with blinding. Other factors can be prospectively identified as covariates for outcome analyses.

6. Blinding

Nonblinded studies risk bias in the administration of ancillary therapies and care. Specification of appropriate ancillary care in the protocol and strict protocol adherence may diminish this source of bias. However, a well-maintained double-blind study design remains the strongest barrier to these confounding factors. When the endpoint is objective, such as mortality, and ancillary treatments and patient assessments are carefully controlled, an unblinded trial may retain adequate credibility for that endpoint. Stroke trials often utilize assessment of impairment or disability as the primary endpoint, however. Such functional assessments may be subjective, and bias may be introduced by patient or investigator unblinding. The potential for bias may be diminished by use of a blinded investigator who serves solely to make the outcome assessment (an "evaluator"). Special precautions may need to be taken to ensure evaluator blinding, such as the sham subclavian bandages utilized in the Hemodilution in Stroke Study [61].

To maintain blinding for therapies requiring adjustment based on a laboratory parameter, a separate "dosing adjustor" may be used. In the Ancrod Stroke Study, ancrod (Arvin) and placebo infusions were adjusted according to a predefined protocol based on fibrinogen levels [6]. The dose adjustor was the only individual to obtain the fibrinogen levels, and provided only the new infusion orders to the other medical staff. Placebo patients received infusion adjustments as well. Adjustments duplicated those made on patients previously treated with ancrod at different study sites.

7. Safety Assessment

As with treatment of acute MI, the single most important safety risk in treatment of ischemic stroke with thrombolytics is generally considered to be ICH. The ICH rate, however, is considerably higher in acute stroke than in AMI, both for untreated (placebo) and for thrombolytic-treated patients. Because stroke and ICH are both brain-damaging events, the efficacy outcome assessment scales account directly for consequences of the ICH. This facilitates assessing the clinical impact of ICH rates and any apparent increases.

Considerations of ICH rates should be included in the dose-optimization component of the overall development plan of new agents. To improve the direction of ICH, trials should include brain imaging at predetermined times, as well as when an ICH is clinically suspected. The NINDS Stroke Study investigators noted that the majority of the increase in ICH associated with alteplase treatment occurred within 36 h of administration. A study that incorporates a CT scan on all patients at 36–48 h after study treatment can expect to ascertain the majority of ICH related to alteplase. The appropriate timing of the CT scan may be different for other agents or treatment regimens, and should be examined during the early pilot studies.

8. The Roles of Brain-Imaging Methods

Brain-imaging methods are an area of intensive investigation, and further advances can be expected. There is presently an important role for some of these methods in stroke trials, and likely to be more as the field advances; CT scans are a critical element of the eligibility screening procedure. Imaging methods may have other roles in the therapeutic development process as well.

a. Brain Imaging as an Activity Endpoint. Some imaging methods may have a valuable role as activity endpoints in the initial clinical trials of thrombolytic agents and as supportive endpoints in pivotal trials. Imaging techniques may be objectively obtained, can be read by a single evaluator to maintain consistency across sites, and can be evaluated in a blinded manner. Some imaging abnormalities can be seen within the first week, which may assist in speeding pilot studies. Quantitative measurements of imaged abnormalities may also provide an improved ability to conduct dose-optimization studies. The objectiveness of these techniques may provide important supportive evidence of treatment effect, particularly when the clinical endpoints rely on subjective components.

Newer techniques, particularly magnetic resonance imaging (MRI) techniques and single-photon emission (SPE)CT imaging, are in early stages of development and hold promise of providing additional objective assessments that may be predictive of clinical outcome. For both CT and these newer techniques the methods for analysis of the scans must be clearly and prospectively defined. At present, imaging techniques are not adequately validated as predictors of clinical outcome to the extent that they could serve as primary endpoints in definitive efficacy trials.

b. Brain Imaging as a Safety Endpoint. Because ICH is the most important safety risk for these classes of agents, ascertainment of ICH is important at all stages of development. CT scans are currently the most sensitive-imaging method for hemorrhage and should be employed in all stroke studies. It is important to gain a thorough understanding of the effect of a prospective therapy on ICH rates and types, including acutely "asymptomatic" ICH, to enable a judgment on the balance of risk to benefit.

9. Informed Consent

Informed consent can be difficult to obtain in this population because of cognitive deficits. Patients who are aphasic or lethargic may be unable to give adequate informed consent. Investigators must work closely with institutional review boards (IRBs) to prospectively devise plans and procedures to ensure valid consent.

V. PERIPHERAL ARTERIAL OCCLUSION

A. Background

Peripheral arterial disease usually begins with mild, intermittent claudication, but may progress to critical ischemia. Critical ischemia usually manifests as rest pain, nonhealing skin ulcerations, or gangrene. Critical limb ischemia is thought to result from an acute vascular occlusion in the setting of chronic atherosclerotic disease, or from an acute embolic phenomenon. If atherosclerotic disease is present, multiple sites in several vessels may be involved, and successful treatments may be difficult. Mild intermittent claudication may carry a less than 10% chance of limb loss over the subsequent decade, whereas critical ischemia often immediately threatens the viability of the affected limb, and amputation will be required in most patients unless perfusion can be restored [62].

When reperfusion therapies are unsuccessful or cannot be accomplished in time, amputation may be required. The perioperative mortality for below-the-knee amputation (BKA) has been quoted at 5–10% and for above-the-knee (AKA) at 15–20% [63]. The prognosis for patients following major amputation is not uniformly favorable; full mobility is achieved in only 50% of BKA and 25% of AKA patients, and an estimated 40% of patients will die within 2 years of their first major amputation procedure [64].

Patients with severe symptomatic peripheral arterial disease (PAD) may have as much as a 15-fold relative risk of death, compared with persons without PAD [65]. One prospective 10-year study revealed a threefold higher relative risk of death for subjects with documented large-vessel PAD when compared with subjects without PAD; however most of this appeared to be due to comorbid cardiovascular disease. More than 50% of the mortality following arterial reconstruction may be due to cardiac disease [66,67].

B. Treatments Available

1. Claudication

Modification of contributing factors, such as cigarette smoking or hyperlipidemia, can help prevent the progression of chronic arterial disease in the patient with intermittent claudication. Pentoxifylline (Trental), an improved treatment for intermittent claudication, decreased symptoms and improved patient functional status in clinical trials. The treatment effect seen in practice has been somewhat unpredictable, however, and the drug has not been reported to be efficacious in the absence of smoking cessation and the modification of other risk factors [66]. Other pharmacological agents have been used to increase peripheral blood flow and relieve claudication; however, benefits have not yet been conclusively demonstrated in controlled clinical trials for most of these agents.

2. Critical Limb Ischemia

a. Operative Intervention.   For patients with an acute embolic occlusion and otherwise normal vessels, surgical embolectomy may be a satisfactory treatment. For patients with critical limb ischemia and underlying atherosclerotic disease, treatment of the acute occlusion may not be successful in restoring blood flow without relief of the underlying chronic obstruction. For many years surgical revascularization with autologous or synthetic grafts has been considered to be the standard of care. Success rates for limb salvage with vascular bypass procedures have been good-to-excellent. Results have been best for proximal vessels and for autologous vein grafts [66], and where there are good distal vessels for anastomosis [63]. Patients with critical ischemia often have poor distal vessels and have a poor prognosis, whatever the treatment selected. Fibrointimal hyperplasia, which can be the result of any manipulation of a blood vessel, is responsible for most early reocclusions (between 2 months and 2 years) [64]. Late reocclusion rates of 20–40% are common, from progressive atherosclerotic disease [68].

b. Percutaneous Transluminal Angioplasty.   Percutaneous transluminal (balloon) angioplasty (PTA) has been applied successfully to some lesions. Early experience found only 50% of patients deriving some benefit at 2 years; more recent estimates of success range from 60 to 90% at 5 years [64,66]. Large proximal vessel occlusions of less than 5 cm in length appear to respond best to angioplasty [69]. The estimated mortality and morbidity of the procedure are low relative to operative treatment [64]. PTA may replace surgical treatment for some patients, or it may be performed as an adjunct to surgery. In one series of 1015 patients treated between 1985 and 1989, 34% of patients were able to be treated with PTA before planned operative intervention; 19% did not require surgery after PTA. The remaining 15% required operative intervention either to treat another lesion not amenable to PTA, or to a failed PTA, or to a complication [69].

Recurrence of stenosis, from fibrointimal hyperplasia, may also be a problem after these procedures, diminishing long-term success. Other endovascular treatments are under investigation, including the use of lasers, rotational atherectomy, and intraluminal stent placement, in an attempt to reduce restenosis rates [70].

c. Thrombolysis.   Thrombolytic treatment has a potential role in the management of acute peripheral arterial occlusion. Although surgical revascularization is frequently the treatment of choice, often comorbid cardiovascular disease makes the patient a poor surgical candidate, and suggests the consideration of an alternative approach. Thrombolytic agents may serve to lyse an acute thrombus, and improve perfusion to an acutely ischemic limb. Thrombolysis may also reveal an underlying atherosclerotic plaque or a more chronic stenosis that may require additional treatment to restore blood flow to the ischemic limb. Treatment with thrombolytic agents may potentially permit the performance of less invasive revascularization procedures or a more minor surgical procedure.

The response to thrombolytic treatment may vary, depending on the age and location of the clot, whether ischemia has been mild or severe, chronic or acute, and whether the clot is de novo or recurrent, embolic or thrombotic, and whether a native artery or grafted vessel is involved. More efficient clot lysis has been seen in vessels with unimpaired blood flow and when there is sufficient surface area of the clot exposed to the plasma to enable contact between the clot and the thrombolytic agent [71].

The time from onset of symptoms to treatment may determine success rates of treatment of acute vascular occlusions. Although fresh thromboses may be amenable to lysis, older clots may contain larger amounts of crosslinked fibrin, and may not respond as well to lytic agents [71]. Data from most patient series suggest that the likelihood of clot lysis is greatest within 6–10 days or 14 days of symptoms' onset, but some small series have demonstrated success with thromboses present for 30 days or more [72–74]. These data are limited to small numbers of patients, and the hypotheses have not been tested in adequately powered controlled trials.

The mode of administration may also influence the outcome. Systemic thrombolytic therapy may have a greater likelihood of bleeding complications; intra-arterial delivery of thrombolytics has achieved efficient clot lysis in some small studies [67], and is thought to have less potential for systemic bleeding [63].

d. Effectiveness of Current Treatments.   Regardless of which treatment is chosen, recurrence of atherosclerotic peripheral vascular disease is common, particularly if contributory risk factors, such as cigarette smoking and hyperlipidemia, are not eliminated. Individual patients frequently develop bilateral disease and in multiple locations in the arterial tree, requiring repeat procedures or long-term pharmacological therapy.

C. Clinical Trial Experience

Streptokinase (Streptase, Kabikinase) was approved in 1980 for treatment of peripheral arterial occlusion on the basis of several small studies indicating both angiographic and clinical improvement, most strikingly for patients treated within 14 days of symptoms' onset [75], yet uncertainty remains about the precise role of thrombolytics in the treatment of peripheral vascular disease. Although clot lysis with urokinase and alteplase has been demonstrated in several clinical studies, severe hemorrhagic complications have been reported [73,76,77]. There have been no large-scale controlled studies clearly demonstrating clinical benefits of treatment.

At present, thrombolytic therapy for acute limb-threatening ischemia is likely to be considered in patients when options for surgical or mechanical intervention are limited or the patient has extensive comorbid disease, yet the patients most likely to benefit from thrombolysis, optimal dosing regimens, optimal delivery methods, and the risk/benefit balance to be expected have not yet been clearly evaluated in prospective, controlled clinical trials. The European Working Group on Critical Leg Ischemia concluded in 1991 that there was "inadequate evidence from published studies to support the routine use of primary pharmacologic treatment in patients with critical leg ischemia" [78]. The group also called for the performance of large, controlled clinical trials to assess all proposed therapies [78,79]. Several problems with reported studies were noted: Few of the reported studies on pharmacotherapeutic agents involved patients with chronic ischemia, patients with a range of severity were included, and the size of most studies was inadequate to evaluate sufficiently the possible differences between treatment and control arms. The group recommended future clinical trials to examine the efficacy of primary medical treatment and of percutaneous catheter procedures in treatment of lower-extremity ischemia. Large-scale studies of thrombolytic therapy in combination with, and compared with, surgical revascularization, angioplasty, or other endovascular treatments have been proposed, but not performed [80].

D. Issues in Clinical Trial Design

1. Controls and Concomitant Therapy

The choice of control treatments for a trial of thrombolytic or antithrombotic therapy for peripheral arterial disease is dependent on whether the agent is being studied for chronic intermittent claudication or acute critical limb ischemia. Operative intervention for revascularization, widely considered the standard of care, would be the most appropriate control for a trial of therapy for critical limb ischemia, although this may change as PTA and endovascular treatments continue to evolve. For a trial in claudication, it may be more appropriate to compare a pharmacological treatment with other medical therapy, or perhaps with placebo and observation.

2. Endpoints

Selection of endpoints for a trial of thrombolytic therapy for peripheral arterial disease is dependent on the potential use of the study agent and for whom the treatment will be indicated. For primary treatment of critical limb ischemia, mortality and amputation rates (or survival and limb salvage) are the most important treatment outcomes. While these are relatively objective endpoints, it is important to ensure, particularly in nonblinded trials, that each arm has comparable supportive care and follow-up, as these factors may affect amputation rates [69]. Avoidance of revascularization procedures may provide substantial benefit to the patient, provided survival and limb salvage rates are comparable between treatment arms and morbidity of the study drug is less than morbidity of the procedure. Thus, when avoidance of revascularization is used as the primary measure of benefit, it is essential that the trial be powered to exclude the possibility of increased mortality or amputation rates, which would outweight revascularization benefits. When treatments are not blinded, care must be taken to avoid bias in endpoint assessment.

For trials of intermittent claudication, when prevention of disease progression is the treatment goal, it is beneficial to use both an objective outcome measure, such as graded exercise testing, and a measure of functional status for patient assessment [81]. Time to required revascularization procedures may also be an appropriate outcome measure in such trials. Criteria should be carefully outlined prospectively to determine that a patient has failed medical therapy and should be considered a candidate for PTA or other revascularization procedures.

The time period for assessment of response is also an important consideration. Restenosis may occur within months after lysis of an acute thrombus. Recurrent ischemia at a later time is common, owing to progression of the underlying vascular disease. Outcome evaluation at 30 days, and at 6, 9, or 12 months after treatment, offers an opportunity for evaluation of both early and late treatment effects.

3. Patient Selection

It may be appropriate to stratify patients or to perform subgroup analysis by treatment site and by location of occlusion, severity of disease, or duration of symptoms. In trials of critical ischemia, the possibility that patients with embolic disease may respond differently to a therapy than patients with thrombosis should be considered. Stratification should be employed only when there is an expectation that a specific parameter will be an important predictor of outcome or a modifier of the treatment effect, and when there will be adequate numbers of patients in each cell for analysis.

4. Safety Parameters and Risk/Benefit Assessment

Evaluation of the rates of stroke, particularly ICH, other major, serious, or life-threatening bleeding complications, and peripheral embolization are key elements in the determination of the risks of treatment of peripheral arterial disease with thrombolytic agents. For an agent that provides significant benefit in a serious disease, such as limb-threatening critical ischemia, agents with some risk (e.g., of bleeding) may be considered acceptable. The potential benefits of the treatment should clearly outweigh any potential risks, however.

5. Areas for Further Study

Critical evaluation of the role of thrombolytic and antithrombotic therapies in treatment of peripheral arterial disease would be enhanced by the performance of adequately powered, randomized, controlled clinical trials. The target population and clinical endpoints should be carefully selected, based on what is known from previous studies. Further study should be devoted to an exploration of the types of lesions that may respond best, the duration of ischemia that will allow successful therapy, the optimal dose regimens, and routes of therapy, and in which patients thrombolytic or antithrombotic therapy might suffice alone, or as an adjunct to percutaneous or surgical treatment. Combination of thrombolytic and antithrombotic agents and of these agents and mechanical devices have constituted an area of recent interest; controlled studies of combination therapies would lend insight into the safety and efficacy of such combined treatment modalities.

Further dose-finding studies would be beneficial to define the optimal thrombolytic doses for local intra-arterial and for intravenous treatment of critical ischemia. Further evaluation of the risk–benefit ratio of treatment with these agents when combined with heparin, aspirin, or other anticoagulants would also be valuable.

REFERENCES

1. Section 312.21 Title 21, U. S. Code of Federal Regulations.
2. Friedman LM, Furberg CD, DeMets DL. Fundamentals of Clinical Trials. 3d ed. St. Louis: Mosby, 1996.
3. Spilker B. Guide to Clinical Trials. New York: Raven Press, 1991.
4. The EPIC Investigators. Use of a monoclonal antibody directed against the platelet glycoprotein IIb/IIIa receptor in high-risk, coronary angioplasty. N Engl J Med 1994; 330:956–961.
5. Ferguson JJ. Meeting highlights: American College of Cardiology, 45th Annual Scientific Session, Orlando, FL, March 24–27, 1996. Circulation 1996; 94:1–5.
6. The Ancrod Stroke Study Investigators. Ancrod for the treatment of acute ischemic brain infarction. Stroke 1994; 25:1755–1759.
7. De Wood MA, Spores, J. Notske R, et al. Prevalence of total coronary occlusion during the early hours of transmural myocardial infarction. N Engl J Med 1980; 303:897–902.
8. Weinstein J. The international registry to support approval of intracoronary streptokinase thrombolysis in the treatment of myocardial infarction. Circulation 1983: 68(suppl 1):61–66.
9. Braunwald E. Thrombolytic therapy in patients with acute myocardial infarction. Circulation 1983; 68(suppl 1):67–69.
10. Brody BA. Ethical Issues in Drug Testing, Approval, and Pricing: The Clot-Dissolving Drugs. New York: Oxford University Press, 1995:29–45.
11. Fibrinolytic Therapy Trialists' Collaborative Group. Indications for fibrinolytic therapy in suspected acute myocardial infarction: collaborative overview of early mortality and major morbidity results from all randomised trials of more than 1000 patients. Lancet 1994; 343:311–322.
12. TIMI Study Group. The thrombolysis in myocardial infarction trial. N Engl J Med 1985; 312:932–936.
13. GISSI Study Group. GISSI-2: a factorial randomized trial of alteplase versus streptokinase and heparin versus no heparin among 12,490 patients with acute myocardial infarction. Lancet 1990; 336:65–71.
14. Third ISIS Collaborative Group. ISIS-3: a randomized comparison of streptokinase vs tissue plasminogen activator vs. antistreplase and of aspirin plus heparin vs aspirin alone among 41,299 cases of suspected acute myocardial infarction. Lancet 1992; 339:753–770.
15. GUSTO Investigators. An international randomized trial comparing four thrombolytic strategies for acute myocardial infarction. N Engl J Med 1993; 329:673–682.

16. Wilcox RG. Randomized, double-blind comparison of reteplase double-bolus administration with streptokinase in acute myocardial infarction (INJECT): trial to investigate equivalence. Lancet 1995; 346:329–336.

17. Passamani E, Hodges M, Herman M, et al. The thrombolysis in myocardial infarction (TIMI) phase II pilot study: tissue plasminogen activator followed by percutaneous transluminal coronary angioplasty. J Am Coll Cardiol 1987; 10:51–64.

18. Anderson HV, Willerson JT. Thrombolysis in acute myocardial infarction. N Engl J Med 1993; 329:703–709.

19. ISIS-2 Collaborative Group. Randomized trial of intravenous streptokinase, oral aspirin, both, or neither among 17,187 cases of suspected acute myocardial infarction: ISIS-2. Lancet 1988; 2:349–360.

20. Dotter CT, Judkins MP. Transluminal treatment of arteriosclerotic obstruction: description of a new technique and a preliminary report of its application. Circulation 964; 30:654–670.

21. Grüntzig A. Die perkutane transluminale Rekanalisation chronischer Arterienverschlüsse mit einer neuen Dilatationstechnik. Baden-Baden: G Witzstrock Verlag, 1977.

22. Grüntzig A. Transluminal dilation of coronary-artery stenosis [letter]. Lancet 1978; 1:263.

23. Landau C, Lange RA, Hillis LD. Percutaneous transluminal coronary angioplasty. N. Eng J Med 1994; 330:981–993.

24. Grüntzig AR, Senning A, Siegenthaler WE. Nonoperative dilatation at coronary-artery stenosis: percutaneous transluminal coronary angioplasty. N Engl J Med 1979; 301:61–68.

25. Barnathan ES, Schwartz JS, Taylor L, et al. Aspirin and dipyridamole in the prevention of acute coronary thrombosis complicating coronary angioplasty. Circulation 1987; 76:125–134.

26. Lembo NJ, Black AJ, Roubin GS, et al. Effect of pretreatment with aspirin versus aspirin plus dipyridamole on frequency and type of acute complications of percutaneous transluminal coronary angioplasty. Am J Cardiol 1990; 65:422–426.

27. McGarry TF Jr, Gottlieb RS, Morganroth J, et al. The relationship of anticoagulation level and complications after successful percutaneous transluminal coronary angioplasty. Am Heart J 1991; 123:1445–1451.

28. Gabliani G, Delegonul U, Kern MJ, Vandormael M. Acute coronary occlusion occurring after successful percutaneous transluminal coronary angioplasty; temporal relationship to discontinuation of anticoagulation. Am Heart J 1988; 116:696–700.

29. Fischell TA, Derby G, Tse TM, Stadius ML. Coronary artery vasoconstriction routinely occurs after percutaneous transluminal coronary angioplasty. A quantitative arteriographic analysis. Circulation 1988; 78:1323–1334.

30. Cowley MJ, Dorros G, Kelsey SF, Van Raden M, Detre KM. Acute coronary events associated with percutaneous transluminal coronary angioplasty. Am J Cardiol 1984; 53:12C–16C.

31. Ellis SG, Rougin GS, King SB III, et al. Angiographic and clinical predictors of acute closure after native vessel coronary angioplasty. Circulation 1988; 77:372–379.

32. Lincoff AM, Popma JJ, Ellis SG, et al. Abrupt vessel closure complicating coronary angioplasty: clinical, angiographic and therapeutic profile. J Am Coll Cardiol 1992; 19:926–935.

33. Simpfendorfer C, Belardi J, Bellamy G, et al. Frequency, management and follow-up of patients with acute coronary occlusions after percutaneous transluminal coronary angioplasty. Am J Cardiol 1987; 59:267–269.

34. Sinclair IN, McCabe CH, Sipperly ME, Baim DS. Predictors, therapeutic options and long-term outcome of abrupt reclosure. Am J Cardiol 1988; 61:61G–66G.

35. Bell MR, Berger PB, Bresnahan JR, et al. Initial and long-term outcome of 354 patients after coronary balloon angioplasty of total coronary artery occlusions. Circulation 1992; 85:1003–1011.

36. Gruentzig AR, King SB III, Schlumpf M, Siegenthaler W. Long-term follow-up after percutaneous transluminal coronary angioplasty. The early Zurich experience. N Engl J Med 1987; 316:1127–1132.

37. Hirschfield JW Jr, Schwartz JS, Jugo R, et al. Restenosis after coronary angioplasty: a multivariate statistical model to relate lesion and procedure variables to restenosis. The M-HEART Investigators. J Am Coll Cardiol 1991; 18:647–656.

38. Leimgruber PP, Roubin GS, Hollman J, et al. Restenosis after successful coronary angioplasty in patients with single-vessel disease. Circulation 1986; 73:710–717.

39. Meier B. Total coronary occlusion: a different animal? J Am Coll Cardiol 1991; 17(6 suppl B):50B–57B.

40. Multicenter European Research Coronary Obstruction and Restenosis (MERCATOR) Study Group. Does the new angiotensin converting enzyme inhibitor cilazapril prevent restenosis after percutaneous transluminal coronary angioplasty? Results of the MERCATOR study: a multicenter, randomized, double-blind, placebo-controlled trial. Circulation 1992; 86:100–110.

41. Coller BS, Scudder LE. Inhibition of dog platelet function by in vivo fusion of F(ab$'$)$_2$ fragments of a monoclonal antibody to the platelet glycoprotein IIb/IIIa receptor. Blood 1985; 66: 1456–1459.

42. Ellis SG, Tcheng JE, Navetta FI, et al. Safety and antiplatelet effect of murine monoclonal antibody 7E3 Fab directed against platelet glycoprotein IIb/IIIa in patients undergoing elective coronary angioplasty. Coron Artery Dis 1993; 4:167–175.

43. Topol EJ, Califf RM, Weisman HF, et al. Randomised trial of coronary intervention with antibody against platelet IIB/IIIa integrin for reduction of clinical restenosis: results at six months. The EPIC Investigators. Lancet 1994; 343:881–886.

44. Ryan TJ, Faxon DP, Gunnary RM, et al. Guidelines for percutaneous transluminal coronary angioplasty. A report of the American College of Cardiology/American Heart Association Task Force on Assessment of Diagnostic and Therapeutic Cardiovascular Procedures (Subcommittee on Percutaneous Transluminal Coronary Angioplasty). Circulation 1988; 78:486–502.

45. Rao AK, Pratt C, Berke A, et al. Thrombolysis in Myocardial Infarction (TIMI) Trial—phase I: hemorrhagic manifestations and changes in plasma fibrinogen and the fibrinolytic system in patients treated with recombinant tissue plasminogen activator and streptokinase. J Am Coll Cardiol 1988; 11:1–11.

46. Landefeld CS, Cook EF, Flatley M, et al. Identification and preliminary validation of predictors of major bleeding in hospitalized patients starting anticoagulant therapy. Am J Med 1987; 82:703–713.

47. del Zoppo GJ, Pessin MS, Mori E, Hacke W. Thrombolytic intervention in acute thrombotic and embolic stroke. Semin Neurol 1991; 11:368–384.

48. Wardlaw JM, Warlow CP. Thrombolysis in acute ischemic stroke: does it work? Stroke 1992; 23:1826–1839.

49. Haley EC Jr. Thrombolytic therapy for acute ischemic stroke. Clin Neuropharm 1993; 16:179–194.

50. Sandercock PAG, van den Belt AGM, Lindley RI, Slattery J. Antithrombotic therapy in acute ischaemic stroke: an overview of the completed randomised trials. J Neurol Neurosurg Psychiatry 1993; 56:17–25.

51. Hommel M, Boissel JP, Cornu C, et al. Termination of trial of streptokinase in severe acute ischemic stroke. Lancet 1995; 345:57.

52. The Multicenter Acute Stroke Trial – Europe Study Group. Thrombolytic therapy with streptokinase in acute ischemic stroke. N Engl J Med 1996; 335:145–150.

53. Donnan GA, Davis SM, Chambers BR, et al. Trials of streptokinase in severe acute ischemic stroke. Lancet 1995; 345:578–579.

54. Multicentre Acute Stroke Trial – Italy Group. Randomized controlled trial of streptokinase, aspirin, and combination of both in treatment of acute ischaemic stroke. Lancet 1995; 346:1509–1514.

55. Hacke W, Kaste M, Fieschi C, et al. Intravenous thrombolysis with recombinant tissue plasminogen activator for acute hemispheric stroke. JAMA 1995; 274:1017–1025.

56. The National Institute of Neurological Disorders and Stroke rt-PA Stroke Study Group. Tissue plasminogen activator for acute ischemic stroke. N Engl J Med 1995; 333:1581–1587.

57. Lenzi GL, Grigoletto F, Gent M, et al. Early treatment of stroke with monosialoganglioside GM-1. Stroke 1994; 25:1552–1558.

58. Food and Drug Administration. Peripheral and Central Nervous System Drugs Advisory Committee Hearing, Bethesda, MD, June 6, 1996.

59. del Zoppo GJ, Ferbert A, Otis S, et al. Local intra-arterial fibrinolytic therapy in acute carotid territory stroke. Stroke 1988; 19:307–313.

60. Solomon NA, Glick HA, Russo CJ, Lee J, Schulman KA. Patient preferences for stroke outcomes. Stroke 1994; 25:1721–1725.

61. The Hemodilution in Stroke Study Group. Hypervolemic hemodilution treatment of acute stroke. Stroke 1989; 20:317–323.
62. Framingham Heart Study and others, cited in Green RM, Ouriel K. Peripheral arterial disease. In: Schwartz SI, Shires TG, Spencer FC, Husser WC, eds. Principles of Surgery. New York: McGraw Hill, 1994.
63. Bell PRF. Peripheral arterial disease. In: Bloom AL, Forbes CD, Thomas DP, Tuddenham EGD, eds. Hemostatis and Thrombosis. Edinburgh: Churchill Livingstone, 1994.
64. Veith FJ, Gupta SK, Wengerter KR, et al. Impact of nonoperative therapy on the clinical management of peripheral arterial disease. Circulation 1991; 83(suppl I):I-137–I-142.
65. Criqui MH, Langer RD, Fronek A, et al. Mortality over a period of 10 years in patients with peripheral arterial disease. N Engl J Med 1992; 326:381–386.
66. Green RM, Ouriel K. Peripheral arterial disease. In: Schwartz SI, Shires TG, Spencer FC, Husser WC, eds. Principles of Surgery. New York: McGraw-Hill, 1994.
67. Pentecost MJ, Criqui MH, Dorros G, et al. American Heart Association Writing Group. Guidelines for peripheral percutaneous transluminal angioplasty of the abdominal aorta and lower extremity vessels. Circulation 1994; 89:511–531.
68. Rutherford RB. Standards for evaluating results of interventional therapy for peripheral vascular disease. Circulation 1991; 83:1-6–I-11.
69. Veith FJ, Gupta SK, Wengerter KR. Changing arteriosclerotic disease patterns and management strategies in lower limb-threatening ischemia. Ann Surg 1990; 112:402–414.
70. Henderson LJ, Kirkland JS. Angioplasty with STENT placement in peripheral arterial occlusive disease. Assoc Operating Room Nurses J 1995; 6:671–685.
71. Bell WR. Thrombolytic therapy: agents, indications and laboratory monitoring. Med Clin North Am 1994; 78:745–765.
72. Quinones-Baldrich WJ, Gomes AS. Thrombolytic therapy. In: Rutherford RB, ed. Vascular Surgery. 3rd ed. Philadelphia: Saunders, 1989.
73. Ouriel K, Shortell CK, DeWeese JA, et al. A comparison of thrombolytic therapy with operative revascularization in the initial treatment of acute peripheral arterial ischemia. J Vasc Surg 1994; 19:1021–1030.
74. Schilling JD, Pond GD, Mulcahy MM, McIntyre KE, Hunter GC, Bernhard JM. Catheter-directed urokinase thrombolysis: an adjunct to PTA/surgery for management of lower extremity thromboembolic disease. Angiology 1994; 45:851–860.
75. PLA 79-115. U. S. Food and Drug Administration, Bureau of Biologics, 1981.
76. Bero CJ, Cardella JF, Reddy K, et al. Recombinant tissue plasminogen activator for treatment of lower extremity peripheral vascular occlusive disease. J Vasc Interv Radiol 1995; 6:571–577.
77. Smith CM, Yellin AE, Weaver AP, Li KM, Siegel AE. Thrombolytic therapy for arterial occlusion: a mixed blessing. Am Surg 1994; 60:371–375.
78. European Working Group on Critical Leg Ischemia. Second European consensus document on chronic critical leg ischemia. Circulation 1991; 84(suppl IV):IV-1–IV-26.
79. Dormandy J. European consensus on critical limb ischemia. Lancet 1989; 1:737–738.
80. Ouriel K. Thrombolytic therapy for acute arterial occlusion. Curr Opin Gen Surg 1994:257–264.
81. Hiatt WR, Hirsch AT, Regensteiner JG, Brass EP, Vascular Clinical Trialists. Clinical trials for claudication: assessment of exercise performance, functional status, and clinical end points. Circulation 1995; 92:614–621.

4

Overview of New Anticoagulant Drugs

Jeffrey I. Weitz and Jack Hirsh
McMaster University and Henderson Research Center, Hamilton, Ontario, Canada

INTRODUCTION

Arterial and venous thrombosis are major causes of morbidity and mortality. Whereas arterial thrombosis is the most common cause of myocardial infarction, stroke, and limb gangrene, venous thrombosis can be complicated by pulmonary embolism, which can be fatal, and by postphlebitic syndrome. Because arterial thrombi consist of platelet aggregates held together by small amounts of fibrin, strategies to inhibit arterial thrombogenesis focus mainly on drugs that block platelet function, but often include anticoagulants to prevent fibrin deposition. In contrast, anticoagulants are the drugs of choice for prevention of cardioembolic events. Anticoagulants are also used for prevention and treatment of venous thrombosis because venous thrombi comprise mainly fibrin and red blood cells. Focusing on new anticoagulant drugs for the prevention and treatment of arterial and venous thrombosis, this chapter (1) reviews arterial and venous thrombogenesis, (2) outlines new anticoagulant strategies, and (3) provides clinical perspective as to which new strategies have the greatest chance of success.

I. THROMBOGENESIS

Arterial thrombi, which form under high-shear conditions, are mainly composed of platelet aggregates joined by fibrin strands. Arterial thrombosis usually is initiated by spontaneous or mechanical rupture of atherosclerotic plaque, a process that exposes thrombogenic material in the lipid-rich core of the plaque to the blood [1]. Intraluminal thrombus superimposed on disrupted atherosclerotic plaque impairs blood flow. Higher shear promotes platelet and fibrin deposition resulting in the formation of an occlusive thrombus that can obstruct blood flow to organs, such as the heart or brain, or to the extremities.

Venous thrombi, which consist mainly of fibrin and red blood cells, develop under low-flow conditions. Often originating in the muscular veins of the calf or in the valve cusp pockets of the deep calf veins, coagulation in these sites is initiated by vascular trauma and is augmented by venous stasis. Damage to the vessel wall is a particularly important predisposing factor to venous thrombosis after major hip or knee surgery.

Initiation of coagulation in veins or arteries is triggered by tissue factor (Fig. 1), a cellular receptor for activated factor VII (factor VIIa) and factor VII [2]. Most nonvascular cells express tissue factor in a constitutive fashion, whereas de novo tissue factor synthesis can be induced in monocytes [3,4]. Injury to the arterial or venous wall exposes nonvascular, tissue factor-expressing cells to blood [2]. Lipid-laden macrophages in the core of atherosclerotic plaques are particularly rich in tissue factor [1], thereby explaining the propensity for thrombus formation at sites of plaque disruption. Factor VIIa, found in small amounts in normal plasma, binds to exposed tissue factor, as does factor VII. Bound factor VII can undergo autoactivation, thereby augmenting the local concentration of factor VIIa [5]. The factor VIIa–tissue factor complex then activates factors IX and X, leading to the generation of factors IXa and Xa, respectively. Factor IXa binds to factor VIIIa on membrane surfaces to form intrinsic tenase, a complex that activates factor X. By feedback activation of tissue factor-bound factor VII, factor Xa amplifies the initiation of clotting [2].

Factor Xa propagates coagulation by binding to factor Va on membrane surfaces to form the prothrombinase complex, which converts prothrombin to thrombin. Once it dissociates from the membrane surface, thrombin converts fibrinogen to fibrin monomer. Fibrin monomers

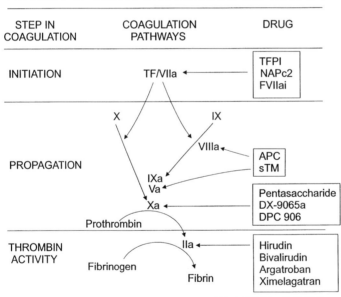

Figure 1 Steps in blood coagulation and sites of action of new anticoagulants: Initiation of coagulation is triggered by the factor VIIa-tissue factor complex (TF/VIIa) which activates factor IX (IX) and factor X (X). Activated factor IX (IXa) propagates coagulation by activating factor X in a reaction that utilizes activated factor VIII (VIIIa) as a cofactor. Activated factor X (Xa), with activated factor V (Va) as a cofactor, converts prothrombin to thrombin (IIa). Thrombin then converts fibrinogen to fibrin. Tissue factor pathway inhibitor (TFPI), nematode anticoagulant peptide (NAPc2), and active–site-blocked factor VIIa (VIIai) and target TF/VIIa, whereas synthetic pentasaccharide, DX-9065a and DCP-906, inactivate Xa. Activated protein C (APC) inhibits the propagation of coagulation by inactivating Va and VIIIa. By catalyzing thrombin-mediated activation of protein C, soluble thrombomodulin (sTM) also promotes the inactivation of Va and VIIIa. Hirudin, bivalirudin, argatroban, and ximelagatran inactivate IIa.

polymerize to form the fibrin mesh, which is stabilized and crosslinked by factor XIIIa, a thrombin-activated transglutaminase. Thrombin amplifies its own generation by feedback activation of factor V and factor VIII, cofactors in the prothrombinase and intrinsic tenase complexes, respectively. Thrombin also can activate factor XI, thereby augmenting factor Xa generation [6].

II. NEW ANTICOAGULANT STRATEGIES

Anticoagulant strategies to inhibit thrombogenesis have focused on blocking initiation of coagulation, preventing the propagation of coagulation, or inhibiting thrombin (see Fig. 1). Initiation of coagulation can be inhibited by agents that target the factor VIIa–tissue factor complex, whereas propagation of coagulation can be blocked by drugs that target factor IXa or factor Xa, or by inactivation of factors Va and VIIIa, key cofactors in coagulation. Finally, thrombin inhibitors prevent fibrin formation and block thrombin-mediated feedback activation of factors V, VIII, and XI. Although there are many candidate drugs to accomplish these tasks, only a few are under development, and even fewer have progressed to clinical testing. Compounds in more advanced stages of clinical development are listed in Table 1.

Table 1 Status of New Anticoagulant Drugs

Target	Drug[a]	Route	Status	Indication
VIIa/TF	TFPI	Intravenous	Phase III	Sepsis
	NAPc2	Subcutaneous	Phase II	Thromboprophylaxis in patients undergoing elective knee arthroplasty; unstable angina
Va/VIIIa	APC	Intravenous	Approved	Sepsis
Xa	Pentasaccharide	Subcutaneous	Approved	Thromboprophylaxis in orthopedic patients
			Phase III	Treatment of venous thromboembolism; treatment of acute coronary syndromes
	DX-9065a	Intravenous	Phase II	Coronary artery disease
	DPC 906	Oral	Phase II	Thromboprophylaxis in patients undergoing elective knee arthroplasty
Xa/IIa	SNAC/heparin	Oral	Phase II/III	Thromboprophylaxis in patients undergoing elective hip or knee arthroplasty
IIa	Hirudin	Intravenous	Approved	Heparin-induced thrombocytopenia
	Bivalirudin	Intravenous	Approved	Alternative to heparin in patients undergoing percutaneous coronary interventions
	Argatroban	Intravenous	Approved	Heparin-induced thrombocytopenia
	Ximelagatran	Oral	Phase III	Thromboprophylaxis in patients undergoing elective hip or knee arthroplasty; treatment of venous thrombosis; alternative to warfarin in patients with atrial fibrillation

[a] APC, activated protein C; NAPc2, nematode anticoagulant peptide c2; SNAC, sodium *N*-(8[2-hydroxybenzoyl]amino) caprylate; TFPI, tissue factor pathway inhibitor.

III. INHIBITORS FOR INITIATION OF COAGULATION

Agents that target the factor VIIa-tissue factor complex block the initiation of coagulation [2]. The drugs in the most advanced stages of development are recombinant tissue factor pathway inhibitor (TFPI) and nematode anticoagulant peptide (NAPc2). Active–site-blocked factor VIIa (factor VIIai) has also been evaluated in humans.

A. TFPI

As a factor Xa-dependent inhibitor of factor VIIa, only small amounts of TFPI circulate in the free state in blood. Most of the circulating TFPI is associated with lipoproteins or is bound to the endothelium; additional TFPI is stored in platelets [6].

Full-length TFPI is released from the endothelium when heparin or low-molecular-weight heparin is given, presumably because these agents displace TFPI bound to endothelial glycosaminoglycans. When administered intravenously, TFPI has a short half-life because it is rapidly cleaved into nonfunctional, truncated forms by an unknown protease. In pigs, TFPI attenuates injury-induced neointimal hyperplasia, and it inhibits smooth muscle cell migration in vitro. TFPI attenuates the coagulopathy and improves survival in sepsis models in baboons or rabbits [7]. Given these results, TFPI has completed phase III evaluation in patients with sepsis. Preliminary reports suggest that TFPI failed to reduce mortality in patients with severe sepsis. Additional studies are needed to determine whether TFPI will be useful for other indications.

B. NAPc2

Small proteins have been isolated from the canine hookworm, *Ancylostoma caninum*, that contain Ascaris-type protease motifs [8]. Some of these proteins directly inhibit factor Xa, whereas others, such as NAPc2, bind to a noncatalytic site on factor X or factor Xa. NAPc2 bound to factor Xa then inhibits factor VIIa within the factor VIIa–tissue factor complex [9]. Because it binds to factor X, in addition to factor Xa, NAPc2 has a half-life of almost 50 h after subcutaneous injection. Functionally, however, NAPc2 behaves similar to TFPI, and attenuates sepsis-induced coagulopathy in laboratory animals. Given promising phase II results when NAPc2 was evaluated as thromboprophylaxis in patients undergoing elective knee arthroplasty [10], the utility of NAPc2 in patients with unstable angina is currently being assessed in a phase II clinical trial.

C. Factor VIIai

By competing with factor VIIa for tissue factor binding, factor VIIai blocks the initiation of coagulation. Based on promising results in animal models of thrombosis [11], factor VIIai is undergoing phase II evaluation in patients having percutaneous coronary interventions.

IV. INHIBITORS OF PROPAGATION OF COAGULATION

Propagation of coagulation can be inhibited by drugs that block factors IXa or factor Xa, or by agents that inactivate factors VIIIa or Va, the cofactors for factors IXa and Xa, respectively.

A. Factor IXa Inhibitors

Strategies to block factor IXa include active–site-blocked factor IXa (factor IXai) and monoclonal antibodies against factor IX/IXa.

1. Factor IXai

By competing with factor IXa for incorporation into the intrinsic tenase complex that assembles on the surface of the activated platelets, factor IXai inhibits clot formation in vitro and blocks coronary artery thrombosis in a canine model [10]. Although factor IXai has yet to be tested in humans, promising results in animals support the concept that agents that target factor IXa will modulate thrombosis.

2. Antibodies Against Factor IX/IXa

Monoclonal antibodies against factor IX/IXa have been described [11–13]. One antibody blocks factor X activation by factor XIa [11], whereas the other binds to the Gla-domains of factor IX and inhibits not only factor XI-mediated activation of factor IX, but also blocks factor IXa activity. A chimeric humanized derivative of the latter antibody has antithrombotic activity in a rat arterial thrombosis model [12,13] and has undergone phase I testing in humans.

B. Factor Xa Inhibitors

Both indirect and direct factor Xa inhibitors are under development. Synthetic pentasaccharide, an analogue of the pentasaccharide sequence of heparin that mediates its interaction with antithrombin [14], is a new indirect factor Xa inhibitor. Direct factor Xa inhibitors, agents that bind directly to factor Xa and block its activity, include recombinant analogues of natural inhibitors, as well as synthetic drugs that target the active site of factor Xa. In contrast to heparin and low-molecular-weight heparins [7,8], which block factor Xa in an antithrombin-dependent fashion and have limited ability to inhibit platelet-bound factor Xa, direct inhibitors of factor Xa inactivate factor Xa bound to phospholipid surfaces, as well as free factor Xa [15].

C. Indirect Factor Xa Inhibitors

1. Synthetic Pentasaccharide

With high affinity for antithrombin, synthetic pentasaccharide (fondaparinux) has greater inhibitory activity against factor Xa than heparin or low-molecular-weight heparin [14]. Because it is too short to bridge antithrombin to thrombin, synthetic pentasaccharide enhances the rate of factor Xa inactivation by antithrombin, but has no effect on the rate of thrombin inhibition. The drug is given subcutaneously on a once-daily basis. In four phase III trials that compared synthetic pentasaccharide with low-molecular-weight heparin for thromboprophylaxis, synthetic pentasaccharide produced a greater reduction in the rates of venous thromboembolism in patients undergoing surgery for hip fracture or elective hip or knee arthroplasty. Based on these findings, synthetic pentasaccharide has been licensed in North America for thromboprophylaxis in high-risk orthopedic patients. Studies comparing synthetic pentasaccharide with low-molecular-weight heparin or heparin for treatment of venous thromboembolism are underway as are investigations into its use in patients with acute coronary syndromes.

D. Direct Factor Xa Inhibitors

Direct inhibitors of factor Xa include recombinant analogues of natural inhibitors of factor Xa and synthetic agents directed against the active site of the enzyme.

1. Natural Inhibitors

Isolated from hematophagous organisms, natural inhibitors of factor Xa include tick anti-coagulant peptide (TAP), antistasin, and lefaxin. Originally isolated from the soft tick, *Ornithodoros moubata*, TAP is a 60-amino–acid polypeptide that forms a stoichiometric complex with factor Xa [15]. Similar to the interaction of hirudin with thrombin, TAP appears to bind to factor Xa in a two-step fashion [15]. An initial low-affinity interaction involves a site distinct from the catalytic site of the enzyme, which may be analogous to exosite 1 of thrombin. This is followed by a high-affinity interaction with the active site, which results in formation of a stable enzyme–inhibitor complex.

Antistasin is a 119-amino–acid polypeptide isolated from the salivary glands of the Mexican leech, *Haementeria officinalis* [17]. Both native and recombinant forms of antistasin are tight-binding, slowly reversible inhibitors of factor Xa [18]. Similar to TAP, antistasin is highly selective for factor Xa. Lefaxin is a 30-kDa polypeptide that was isolated from the saliva of the *H. depressa* leech [19]. Although the gene encoding this protein has yet to be cloned, limited sequence analysis shows no homology between lefaxin and other natural inhibitors of factor Xa.

2. Synthetic Factor Xa Inhibitors

Nonpeptidic, low-molecular-weight, reversible inhibitors of factor Xa include DX-9065a [16] and DPC 906. Intravenous DX-9065a is currently undergoing phase II testing in patients with coronary artery disease. DPC 906 is an aminobenzisoxazole that binds factor Xa with high affinity. With good oral bioavailability, DPC 906 has a half-life of about 12 h. A phase II trial comparing various doses of twice-daily oral DPC 906 with subcutaneous low-molecular-weight heparin for thromboprophylaxis in knee arthroplasty patients is underway.

E. Inhibitors of Factors Va and VIIIa

As key cofactors for intrinsic tenase and prothrombinase, respectively, factors Va and VIIIa are critical for propagation of coagulation. Factors Va and VIIIa are inactivated by activated protein C, a naturally occurring anticoagulant that is generated when the thrombin–thrombomodulin complex activates protein C. Strategies aimed at enhancing the protein C anticoagulant pathway include administration of (1) protein C or activated protein C concentrates, or (2) soluble thrombomodulin.

1. Protein C Derivatives

Both plasma-derived and recombinant forms of protein C and activated protein C are available. Intravenous recombinant activated protein C has recently been shown to reduce mortality in patients with sepsis-induced coagulopathy [20], and has been approved for this indication.

2. Soluble Thrombomodulin

An analogue of the extracellular portion of membrane-bound thrombomodulin, soluble throm-bomodulin complexes thrombin and induces a conformational change in the active site of the enzyme that abolishes its procoagulant activity and converts it into a potent activator of protein C [7]. Now available by recombinant DNA technology [21], soluble thrombomodulin is an effective antithrombotic agent in a variety of animal models [22,23]. Subcutaneous thrombo-modulin, which has a long half-life, is undergoing phase II evaluation for thromboprophylaxis in patients undergoing elective hip arthroplasty.

V. THROMBIN INHIBITORS

Thrombin can be inhibited indirectly by agents that activate naturally occurring thrombin inhibitors (namely, antithrombin or heparin cofactor II), or directly, by drugs that bind to thrombin and prevent its interaction with substrates. Unfractionated heparin and low-molecular-weight heparins are examples of indirect thrombin inhibitors. These agents act as anticoagulants by activating antithrombin, which then complexes and inhibits thrombin and factor Xa, thereby blocking thrombin generation as well as thrombin activity [24,25]. Likewise, dermatan sulfate also is an indirect thrombin inhibitor that activates heparin cofactor II, a selective inhibitor of thrombin [26]. A number of direct thrombin inhibitors have been developed. Of these, three parentral agents, hirudin, argatroban, and bivalirudin, have been approved for use, whereas ximelagatran, an orally active drug, is undergoing phase III evaluation.

A. Indirect Thrombin Inhibitors

Unfractionated heparin and low-molecular-weight heparin are cornerstones for prevention and treatment of venous thrombosis and are widely used in combination with antiplatelet drugs, such as aspirin and glycoprotein IIb/IIIa antagonists, and/or thrombolytic agents in patients with acute coronary ischemic syndromes. Because it produces a more predictable anticoagulant profile than heparin, low-molecular-weight heparin can be given without laboratory monitoring, making it a useful drug for out-of-hospital treatment [25]. Consequently, low-molecular-weight heparin is gradually replacing heparin for treatment of patients with venous thrombosis, and is rapidly establishing a niche for treatment of unstable angina.

Recently, delivery systems have been developed that make it possible to give heparin or low-molecular-weight heparin orally. These delivery systems utilize synthetic amino acids such as sodium N-(8[2-hydroxybenzoyl]amino) caprylate (SNAC) to facilitate heparin absorption by the gut [27]. Although absorption is limited and somewhat variable, sufficient amounts of heparin can be delivered orally to prolong the activated partial thromboplastin time [27]. With phase I and phase II trials completed [28,29], phase III studies comparing SNAC–heparin with low-molecular-weight heparin for thromboprophylaxis in patients undergoing elective hip or knee arthroplasty are now underway.

Dermatan sulfate, which acts as an anticoagulant by activating heparin cofactor II [26], was more effective than low-dose heparin for thromboprophylaxis in cancer patients [30]. Because its low specific activity and poor solubility limit the amount of drug that can be given by subcutaneous injection, dermatan sulfate has yet to be evaluated in the treatment setting. A low-molecular-weight form of dermatan sulfate has been generated to improve bioavailability after subcutaneous injection [31], and various physical methods have been used to enhance specific activity [32]. Whether these maneuvers will render dermatan sulfate a clinically viable anticoagulant remains to be established.

B. Direct Thrombin Inhibitors

Direct thrombin inhibitors have potential advantages over heparin. Whereas thrombin bound to fibrin, or fibrin degradation products, is relatively protected from inactivation by heparin [33–35], bound thrombin is readily inhibited by direct thrombin inhibitors [34,35]. Direct thrombin inhibitors produce a more predictable anticoagulant response than heparin because, unlike heparin, they do not bind to plasma proteins. Likewise, direct thrombin inhibitors are not neutralized by platelet factor 4, a highly cationic, heparin-binding protein released from activated platelets [36].

The most extensively evaluated direct thrombin inhibitors include (1) hirudin, an agent originally isolated from the saliva of the medicinal leech; (2) bivalirudin, a synthetic hirudin analogue; (3) argatroban, a noncovalent inhibitor that reacts with the active site of thrombin; and (4) ximelagatran, an orally available prodrug form of melagatran that reversibly inhibits the active site of thrombin.

1. Hirudin

Hirudin, a 65-amino–acid polypeptide, originally isolated from the salivary glands of the medicinal leech *Hirudo medicinalis*, is now available through recombinant DNA technology [37]. Hirudin is a potent and specific inhibitor of thrombin that forms a stoichiometric, slowly reversible complex with the enzyme [38]. Analysis of the crystal structure of the hirudin–thrombin complex illustrates how the globular amino-terminal domain of hirudin interacts with the active site of thrombin, whereas its carboxy-terminal domain binds to exosite 1 on the enzyme [39].

The almost irreversible nature of the hirudin–thrombin complex may be considered a potential weakness of this drug, as no antidote is available should bleeding occur. Hirudin is cleared predominantly by the kidneys and undergoes little hepatic metabolism [40]. It has a plasma half-life of 40 min after intravenous administration, and approximately 120 min after subcutaneous injection.

Hirudin has been used successfully to treat patients with arterial or venous thrombotic complications of heparin-induced thrombocytopenia [41,42]. It also has been used effectively as an alternative to heparin during cardiopulmonary bypass in a small number of patients with heparin-induced thrombocytopenia [43,44]. On the basis of these data, hirudin has been licensed for the treatment of heparin-induced thrombocytopenia in North America [45].

Subcutaneous hirudin has been shown to be superior to low-dose subcutaneous heparin or low-molecular-weight heparin for thromboprophylaxis in patients undergoing elective hip arthroplasty, and does not increase the risk of bleeding in this high-risk setting [46,47]. In patients with unstable angina and non–ST-elevation myocardial infarction, hirudin appears to be more effective than heparin at reducing recurrent ischemia [48,49]. Although hirudin increases the risk of major bleeding in these patients, there is no increase in life-threatening bleeds [49].

2. Bivalirudin

A synthetic bivalent thrombin inhibitor, bivalirudin comprises a dodecapeptide analogue of the carboxy-terminal of hirudin that binds to exosite 1 on thrombin linked to an active–site-directed moiety, D-Phe-Pro-Arg-Pro, by four glycine residues [50]. Unlike hirudin, bivalirudin produces only transient inhibition of the active site of thrombin because once bound to thrombin, the Arg-Pro bond on the amino-terminal extension of bivalirudin is cleaved, converting bivalirudin into a lower-affinity inhibitor [51]. The shorter half-life of bivalirudin may render it safer than hirudin. In phase III trials, bivalirudin showed enhanced safety relative to heparin in patients undergoing coronary angioplasty [52,53]; bivalirudin has been licensed in North America for this indication. In contrast to hirudin, only a fraction of bivalriudin is renally excreted, suggesting that hepatic metabolism and proteolysis at other sites contribute to its clearance [54]. Bivalirudin has a plasma half-life of 25 min.

3. Argatroban

As a carboxylic acid derivative, argatroban binds noncovalently to the active site of thrombin [55]. Argatroban is an effective alternative to heparin in patients with heparin-induced thrombocytopenia and is approved for this indication. Studies are now underway to evaluate argatroban for the treatment of arterial thrombosis.

4. Ximelagatran

Ximelagatran, a prodrug form of melagatran, is an uncharged lipophilic drug with little intrinsic activity against thrombin. It is well absorbed from the gastrointestinal tract and undergoes rapid biotransformation to melagatran, an active–site-directed thrombin inhibitor [56,57]. The drug produces a predictable anticoagulant response after oral administration, and little or no laboratory monitoring appears to be necessary. Phase II studies with ximelagatran for prevention and treatment of venous thrombosis have been completed [58–61], and phase III trials for these indications are underway. In addition, given promising phase II data [62], ximelagatran is being compared with warfarin for prevention of cardioembolic events in patients with nonvalvular atrial fibrillation.

VI. CHALLENGES AND OPPORTUNITIES FOR NEW ANTICOAGULANT DRUGS

Further clinical testing is needed to define the role of new anticoagulants in the prevention and treatment of venous and arterial thrombosis. In addition to establishing the benefit/risk profiles of new agents, cost-effectiveness analyses will be critical when evaluating drugs with marginal advantages over existing agents. The challenges for the development of drugs for venous thromboembolism will be different from those for arterial thrombosis.

A. New Drugs for Venous Thromboembolism

Although hirudin has been shown to be superior to low-dose heparin or low-molecular-weight heparin for thromboprophylaxis in patients undergoing major orthopedic surgery of the lower limbs [46,47], hirudin is unlikely to gain wide acceptance for this indication unless its cost is comparable with that of low-molecular-weight heparin. Cost considerations may also limit widespread use of synthetic pentasaccharide in this setting, despite its recent approval.

The success of hirudin for thromboprophylaxis in high-risk patients bodes well for orally available agents in this class. With progressive reductions in hospital stay, and evidence that the risk of thrombosis remains high for several weeks after major orthopedic surgery to the lower limbs [63–66], orally available drugs that have a rapid onset of action and need little or no laboratory monitoring may prove to be more convenient than low-molecular-weight heparin, or coumarin derivatives. Although oral delivery systems for heparin or low-molecular-weight heparin are promising [28,29], variable absorption may limit the utility of this approach. In contrast, ximelagatran exhibits good bioavailability after oral administration [56,57] and has undergone promising phase II testing for thromboprophylaxis in orthopedic patients.

The effectiveness of orally available drugs that target factor Xa, or clotting enzymes higher in the coagulation cascade, remains to be established. However, the success of synthetic pentasaccharide in phase III thromboprophylaxis trials suggests that factor Xa inhibitors may also be effective in this setting.

Only limited information is available on the use of hirudin for treatment of venous thrombosis. Despite apparent efficacy, cost considerations are likely to limit the usefulness of hirudin, or other parenteral thrombin inhibitors, as replacements for low-molecular-weight heparin for brief treatment of patients with established venous thromboembolism.

There remains a need for orally active anticoagulants that are safer than coumarin derivatives, given the mounting evidence that patients who develop venous thromboembolism in the absence of identifiable risk factors require longer-term anticoagulation [67–70]. Orally active drugs that target thrombin or factor Xa have the potential to be superior to coumarins for this indication, if they can be administered safely with little or no laboratory monitoring.

B. New Anticoagulants for Arterial Thrombosis

Direct thrombin inhibitors have yet to find a place in the treatment of arterial thrombosis. As an adjunct to thrombolytic therapy, the narrow therapeutic window with hirudin limits its usefulness. Large phase III trials comparing hirudin with heparin as adjuncts to thrombolytic therapy, showed no significant differences in 30-day mortality or reinfarction with the two drugs [71–73]. In contrast, hirudin appears to be superior to heparin in patients with acute coronary syndromes without ST elevation [48,49]. The benefit/risk profile of hirudin relative to low-molecular-weight heparin or parenteral GPIIb/IIIa antagonists, agents that also show promise in these patients, has yet to be established.

Bivalirudin is safer than heparin in patients undergoing coronary angioplasty, or when used as an adjunct to streptokinase in patients with acute myocardial infarction [68]. Approval for bivalirudin as an alternative to heparin in patients undergoing coronary angioplasty is pending, but further trials are needed to determine whether bivalirudin obviates the need for GPIIb/IIIa antagonists in all but the highest risk patients undergoing percutaneous coronary interventions.

Inhibition of clotting enzymes higher than thrombin in the coagulation cascade may be effective, but safety will be a major consideration. Although the factor VIIa–tissue factor complex is an attractive target for inhibition because it initiates coagulation at sites of arterial injury, tissue factor is essential for hemostasis. Consequently, the safety of this approach requires careful evaluation.

Given that atherothrombotic disease develops over decades, long-term therapy is likely to be needed to prevent thrombosis at sites of plaque rupture. Drugs that enhance the activity of natural anticoagulants, such as protein C or TFPI, are likely to be safe. The challenge will be development of orally available small molecules that accomplish these tasks.

ACKNOWLEDGMENTS

The authors thank S. Crnic for her help in preparing this manuscript. Dr. Weitz is a Career Investigator of the Heart and Stroke Foundation of Canada and holds the Canada Research Chair in Thrombosis and the Heart and Stroke Foundation of Ontario/J. Fraser Mustard Chair in Cardiovascular Research at McMaster University.

REFERENCES

1. Fuster V, Badimon L, Badimon JJ, Chesebro JH. The pathogenesis of coronary artery disease and the acute coronary syndromes. N Engl J Med 1992; 326:310–318.
2. Furie B, Furie BC. Molecular and cellular biology of blood coagulation. N Engl J Med 1992; 326:800–806.
3. van den Eijnden MM, Steenhauer SI, Reitsma PH, Bertina RM. Tissue factor expression during monocyte–macrophage differentiation. Thromb Haemost 1997; 77:1129–1136.

4. Neumann FJ, Ott I, Marx N, et al. Effect of human recombinant interleukin-6 and interleukin-8 on monocyte procoagulant activity. Arterioscler Thromb Vasc Biol 1997; 17:3399–3405.
5. Yamamoto M, Nakagaki T, Kisiel W. Tissue factor-dependent autoactivation of human blood coagulation factor. J Biol Chem 1992; 267:19089–19094.
6. Broze GJ Jr. Tissue factor pathway inhibitor. Thromb Haemost 1995; 74:90–93.
7. Hirsh J. Heparin. N Engl J Med 1991; 324:1565–1574.
8. Weitz JI. Low molecular weight heparins. N Engl J Med 1997; 337:688–698.
9. Stassens P, Bergum PW, Gansemans Y, et al. Anticoagulant repertoire of the hookworm *Ancylostoma caninum*. Proc Natl Acad Sci USA 1996; 93:2149–2154.
10. Lee A, Agnelli G, Buller H, et al. Dose–response study of recombinant factor VIIa/tissue factor inhibitor recombinant nematode anticoagulant protein c2 in prevention of post-operative venous thromboembolism in patients undergoing total knee replacement. Circulation 2001; 104:74–78.
11. Benedict CR, Ryan J, Wolitzky B, et al. Active site-blocked factor IXa prevents intravascular thrombus formation in the coronary vasculature without inhibiting extravascular coagulation in a canine thrombosis model. J Clin Invest 1991; 88:1760–1765.
12. Bajaj SP, Rapaport SI, Maki SL. A monoclonal antibody to factor IX that inhibits the factor VIII:Ca potentiation of factor X activation. J Biol Chem 1985; 260:11574–11580.
13. Feuerstein GZ, Toomey JR, Valocik R, Koster P, Patel A, Blackburn MN. An inhibitory anti-factor IX antibody effectively reduces thrombus formation in a rat model of venous thrombosis. Thromb Haemost 1999; 82:1443–1450.
14. Feuerstein GZ, Patel A, Toomey JR, et al. Antithrombotic efficacy of a novel murine antihuman factor IX antibody in rats. Arterioscler Thromb Vasc Biol 1999; 19:2554–2562.
15. Herbert JM, Herault JP, Bernat A, et al. Biochemical and pharmacological properties of SANORG 340006, a potent and long-acting synthetic pentasaccharide. Blood 1998; 91:4197–4205.
16. Vlasuk GP. Structural and functional characterization of tick anticoagulant peptide (TAP): a potent and selective inhibitor of blood coagulation factor Xa. Thromb Haemost 1993; 70:212–216.
17. Herbert JM, Bernat A, Dol F, Herault JP, Crepon B, Lormeau JC. DX-9065a, a novel, synthetic, selective and orally active inhibitor of factor Xa: in vitro and in vivo studies. J Pharmacol Exp Ther 1996; 276:1030–1038.
18. Tuszyuski G, Gasic TB, Gasic GJ. Isolation and characterization of antistasin. J Biol Chem 1987; 262:9718–9723.
19. Dunwiddie C, Thornberry NA, Bull HG, et al. Antistasin: a leech-derived inhibitor of factor Xa: kinetic analysis of enzyme inhibition and identification of the reactive site. J Biol Chem 1989; 264:16694–16699.
20. Faria F, Kelen EM, Sampaio CA, Bon C, Duval N, Chudzinski–Tavassi AM. A new factor Xa inhibitor (lefaxin) from the *Haementeria depressa* leech. Thromb Haemost 1999; 82:1469–1473.
21. Bernard GR, Vincent JL, Laterre PF et al. Efficacy and safety of recombinant hirudin activated protein C for severe sepsis. New Engl J Med 2001; 344:699–709.
22. Parkinson JF, Grinnell BW, Moore RE, Hoskins J, Vlahos CJ, Bang NU. Stable expression of a secretable deletion mutation of recombinant human thrombomodulin in mammalian cells. J Biol Chem 1990; 265:12602–12610.
23. Gomi K, Zushi M, Honda G, et al. Antithrombotic effect of recombinant human thrombomodulin on thrombin-induced thromboembolism in mice. Blood 1990; 75:1369–1399.
24. Aoki Y, Ohishi R, Takei R, et al. Effects of recombinant human soluble thrombomodulin (rhs-TM) on a rat model of disseminated intravascular coagulation with decreased levels of plasma antithrombin III. Thromb Haemost 1994; 71:452–455.
25. Tollefsen DM. Insight into the mechanism of action of heparin cofactor II. Thromb Haemost 1995; 74:1209–1214.
26. Rivera TM, Leone–Bay A, Paton DR, Leipold HR, Baughman RA. Oral delivery of heparin in combination with sodium N-[8-(2-hydroxybenzoyl)amino] caprylate: pharmacological considerations. Pharm Res 1997; 14:1830–1834.

27. Baughman RA, Kapoor SC, Agarwal RK, et al. Oral delivery of anticoagulant doses of heparin. A randomized, double-blind controlled study in humans. Circulation 1998; 98:1610–1615.

28. Gonze MD, Manord JD, Leone–Bay A, et al. Orally administered heparin for preventing deep venous thrombosis. Am J Surg 1998; 176:176–178.

29. DiCarlo V, Agnelli G, Prandoni P, et al. Dermatan sulphate for the prevention of postoperative venous thromboembolism in patients with cancer. DOS (Dermatan sulphate in Oncologic Surgery) Study Group. Thromb Haemost 1999; 82:30–34.

30. Miglioli M, Pironi L, Ruggeri E, et al. Bioavailability of Desmin, a low molecular weight dermatan sulphate, after subcutaneous administration to healthy volunteers. Int J Clin Lab Res 1997; 27:195–198.

31. Linhardt RJ, al-Hakim A, Liu JA, et al. Structural features of dermatan sulfates and their relationship to anticoagulant antithrombotic activities. Biochem Pharmacol 1991; 42:1609–1619.

32. Hogg PJ, Jackson CM. Fibrin monomer protects thrombin from inactivation by heparin-antithrombin III: implications for heparin efficacy. Proc Natl Acad Sci USA 1989; 86:3619–3623.

33. Weitz JI, Hudoba M, Massel D, Maraganore J, Hirsh J. Clot-bound thrombin is protected from inhibition by heparin–antithrombin III but is susceptible to inactivation by antithrombin III-dependent inhibitors. J Clin Invest 1990; 86:385–391.

34. Weitz JI, Leslie B, Hudoba M. Thrombin binds to soluble fibrin degradation products where it is protected from inhibition by heparin–antithrombin but susceptible to inactivation by antithrombin-independent inhibitors. Circulation 1998; 97:544–552.

35. Lane DA, Pejler J, Flynn AM, Thompson EA, Lindahl U. Neutralization of heparin-related saccharides by histidine-rich glycoprotein and platelet factor 4. J Biol Chem 1986; 261:3980–3986.

36. Harvey RP, Degryse E, Stefani L, et al. Cloning and expression of cDNA coding for the anticoagulant hirudin from blood sucking leech, *Hirudo medicinalis*. Proc Natl Acad Sci USA 1986; 83:1084–1088.

37. Stone SR, Hofsteenge J. Kinetics of inhibition of thrombin by hirudin. Biochemistry 1986; 25:4622–4628.

38. Rydel TJ, Ravichandran KG, Tulinsky A, et al. The structure of a complex of recombinant hirudin and human α-thrombin. Science 1990; 249:277–280.

39. Stringer KA, Lindenfeld J. Hirudins: antithrombin anticoagulants. Ann Pharmacother 1992; 26:1535–1540.

40. Schiele F, Vuillemenot A, Kramarz P, et al. Use of recombinant hirudin as antithrombotic treatment in patients with heparin-induced thrombocytopenia. Am J Hematol 1995; 50:25–29.

41. Nand S. Hirudin therapy for heparin-associated thrombocytopenia and deep venous thrombosis. Am J Hematol 1993; 43:310–311.

42. Riess FC, Lower C, Seelig C. Recombinant hirudin as a new anticoagulant during cardiac operations instead of heparin: successful for aortic valve replacement in man. J Thorac Cardiovasc Surg 1995; 110:265–267.

43. Potzsch B, Iversen S, Riess FC. Recombinant hirudin as an anticoagulant in open-heart surgery; a case report. Ann Hematol 1994; 68:A53.

44. Ortel TL, Chong BH. New treatment options for heparin-induced thrombocytopenia. Semin Hematol 1998; 35:26–34.

45. Eriksson BI, Ekman S, Kalebo P, Zachrisson B, Bach D, Close P. Prevention of deep-vein thrombosis after total hip replacement: direct thrombin inhibition with recombinant hirudin, CGP 39393. Lancet 1996; 347:635–639.

46. Eriksson BI, Wille–Jorgensen P, Kalebo P, et al. A comparison of recombinant hirudin with a low-molecular-weight heparin to prevent thromboembolic complications after total hip replacement. N Engl J Med 1997; 337:1329–1335.

47. OASIS Investigators. Comparison of the effects of two doses of recombinant hirudin compared with heparin in patients with acute myocardial ischemia without ST elevation: a pilot study. Circulation 1997; 96:769–777.

48. The OASIS-2 Investigators. Effects of recombinant hirudin (lepirudin) compared with heparin on death, myocardial infarction, refractory angina, and revascularization procedures in patients with acute myocardial ischemia without ST elevation: a randomized trial. Lancet 1998; 353:429–448.

49. Maraganore JM, Bourdon P, Jablonski J, Ramachandran KL, Fenton JW. Design and characterization of hirulogs: a novel class of bivalent peptide inhibitors or thrombin. Biochemistry 1990; 29:7095–7101.

50. Witting JI, Bourdon P, Brezniak DV, Maraganore JM, Fenton JW. Thrombin-specific inhibition by and slow cleavage of hirulog-1. Biochem J 1992; 283:737–743.

51. Bittl JA, Strony J, Brinker JA, et al. Treatment with bivalirudin (Hirulog) as compared with heparin during coronary angioplasty for unstable or postinfarction angina. Hirulog Angioplasty Study Investigators. N Engl J Med 1995; 333:764–769.

52. Bittl JA, Feit F. A randomized comparison of bivalirudin and heparin in patients undergoing coronary angioplasty for postinfarction angina. Hirulog Angioplasty Study Investigators. Am J Cardiol 1998; 82:43–49.

53. Fox I, Dawson A, Loynds P, et al. Anticoagulant activity of hirulog, a direct thrombin inhibitor, in humans. Thromb Haemost 1993; 69:157–163.

54. Fitzgerald D, Murphy N. Argatroban: a synthetic thrombin inhibitor of low relative molecular mass. Coronary Artery Dis 1996; 7:455–458.

55. Eriksson UG, Johansson L, Frison L, et al. Single and repeated oral dosing of H376/95, a prodrug of the direct thrombin inhibitor melagatran, to young healthy male subjects. Blood 1999; 94:26a [abstr 101].

56. Gustafsson D, Nystrom J–E, Carlsson S, et al. Pharmacodynamic properties of H376/95, a prodrug of the direct thrombin inhibitor melagatran, intended for oral use. Blood 1999; 94:26a [abstract 102].

57. Eriksson BI, Lindbratt S, Kalebo P, et al. METHRO II: dose–response study of the novel oral, direct thrombin inhibitor, H376/95 and its subcutaneous formulation, melagatran, compared with dalteparin as thromboembolic prophylaxis after total hip or total knee replacement, [abstr]. Haemostasis 2000; 30:(S1)183.

58. Eriksson BI, Ogren M, Agnelli G, et al. The oral direct thrombin inhibitor ximelagatran and its subcutaneous form melagatran compared with enoxaparin as prophylaxis after total hip or knee joint replacement. Thromb Haemost ximelagatran [supplement] [abstr. 58] 2001.

59. Heit JA, Colwell CWJ, Francis CW, et al. Comparison of the oral direct thrombin inhibitor with enoxaparin as prophylaxis against venous thromboembolism after total knee replacement: a phase 2 dose-finding study, Arch Intern Med 2001; 161:2215–2222.

60. Francis CW, Davidson BL, Berkowitz SD, et al. Randomized, double-blind, comparative study of ximelagatran, an oral direct thrombin inhibitor, and warfarin to prevent venous thromboembolism (VTE) after total knee arthroplasty (TKA). Thromb Haemost [supplement] [abstr 60] 2001.

61. Crowther MA. Oral direct thrombin inhibitors. In: New Therapeutic Agents in Thrombosis and Thrombolysis. 2002; in press.

62. Planes A, Vochelle N, Darmon J–Y, Fagola M, Bellaud M, Huet Y. Risk of deep venous thrombosis after hospital discharge in patients having undergone total hip replacement: double-blind randomized comparison of enoxaparin and placebo. Lancet 1996; 348:28–31.

63. Bergqvist D, Benoni G, Bjurgell O, et al. Low-molecular-weight heparin (enoxaparin) as prophylaxis against venous thromboembolism after total hip replacement. N Engl J Med 1996; 335:696–700.

64. Dahl OE, Andreassen G, Aspelin T, et al. Prolonged thromboprophylaxis following hip replacement surgery—results of a double-blind, prospective, randomized, placebo-controlled study with dalteparin (Fragmin). Thromb Haemost 1997; 77:26–31.

65. Levine MN, Hirsh J, Gent M, et al. Optimal duration of oral anticoagulant therapy: a randomized trial comparing four weeks with three months of warfarin in patients with proximal deep vein thrombosis. Thromb Haemost 1995; 74:606–611.

66. Schulman S, Rhedin A–S, Lindmarker P, et al. A comparison of six weeks with six months of oral anticoagulant therapy after a first episode of venous thromboembolism. N Engl J Med 1995; 332:1661–1665.

67. Prandoni P, Lensing AWA, Cogo A, et al. The long-term clinical course of acute deep venous thrombosis. Ann Intern Med 1996; 125:1–7.

68. Kearon C, Gent M, Hirsh J, et al. A comparison of three months of anticoagulation with extended anticoagulation for a first episode of idiopathic venous thromboembolism. N Engl J Med 1999; 340:901–907.

69. Antman EM, for the TIMI 9B Investigators. Hirudin in acute myocardial infarction: thrombolysis and thrombin inhibition in myocardial infarction (TIMI) 9B trial. Circulation 1996; 94:911–921.

70. GUSTO IIb Investigators. A comparison of recombinant hirudin with heparin for the treatment of acute coronary syndromes. N Engl J Med 1996; 335:775–782.

71. Metz BK, White HD, Granger CB, et al. Randomized comparison of direct thrombin inhibition versus heparin in conjunction with fibrinolytic therapy for acute myocardial infarction: results from the GUSTO IIb trial. J Am Coll Cardiol 1998; 31:1493–1498.

72. White HD, Aylward PE, Frey MJ, et al. Randomized, double-blind comparison of hirulog versus heparin in patients receiving streptokinase and aspirin for acute myocardial infarction (HERO). Circulation 1997; 96:2155–2161.

5

Low-Molecular-Weight Heparins in Acute Coronary Syndromes

David A. Morrow and Elliott M. Antman
Brigham and Women's Hospital, Boston, Massachusetts, U.S.A.

SUMMARY

Effective antiplatelet and antithrombin therapy are central to the management of unstable coronary heart disease. Unfractionated heparin (UFH) has been the mainstay of antithrombin therapy, but has practical and therapeutic disadvantages. The low-molecular-weight heparins (LMWHs) overcome several of these disadvantages, achieving highly predictable levels of anticoagulation with weight-based subcutaneous dosing. Prospective studies support the efficacy of LMWHs compared with aspirin alone for the treatment of patients with non-ST elevation acute coronary syndromes, and have led to a series of randomized clinical trials comparing LMWH with UFH.

The results of five randomized trials support the use of LMWH as a convenient, safe, and effective alternative to UFH for the acute-phase management of unstable angina and non-ST elevation myocardial infarction (MI). Different efficacy results with various LMWHs may partly relate to variation in their relative anti-Xa/anti-IIa ratios, or differences in the study populations or outcomes. Several trials evaluating extended use of fixed dose LMWH after discharge demonstrated no advantage over placebo and higher rates of major hemorrhage. Subgroup analyses, however, have identified selected high-risk patients (e.g., those with elevated cardiac troponins) who may benefit from prolonged treatment.

Preliminary work testing the safety and efficacy of LMWHs as adjunctive therapy for fibrinolysis in ST-elevation MI has produced promising results. In addition, LMWHs appear to be safe when used in combination with platelet glycoprotein IIb/IIIa inhibitors for medical or invasive therapy. Further study in these areas will be important for optimizing the use of LMWHs in the contemporary management of acute coronary syndromes.

I. INTRODUCTION

The genesis of an acute coronary syndrome (ACS) is typically marked by rupture or erosion of atherosclerotic plaque, with ensuing formation of intravascular thrombus [1,2]. Disruption of the protective fibrous cap exposes the highly procoagulant contents of the atheroma core to the circulating bloodstream. The resulting activation of the coagulation cascade and aggregation of platelets culminates in the formation of a flow-limiting thrombus in the coronary circulation [3]. Aimed at halting the propagation of unstable thrombus, antithrombin and antiplatelet therapies are fundamental to the management of unstable coronary artery disease [4,5]. Although unfractionated heparin (UFH) has been a mainstay of anticoagulant therapy, it has several important disadvantages. Thus, the introduction of a novel class of heparins, the LMWHs, that overcome many of these disadvantages, represents an important advance in the therapeutic options for acute coronary syndromes.

II. THE COAGULATION CASCADE AS A TARGET FOR THERAPY IN ACS

Damage to the coronary arterial intima initiates a cascade of prothrombotic events [3,6]. In particular, exposure of tissue factor, a protein present in the subendothelial matrix and expressed by inflammatory cells predominant in vulnerable atheroma, activates the extrinsic coagulation pathway through interaction with factor VII and leads to the generation of activated factor X (Xa) [7–11]. Through a multiplier effect, a single molecule of factor Xa produces multiple molecules of thrombin (factor IIa), which may exist in both the fluid and the fibrin-bound phase. Thrombin catalyzes not only the transformation of soluble fibrinogen into fibrin monomers, but also plays an important role in promoting platelet activation, adhesion, and aggregation, and exerts feedback interactions that stimulate further production of factor Xa [11,12]. Thrombin also stimulates the release of vasoactive mediators that may alter vascular reactivity, further reducing intracoronary blood flow in the setting of ACS [12,13].

This cascade of coagulation proteins is controlled by several inhibitory mechanisms, including the protein C system, tissue factor pathway inhibitor, and the serine protease inhibitor, antithrombin. Antithrombin irreversibly inactivates factors XIIa, XIa, IXa, Xa, as well as thrombin in a reaction catalyzed by both UFH and LMWH.

III. UNFRACTIONATED HEPARIN

The antithrombin agent used most often in the management of ACS is unfractionated heparin (UFH), a mixture of polysaccharide chains of varying length and molecular weight (3000–30,000 Da), consisting of alternating residues of D-glucosamine and uronic acid [14]. The use of UFH for patients with non-ST elevation ACS is supported by pooled data from six trials suggesting that UFH plus aspirin produces a 33% reduction in the risk of death or MI (RR 0.67, 95% CI 0.44–1.02) compared with aspirin alone [4,15]. Also, UFH is often used as an adjunct to fibrin-specific plasminogen activators in patients with ST elevation myocardial infarction (MI) [5,16]. Moreover, UFH is administered in those undergoing percutaneous coronary interventions.

Clinical trials of fibrinolytics in ST elevation ACS have emphasized the need for tight control of the level of anticoagulation achieved with UFH, and the substantial increase in the risk of intracranial hemorrhage with excessive dosing of UFH [17]. However, concurrent evaluation of the range of activated partial thromboplastin times observed in such studies has highlighted the difficulty in achieving predictable levels of anticoagulation with UFH [18]. Variability in anticoagulant effect is one of several important disadvantages of UFH.

Because it binds nonspecifically to plasma proteins, many of which are acute-phase reactants the levels of which are variably increased in ill patients, the anticoagulant response to

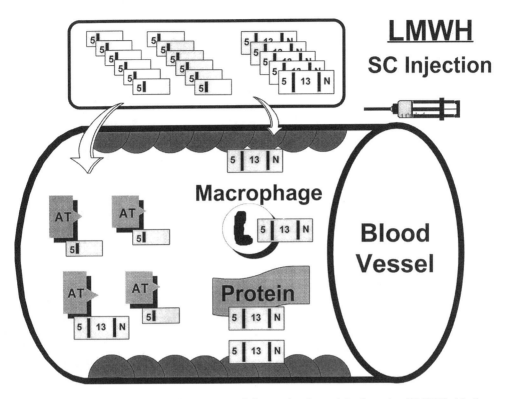

Figure 1 Cartoon illustrating the pattern of low-molecular-weight heparin (LMWH) binding to antithrombin (AT). (A) UFH is a heterogeneous mixture with longer chains containing both the key AT-binding pentasaccharide and 13-saccharide segment necessary to simultaneously bind to AT and thrombin, resulting in a ~1 : 1 ratio of AT bound to short- and long-chain heparin, with consequent 1 : 1 anti-Xa/anti-IIa activity. Nonspecific binding of a proportion of the UFH injected to macrophages and proteins results in variable bioavailability. LMWH preparations (above) consist of a greater proportion of small chains without the full 13-saccharide segment necessary for binding thrombin, resulting in an increased ratio of AT bound to short versus long chains and consequent anti-Xa/anti-IIa ratio > 1. The small chains of LMWH are relatively resistant to nonspecific binding; thus, they have more predictable bioavailability.

UFH is unpredictable. Consequently, frequent monitoring is needed to maintain levels within the therapeutic target range (Fig. 1A) [14,19,20]. UFH also has less inhibitory activity against fibrin-bound thrombin than against circulating thrombin. In addition, a "rebound" increase in thrombotic events occurs on discontinuation of UFH and UFH can cause heparin-induced thrombocytopenia, which can be complicated by thrombosis [21–24]. Thus, in spite of the widespread clinical acceptance of UFH, its multiple practical and therapeutic limitations highlight the need for alternative antithrombotic therapies.

IV. LOW-MOLECULAR-WEIGHT HEPARINS: ADVANTAGES OVER UFH

The LMWHs overcome several disadvantages of UFH as well as offering additional theoretical advantages for the management of patients with ACS (Table 1). With fewer molecules of sufficient length to bring the key binding regions of antithrombin and thrombin into contact,

Table 1 Comparison of Unfractionated Versus Low-Molecular Weight Heparins

	Unfractionated heparin	Low-molecular-weight heparin
Anti-Xa/anti-IIa activity ratio	1	>1
Inhibits thrombin	Yes	Yes
Inhibits thrombin production	Yes	Yes
Bioavailability	Low	High
Requires monitoring of aPTT	Yes	No
Neutralized by platelet factor 4	Yes	No

Source: Ref. 67.

LMWHs have a greater relative activity against factor Xa (i.e., a higher anti-Xa/anti-IIa ratio, than UFH (see Fig. 1B). Theoretically, the increased anti-Xa activity of LMWHs may provide greater "upstream" inhibition of the coagulation cascade, thereby reducing the production of new thrombin [13,14,25].

Further, LMWHs exhibit less susceptibility to inhibition by platelet factor 4, a greater capacity to release tissue factor pathway inhibitor and less nonspecific binding to plasma proteins [26–29]. Each of these factors contributes to a greater stability of anticoagulant effect. Moreover, LMWHs may also have less propensity to stimulate, and may even act to suppress platelet activation and aggregation [13,30–32]. Finally, with high degrees of bioavailability across the various preparations, LMWH may be administered subcutaneously (s.c.), yielding a predictable level of anticoagulation without the need for an infusion pump or hematological monitoring.

Of potential importance to their clinical use, available preparations of LMWH vary in their average length of glycosaminoglycan chains and, consequently, in their relative anti-Xa/anti-IIa ratios. In addition, the LMWHs differ in their ionic form, ability to release tissue factor pathway inhibitor, and potential to cause bleeding in experimental models [33,34]. Together, these differences in structure and function may be of clinical importance and may partly account for variation in the results of clinical trials evaluating these agents in ACS.

V. CLINICAL EVALUATION OF LMWH IN ACS

A. Unstable Angina and Non-ST Elevation MI

1. Acute-Phase Management

Several of the LMWHs have been studied extensively in the management of non-ST elevation acute coronary syndromes. Consistent with the aggregate evaluation of UFH, the combination of LMWH and aspirin offers a benefit over treatment with aspirin alone. In the first large trial of a LMWH in unstable angina, the FRISC (Fragmin During Instability in Coronary Artery Disease) study, dalteparin (120 IU/kg s.c. twice daily) plus aspirin, significantly reduced the risk of death or MI over the first 6 days compared with aspirin alone (Fig. 2) [35]. Similar results have been observed with nadroparin [36].

The results of trials comparing LMWHs with active therapy with UFH, however, have not been uniform and are challenging to interpret [37–40]. In addition to the chemical differences in the LMWHs, variation in the dosing algorithms, risk profiles of the study populations, and definitions of the primary outcomes require individual consideration of each of these major

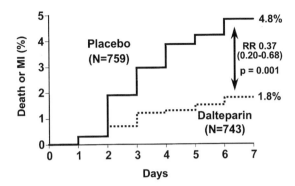

Figure 2 Kaplan–Meier plots of time to first event of the primary endpoint of death or myocardial infarction (MI) over the first 6 days of treatment with dalteparin and placebo in the FRISC trial. (From Ref. 35.)

clinical trials. Caution should be exercised in pooling the results of these heterogeneous LMWH trials [41,42].

Following initial promising work demonstrating a reduction in the risk of major cardiac events or bleeding with use of nadroparin compared with UFH among patients with unstable angina treated with aspirin [36], several phase III trials testing the superiority of LMWHs to UFH were performed (Table 2). Each of these has evaluated LMWHs both for management in the acute phase as well as prevention of recurrent events with extended therapy versus placebo.

In the acute phase of the Fragmin in Unstable Coronary Artery Disease (FRIC) trial, investigators randomly allocated patients within 72 h of symptom onset to treatment for 6 days with open-label dalteparin (120 IU/kg s.c. twice daily) or UFH (intravenously for ≥ 48 h followed by 12,500 IU s.c. twice daily) [37]. Evaluated in this fashion against active therapy with UFH, dalteparin showed no reduction in a composite of death, new MI, or recurrent ischemia (13.0 vs. 12.5%, p = 0.99). With very few episodes of major bleeding and no difference in minor

Table 2 Randomized Clinical Trials Evaluating the Efficacy of Low-Molecular-Weight Heparins in the Acute Management of Patient with Unstable Angina and Non–ST Elevation Myocardial Infarction

Investigator/trial	Size	LMWH	Duration of acute phase	Endpoint	Timepoint	Event rates (LMWH vs. UFH)
Gurfinkel, 1997	219	Nadroparin	5–7 d	MI, RA, UR, or major bleed	7 d	22 vs. 63%, p = 0.0001
Klein, 1997 (FRIC)	1482	Dalteparin	6 d	Death or MI	6 d	3.9 vs. 3.6%, p = NS
Cohen, 1997 (ESSENCE)	3171	Enoxaparin	2–8 d	Death, MI, or UR	14 d	16.6 vs. 19.8%, p = 0.019
Antman, 1999 (TIMI 11B)	3910	Enoxaparin	3–8 d	Death, MI, or UR	8 d	12.4 vs. 14.5%, p = 0.048
FRAXIS Investig, 1999	3468	Nadroparin	6 d	Death, MI, RA, UA	6 d	14.8 vs. 14.9%, p = NS

LMWH, low-molecular-weight heparin; UFH, unfractionated heparin; MI, myocardial infarction; RA, refractory angina; UR, urgent revascularization; d, days.

bleeding between dalteparin and UFH, the FRIC investigators concluded that dalteparin was a safe and convenient alternative to UFH in the early management of non-ST elevation ACS. Consistent with the findings in FRIC, but in distinction to prior work with nadroparin, the Fraxiparine in Ischemic Syndrome (FRAX.I.S) trial enrolled patients within 48 h of onset of unstable angina and demonstrated comparable, but not superior, efficacy to UFH with 6 or 14 days of treatment with nadroparin [40]. Extended therapy (14 days) with nadroparin was, however, associated with an increased risk of major hemorrhage compared with UFH (3.5 vs. 1.6%, p = 0.004).

Two randomized, double-blind, parallel group trials have evaluated enoxaparin for the early management of non-ST elevation ACS. In the Efficacy and Safety of Subcutaneous Enoxaparin in Non–Q-Wave Coronary Events (ESSENCE) trial, patients with rest symptoms in the prior 24 h were treated with aspirin and allocated to either enoxaparin 1 mg/kg s.c. twice daily or intravenous (i.v.) UFH [38]. Treatment with enoxaparin for 2–8 days was associated with a lower risk of death, MI, or recurrent angina through 14 days (16.6 vs. 19.8%, p = 0.019). This benefit was sustained at 30 days and 1 year (13% relative risk reduction, p = 0.016). The reduction in major cardiac events with enoxaparin was associated with an increase in minor, but not major, bleeding (6.5% with enoxaparin vs. 7.0% with UFH).

The TIMI 11B trial [43] supported and extended these findings during the early phase of therapy with the addition of an i.v. bolus of enoxaparin (30 mg) immediately before starting 1 mg/kg s.c. every 12 h. As such, TIMI 11B showed a 23.8% reduction in the composite of death, nonfatal MI, or urgent revascularization at 48 h (Fig. 3) with a persistent advantage at 8 days (Table 3) and similar rates of major bleeding compared with UFH (0.8 vs. 0.7% through 72 h). The treatment benefit of enoxaparin was evident during the period of direct concurrent comparison with UFH (0–48 h) and was of similar magnitude among patients treated medically and those who underwent percutaneous coronary revascularization after initial medical stabilization. Notably, the very early advantage of enoxaparin was less striking and did not achieve statistical significance in ESSENCE. This early benefit may be related to the administration of the i.v. bolus and the higher risk profile of patients in TIMI 11B.

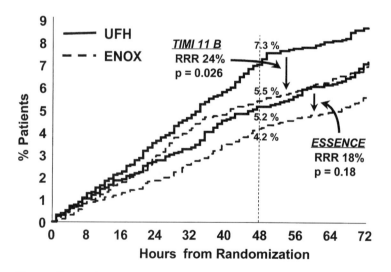

Figure 3 Kaplan–Meier plots of time to first event of the primary endpoint of death, myocardial infarction (MI), or urgent revascularization during head-to-head treatment with enoxaparin (Enox) and UFH in TIMI 11B and ESSENCE. RRR, relative risk reduction.

Table 3 Clinical Trials Evaluating the Safety and Efficacy of Extended Therapy with Low-Molecular-Weight Heparin in the Management of Patients with Unstable Angina, and Non–ST-Elevation Myocardial Infarction

Investigator	Size	LMWH	Duration of chronic phase	Comparator	Endpoint	Timepoint	Event rates (LMWH vs. comparator)
FRISC Study Group, 1996	1506	Dalteparin	40 d	Placebo	Death or MI	40 d	8.0 and 10.7%, p = 0.07
Klein, 1997 (FRIC)	1482	Dalteparin	45 d	Placebo	Death, MI, or UR	45 d	12.3 vs. 12.3%, p = NS
Antman, 1999 (TIMI 11B)	3910	Enoxaparin	43 d	Placebo	Death, MI, or UR	43 d	17.3 vs. 19.7%, p = 0.048
FRISC II, 1999	2267	Dalteparin	90 d	Placebo	Death, or MI	30 d	3.1 vs. 5.9%, p = 0.002
FRAXIS Investig, 1999	3468	Nadroparin × 14 d	Nadroparin × 14 d	UFH×6 d / Nadroparin 6 d	Death, MI, RA, UA	14 d	20.0 vs. 18.1%, p = NS / 20.0 vs. 17.8%, p = NS

LMWH, low-molecular-weight heparin; MI, myocardial infarction; UR, urgent revascularization; NS, nonsignificant; UFH, unfractionated heparin; RA, refractory angina; d, days.

A prespecified metanalysis combining data from ESSENCE and TIMI 11B demonstrated a stable 20% reduction in the composite of death, MI, and urgent revascularization at 48 h and 8 days, with a persistent benefit of enoxaparin at 6 weeks and 1 year (23.3 vs. 25.8%, p = 0.008) [39,44]. In addition, a consistent pattern of proportionate reductions in each element of the composite endpoint was evident. Rates of major bleeding were similar in patients treated with enoxaparin or UFH, but minor episodes, such as ecchymoses at the injection site, were more common with enoxaparin. Together, data from ESSENCE and TIMI 11B provide consistent evidence for a modest, but statistically significant, benefit of enoxaparin over UFH for the short-term management of patients with non-ST elevation ACS. In addition, data from TIMI 11B suggest that an i.v. bolus of 30 mg enoxaparin may be considered for high-risk patients (e.g., ST segment depression or elevated cardiac markers) with rest symptoms in the prior 24 h. Economic analysis performed using data from ESSENCE demonstrate that while the unit cost of treatment with enoxaparin is greater than that of UFH, by reducing the rate of events and the need for invasive procedures, enoxaparin therapy produces a cost reduction of 1172 dollars per patient treated [45,46].

The aggregate data from multiple clinical trials establish LMWHs as safe and practical alternatives to UFH for therapeutic anticoagulation of patients with non-ST elevation ACS, with no difference in major bleeding observed during the acute phase of management. In particular, enoxaparin offers a therapeutic benefit over UFH in the treatment of high-risk patients with unstable angina and non-ST elevation MI. Differences in the results of the five major clinical trials caution against extrapolating these results across the class of LMWHs. However, clear differences in efficacy between LMWH preparations have not been established and will require direct comparison in randomized clinical trials. Nevertheless, pooling of trials using different LWMHs similarly may lead to misleading conclusions. Potential reasons for the absence of detected benefit in FRIC and FRAXIS should be considered. One potential explanation is that enoxaparin, with its high relative anti-Xa/anti-IIa activity and extension of its antithrombotic actions to include inhibition of platelet aggregation [13], achieved a greater early reduction in thrombus burden that translated into fewer clinical events during subsequent follow-up. Alternatively, differences in the acuity of illness of the patients enrolled or the pattern of dosing may be important to the divergence between trial results.

2. Evaluation of Prolonged Treatment with LMWH

Patients stabilized after presentation with unstable ischemic heart disease remain at particular risk for recurrent events in the next 6–12 weeks. Persistent activation of the coagulation cascade has been documented up to several months after an index coronary event [47]. Such clinical and experimental observations, together with the "rebound" increase in thrombotic events after discontinuation of UFH, have led investigators to explore the benefits of prolonged antithrombotic therapy (21). Given the ease and reliability of s.c. dosing of the LMWHs, they are particularly appealing for this purpose and have been assessed for prolonged therapy in several randomized trials (see Table 3).

Both FRISC and FRIC were configured with a placebo-controlled chronic phase in which dalteparin was continued at reduced dosing (7500 IU s.c. daily) after 6 days of a weight-based regimen. Results were similar in both studies, with loss of the initial benefit in FRISC by 40 days and no benefit from 6 to 45 days in FRIC, but increased risk of minor bleeding (e.g., 5.1 vs. 2.8% in FRIC). TIMI 11B also tested the efficacy of extended treatment with LMWH and detected no additional benefit with therapy between 8 and 43 days (5.2 vs. 4.9%, p =NS). However, prolonged treatment with enoxaparin did carry an excess risk of major bleeding (2.9 vs. 1.5%, p = 0.02) in TIMI 11B.

Although no advantage of prolonged dalteparin was seen in FRISC or FRIC, investigators raised the possibility that more frequent dosing might have resulted in a benefit. The Long-Term Low-Molecular-Mass Heparin in Unstable Coronary Artery Disease Trial was thus implemented by the FRISC II investigators to assess the efficacy of 3 months of dalteparin dosed twice daily in two tiers based on body weight (5000 IU or 7500 IU) for high-risk patients with non-ST elevation acute coronary syndromes [48]. Over 2000 patients with symptoms in the prior 48 h and ST/T-wave changes or elevated serum cardiac markers were treated with open-label dalteparin and randomized in a 2 × 2-factorial design to prolonged dalteparin (3 months) or placebo, and an invasive or noninvasive strategy. Among patients in the noninvasive arm, dalteparin conferred a 2.8% absolute reduction in the risk of death or MI by 30 days which was sustained at 60, but not 90 days after randomization (Fig. 4). Patients randomized to the invasive arm had no benefit from continuation of dalteparin after revascularization. These results suggest that with more frequent dosing, sustained therapy with dalteparin may reduce recurrent events during the first month among high-risk patients managed with a conservative strategy or awaiting a delayed invasive evaluation. These data also raise the possibility that the absence of additional benefit with continued enoxaparin in TIMI 11B may be partly explained by the predominant strategy of revascularization for high-risk patients during the index hospitalization.

3. Targeting LMWH Therapy

Although none of the clinical trials with LMWHs were sufficiently powered to detect significant differences in therapeutic efficacy among individual subgroups, additional analyses from several of these trials have revealed subgroups that may derive particular benefit from LMWHs. Data from FRISC [49] and FRISC II [50] suggest that prolonged dalteparin may be of benefit for high-risk patients with elevated cardiac troponin T. Additionally, among patients with unstable angina (normal CKMB) in TIMI 11B, elevated levels of troponin I identified patients who had derived particular benefit from acute-phase treatment with enoxaparin over UFH (Fig. 5) [51].

Clinical risk indicators other than cardiac markers may also be useful for therapeutic decision-making relative to LMWHs. For example, application of a simple clinical score for risk

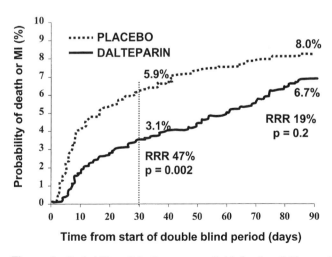

Figure 4 Probability of death or myocardial infarction (MI) over 3 months of therapy with dalteparin or placebo during the blinded treatment phase of the FRISC II trial. RRR, relative risk reduction. (From Ref. 48.)

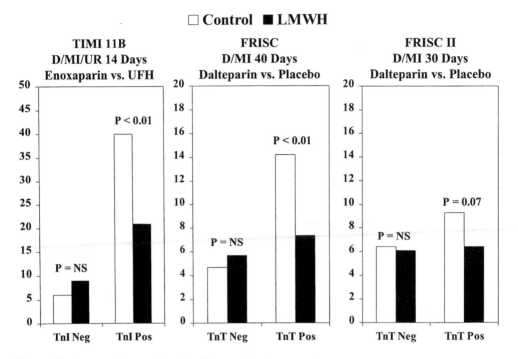

Figure 5 Pattern of greater benefit of low-molecular-weight heparin versus control (UFH or placebo) among troponin-positive patients in three clinical trials: D, death; MI, myocardial infarction; UR, urgent revascularization; Neg, negative; Pos, positive. (Data from Refs. 48, 49, and 51.)

assessment (TIMI Risk Score for Unstable Angina/Non–ST Elevation MI) identifies an increasing gradient of benefit with enoxaparin versus UFH with rising risk score (Fig. 6) [52]. These data suggest that enoxaparin offers its greatest benefit over UFH among high-risk patients. However, even among lower-risk patients where efficacy of enoxaparin and UFH appear similar, there may be practical advantages to the use of the LWMH.

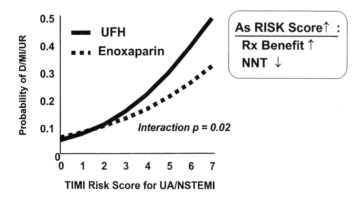

Figure 6 Relation between patient risk group (stratified by the TIMI Risk Score for unstable angina/non–ST elevation MI) and the benefit of treatment with enoxaparin versus unfractionated heparin (UFH). Rx, treatment; NNT, number needed to treat to avoid one event.

B. ST Elevation ACS

Trials of LMWH in ST-elevation MI treated with thrombolytic therapy are also underway. Compared with placebo, dalteparin may facilitate fibrinolysis with streptokinase (SK) with a trend toward higher rates of TIMI 3 flow at angiography in the first 20–28 h (68 vs. 51%, p = 0.10) and lower incidence of recurrent ischemic episodes on continuous ECG monitoring (16 vs. 38%, p = 0.04), coupled with acceptable safety [53]. When administered at presentation and continued for 3–8 days after fibrinolysis with SK, enoxaparin (30 mg i.v. bolus followed by 1 mg/kg s.c. every 12 h for 3–8 days) is associated with higher rates of patency (87.6 vs. 71.7%, p = 0.001) and TIMI 3 flow (70.3 vs. 57.8%) compared with placebo on angiographic evaluation at 8 days [54]. In addition, this study of 496 patients showed a favorable effect of enoxaparin relative to the composite clinical outcome of death, MI, or recurrent angina through 30 days (13.4 vs. 21.0%, p = 0.03) [54]. Preliminary work comparing LMWHs with UFH also appears promising.

When compared with UFH in the HART II trial, treatment with enoxaparin as an adjunct to t-PA showed comparable safety and was associated with a trend toward higher rates of patency of the infarct-related artery (81.1 vs. 75.1% at 90 min) [55]. Angiographic reevaluation at 5–7 days also demonstrated a trend toward lower rates of reocclusion among patients treated with enoxaparin (5.9 vs. 9.8%, p = NS). Consistent encouraging data have come from comparison of dalteparin versus UFH as an adjunct to fibrinolysis with t-PA in the ASSENT PLUS trial [56]. Although angiography performed at 4–7 days showed a nonsignificant trend toward higher rates of TIMI 3 flow (69.3 vs. 62.5%, p = 0.16) and less visible thrombus (18.9 vs. 27.3%, p = 0.05), the incidence of reinfarction was reduced among patients treated with dalteparin (1.4 vs. 5.4%, p = 0.02) [56]. One intracranial hemorrhage was observed in the LMWH-treated group (N = 221) [56]. Furthermore, in a study of 300 patients treated with thrombolysis and randomized to i.v. UFH or enoxaparin for 4 days (40 mg i.v. bolus, followed by 40 mg s.c. every 8 h), a reduction in the cumulative incidence of death, MI, or readmission for ACS was suggested in the enoxaparin group (25.5 vs. 36.4%, p = 0.04) [57]. In particular, early reinfarction between days 4 and 6, potentially related to "rebound" after discontinuation of heparin, was reduced in the enoxaparin group (2.2 vs. 6.6%, p = 0.05) [57].

Ongoing evaluations of LMWHs versus UFH include an angiographic study of enoxaparin in patients receiving either full-dose TNK-t-PA or reduced dose TNK-t-PA in combination with abciximab (ENTIRE–TIMI 23 trial, Fig. 7), and a comparison of clinical events with full-dose TNK-t-PA (ASSENT 3 and ASSENT 3 PLUS studies). In addition, combined therapy with enoxaparin and tirofiban is being evaluated for management of patients ineligible for reperfusion therapy (TETAMI trial) [58].

C. Special Issues: Periprocedural Use and Combination with GPIIb/IIIa Inhibition

Some clinicians have delayed the switch from UFH to LMWHs because of uncertainty about administration of LMWHs in patients undergoing catheterization and those receiving intravenous GP IIb/IIIa inhibitors. However, the emerging experience with these combinations is encouraging. Pilot data suggest that LMWHs are safe and effective for routine anticoagulation during percutaneous coronary intervention (PCI). Either when used alone or in combination with abciximab during PCI, enoxaparin has performed with safety comparable with historical experience with UFH [59]. Specifically, results from the National Investigators Collaborating on Enoxaparin (NICE) 4 Study [60] suggest that with 75% of the usual enoxaparin dose (0.75 mg/kg) administered i.v. in combination with a standard dose of abciximab, rates of major

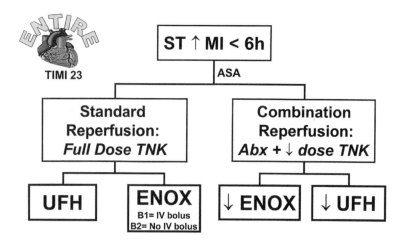

Primary Endpoint: TIMI 3 Flow at 60 min
Secondary Endpoints: ST Res, Clin. Events, anti-Xa

Figure 7 Protocol design for the ENTIRE–TIMI 23: Abx, abciximab; UFH, unfractionated; Enox, enoxaparin; IV, intravenous; ST Res, ST-segment resolution; Clin, clinical.

hemorrhage (0.6%), transfusion (1.8%), and thrombocytopenia (2.3%) are similar or lower than those reported in other contemporary interventional trials with abciximab and UFH [61,62]. The NICE 3 study followed patients treated with enoxaparin (1 mg/kg s.c. Q12) in combination with either tirofiban, eptifibatide, or abciximab through catheterization and percutaneous intervention. Observed bleeding rates (non-CABG major bleeding 1.9%) were comparable with those from prior studies of GPIIb/IIIa inhibitors alone [63]. In this study, no additional heparin was administered if the procedure was performed within 8 h of the last dose of enoxaparin, and 0.3 mg/kg enoxaparin was given i.v. if more than 8 h since the most recent s.c. dose [63]. In the event of an urgent need to reverse anticoagulation with a LMWH, stoichiometric neutralizing doses of protamine may be used to reverse 100% of the anti-IIa effect of LMWHs and about two-thirds of the anti-Xa effect [64].

An additional evolving area of clinical importance is the safety and efficacy of combining LMWHs with GP IIb/IIIa inhibitors in the medical management of ACS. Studied in the ACUTE I and II trials, the coadministration of enoxaparin with tirofiban was associated with more consistent inhibition of platelet aggregation than with UFH [65] with comparable low rates of major bleeding (0.6% with enoxaparin vs. 0.5% with UFH) [66]. Such data provide evidence for a possible advantage of LMWHs in combined antithrombin and antiplatelet therapy. Ongoing studies, such as the Aggrastat to Zocor (AtoZ) Trial, will provide further valuable information on the safety and clinical efficacy of LMWHs in combination with GP IIb/IIIa inhibitors for medical therapy. These data will be important to clinicians as the proportion of patients with acute coronary syndromes treated with LMWHs continues to increase.

VI. CONCLUSIONS: ROLE OF LMWHS IN THE MANAGEMENT OF UNSTABLE CAD

With predictable pharmacokinetics and high bioavailability, LMWHs are able to achieve a stable, durable anticoagulant effect without the need for continuous intravenous administration and frequent laboratory monitoring. The safety and efficacy of the LMWHs for the immediate management of non-ST elevation ACS have been demonstrated across multiple randomized clinical trials. On the basis of these data, enoxaparin and dalteparin have been approved for brief treatment of patients with unstable angina and non-ST elevation MI. In addition, prolonged therapy with some LMWHs may be useful in reducing the risk of recurrent coronary events among selected high-risk populations, or those awaiting delayed invasive evaluation. Given promising pilot data, clinical evaluation of the LMWHs as an adjunct to fibrinolysis is ongoing. Future research carefully evaluating the correlation of anti-Xa and anti-IIa activity, with biochemical markers of platelet and coagulation cascade activation may help elucidate some of the variation in outcomes seen between studies. In addition, questions about the safety and efficacy of combined therapy with glycoprotein IIb/IIIa receptor antagonists, and the optimal use of LMWHs during percutaneous coronary interventional procedures will be addressed.

REFERENCES

1. Fuster V, Badimon L, Badimon JJ, Chesebro JH. The pathogenesis of coronary artery disease and the acute coronary syndromes (1). N Engl J Med 1992; 326:242–250.
2. Fuster V, Badimon L, Badimon JJ, Chesebro JH. The pathogenesis of coronary artery disease and the acute coronary syndromes (2). N Engl J Med 1992; 326:310–318.
3. Weitz JI. Activation of blood coagulation by plaque rupture: mechanisms and prevention. Am J Cardiol 1995; 75:18B–22B.
4. Braunwald E, Antman EM, Beasley JW, Califf RM, Cheitlin MD, Hochman JS, Jones RH, Kereiakes D, Kupersmith J, Levin TN, Pepine CJ, Schaeffer JW, Smith EEI, Steward DE, Theroux P. ACC/AHA guidelines for the management of patients with unstable angina and non–ST-segment elevation myocardial infarction: a report of the American College of Cardiology/American Heart Association Task Force on Practice Guidelines (Committee on the Management of Patients with Unstable Angina). J Am Coll Cardiol 2000; 36:970–1062.
5. Ryan TJ, Antman EM, Brooks NH, Califf RM, Hillis LD, Hiratzka LF, Rapaport E, Riegel B, Russell RO, Smith EE 3rd, Weaver WD, Gibbons RJ, Alpert JS, Eagle KA, Gardner TJ, Garson A Jr, Gregoratos G, Smith SC Jr. 1999 update: ACC/AHA Guidelines for the Management of Patients With Acute Myocardial Infarction: Executive Summary and Recommendations: a report of the American College of Cardiology/American Heart Association Task Force on Practice Guidelines (Committee on Management of Acute Myocardial Infarction). Circulation 1999; 100:1016–1030.
6. Morrow DA, Ridker PM. Inflammation in cardiovascular disease. In: Topol E, ed. Textbook of Cardiovascular Medicine Updates. Vol. 2. Cedar Knolls: Lippincott Williams & Wilkins, 1999:1–12.
7. Wilcox JN, Smith KM, Schwartz SM, Gordon D. Localization of tissue factor in the normal vessel wall and in the atherosclerotic plaque. Proc Natl Acad Sci USA 1989; 86:2839–2843.
8. Camerer E, Kolsto AB, Prydz H, Kolst AB. Cell biology of tissue factor, the principal initiator of blood coagulation. Thromb Res 1996; 81:1–41.
9. Moreno PR, Bernardi VH, Lopez–Cuellar J, Murcia AM, Palacios IF, Gold HK, Mehran R, Sharma SK, Nemerson Y, Fuster V, Fallon JT. Macrophages, smooth muscle cells, and tissue factor in unstable angina. Implications for cell-mediated thrombogenicity in acute coronary syndromes. Circulation 1996; 94:3090–3097.
10. Toschi V, Gallo R, Lettino M, Fallon JT, Gertz SD, Fernandez–Ortiz A, Chesebro JH, Badimon L, Nemerson Y, Fuster V, Badimon JJ. Tissue factor modulates the thrombogenicity of human athero-sclerotic plaques. Circulation 1997; 95:594–599.
11. Dahlback B. Blood coagulation. Lancet 2000; 355:1627–1632.
12. Harker LA, Hanson SR, Runge MS. Thrombin hypothesis of thrombus generation and vascular lesion formation. Am J Cardiol 1995; 75:12B–17B.

13. Antman EM, Handin R. Low-molecular-weight heparins: an intriguing new twist with profound implications. Circulation 1998; 98:287–28.
14. Weitz JI. Low-molecular-weight heparins. N Engl J Med 1997; 3:688–698.
15. Oler A, Whooley MA, Oler J, Grady D. Adding heparin to aspirin reduces the incidence of myocardial infarction and death in patients with unstable angina. JAMA 1996; 276:811–815.
16. Mahaffey KW, Granger CB, Collins R, O'Connor CM, Ohman EM, Bleich SD, Col JJ, Califf RM. Overview of randomized trials of intravenous heparin in patients with acute myocardial infarction treated with thrombolytic therapy. Am J Cardiol 1996; 77:551–556.
17. Giugliano RP, McCabe CH, Antman EM, Cannon CP, Van de Werf F, Wilcox RG, Braunwald E, for the Thrombolysis in Myocardial Infarction (TIMI) Investigators. Lower dose heparin with fibrinolysis is associated with lower rates of intracranial hemorrhage. Am Heart J 2001; 141:742–750.
18. Granger CB, Hirsh J, Califf RM, Col J, White HD, Betriu A, Woodlief LH, Lee KL, Bovill EG, Simes RJ, Topol EJ. Activated partial thromboplastin time and outcome after thrombolytic therapy for acute myocardial infarction: results from the GUSTO-I trial. Circulation 1996; 93:870–878.
19. Hirsh J. Heparin. N Engl J Med 1991; 324:1565–1574.
20. Young E, Prins M, Levine MN, Hirsh J. Heparin binding to plasma proteins, an important mechanism for heparin resistance. Thromb Haemost 1992; 67:639–643.
21. Theroux P, Waters D, Lam J, Juneau M, McCans J. Reactivation of unstable angina after the discontinuation of heparin. N Engl J Med 1992; 327:141–145.
22. Granger CB, Miller JM, Bovill EG, et al. Rebound increase in thrombin generation and activity after cessation of intravenous heparin in patients with acute coronary syndromes. Circulation 1995; 91:1929–1935.
23. Smith AJ, Holt RE, Fitzpatrick JB, Palacios IF, Gold HK, Werner W, Bovill EG, Fuster V, Jang IK. Transient thrombotic state after abrupt discontinuation of heparin in percutaneous coronary angioplasty. Am Heart J 1996; 131:434–439.
24. Warkentin TE, Levine MN, Hirsh J, Horsewood P, Roberts RS, Gent M, Kelton JG. Heparin-induced thrombocytopenia in patients treated with low-molecular-weight heparin or unfractionated heparin. N Engl J Med 1995; 332:1330–1335.
25. Ernofsson M, Strekerud F, Toss H, Abildgaard U, Wallentin L, Siegbahn A. Low-molecular weight heparin reduces the generation and activity of thrombin in unstable coronary artery disease. Thromb Haemost 1998; 79:491–494.
26. Lane DA, Denton J, Flynn AM, Thunberg L, Lindahl U. Anticoagulant activities of heparin oligosaccharides and their neutralization by platelet factor 4. Biochem J 1984; 218: 725–732.
27. Hansen JB, Sandset PM. Differential effects of low molecular weight heparin and unfractionated heparin on circulating levels of antithrombin and tissue factor pathway inhibitor (TFPI): a possible mechanism for difference in therapeutic efficacy. Thromb Res 1998; 91:177–181.
28. Hansen JB, Sandset PM, Huseby KR, Huseby NE, Bendz B, Ostergaard P, Nordoy A. Differential effect of unfractionated heparin and low molecular weight heparin on intravascular tissue factor pathway inhibitor: evidence for a difference in antithrombotic action. Br J Haematol 1998; 101:638–646.
29. Young E, Cosmi B, Weitz J, Hirsh J. Comparison of the non-specific binding of unfractionated heparin and low molecular weight heparin (enoxaparin) to plasma proteins. Thromb Haemost 1993; 70:625–630.
30. Schneider DJ, Tracy PB, Mann KG, Sobel BE. Differential effects of anticoagulants on the activation of platelets ex vivo. Circulation 1997; 96:2877–2883.
31. Xiao Z, Theroux P. Platelet activation with unfractionated heparin at therapeutic concentrations and comparisons with a low-molecular-weight heparin and with a direct thrombin inhibitor. Circulation 1998; 97:251–256.
32. Montalescot G, Philippe F, Ankri A, Vicaut E, Bearez E, Poulard JE, Carrie D, Flammang D, Dutoit A, Carayon A, Jardel C, Chevrot M, Bastard JP, Bigonzi F, Thomas D. Early increase of von Willebrand factor predicts adverse outcome in unstable coronary artery disease: beneficial effects of enoxaparin. French Investigators of the ESSENCE Trial. Circulation 1998; 98:294–299.

33. Hoppensteadt DA, Jeske W, Fareed J, Bermes EW Jr. The role of tissue factor pathway inhibitor in the mediation of the antithrombotic actions of heparin and low-molecular-weight heparin. Blood Coagul Fibrinolysis 1995; 6(suppl 1):S57–64.

34. Fareed J, Hoppensteadt DA, Bick RL. An update on heparins at the beginning of the new millennium. Semin Thromb Hemost 2000; 26:5–21.

35. FRISC Study Group. Low-molecular-weight heparin during instability in coronary artery disease, Fragmin during Instability in Coronary Artery Disease (FRISC). Lancet 1996; 347:561–568.

36. Gurfinkel EP, Manos EJ, Mejail RI, Cerda MA, Duronto EA, Garcia CN, Daroca AM, Mautner B. Low molecular weight heparin versus regular heparin or aspirin in the treatment of unstable angina and silent ischemia. J Am Coll Cardiol 1995; 26:313–318.

37. Klein W, Buchwald A, Hillis SE, Monrad S, Sanz G, Turpie AG, van der Meer J, Olaisson E, Undeland S, Ludwig K. Comparison of low-molecular-weight heparin with unfractionated heparin acutely and with placebo for 6 weeks in the management of unstable coronary artery disease. Fragmin in unstable coronary artery disease study (FRIC). Circulation 1997; 96:61–68.

38. Cohen M, Demers C, Gurfinkel EP, Turpie AG, Fromell GJ, Goodman S, Langer A, Califf RM, Fox KA, Premmereur J, Bigonzi F. A comparison of low-molecular-weight heparin with unfractionated heparin for unstable coronary artery disease. Efficacy and safety of subcutaneous enoxaparin in non–Q-wave coronary events study group. New Engl J Med 1997; 337:447–452.

39. Antman EM, Cohen M, Radley D, McCabe C, Rush J, Premmereur J, Braunwald E. Assessment of the treatment effect of enoxaparin for unstable angina/non–Q-wave myocardial infarction. TIMI 11B-ESSENCE meta-analysis. Circulation 1999; 100:1602–1608.

40. The FRAXIS Study Group. Comparison of two treatment durations of a low molecular weight heparin in the initial management of unstable angina of non–Q wave myocardial infarction: FRAX.I.S. Eur Heart J 1999; 20:1553–1562.

41. Eikelboom JW, Anand SS, Malmberg K, Weitz JI, Ginsberg JS, Yusuf S. Unfractionated heparin and low-molecular-weight heparin in acute coronary syndrome without ST elevation: a meta-analysis. Lancet 2000; 355:1936–1942.

42. Antman EM. The search for replacements for unfractionated heparin. Circulation 2001; 103:2310–2314.

43. Antman EM, McCabe CH, Gurfinkel EP, Turpie AG, Bernink PJ, Salein D, Bayes De Luna A, Fox K, Lablanche JM, Radley D, Premmereur J, Braunwald E. Enoxaparin prevents death and cardiac ischemic events in unstable angina/non–Q-wave myocardial infarction. Results of the thrombolysis in myocardial infarction (TIMI) 11B trial. Circulation 1999; 100:1593–1601.

44. Antman EM, Cohen M, McCabe CH, Radley D, Braunwald E. Enoxaparin is superior to unfractionated heparin for preventing clinical events at one year follow-up in TIMI 11B and ESSENCE [abstr]. Circulation 2000; 102:II-429.

45. Mark DB, Cowper PA, Berkowitz SD, Davidson–Ray L, DeLong ER, Turpie AG, Califf RM, Weatherley B, Cohen M. Economic assessment of low-molecular-weight heparin (enoxaparin) versus unfractionated heparin in acute coronary syndrome patients: results from the ESSENCE randomized trial. Circulation 1998; 97:1702–1707.

46. O'Brien BJ, Willan A, Blackhouse G, Goeree R, Cohen M, Goodman S. Will the use of low-molecular-weight heparin (enoxaparin) in patients with acute coronary syndrome save costs in Canada? Am Heart J 2000; 139:423–429.

47. Merlini PA, Bauer KA, Oltrona L, Ardissino D, Cattaneo M, Belli C, Mannucci PM, Rosenberg RD. Persistent activation of coagulation mechanism in unstable angina and myocardial infarction. Circulation 1994; 90:61–68.

48. FRISC II Investigators. Long-term low-molecular-mass heparin in unstable coronary-artery disease: FRISC II prospective randomised multicentre study. Lancet 1999; 354:701–707.

49. Lindahl B, Venge P, Wallentin L. Troponin T identifies patients with unstable coronary artery disease who benefit from long-term antithrombotic protection. Fragmin in Unstable Coronary Artery Disease (FRISC) Study Group. J Am Coll Cardiol 1997; 29:43–48.

50. Lindahl B, Diderholm E, Kontny F, Lagerqvist B, Husted S, Stahle E, Swahn E, Wallentin L. Long term treatment with low molecular weight heparin (dalteparin) reduces cardiac events in unstable coronary disease with troponin-T elevation: a FRISC II substudy [abstr]. Circulation 1999; 100:I-498.

51. Morrow DA, Antman EM, Tanasijevic J, Rifai N, de Lemos JA, McCabe CH, Cannon CP, Braunwald E. Cardiac troponin I for stratification of early outcomes and the efficacy of enoxaparin in unstable angina: a TIMI 11B sub-study. J Am Coll Cardiol 2000; 36:1812–1817.

52. Antman EM, Cohen M, Bernink PJ, McCabe CH, Horacek T, Papuchis G, Mautner B, Corbalan R, Radley D, Braunwald E. The TIMI risk score for unstable angina/non–ST elevation MI: a method for prognostication and therapeutic decision making. JAMA 2000; 284:835–842.

53. Frostfeldt G, Ahlberg G, Gustafsson G, Helmius G, Lindahl B, Nygren A, Siegbahn A, Swahn E, Venge P, Wallentin L. Low molecular weight heparin (dalteparin) as adjuvant treatment of thrombolysis in acute myocardial infarction—a pilot study: biochemical markers in acute coronary syndromes (BIOMACS II). J Am Coll Cardiol 1999; 33:627–633.

54. Simoons M. Antithrombin adjuncts to fibrinolysis, the Dutch SK-Enoxaparin Study, Thrombolysis and Interventional Therapy in Acute Myocardial Infarction, New Orleans, 2000.

55. Villareal RP, Kim P, Mahmood H, Civitello A, Ferguson JJ 3rd. Meeting highlights: Highlights of the 49th Scientific Sessions of the American College of Cardiology. Circulation 2000; 102:E53–60.

56. Wallentin L. Dalteparin and tPA: the ASSENT-Plus Trial, Thrombolysis and Interventional Therapy in Acute Myocardial Infarction, New Orleans, 2000.

57. Baird SH, McBride SJ, Trouton TG, Wilson C. Low-molecular-weight heparin versus unfractionated heparin following thrombolysis in myocardial infarction [abstr.]. J Am Coll Cardiol 1998; 31(suppl A):191A.

58. Cohen M, Gensini GF, Maritz F, Bremer K, Timerman A, Pazzanese D, Danchin N, Huber K, Gurfinkel EP, White HD, Fox KAA, Vittori L, Le-Louer V, Bigonzi F. Characteristics and outcome of patients presenting with ST elevation MI ineligible for reperfusion therapy in the TETAMI study (Safety and Efficacy of Subcutaneous Enoxaparin versus Unfractionated Heparin and of Tirofiban versus Placebo in the Treatment of Acute MI) [abstr.]. Circulation 2000; 102:II–795.

59. Kereiakes DJ, Grines C, Fry E, Esente A, Barr L, Matthai W, Shimshak T, Broderick T, Cohen M. Combination enoxaparin and abciximab during percutaneous coronary intervention: a new standard of care? Curr Interv Cardiol Rep 2000; 2:157–164.

60. Kereiakes DJ, Grines C, Fry E, Barr L, Matthai W, Broderick T, Lengerich R, Cohen M, Esente P. Abciximab–enoxaparin interaction during percutaneous coronary intervention: results of the NICE-1 and 4 trials [abstr.]. J Am Coll Cardiol 2000; 35.

61. The EPILOG Investigators. Platelet glycoprotein IIb/IIIa receptor blockade and low-dose heparin during percutaneous coronary revascularization. N Engl J Med 1997; 336:1689–1696.

62. The EPISTENT Investigators. Randomised placebo-controlled and balloon-angioplasty-controlled trial to assess safety of coronary stenting with use of platelet glycoprotein–IIb/IIIa blockade. Evaluation of platelet IIb/IIIa inhibitor for stenting (EPISTENT). Lancet 1998; 352:87–92.

63. Ferguson JJ 3rd. NICE-3 preliminary results. 22nd Congress of the European Society of Cardiology, Amsterdam, 2000.

64. Holst J, Lindblad B, Bergqvist D, Garre K, Nielsen H, Hedner U, Ostergaard PB. Protamine neutralization of intravenous and subcutaneous low-molecular-weight heparin (tinzaparin, Logiparin). An experimental investigation in healthy volunteers. Blood Coagul Fibrinolysis 1994; 5:795–803.

65. Cohen M, Theroux P, Weber S, Laramee P, Huynh T, Borzak S, Diodati JG, Squire IB, Deckelbaum LI, Thornton AR, Harris KE, Sax FL, Lo MW, White HD. Combination therapy with tirofiban and enoxaparin in acute coronary syndromes. Int J Cardiol 1999; 71:273–281.

66. Cohen M, Theroux P, Frey MJ, White HD, Borzak S, Weber S, Senatore F, Mukherjee R, Thornton A, Bigonzi F, Sax FL. Anti-thrombotic combination using tirofiban and enoxaparin: the ACUTE II study [abstr.]. Circulation 2000; 102:II–826.

67. Morrow DA, Antman E. Low molecular weight heparin in non–ST elevation acute coronary syndromes. In: Braunwald E, ed. Harrison's Principles of Internal Medicine Online. New York: McGraw-Hill, 2000.

6

Low-Molecular-Weight Heparin Use in Pregnancy

Wee Shian Chan
University of Toronto, Toronto, Ontario, Canada

Jeffrey S. Ginsberg
McMaster University, Hamilton, Ontario, Canada

SUMMARY

Low-molecular-weight heparin (LMWH) is rapidly replacing unfractionated heparin (UFH) as the treatment of choice for the management of women requiring anticoagulant therapy during pregnancy. There is convincing evidence that LMWH is safe for the developing fetus and the mother, and that it might also be associated with a lower risk of osteoporosis, bleeding, and heparin-induced thrombocytopenia.

LMWH is likely to be as effective as UFH for treatment and prevention of venous thromboembolism (VTE) during pregnancy, and prevention of recurrent pregnancy loss associated with antiphospholipid antibodies. LMWH has also been successfully used for arterial thrombosis prevention in women with prosthetic heart valves; a problematic group because there are reports of failure with UFH, and embryopathy and fetal hemorrhage can occur with coumarin derivatives. However, definitive conclusions about the efficacy and safety of LMWH in pregnancy must be tempered, because particularly for treatment of VTE and prevention of cardioembolic events in those with prosthetic heart valves, LMWH has yet to be tested in rigorous studies. Furthermore, appropriate LMWH dosing for each of these indications remains to be defined.

I. INTRODUCTION

Use of LMWH is effective for the treatment and prevention of VTE [1]. Owing to its predictable bioavailability relative to UFH, dosing of LMWH in nonpregnant subjects is simple and is based on a patient's weight [2]. The lack of requirement for laboratory monitoring in nonpregnant patients makes LMWH more convenient than UFH.

In this chapter, we will review the available data on pharmacokinetics, safety, efficacy, and indications for LMWH use in pregnancy. Unfortunately, the quality of most studies on the use of

LMWH in pregnancy is poor. However, by combining the available studies in pregnant women and extrapolating from studies performed in nonpregnant patients, we will attempt to make sensible recommendations about the use of LMWH during pregnancy.

II. PHARMACOKINETICS OF LMWH IN PREGNANCY

Compared with UFH, LMWH binds less to plasma proteins and cell surfaces [2]. This lack of binding contributes to its excellent and predictable bioavailability making it suitable for administration in fixed–weight-adjusted doses for the treatment of VTE and prosthetic heart valves. The primary issue surrounding the appropriate dosing of LMWH in pregnant women arises because during pregnancy, two major physiological changes occur: an increase in glomerular filtration rate [3] and an increase in plasma volume [4]. Both of these have the potential to necessitate modification of the dose to achieve a constant anticoagulant level, as evaluated by antifactor Xa levels. Shortly after conception, and peaking at 9–11 weeks of gestation, the glomerular filtration rate (GFR) increases by 35–50% [3]. This increase is sustained until about 36 weeks of gestation, after which a decrease may occur. The plasma volume increases by about 50% [4], beginning in the first trimester and peaking at 32 weeks of gestation. Owing to these two changes and assuming that increased GFR causes increased renal clearance of LMWH, the dose of LMWH would be expected to require adjustment to achieve a consistent antifactor Xa activity level during pregnancy. However, despite these physiological changes and maternal weight gain, the need for continued dose-adjustment as pregnancy progresses is uncertain. Several small case-series of pregnant women treated with prophylactic doses of LMWH [5–8] showed that the antifactor Xa activity measured 3 h after administration of fixed doses of LMWH did not change throughout pregnancy, suggesting that dose adjustment may not be necessary.

Although the "time-to-peak" concentration after injection of prophylactic doses of LMWH in pregnant women is not significantly different from that in nonpregnant patients, maximum and trough antifactor Xa activities are both significantly lower in pregnancy [8]. In other words, low doses of LMWH show less bioavailability and are cleared faster in pregnant women than in nonpregnant subjects. These findings suggest that twice-daily, rather than once-daily, dosing and higher doses of LMWH may be needed during pregnancy. It is unknown whether there are differences in efficacy and safety among various LMWH preparations.

There are no published studies investigating the pharmacokinetics of therapeutic doses of LMWH in pregnancy. For treatment of venous thromboembolism, we recommend starting with a weight-adjusted dose and targeting a postinjection antifactor Xa level of 0.5–1.2 U/mL. This recommendation is empiric and underlines the need for well-designed trials to determine appropriate dosing in these patients.

III. SAFETY OF LMWH IN PREGNANCY

A. Fetal Safety

The mean molecular weight of LMWHs is approximately 5000 Da; because of their size, LMWHs are not expected to cross the placenta [9]. Although a study performed over 15 years ago using sheep placentae and labeled heparins suggested that transplacental passage of LMWH could occur [10], several studies in pregnant women given LMWH showed no measurable antifactor Xa activity in the cord blood during both second and third trimesters of pregnancy [11–18]. These studies suggest that there is no transplacental passage of LMWH in humans.

Exposure of the developing fetus to LMWH during pregnancy has not been linked to an increased risk of congenital anomalies or adverse fetal outcomes [19–21]. In a review of LMWH use in pregnant women, Sanson and co-workers [20] pooled published case reports and case series on a total of 486 women exposed to LMWH during pregnancy. No congenital malformations were reported in these individuals. In a retrospective analysis of 184 women given LMWH during pregnancy [19], the rate of congenital malformations was reported to be 3.3%, a rate similar to that in women not receiving LMWH. Further evidence that LMWH use in pregnancy does not increase the risk of congenital malformations comes from a population-based cohort study [20] during which no increase in the rate of congenital malformations was found (3.0% in LMWH users vs. 4.5% in pregnant controls).

There is no evidence that LMWH use in pregnancy results in other adverse outcomes, such as preterm deliveries, spontaneous pregnancy losses, or stillbirths [20,21].

Similar to UFH, women treated with LMWH during pregnancy often have underlying comorbid conditions that may predispose them to adverse pregnancy outcomes such as connective tissue diseases and a history of previous pregnancy losses. From a series of detailed analyses, Ginsberg and colleagues [22] reported that, in the absence of concurrent maternal comorbid conditions, the use of UFH in pregnancy did not increase the risk of spontaneous abortions, stillbirths, or neonatal deaths. In a similar review by Sanson and co-workers, the risk of adverse pregnancy outcomes in women without comorbid conditions exposed to LMWH was 3.1% (95% confidence interval [CI]; 1.1–6.6%). This rate is low, and despite the absence of concurrent control groups, it is similar to that reported in historical controls. These data suggest that similar to UFH, LMWH does not adversely affect the fetus.

B. Breastfeeding

UFH is not excreted into breast milk because of its high molecular weight [23]. Although there is no direct evidence that LMWH is not excreted in breast milk, its relatively large molecular weight (mean of approximately 5000 Da) makes this unlikely. Even if LMWH was excreted in the breast milk, it would not be absorbed by the nursing infant [2]. Consequently, the risk of an anticoagulant effect in the infant is highly unlikely.

C. Maternal Safety

The use of UFH and LMWH is associated with bleeding [24–29], thrombocytopenia [30], and osteoporosis [31–34].

1. Bleeding

The risk of bleeding associated with treatment doses of LMWH is probably slightly less than the rate in patients treated with UFH [28,29]. In one metanalysis [28], the relative risk of major bleeding associated with LMWH, compared with UFH, was 0.65 (95% CI; 0.37–1.05); in a second metanalysis [29], this risk was 0.57 (95% CI; 0.33–0.99) in favor of LMWH.

There are currently no prospective studies comparing the bleeding risks of UFH and LMWH in pregnancy. It is likely, however, that the overall risk of bleeding in pregnancy is low, as most pregnant women are young and do not often have comorbid conditions that predispose to bleeding. In a retrospective cohort study of pregnant women treated with UFH, the rate of major bleeding was 2% [35]; in a systematic review, the pooled rate of bleeding in women treated with LMWH was estimated to be 2.7% (95% CI; 1.4–4.5%) [21].

The risk of bleeding is greatest at the time of delivery. Women treated with LMWH have been reported to have increased blood loss compared with controls (473 mL vs. 365 mL, p = 0.02) [36]; although this difference is statistically significant, it is of dubious clinical importance.

Another consideration with LMWH during pregnancy is its use in conjunction with epidural analgesia at the time of delivery. The overall risk of bleeding complications from neuraxial procedures (spinal or epidural) in young obstetrical patients has been reported to be 1 : 10,000–1 : 100,000 [37,38]. Several small studies involving more than a 100 women given LMWH [7,39–40] report no neurological complications. Data from the general population suggest that the risk of spinal bleeding in patients given LMWH is low; no cases were reported in two large reviews that included 9,000 and more than 15,000 patients [41,42] given epidural analgesia.

Despite the rarity of this event, case reports of nonobstetrical patients developing spinal hematomas while receiving LMWH have heightened physician and patient concerns. Thus, elective induction of delivery near term should be considered, so that LMWH can be discontinued 24 h before delivery and epidural analgesia can be safely given, if desired. Because women treated with subcutaneous UFH can have persistent prolongation of the activated partial thromboplastin time (aPTT) at the time of delivery [43], we encourage discontinuation of subcutaneous UFH or LMWH at least 24 h before a planned induction of labor.

2. Heparin-Induced Thrombocytopenia

Heparin-induced thrombocytopenia occurs in approximately 3% of patients exposed to UFH [30]; this risk is lower with LMWH [30].

Heparin-induced thrombocytopenia has been reported infrequently during pregnancy in subjects receiving either UFH or LMWH [21,44]. In the review by Sanson and colleagues [21], heparin-induced thrombocytopenia did not occur in any of the 486 pregnancies in which LMWH was given.

If heparin-induced thrombocytopenia develops during pregnancy, LMWH should be discontinued. Danaparoid sodium or hirudin can be used as alternative anticoagulants [2]. We prefer the former because it does not cross the placenta and there is considerable experience with its use, albeit not in pregnancy.

3. Osteoporosis

The development of osteoporosis with heparin-related compounds is a particular problem in pregnancy because these patients often require extended treatment. Studies in rats suggest that bone loss induced by UFH reflects both decreased bone formation and increased bone resorption [31]. Bone loss in this model is not readily reversible [33], and LMWH causes less bone loss than UFH [32].

From the results of a retrospective cohort study, the rate of osteoporotic fractures in women given long-term (≥ 1 month) UFH during pregnancy was 2% [34]. Using serial measures of bone density endpoints, several small studies suggest that subclinical bone loss occurs more frequently in pregnant women given UFH than in untreated controls [36,37]. In a small prospective study [37], 36% (5/14) of women treated with UFH had a 10% or higher decrease in bone density. In contrast, none of the matched controls had such a decrease (p = 0.03). Although a relation between the dose of heparin administered in pregnancy and the extent of bone loss has not been demonstrated [36,37], this may reflect the small number of patients included in these studies.

Bone loss associated with UFH exposure may be partially reversible when treatment is stopped. It is uncertain whether UFH-induced bone loss increases the subsequent risk [49] of osteoporosis.

LMWH may produce less bone loss than UFH. Although there are case reports of osteoporotic fractures in women treated with LMWH during pregnancy [43,49], several small prospective studies did not detect a decrease in bone density in women given LMWH throughout pregnancy [50,51].

Small studies of patients treated with UFH or LMWH have reported no differences in bone densities between the UFH- or LMWH-treated groups [35,52]. A cohort study of pregnant women treated with either UFH or LMWH failed to show a difference in bone density between the two groups [51]. One study, in which 80 elderly patients were randomly allocated to receive UFH or LMWH [35], demonstrated more vertebral fractures in those given UFH, even though bone densities were similar in the two groups. With the limited data available, women receiving extended therapy with either UFH or LMWH should be considered to have an increased risk of osteoporosis. Consequently, we empirically prescribe supplemental calcium and vitamin D throughout pregnancy to these women.

4. Skin Reactions

In addition to local bruising at injection sites, heparin-associated cutaneous reactions have been reported with both LMWH and UFN [2]. Severe immediate-type hypersensitivity, skin necrosis related to heparin-induced thrombocytopenia, as well as delayed type IV skin reactions can occur with heparin. Delayed type IV skin reactions have been reported more frequently in women than in men (10 : 1) [53]. This condition is characterized by well-circumscribed erythematous plaques at subcutaneous injection sites. These occur approximately 10 days after initiation of therapy. A switch to a different LMWH preparation is safe if skin provocation tests are negative [53], but administration of intravenous heparin in these women should be avoided until more is known about this side effect.

IV. INDICATIONS OF LMWH USE IN PREGNANCY

A. Prophylaxis and Treatment of Venous Thromboembolism

There are no randomized trials investigating the efficacy of LMWH for the prevention or treatment of VTE during pregnancy. Recommendations for its use in pregnancy are derived from randomized trials of nonpregnant patients and case–series of pregnant patients.

1. Treatment of VTE

A randomised, controlled trial in nonpregnant patients has demonstrated the effectiveness of treatment of VTE with intravenous UFH followed by subcutaneous adjusted-dose UFH for 3 months [54]. In addition, several large, randomized-controlled studies [55,56] demonstrate that LMWH is at least as effective, and possibly safer, than intravenous UFH for the initial treatment of VTE. Extrapolating from these studies, LMWH is likely to be as effective as UFH for initial and long-term treatment of pregnant women with VTE.

The optimal duration of anticoagulant therapy for treatment of VTE during pregnancy has not been determined [57,58]. Anticoagulant therapy should be given for at least 3 months and probably for the duration of the pregnancy, because it is likely that the risk factors that triggered the initial episode remain operative throughout pregnancy. Reduction of the dose of UFH or

LMWH after the initial 3 months of therapy may be a reasonable compromise to reduce the risk of bleeding and osteoporosis. In any case, a 4 to 6-week course of warfarin after delivery should be given because women in the postpartum period are at risk of thrombosis.

The appropriate dosing LMWH regimen during pregnancy remains unclear. If possible, antifactor Xa levels should be measured to ensure that the appropriate dose is given, particularly as the pregnancy progresses. For treatment of VTE, an antifactor Xa range of 0.5–1.2 U/mL measured 4 h after subcutaneous LMWH administration can be considered therapeutic. It is our practice to administer LMWH twice-daily during pregnancy because there is a possibility that LMWH is cleared more rapidly as a result of the increased glomerular filtration rate.

Although nonpregnant patients with VTE are often treated out-of-hospital, in the absence of supporting data from trials, initial hospitalization should be considered in pregnant women who present with extensive VTF or symptomatic pulmonary embolism.

2. Prophylaxis of VTE

Women with previous VTE have an increased risk of recurrence during pregnancy [59]. In a recent cohort study, women with a previous single episode of VTE were not anticoagulated during pregnancy, but were treated with warfarin for 4–6 weeks postpartum. The risk of recurrence in the antepartum period was 2.4% (95% CI; 0.2–6.9%) [59], suggesting that clinical surveillance, combined with appropriate investigation of suspected events, is a safe approach.

Women with asymptomatic thrombophilia (deficiencies of protein S, protein C, or anti-thrombin III, or heterozygotes for factor V Leiden or prothrombin gene mutation) likely also have an increased risk of VTE during pregnancy [60–62]. Antepartum prophylaxis with UFH or LMWH is reasonable, but clinical surveillance alone may be sufficient. Regardless of the antepartum approach taken, strong consideration should be given to the use of warfarin for 4–6 weeks postpartum. Women with antiphspliolipid antibodies and no previous history or VTE are candidates for LMWH or UFH prophylaxis because they probably have an increased risk of VTE [63]. In the absence of data from properly designed studies, treatment should be individualized for women with thrombophilia.

If LMWH is used in place of UFH for VTE prophylaxis during pregnancy, once-daily–dosing is probably adequate. The most frequently used LMWI-I preparations for this indication are dalteparin and enoxaparin [64].

B. Recurrent Pregnancy Losses and Adverse Pregnancy Outcomes

Women with antiphospholipid antibodies have an increased risk of pregnancy loss [65]. Based on the results of two prospective studies [66,67], one of which was a randomized controlled trial [66], low-dose aspirin together with low-dose UFH improves the rate of successful pregnancy outcomes. Thus, compared with aspirin alone, the combination improved the rate of successful pregnancy outcomes from 42 to 71% (p = 0.01). Based on these data, low-dose UFH and aspirin is a reasonable option in this setting. Whether LMWH is as effective as UFH for this purpose is currently under evaluation.

Several retrospective studies suggest that women with inherited thrombophilia also have an increased risk of adverse pregnancy outcomes, including pregnancy loss, preeclampsia, placental abruption, fetal growth retardation, and stillbirths [67,68]. Several small, uncontrolled studies [69–72] suggest that antepartumn LMWH reduces the risk of these complications.

C. Prosthetic Heart Valves

Women with prosthetic heart valves require ongoing anticoagulation during pregnancy to prevent valve thrombosis. Coumarins are contraindicated between 6 and 12 weeks of gestation because their use is associated with an increased risk of warfarin embryopathy. Likewise, these agents should be avoided in the third trimester because of the risk of fetal bleeding at the time of delivery [73]. During these periods, full-dose UFH (30–40,000 U/24 h) is required to maintain adequate anticoagulation. Lower doses of UFH are associated with valve thrombosis [74,76], raising concerns about the use of UFH for thromboprophylaxis of arterial thrombosis in pregnant women with mechanical prosthetic heart valves during pregnancy. However, many UFH failures were undoubtedly due to inadequate starting doses ($\leq$ 15,000 U/day), as well as the use of an inappropriately low target therapeutic range. A commonly used therapeutic range for UFH is 1.5–2.5 times control. Different aPTT reagents have varying responses to UFH, and, therefore, the corresponding heparin levels differ for a given aPTT, depending on the reagent used [77]. Moreover, a fixed ratio of 1.5 limes control as the lower limit of the therapeutic range corresponds to subtherapeutic heparin levels for virtually all aPTT reagents. Therefore, if a clinician targets an aPTT result of 1.5 times control, the dose of UFH is likely to be inadequate. Owing to the reports of high rates of bad outcomes with UFH and the reluctance of physicians (particularly in North America) to use warfarin during pregnancy, LMWH has become an attractive alternative to UFH for such women because it probably causes less bleeding. Consequently, doses of LMWH that produce a relatively greater antithrombotic effect than UFH can be used, which is likely to result in fewer failures. Experience with LMWH is, however, still limited to small case–series [78,79].

Although empiric, and dependent on the individual, we recommend doses of LMWH adjusted to maintain an antifactor Xa target of 1.0–1.5 U/mL measured between 3 and 4 h after administration. In patients at high-risk for thrombosis, such as those with valves of high thrombogenic potential (e.g., mitral valves with concomitant atrial fibrillation or older generation valve types), the addition of low-dose aspirin, 80 mg/day, which increases efficacy (as well as bleeding) in nonpregnant subjects, should be considered [80].

V. MANAGEMENT OF WOMEN RECEIVING LMWH AT TERM

The management of women receiving LMWH requires the coordinated efforts of the obstetrician, the anesthesiologist, and the hematologist at the time of labor and delivery because of a concern about epidural hematomas associated with epidural analgesia. If prophylactic doses of LMWH are given, the drug should be discontinued 24 h before planned elective induction of labor. This protocol is expected to result in no detectable anticoagulant activity so that epidural analgesia can be safely administered. If spontaneous labor occurs within 24 h of a dose of prophylactic LMWH, the risk of epidural hematoma is likely to be extemely low. Accordingly, three options are available: (1) proceed with the epidural; (2) measure an antifactor Xa level, and if it is undetectable or low (<0.2 U/mL), proceed with the epidural (3) avoid epidural analgesia and use an alternative.

In situations for which the risk of thromboembolism is high (e.g., in a woman with a prosthetic heart valve), hospitalization at term and conversion to UFH should be considered. The ease of measuring the aPTT as a surrogate for the anticoagulant effect of UFH and the rapid reversibility of UFH with protamine sulfate [2] are important considerations for such change. If spontaneous labor occurs within 12–24 h of a "treatment" dose of LMWH, epidural analgesia should probably be avoided.

In the postparturn period, LMWH can safely be given 8–12 h [45] after the epidural catheter is removed. For ongoing treatment, either LMWH or warfarin can be used. LMWH has the advantage of not requiring laboratory monitoring.

VI. CONCLUSION

LMWH will almost certainly replace UFH as the anticoagulant choice during pregnancy. LMWH is probably as effective as UFH for the treatment and prophylaxis of VTE during pregnancy, but LMWH is easier to administer and its use may be associated with a lower incidence of heparin-induced thrombocytopenia and osteoporosis.

Further work is needed to determine the optimal dose and appropriate dosing schedule for LMWH during pregnancy. The efficacy of LMWH for the prevention of recurrent pregnancy losses and adverse pregnancy outcomes in women with thrombophilia remains to be established. Likewise, the efficacy, safety, and appropriate dosing of LMWH in women with prosthetic valves also needs to be elucidated.

REFERENCES

1.   Hyers TM, Agnelli G, Hull RD, Weg JG, Morris TA, Samana M, Tapson VF. Antithrombotic therapy for venous thromboembolism. Chest 1998; 114:561S–578S.
2.   Hirsh J, Warkentin TE, Raschke R, Granger C, Ohman EM, Dalen JE. Heparin and low-molecular heparin: mechanisms of action, pharmacokinetics, dosing considerations, monitoring, efficacy, and safety. Chest 1998; 114:489S–510S.
3.   Lindheimer MI), Katz Al. Renal physiology and disease in pregnancy. In: Sedin DW, Giebisch G, eds. The Kidney: Physiology and Pathophysiolgy. New York: Raven Press, 1992; 3371–3431.
4.   Metcalfe J, Ueland K. Maternal cardiovascular adjustments to pregnancy. Prog Cardiovasc Dis 1974; 16:363–374.
5.   Ellinson J, Walker ID, Greer IA. Antenatal use of enoxaparin for prevention and treatment of thromboembolism in pregnancy. 2000; 107:1 116–1121.
6.   Brennand JE, Walker ID, Greer IA. Anti-activated factor X profiles in pregnant women receiving antenatal thromboprophylaxis with enoxaparin. Acta Haematol 1999; 101:53–55
7.   Nelson–Piercy C, Letsky EA, de Swiet M. Low-molecular-weight heparin for obstetric thromboprophylaxis: experience of sixty-nine pregnancies in sixty-one women at high risk. Am J Obstet Gynecol l997; 176:1062–1068.
8.   Casele HL, Laifer SA, Woelkers DA, Venkataramanan R. Changes in the pharmacokinetics of the low-molecular weight heparin enoxaparin sodium during pregnancy. Am J Obstet Gynecol 1999; 181:1113–1117.
9.   Koren G, Pastuszak A, Ito S. Drugs in pregnancy. N Engl J Med 1998; 338:1128–1137.
10.   Andrew M, Ofosu F, Fernandez F, Jefferies A, Hirsh J, Mitchell L, Buchanan MR. A low molecular heparin alters the fetal coagulation system in the pregnant sheep. Thromb Haemost 1986; 55:342–346.
11.   Saivin S, Giroux M, Dumas JC, Faure F, Rekik L, Grandjean H, Boneu B, Houin G. Placental transfer of glycosaminoglycans in the human perfused placental cotyledon model. Eur J Obstet Gynecol Reprod Biol 1992; 22:221–225.
12.   Forestier F, Daffos F, Capell–Pavlovsky M. Low molecular weight heparin (PK 10169) does not cross the placenta during the second trimester of pregnancy. Study by direct fetal blood sampling under ultrasound. Thromb Res 1984; 34:557–560.
13.   Rainaut M, Forestier F, Daffos S, Forestier F. [Prenatal pharmacology of LMW heparin and pentosan polysulfate]. J Mal Vase l987; 12(suppl):119–122. [French].
14.   Forestier F, Daffos F, Rainaut M, Toulemonde F. Low molecular weight heparin (CY 216 does not cross the placenta during the second trimester of pregnancy. Study by direct fetal blood sampling under ultrasound. Thromb Haemost 1987; 57:234.
15.   Otnri A, Dellaloye JF, Anderson H, Bachmann F. Low molecular weight heparin novo (LHN-1) does not cross the placenta during the second trimester of pregnancy. Thromb Haemos 1989; 1:55–56.

16. Harenberg J, Schneider D, Heilmann L, Wolf H. Lack of anti-factor Xa activity in umbilical cord vein samples after subcutaneous administration of heparin or low molecular mass heparin in pregnant women. Haemostasis 1993; 23:314–320.

17. Melissari E, Parker CJ, Wilson NV, Monte G, Kanthou C, Pemberton KD, Nicolaides KH, Barrett JJ, Kakkar VV. Use of low molecular weight heparin in pregnancy. Thromb Haemost 1992; 68:652–656.

18. Schneider DM, Heililnann L, Harenberg J. Placental passage of low molecular weight heparin. Geburtshilfe Fruenheilkd 1995; 55:93–98.

19. Wahlberg TB, Kher A. Low molecular weight heparin as thromboprophylaxis in pregnancy. Hemostasis 1994; 24:55–56.

20. Sorenson HT, Johnsen SP, Larsen H, Pederson L, Nielson GL, Moller M. Birth outcomes in pregnant women treated with low-molecular-weight heparin. Acta Obstet Gynecol Scand 2000; 79:655–659.

21. Sanson BJ, Lensing AWA, Prins MH, Ginsberg JS, Barkagan ZS, Lavene–Pardonge E, Brenner B, Dulitzky M, Nielson JD, Boda Z, Turi S, MacGillavry MR, Hamulyak K, Theunissen IM, Hunt BJ, Buller HR. Safety of low-molecular-weight heparin in pregnancy: a systematic review. Thromb Haemost 1999; 81:668–672.

22. Ginsberg JS, Hirsh J. Anticoagulants during pregnancy. Annu Rev Med 1989; 40:79–86.

23. O'Reilly RA. Anticoagulant, antithrombotic, and thrombolytic drugs. In: Gilman AG, Goodman LS, Gilman A, eds. The Pharmacological Basis of Therapeutics. 6th ed. New York: Macmillian, 1980; 1350.

24. Leizorovicz A, Simonneau G, Decousus H, Boissel JP. Comparison of efficacy and safety of low molecular weight heparins and unfractionated heparin in initial treatment of deep vein thrombosis: a meta-analysis. Br Med J 1994; 309:299–304.

25. Lensing AW, Prins MH, Davidson BL, Hirsh J. Treatment of deep venous thrombosis with low molecular weight heparins: a meta-analysis. Arch Intern Med 1995; 155:601–607.

26. Siragusa S, Cosmi B, Piovella F, Hirsh J, Ginsberg JS. Low-molecular-weight heparins and unfractionated heparin in the treatment of patients with acute venous thromboembolism: results of a metanalysis. Am J Med 1996; 100:269–277.

27. Koopman MM, Prandoni P, Piovella F, Ockelford PA, Bandjes DP, van der Meer J, Gallus AS, Simmonneau G, Chesterman CH, Prins MH. Treatment of venous thrombosis with intravenous unfractionated heparin administered in the hospital as compared with subcutaneous low-molecular-weight heparin administered at home. The Tasman Study Group. N Engl J Med 1996; 334:682–687.

28. Dolovich LR, Ginsberg JS, Douketis ID, Holbrook AM, Cheah G. A meta-analysis comparing low-molecular-weight heparins with unfractionated heparin in the treatment of venous thromboembolism: examining some unanswered questions regarding location of treatment, product type, and dosing frequency. Arch Intern Med 2000; 160:181–188.

29. Gould MK, Dembitzer AD, Doyle RL, Hastie TJ, Garber AM. Low-molecular-weight heparins compared with unfractionated heparin for treatment of acute deep venous thrombosis. A meta-analysis of randomized, controlled trials. Ann Intern Med 1999; 130:800–809.

30. Warkentin TE, Levine MN, Hirsh J, Horsewood P, Roberts RS, Gent M, Kelton JG. Heparin induced thrombocytopenia in patients treated with low-molecular-weight heparin or unfractionated heparin. N Engl J Med 1995; 332:1330–1335.

31. Muir JM, Andrew M, Hirsh J, Weitz JL, Young E, Deschamps P, Shaughnessy SG. Histomorphometric analysis of the effects of standard heparin on trabecular bone *in vivo*. Blood 1996; 88:1314–1320.

32. Muir JM, Hirsh J, Weitz JI, Andrew M, Young E, Shaughnessy SG. A histomorphometric comparison of the effects of heparin and low-molecular weight heparin on cancellous bone in rats. Blood 1997; 89:3236–3242.

33. Shaughnessy SG, Hirsh J, Bhandari M, Muir JM, Young E, Weitz JI. Histomorphometric evaluation of heparin-induced bone loss after discontinuation of heparin treatment in rats. Blood 1999; 93:1231–1236.

34. Dahlman TC. Osteoporotic fractures and recurrence of thromboembolism during pregnancy and the puerperium in 184 women undergoing thromboprophylaxis with heparin. Am J Obstet Gynecol 1993; 168:1265–1270.

35. Monreal M, Lafoz E, Olive A, del Rio L, Vedia C. Comparison of subcutaneous unfractionated heparin with a low molecular heparin (Fragmin) in patients with venous thromboembolism and contra-indications to coumarin. Thromb Haemost 1994; 71:7–11.

36. Ginsberg JS, Kowalchuk G, Hirsh J, Brill–Edwards, Burrows R, Coates G, Webber C. Heparin effect on bone density. Thromb Haemost 1990; 64:286–289.

37. Barbour L, Kick SD, Steiner JF, LoVerde MIS, Heddleston LN, Lear JL, Baron AE, Barton PL. A prospective study of heparin-induced osteoporosis in pregnancy using bone densitometry. Am J Obstet Gynecol 1994; 170:862–869.

38. Ginsberg JS, Kowalchuk G, Hirsh J, Brill–Edwards P, Burrows R. Heparin therapy during pregnancy. Arch Intern Med 1989; 149:2233–2236.

39. Lindqvist GP, Dahlback B. Bleeding complications associated with low molecular weight heparin prophylaxis during pregnancy. Thromb Haemost 2000; 84:140–141.

40. Scott DB, Hibbard BM. Serious non-fatal complications associated with extradural block in obstetric practice. Br J Anaesth 1990; 64:537–541.

41. Scott DB, Tunstall ME. Serious complications associated with epidural/spinal blockade in obstetrics: a two-year prospective study. Int J Obstet Anesth 1995; 4:133–139.

42. Dulitzki M, Pauzner R, Langevitz P, Pras M, Many A, Schiff E. Low molecular weight heparin during pregnancy and delivery: preliminary experience with 41 pregnancies. Obstet Gynecol 1996; 87:380–383.

43. Hunt BJ, Doughty HA, Majumbar G, Copplestone A, Kerslake S, Buchanan N, Hughes G, Khamashta M. Thromboprophylaxis with low molecular weight heparin (Fragmin) in high risk pregnancies. Thromb Haemost 1997; 77:39–43.

44. Bergqvist D, Lindblad B, Matzsch T. Risk of combining low molecular weight heparin for thromboprophylaxis and epidural or spinal anesthesia. Semin Thromb Hemost 1993; 19(suppl 1): 147–151.

45. Horlocker TT, Heit JA. Low molecular weight heparin: Biochemistry, pharmacology, perioperative prophylaxis regimens, and guidelines for regional anesthetic mangement. Anesth Analg 1997; 85: 874–885.

46. Anderson DR, Ginsberg JS, Burrows R, Brill–Edwards P. Subcutaneous heparin therapy during pregnancy: a need for concern at the time of delivery. Thromb Haemost 1991; 65:48–250.

47. Fausett MB, Vogtlandler M, Burgett D, Lee RM, Larkin A, Branch DW, Silver RM. Heparin induced thrombocytopenia is rare in pregnancy. Am J Obstet Gynecol 1998; 178:S66.

48. Douketis JD, Ginsberg JS, Burrows R, Duku EK, Weber CE, Brill–Edwards P. The effects of long-term heparin therapy during pregnancy on bone density. A prospective matched cohort study. Thromb Hemost 1996; 75:254–257.

49. Lima F, Khamashta MA, Buchanan NM, Kerslake S, Hunt BJ, Hughes GR. A study of sixty pregnancies in patients with the antiphospholipid syndrome. Clin Exp Rheumatol 1996; 14:131–136.

50. Casele H, Laifer S. Prospective evaluation of bone density changes in pregnant women on low molecular weight heparin [abstr]. Am J Obstet Gynecol 1998; 178:S65.

51. Shefras J, Farquharson RG. Bone density studies in pregnant women receiving heparin. Eur J Obstet Gynecol 1996; 65:171–174.

52. Backos M, Rai R, Thomas E, Murphy M, Dore C, Regan L. Bone density changes in pregnant women treated with heparin: a prospective, longitudinal study. Hum Reprod 1999; 14:2876–2880.

53. Wutschert R, Piletta P, Bounameaux H. Adverse skin reactions to low molecular weight heparins. Drug Safety 1999; 20:515–525.

54. Hull RD, Raskob GE, Pineo GF, Green D, Trowbridge AA, Elliott CG, Lerner RG, Hall J, Sparling T, Bretell HR, Norton J, Carter CJ, George R, Merli G, Ward J, Mayo W, Rosenbloom D, Brant R. Subcutaneous low-molecular-weight heparin compared with continuous heparin in the treatment of proximal vein thrombosis. N Engl J Med 1992; 326:975–982.

55. The Columbus Investigators. Low-molecular-weight heparin in the treatment of patients with venous thromboembolism. N Engl J Med 1997; 337:657–662.

56. Simonneau G, Sors H, Charbonnier B, Page Y, Laaban JP, Azarian R, Laurent M, Hirsch JL, Ferrari E, Bosson JL, Mottler D, Beau B. A comparison of low-molecular-weight heparin with unfractionated

heparin for active pulmonary embolism. The THESEE Study. N Engl J Med 1997; 332:663–669.

57. Schulman S, Rhedin AS, Lindmaker P, Carlsson A, Larfars G, Nicol P, Loogna E, Svensson E, Ljungberg B, Walter H. A comparison of six weeks with six months of oral anticoagulant therapy after a first episode of venous thromboembolism. Duration of anticoagulation trial study group. N Engl J Med 1995; 332:1661–1665.

58. Kearon C, Gent M, Hirsh J, Kovacs MJ, Anderson DR. Turpie AG, Green D, Ginsberg JS, Wells P, MacKinnon B, Julian JA. A comparison of three months of anticoagulation with extended anticoagulation for a first episode of idiopathic venous thromboembolism. N Engl J Med 1999; 340: 901–907.

59. Brill–Edwards P, Ginsberg JS, Gent M, Hirsh J, Burrows R, Kearon R, Geerts W, Kovacs M, Weitz JI, Robinson KS, Whittom R, Couture G. Safety of withholding heparin in pregnant women with a history of venous thromboembolism. N Engl J Med 2000; 343: 1439–1444.

60. Conrad J, Horellou M, Sarnama MM. Management of pregnancy in women with thrombophilia. Hemostasis 1999; 29(suppl):98–104.

61. Lindqvist PG, Svensson PJ, Marsaal K, Grennert L, Luterkort M, Dahlback B. Activated protein C resistance (FV:Q506) and pregnancy. Thromb Haemost 1999; 81:532–537.

62. Simioni P. Sanson BJ, Prandoni P, Tormene D, Friederich PW, Girolami B, Gavasso S, Huisman MV, Buller HR, Wouter ten Cate J, Girolami A, Rrins MH. Incidence of venous thromboembolism in families with inherited thrombophilias. Thromb Haemost 1999; 81:198–202.

63. Ginsberg JS, Hirsh J. Use of antithrombotic agents during pregnancy. Chest 1998; 114:524S–530S.

64. WS Chan, Ray J. Low molecular weight heparin use in pregnancy: issues of safety and practicality. Obstet Gynecol Surv 1999: 54:649–654.

65. Finazzi G, Brancaccio V, Moia M, Ciaverella N, Mazzucconi MG, Schinco PC, Ruggeri M, Pogliani EM, Gamba G, Rossi E, Baudo F, Manotti C, D'Angelo A, Palareti G, De Stefano V, Berrettini M, Barbui T. Natural history and risk factors for thrombosis in 360 patients with antiphospholipid antibodies: a four-year prospective study from the Italian Registry. Am J Med 1996; 100:530–536.

66. Rai R, Cohen H, Dave M, Regan L. Randomised controlled trial of aspirin and aspirin plus heparin in pregnant women with recurrent miscarriage associated with phospholipid antibodies (or antiphospholipid antibodies). Br J Med 1997; 314:253–257.

67. Kutteh WH. Antiphospholipid antibody-associated recurrent pregnancy loss: treatment with heparin and low-dose aspirin is superior to low-dose aspirin alone. Am J Obstet Gynecol 1996; 174:1584–1589.

68. Brenner B. Inherited thrombophilia and pregnancy loss. Thromb Haemost 1999; 82:634–640.

69. Brenner B, Hoffman R, Blumenfeld Z, Weiner Z, Younis JS. Gestational outcome in thrombophilic women with recurrent pregnancy loss treated by enoxaparin. Thromb Haemost 2000; 83:693–697.

70. Riyazi N, Leda M, de Vries JIP, Huijgens PC, van Gejin HP, Dekker GA. Low-molecular-weight heparin combined with aspirin in pregnant women with thrombophilia and history of preeclampsia or fetal growth restriction: a preliminary study. Eur J Obstet Gynecol 1998; 80:49–54.

71. Bar J, Cohen–Sacher B, Hod M, Blickstein D, Lahav J, Merlob P. Low-molecular-weight heparin for thrombophilia in pregnant women. Int J Gynecol Obstet 2000; 69:209–213.

72. Younis JS, Ohel G, Brenner B, Haddad S, Lanir N, Ben-Ami M. The effect of thromboprophylaxis on pregnancy outcome in patients with recurrent pregnancy loss associated with factor V Leiden mutation. Br J Obstet Gynaecol 2000; 107:415–419.

73. WS Chan, Ginsberg, JS. Anticoagulation of pregnant women with mechanical heart valves: a systemic review of the literature. Arch Intern Med, 2000; 160:191–196.

74. Salazar E, Izaguirre R, Verdejo J, Mutchinick O. Failure of adjusted doses of subcutaneous heparin to prevent thromboembolic phenomena in pregnant patients with mechanical cardiac valve prostheses. J Am Coll Cardiol 1996; 27:1698–1703.

75. Ayhan A, Yapar EG, Yuce K, Kisnisci HA, Nazli N, Ozmen F. Pregnancy and its complications after cardiac valve replacement. Int J Gynecol Obstet 1991; 35:117–122.

76. Ben Ismail M, Abid F, Trabelsi S, Taktak M, Fekih M. Cardiac valve prostheses, anticoagulation, and pregnancy. Br Heart J 1986; 55:101–105.

77. Brill–Edwards P, Ginsberg JS, Johnston M, Hirsh J. Establishing a therapeutic range for heparin therapy. Ann Intern Med 1993; 119:104–109.

78. Lee LH, Liauw PC, Ng AS. Low molecular weight heparin for thromboprophylaxis during pregnancy in 2 patients with mechanical mitral valve replacement. Thromb Haemost 1996; 76:628–630.

79. Arnaout MS. Kazma H, Khalil A, Shasha N, Nasrallah A, Karam K, Alam SE. Is there a safe anticoagulation protocol for pregnant women with prosthetic heart valves? Clin Exp Obstet Gynecol 1998; 25:101–104.

80. Turpie AG, Gent M, Laupacis A, Latour Y, Gunstensen J, Basile F, Klimek M, Hirsh J. A comparison of aspirin with placebo in patients treated with warfarin after heart valve replacement. N Engl J Med 1993; 329:524–529.

7

Antithrombotic Therapy and Cancer

Gloria Petralia and Ajay K. Kakkar
Hammersmith Hospital, Imperial College, London, England

SUMMARY

Thromboprophylaxis for patients undergoing surgery for cancer should include the use of graduated compression stockings associated with either unfractionated heparin (UFH) or low-molecular-weight heparin (LMWH).

In patients receiving chemotherapy or radiotherapy, and considered to be at high risk for venous thromboembolism (VTE), thromboprophylaxis can be achieved by warfarin titrated to maintain an international normalized ratio (INR) between 1.3 and 1.9. The value of prophylaxis with LMWH in nonsurgical cancer patients is the subject of current prospective clinical trials.

In cancer patients with central venous catheters, either the LMWH dalteparin 2500 once daily or the oral anticoagulant warfarin in a dose of 1 mg can be used for the prevention of line-associated thrombosis.

Primary treatment of established VTE in those with cancer is identical with that recommended for noncancer patients (i.e., treatment with intravenous UFH or subcutaneous LMWH). Prevention of recurrent VTE is more difficult in the presence of malignant disease. Warfarin is the established first-line approach, failing which, UFH and LMWH are employed to prevent symptomatic recurrences.

I. INTRODUCTION

The association between thrombosis and malignant disease was first described by Armand Trousseau in 1865 [1].

Since his original description of the syndrome of thrombophlebitis migrans, a clinical entity now recognized as pathognomonic for underlying cancer, there has been a growing recognition that thromboembolic events may be the first clinical manifestation of undiagnosed malignancy [2–4]. As a corollary, patients with established cancer have an increased risk of venous thromboembolic disease (VTE). Cancer patients are often debilitated, are frequently immobile, and may require surgery or chemotherapy. All these factors contribute to increased VTE risk, which may be compounded by a hypercoagulable state associated with the cancer itself. Venous thromboembolism, manifesting in a spectrum from symptomatic deep-vein thrombosis to fatal pulmonary embolism, is much more likely in the cancer patient, and it is estimated that up to 60% of thromboembolic deaths occur at an otherwise favorable time in the natural history of the cancer. Thus, VTE is a major concern for the cancer physician and antithrombotic therapy for the prevention and treatment forms a key component of cancer management with important implications for patient outcome.

II. PATHOGENESIS

Virchow, working in the early 1800s, identified a triad of factors that influence the pathogenesis of VTE. These factors—venous stasis, coupled with vascular trauma, and blood hypercoagulability—are also the central features of thrombus formation in cancer patients.

A. Tumor-Associated Hypercoagulability

A hypercoagulable state occurs in malignancy and appears to be partly associated with the expression of procoagulant molecules by tumor cells. Tumor secretion of the physiological tissue factor (TF) plays a significant role in the generation of the hypercoagulable state, causing activation of the extrinsic coagulation pathway, which may lead to overt thrombosis or a subclinical disseminated intravascular coagulation (DIC) [6–8]. Tumor cells may also secrete cysteine and serine proteases that exert coagulation activation indirectly by secreting tumor necrosis factor (TNF) or interleukin (IL)-like proteins [2] that act on endothelial and mononuclear cells, with resultant secretion of procoagulant molecules that may have a role in platelet activation [9].

B. Vascular Trauma and Venous Stasis

A hypercoagulable state may occur as a result of vascular trauma or venous stasis caused directly or indirectly by the pressure of a tumor. Invasion into blood vessels by cancer cells, which, for example, occurs in thrombosis of the inferior vena cava in renal cell carcinoma [9], results directly in a prothrombotic state that may be further enhanced by local secretion of vascular permeability factors [10]. Mechanical causes that can lead to vascular stasis include vessel compression by bulky tumor masses and introduction of a central line, resulting in mechanical insult and subsequent slowing of blood flow. Certain chemotherapeutic agents exert a prothrombotic effect, part of which may be mediated by damage caused to the endothelial cells [11]. Tumor-induced angiogenesis creates a network of aberrant vessels in which flow is disordered, resulting in impaired clearance of activated coagulation factors and hypoxic alterations, which can be responsible for a procoagulant state [2].

III. VENOUS THROMBOEMBOLIC DISEASE IN CANCER PATIENTS

The clinical manifestations of VTE range from asymptomatic calf vein thrombosis, through to acute, life-threatening massive pulmonary embolism.

Several studies have shown that cancer patients undergoing surgery have a substantially higher risk of postoperative deep-vein thrombosis (DVT) and pulmonary embolism (PE) compared with noncancer patients. Cancer patients who were undergoing major abdominal surgery had a significantly higher incidence of DVT compared with noncancer patients (41 compared with 26%; RR 1.96; p = 0.04) [12].

Similarly, other studies showed the rate of fatal PE after major surgery was significantly higher in cancer patients than in noncancer patients (1.6 vs. 0.4%; p =<0.05) [13]. Rates of VTE in studies that have reported outcome for cancer and non cancer subjects separately are detailed in Table 1.

In patients with malignant disease, VTE is estimated to be the second most common cause of death [9,14], and its treatment accounts for 6% of inpatient bed use in medical oncology wards [15]. Up to 15% of cancer patients will experience a symptomatic thromboembolic event [9,14,15]. Risk of PE seems to be dependent on tumor histology. In a necroscopic study [16], the highest rates were found in ovarian cancer (34.6%), followed by malignancies of the extrahepatic biliary system (31.7%), and of the stomach (15.2%); whereas the lowest rates (0.5–6%) were in cancer of the esophagus and larynx, myelomatosis, and lymphoma.

Risk of bleeding is also higher in patients with cancer who are receiving anticoagulant therapy than in non-cancer patients (16.1 vs. 7.4%) [17]. In addition, the incidence of disseminated intervascular coagulation (DIC) requiring intervention in patients with cancer has been estimated to be between 9 and 15% [15].

The risk of VTE associated with the use of chemotherapeutic agents has been well documented in trials relating to the treatment of breast cancer (Table 2), with the incidence of thrombotic events ranging from 1.7 to 17.6%. Furthermore, Levine's review of 205 women with breast cancer (stage II) showed an increased risk of DVT while combination chemotherapy was administered [18]. Chalsen et al. compared postmenopausal women with breast cancer (stages I and II) undergoing surgery alone with those receiving postoperative chemotherapy and showed an increased risk associated with adjuvant therapy (0.7 vs. 2.3%; p = 0.001) [19]. Tamoxifen increases DVT risk in both premenopausal (2.3 vs. 0.8%; p = 0.003) and postmenopausal (8.0 vs. 2.3%, p = 0.003) women [20]. Chemotherapy associated with tamoxifen increases DVT risk when compared with tamoxifen alone in a group of women with stage II breast cancer (from 1.4 to 9.6%: (p = 0.0001) [21].

Radiotherapy similarly increases VTE risk. In a study of patients receiving neoadjuvant radiotherapy for rectal carcinoma, an increased rate of thromboembolic events was reported in the first 30 days following surgery [22]. Comparable results were found in a 5-year follow-up study in similar patients (7.5 vs. 3.6%; p = 0.001) [23].

Table 1 Incidence of Postoperative VTE in Patients with and without Malignant Disease (Differing Methods of Diagnosis)

Study ref.	Cancer patients (%)	Noncancer patients (%)
12	24/59 (41%)	38/144 (26%)
60	8/16 (50%)	7/34 (21%)
61	16/45 (35%)	22/217 (10%)
27	28/66 (42%)	29/128 (23%)
62	16/30 (53%)	16/65 (28%)
63	17/76 (22%)	49/36 (16%)
30	41/100 (31%)	21/100 (21%)
64	62/304 (20%)	113/707 (16%)
65	21/310 (6.7%)	10/597 (1.6%)
66	12/23 (52%)	16/62 (26%)
15	25/1407 (1.8%)	16/2402 (0.7%)
Total	270/2436 (11%)	337/3898 (8.6%)

Table 2   Incidence of VTE Patients with Breast Cancer Undergoing Chemotherapy

Study ref.	Stage	Number of patients	Thrombosis (%)	Type of thrombosis
71	II	433	5.0	Venous
68	IV	159	17.6	Venous and arterial
18	II	205	6.8	Venous and arterial
69	II, III	1014	1.3	Arterial
70	II	383	3.1	Venous
20	I, II	2352	5.4	Venous and arterial
19	I, II	1292	2.1	Venous
71	II	603	2.5	Venous and arterial
43	IV	159	4.4	Venous and arterial
21	II	353	9.6	Venous and arterial
72	II	50	10	Venous
73	Various	182	7.7	Venous

The increasing use of central lines in cancer patients to deliver chemotherapy, parenteral nutrition, blood and its derivatives, or simply as access, further contributes to the thromboembolic risk (Table 3).

From a reverse point of view VTE can be the first manifestation of an occult malignancy. Two recent population-based analyses of cancer risk, performed in Scandinavia [24,25], involving about 86,000 patients with venous thromboembolism (4,200 of whom had cancer), observed that the incidence of cancer in patients with VTE was 1.3 times and 3.2 times higher than among the Danish and Swedish population without thrombosis.

IV. PREVENTION OF VENOUS THROMBOEMBOLIC DISEASE IN CANCER PATIENTS

The effective prevention of VTE is especially important in cancer patients, given that the diagnosis is more difficult, the treatment of an acute thromboembolic event is less satisfactory, and there is a higher risk of bleeding complications. Thromboprophylaxis is essential as a means of achieving reduced rates of mortality and morbidity and to maintain the quality of life in those patients whose life expectancy may be short. An effective prevention program needs to target underlying factors that predispose to VTE, to minimize any secondary effects, be well tolerated by the patient, and be feasible both from a logistic and economic point of view [26].

Table 3   Incidence of VTE in Cancer Patients with Venous Central Line not Receiving Thromboprophylaxis

Study ref.	% (no. of patients)
45	37.5%
74	62% (8/13)
75	66%
11	13% (15/115)

A. Prevention in Surgical Patients

In patients undergoing surgery, several strategies can be adopted to reduce the risk of thromboembolism, including elevation of the lower extremities, leg exercise, early ambulation, and pressure prevention during the operation. However, more specific measures, including mechanical and pharmacological modes of prevention, are recommended.

1. Mechanical Modes of Prevention

The use of electrical stimulation of the calf muscles during surgery has been described and has been of benefit in reducing stasis-related problems, but not in patients with malignancy [27]. Intermittent pneumatic compression (IPC) presents certain attractive features as a method of thromboprophylaxis because there is no associated hemorrhagic risk, but it has not been as thoroughly investigated as other methods. In a study of pneumatic compression of the calf evaluated in cancer patients, the incidence of VTE was 9% (2/23) in patients receiving the treatment, compared with 40% (8/20) in the control group [28]. However, the number of patients enrolled was small with the confidence intervals extremely wide, making it difficult to draw a firm conclusion on efficacy.

In a metanalysis of 355 patients [29] intermittent compression of the calf showed a reduced rate of VTE compared with no treatment (21 vs. 12.8%) but any decrease in the risk of fatal PE has yet to be proved with this method.

The use of a graduated compression stocking reduces the incidence of postoperative VTE [30] and enhances the protection provided by low-dose UFH, although the measure appears to be less effective in cancer patients undergoing surgery compared with noncancer patients.

In patients with brain metastases, the use of inferior vena cava (IVC) filters has been proposed. Studies have described widely varying rates of recurrent PE (3–20%) [31,32] and of local thrombotic complication (5–57%) [33] in patients with IVC filters.

2. Aspirin

Aspirin, whose mechanism of action involves inactivation of platelet cyclooxygenase, has attractive features as an antithrombotic agent in cancer patients. It is relatively inexpensive, easy to administer, and has few side effects. A recent study reviewed 145 trials and suggested that low-dose aspirin reduced the incidence of vascular events by about one-third [34]. However, aspirin has been generally ineffective in preventing VTE in surgical patients and, therefore, is not recommended for that purpose in cancer patients.

3. Dextran

Dextran is used to expand blood volume, especially in cases of hypovolemic shock and in situations during which blood flow is slowed. It has been used in the prevention of postoperative VTE and acts by being absorbed onto the platelet surface, increasing the negative charge and leading to the formation of a blood clot that is more susceptible to lysis by plasmin. It is relatively expensive, requires intravenous administration; and offers no advantages over oral anticoagulants in terms of bleeding.

4. Unfractioned Heparin

Unfractionated heparin (UFH) is widely used as a thromboprophylactic agent in patients undergoing surgery. It is a heterogeneous mix of heparins that contain a pentasaccharide sequence. This sequence binds to the endogenous anticoagulant protein antithrombin III (ATIII) and greatly increases the ability of ATIII to inhibit thrombin and factor Xa. However, ATIII is unable to inhibit thrombin that is bound to fibrin and platelet-bound factor X.

Treatment with low-dose UFH (5000 U) is administered subcutaneously, starting 2 h before surgery and continuing every 8–12 h thereafter. In a metanalysis of 29 trials describing the use of heparin thromboprophylaxis, results from cancer patients were presented separately in 10 of the trials. The metanalysis showed that the incidence of VTE in 919 patients with cancer was significantly reduced in those receiving UFH, compared with that of placebo (13.6 vs. 30.6%; $p<0.001$) [35]. The efficacy of the treatment is still less when compared with noncancer patients (Table 4).

Studies also show that UFH is effective in the prevention of PE. In an international randomized trial, heparin reduced mortality from 1.6% in the control group receiving no thromboprophylaxis to 0.4% after treatment with UFH [36].

5. Low-Molecular-Weight Heparin

The use of low-dose LMWH has been recommended for patients with cancer undergoing minor operations, or in those who, for whatever reason, are confined to bed [37]. LMWH has a mechanism of action similar to UFH, but with diminished inhibition of thrombin. It has several potential advantages when compared with UFH, including a longer half-life, simple subcutaneous administration, and no requirement for dose monitoring; making it suitable for the outpatient setting. In addition, LMWH has a more limited effect on platelets, with a reduced incidence of heparin-induced thrombocytopenia, and it has not been associated with osteoporosis [38]. Although LMWH thromboprophylaxis has been extensively investigated in noncancer surgical patients, very few studies have specifically investigated VTE prophylaxis in patients with cancer. However, LMWH was more effective and as safe as UFH in studies containing a high percentage of cancer patients (Table 5). Bergqvist et al. [39] randomized 2097 surgical patients, 66.4% of whom had malignant disease, to receive prophylactic treatment for VTE with LMWH (2500 U) versus LMWH dalteparin (5000 U). Thromboembolic rates decreased in the group receiving the higher dose (8.5 vs. 14.9%; $p = 0.001$) demonstrating for the first time that efficacy can be improved by a higher dose, in cancer patients, without an increased rate of bleeding.

In a study [40] of over 300 patients undergoing neurosurgery and receiving thromboprophylaxis by means of graduated compression stockings, LMWH was randomized against placebo. About 85% of these patients suffered from tumors of the central nervous system, which itself is an independent risk factor for VTE and intracranial bleeding. The results proved that LMWH effectively reduced thromboembolic risk ($p = 0.004$) without increasing the risk of bleeding complications.

Table 4 Incidence of VTE in Patients Receiving Unfractionated Heparin Prophylaxis

Study ref.	Group	UFH patient no. (%)	Control patient no. (%)	Relative risk
62	Benign	4/59 (7%)	18/65 (28%)	25
	Malignant	7/24 (30%)	16/30 (53%)	55
63	Benign	8/304 (3%)	49/36 (16%)	18
	Malignant	5/58 (9%)	17/76 (22%)	39

Table 5 DVT Rates in Cancer Surgical Patients: Comparison of Thromboprophylaxis with LMWH and UFH

Study ref.	Type of LMWH	Cancer (%)	LMWH (%)	UFH (%)
77	Dalteparin	45	6.4	4.3
78	Nadroparin	100	4.2	5.4
79	Dalteparin	63.3	5.5	8.3
80	Enoxaparin	30	3.2	5.0
81	Tinzaparin	38.5	5.8	4.2
17	Fragmin	37.6	1.26	1.30
82	Reviparin	52.3	4.6	4.2
83	Eparinoid	100	10.4	14.9
84	Enoxaparin	100	13.6	8.7
39	Enoxaparin	100	14.7	18.2

Source: Ref. 76.

6. Dermatan Sulfate

There are limited trial data examining the efficacy of dermatan sulfate as a thromboprophylactic agent. Dermatan sulfate is a glycosaminoglycan that selectively inhibits heparin cofactor II. It is effective on both fibrin-bound and free thrombin. In a study by Di Carlo [41], the efficacy of dermatan sulfate for the prevention of VTE was compared with heparin in 842 patients with cancer. The incidence of VTE in the dermatan sulfate and heparin group was 15.0 and 22.0%, respectively.

B. Oral Anticoagulants

1. Prevention in Medical Oncological Patients

Oral anticoagulants, such as warfarin, are vitamin K antagonists and interfere with the production of factors II, VII, IX, and X in the liver. Prophylactic levels of anticoagulation are achieved by adjusting the dose to maintain an international normalized ratio (INR) of between 2.0 and 3.0.

Even at low levels of anticoagulation there may be an unacceptable risk of bleeding in cancer patients. In addition anticoagulation is more difficult to control in cancer than in noncancer patients, and prophylactic INR levels are more difficult to achieve (43.3% of the time vs. 56.9%; p<0.0001) [42].

In a study by Levine and colleagues [43], 311 patients undergoing chemotherapy for stage IV breast cancer were randomized to receive very low-dose warfarin, targeted to achieve an INR between 1.3 and 1.9, and placebo. The study showed a significant 85% reduction in VTE risk for the group receiving warfarin (0.6 vs. 4.4%; p = 0.031) with no significant increase in bleeding rates.

When analyzed in a cohort of over 100 patients undergoing postoperative radiotherapy for gynecological tumors, thromboprophylaxis with warfarin showed a VTE rate of 7.5%, with a 3.8% rate of PE, and with bleeding complications in 5.3% of the patients [44].

2. Prevention in Patients with Indwelling Central Line Catheters

The use of oral anticoagulants for thromboprophylaxis has been advocated for cancer patients with indwelling central catheters. In a study of 84 patients randomised to receive warfarin (1 mg)

or placebo, the incidence of VTE was significantly reduced in the group receiving warfarin (9 vs. 37%; p = 0.001) [45]. Similar results have been obtained with low-dose oral anticoagulation in the prophylaxis of line-associated thrombosis, [11,75], and with the low-molecular-weight heparin, dalteparin, given in a dose of 2500 U/day, VTE rates were reduced from 60 to 6%, [74].

V. TREATMENT

The objectives of therapy for established VTE are to prevent PE, reduce recurrence rates and minimize the morbidity from deep-vein thrombosis (DVT). In patients with malignant diseases, an increased risk of recurrence (1.72-fold) [46] (Table 6), and bleeding complicates the treatment. In a recent study [47], which compared the outcome of secondary prophylaxis with oral anticoagulants, the incidence of bleeding episodes and rates of recurrence of VTE were lower in the noncancer group than in the cancer patients: total bleeding 21.6 versus 4.5% (RR, 4.5; 95% CI, 2.6–7.8; p<0.0001); whereas VTE recurrence was 6.8 versus 2.7% (RR, 2.5; 95% CI, 0.96 – 6.5; p = 0.059).

A. Primary Thrombosis

Until recently, UFH was the most commonly used initial treatment for DVT. It is administered as an initial dose of 5000 U, followed by continuous infusion to maintain an activated partial thromboplastin time (aPTT) of 1.5–2.0 times the control value [48]. UFH can increase circulating levels of tissue plasminogen activator and tissue factor pathway inhibitor (TFPI) by causing them to be released from binding sites on the surface of endothelial cells. Specifically, TFPI is a tridomain protein that binds to the tissue factor FVIIa–FX complex that suppresses the generation of factor Xa by tissue factor [49]. As tissue factor plays a major role in the coagulation process in cancer patients this may account for its some of activity in these patients.

In a large retrospective study [50] of patients with adenocarcinoma and Trousseau's syndrome, UFH was beneficial in 65% of the patients compared with only 19% of patients given warfarin. Recurrence rates of VTE in cancer patients have been 22% with warfarin treatment and only 7% when UFH or LMWH was used [51].

Following the numerous studies that proved its safety and efficacy [52–55], the use of subcutaneous LMWH has become widely accepted. Prepared by chemical or enzymatic degradation of unfractionated heparin, LMWH has a narrower molecular-weight range, is effectively absorbed from the subcutaneous tissue, has an half-life of 3.5–4.5 h and a bioavailability of over 85% owing to low plasma protein concentrations and cellular-binding properties. These factors allow LMWH to be given in a twice-a-day or once daily regimen, simplifying administration. In addition dose monitoring of LMWH is not required. This offers the

Table 6 Incidence of Recurrent Venous Thromboembolism in Patients With and Without Malignant Disease

Study ref.	Cancer patients (%)	Noncancer patients (%)
42	4/44 (9.1%)	3/64 (4.6%)
85	20/232 (8.6%)	32/789 (4.1%)
86	14/264 (5%)	21/1039 (2%)

opportunity to treat most patients who have uncomplicated DVT, safely, and effectively at home, improving quality of life.

B. Prevention of Secondary Recurrence

Following initial treatment with heparin (either UFH and LMWH) prevention of recurrence can be achieved by oral anticoagulation. Recurrent venous thromboembolic disease occurs more frequently in cancer patients and the duration of oral anticoagulation in cancer patients remains unclear. Current recommendations suggest that oral anticoagulation therapy be continued as long as there is active cancer or active cancer therapy. The potential value of prolonged LMW therapy for prevention of recurrent VTE in cancer patients is currently being evaluated in clinical trials.

VI. ANTITHROMBOTIC THERAPY AND CANCER SURVIVAL

An interesting question that has surfaced in the literature is whether antithrombotic treatment might help improve survival rates in patients with cancer.

Retrospective analyses of studies undertaken to compare the safety and efficacy of UFH and LMWH in the treatment of DVT have examined 3–6 month survival rates in cancer patients with DVT who were randomized for these trials. These analyses have demonstrated a trend toward a mortality benefit in those cancer patients receiving LMWH [57,58]. In a metanalysis [59] of nine randomized clinical trials, including data from 629 cancer patients in these DVT studies, the effects of UFH or LMWH as initial treatment of DVT demonstrated a statistically significant difference in the 3-month–mortality rate of approximately 40% in favor of LMWH (OR = 0.39; 95% CI; 0.15–1.02). These findings are difficult to explain, given that the cancer patients with DVT received only a short course (7–10 days) of LMWH for initial treatment of their DVT. These data must be interpreted with caution because the original studies were not designed to evaluate long-term cancer mortality. A recent prospective study evaluating perioperative LMWH prophylaxis in surgery for breast or gynecological malignancy [87], demonstrated a late survival benefit for patients with pelvic malignancy who received thromboprophylaxis with LMWH for up to 2 years after surgery. It appears that LMWH, either by effectively preventing VTE, or by directly influencing tumor biology, can improve outcome in cancer patients. If the results of prospective studies currently assessing the value of prolonged LMWH therapy in cancer patients, without thrombosis, confirm the previous retrospective analyses, use of these agents may become routine.

REFERENCES

1. Cormack JR, trans. *Plegmasia alba dolens*. In: Trousseau A. Lectures on Clinical Medicine (delivered at the Hotel-Dieu, Paris, France). London: New Sydenham Society, 1872; 282–332.
2. Prandoni P, Piccioli A. Venous thromboembolism and cancer: a two-way clinical association. Frontiers Biosci 1997; 2:e12–20.
3. Kakkar AK, Williamson RCN. Antithrombotic therapy in cancer: low molecular weight heparins may have a direct effect on tumors. Br Med J 1999; 318:1571–1572.
4. Di-Carlo V, Agnelli G, Prandoni P, Coccheri S, Gensini GF, Gianese F, Mannucci PM. Dermatan sulphate for the prevention of postoperative venous thromboembolism in patients with cancer. DOS (dermatan sulphate in oncologic surgery) study group. Thromb Haemost 1999; 82:30–4.

5. Shen VS, Pollack EW. Fatal pulmonary embolism in cancer patients: is heparin prophylaxis justified? South Med J 1980; 73:841–843.

6. Kakkar AK, DeRuvo N, Chinswangwatanakul V, Tebbutt S, Williamson RCN. Extrinsic-pathway activation in cancer with high factor VIIa and tissue factor. Lancet 1995; 346:1004–1005.

7. Kakkar AK, Lemoine NR, Scully MF, Tebbutt S, Williamson RCN. Tissue factor expression correlates with histological grade in human pancreatic carcinoma. Br J Surg 1995; 82:1101–04.

8. Gordon SG. Cancer cell procoagulants and their implications. Hematol Clin North Am 1992; 6:1359–1374.

9. Letai A, Kutera DJ. Cancer, coagulation, and anticoagulation. Oncologist, 1999; 4:443–449.

10. Edwards RL, Rickles FR. Thrombosis and cancer. In: Hull R, Pineo GF, eds. Disorders of Thrombosis. Philadelphia: WB Saunders, 1996; 374–382.

11. Boraks P, Seale J, Price J, Bass G, Ehtel M, Keeling D, Mahendra P, Baglin T, Marcus R. Prevention of central venous catheter associated thrombosis using minidose warfarin in patients with hematological malignancies. Br J Haematol 1998; 101:483–486.

12. Kakkar VV, Howe CT, Nicolaides AN, Renney JTG, Clarke MB. Deep vein thrombosis of the leg. Is there a "high risk" group? Am J Surg 1970; 120:527–530.

13. Rahr HB, Sorensen JV. Venous thromboembolism and cancer. Blood Coagul Fibrin 1992; 3:451–460.

14. Rickles FR, Edwards RL. Activation of blood coagulation in cancer: Trousseau's syndrome revisited. Blood 1983; 62:14–31.

15. Harrington KJ, Bateman AR, Syrigos KN, Rintoul R, Bhidayasiri R, McCormack M, Thomas H. Cancer-related thromboembolic disease in patients with solid tumors: a retrospective analysis. Ann Oncol 1997; 8:669–673.

16. Svendsen E, Karwinski B. Prevalence of pulmonary embolism at necroscopy in patients with cancer. J Clin Pathol 1989; 42:805–809.

17. Kakkar VV, Cohen AT, Edmondson RA, Philips MJ, Cooper DJ, Das SK, Maher KT, Sanderson RM, Ward VP, Kakkar S. Low molecular weight versus standard heparin for prevention of venous thromboembolism after major abdominal surgery. Lancet 1993; 341:259–265.

18. Levine M, Gent M, Hirsh J, Arnold A, Goodyear MD, Hryniuk W, De Pauw S. The thrombogenic effect of anticancer drug therapy in women stage II breast cancer. N Engl J Med. 1988; 318:404–407.

19. Clahsen PC, Van de Velde CJH, Julien JP, Floiras Mignolet JL. Thromboembolic complications after perioperative chemotherapy in women with early breast cancer: a European Organization for Research and Treatment of Breast Cancer Cooperative Group Study. J Clin Oncol 1994; 12:1266–1271.

20. Saphner T, Tormey DC, Gray R. Venous and arterial thrombosis in patients who received adjuvant therapy for breast cancer. J Clin Oncol 1991; 9:286–294.

21. Pritchard KI, Paterson AH, Paul NA, Zee B, Fine S, Pater J. Increases in thromboembolic complications with current tamoxifen and chemotherapy in a randomized trial of adjuvant therapy for women with breast cancer. National Cancer Institute of Canada Clinical Trials Group Breast Cancer Site Group. J Clin Oncol 1996; 14:2731–2737.

22. Goldberg PA, Nicholls FJ, Porter NH, Love S, Grimsey KE. Long-term results of a randomised trial of short-course low-dose adjuvant preoperative radiotherapy for rectal cancer: reduction in local treatment failure. Eur J Cancer 1994; 11:1602–1606.

23. Holm T, Singnomklao T, Rutqvist LE, Cedermark D. Adjuvant preoperative radiotherapy in patients with rectal carcinoma. Adverse effects during long-term follow-up of two randomised trials. Cancer 1996; 78:968–976.

24. Sorensen HT, Mellemkjaer L, Steffensen FH, Olsen JH, Nielsen GL. The risk of a diagnosis of cancer after primary deep venous thrombosis or pulmonary embolism. N Engl J Med 1998; 338:1169.

25. Baron JA, Gridley G, Weiderpass E, Nyren O, Linet M. Venous thromboembolism and cancer. Lancet 1998; 351:1077–1080.

26. Kakkar VV. Prevention of venous thromboembolism. In: Bloom AL, et al., eds. Haemostasis and Thrombosis. Edinburgh: Churchill Livingstone, 1994; 1361–1379.

27. Rosemberg IL, Evans M, Pollock AV. Prophylaxis of postoperative leg vein thrombosis by low dose subcutaneous heparin or perioperative calf muscles stimulation: a controlled clinical trial. Br Med J 1975; 1:649–651.

28. Roberts VS, Cotton LT. Prevention of postoperative deep vein thrombosis in patients with malignant disease. Br Med J 1974; 1:435–448.

29. Clagett GP, Anderson FA, Heith J, Levine MN. Prevention of venous thromboembolism. Chest 1995; 108:312–324.

30. Allan A, Williams JT, Bolton JP, Le Quesne LP. The use of graduated compression stockings in the prevention of postoperative deep vein thrombosis. Br J Surg 1983; 70:172–174.

31. Schwarz RE, Marrero AM, Conlon KC, et al. Inferior vena cava filters in cancer patients: indications and outcome. J Clin Oncol 1996; 14:652–657.

32. Levin JM, Schiff D, Loeffler JS, et al. Complications of therapy for venous thromboembolic disease in patients with brain tumors. Neurology 1993; 43:1111–1114.

33. Letaia A, Kutera DJ. Cancer, coagulation and anticoagulation. Oncologist, 1999; 4:443–449.

34. Elwood PC, Hughes C, O'Brien JR. Platelets, aspirin, and cardiovascular disease. Postgrad Med J. 1998; 74:587–591.

35. Clagett PG, Reisch JS. Prevention of venous thromboembolism in general surgical patients. Result of a meta-analysis. Ann Surg 1988; 208:227–240.

36. International Multicentre Trial. Prevention of fatal postoperative pulmonary embolism by low doses of heparin. Lancet 1975; 2:45–51.

37. European Consensus Statement. Prevention of venous thromboembolism. Int Angiol 1992; 11:151–159.

38. Kakkar AK, Williamson RC. Prevention of venous thromboembolism in cancer using low-molecular-weight heparins. Haemostasis 1997; 27 (suppl 1):32–37.

39. Bergqvist, D, Burmark, US, Flordal PA, Frisell J, Hallbook T, Hedberg M, Horn A, Kelty E, Kvittiing P, Lindhagen A, Ljungstrom KG, Matzsch T, Risberg B, Syk I, Torngren S, Wellander E, Ortenwall P. Low molecular weight heparin started before surgery as prophylaxis against deep vein thrombosis: 2500 versus 5000 XaI units in 2070 patients. Br J Surg 1995; 82:496–501.

40. Agnelli G, Piovella F, Buoncristiani P, Severi P, Pini M, D'Angelo A, Beltrametti C, Damiani M, Andrioli GC, Pugliese R, Lorio A, Brambilla G. Enoxaparin plus compression stocking compared with compression stockings alone in the prevention of venous thromboembolism after elective neurosurgery. N Engl J Med 1998; 339:80–85.

41. Di-Carlo V, Agnelli G, Prandoni P, Coccheri S, Gensini GF, Gianese F, Mannucci PM. Dermatan sulphate for the prevention of postoperative venous thromboembolism in patients with cancer. DOS (dermatan sulphate in oncologic surgery) study group. Thromb Haemost 1999; 82:30–34.

42. Bona RD, Sivjee KY, Hickey AD, Wallace DM, Wajcs SB. The efficacy and safety of oral anticoagulation in patients with cancer. Thromb Haemost 1995; 74:1055–1058.

43. Levine M, Hirsh J, Gent M, Arnold A, Warr D, Falanga A, Samosh M, Bramwell V, Pritchard KI, Stewart D, Goodwin, P. Double-blind randomised trial of a very-low-dose warfarin for prevention of thromboembolism in stage IV breast cancer. Lancet 1994; 343:886–889.

44. Graf AH, Graf B, Brandis MG, Kogelnik HD, Staudach A, Traun H. Oral anticoagulation in patients with gynaecological cancer and radiotherapy: a retrospective analysis of 132 patients. Anticancer Res 1998; 18(3B):2047–2051.

45. Bern MM, Lokich JJ, Wallach SR Jr, Bothe A, Benotti PN, Arkin CF, Greco FA, Huberman M, Moore C. Very low doses of warfarin can prevent thrombosis in central venous catheters. Ann Intern Med 1990; 112:423–428.

46. Prandoni P, Lensing AWA, Cogo A, et al. The long-term clinical course of acute deep venous thrombosis. Ann Intern Med 1996; 125:1–7.

47. Palareti G, Legnani C, Lee A, Manotti C, Hirsk J, D'Angelo A, Pengo V, Moia M, Coccheri S. A comparison of the safety and efficacy of oral anticoagulation for the treatment of venous thromboembolic disease in patients with or without malignancy. Thromb Haemost 2000; 84:805–810.

48. Kakkar AK, de Lorenzo F, Pineo GF, Williamson RC. Venous thromboembolism and cancer. Baillieres Clin Haematol 1998; 11:675–687.

49. Baugh RJ, Broze GJ, Krishnaswamy S. Regulation of extrinsic pathway factor Xa formation by TFPI. J Biol Chem 1998; 273:4378–4386.

50. Sack GH, Levin J, Bell W. Trousseau's syndrome and other manifestations of chronic disseminated coagulopathy in patients with neoplasms: clinical, pathologic, and therapeutic features. Medicine 1977; 56:1–37.

51. Martins RG, Colowick AB, Ewenstein BM, et al. Anticoagulation in cancer patients with venous thromboembolic disease. Blood 1997; 909 (suppl 1):297a.

52. Levine M, Gent M, Hirsh, Leclerc J, Anderson D, Weitz J, Ginsberg J, Turpie AG, Demers C, Kovacs M, Geerts W, Kassis J, Desjardins L, Cusson J, Cruickshank M, Powers P, Brien W, Haley S, Willan A. A comparison of low-molecular-weight heparin administered primarily at home with unfractionated heparin administered in the hospital for proximal deep vein thrombosis. N Engl J Med 1996; 334:677–681.

53. Hull RD, Raskob GE, Pineo GF, Green D, Trowbridge AA, Elliott CG, Lerner RG, Hall J, Sparling T, Bretell HR. Subcutaneous low-molecular weight heparin compared with continuous intravenous heparin in the treatment of proximal-vein thrombosis. N Engl J Med 1992; 326:975–982.

54. Koopman MMW, Prandoni P, Piovella F, et al. Treatment of venous thrombosis with intravenous unfractionated heparin administrated in the hospital as compared with subcutaneous low-molecular weight heparin administered at home. N Engl J Med 1996; 334:682–687.

55. Rodgers GM, Spiro TE. Treatment of cancer-associated deep vein thrombosis with enoxaparin: comparison with unfractionated heparin therapy. Proc Am Soc Clin Oncol 1999; 18:193a.

56. Breddin HK, Hach-Wunderle V, Nakov R, Kakkar VV. Effects of low-molecular-weight-heparin on thrombus regression and recurrent thromboembolism in patients with deep vein thrombosis. N Eng J Med 2001; 334:626–631.

57. Walsh–McMonagle D, Green D. Low-molecular-weight heparin in the management of Trousseau's syndrome. Cancer 1997; 80:649–655.

58. Green D, Hull RD, Brant R, et al. Lower mortality in cancer patients treated with low-molecular weight versus standard heparin. Lancet 1992; 339:1476.

59. Buller HR, Hettiarachchi RJK, Smorenberg S, Ginsberg J, Levine M, Prins MH. Do heparins do more than just treat thrombosis? The influence of heparins on cancer spread. In: Abstract Book Simposio Eparina 2000 (Bologna 29–30 September 2000). Itlalfarmaco Editors. pp 7–11.

60. Hills NH, Pflug JJ, Jeyasingh K, Boardman L, Calnan JS. Prevention of deep vein thrombosis by intermittent pneumatic compression of calf. Br Med J 1972; 1:131–135.

61. Walsh JJ, Bonnar J, Wright FW. A study of pulmonary embolism and deep vein thrombosis after major gynaecological surgery using labelled fibrinogen–phlebography and lung scanning. J Obstet Gynaecol Br Commonw 1974; 81:311–316.

62. Rem J, Duckert F, Friedrich R, Gruber UK, Subkutane kleine Heparindosen zur Thromboseprophylaxe in der allgemeinen Chirurgie and Urologie. Schweiz Med Wschr 1975; 105:827–835.

63. Gallus AS, Hirsh J, O'Brien SE, McBride JA, Tuttle RJ, Gent M. Prevention of venous thrombosis with small subcutaneous dose heparin. JAMA 1976; 235:1980–1982.

64. The Multicentre Trial Committee. Dihydroergotamine–heparin prophylaxis of postoperative deep vein thrombosis: a multicentre trial. JAMA 1984; 251:2960–2966.

65. Kakkar VV, Murray WJG. Efficacy and safety of low molecular weight heparin (CY216) in preventing postoperative venous thromboembolism: a cooperative study. Br J Surg 1985; 82:724–725.

66. Sue–Ling HM, Johnston D, McMahon MU, Philips PR, Davies JA. Preoperative identification of patients at high risk of deep venous thrombosis after elective major abdominal surgery. Lancet 1986; 1:1173–1176.

67. Weiss RB, Tormey DC, Holland JF, Weinberg VE. Venous thrombosis during multinodal treatment of primary breast carcinoma. Cancer Treat Rep 1981; 65:677–679

68. Goodnough LT, Saito H, Manni A, Jones PK, Pearson OH. Increased incidence of thromboembolism in stage IV breast cancer patients treated with a five-drug chemotherapy regimen. Cancer 1984; 54:1264–1268.

69. Wall JC, Weiss RB, Norton L, Perloff M, Rice MA, Korzun AH, Wood WC. Arterial thrombosis associated with adjuvant chemotherapy for breast cancer: a Cancer and Leukaemia Group B Study. Am J Med 1989; 87:501–504.

70. Fisher B, Redmond C, Legault–Poisson R. Postoperative chemotherapy and tamoxifen compared with tamoxifen alone in treatment of positive node breast cancer patients aged 50 years and older with tumors responsive to tamoxifen: results from national adjuvant breast and bowel project B. J Clin Oncol 1990; 8:1005–1018.

71. Rifkin SE, Green S, Metch B, Jewell WR, Costanzi JJ, Ahman SJ, Minton JP, O'Bryan RM, Osborne CK. Adjuvant CMFVP versus tamoxifen versus concurrent CMFVP and tamoxifen for postmenopausal node positive and oestrogen receptor positive breast cancer patients: a Southwest Oncology Group study. J Clin Oncol 1994; 12:2078–2085.

72. Von Tempelhoff GF, Dietrich M, Hommel G, Heilman L. Blood coagulation during adjuvant epirubicin/cyclophosphamide chemotherapy in patients with primary operable breast cancer. J Clin Oncol 1996; 14:2560–2568.

73. Orlando L, Colleoni M, Nole F, Biffi R, Rocca A, Curigliano G, Ferretti G, Peruzzotti G, de Braud F, Masci G, Goldhirsch A. Incidence of venous thromboembolism in breast cancer patients during chemotherapy with vinorelbine, cisplatin, 5-fluorouracil as continuous infusion (ViFuP regimen): is prophylaxis required? Ann Oncol. 2000; 11:117–118.

74. Monreal M, Alastrue A, Rull M, Mira X, Muxart J, Rosell R, Abad A. Upper extremity deep venous thrombosis in cancer patients with venous access devices—prophylaxis with a low molecular weight heparin (Fragmin). Thromb Haemost. 1996; 75:251–253.

75. DeCicco M, Matovic M, Balesterri L, Panarello G, Fantin D, Morassut S, Testa V. Central venous thrombosis: an early and frequent complication in cancer patients bearing long-term Silastic catheter. A prospective study. Thromb Res 1997; 86:101–113.

76. Gallus AS. Prevention of post-operative deep leg vein thrombosis in patients with cancer. Thromb Haemost 1997; 78:126–132.

77. Bergqvist D, Burmark US, Frisell J, et al. Low molecular weight heparin once daily compared with conventional low-dose heparin twice daily. A prospective double-blind multicentre trial on prevention of postoperative thrombosis. Br J Surg 1986; 73:204–208.

78. The European Fraxiparin Study (EFS) Group. Comparison of a low molecular weight heparin and unfractionated heparin for the prevention of deep vein thrombosis in patients undergoing abdominal surgery. Br J Surg 1988; 75:1058–1063.

79. Bergqvist D, Matzsch T, Burmark US, et al. Low molecular weight heparin given the evening before surgery compared with conventional low dose heparin in the prevention of thrombosis. Br J Surg 1988; 75:888–891.

80. Samama M, Bernard P, Bonnardot JP, Combe–Tamzali S, Lanson Y, Tissot E. Low molecular weight heparin compared with unfractionated heparin in prevention of postoperative thrombosis. Br J Surg 1988; 75:128–31.

81. Liezorovicz A, Picolet H, Peyrieux JC, Boissel JP, HBPM Research Group. Prevention of perioperative deep vein thrombosis in general surgery: a multicentre double blind study comparing two doses of Logiparin and standard heparin. Br J Surg 1991; 78:412–416.

82. Boneu B. An international multicentre study: clivarin in the prevention of thromboembolism in patients undergoing general surgery. Blood Coagul Fibrinolysis 1993; 4:S21–S22.

83. Gallus A, Cade J, Ockelford P, Hepburn S, Maas M, Magnani H, Bucknall T, Stevens J, Porteous F. Orgaran (Org 10172) or heparin for preventing venous thrombosis after elective surgery for malignant disease? A double-blind, randomised, multicentre comparison. ANZ-Organon Investigators' Group. Thromb Haemost. 1993; 70:562–567.

84. Nurmohamed MT, Verhaege R, Haas, S et al. A comparative trial of a low molecular weight heparin (enoxaparin) versus standard heparin for the prophylaxis of postoperative deep vein thrombosis in general surgery. Am J Surg 1995; 169:567–571.

85. The Columbus Investigators. Low-molecular-weight heparin in the treatment of patients with venous thromboembolism N Engl J Med 1997; 337:657–662.

86. Hutten BA, Prins MH, Gent M, Ginsberg J, Tijssen JGP, Buller HR. Incidence of recurrent thromboembolic and bleeding complications among patients with venous thromboembolism in relation to both malignancy and achieved international normalized ratio: a retrospective study analysis. J Clin Oncol 2000; 18:3078–3083.

87. von Tempelhof GF, Harenberg J, Niemann F, Hommel G, Kirkpatrick CJ, Heilmann J. Effect of low molecular weight heparin (Certoparin) versus unfractionated heparin on cancer survival following breast or pelvic cancer surgery: a prospective randomised double-blind trial. Int J Oncol 2000; 16:815–824.

8

Thrombosis Prophylaxis with Low-Molecular-Weight Heparin in Medical Patients

Walter Ageno
University of Insubria, Varese, Italy

Alexander G. G. Turpie
McMaster University and Hamilton Health Sciences Corporation, Hamilton, Ontario, Canada

SUMMARY

Autopsy studies and epidemiological data have shown that the risk of venous thromboembolism in medical patients is comparable with the risk in surgical patients in whom there is a large amount of data to support the use of thrombosis prophylaxis. Indeed, 75% of all inhospital deaths for pulmonary embolism occur in nonsurgical patients. Thus, there is increasing evidence for the need for prophylaxis of venous thromboembolism in medical patients. However, hospitalized medical patients represent a very heterogeneous population, and the indications for thromboprophylaxis have remained controversial despite evidence of a substantial risk. Patients with medical disorders who should be considered for prophylaxis include those with heart failure, acute respiratory failure, acute infectious diseases, acute rheumatic disorders, inflammatory bowel diseases, and cancer. Several consensus conferences have produced detailed recommendations for thrombosis prophylaxis in both surgical and medical patients. Unfractionated heparin (UFH) and low-molecular-weight heparins (LMWH) have been evaluated in medical patients. Both have been effective when compared with placebo and are recommended in high-risk medical patients. When LMWHs were compared with UFH, they were shown to have equivalent efficacy and greater safety than the parent compound.

I. INTRODUCTION

A. Epidemiology of Thrombosis

Venous thromboembolism (VTE) is a common cause of morbidity and mortality in the United States and approximately 200,000 patients die from pulmonary embolism as a direct or a contributing cause [1]. Pulmonary embolism is responsible for 10% of overall deaths in hospitalized patients [2] and, each year, 170,000 new episodes and 90,000 recurrent cases of venous thromboembolism are diagnosed [3]. However, the real incidence, prevalence and mortality rates of venous thromboembolism are likely to be underestimated because the disease is often clinically silent and because autopsy data are limited [3]. When autopsy data were available and pulmonary embolism identified as the cause of death, it was often observed that the preceding thrombosis was not clinically recognized [2]. Failure to recognize venous thrombo-embolism reflects the unreliability of the clinical diagnosis and the poor sensitivity of screening tests providing the rationale for the recommendation for routine prophylaxis in patients identified to be at risk of VTE [4]. The choice of treatment requires careful evaluation of the risk of thrombosis and the hazards, inconveniences, and costs of prophylaxis.

1. Risk Factors and Prophylactic Methods

Knowledge of specific clinical risk factors is essential to identify the degree of risk in hospital patients and to address the most appropriate prophylactic strategy. The risk factors for the development of deep-venous thrombosis are determined both by the patient characteristics and by the clinical setting. Patients undergoing surgical procedures, particularly orthopedic surgery, cancer surgery, and neurosurgery are at highest risk for developing VTE [5]. Patients with major illnesses, such as malignancy, especially when treated with chemotherapy, or lower-limb paresis from stroke or spinal cord disorders, are also at very high risk of developing VTE [6]. Individual patient characteristics also contribute to the risk. Age older than 40 years, obesity, prolonged bed rest, varicose veins, and previous deep-vein thrombosis or pulmonary embolism, are significant risk factors, as well as congenital or acquired thrombophilic states, such as antithrombin, protein C, or protein S deficiencies; mutations in factor V or factor II; hyperhomocysteinemia; and the antiphospholipid antibodies syndrome (Table 1). The effects of these risk factors are cumulative, with the risk increasing with the number of risk factors [7,8]. It has been reported that 80% of hospitalized patients with an initial episode of deep-vein thrombosis and 85% with an initial episode of pulmonary embolism have three or more concomitant risk factors [3]. A useful classification of the degree of risk in hospital patients has been proposed allowing appropriate prophylaxis to be tailored according to risks [9]. Four groups were identified, ranging from low-risk patients, those younger than 40 years, and undergoing minor surgery without associated risk

Table 1 Risk Factors for Venous Thromboembolism

Individual factors	Disease or surgical procedure
Age >40	Trauma or surgery
Obesity	Malignancy
Varicose veins	Heart failure
Immobility (bed rest over 4 days)	Paralysis of lower limb
High-dose estrogen therapy	Recent myocardial infarction
Previous episode of venous thromboembolism	Infection
Thrombophilia	Inflammatory bowel disease
Antithrombin, protein C, protein S deficiencies	
Factor V, factor II mutations	Nephrotic syndrome
Hyperhomocysteinemia	
Antiphospholipid antibody	

Source: Ref. 7.

factors, to very high-risk patients, those older than 40 years undergoing major surgery and with previous venous thromboembolism or a history of malignant disease; patients undergoing orthopedic surgery; or patients suffering a stroke or a spinal cord injury. Without prophylaxis, proximal deep-vein thrombosis occurs in 0.4% low-risk patients, and in 10–20% very high risk patients, and with corresponding rates of clinical pulmonary embolism of 0.2 and 5–10%, respectively.

Guidelines on most appropriate prophylactic strategies have been developed based on the risk categories into which the patients fall, including physical methods such as early ambulation, graduated compression stockings, and intermittent pneumatic compression (IPC) devices, and pharmacological agents such as low-dose or adjusted-dose unfractionated heparin, low molecular weight heparins, and warfarin. Pharmacological measures have become the most widely used methods based on results of a large international trial that showed a clear reduction in the rate of fatal pulmonary emboli when surgical patients received unfractionated heparin three times daily as compared with placebo [10]. Subsequently, more than 100,000 patients have been included in clinical trials of VTE prophylaxis in surgical patients [11], and a number of consensus conferences have produced clinical guidelines based on the results of the most rigorously designed studies [4,7].

2. Epidemiology of Thrombosis in Medical Patients

The prevention of VTE has been less extensively studied in medical patients than in surgical patients and until recently, clear indications for prophylaxis have only applied in two clinical settings. These are patients with myocardial infarction or acute ischemic stroke in whom there is a well-established risk of thrombosis similar to that observed in surgical patients. However, it has been reported that 75% of all inhospital deaths caused by pulmonary embolism occur to nonsurgical patients [2]. Thus, although the incidence of venous thromboembolism has not been clearly defined, other medical patients in addition to those with myocardial infarction should be considered for routine prophylaxis. More recent data suggest that thromboembolism rates in a broad spectrum of medical patients are comparable with those of general surgical or even orthopedic patients. Data from epidemiological and clinical studies showed a risk for deep-vein thrombosis of 60% in ischemic stroke patients [12], 24% in myocardial infarction patients [4], and 19% in other medical patients [11]. In addition, two autopsy studies in general medical patients [13,14] revealed an incidence of deep-vein thrombosis 23% and pulmonary embolism of 24%, one-third of which were fatal.

3. Thrombosis Prophylaxis in Medical Patients

The first studies on prophylaxis in medical patients were conducted in those with acute myocardial infarction, or patients with stroke in whom unfractionated heparin, was effective when it was administered subcutaneously in low doses. In myocardial infarction patients, the benefits of either low-dose unfractionated heparin (5000 IU every 8–12 h or 7500 IU every 12 h) evaluated in four studies [15–18], or high-dose heparin, evaluated in two studies [19,20] were substantial, with 71 and 86% relative risk reductions, respectively, in the occurrence of deep-vein thrombosis, when compared with no prophylaxis. Stroke patients are at very high risk of developing VTE. Three studies [21–23] have compared low-dose heparin, administered in 5000-IU doses every 8 or 12 h, with no treatment, which showed an overall relative risk reduction of 63% incidence of VTE without clinically important bleeding. Data from the International Stroke Trial [24], which was primarily aimed at evaluating the treatment of ischemic stroke also showed a significant reduction in the occurrence of fatal and nonfatal pulmonary embolism with 5000 or 12,500 IU of unfractionated heparin twice daily as compared with no heparin.

Three studies have evaluated low-dose heparin in the general medical population [25–27] and one in patients with infectious diseases [28]. The studies were heterogeneous in design and included poorly defined patient populations. The first trial [25] was conducted on 100 patients with congestive heart failure or chest infection or both. In this study, low-dose heparin (5000 IU three times daily) resulted in a significant reduction of deep-vein thrombosis from 26% among nontreated patients to 4% in the heparin-treated patients, without any increase in major bleeding. The second larger study of 1358 general medical patients admitted to an acute care hospital [26] demonstrated a 31% reduction in the incidence of VTE from 10.9 to 7.8% in the group treated with 5200 IU of heparin twice daily as compared with no treatment. The third study was carried out in patients from both the intensive care and general medical ward settings. In this study, there was an overall reduction in the occurrence of deep-vein thrombosis from 29 to 13%. However the benefit was observed only in the group admitted to the intensive care unit [27]. Finally, a more recent study from Sweden compared 5000 IU of unfractionated heparin administered every 12 h with no treatment in patients with infectious disease [28]. In this study, there was no difference in the primary outcome of mortality, which occurred in 5.3 and 5.6% of the heparin-treated and control patients, respectively. There was however, significant reduction in nonfatal thromboembolic events, but this finding was considered to be inconclusive because diagnostic methods were not standardized among the participating centers.

4. Low-Molecular-Weight Heparin

The development of low-molecular-weight heparins, with pharmacological advantages over standard heparin, has led to their widespread use in a broad spectrum of thromboembolic disorders including thrombosis prophylaxis. The LMWHs have fewer saccharide units than UFH, resulting in the antithrombotic activity being mainly from inactivation of factor Xa [29]. Moreover, the LMWHs do not bind to endothelium and have a lower affinity for plasma proteins. They also have a minimal interaction with platelets when compared with UFH. These features result in LMWH having greater bioavailability, a substantially longer half-life, and potentially more antithrombotic than hemorrhagic activity than the parent compound [29]. Low-molecular-weight-heparins also have a stable dose–response when injected subcutaneously.

Evidence has accumulated that the LMWHs are more effective and safer than standard heparin for prophylaxis in patients at high risk for thrombosis, such as patients undergoing major orthopedic surgery [4]. Low molecular weight heparins or heparinoids have been evaluated in venous thromboembolism prophylaxis in stroke patients and in general medical patients.

Two studies [30,31] with dalteparin and two with the heparinoids, danaparoid [32,33], have been carried out in stroke patients. The results are summarized in Table 2. The first LMWH study compared dalteparin, in a dose of 2500 antifactor Xa units twice a day, with placebo [30]

Table 2 LMWH or Heparinoid in the Prevention of Deep-Vein Thrombosis in Stroke Patients

Ref.	Agent	LMWH/heparinoid	Control/Heparin
30	Dalteparin	6/27 (22.2%)	15/30 (50.0%)
31	Dalteparin	5/42 (35.7%)	17/50 (34.0%)
32	Danaparoid	2/50 (4.0%)	7/25 (28.0%)
33	Danaparoid	4/45 (8.9%)	13/42 (30.9%)[a]
34	Danaparoid	13/89 (14.6%)	17/86 (19.8%)[a]

[a]Heparin.

and demonstrated a reduction in the rate of venous thrombosis from 15 of 30 patients (50%) to 6 of 27 patients (22%). In the second study [31], dalteparin was given in a dose of 50–65 antifactor Xa units per kilogram of body weight once daily. In this study, there was no difference in the rate of deep-vein thrombosis between placebo-treated patients (34%) and dalteparin-treated patients (36%). The reason for the inconsistent results between the two trials is unclear, but may be related to the doses used in the trials. Larger trials in stroke patients have been conducted with the heparinoid danaparoid, a mixture of glycosaminoglycans characterized by an antifactor Xa/antithrombin ratio of greater than 28. Previously, danaparoid had been effective in preventing venous thromboembolism in high-risk orthopedic patients. In the first study [32] danaparoid was given in doses of 750 anti-Xa units twice daily subcutaneously, which reduced the incidence of deep-vein thrombosis from 28% in the placebo group to 4% in the danaparoid group, and proximal vein thrombosis from 16 to 0%, respectively, without an increased risk of bleeding. In the second study [33], the same dose of danaparoid was compared with unfractionated heparin (5000 IU twice daily). In this study, there was a significant reduction in the occurrence of deep-vein thrombosis from 31 to 8.9% and a corresponding rate of proximal deep-vein thrombosis of 11.9 and 4.4% in the heparin- and danaparoid-treated patients, respectively, with no difference in bleeding rates. The third study [34] assessed the efficacy of danaparoid given in a dose of 1250 anti-Xa units once daily compared with unfractionated heparin 5200 IU twice daily. Deep-vein thrombosis was diagnosed in 14.6% of the patients in the danaparoid group and in 19.8% of the patients treated with heparin. Hemorrhagic transformation of the infarct occurred in two patients in each group. The results of the prophylaxis studies with danaparoid demonstrated low rates of deep-vein thrombosis with significantly greater efficacy of danaparoid over unfractionated heparin without excess bleeding.

A number of clinical trials have been conducted on general medical patients with the LMWHs dalteparin, nadroparin, and enoxaparin. Dalteparin was evaluated in two small trials in general medical patients [35,36]. In both studies, which were conducted on small numbers of medical patients (192 and 166 patients), dalteparin administered in a 2500-IU once-daily dose was equivalent to unfractionated heparin given in doses of 5000 IU twice or three times daily Four studies have been carried out with nadroparin in medical patients [37–40]. All of the studies used the same dose of 3075 IU nadroparin given once daily. In all but one of the studies, nadroparin was compared with UFH given two or three times daily [37–39], and the remaining study was compared with placebo [40]. Each of the studies enrolled patients with a broad spectrum of medical conditions. Patients were screened for deep-vein thrombosis by ultrasonography [37–39] or by fibrinogen uptake [40]. There was a significant difference in the duration of treatment among the trials, which varied from 28 days [37], 10 days [38], 90 days [39], and 21 days [40]. There was no difference in efficacy between nadroparin and UFH in all three studies that compared the two treatments directly [37–39]. However, the rate of major bleeding was lowest in two of the studies in the LMWH-treated patients [37,39]. The placebo-controlled trial reported the rates of the overall mortality and autopsy detected pulmonary embolism, and no beneficial effect of nadroparin was found. The results of the studies with dalteparin and nadroparin are shown in Table 3.

Five studies in the prevention of VTE in medical patients have been carried out with enoxaparin. Again, the designs and results of these studies were heterogeneous. The results are shown in Table 4. The first trial [41] randomized 270 elderly patients suffering from various medical disorders to enoxaparin given in doses of 60 mg once daily or to placebo. After 10 days, enoxaparin resulted in a statistically significant reduction in the incidence of deep-vein thrombosis diagnosed by ^{125}I-fibrinogen leg scanning, from 9.2 to 3.0%, without any excess in major bleeding rates. In the subsequent three studies [42–44], enoxaparin was compared with the standard prophylactic doses of unfractionated heparin. Treatment with 20 [43] or 40 mg

Table 3 Dalteparin or Nadroparin in the Prevention of VTE in Medical Patients

Ref.	Agent	Outcome	LMWH	Heparin/placebo
35	Dalteparin	PE	0.100 (0.0%)	0/100 (0.0%)
36	Dalteparin	DVT	3/84 (3.6%)	4/82 (4.9%)
37	Nadroparin	DVT	3/146 (2.0%)	3/149 (2.0%)
38	Nadroparin	DVT	6/726 (0.8%)	4/710 (0.6%)
39	Nadroparin	DVT	0/129 (0.0%)	1/127 (0.8%)
40	Nadroparin	PE	0/1230 (0.8%)	17/1244 (1.4%)[a]

[a]Placebo.

[42,44] of enoxaparin was administered for 7 [42] to 10 days [43,44], and deep-vein thrombosis was assessed with ultrasonography [42], fibrinogen-uptake test [43], or venography [44]. Patients with a variety of medical disorders were recruited into two studies [42,43], and patients with cardiac or respiratory diseases to the other [44]. In all three studies enoxaparin and unfractionated heparin were equivalent, with a trend in favor of the LMWH in one [42]. Relative to safety, there was a reduction in major bleeding events in one study, with enoxaparin [42], but no difference in the other two studies [43,44]. A large, placebo-controlled trial evaluating enoxaparin in well-defined medical patients was recently completed [45]. In this study, two dosages of enoxaparin, 20 and 40 mg, administered for 6–14 days, were compared with placebo in 1102-bedridden medical patients. In contrast to most of the previous studies, which did not clearly define the patient population or included patients at very different risks for venous thrombosis, this trial included well-defined categories of patients, such as patients with congestive heart failure, acute respiratory failure, acute infection without septic shock, acute rheumatic disorders, or inflammatory bowel disease, all disorders that are considered to be at a moderate risk for VTE. In this study, the occurrence of deep-vein thrombosis was systematically evaluated with venography at the end of the treatment. After 14 days, there was a statistically significant reduction in venous thromboembolic events in the group treated with enoxaparin 40 mg as compared with placebo, but there was no reduction with enoxaparin 20 mg. Major bleeding rates and mortality rates were comparable among the three groups. At 110 day follow-up, there was no evidence of rebound in clinically detected thromboembolic events. This study is the largest study of prophylaxis in medical patients using appropriate methodology, and it clearly demonstrated the significant risk of VTE in this patient population and the effectiveness of prophylaxis with the LMWH enoxaparin given in doses of 40 mg, once daily, by subcutaneous injection.

Table 4 Enoxaparin in the Prevention of Deep-Vein Thrombosis in Medical Patients

Ref.	Enoxaparin dose (mg)	LMWH	Control/placebo[a]/heparin
41	60	4/132 (3.0%)	12/131 (9.2%)[a]
42	40	1/477 (0.2%)	4/482 (0.8%)
43	20	9/207 (4.3%)	10/216 (4.6%)
44	40	19/239 (7.9%)	22/212 (10.4%)
45	20	42/287 (14.6%)	40/288 (13.9%)
45	40	16/291 (5.5%)	40/288 (13.9%)

[a]Enoxaparin, 40-mg group.

III. CONCLUSION

The extensive knowledge of the epidemiology of VTE in surgical patients and a large amount of data supporting the use of pharmacological prophylaxis, have resulted in risk assessment models and clinical guidelines for safe and effective prophylaxis. Hitherto, the heterogeneity of the medical conditions and the lack of large, methodologically rigorous clinical trials has limited the application of prophylaxis to medical patients. The risk for venous thromboembolism is now adequately defined and thromboprophylaxis is recommended for specific medical patients. The results of a metanalysis evaluating all clinical trials conducted in medical patients [11] have confirmed that the risk of deep-vein thrombosis in medical patients is similar to that found in general surgery and lies between the moderate and high-risk groups [9]. Second, the use of pharmacological prophylaxis, either UFH or LMWH has clearly reduced the risk of deep-vein thrombosis by between 50 and 60% and the risk of clinical and fatal pulmonary embolism by about 50%, compared with placebo or no treatment. Unfractionated heparin and LMWH appear to be similar in efficacy, but the LMWHs are safer, with an approximately 50% reduction in the risk of major bleeding [11].

However, many questions remain to be answered. Given current evidence, the LMWHs appear to be equally effective, but are safer, and more practical (once-daily administration versus twice or three times daily) than UFH, and their use can be recommended in medical patients. However, each LMWH must be tested individually for every clinical indication. Clinical trials have evaluated three LMWHs—enoxaparin, nadroparin, and dalteparin—in medical patients, but owing to methodological limitations of some of the studies, the efficacy of all three drugs cannot be considered to be the same in all patient groups. In addition, the optimal doses of LMWH remain to be clarified. Doses commonly used in surgical patients have been tested, but the results have not been consistent; the results of the study with enoxaparin [45] provided important evidence that prophylactic doses that are effective in surgical patients may not be effective in medical patients. Finally, the optimal duration of treatment is unknown. Most studies were conducted over an average 10 days, based on the average inhospital stay. It is not known how long medical patients are at risk, although it is apparent that the risk is highest during the acute phase of the illness during initial hospitalization. However, patients confined to a nursing home or a chronic care facility also have an increased risk for VTE [6] and further studies are required in this setting.

Current recommendations for thrombosis prophylaxis in medical patients are summarized in the Sixth Consensus Conference of the American College of Chest Physicians on anti-thrombotic therapy and include low-dose UFH or LMWH [4].

REFERENCES

1. Alpert JS, Dalen JE. Epidemiology and natural history of venous thromboembolism. Prog Cardiovasc Dis 1994; 36:417–422.
2. Sandler DA, Martin JF. Autopsy proven pulmonary embolism in hospital patients: are we detecting enough deep vein thrombosis? J R Soc Med 1989; 82:203–205.
3. Anderson FA, Wheeler HB, Goldberg RJ, Hosmer DW, Patwardhan NA, Jovanovic B, Forcier A, Dalen JE. A population-based perspective of the hospital incidence and case–fatality rates of deep vein thrombosis and pulmonary embolism. The Worcester DVT study. Arch Intern Med 1991; 151:933–938.
4. Geerts WH, Heit JA, Clagett GP, Pineo GF, Colwell CW, Anderson FA Jr, Wheeler HB. Prevention of venous thromboembolism. Chest 2001; 119(supp.):1325–1755.

5. Agnelli G, Sonaglia F. Prevention of venous thromboembolism. Thromb Res 2000; 97:V49–V62.
6. Heit JA, Silverstein MD, Mohr DN, Petterson TM, O'Fallon M, Melton LJ III. Risk factors for deep vein thrombosis and pulmonary embolism. Arch Intern Med 2000; 160:809–815.
7. Thromboembolic Risk Factors (THRIFT) Consensus Group. Risk of and prophylaxis for venous thromboembolism in hospital patients. Br Med J 1992; 305:567–574.
8. Flordal PA, Bergqvist D, Burmark US, Ljungstrom KG, Torngren, for the Fragmin Multicentre Study Group. Risk factors for major thromboembolism and bleeding tendency after elective general surgical operations. Eur J Surg 1996; 162:783–789.
9. Gallus AS, Salzman EW, Hirsh J. Prevention of venous thromboembolism. In: Colman RW, Hirsh J, Marder VJ, Salzman EW, eds. Hemostasis and Thrombosis: Basic Principles and Clinical Practice. 3rd ed. Philadelphia: JB Lippincott, 1994; 1331–1345.
10. Kakkar VV, Corrigan TP, Fossard DP, Sutherland I, Shelton MG, Thirlwall J. Prevention of fatal postoperative pulmonary embolism by low doses of heparin. An International Multicentre Trial. Lancet 1975; 2:45–51.
11. Mismetti P, Laporte–Simitsidis S, Tardy B, Cucherat M, Buchmuller A, Juillard–Delsart D, Decousous H. Prevention of venous thromboembolism in internal medicine with unfractionated or low molecular weight heparins: a meta-analysis of randomised clinical trials. Thromb Haemost 2000; 83:14–19.
12. Antiplatelet Trialists Collaboration. Collaborative overview of randomized trials of antiplatelet therapy: III. Reduction in venous thrombosis and pulmonary embolism by antiplatelet prophylaxis among surgical and medical patients. Br Med J 1994; 308:1213–1215.
13. Gross JS, Neufeld RR, Libow LS, Gerber I, Rodstein M. Autopsy study of the elderly institutionalized patient. Review of 234 autopsies. Arch Intern Med 1988; 148:173–176.
14. Lindblad B, Sternby NH, Bergqvist D. Incidence of venous thromboembolism verified by necropsy over 30 years. Br Med J 1991; 302:709-711.
15. Handley AJ. Low dose heparin after myocardial infarction. Lancet 1972; 2:623–624.
16. Gallus AS, Hirsh J, Tuttle RJ, et al. Small subcutaneous doses of heparin in prevention of venous thrombosis. N Engl J Med 1973; 288:545–551.
17. Warlow C, Beattie AG, Terry G, Ogston D, Kenmure ACF, Douglas AF. A double blind trial of low doses of subcutaneous heparin in the prevention of deep vein thrombosis after myocardial infarction. Lancet 1973; 1:934–936.
18. Emerson PA, Marks P. Preventing thromboembolism after myocardial infarction: effect of low dose heparin or smoking. Br Med J 1977; 1:18–20.
19. Handley AJ, Emerson PA, Fleming PR. Heparin in the prevention of deep vein thrombosis after myocardial infarction. Br Med J 1972; 2:436–438.
20. Wray R, Maurer B, Shillingford J. Prophylactic anticoagulant therapy in the prevention of calf vein thrombosis after myocardial infarction. N Engl J Med 1973; 288:815–817.
21. McCarthy ST, Robertson D, Turner JJ, Hawkey CJ. Low dose heparin as a prophylaxis against deep vein thrombosis after acute stroke. Lancet 1977; 2:800–801.
22. McCarthy ST, Turner J. Low dose subcutaneous heparin in the prevention of deep vein thrombosis and pulmonary emboli following acute stroke. Age Ageing 1986,15:84–88.
23. Czechanowski B, Heinrich F. Prophylaxe venoeser Thrombosen bei frischem ischaemischen zerebro-vasculaeren Insult. Dtsch Med Wochenschr 1981; 106:1254–1260.
24. International Stroke Trial Collaborative Group. The International Stroke Trial (IST): a randomized trial of aspirin, subcutaneous heparin, both, or neither among 19,435 patients with acute ischemic stroke. Lancet 1997; 349:1569–1581.
25. Belch JJ, Lowe GDO, Ward AG, Forbes CD, Prentice CR. Prevention of deep vein thrombosis in medical patients by low dose heparin. Scott Med J 1981; 26:115–117.
26. Halkin H, Golberg J, Modan M, Modan B. Reduction in mortality in general medical in-patients by low dose heparin prophylaxis. Ann Intern Med 1982; 96:561–565.
27. Cade JF. High risk of the critically ill for venous thromboembolism. Crit Care Med 1982; 10:448–450.
28. Gardlund B, Heparin Prophylaxis Study Group. Randomised, controlled trial of low dose heparin for prevention of fatal pulmonary embolism in patients with infectious diseases. Lancet 1996; 347:1357–1361.

29. Hirsh J, Levine MN. Low molecular weight heparin. Blood 1992; 79:1–17.

30. Prins MH, Gelsema R, Sing AK, van Heerde LR, den Ottolander GJH. Prophylaxis of deep venous thrombosis with a low molecular weight heparin (Kabi 2165/ Fragmin) in stroke patients. Haemostasis 1989; 19:245–250.

31. Sandset PM, Dahl T, Stiris M, Rostad B, Scheel B, Abilgaard U. A double blind and randomized placebo controlled trial of low molecular weight heparin once daily to prevent deep vein thrombosis in acute ischemic stroke. Semin Thromb Haemost 1990; 16:25–33.

32. Turpie AGG, Levine MN, Hirsh J, Carter CJ, Jay RM, Powers PJ, Andrew M, Magnani HN, Hull RD, Gent M. A double-blind randomized trial of Org 10172 low molecular weight heparinoid in the prevention of deep vein thrombosis in patients with thrombotic stroke. Lancet 1987; 1:523–526.

33. Turpie AGG, Gent M, Cote R, Levine MN, Ginsberg JS, Powers PJ, Leclerc J, Geerts W, Jay R, Neemeh J, Klimek M, Hirsh J. A low molecular weight heparinoid compared with unfractionated heparin in the prevention of deep vein thrombosis in patients with acute ischemic stroke. Ann Intern Med 1992; 117:353–357.

34. Dumas R, Woitinas F, Kutnowski M, Nikolic I, Berberich R, Abedinpour F, Zoeckler S, Gregoire F, Jerkovic M, Egberts JFM, Stiekema JCJ. A multicenter, double-blind, randomized study to compare the safety and efficacy of once daily ORG 10172 and twice daily low-dose heparin in preventing deep vein thrombosis in patients with acute ischemic stroke. Age and Aging 1994; 23:512–516.

35. Poniewierki M, Barthels M, Kuhn M, Poliwoda H. Uber die Wirksamkeit niedermolekularen Heparins (Fragmin) in der Thromboembolieprophylaxe bei internistischen Patienten: eine randomisierte Doppelblindstudie. Med Klin 1988; 83:241–245.

36. Harenberg J, Kallenbach B, Martin U, Dempfle CE, Zimmermann R, Kubler W, Heene DL. Randomized controlled study of heparin and low molecular weight heparin for prevention of deep vein thrombosis in medical patients. Thromb Res 1990; 59:639–650.

37. Forette B, Wolmark Y. Calcium nadroparin in the prevention of thromboembolic disease in elderly subjects. Study of tolerance. Press Med 1995; 24:567–571.

38. Harenberg J, Roebruck P, Heene DL. Subcutaneous low molecular weight heparin versus standard heparin and the prevention of thromboembolism in medical inpatients. The Heparin Study in Internal Medicine (HESIM) Group. Haemostasis 1996; 26:127–139.

39. Manciet G, Vergnes C, Vaissié JJ, Boisseau MR. Etude de l'Efficacité et de la Tolérance de Fraxiparine Administrée au Long Cours Chez le Sujet Agé: Étude Randomisée de Double Insu (APTE). Bounameaux H, Samama MM, Ten Cate JW, eds. New York: Schattauer, 1990; 55–59.

40. Bergmann JF, Caulin C. Heparin prophylaxis in bedridden patients. Lancet 1996; 348–205–206.

41. Dahan R, Houlbert D, Caulin C, Cuzin E, Viltart C, Woler M, Segrestaa JM. Prevention of deep vein thrombosis in elderly medical in-patients by a low molecular weight heparin: a randomized double blind trial. Haemostasis 1986; 16:159–164.

42. Lechler E, Schramm W, Flosbach CW. The venous thrombotic risk in non-surgical patients: epidemiological data and efficacy/safety profile of a low molecular weight heparin (enoxaparin). Haemostasis 1996; 26(suppl 2):49–56.

43. Bergmann JF, Neuhart E. A multicenter randomized double blind study of enoxaparin compared with unfractionated heparin in the prevention of venous thromboembolic disease in elderly in-patients bedridden for an acute medical illness. Thromb Haemost 1996; 76:529–534.

44. Kleber FX, Witt C, Flosbach CW, Koppenhagen K, Vogel G, PRINCE Study Group. Study to compare the efficacy and safety of the LMWH enoxaparin and standard heparin in the prevention of thromboembolic events in medical patients with cardiopulmonary diseases. Ann Hematol 1998; 76(suppl 1):P261.

45. Samama MM, Cohen AT, Darmon JY, Desjardins L, Eldor A, Janbon C, Leizorovicz A, Nguyen H, Olsson CG, Turpie AG, Weisslinger N, Prophylaxis in Medical Patients with Enoxaparin Study Group. A comparison of enoxaparin with placebo for the prevention of venous thromboembolism in acutely ill medical patients. N Engl J Med 1999; 341:793–800.

9

Low-Molecular-Weight Heparins in Prevention and Treatment of Venous Thromboembolism

Richard M. Jay and William H. Geerts
University of Toronto, Toronto, Ontario, Canada

SUMMARY

The low-molecular-weight heparins (LMWHs) were initially developed and evaluated as antithrombotic agents for the prevention of venous thromboembolism (VTE). More than 25 years later, these drugs are still the most extensively studied class of anticoagulants [1–3]. Demonstration of the efficacy of the LMWHs has transformed the prevention and treatment of thromboembolic disorders. There is now substantial evidence that LMWHs are as effective as unfractionated heparin (UFH) in the prevention of VTE in moderate-risk surgical and medical patients, and is more effective than heparin or warfarin in high-risk surgical groups, including major orthopedic surgery and multiple trauma patients. The most dramatic clinical impact of LMWHs has been on the initial treatment of VTE. Numerous clinical trials and subsequent metanalyses have clearly demonstrated that LMWHs are an effective and safe alternative to UFH for treatment of deep-vein thrombosis. Further clinical trials have demonstrated the feasibility and safety of LMWHs for the outpatient management of VTE, and several cost-effectiveness analyses have indicated the potential for substantial financial savings for the health care system. These findings have revolutionized the initial management of VTE. In many countries, outpatient LMWH is now the treatment of choice for most patients with acute VTE. Recent clinical trials have explored the use of LMWHs for the long-term treatment of VTE as an alternative to oral anticoagulants.

I. LMWHs AS THROMBOPROPHYLAXIS AGENTS

A. Introduction

Over the past three decades, a vast amount of research has helped to establish the risks of VTE in various groups of hospitalized patients (Table 1). It is now recognized that deep vein thrombosis (DVT) is very common in a large proportion of patients, whereas pulmonary embolism is the most common preventable cause of hospital death. The routine use of thromboprophylaxis for

Table 1 Deep-Vein Thrombosis in Hospitalized Patients

Risk group	DVT prevalence[a] (%)
Medical patients	10–20
Major gynecological surgery	15–40
Major urological surgery	15–40
Neurosurgery	15–40
Major general surgery	20–40
Isolated lower extremity fracture	20–45
Stroke	20–50
Critical care patients	15–80
Hip fracture surgery	40–60
Hip or knee arthroplasty	40–70
Major trauma	40–80
Spinal cord injury	60–80

[a]DVT rates in patients not receiving thromboprophylaxis and who were screened using routine, objective surveillance methods (generally with fibrinogen leg scanning or contrast venography).

patients at moderate and high risk has repeatedly been shown to reduce thromboembolic complications [4–8]. Prophylaxis, therefore, provides clinicians with an opportunity to both improve patient outcomes and reduce costs.

The biological properties of LMWH, discussed elsewhere in this book, result in several clinical advantages over other antithrombotic agents (Table 2). There is strong evidence that the LMWHs are highly efficacious and safe in a wide variety of patient groups, and they are simple to use. Furthermore, numerous economic evaluations support the use of LMWHs, at least in moderate and high-risk patients [9–15].

B. General Surgery, Gynecology, and Major Urology

With fibrinogen leg scanning as the screening modality, the risk of DVT in unprophylaxed general surgery patients has been 15–40%, with an average of 25%. [8]. Low-dose unfractionated heparin (LDUH) and LMWH have each been formally evaluated in more than 10,000 patients, and both agents reduce the risk of DVT by approximately 70%, compared with no prophylaxis, in a wide spectrum of general surgery, gynecology, and urology patient groups [8]. Both LDUH and LMWH also reduce fatal pulmonary embolism and all-cause mortality in surgical patients [16,17]. There is evidence that the incidence of wound-related bleeding is

Table 2 Clinical Advantages of Low-Molecular-Weight-Heparins

1. Highly efficacious in the prevention of venous thromboembolism
2. Low risk of bleeding
3. Lower risk of heparin-induced thrombocytopenia than heparin
4. Fixed dose
5. Preloaded syringes
6. Once- or twice-daily dosing } Highly convenient
7. Postoperative initiation
8. No laboratory monitoring

increased with use of anticoagulant prophylaxis, although rates of major bleeding are not [16,18].

Selection of a thromboprophylaxis method for general surgery patients essentially involves a choice between LDUH and LMWH. For both anticoagulants, efficacy and bleeding are dose-related. [18–20]. The potential advantages of LMWH over LDUH in general surgery include once-daily dosing and reduced risk of heparin-induced thrombocytopenia, while the chief disadvantage is greater cost, at least in North America. Metanalyses of studies, in which LDUH and LMWH have been directly compared, demonstrate no significant differences in either efficacy or bleeding. [8,21–24]. Furthermore, recent individual large trials in a spectrum of general surgical patients also show no differences in efficacy or safety when LDUH and LMWH are both included in the same study. [25–30].

Patients undergoing major gynecological or urological procedures have a thrombosis risk comparable with that seen in general surgery [31–34]. Surgery for genitourinary malignancy is associated with an important risk for symptomatic VTE, and the routine use of thrombo-prophylaxis is warranted. Unfortunately, there are no methodologically rigorous clinical trials in gynecological or urological surgery in which LMWHs have been assessed using accurate screening tests for DVT. However, the available indirect evidence suggests that LDUH and LMWH would be expected to have similar effects in these patients as in general surgery [8,35].

C. Hip and Knee Arthroplasty and Hip Fracture

Hip and knee arthroplasty patients and those having surgery to repair hip fractures have high risks for VTE, with DVT rates of 45–70%, proximal DVT rates of 10–30%, and fatal pulmonary embolism (PE) rates of 0.1–5%, without prophylaxis [8]. Routine use of thromboprophylaxis, therefore, is recommended for these three patient groups [4–8].

Low-molecular-weight heparins are the most extensively studied prophylaxis interventions in major orthopedic surgery, with more than 45-randomized trials involving over 11,000 patients [8]. Compared with no prophylaxis, LMWH use is associated with a 44–78% relative risk reduction in DVT rates following hip and knee arthroplasty or hip fracture surgery [8]. LMWH, at doses approximately twice that used in general surgery trials, is more efficacious than LDUH in hip and knee arthroplasty without increased bleeding [8,21,22,36]. The most relevant alternative to LMWH in these patients is oral anticoagulation with warfarin. When the results of the five studies in which patients with hip replacement were randomized to LMWH, or warfarin were pooled, the DVT rates were 14 and 21%, respectively, whereas the pooled proximal DVT rates were 3 and 5%, respectively [37–41]. These studies, therefore, demonstrate that LMWH is more efficacious than warfarin in total hip replacement (THR) using asymptomatic venographic DVT outcomes. However, a recent randomized 3000-patient trial of these two interventions found no difference in the rates of symptomatic VTE [36].

In patients undergoing orthopedic surgery, LMWH prophylaxis has traditionally commenced before surgery in European studies and clinical practice, whereas, in North America, postoperative initiation has been the norm. This controversy was recently resolved by a large randomized trial in which hip replacement patients were allocated to dalteparin, 2500 U, starting about 1 h before surgery, with a second dose given about 7 h after surgery, followed by 5000 U once daily, or to dalteparin 5000 U started about 7 h postoperatively and then once daily [41]. There were slightly fewer DVT when the LMWH was started preoperatively (10.7 vs. 13.1%), whereas there was also a trend toward more bleeding in the group that started dalteparin before surgery. Another controversial issue is the relative benefits and safety of different LMWHs. Planes et al. have conducted two trials in which hip arthroplasty patients were randomized to either enoxaparin or reviparin in one trial and either enoxaparin or tinzaparin in the other [42,43].

These studies demonstrate that the differences in outcomes between LMWHs are comparable with the differences for the same LMWH used in different trials in the same types of patients.

In contrast to patients undergoing hip arthroplasty, knee replacement patients have an even greater risk of DVT. The prophylaxis interventions which are so efficacious in hip surgery are much less efficacious following knee replacement, and bleeding is potentially a more significant problem. In knee arthroplasty, LMWH and warfarin are again the most extensively evaluated prophylaxis modalities with relative risk reductions compared with no prophylaxis of 52 and 27%, respectively [8]. Mechanical prophylaxis also appears to be protective in these patients although there are only a few small trials and, in the only direct comparison of LMWH and the venous foot pump, LMWH provided significantly greater protection [44]. There have been six randomized trials, including a total of 2300 patients, that have directly compared LMWH and warfarin in knee arthroplasty [37–39,45–47] When the results of these trials are pooled, the DVT and proximal DVT rates for patients receiving LMWH and warfarin are 32 vs. 47% and 7 vs. 10%, respectively. Therefore, LMWH is more efficacious than warfarin in knee arthroplasty using venographic DVT as the primary outcome. There are no comparative studies using symptomatic events as the outcome.

Unfortunately, there are few high-quality prophylaxis trials in patients with hip fractures, and there are no large studies of LMWH use. Although one study found a trend toward greater efficacy without more bleeding when patients with a hip fracture received enoxaparin 40 mg daily rather than 20 mg, only 103 patients were randomized [48]. Another trial observed similar rates of DVT when LDUH or LMWH were administered [49]. The most relevant prophylaxis methods in patients with hip fractures are LDUH, LMWH, and adjusted-dose warfarin. There is insufficient evidence to definitively recommend one of these modalities over the others.

Over the past decade, there has been a progressive reduction in length of hospital stay for patients undergoing major orthopedic surgery. It is now common for patients to be discharged home or to a rehabilitation unit 4–6 days after surgery. Most published studies of thromboprophylaxis in these patient groups have provided 10–14 days of prophylaxis, commensurate with the more prolonged hospital stays when these trials were conducted. Several recent randomized trials have assessed the optimal length of prophylaxis with LMWH following hip replacement. All of these studies have had a similar design; namely, a comparison of inhospital prophylaxis (with LMWH in five trials and warfarin in the sixth) to postdischarge LMWH prophylaxis for an additional 4 weeks and using routine venography at about 5 weeks in both groups. When the results of these six trials are pooled, the DVT rates in the inhospital and postdischarge LMWH prophylaxis groups were 28 and 14%, respectively, a 50% relative risk reduction associated with extended prophylaxis [50–55]. Proximal DVT rates were 12 and 4%, respectively, a 67% risk reduction. In the one study that assessed symptomatic, objectively confirmed thromboembolic events, these outcomes were encountered in ten patients given inhospital prophylaxis (7.6%) and in two patients who received postdischarge prophylaxis (1.5%) [50]. These data provide compelling evidence to continue thromboprophylaxis following major orthopedic surgery for at least 10 days (and perhaps even up to 1 month).

D. Major Trauma or Spinal Cord Injury

Among hospital patient groups, major trauma patients have the highest risk of VTE [8,56]. Despite this, there are few methodologically rigorous prophylaxis trials in these patients. We have conducted a double-blind, randomized trial comparing heparin 5000 U b.i.d with enoxaparin 30 mg b.i.d. in 344 major trauma patients [57]. The prophylaxis interventions commenced an average of 30 h after injury, and patients underwent routine contrast venography 10–14 days later. Compared with the predicted rates for patients not receiving any prophylaxis, LDUH reduced the rates of DVT and proximal DVT by only 19 and 14%, respectively. LMWH further decreased the DVT and proximal DVT rates by 30 and 58%, respectively, compared with LDUH. There were no significant differences in any of the bleeding parameters in the trial, although there was a trend toward more bleeding in the patients who received LMWH. Other studies have repeatedly demonstrated the poor efficacy of mechanical prophylaxis methods in these high-risk patients, even though they are widely used. There are no direct comparisons of LMWH with mechanical prophylaxis in trauma.

Without prophylaxis, the overwhelming majority of patients with acute spinal cord injury develop DVT, and pulmonary embolism is one of the most common causes of death in this condition [58]. Low-dose heparin is not efficacious in these patients, whereas there is some evidence that LMWH is protective [59,60].

Given the high thrombosis risk in major trauma and spinal cord injury patients, we feel that prophylaxis should be used in all of these patients. LMWH appears to be the prophylaxis of choice since it is the simplest, most efficacious option for most patients. The LMWH should commence as early as the bleeding risk allows, usually within 36 h after injury. In the presence of intracranial bleeding or active bleeding at other sites, mechanical prophylaxis with either graduated compression stockings or intermittent pneumatic compression devices, or both, should be considered until it is safe to use LMWH.

Patients with isolated lower extremity injuries appear to have a DVT risk of 20–45% [8,61]. Two studies from Germany randomized outpatients with plaster casts for lower extremity injuries to no prophylaxis or a LMWH during the period of cast therapy [62,63]. Using routine duplex ultrasonography at the time of cast removal, significant protection by the LMWH was demonstrated in both trials. No clinically important bleeding event was found in the 350 patients who received LMWH.

E. Neurosurgery

A 15–40% risk of thromboembolism following major neurosurgical procedures warrants the use of prophylaxis in these patients. Fear of the potential for intracranial bleeding has prompted several small studies of mechanical methods of prophylaxis [8]. LMWH has also been evaluated in these patients. Three randomized trials have compared graduated compression stockings alone with the combination of stockings and LMWH using contrast venography as the primary efficacy outcome [64–67]. When these trials are pooled, the DVT rates in the patients given stockings alone and those who received stockings plus LMWH were 28 and 18%, respectively, a 38% risk reduction favoring the combined therapy. However, when LMWH is given before craniotomy, increased intracranial bleeding is observed [68]. No studies have compared LMWH with LDUH or with intermittent pneumatic compression devices in neurosurgery. If LMWH is used in these patients, it should probably commence no sooner than 12–24 h after surgery to allow time for primary hemostasis to occur.

F. Medical Patients

Deep-vein thrombosis prevention has been studied to a much lesser extent in medical groups than in surgical populations. However, it is clear that medical patients with additional risk factors for thromboembolism, including active cancer, paralysis, immobilization, heart or respiratory failure, or inflammatory bowel disease, have at least a moderate risk for DVT. For example, DVT is seen in 20–50% of patients who are recovering from an acute ischemic stroke, with the overwhelming majority occurring in the paretic or dysfunctional limb. Low-dose heparin, LMWH, and the low molecular weight heparinoid, danaparoid, are each efficacious in the prevention of DVT in stroke patients, although LMWH and danaparoid appear to be more efficacious than LDUH [8].

A recent metanalysis of thromboprophylaxis in medical patients included seven trials, with a total sample of more than 15,000 patients [69]. The use of LDUH or LMWH reduced the risk of DVT or PE by more than 50% compared with no prophylaxis. When the effects of LDUH were compared with LMWH, there were no significant differences in thromboembolic outcomes or mortality, but bleeding was less common in the LMWH patients. The MEDENOX trial randomized 1102 medical patients, older than age 40, to placebo or to two different doses of enoxaparin for 6–14 days [70]. Enoxaparin 20-mg daily was no better than control, but 40-mg daily was associated with a 63% risk reduction for venographic DVT and no significant increase in bleeding.

G. Critical Care Patients

Virtually every medical and surgical patient in a critical care unit has at least one risk factor for VTE and most have multiple factors. The DVT rates in critical care patients are generally in the moderate- or high-risk categories, certainly high enough to warrant the routine use of thromboprophylaxis [8]. Only one study has evaluated LMWH in critical care [71]. In this trial, patients requiring mechanical ventilation for exacerbations of chronic obstructive pulmonary disease received either placebo or nadroparin and then underwent venography. DVT was detected in 28% of the patients given placebo and 16% of those who received the LMWH (p = 0.045). Bleeding was not significantly increased in the nadroparin group.

H. Summary of Prophylaxis Recommendations

The LMWHs are the most effective thromboprophylactic agents currently available. Among moderate-risk surgical or medical patients, it appears that LDUH and LMWH have approximately equal efficacy and safety, and either of these prophylactic agents is recommended (Table 3). Among high-risk groups, including major orthopedic surgery and trauma patients, LMWH is more efficacious than LDUH or warfarin. Prophylaxis with LMWH is recommended in these patients. Warfarin is an acceptable alternative in high-risk orthopedic patients on the basis of low rates of symptomatic thromboembolic events following hip arthroplasty. The future clinical role of newer antithrombotic agents such as recombinant hirudin, pentasaccharide, and oral direct thrombin inhibitors is uncertain, for they must now demonstrate significantly greater efficacy or safety and improved cost-effectiveness when compared with LMWH. At the same time, there are still a number of unresolved issues related to the use of the LMWHs in the prevention of venous thromboembolism (Table 4).

II. LMWHS IN THE TREATMENT OF VTE

The objectives of anticoagulant therapy in patients with VTE are:

To prevent further extension of local thrombus
To prevent morbidity and mortality from PE [72]
To prevent recurrent thrombosis [73–75]
To minimize the development of the postphlebitic syndrome

The traditional initial treatment for acute VTE involves inhospital administration of continuous intravenous UFH for 5–7 days, followed by long-term secondary prophylaxis with

Table 3 Summary of Prophylaxis Recommendations

Patient group	Subgroups	Recommended prophylaxis options
General surgery Major gynecology surgery	Usual risk	Heparin 5000 U q12h LMWH<4000 U/24h
Major urology surgery	High-risk (previous VTE, extensive surgery for cancer especially in elderly)	Heparin 5000 U q8h LMWH ≥ 4000 U/24h LDUH or LMWH + mechanical prophylaxis with GCS or IPC
Major orthopedic surgery	Hip arthroplasty Knee arthroplasty Hip fracture repair	LMWH Warfarin (INR 2–3)
Major trauma	Multiple injuries Lower extremity fractures Spinal cord injuries	LWMH when hemostasis has been demonstrated Mechanical prophylaxis initially in patients with intracranial or other active bleeding
Neurosurgery	Craniotomy	Postoperative LDUH or LMWH Perioperative IPC
Medical patients	With additional risk factors such as paresis, cancer, stroke, heart, or respiratory failure, prolonged bed rest	LDUH LMWH
Critical care patients	Low bleeding risk; moderate thrombosis risk	LDUH
	Low bleeding risk; high thrombosis risk	LMWH
	High bleeding risk; moderate thrombosis risk	Mechanical prophylaxis initially followed by LDUH when bleeding risk is down
	High bleeding risk; high thrombosis risk	Mechanical prophylaxis initially, followed by LMWH when bleeding risk is down

GCS, graduated compression (elastic) stockings; IPC, intermittent pneumatic compression devices; LDUH, low dose unfractionated heparin; LMWH, low-molecular-weight heparin; VTE, venous thromboembolism.

oral anticoagulants for at least 3–6 months to prevent recurrences [73,75,76]. Hospitalization has been required both to administer intravenous heparin and to facilitate frequent laboratory monitoring and dose adjustments of the anticoagulants. Laboratory monitoring and heparin dose adjustments are necessary because of the marked variability in anticoagulant response among patients with VTE and from day to day in the same patient as well as to reduce the potential risks of bleeding or further thrombosis resulting from excessive or inadequate initial anticoagulation. [77–79].

Over the last 25 years, LMWHs have undergone preclinical studies that demonstrated several distinct advantages over UFH, the most important being the following:

Superior bioavailability by subcutaneous injection, which allows therapeutic anticoagulation by the subcutaneous route

Dose-independent clearance and longer half-life, which allows therapeutic anticoagulation to be given as a once-daily or twice-daily dose

Table 4 Some Unresolved Issues in the Prevention of Venous Thromboembolism with Low-Molecular-Weight Heparins

---

Quantitation of the various mechanisms of antithrombotic action of LMWH
Development of a method to standardize the various LMWHs relative to dosing
Effect of LMWHs on clinically important venous thromboembolism
Preoperative vs. postoperative initiation of prophylaxis in moderate-risk patients
Optimal doses of LMWHs in various patient groups
Optimal dosing in very low-weight and markedly overweight patients
Predictors of failed prophylaxis and bleeding with LMWH
Optimal duration of prophylaxis in moderate- and high-risk patients, especially in orthopedic surgery,
    trauma, and patients with cancer
Cost-effectiveness of prolonged prophylaxis in high-risk patients
Comparisons between LDUH and LMWH in medical patients
Comparisons between various LMWHs in different patient groups
Role of LMWHs as primary prophylaxis in certain malignancies
Role of LMWHs in gynecological oncology and urological oncology
Role of LMWHs in laparoscopic surgery
Role of LMWHs in hip fracture surgery
Role of LMWHs in major trauma and spinal cord injury
Role of LMWHs in isolated lower extremity fractures
Role of LMWHs in critical care patients

Predictable anticoagulant dose–response which eliminates the need for laboratory monitoring

Other clinically relevant advantages of LMWH include a low-bleeding potential [80], reduced risk of heparin-induced thrombocytopenia [81], and decreased effects on bone metabolism [82,83].

A. Efficacy and Safety of LMWH for Treatment of Acute VTE

1. Venographic Endpoints

In early clinical trials, comparing LMWHs given by subcutaneous or intravenous injection to continuous intravenous UFH for the treatment of established DVT, the change in size of the thrombus by repeat venography after 5–10 days of treatment was used as the outcome measure [84–92]. Metanalyses of these radiological endpoint studies demonstrate that LMWHs prevented further thrombus extension and increased thrombus resolution more effectively than UFH [93,94]. A reduction in thrombus size was demonstrated in 65% of LMWH-treated patients compared with 52% of UFH-treated patients, and an increase in thrombus size was found in only 5.6% of LMWH patients compared with 10.3% of UFH patients (p<0.001) [93].

A metanalysis performed by the Cochrane Collaboration included more recent venographic endpoint studies and confirmed the earlier observations. Reduction in thrombus size was demonstrated in 60% of LMWH patients compared with 54% of UFH patients (odds ratio 0.77, 95% confidence intervals [CI]; 0.61–0.97) [94].

2. Clinical Endpoints

Multiple large, randomised, controlled trials have prospectively assessed clinical endpoints including recurrent VTE, major bleeding, and death. Several of these trials have addressed other issues, including outpatient treatment of VTE, treatment of pulmonary embolism, and the frequency of drug administration (once-daily vs. twice-daily subcutaneous injections). Several metanalyses have pooled the results of these studies to assess the efficacy and safety of LMWH therapy [93–98]. The Cochrane Collaboration metanalysis included 14 randomized trials, published between 1988 and 1998 with a total of 4754 patients [94]. In all of the trials, VTE and recurrent VTE were diagnosed by objective testing. One trial included only patients with PE [99]. Fixed-dose subcutaneous LMWH, given once daily [99–103] or twice daily [86,90–92,04–108] was compared with adjusted dose intravenous [90,92,99–108] or subcutaneous [86,91] unfractionated heparin. No individual trial demonstrated a statistically significant reduction in the risk of recurrent VTE with LMWH, and only one study demonstrated a significant reduction in major bleeding and mortality with LMWH treatment [100].

B. Results of the Cochrane Metanalysis (Table 5)

1. Recurrent Venous Thromboembolism

In the Cochrane Collaboration metanalysis, the incidence of recurrent VTE was assessed during the initial treatment period and for variable periods of follow-up (3–6 months). Combining the ten trials with long-term follow-up, symptomatic recurrent thromboembolic events occurred in 4.3% (86/1998) LMWH-treated patients, compared with 5.6% (113/2021) UFH patients (odds ratio 0.76: 95% CI; 0.57–1.01). This represents a statistically nonsignificant reduction in favor of LMWH. There was also no significant difference in recurrent venous thromboembolic events in patients with PE (odds ratio 0.91; 95% CI; 0.42–1.97).

2. Major Bleeding

All 14 trials assessed the incidence of major bleeding during the initial treatment period. Analysis of the pooled data demonstrated a statistically significant reduction in major bleeding events in favor of LMWH. At the end of the initial treatment period, 1.3% (30/2353) LMWH patients compared with 2.1% (51/2401) UFH patients had suffered a major bleed (odds ratio 0.60: 95% CI; 0.39–0.93).

3. Mortality

Overall mortality was assessed prospectively in 11 studies. A statistically significant reduction in overall mortality was observed in favor of LMWH. By the end of the follow-up period, 6.4%

Table 5 Metanalysis Comparing LMWH with UFH for VTE Treatment: The Cochrane Systematic Review (Studies that included all patients with VTE)[a]

Outcomes	LMWH (%)	UFH (%)	Odds ratio (95% CI)
Recurrent VTE	4.3	5.6	0.76 (0.57–1.01)
Major bleeding	1.3	2.1	0.60 (0.39–0.93)
Death	6.4	8.0	0.78 (0.62–0.99)
Death (cancer patients)	14.0	24.0	0.53 (0.33–0.85)

[a]Fourteen randomized trials including 4754 patients.
Source: Ref. 94.

(135/2108) LMWH patients had died compared with 8.0% (172/2137) unfractionated heparin patients (odds ratio 0.78: 95% CI;. 0.62–0.99).

4. Mortality in Cancer Patients

Six of the trials [91,99–101,104,107] assessed the mortality rates in patients with cancer. Pooled data from these studies demonstrated a statistically significant reduction in mortality in the cancer patients treated with LMWH. By the end of follow-up, 14% (31/221) LMWH patients compared with 24% (54/225) UFH patients had died (odds ratio 0.53: 95% CI; 0.33–0.85). In these trials, there was no significant difference in mortality among patients without cancer. By the end of follow-up, 3.2% (35/1066) LMWH patients compared with 3.3% (36/1073) UFH patients had died (odds ratio 0.97, 95% CI; 0.61–1.56).

5. Proximal DVT (Table 6)

Five studies included only patients with proximal DVT [92,100,104–106]. They involved 1636 patients, of whom 814 were treated with LMWH and 822 were treated with UFH. At the end of the follow-up period, 4.8% (39/814) LMWH patients had suffered a symptomatic recurrent venous thromboembolic event, compared with 7.8% (64/822) UFH patients (odds ratio 0.60 in favor of LMWH: 95% CI; 0.40–0.89). There was also a significant reduction in major bleeding in favor of LMWH. At the end of the initial treatment period, 1.0% (8/814) LMWH patients compared with 2.3% (19/822) UFH patients had suffered a major bleeding event (odds ratio 0.44: 95% CI; 0.21–0.95). By the end of the follow-up period 5.4% (44/814) LMWH patients had died compared with 8.3% (68/822) UFH patients (odds ratio 0.64: 95% CI; 0.43–0.93).

The metanalysis of these 14 studies demonstrates improved efficacy with LMWH treatment as well as statistically significant reductions in major bleeding events and overall mortality. Among patients with malignancy treated with LMWH, there was a highly significant reduction in mortality compared with UFH-treated patients. In those studies for which proximal DVT was the primary reason for treatment, LMWH clearly demonstrates superior safety, efficacy, and reduction in overall mortality.

C. TREATMENT OF PULMONARY EMBOLISM

Four clinical trials have addressed the treatment of submassive pulmonary embolism with LMWH [99,107,109,110].

Meyer et al. randomized 60 patients with pulmonary embolism to receive continuous intravenous UFH or LMWH (dalteparin). No recurrence of PE or major bleeding was observed

Table 6 Metanalysis Comparing LMWH with UFH for VTE Treatment: The Cochrane Systematic Review (Studies that included only patients with proximal DVT)[a]

Outcomes	LMWH (%)	UFH (%)	Odds ratio (95% CI)
Recurrent VTE	4.8	7.8	0.60 (0.40–0.89)
Major bleed	1.0	2.3	0.44 (0.21–0.95)
Death	5.4	8.3	0.64 (0.43–0.93)

[a]Five randomized trials including 1636 patients.
Source: Ref. 94.

in either group during the initial therapy or the 3-month follow-up period [109]. In the Columbus trial, 1021 patients with VTE were treated with either UFH or LMWH (reviparin) [107]. Twenty-six percent of the study population presented with PE. Symptomatic recurrent VTE occurred in 6.0% of the UFH and 5.8% of the LMWH patients. The THESEE Study Group randomized 612 patients with symptomatic PE to tinzaparin or adjusted-dose heparin [99]. At the end of the initial 8-day treatment period, 2.9% of the UFH patients, compared with 3.0% of the LMWH patients, had suffered at least one of the clinical endpoints (recurrent thromboembolism, major bleeding, or mortality). At the end of the 90-day follow-up period, 7.1% of UFH patient and 5.9% of LMWH patients had reached at least one of the endpoints ($p = 0.54$). The risks of major bleeding were similar in both treatment groups. Finally, the American–Canadian Thrombosis Study Group compared subcutaneous tinzaparin with adjusted-dose intravenous heparin for the treatment of patients with proximal DVT and PE [110]. Recurrent episodes of VTE occurred in 6.8% (7/103) UFH patients compared with 0/97 LMWH patients ($p = 0.009$). Major bleeding during the initial treatment period was seen in 1.9% (2/103) UFH patients compared with 1.0% (1/97) LMWH patients. Mortality at 3 months occurred in 8.7% (9/103) UFH patients compared with 6.2% (6/97) LMWH patients.

These studies consistently demonstrate that fixed-dose body-weight-determined subcutaneous LMWH is as effective and safe as adjusted-dose heparin for the initial management of submassive PE. No clinical studies have yet addressed the use of LMWH for treatment of patients with massive PE who are hemodynamically unstable.

D. Outpatient Treatment of VTE

Many clinical trials and metanalyses of these trials [93–98] have demonstrated that body-weight-determined, unadjusted, subcutaneous LMWH is at least as efficacious and safe as standard adjusted-dose intravenous UFH for the treatment of VTE in a hospital setting. The effectiveness and simplicity of LMWH therapy provides the potential for outpatient treatment of a high proportion of patients with symptomatic VTE [105–107,111].

Lindmarker and Holstrom evaluated the safety and feasibility of treating acute DVT in an outpatient setting using dalteparin [111]. Of the 434 patients, 80% were treated as outpatients for at least part of their initial treatment period (35% were discharged home within the first 24 h to continue treatment on an outpatient basis).The overall incidence of serious complications was 0.92% (three pulmonary emboli, one major bleed) during the initial LMWH treatment period. During the 3-month follow-up period, three additional recurrent DVTs and one PE occurred while patients were taking oral anticoagulants. Therefore, 7 of 434 patients (1.6%) developed recurrent VTE during the 3-month study period while receiving anticoagulant therapy. The Columbus study allowed patients with venous thrombosis who were assigned to the LMWH group to be treated as outpatients at the discretion of the treating physician [107]. One hundred patients (27%) were treated entirely as outpatients and another 56 (15%) were discharged within the first 3 days to continue treatment at home. Although the results for this subgroup were not separately reported, the entire LMWH treatment group showed no significant increases in recurrent VTE, major bleeding, or mortality, when compared with the UFH treatment group. Two large multicenter randomized studies have demonstrated the potential feasibility, safety, and effectiveness of outpatient LMWH as the initial treatment of selected patients with acute proximal DVT [105,106]. Each study compared intravenous heparin administered in hospital with subcutaneous LMWH (nadroparin or enoxaparin) administered primarily at home. Each study allowed outpatients to go home immediately with LMWH, whereas hospitalized patients could be discharged home early with LMWH. Both studies demonstrated similar rates of recurrent VTE, major bleeding and death between inhospital UFH and outpatient LMWH groups

(Table 7). If these studies are pooled, the main outcomes for the 451 intravenous heparin patients and the 449 LMWH patients are, respectively, 7.5 and 6.0% for recurrent VTE, 1.6 and 1.3% for major bleeding, and 7.3 and 5.6% for death. With the potential for outpatient treatment using LMWH, a substantial number of patients did not require hospital admission and could be treated entirely at home (36% in the Koopman study [105], 49% in the Levine study [106]). The mean duration of hospital stay was only 2.7 days in the Koopman study and 1.1 days in the Levine study in patients treated with LMWH.

The consistent results of these two trials as well as the extensive experience in numerous centers indicate that outpatient treatment of proximal venous thrombosis is feasible and is as effective and as safe as inhospital heparin therapy.

1. Effect on Clinical Practice

These trials have prompted many clinicians to consider the use of outpatient LMWH as treatment for VTE outside the structured framework of an well-organized clinical study carried out by expert thrombosis physicians [112–115].

A study by Wells et al. [112] demonstrated that 83% of 233 patients with DVT or submassive PE were treated as outpatients with LMWH. Of these, 95% were treated entirely at home. Two models of patient care delivery were assessed: daily drug administration by home visit nurses and patient or family member administration. The incidence of recurrent VTE and bleeding were comparable with the results obtained from major clinical trials [105,106]: VTE recurrence 3.6%, major bleeds 2%, and deaths 7%. There were no differences between the two care-delivery models relative to these outcome measures. A prospective study to assess the quality of life and patient compliance aspects of outpatient treatment demonstrated that 79% of 113 patients with VTE could be treated as outpatients [113]. Of these, 75% were able to manage self-injection or have a family member administer the injections. More than 90% were satisfied with treatment at home and the support provided by the supervising thrombosis center. Two recent studies have also assessed the use of LMWH as outpatient treatment of upper extremity venous thrombosis [114] and submassive PE [115]. In a prospective cohort study, 46 patients (75% had cancer and 35% had a central venous catheter) with upper extremity DVT were treated with an initial course of therapeutic dalteparin for 5–7 days with subsequent long-term warfarin therapy in 40 patients [114]. Treatment with LMWH was continued in 6 patients (10 days to 3 months) because of persistent symptoms or patient preference. While receiving LMWH therapy, there were no episodes of PE or bleeding, although one patient had extension of existing DVT. The prospective cohort study by Kovacs et al. evaluated the management of 158 patients, who

Table 7 LMWH in Outpatient Treatment of DVT

| | Koopman[a] | | Levine[b] | |
| | No. of patients (%) | | | |
	LMWH	UFH	LMWH	UFH
No. of patients	202	198	247	253
Not admitted	72 (36%)		120 (49%)	
Mean length of hospital stay (days)	2.7	8.1	1.1	6.5
Recurrent VTE	14 (6.9%)	17 (8.6%)	13 (5.3%)	17 (6.7%)
Major bleed	1 (0.5%)	4 (2.0%)	5 (2.0%)	3 (1.2%)
Death	14 (6.9%)	16 (8.1%)	11 (4.5%)	17 (6.7%)

Source: Ref. [a]105; [b]106.

had hemodynamically stable PE, on an outpatient basis with dalteparin [115]. Sixty-eight percent were managed as outpatients, and 75% of these patients were managed entirely as outpatients. The overall outcomes, symptomatic VTE recurrence (5.6%), major bleeding (1.9%), and deaths (4.9%—none by PE or bleeding), suggest that outpatient treatment of selected patients with submassive PE is safe, effective and feasible.

These studies demonstrate the feasibility of home treatment of VTE, including upper extremity thrombosis and submassive PE, in a large proportion of patients. Most of these patients are capable of self-injection. However, careful medical supervision to teach and support home therapy and to monitor the conversion of initial LMWH therapy to ongoing oral anticoagulant is a mandatory requirement.

2. Cost Effectiveness of LMWH Treatment

Because LMWH treatment of VTE has been demonstrated to be at least equivalent to UFH in safety and effectiveness, both for inpatient and outpatient use, the question of relative cost differences between LMWH and UFH therapy has been explored [111,116–119].

Lindmarker demonstrated a 35% potential reduction in treatment costs between outpatient dalteparin therapy and traditional inhospital heparin treatment by using a hypothetical model based on the result of their clinical trial and cost calculations at two representative study hospitals [111] Hull et al. performed a cost-effectiveness analysis of the patients in their LMWH treatment study from the economic perspective of a third-party payer in Canada or the United States [116]. They demonstrated that, despite higher drug cost, LMWH was more cost-effective than UFH in both health economy systems. The comparative cost savings per patient treated in hospital with LMWH instead of with intravenous heparin was $150 (Canada) or $400 (USA). They estimated that 37% of their patients could have been treated as outpatients, increasing the average potential cost savings to $960 and $910 per patient in Canada and the United States, respectively. The TASMAN study group demonstrated a 59% reduction in the average number of hospital days for initial treatment period (4.0 days vs. 9.4 days) with LMWH compared with intravenous heparin [117]. A cost-minimization analysis demonstrated a 64% reduction in costs with outpatient LMWH. This cost reduction was primarily achieved through a decreased duration of hospital stay and was not offset by the costs associated with outpatient and professional home care services. Rodgers et al. performed an incremental cost-effectiveness analysis on four treatment strategies for DVT [118]. Cost data were derived from case-costing data for actual patients treated for DVT at their tertiary care institution in Canada. The cost to treat one DVT patient was $3048 for inpatient UFH, $2993 for inpatient LMWH, and $1641 for outpatient LMWH. Tillman et al. analyzed the clinical and economic effect associated with an outpatient LMWH treatment program in a regional health maintenance organization (HMO) [119]. Of the 391 patients treated in this program, 95% completed treatment without recurrent VTE or major bleeding. The mean incremental cost savings associated with outpatient therapy (mean cost per patient $1868) compared with the potential costs that the HMO would have incurred for inhospital UFH treatment (mean cost per patient $4696) was $2828 per patient [119].

In summary, LMWH is significantly more cost-effective than UFH both for inhospital and for outpatient treatment of VTE. The increased costs of the medication and the costs of the outpatient support mechanisms do not offset these cost savings. The actual cost savings in each health care jurisdiction will be determined by the medication costs, the specific costs of local health care delivery, and by the subsequent use of the reduced number of hospital bed-days.

3. Outpatient Treatment Program for VTE

Although outpatient treatment of acute VTE with LMWH offers the opportunity to provide safe and effective treatment at home and, at the same time, to reduce the major health care costs and inconvenience associated with inhospital treatment, several factors must be considered to optimize this therapy.

a. Appropriate Patient Selection

The objective diagnosis of DVT or PE must be confirmed by medical imaging investigations (Doppler ultrasound, venography, nuclear scans, spiral computerized tomography, or other) in every patient to avoid unnecessary anticoagulant therapy.

Once the diagnosis has been reliably confirmed, the patient must be assessed for the safety and feasibility of home treatment or whether inhospital care is required. Several factors will influence this decision:

1. The presence of concomitant medical or surgical illness requiring hospitalization.
2. Patients must be clinically stable with no evidence of physiologically major PE (hypotension, oxygen saturation less than 90% on room air, or right heart failure).
3. Extensive, severely symptomatic DVT (e.g., phlegmasia, extensive iliofemoral thrombosis) may require hospitalization for catheter-directed thrombolysis or pain management.
4. Active or recent bleeding warrants close inhospital observation during initial anticoagulant therapy or consideration of a vena caval filter device.
5. High bleeding risks including a history of a bleeding disorder, recent history of a hemorrhagic stroke, severe uncontrolled hypertension, renal or hepatic failure may warrant inhospital observation during initial anticoagulant therapy.
6. Proper arrangements for the administration of LMWH (if the patient or a family member is unable to do this) must be instituted before the patient is discharged from the office, emergency department, or hospital.

We feel that the following are not necessarily reasons to preclude outpatient LMWH therapy:

Extensive DVT
Reduced cardiopulmonary reserve
Pregnancy
Marked obesity
Cancer
Pediatric thrombosis
Patient inability or refusal to do their own injections

b. Patient Education, Support, and Supervision

Patients suitable for home treatment require adequate education by the physician, dedicated nurse clinician, pharmacist, or any combination thereof. Patients should be instructed in the proper technique of LMWH subcutaneous administration. They should also receive information and counseling about venous thrombosis in general, the anticoagulant treatment plan including both the initial LMWH and the oral anticoagulant phases, and the symptoms and signs of possible recurrence of VTE and significant bleeding. A support system must be available by telephone or return clinic visits for supervision of these patients in the early phase of treatment and to deal with any difficulties or concerns that the patient or family member or caregiver may encounter. Experienced medical personnel (physician, nurse clinician) must be available on a 24-h basis to address any concerns about home injections, as well as complications including possible thrombosis recurrences, bleeding, or side effects of treatment. Careful medical supervision is required to monitor the conversion of initial LMWH therapy to ongoing oral anticoagulation. Once the patient's oral anticoagulation status is stable, ongoing supervision of therapy can be transferred to the primary physician. At some point, the patient should be formally assessed for possible risk factors or precipitating causes for the thrombosis episode. If warranted, further investigations for possible malignancy or thrombophilic states should be initiated.

E. Once-Daily vs. Twice Daily LMWH Dose Regimen

Because of the longer plasma half-life of LMWH, a once-daily injection could provide sustained therapeutic anticoagulant effect over a 24-h period. A once-daily administration regimen would simplify the use of LMWH for outpatient therapy of VTE; especially in those patients requiring professional home visits for medication administration, as well as improve patient acceptability and compliance.

In a metanalysis, Dolovich and colleagues performed a subgroup analysis comparing once-daily vs. twice-daily administration of LMWH. Once-daily LMWH appeared to be as effective and safe as twice-daily LMWH in comparison with UFH (Table 8) [98]. Spiro et al. compared UFH with once-daily enoxaparin (1.5 mg/kg o.d.) or twice-daily enoxaparin (1.0 mg/kg b.i.d.) for the treatment of VTE in 900 patients [120]. Enoxaparin either once or twice daily was as effective as UFH for VTE treatment and the frequency of bleeding events was similar (Table 9). A recent clinical trial of 651 patients with DVT directly compared once-daily with twice-daily nadroparin therapy in a randomized double-blind study [121]. The once-daily dosage regimen was as safe and effective as the same total daily dose of LMWH divided into two injections (Table 10).

In summary, both indirect and direct comparisons suggest that once-daily administration is as effective and safe as twice-daily administration of therapeutic doses of LMWH. A once-daily regimen has the advantage of a simpler, more convenient schedule for medication administration, making outpatient VTE treatment both more feasible and more acceptable to patients.

Table 8 Once-Daily LMWH Versus Twice-Daily LMWH for Treatment of VTE

Outcomes	Once-daily LMWH $N = 1846$ patients—5 studies Relative risk[a] (95% CI)	Twice-daily LMWH $N = 2601$ patients—8 studies Relative risk[a] (95% CI)
Recurrent VTE	0.98 (0.49–1.93)	0.84 (0.62–1.14)
PE	1.06 (0.38–2.92)	1.01 (0.60–1.70)
Major bleeding	0.46 (0.20–1.07)	0.70 (0.36–1.37)
Death	0.61 (0.37–0.99)	0.82 (0.61–1.11)

[a]Relative risks: comparisons between LMWH and intravenous heparin treatment.
Source: Ref. 98.

Table 9 Once-Daily LMWH Versus Twice-Daily LMWH for Treatment of VTE

	IV heparin	Enoxaparin (1 mg/kg b.i.d.)	Enoxaparin (1.5 mg/kg o.d.)
No. of patients	290	312	298
Outcomes			
Recurrent VTE (3 months)	4.3%	2.9%	4.4%
Major bleed	2.1%	1.3%	1.7%
Death	3.1%	2.2%	3.7%

Source: Ref. 120.

F. Fixed-Dose LMWH

Although weight-adjusted-dose LMWH has been equally as effective and safe as dose-adjusted UFH for VTE treatment [99,105–107], the need for LMWH dosage adjustment based on body weight has never been clearly demonstrated by pharmacokinetic or clinical studies.

A recent clinical study compared fixed-dose certoparin (8000 anti-Xa IU b.i.d. for 11.8 ± 2.8 days) to adjusted-dose intravenous UFH (for 10.7 ± 2.7 days) for initial treatment in 538 patients with venographically demonstrated DVT [122]. The principal outcome measures were a 30% or greater reduction in thrombus size at repeat venography on day 12, and a composite outcome measure that included recurrent VTE, bleeding, and mortality (Table 11). Fixed-dose certoparin was as effective as UFH in resolving DVT. The results of this study demonstrate that a fixed, weight-independent dose of certoparin is as effective in facilitating thrombus regression and is significantly more effective and safer than UFH for VTE treatment. A fixed-dose regimen for LMWH may avoid medication errors and confusion associated with different doses and also further simplifies LMWH treatment of VTE. However more studies need to be performed, before this approach can be adopted

III. LONG-TERM TREATMENT OF VTE: LMWH VS. ORAL ANTICOAGULANTS

Following a short initial period of therapy with LMWH or heparin, patients with acute thromboembolism require long-term anticoagulant therapy, usually with oral anticoagulants for at least 3–6 months to prevent recurrent VTE [73–74,123–125]. Although oral anticoagulants, including warfarin sodium and acenocoumarol, are effective in preventing recurrent

Table 10 Once-Daily LMWH Versus Twice-Daily LMWH for Treatment of VTE

Outcome	Once-daily nadroparin 20,500 IU anti-Xa o.d. $N = 316$ patients	Twice-daily nadroparin 10,250 IU anti-Xa b.i.d. $N = 335$ patients
Recurrent VTE	4.1%	7.2%
Major bleed[a]	1.3%	1.2%
Death	2.8%	3.9%

[a]During LMWH treatment.
Source: Ref. 121.

Table 11 Fixed-Dose, Weight-Independent LMWH for Treatment of DVT

	i.v. Heparin	Certoparin 8000 IU Anti-Xa s.c. b.i.d.	p-Value
Number of patients	273	265	—
Outcomes			
30% improvement in venogram scores (Marder)	25%	30%	0.26
Recurrent VTE (<6 months)	6%	2%	0.07
Major bleeding (initial therapy)	4%	2%	0.11
Composite outcome (<6 months)	13%	7%	0.02

Source: Ref. 122.

VTE [73–74,123] and, therefore, are the most widely used form of long-term anticoagulant therapy, there are several limitations to their use. On-going treatment with these drugs necessitates regular laboratory monitoring and often frequent drug dosage adjustments. The fluctuating anticoagulant levels of the coumarin drugs reflects the influence of various factors on the drug's metabolism, including genetic factors, diet, intestinal absorption, alcohol intake, interactions with other medications, exercise, and acute illnesses. There is a substantial risk of bleeding complications associated with long-term oral anticoagulant use [80]. These drugs are contraindicated during pregnancy because of congenital abnormalities and the potential for intrauterine intracranial bleeding [126,127]. Finally, several studies have indicated that cancer patients have a higher risk of recurrent VTE, despite adequate coumarin therapy ("warfarin failures") [128].

Previous clinical trials comparing warfarin with subcutaneous UFH injections have demonstrated that adjusted-dose UFH, but not fixed-low–dose UFH, is as effective as warfarin for the long-term treatment of VTE [73,123]. However, UFH has not been widely adopted because of the twice-daily injection regimen, the need for monitoring and dose adjustment, and the potential for osteopenia with prolonged use [127]. The demonstrated effectiveness and safety of LMWH in the initial treatment of VTE and its superior pharmacokinetics allowing once-daily dosing without laboratory monitoring makes LWMH a practical alternative to oral anticoagulants for the long-term treatment of VTE as well.

Several clinical trials have evaluated fixed-dose LMWH for the long-term treatment of VTE, including five studies in which LMWH has been compared with oral anticoagulants (Table 12) [129–134]. Monreal and co-workers compared the efficacy and safety of dalteparin (5,000 anti-Xa IU b.i.d.) and subcutaneous UFH (10,000 IU b.i.d.) in the long-term treatment of 80 patients with VTE in whom coumarin drugs were felt to be contraindicated [129]. No LMWH patient and two UFH patients suffered PE during follow-up. There were no recurrent DVTs or major bleeding episodes in either group. However, there were seven cases of spinal fracture, six in UFH patients, and one in a LMWH patient.

Two clinical trials have compared prophylactic doses of LMWH to warfarin for the long-term treatment of DVT following initial therapy with full doses of intravenous UFH [130,131]. The first study used enoxaparin (4000 IU anti-Xa once daily) [130] and the other used dalteparin (5000 IU anti-Xa once daily) [131]. Although both studies demonstrated fewer bleeding complications with LMWH, there was a small nonsignificant trend toward a higher incidence of recurrent VTE with LMWH given in prophylactic doses. Another clinical trial evaluated the rate of thrombus regression on repeated venography following 3 months of LMWH, compared

Table 12 Long-Term Treatment of VTE: LMWH Vs. Oral Anticoagulant

Trial [ref]	Therapy	No. of Pts.	Recurrent VTE	Bleeding
Pini [130]	LMWH	93	6 (6%)	4 (4%) 3 major
	Warfarin	94	4 (4%)	15 (16%) 3 major
			p = 0.5	p = 0.04
Das [131]	LMWH	50	5 (10%)	0 (0%)
	Warfarin	55	2 (4%)	5 (10 %)
			p = 0.43	p = 0.06
Gonzalez [132]	LMWH	85	8 (10%)	1 (1%) 1 major
	Warfarin	80	19 (24%)	8 (10%) 2 major
			p = 0.02	p = 0.02
Lopaciuk [133]	LMWH	101	2 (2%)	4 (4%) 1 major
	Acenocoumarol	101	7 (7%)	7 (7%) 1 major
			p = 0.1	p = 0.37
Viega [134]	LMWH	50	2 (4%)	1 (2%)
	Acenocoumarol	50	1 (2%)	6 (12%) 1 major
			p = 0.9	p = 0.1

Pini	Enoxaparin:	4000 IU anti-Xa o.d.
Das	Dalteparin:	5000 IU anti-Xa o.d.
Gonzalez	Enoxaparin:	4000 IU anti-Xa o.d.
Lopaciuk	Nadroparin:	85 IU anti-Xu/kg o.d.
Viega	Enoxaparin:	4000 IU anti-Xa o.d.

with warfarin [132]. Secondary outcome measures included recurrent VTE and bleeding events. Eighty-five patients initially treated for 7 days with enoxaparin (4000 IU anti-Xa twice daily), continued on 4000 IU anti-Xa once-daily for 3 months and were compared with 80 patients who received standard UFH therapy followed by warfarin for 3 months. There was a significantly greater reduction in the quantitative venographic score on repeat venography at the end of treatment, in favor of LMWH with a 49% reduction in thrombus size compared with warfarin with a 25% reduction (p<0.001). There were also significantly lower rates of VTE recurrence and bleeding with LMWH. A more recent clinical trial compared nadroparin 85 IU of anti-Xa per kilogram once-daily with acenocoumarol for long-term treatment in 202 VTE patients, all of whom were initially treated with nadroparin in therapeutic doses (85 IU/kg anti-Xa b.i.d. s.c.) [133]. This trial demonstrated that weight-adjusted fixed-dose LMWH was as safe and at least as effective as oral anticoagulants for the long-term treatment of DVT. Elderly patients who require long-term oral anticoagulants represent a high-risk group for bleeding complications and could particularly benefit from LMWH if it were a safer alternative. A recent study evaluated enoxaparin 4000 IU anti-Xa once daily and acenocoumarol in 100 elderly patients (>75 years old) for the long-term treatment of proximal DVT, following initial intravenous UFH therapy [134]. This trial demonstrated that fixed-dose LMWH appears to be as effective and as safe as oral anticoagulants in long-term treatment of DVT in the elderly. The results also suggest that LMWH therapy may have fewer bleeding complications than oral anticoagulants (2% in LMWH patients and 12% in warfarin patients; p = 0.1: 95% CI; 1.8–21.8), although the wide confidence levels around these differences makes this finding inconclusive.

Other patient groups in which LMWH may offer a safe, effective, and practical alternative to oral anticoagulants for long-term therapy include: pregnant patients, cancer patients, patients in whom oral anticoagulants cannot be given because of medical contraindications, or technical and logistical reasons.

Table 13 Some Unresolved Issues in the Treatment of Venous Thromboembolism with LMWHs

---

Direct comparisons of different LMWHs
Dosing in patients with marked obesity
Fixed-dose or weight-adjusted dosing of LMWH treatment
Need for anti-Xa monitoring in certain patient groups
Efficacy and safety of LMWH in pregnant and pediatric patients
Rapid neutralization of anticoagulant effect of LMWHs
Effect of LMWH on the future risk of postthrombotic syndrome
Optimal dose and duration of LMWH for secondary prophylaxis after a thromboembolic event
Benefits and risks of long-term therapy with LMWHs
Effect of LMWH on bone metabolism with long-term use
Effect of LMWH on all-cause and cancer mortality
Potential anticancer effect of treatment with LMWHs

In summary, oral anticoagulants remain the cornerstone of long-term anticoagulant treatment for most patients who do not have contraindications. The evidence now available does not demonstrate any clear advantages to the average VTE patient for LMWH in terms of safety and efficacy, although there is a trend toward less bleeding with LMWH. Larger studies using higher doses of LMWH are required to clearly define the relative safety and efficacy of this therapy and its use in specific patient groups.

IV. SUMMARY OF TREATMENT OF VTE

Low-molecular-weight heparins have distinct pharmacokinetic advantages that make possible the administration of therapeutic anticoagulation with greater predictability and simplicity than UFH. A large number of clinical studies and metanalyses have clearly established LMWHs as effective, safe alternatives to UFH for the treatment of acute VTE. Several of these studies have demonstrated the feasibility, safety, and cost-effectiveness of the outpatient treatment of VTE with LMWH. This has revolutionized the management of acute DVT and PE. The simplicity, convenience, and potential economic savings to health care delivery have made home treatment with LMWH, the management of choice in a large proportion of VTE patients. Recent studies have indicated that once-daily and fixed-dose LMWH administration are effective treatment regimens for VTE. These approaches would further simplify LMWH treatment but additional studies are required. Several studies have suggested that LMWHs may be an effective alternative to oral anticoagulants for long-term treatment of VTE. The practical and clinical advantages of a once-daily injection of unmonitored anticoagulant therapy for specific patient groups need more delineation by further clinical studies. Finally, there remain several unresolved issues that should be addressed to fully optimize the treatment of VTE with LMWH (Table 13).

REFERENCES

1. Nurmohamed MT, ten Cate H, ten Cate JW. Low molecular weight heparin(oid)s. Clinical investigations and practical recommendations. Drugs 1997; 53:736–751.
2. Weitz JI. Low-molecular-weight heparins. N Engl J Med 1997; 337:688–698.

3. Sarret M, Kher A, Toulemonde F. Low Molecular Weight Heparin Therapy. An Evaluation of Clinical Trials Evidence. New York: Marcel Dekker, 1999.
4. Nicolaides AN, Bergqvist D, Hull R. Prevention of venous thromboembolism. International Consensus Statement. Int Angiol 1997; 16:3–38.
5. Clagett GP, Anderson FA, Geerts W, Heit JA, Knudson M, Lieberman JR, Merli GJ, Wheeler HB. Prevention of venous thromboembolism. Chest 1998; 114(suppl):531S–560S.
6. Second Thromboembolic Risk Factors (THRiFT II) Consensus Group. Risk of and prophylaxis for venous thromboembolism in hospital patients. Phlebology 1998; 13:87–97.
7. Agnelli G, Sonaglia F. Prevention of venous thromboembolism. Thromb Res 2000; 97:V49-V62.
8. Geerts WH, Heit JA, Clagett GP, Pineo GF, Colwell CW, Anderson FA, Wheeler HB. Prevention of venous thromboembolism. Chest. 2001; 119: 132S–175S.
9. Anderson DR, O'Brien BJ, Levine MN, Roberts R, Wells PS, Hirsh J. Efficacy and cost of low-molecular-weight heparin compared with standard heparin for the prevention of deep vein thrombosis after total hip arthroplasty. Ann Intern Med 1993; 119:1105–1112.
10. Bergqvist D. Cost-effectiveness of venous thromboembolism prophylaxis in surgery. Eur J Surg 1994; 571(suppl):49–53.
11. Drummond M, Aristides M, Davies L, Forbes C. Economic evaluation of standard heparin and enoxaparin for prophylaxis against deep vein thrombosis in elective hip surgery. Br J Surg 1994; 81:1742–1746.
12. Menzin J, Colditz GA, Regan MM, Richner RE, Oster G. Cost-effectiveness of enoxaparin vs. low-dose warfarin in the prevention of deep-vein thrombosis after total hip replacement surgery. Arch Intern Med 1995; 155:757–764.
13. Bergqvist D, Lindgren B, Matzsch T. Comparison of the cost of preventing postoperative deep vein thrombosis with either unfractionated or low molecular weight heparin. Br J Surg 1996; 83:1548–1552.
14. Hull RD, Raskob GE, Pineo GF, Feldstein W, Rosenbloom D, Gafni A, Green D, Feinglass J, Trowbridge AA, Elliott CG, Lerner RG, Brant R. Subcutaneous low-molecular-weight heparin vs. warfarin for prophylaxis of deep vein thrombosis after hip or knee implantation. An economic perspective. Arch Intern Med 1997; 157:298–303.
15. Friedman RJ, Dunsworth GA. Cost analyses of extended prophylaxis with enoxaparin after hip arthroplasty. Clin Orthop 2000; 370:171–182.
16. Collins R, Scrimgeour A, Yusuf S, Peto R. Reduction in fatal pulmonary embolism and venous thrombosis by perioperative administration of subcutaneous heparin: overview of results of randomized trials in general, orthopedic, and urologic surgery. N Engl J Med 1988; 318:1162–1173.
17. Pezzuoli G, Neri Serneri GG, Settembrini P, Coggi G, Olivari N, Buzzetti G, Chierichetti S, Scotti A, Scatigna M, Carnovali M, the STEP-Study Group. Prophylaxis of fatal pulmonary embolism in general surgery using low-molecular weight heparin Cy 216: a multicentre, double-blind, randomized, controlled, clinical trial versus placebo (STEP). Int Surg 1989; 74:205–210.
18. Levine MN, Hirsh J, Gent M, Turpie AG, Leclerc J, Powers PJ, Jay RM, Neemeh J. Prevention of deep vein thrombosis after elective hip surgery. A randomized trial comparing low molecular weight heparin with standard unfractionated heparin. Ann Intern Med 1991; 114:545–551.
19. Bergqvist D, Burmark US, Flordal PA, Frisell J, Hallbook T, Hedberg M, Horn A, Kelty E, Kvitting P, Lindhagen A, Ljungstrom KG, Matzsch T, Risberg B, Syk I, Torngren S, Wellander E, Ortenwall P. Low molecular weight heparin started before surgery as prophylaxis against deep vein thrombosis: 2500 versus 5000 XaI units in 2070 patients. Br J Surg 1995; 82:496–501.
20. Koch A, Bouges S, Ziegler S, Dinkel H, Daures JP, Victor N. Low molecular weight heparin and unfractionated heparin in thrombosis prophylaxis after major surgical intervention: update of previous meta-analyses. Br J Surg 1997; 84:750–759.
21. Leizorovicz A, Haugh MC, Chapuis F–R, Samama MM, Boissel J–P. Low molecular weight heparin in prevention of perioperative thrombosis. Br Med J 1992; 305:913–920.
22. Nurmohamed MT, Rosendaal FR, Buller HR, Dekker E, Hommes DW, Vandenbroucke JP, Briet E. Low-molecular-weight heparin versus standard heparin in general and orthopaedic surgery: a metanalysis. Lancet 1992; 340:152–156.

23. Jorgensen LN, Wille–Jorgensen P, Hauch O. Prophylaxis of postoperative thromboembolism with low molecular weight heparins. Br J Surg 1993; 80:689–704.

24. Palmer AJ, Schramm W, Kirchhof B, Bergemann R. Low molecular weight heparin and unfractionated heparin for prevention of thrombo-embolism in general surgery: a metanalysis of randomised clinical trials. Haemostasis 1997; 27:65–74.

25. Gazzaniga GM, Angelini G, Pastorino G, Santoro E, Lucchini M, Dal Pra MLA, and the Italian Study Group. Enoxaparin in the prevention of deep venous thrombosis after major surgery: multicentric study. Int Surg 1993; 78:271–275.

26. Kakkar VV, Cohen AT, Edmonson RA, Phillips MJ, Cooper DJ, Das SK, Maher KT, Sanderson RM, Ward VP, Kakkar S, on behalf of the Thromboprophylaxis Collaborative Group. Low molecular weight versus standard heparin for prevention of venous thromboembolism after major abdominal surgery. Lancet 1993; 341:259–265.

27. Nurmohamed MT, Verhaeghe R, Haas S, Iriarte JA, Vogel G, van Rij AM, Prentice CRM, ten Cate JW, the Surgex Study Group. A comparative trial of a low molecular weight heparin (enoxaparin) versus standard heparin for the prophylaxis of postoperative deep vein thrombosis in general surgery. Am J Surg 1995; 169:567–571.

28. ENOXACAN Study Group. Efficacy and safety of enoxaparin versus unfractionated heparin for prevention of deep vein thrombosis in elective cancer surgery: a double-blind randomized multicentre trial with venographic assessment. Br J Surg 1997; 84:1099–1103.

29. Kakkar VV, Boeckl O, Boneu B, Bordenave L, Brehm OA, Brucke P, Coccheri S, Cohen AT, Galland F, Haas S, Jarrige J, Koppenhagen K, LaQuerrec A, Parraguette E, Prandoni P, Roder JD, Roos M, Ruschemeyer C, Siewert JR, Vinazzer H, Wenzel E. Efficacy and safety of a low-molecular-weight heparin and standard unfractionated heparin for prophylaxis of postoperative venous thromboembolism: European Multicenter Trial. World J Surg 1997; 21:2–9.

30. Etchells E, McLeod RS, Geerts W, Barton P, Detsky AS. Economic analysis of low-dose heparin vs. the low-molecular-weight heparin enoxaparin for prevention of venous thromboembolism after colorectal surgery. Arch Intern Med 1999; 159:1221–1228.

31. Brennand JE, Greer IA. Thromboembolism in gynaecological surgery. Curr Obstet Gynaecol 1998; 8:44–48.

32. Dubuc–Lissoir J, Ehlen T, Heywood M, Plante M. Prevention and treatment of thrombo-embolic disease in gynaecological surgery. J Soc Obstet Gynaecol Can 1999; 21:1087–1094.

33. von Tempelhoff G–F, Heilmann L. Antithrombotic therapy in gynecologic surgery. Hematol Oncol Clin N Am 2000; 14:1151–1169.

34. Kibel AS, Loughlin KR. Pathogenesis and prophylaxis of postoperative thromboembolic disease in urological pelvic surgery. J Urol 1995; 153:1763–1774.

35. Heilmann L, von Tempelhoff G–F, Kirkpatrick C, Schneider DM, Hommel G, Pollow K. Comparison of unfractionated versus low molecular weight heparin for deep vein thrombosis prophylaxis during breast and pelvic cancer surgery: efficacy, safety, and follow-up. Clin Appl Thromb Hemos 1998; 4:268–273.

36. Colwell CW, Collis DK, Paulson R, McCutcheon JW, Bigler GT, Lutz S, Hardwick ME. Comparison of enoxaparin and warfarin for the prevention of venous thromboembolic disease after total hip arthroplasty. J Bone Joint Surg 1999; 81A:932–940.

37. Hull R, Raskob G, Pineo G, Rosenbloom D, Evans W, Mallory T, Anquist K, Smith F, Hughes G, Green D, Elliott CG, Panju A, Brant R. A comparison of subcutaneous low-molecular-weight heparin with warfarin sodium for prophylaxis against deep-vein thrombosis after hip or knee implantation. N Engl J Med 1993; 329:1370–1376.

38. RD Heparin Arthroplasty Group. RD heparin compared with warfarin for prevention of venous thromboembolic disease following total hip or knee arthroplasty. J Bone Joint Surg 1994; 76A:1174–1185.

39. Hamulyak K, Lensing AWA, van der Meer J, Smid WM, van Ooy A, Hoek JA, the Fraxiparine Oral Anticoagulant Study Group. Subcutaneous low-molecular weight heparin or oral anticoagulants for the prevention of deep-vein thrombosis in elective hip and knee replacement? Thromb Haemost 1995; 74:1428–1431.

40. Francis CW, Pellegrini VD, Totterman S, Boyd AD, Marder VJ, Liebert KM, Stulberg BN, Ayers DC, Rosenberg A, Kessler C, Johanson NA. Prevention of deep-vein thrombosis after total hip arthroplasty. Comparison of warfarin and dalteparin. J Bone Joint Surg 1997; 79A:1365–1372.

41. Hull RD, Pineo GF, Francis C, Bergqvist D, Fellenius C, Soderberg K, Holmqvist A, Mant M, Dear R, Baylis B, Mah A, Brant R, the North American Fragmin Trial Investigators. Low-molecular-weight heparin prophylaxis using dalteparin in close proximity to surgery vs. warfarin in hip arthroplasty patients. A double-blind, randomized comparison. Arch Intern Med 2000; 160:2199–2207.

42. Planes A, Vochelle N, Fagola M, Bellaud M, the Reviparin Study Group. Comparison of two low-molecular-weight heparins for the prevention of postoperative venous thromboembolism after elective hip surgery. Blood Coagul Fibrinolysis 1998; 9:499–505.

43. Planes A, Samama MM, Lensing AWA, Buller HR, Barre J, Vochelle N, Beau B. Prevention of deep vein thrombosis after hip replacement. Comparison between two low-molecular-heparins, tinzaparin and enoxaparin. Thromb Haemost 1999; 81:22–25.

44. Blanchard J, Meuwly J–Y, Leyvraz P–F, Miron M–J, Bounameaux H, Hoffmeyer P, Didier D, Schneider P–A. Prevention of deep-vein thrombosis after total knee replacement. Randomised comparison between a low-molecular-weight heparin (nadroparin) and mechanical prophylaxis with a foot-pump system. J Bone Joint Surg 1999; 81B:654–659.

45. Spiro TE, Fitzgerald RH, Trowbridge AA, Overdyke WL, Gardiner GA, Young TR, Ohar JA, Gustilo RB, Whitsett TL. Enoxaparin a low molecular weight heparin and warfarin for the prevention of venous thromboembolic disease after elective knee replacement surgery [abstr]. J Bone Joint Surg 1995; 77B(suppl III):317.

46. Leclerc JR, Geerts WH, Desjardins L, Laflamme GH, l'Esperance B, Demers C, Kassis J, Cruickshank M, Whitman L, Delorme F. Prevention of venous thromboembolism after knee arthroplasty. A randomized, double-blind trial comparing enoxaparin with warfarin. Ann Intern Med 1996; 124:619–626.

47. Heit JA, Berkowitz SD, Bona R, Cabanas V, Corson JD, Elliott CG, Lyons R, (Ardeparin Arthroplasty Study Group). Efficacy and safety of low molecular weight heparin (ardeparin sodium) compared to warfarin for the prevention of venous thromboembolism after total knee replacement surgery: a double-blind, dose-ranging study. Thromb Haemost 1997; 77:32–38.

48. Barsotti J, Gruel Y, Rosset P, Favard L, Dabo B, Andreu J, Delahousse B, Leroy J. Comparative double-blind study of two dosage regimens of low-molecular weight heparin in elderly patients with a fracture of the neck of the femur. J Orthop Trauma 1990; 4:371–375.

49. Borris LC, Lassen MR, Poulsen KA, Jensen HP. Thromboembolic complications after hip fracture—prophylaxis with low molecular weight vs. unfractionated heparin [abstr]. Thromb Haemost 1995; 73:1104.

50. Bergqvist D, Benoni G, Bjorgell O, Fredin H, Hedlundh U, Nicolas S, Nilsson P, Nylander G. Low-molecular-weight heparin (enoxaparin) as prophylaxis against venous thromboembolism after total hip replacement. N Engl J Med 1996; 335:696–700.

51. Planes A, Vochelle N, Darmon J–Y, Fagola M, Belland M, Yuet Y. Risk of deep-venous thrombosis after hospital discharge in patients having undergone total hip replacement: double-blind randomized comparison of enoxaparin versus placebo. Lancet 1996; 348:224–228.

52. Dahl OE, Andreassen G, Aspelin T, Muller C, Mathiesen P, Nyhus S, Abdelnoor M, Solhaug J–H, Arnesen H. Prolonged thromboprophylaxis following hip replacement surgery—results of a double-blind, prospective, randomised, placebo-controlled study with dalteparin (Fragmin). Thromb Haemost 1997; 77:26–31.

53. Spiro TE. A double-blind multicenter clinical trial comparing long term enoxaparin and placebo treatments in the prevention of venous thromboembolic disease after hip and knee replacement surgery [abstr]. Blood. 1997; 90(suppl 1):295a.

54. Lassen MR, Borris LC, Anderson BS, Jensen HP, Skejo Bro HP, Andersen G, Petersen AO, Siem P, Horlyck E, Jensen BV, Thomsen PB, Hansen BR, Erin–Madsen J, Moller JC, Rotwitt L, Christensen F, Nielsen JB, Jorgensen PS, Paaske B, Torholm C, Hvidt P, Jensen NK, Nielsen AB, Appelquist F, Hansen OG, Mortensen D, Tjalve E. Efficacy and safety of prolonged thromboprophylaxis with a low

molecular weight heparin (dalteparin) after total hip arthroplasty—the Danish Prolonged Prophylaxis (DaPP) Study. Thromb Res 1998; 89:281–287.

55. Hull RD, Pineo GF, Francis C, Bergqvist D, Fellenius C, Soderberg K, Holmqvist A, Mant M, Dear R, Baylis B, Mah A, Brant R, the North American Fragmin Trial Investigators. Low-molecular-weight heparin prophylaxis using dalteparin extended out-of-hospital vs in-hospital warfarin/ out-of-hospital placebo in hip arthroplasty patients. A double-blind, randomized comparison. Arch Intern Med 2000; 160:2208–2215.

56. Geerts WH, Code KI, Jay RM, Chen E, Szalai JP. A prospective study of venous thromboembolism after major trauma. N Engl J Med 1994; 331:1601–1606.

57. Geerts WH, Jay RM, Code KI, Chen E, Szalai JP, Saibil EA, Hamilton PA. A comparison of low-dose heparin with low-molecular-weight heparin as prophylaxis against venous thromboembolism after major trauma. N Engl J Med 1996; 335:701–707.

58. Consortium for Spinal Cord Medicine. Prevention of thromboembolism in spinal cord injury. J Spinal Cord Med 1997; 20:259–283.

59. Green D, Lee MY, Ito VY, Cohn T, Press J, Filbrandt PR, VandenBerg WC, Yarkony GM, Meyer PR. Fixed- vs. adjusted-dose heparin in the prophylaxis of thromboembolism in spinal cord injury. JAMA 1988; 260:1255–1258.

60. Green D, Lee MY, Lim AC, Chmiel JS, Vetter M, Pang T, Chen D, Fenton L, Yarkony GM, Meyer PR. Prevention of thromboembolism after spinal cord injury using low-molecular-weight heparin. Ann Intern Med 1990; 113:571–574.

61. Abelseth G, Buckley RE, Pineo GE, Hull R, Rose MS. Incidence of deep-vein thrombosis in patients with fractures of the lower extremity distal to the hip. J Orthop Trauma 1996; 10:230–235.

62. Kujath P, Spannagel U, Habscheid W. Incidence and prophylaxis of deep venous thrombosis in outpatients with injury of the lower limb. Haemostasis 1993; 23(suppl 1):20–26.

63. Kock H–J, Schmit–Neuerburg KP, Hanke J, Rudofsky G, Hirche H. Thromboprophylaxis with low-molecular-weight heparin in outpatients with plaster-cast immobilisation of the leg. Lancet 1995; 346:459–461.

64. Melon E, Keravel Y, Gaston A, Huet Y, Combes S, the "NEURONOX" group. Deep venous thrombosis prophylaxis by low molecular weight heparin in neurosurgical patients [abstr]. Anesthesiology 1991; 75:A214.

65. Nurmohamed MT, van Riel AM, Henkens CMA, Koopman MMW, Que GTH, d'Azemar P, Buller HR, ten Cate JW, Hoek JA, van der Meer J, van der Heul C, Turpie AGG, Haley S, Sicurella J, Gent M. Low molecular weight heparin and compression stockings in the prevention of venous thromboembolism in neurosurgery. Thromb Haemost 1996; 75:233–238.

66. Agnelli G, Piovella F, Buoncristiani P, Severi P, Pini M, D'Angelo A, Beltrametti C, Damiani M, Andrioloi GC, Pugliese R, Iorio A, Brambilla G. Enoxaparin plus compression stockings compared with compression stockings alone in the prevention of venous thromboembolism after elective neurosurgery. N Engl J Med 1998; 339:80–85.

67. Iorio A, Agnelli G. Low-molecular-weight and unfractionated heparin for prevention of venous thromboembolism in neurosurgery: a meta-analysis. Arch Intern Med 2000; 160:2327–2332.

68. Dickinson LD, Miller LD, Patel CP, Gupta SK. Enoxaparin increases the incidence of postoperative intracranial hemorrhage when initiated preoperatively for deep venous thrombosis prophylaxis in patients with brain tumors. Neurosurgery 1998; 43:1074–1081.

69. Mismetti P, Laporte–Simitsidis S, Tardy B, Cucherat M, Buchmuller A, Juillard–Delsart D, Decousus H. Prevention of venous thromboembolism in internal medicine with unfractionated or low-molecular-weight heparins: a meta-analysis randomised clinical trials. Thromb Haemost 2000; 83:14–19.

70. Samama MM, Cohen AT, Darmon Y–J, Desjardins L, Eldor A, Janbon C, Leizorovicz A, Nguyen H, Olsson C–G. Turpie AG, Weisslinger N, the Prophylaxis in Medical Patients with Enoxaparin Study Group. A comparison of enoxaparin with placebo for the prevention of venous thromboembolism in acutely ill medical patients. N Engl J Med 1999; 341:793–800.

71. Fraisse F, Holzapfel L, Couland J–M, Simonneau G, Bedock B, Feissel M, Herbecq P, Pordes R, Poussel J–F, Roux L, The Association of Non-University Affiliated Intensive Care Specialist

Physicians of France. Nadroparin in the prevention of deep vein thrombosis in acute decompensated COPD. Am J Respir Crit Care Med 2000; 161:1109–1114.

72. Barritt DW, Jordan SC. Anticoagulant drugs in the treatment of pulmonary embolism: a controlled trial. Lancet 1960; 1:1309–1312.

73. Hull R, Delmore T, Genton E, Hirsh J, Gent M, Sackett D, McLaughlin D, Armstrong P. Warfarin sodium versus low-dose heparin in the long-term treatment of venous thrombosis. N Engl J Med 1979; 301:855–858.

74. Lagerstedt C, Olsson C, Fagher B, Oqvist B, Albrechtsson U. Need for long-term anticoagulant treatment in symptomatic calf-vein thrombosis. Lancet 1985; 2:515–518.

75. Brandjes DPM, Heijboer H, Buller H, de Rijk M, Jagt H, ten Cate JW. Acenocoumarol and heparin compared with acenocoumarol alone in the initial treatment of proximal vein thrombosis. N Engl J Med 1992; 327:1485–1489.

76. Hyers T, Agnelli G, Hull RD, Weg JG, Morris T, Samama M, Tapson V. Chest 1998; 114:561S–578S.

77. Hull RD, Raskob GE, Hirsh J, Jay RM, Leclerc JR, Geerts WH, Rosenbloom D, Sackett D, Anderson C, Harrison L, Gent M. Continuous intravenous heparin compared with intermittent subcutaneous heparin in the initial treatment of proximal-vein thrombosis. N Engl J Med 1986; 315:1109–1114.

78. Basu D, Gallus A, Hirsh, Cade J. A prospective study of the value of monitoring heparin treatment with activated partial thromboplastin time. N Engl J Med 1972; 287:324–327.

79. Hirsh J. Heparin. N Engl J Med 1991; 324:1565–1574.

80. Levine M, Raskob G, Landefeld S, Kearon C. Hemorrhagic complications of anticoagulant treatment. Chest 1998; 114(suppl. 5):511S–523S.

81. Warkentin T, Levine M, Hirsh J, Horsewood P, Roberts R, Gent M, Kelton J. Heparin-induced thrombocytopenia in patients treated with low-weight-heparin or unfractionated heparin. N Engl J Med 1995; 332:1330–1335.

82. Bhandari M, Hirsh J, Weitz JI, Young E, Venner TJ, Shaughnessy SG. The effect of standard and low molecular weight heparin on bone nodule formation. Thromb Haemost 1998; 80:413–417.

83. Bhandari M, Hirsh J, Weitz JI, Shaughnessy SG. The effect of standard and low molecular weight heparin on osteoblastogenesis in vitro. Blood 1998; 92(suppl 1):358a.

84. Bratt G, Tornebohm E, Granqvist S, Aberg W, Lockner D. A comparison between low molecular weight heparin (KABI 2165) and standard heparin in the intravenous treatment of deep venous thrombosis. Thromb Haemost 1985; 54:813–817.

85. Holm H, Ly B, Handeland G, Abildgaard U, Arnesen K, Gottschalk P. Subcutaneous heparin treatment of deep venous thrombosis: a comparison of unfractionated and low molecular weight heparin. Haemostasis. 1986; 16(suppl 2):30–37.

86. Faivre R, Neuhart Y, Kieffer Y, Apfel F, Magnin D, Didier D, Toulemonde F, Bassand JP, Maurat JP. Un nouveau traitement des thromboses veineuses profondes: les fractions d'heparine de bas poids moleculaire. Etude randomisee. Presse Med 1988; 17:197–200.

87. Albada J, Nieuwenhuis H, Sixma J. Treatment of acute thromboembolism with low molecular weight heparin (Fragmin). Circulation 1989; 80:935–940.

88. Bratt G, Aberg W, Johansson M, Tornebohm E, Granqvist S, Lockner D. Two daily subcutaneous injections of Fragmin as compared with intravenous standard heparin in the treatment of deep venous thrombosis. Thromb Haemost 1990; 64:506–510.

89. Harenberg J, Huck K, Bratsch H, Stehle G, Dempple C, Mall K. Therapeutic application of subcutaneous low-molecular-weight heparin in acute venous thrombosis. Haemostasis. 1990; 20(suppl 1):205–219.

90. Duroux P, Beclere A. A Collaborative European Multicentre Study: a randomized trial of subcutaneous low molecular weight heparin (CY 216) compared with intravenous unfractionated heparin in the treatment of deep vein thrombosis. Thromb Haemost 1991; 65:251–256.

91. Lopaciuk S, Meissner AJ, Filipeci S, Zawilska K, Sowier J, Ciesielski L, Bielawiec M, Glowinski S, Czestochowska E. Subcutaneous low molecular weight heparin versus subcutaneous unfractionated heparin in the treatment of deep vein thrombosis: a Polish multicenter trial. Thromb Haemost 1992; 68:14–18.

92. Simonneau G, Charbonnier B, Decousus H, Planchon B, Ninet J, Sie P, Silsiguen M, Combe S. Subcutaneous low-molecular-weight heparin compared with continuous intravenous heparin in the treatment of proximal deep vein thrombosis. Arch Intern Med 1993; 153:1541–1546.
93. Siragusa S, Cosmi B, Piovella F, Hirsh J, Ginsberg JS. Low-molecular-weight heparins and unfractionated heparin in the treatment of patients with acute venous thromboembolism: results of a meta-analysis. Am J Med 1996; 100:269–277.
94. van den Belt AGM, Prins MH, Lensing AWA, Castro AA, Clark OAC, Atallah AN, Burihan E. Fixed dose subcutaneous low molecular heparins versus adjusted dose unfractionated heparin for venous thromboembolism (review) In: The Cochrane Database of Systematic Reviews. 2000; 3, Oxford: Update Software.
95. Leizorovicz A, Simonneau G, Decousus H, Boissel J. Comparison of efficacy and safety of low molecular weight heparins and unfractionated heparin in the initial treatment of deep venous thrombosis: a metanalysis. Br J Med 1994; 309:299–304.
96. Lensing A, Prins M, Davidson B, Hirsh J. Treatment of deep venous thrombosis with low-molecular-weight heparins: a metanalysis. Arch Intern Med 1995; 155:601–607.
97. Gould M, Dembitzer A, Doyle R, Hastie T, Garber A. Low-molecular-weight heparins compared with unfractionated heparin for the treatment of acute deep venous thrombosis: a meta-analysis of randomized, controlled trials. Ann Intern Med 1999; 130:800–809.
98. Dolovich L, Ginsberg J, Douketis J, Holbrook A, Cheah G. A meta-analysis comparing low-molecular-weight heparins with unfractionated heparin in the treatment of venous thromboembolism. Arch Intern Med 2000; 160:181–188.
99. Simonneau G, Sors H, Charbonnier B, Page Y, Laaban JP, Azarian R, Laurent M, Hirsch JL, Ferrari E, Bosson JL, Mottier D, Beau B, the THESEE Group. A comparison of low-molecular-weight heparin with unfractionated heparin for acute pulmonary embolism. N Engl J Med 1997; 337:663–669.
100. Hull RD, Raskob GE, Pineo G, Green D, Trowbridge A, Elliott G, Lerner R, Hall J, Sparling T, Brettell HR, Norton J, Carter CJ, George R, Merli G, Ward J, Mayo W, Rosenbloom D, Brant R. Subcutaneous low-molecular-weight heparin compared with continuous intravenous heparin in the treatment of proximal-vein thrombosis. N Engl J Med 1992; 326:975–982.
101. Lindmarker P, Holmstrom M, Granqvist S, Johnsson H, Lockner D. Comparison of once-daily subcutaneous Fragmin with continuous intravenous heparin in the treatment of deep vein thrombosis. Thromb Haemost 1994; 72:186–190.
102. Fiessinger JN, Lopez–Fernandez M, Gatterer E, Granqvist S, Kher A, Olsson CG, Soderberg K. Once-daily subcutaneous dalteparin, a low molecular weight heparin, for the initial treatment of acute deep vein thrombosis. Thromb Haemost 1996; 76:195–199.
103. Luomanmaki K, Grankvist S, Hallert C, Jauro I, Ketola K, Kim HC, Kiviniemi H, Koskivirta H, Sorskog L, Vilkko P. A multicentre comparison of once-daily subcutaneous dalteparin (low molecular weight heparin) and continuous intravenous heparin in the treatment of deep vein thrombosis. J Intern Med 1996; 240: 85–92.
104. Prandoni P, Lensing AWA, Buller HR, Carta M, Cogo A, Vigo M, Casara D, Ruol A, ten Cate JW. Comparison of subcutaneous low-molecular-weight heparin with intravenous standard heparin in proximal deep-vein thrombosis. Lancet 1992; 339:441–445.
105. Koopman M, Prandoni P, Piovella F, Ockelford P, Brandjes D, van der Meer J, Gallus A, Simonneau G, Chesterman C, Prins M, Bossuyt P, de Haes H, van den Belt A, Sagnard L, d'Azemar P, Buller H, the Tasman Study Group. Treatment of venous thrombosis with ntravenous unfractionated heparin administered in the hospital as compared with subcutaneous low-molecular-weight heparin administered at home. N Engl J Med 1996; 334:682–687.
106. Levine M, Gent M, Hirsh J, Leclerc J, Anderson D, Weitz J, Ginsberg J, Turpie AG, Demers C, Kovacs M, Geerts W, Kassis J, Desjardins L, Cusson J, Cruickshank M, Powers P, Brien W, Haley S, Willan A. A comparison of low-molecular-weight heparin administered primarily at home with unfractionated heparin administered in the hospital for proximal deep-vein thrombosis. N Engl J Med 1996; 334:677–681.
107. The Columbus Investigators. Low-molecular weight heparin in the treatment of patients with venous thromboembolism. N Engl J Med 1997; 337:657–662.

108. Decousus H, Leizorovicz A, Parent F, Page Y, Tardy B, Girard P, Laporte S, Faivre R, Charbonnier B, Barral F–G, Huet Y, Simonneau G. A clinical trial of vena caval filters in the prevention of pulmonary embolism in patients with proximal deep-vein thrombosis. N Engl J Med 1998; 338:409–415.

109. Meyer G, Brenot F, Pacouret G, Simonneau G, Gillet Juvin K, Charbonnier B, Sors H. Subcutaneous low-molecular-weight heparin Fragmin versus intravenous unfractionated heparin in the treatment of acute non massive pulmonary embolism: an open randomized pilot study. Thromb Haemost 1995; 74:1432–1435.

110. Hull RD, Raskob G, Brant R, Pineo G, Elliott G, Stein P, Gottschalk A, Valentine K, Mah A, The American–Canadian Thrombosis Study Group. Low-molecular-weight heparin vs. heparin in the treatment of patients with pulmonary embolism. Arch Intern Med 2000; 160:229–236.

111. Lindmarker P, Holmstorm M, The Swedish Venous Thrombosis Dalteparin Trial Group. Use of low molecular weight heparin (dalteparin), once daily, for the treatment of deep vein thrombosis. A feasibility and health economic study in an outpatient setting. J Intern Med 1996; 240:395–401.

112. Wells P, Kovacs M, Bormanis J, Forgie M, Goudie D, Morrow B, Kovacs J. Expanding eligibility for outpatient treatment of deep venous thrombosis and pulmonary embolism with low-molecular-weight heparin. Arch Intern Med 1998; 158:1809–1812.

113. Harrison L, McGinnis J, Crowther M, Ginsberg J, Hirsh J. Assessment of outpatient treatment of deep-vein thrombosis with low-molecular-weight heparin. Arch Intern Med 1998; 158:2001–2003.

114. Savage K, Wells P, Schulz V, Goudie D, Morrow B, Cruickshank M, Kovacs M. Outpatient use of low molecular weight heparin (dalteparin) for the treatment of deep vein thrombosis of the upper extremity. Thromb Haemost 1999; 82:1008–1010.

115. Kovacs M, Anderson D, Morrow B, Gray L, Touchie D, Wells P. Outpatient treatment of pulmonary embolism with dalteparin. Thromb Haemost 2000; 83:209–211.

116. Hull R, Raskob G, Rosenbloom D, Pineo G, Lerner R, Gafni A, Trowbridge A, Elliott G, Green D, Feinglass J, Feldstein W, Brant R. Treatment of proximal vein thrombosis with subcutaneous low-molecular-weight heparin vs. intravenous heparin: an economic perspective. Arch Intern Med 1997; 157:289–294.

117. van den Belt A, Bossuyt P, Prins M, Gallus A, Buller H, The TASMAN Study Group. Replacing inpatient care by outpatient care in the treatment of deep venous thrombosis—an economic evaluation. Thromb Haemost 1998;79:259–263.

118. Rodgers M, Bredeson C, Wells P, Beck J, Kearns B, Huebsch L. Cost-effectiveness of low-molecular weight heparin and unfractionated heparin in the treatment of deep vein thrombosis. Can Med Assoc J 1998; 159:931–938.

119. Tillman D, Charland S, Witt D. Effectiveness and economic impact associated with a program for outpatient management of acute deep vein thrombosis in a group model health maintenance organization. Arch Intern Med 2000; 160:2926–2932.

120. Spiro T, The Enoxaparin Clinical Trial Group [abstr]. Thromb Haemost 1997; 78(suppl):373–374.

121. Charbonnier B, Fiessinger J, Banga J, Wenzel E, d'Azemar P, Sagnard L, The FRAXODI Group. Comparison of a once daily with a twice daily subcutaneous low molecular weigh heparin regimen in the treatment of deep vein thrombosis. Thromb Haemost 1998; 79:897–901.

122. Harenberg J, Schmidt J, Koppenhagen K, Toile A, Huisman M, Buller H, The EASTERN Investigators. Fixed-dose, body weight-independent subcutaneous LMW heparin versus adjusted dose unfractionated intravenous heparin in the initial treatment of proximal venous thrombosis. Thromb Haemost 2000; 83:652–656.

123. Hull R, Delmore T, Carter C, Hirsh J, Genton E, Gent M, Turpie G, McLaughlin D. Adjusted subcutaneous heparin versus warfarin sodium in the long-term treatment of venous thrombosis. N Engl J Med. 1982; 306:189–194.

124. Schulman S, Rhedin AS, Lindmarker P, Carlsson A, Larfars G, Nicol P, Loogna E, Svensson E, Ljuneberg B, Walter H, Viering S, Nordlander S, Leijd B, Jonsson K–A, Hjorth M, Linder O, Boberg J, The Duration of Anticoagulation Trial Study Group. A comparison of six weeks with six months of oral anticoagulant therapy after a first episode of venous thromboembolism. N Engl J Med 1995; 332:1661–1665.

125. Kearon C, Gent M, Hirsh J, Weitz J, Kovacs M, Anderson D, Turpie A, Green D, Ginsberg J, Wells P, MacKinnon B, Julian J. A comparison of three months of anticoagulation with extended antic-oagulation for a first episode of idiopathic venous thromboembolism. N Engl J Med 1999; 340:901–907.

126. Hall J, Pauli R, Wilson K. Maternal and fetal sequelae of anticoagulant during pregnancy. Am J Med 1980; 68:122–140.

127. Ginsberg J, Hirsh J. Use of antithrombotic agents during pregnancy. Chest 1998; 114:524S–530S.

128. Levine M, Lee A. Treatment of venous thromboembolism in cancer patients. Semin Thromb Haemost 1999; 25:245–249.

129. Monreal M, Lafoz E, Olive A, del Rio L, Vedia C. Comparison of subcutaneous unfractionated heparin with a low molecular weight heparin (Fragmin) in patients with venous thromboembolism and contraindications to coumarin. Thromb Haemost 1994; 71:7–11.

130. Pini M, Aiello C, Manotti C, Pattacini C, Quintavalla R, Poli T, Tagliaferri A, Dettori A. Low molecular weight heparin versus warfarin in the prevention of recurrences after deep vein thrombosis. Thromb Haemost 1994; 72:191–197.

131. Das S, Cohen A, Edmondson R, Melissari E, Kakkar VV. Low-molecular-weight heparin versus warfarin for prevention of recurrent venous thromboembolism: a randomized trial. World J Surg 1996; 20:521–527.

132. Gonzalez–Fajardo J, Arreba E, Castrodeza J, Perez J, Fernandez L, Agundez I, Mateo M, Carrera S, Gutierrez V, Vaquero C. Venographic comparison of subcutaneous low-molecular weight heparin with oral anticoagulant therapy in the long-term treatment of deep venous thrombosis. J Vasc Surg 1999; 30:283–292.

133. Lopaciuk S, Bielska–Falda H, Noszczyk W, Bielawiec M, Witkiewicz W, Filipecki S, Michalak J, Ciesielski L, Mackiewicz Z, Czestochowska E, Zawilska K, Cencora A. Low molecular weight heparin versus acenocoumarol in the secondary prophylaxis of deep vein thrombosis. Thromb Haemost 1999; 81:26–31.

134. Veiga F, Escriba A, Maluenda M, Lopez Rubio M, Margalet I, Lezana A, Gallego J, Ribera J. Low molecular weight heparin (enoxaparin) versus oral anticoagulant therapy (acenocoumarol) in the long-term treatment of deep venous thrombosis in the elderly: a randomized trial. Thromb Haemost 2000; 84:559–564.

10

Low-Molecular-Weight Heparin in the Pediatric Population

Manuela Albisetti
University Children's Hospital, Zurich, Switzerland

Maureen Andrew*
The Hospital for Sick Children, Toronto, Ontario, Canada

SUMMARY

Over the last two decades, several large randomized clinical trials have demonstrated advantages of low-molecular-weight heparin (LMWH) over unfractionated heparin (UFH) for the prevention and treatment of thromboembolic events (TEs) in adults. These advantages include predictable pharmacokinetics; subcutaneous administration; no need for, or minimal, monitoring; decreased risk of heparin-induced thrombocytopenia; and decreased risk of osteoporosis.

Children also are at risk for TEs and require anticoagulants. For treatment, the most common approach is a short course of intravenous UFH followed by oral anticoagulants (OA). Both of these drugs have disadvantages that limit optimal prevention and treatment of TEs in children. The major limitations include age-dependent pharmacokinetics; a need for frequent monitoring, despite poor venous access; difficulties in achieving and maintaining adequate anticoagulation; a risk of bleeding and of osteoporosis; and a risk of heparin-induced thrombocytopenia (HIT) with UFH. Low-molecular-weight heparins have advantages over UFH and OA in children, and several studies have assessed the use of LMWHs in children. This chapter will summarize the available information on LMWHs relative to pharmacokinetics, dose requirements, efficacy, and safety in children.

I. MECHANISMS OF ACTION OF LMWHs

Low-molecular-weight heparins act as anticoagulants by catalyzing the inhibitory effects of antithrombin (AT) on factor (F)Xa and thrombin [1]. In contrast to UFH, which possesses equal anticoagulant activity against both FXa and thrombin, LMWHs have greater activity against FXa

---

*Deceased

than against thrombin [2]. At birth and during early infancy, plasma concentrations of some coagulation components including prothrombin, FVII, FIX, FX, and AT are decreased compared with adults, resulting in both a decrease and delay in thrombin generation relative to adults. Studies assessing the effects of LMWHs on thrombin generation indicate that LMWHs produce greater inhibition of thrombin generation in plasma from newborns than in plasma from adults [4]. This reflects increased levels of AT relative to prothrombin in newborns (ratio, 1.5 : 1) compared with adults (ratio, 1 : 1) because the sensitivity of newborn plasma to LMWH can be enhanced or reduced by increasing plasma concentrations of AT or prothrombin, respectively (Fig. 1) [4].

A. Pharmacokinetics

The pharmacokinetics of several LMWHs have been assessed in animal models and during infancy and childhood.

1.   Animal Models

The pharmacokinetics and pharmacodynamics of the LMWH, CY 222 (Choay Laboratoires, Paris, France), were studied in a porcine model by monitoring the clearance of ^{125}I–radiolabeled CY 222 and anti-FXa levels, respectively [5]. The porcine model was selected because, similar to humans, newborn piglets have plasma AT concentrations approximately 50% of adult values. CY 222 was administered by bolus injection in doses of 5, 25, or 100 U/kg to adult pigs, newborn piglets, and newborn piglets supplemented with AT. The half-life of CY 222, measured as either ^{125}I-radioactivity or anti-FXa activity, was not dose-dependent and was similar in pigs and piglets, reflecting a similar linear nonsaturable clearance mechanism. The overall clearance of CY 222 in piglets was faster than in pigs, reflecting the larger volume of distribution in newborn

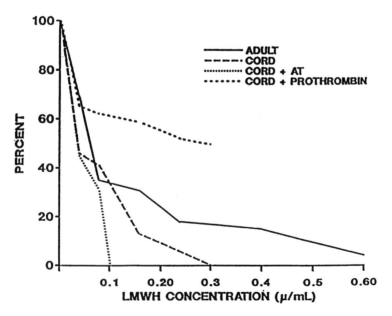

Figure 1 Dose–response curves of thrombin activity (expressed as area under the curve) versus the concentration of LMWH, CY 222 (Choay Laboratoires, Paris, France). Abbreviations: LMWH, low molecular weight heparin; AT, antithrombin; U, unit; mL, milliliter. (From Ref. 4.)

piglets. AT supplementation did not alter CY 222 clearance in piglets [5]. The half-life of CY 222 in piglets and pigs was approximately twice as long as that reported for UFH in the same porcine model [5,6].

2. Infants and Children

The pharmacodynamics of two LMWHs, enoxaparin (Rhone-Poulenc Rorer), and reviparin-sodium (Knoll Pharma, Inc.) have been evaluated in children.

   a. Enoxaparin. The pharmacodynamics of therapeutic and prophylactic doses of enoxaparin were assessed in infants and children in two studies [7,8]. In the first study, therapeutic doses of enoxaparin were administered to 14 children older than 2 months of age, and 9 infants younger than 2 months of age [7]. The target therapeutic anti-FXa range of 0.5–1.0 U/mL was achieved after a subcutaneous enoxaparin dose of 1.0 mg/kg every 12 h in children older than 2 months of age, and after a mean dose of 1.6 mg/kg every 12 h in infants younger than 2 months of age [7]. In the second study, therapeutic doses of enoxaparin were administered to 12 children older than 2 months of age and to 2 infants younger than 2 months of age [8]. The adult target therapeutic anti-FXa range of 0.5–1.2 U/mL was achieved after a subcutaneous enoxaparin dose of 1.0 mg/kg every 12 h in children older than 2 months of age. No recommendations on dose requirements in infants younger than 2 months of age can be made on the basis of this study because few patients in this age group were included [8]. In both studies, therapeutic anti-FXa peak levels were achieved 3–4 h after the first subcutaneous injection of enoxaparin [7,8].

   Prophylactic doses of enoxaparin were studied in only a small number of patients. In one study, two children given a subcutaneous enoxaparin dose of 0.5 mg/kg every 12 h achieved anti-FXa levels of 0.35±0.03 U/mL [7]. In the second study, five patients given a therapeutic subcutaneous enoxaparin dose of 1.0 mg/kg once daily achieved peak anti-FXa levels ranging from 0.43–1.38 U/mL, levels that were within the therapeutic range [8].

   b. Reviparin Sodium. The pharmadynamics of therapeutic and prophylactic doses of reviparin sodium have been assessed in infants and children in two studies [9,10]. In the first study, therapeutic doses of reviparin sodium were administered to 12 children weighing more than 5 kg [9]. Therapeutic anti-FXa peak levels were achieved approximately 4 h after the first subcutaneous injection of 100 U/kg of reviparin sodium. The target therapeutic anti-FXa range of 0.5–1.0 U/mL was achieved in 75% of these children [9]. Currently, no data on therapeutic doses of reviparin sodium in infants weighing less than 5 kg are available.

   In a second study, a detailed pharmacodynamics assessment of prophylactic doses of reviparin sodium was made in nine children less than 5 kg and in ten children more than 5 kg [10]. After the first subcutaneous dose, peak anti-FXa levels were achieved at 1–4 h in children less than 5 kg, and at 2 h in children more than 5 kg. With a dose of 50 U/kg for children less than 5 kg and 30 U/kg for children more than 5 kg, peak anti-FXa levels of approximately 0.27 U/mL and trough levels of 0.13 U/mL were obtained [10].

II. EFFICACY AND SAFETY

Data on the efficacy and safety of LMWH in the pediatric population are currently available for enoxaparin (Rhone–Poulenc Rorer), reviparin sodium (Knoll Pharma, Inc.), and dalteparin (Pharmacia Upjohn). All three agents appear to be effective and safe prevention for and treatment of TEs in children.

Table 1   Studies on Efficacy and Safety of Enoxaparin in Pediatric Patients

Study ref.	N^a	New TEs[b]	Bleeding		
			Minor	Major	Fatal
Therapeutic doses					
7	23	0	0	2 (8.6%)	0
11	143	2 (1.3%)	26 (17%)	6 (4%)	1 (0.6%)
Prophylactic doses					
11	30	1 (3%)	2 (6.6%)	0	0
12	46	1 (2%)	5 (10%)	7 (15%)	0

[a]N, number of patients; [b]TEs, thromboembolic events.

A.   Enoxaparin

The efficacy and safety of therapeutic and prophylactic doses of enoxaparin have been evaluated in infants and children in three studies [7, 11–12]. The results of these studies are summarized in Table 1.

1.   Therapeutic Doses

In a prospective cohort study, therapeutic doses of enoxaparin were administered to 23 children with deep-vein thrombosis (DVT) or pulmonary embolism (PE), all of whom were at significant risk for bleeding because of underlying diseases, such as cancer or congenital heart disease. Enoxaparin was administered at a dose of 1 mg/kg every 12 h in children older than 2 months of age, and at an average dose of 1.6 mg/kg every 12 h in newborns and infants younger than 2 months of age. The duration of enoxaparin therapy, which depended on the indication for anticoagulation and the feasibility of initiating oral anticoagulation therapy with warfarin, ranged from a few days to more than 60 days. Of the 23 children entered in this study, 12 were given enoxaparin through an indewelling subcutaneous catheter (Insuflon; Viggo-Spectramed, Singapore). There were no episodes of recurrent TEs during treatment. Two children had bleeds from previously identified gastrointestinal ulcers and required blood transfusions (see Table 1) [7].

In another prospective cohort study, therapeutic doses of enoxaparin were administered to 143 children. Of these, approximately 33% were younger than 3 months of age, and 84% presented with serious underlying diseases or associated conditions such as cancer or congenital heart disease. Indications for enoxaparin therapy are reported in Figure 2. The observed mean

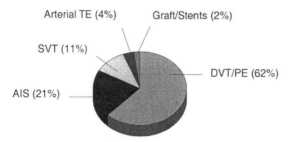

Figure 2   Indications for enoxaparin therapy in the study by Dix et al. [11]: DVT, deep-vein thrombosis; PE, pulmonary embolism; AIS, arterial ischemic stroke; SVT, sinovenous thrombosis; TE, thromboembolic event.

dose that achieved the target therapeutic anti-FXa range of 0.5–1.0 U/mL was 1.76 mg/kg every 12 h in infants younger then 2 months of age, and 1.05 mg/kg every 12 h in patients older then 2 months of age. Fifty percent of patients, including all of the neonates, received enoxaparin for 20 days or less. Eighty-seven percent of patients had enoxaparin administered through an indwelling subcutaneous catheter. Clinical resolution of TEs was reported in 94% of children receiving therapeutic doses of enoxaparin. Two patients (3%) had progression of TE despite treatment. Both were premature infants with multiple medical problems who had subtherapeutic anti-FXa levels at the time of TE extension. Clinically significant bleeding, including gastrointestinal bleeds, intracranial bleeds, and thigh hematomas at the Insuflon injection sites, occurred in seven (4%) patients. Intracranial bleeding occurred in two sick neonates with structural cerebral abnormalities, and at the site of a previous cerebral infarct in an infant with congenital heart disease. Thigh hematomas at the Insuflon injection sites occurred in two premature infants, both with a gestational age of less then 30 weeks. Minor bleeding, which included oozing from central venous line (CVL) sites, gastric tubes, and an abscess site, occurred in 26 (18%) patients (see Table 1) [11].

2. Prophylactic Doses

In a prospective cohort study, prophylactic doses of enoxaparin were administered to 30 children. Of these, 7% were younger than 3 months of age, and all presented with serious underlying diseases or associated conditions including cancer, congenital heart disease, renal disorders, surgery, or trauma. The observed mean enoxaparin dose that achieved the target prophylactic anti-FXa range of 0.1–0.3 U/mL was 0.83 mg/kg every 12 h in infants younger then 2 months of age, and 0.62 mg/kg every 12 h in patients older then 2 months of age. Forty-eight percent of patients received enoxaparin for 7 days or less. Sixty-four percent of patients had enoxaparin administered through a subcutaneous catheter. Symptomatic recurrence of TE occurred in one (3%) sick premature neonate who required multiple CVLs. There were no major bleeding complications, and minor bleeding, including oozing at the Insuflon site and epistaxis, occurred in two patients (see Table 1) [11].

In another study, prophylactic doses of enoxaparin were administered to 46 children with identified risk factors for venous TE following kidney transplantation. Enoxaparin was administered subcutaneously during pretransplant dialysis at a dose of 0.5 mg/kg and started again after grafting at a dose of 0.4 mg/kg with subsequent dose adjustment to achieve a target anti-FXa level of 0.2 U/mL. Historical controls were 73 consecutive patients undergoing kidney transplantation without enoxaparin prophylaxis in the year before the study. Only 1 patient given prophylactic enoxaparin developed graft failure owing to venous TE. In contrast, 9 children in the control group developed venous TEs after transplantation. Hemorrhagic complications occurred in 12 (26%) of 46 patients, and 7 required blood transfusion. Bleeding was mainly observed at the operative site and included perirenal, ureteral, and perivesical hematomas (see Table 1) [12].

B. Reviparin Sodium

Only prophylactic doses of reviparin sodium have been evaluated in children to-date [10,13]. Results of these studies are summarized in Table 2.

1. Prophylactic Doses

In a dose-finding and pharmadynamic study, 47 children with serious underlying disorders and a CVL in place received reviparin sodium subcutaneously at prophylactic doses of 30 U/kg every

Table 2   Studies on Efficacy and Safety of Prophylactic Doses of Reviparin Sodium in Pediatric Patients

Study ref.	N^a	Treatment	New TEs[b]	Bleeding		
				Minor	Major	Fatal
10	47	Reviparin sodium	No data	0	3 (6.3%)	0
13	78	Reviparin-sodium	11 (14%)	0	0	0
	80	Standard of care	10 (12.5%)	0	1 (1.2%)	0

[a]N, number of patients; [b], TEs thromboembolic events.

12 h for children older than 3 months of age, and 50 kg every 12 h for newborns and infants younger than 3 months of age. Clinically significant bleeding occurred in 5 patients. In 2 of 5 patients, bleeding episodes, which included epistaxis and intracardiac hemorrhage, were not related to reviparin sodium therapy because they occurred more then 3 weeks after discontinuation of the drug. The other three bleeding episodes, which included gastrointestinal bleed, an intracranial hemorrhage, and hemorrhage during cardiac surgery, occurred during reviparin prophylaxis, but were more likely related to the complex underlying disease of these patients (see Table 2) [10].

In a randomized controlled, multicenter trial (PROTEKT), 158 children with newly placed CVLs, aged between 3 months and 16 years, and weighing more than 5 kg were randomly assigned to either prophylactic doses of 30 U/kg of reviparin sodium given subcutaneously every 12 h or to standard of care. Venous TEs occurred in 11 (14.1%) of the 78 patients given reviparin sodium, and in 10 (12.5%) of the 80 control patients. Major bleeding occurred in only 1 patient randomized in the control arm (see Table 2) [13].

C.   Dalteparin

The efficacy and safety of therapeutic and prophylactic doses of dalteparin have been studied in infants and children in one study [14].

1.   Therapeutic Doses

Therapeutic doses of dalteparin were administered to 38 children with venous TEs (76%), arterial thrombosis (19%), pulmonary veno occlusive disease (2.5%), or primary pulmonary hypertension (2.5%). The target anti-FXa range was 0.4–1.0 U/mL, with doses administered every 12 h. A recanalization rate of 60% was observed in patients with TEs receiving primary antithrombotic therapy with dalteparin. Complete recanalization was proved by lung biopsy in the patient with pulmonary venoocclusive disease, while improvement of right heart function was observed in the patient with primary pulmonary hypertension [14].

2.   Prophylactic Doses

Prophylactic doses of dalteparin were administered to ten children with indications that included obesity, protein C deficiency, and cancer. The target anti-FXa range for prophylaxis with dalteparin was 0.2–0.4 U/mL, with doses administered every 12 h. There were no recurrent TEs. Only minor bleeding episodes, including recurrent epistaxis and hemorrhage after venipuncture, occurred in two (4%) patients, but no information is available on whether these bleeding episodes occurred in patients receiving therapeutic or prophylactic doses of dalteparin [14].

III. DOSAGE

Based on the previously described studies, the recommended therapeutic and prophylactic doses of enoxaparin, or reviparin sodium for children are listed in Table 3. Low-molecular-weight heparins can be administered by indwelling subcutaneous catheters that can remain in place for 7 days. Because they have little subcutaneous tissue, subcutaneous catheters should not be used in premature newborns.

IV. MONITORING

Low-molecular-weight heparins are monitored using anti-FXa levels.

A. Monitoring for Therapeutic Doses of LMWHs

Studies in adults indicate that unmonitored subcutaneous LMWH is as safe and effective as intravenous UFH for the treatment of DVT and PE [16–18]. In children, laboratory monitoring of therapeutic doses of LMWHs is more important because the clearance of LMWH is age- and weight-dependent so that newborns and young infants require higher doses than older children or adults. In addition, children with serious underlying disorders can develop renal insufficiency or acquired coagulopathies that may increase the risk of bleeding during LMWH therapy.

For treatment, the target therapeutic anti-FXa range is 0.5–1.0 U/mL. The anti-FXa level should be measured at 4 h after subcutaneous injection early in therapy, and after subsequent injections if dose-adjustments are required. Once the target anti-FXa range is achieved, anti-FXa levels should be monitored after 24 h, then 1 week later, and monthly thereafter. A nomogram for the adjustment of therapeutic doses of LMWHs is provided in Table 4.

B. Monitoring Prophylactic Doses of LMWHs

There is no need for monitoring when LMWHs are given in prophylactic doses. The anti-FXa range of 0.1–0.3 U/mL reflects values achieved in adults given prophylactic doses of LMWH.

V. INDICATIONS

LMWHs are increasingly being used for the treatment and prevention of TEs in children.

Table 3 Therapeutic and Prophylactic Doses of Enoxaparin and Reviparin Sodium in Pediatric Patients

	Therapeutic dose	Prophylactic dose
Enoxaparin		
Age < 2 months	1.5 mg/kg/dose q12h	0.75 mg/kg/dose q12h
Age > 2 months	1.0 mg/kg/dose q12h	0.50 mg/kg/dose q12h
Reviparin sodium		
Weight < 5 kg	150 U/kg/dose q12h	50 U/kg/dose q12h
Weight > 5 kg	100 U/kg/dose q12h	30 U/kg/dose q12h

U, units; kg, kilogram; mg, milligram; h, hours.
Source: Ref. 15.

Table 4 Nomogram for Monitoring LMWHs in Pediatric Patients

Antifactor Xa level (U/mL)	Hold next dose	Dose change	Repeat antifactor Xa level
< 0.35	—	Increase by 25%	4 h after next-morning dose
0.35–0.49		Increase by 10%	4 h after next-morning dose
0.5–1.0	—	—	Next day, then 1 week later and monthly thereafter while receiving reviparin sodium (at 4 h after AM dose)
1.1–1.5	—	Decrease by 20%	Before next-morning dose
1.6–2.0	3 h	Decrease by 30%	Before next-morning dose
>2.0	Until antifactor Xa is 0.5 U/mL	Decrease by 40%	Before next dose

Abbreviations: LMWHs, low-molecular-weight heparins; U, unit; mL, milliliter.
Source: Ref. 15.

A. Indications for Therapy with LMWHs

LMWHs are increasingly being used as an alternative to UFH and OA for the treatment of both venous and arterial TEs including PE, thrombosis of either the upper or lower venous system owing to indwelling central venous lines, renal vein thrombosis, sinovenous thrombosis, or arterial ischemic stroke in newborns and children [7–11,19].

1. Venous Thromboembolic Events

Venous TEs in pediatric patients are usually secondary complications of a primary illness or therapy. Ninety percent of neonatal venous TEs and approximately 60% of childhood venous TEs are associated with CVLs [20]. Idiopathic venous TEs occur in less than 1% of newborns, and in less than 5% of children [21–22]. Secondary venous TEs in children older than 2 months of age are initially treated with therapeutic doses of LMWH or UFH for 5–10 days, followed by 3 months of either therapeutic doses of LMWH or OA. Idiopathic venous TEs are treated with initial therapeutic doses of LMWH or UFH for 5–10 days, followed by at least 6 months of either therapeutic doses of LMWH or OA (see Tables 3, and 4). If OAs are used, they should be overlapped with LMWH until the international normalized ratio (INR) is therapeutic (2.0–3.0) on 2 consecutive days. Recommendations for treatment of patients with recurrent venous TEs include the administration of therapeutic doses of LMWH or OA for an indefinite period.

2. Venous Thromboembolic Events in Newborn

There is insufficient information to provide recommendations for the optimal use of antithrombotic agents in newborns. If LMWHs are used, one option is to administer treatment for 10–14 days to achieve anti-FXa levels at the low end of the target therapeutic range (see Tables 3 and 4). If the thrombus extends after discontinuation of short-term therapy, administration of LMWH for 3 months should be considered. In general, OA should be avoided in newborns.

3. Pulmonary Embolism

Pulmonary embolism in children often arises from DVT in the upper or central venous systems and is commonly related to indwelling CVLs [20]. Options for anticoagulation therapy include the administration of therapeutic doses of LMWH or UFH for 7–10 days, followed by either therapeutic doses of LMWH or OA for a minimum of 3 months. A longer course of treatment is given for more extensive PE (see Tables 3 and 4). If OA are used, they should be started after 1–2 days of therapeutic LMWH or UFH administration is completed.

4. Renal Vein Thrombosis

Renal vein thrombosis (RVT) is the most common noncatheter-related venous TE seen in infancy and is responsible for approximately 10% of all venous TEs in newborns [22]. Besides supportive care, anticoagulation therapy with LMWH or UFH should be considered for unilateral RVT that extends into the inferior vena cava, and for bilateral RVT (see Tables 3 and 4). If the patient has renal failure, UFH is preferable to LMWH because the latter is cleared by the kidneys.

5. Venous Thromboembolic Events in Nephrotic Syndrome

Children with relapsed, refractory, or untreated nephrotic syndrome are at risk for TEs. In these children, therapeutic doses of LMWH or OA should be considered, following the guidelines outlined in Tables 3 and 4.

6. Venous Thromboembolic Events in Systemic Lupus Erythematosus

Venous TEs in children with systemic lupus erythematosus can be treated initially with LMWHs or UFH, and subsequently with either LMWH or OA (see Tables 3 and 4). The duration of therapy depends on the persistence of antiphospholipid antibodies (APLA) and, to a lesser extent, the location of VTEs. Indefinite anticoagulant therapy with LMWH or OA is indicated as long as APLA are present. In children with recurrent TE in the setting of APLA, lifelong anticoagulant therapy with LMWH or OA is recommended.

7. Venous Thromboembolic Events During Bone Marrow Transplant

Successful treatment of venous TEs with therapeutic doses of LMWH has been reported in nine patients undergoing bone marrow transplant [23].

8. Thromboembolic Events Resulting from Peripheral Artery, Umbilical Artery, or Cardiac Catheterization

Arterial TEs in children usually occur secondary to arterial catheterizations. Thrombolytic therapy is given if extensive thrombosis compromises a limb or organ. Therapeutic doses of LMWH can be used after thrombolytic therapy or as primary therapy in those patients who are not candidates for thrombolysis (see Tables 3 and 4).

B. Indications for Prophylaxis with LMWHs

1. Homozygous Protein C Deficiency

Successful administration of long-term prophylactic doses of LMWH has been reported in two sisters with homozygous protein C deficiency [24].

2. Nephrotic Syndrome

Prophylactic doses of LMWH should be considered in children with uncontrolled nonminimal change nephrotic syndrome (see Table 3).

3. Hemodialysis in Children

LMWHs offer a safe and effective alternative to UFH for the prevention of TE complications in children undergoing hemodialysis [12,25]. In one crossover, dose-finding study in six children receiving chronic hemodialysis, LMWH administered at an initial bolus dose of 24 U/kg followed by an infusion of 15 U/kgh^{-1} was as safe and effective as UFH in preventing clotting in the extracorporal circuit [25]. In the other study, LMWH was administered to 46 children undergoing kidney transplantation at a dose of 0.5 mg/kg during the pretransplant dialysis, and at a dose of 0.4 mg/kg following grafting, with subsequent dose adjustment to achieve an anti-FXa level of 0.2 U/mL. Only 1.5% lost the kidney owing to a TE, as compared with an incidence of 12% in untreated patients. Minor bleeding occurred in 12 (26%) of the 46 patients [12].

4. Bone Marrow Transplant

LMWH thromboprophylaxis with a target anti-FXa range of 0.1–0.4 U/mL successfully prevented TEs in five patients undergoing bone marrow transplant [23].

VI. ADVERSE EFFECTS

Important adverse effects of LMWHs include hemorrhagic complications, osteoporosis, and HIT. Other rarer complications include allergic skin reactions, skin necrosis at the injection site, and hyperkalemia caused by hypoaldosteronism [26–28]. Recently, alopecia secondary to dalteparin therapy has been reported in a 9-year-old girl [29].

A. Hemorrhagic Complications

Metanalyses of several randomized clinical trials comparing the safety and efficacy of LMWHs and UFH for the prevention and treatment of DVT in adults suggest that LMWHs cause less bleeding than UFH [30,31]. In the largest pediatric study, major bleeding during LMWH therapy occurred in 4% of patients, a rate similar to that observed in adults or in children receiving UFH or OA [11,18].

In 1997, the U.S. Food and Drug Administration (FDA) Public Health Advisory noted that there was a small risk of spinal hematoma formation when prophylactic doses of LMWH were given to patients with epidural catheters. For children receiving therapeutic doses of LMWH who require lumbar puncture, two doses should be omitted, and an anti-FXa level should be obtained before the procedure.

1. Reversal of LMWH Therapy

Protamine sulfate completely neutralizes the anti-thrombin activity of LMWH, but reverses only 60–75% of the anti-FXa activity [32]. The affinity of LMWH for protamine is lower than that of UFH because LMWH has a reduced sulfate-charged density. Consequently, protamine does not bind to the smaller LMWH chains [33]. Despite the inability of protamine sulfate to completely neutralize the anti-FXa activity of LMWH, studies in animals suggest that protamine sulfate attenuates LMWH-induced bleeding [32]. The dose of protamine sulfate is based on the amount of LMWH received in the previous 8 h. Usually, 1 mg of protamine sulfate neutralizes 100 U of LMWH. Because LMWHs are administered subcutaneously, there will be ongoing LMWH delivery into the circulation. Consequently, protamine sulfate can be administered by repeated small doses or as a low-dose infusion.

2. Osteoporosis

Retrospective and case–control studies in adults suggest that LMWHs cause less osteoporosis than UFH [34,35]. Relatively little information on LMWH-induced osteoporosis in children is available. Two siblings with homozygous protein C deficiency continue to have normal bone density despite 3 years of subcutaneous LMWH prophylaxis [24].

3. Heparin-Induced Thrombocytopenia

Heparin-induced thrombocytopenia is a serious complication of heparin therapy caused by antibodies directed against heparin–platelet factor 4 complexes that activate platelets [36]. The incidence of HIT is less with LMWHs than UFH [37,38]. There are no data on the incidence of HIT with LMWH in children. LMWH should not be used in patients with established HIT. Two patients who developed HIT while receiving hemodialysis had progression of their disease when switched to dalteparin [39].

Currently, danaparoid sodium is the treatment of choice for children with HIT. Danaparoid sodium is administered at a 30 U/kg loading dose followed by an initial maintenance dose of 1.2–2.0 U/kgh^{-1}. The dose is then adjusted to achieve an anti-FXa level of 0.4–0.8 U/mL. Because danaparoid sodium is excreted by the kidneys, this drug is contraindicated in children with impaired renal function [40].

VII. CONCLUSIONS

Based on data now available, LMWHs have advantages over UFH and OA for the treatment and prevention of venous TEs in children. Results of ongoing large international clinical trials comparing LMWHs with UFH in children will provide more definitive data on the role of LMWHs in the pediatric population.

ACKNOWLEDGMENTS

This study was supported by a grant-in-aid from the Medical Research Council of Canada. M. Andrew is a career scientist of the Heart and Stroke Foundation of Canada. M. Albisetti is the recipient of a Stipendium zur Foerderung des Akademischen Nachwuchses of the University of Zuerich, Switzerland.

REFERENCES

1. Harenberg J. Pharmacology of low molecular weight heparins. Semin Thromb Hemost 1990; 16(suppl):12–18.
2. Jordan RE, Oosta GM, Gardner WT, Rosenberg RD. The kinetics of hemostatic enzyme–antithrombin interactions in the presence of low molecular weight heparin. J Biol Chem 1980; 255:10081–10090.

3. Andrew M, Vegh P, Johnston M, Bowker J, Ofosu F, Mitchell L. Maturation of the hemostatic system during childhood. Blood 1992; 80:1998–2005.
4. Vieira A, Berry L, Ofosu F, Andrew M. Heparin sensitivity and resistance in the neonate: an explanation. Thromb Res 1991; 63:85–98.
5. Andrew M, Ofosu F, Brooker LA, Buchanan MR. The comparison of the pharmacokinetics of a low molecular weight heparin in the newborn and adult pig. Thromb Res 1989; 56:529–539
6. Andrew M, Ofosu F, Schmidt B, Brooker LA, Hirsch J, Buchanan MR. Heparin clearance and ex vivo recovery in newborn piglets and adult pigs. Thromb Res 1988; 52:517–527.
7. Massicotte P, Adams M, Marzinotto V, Brooker LA, Andrew M. Low-molecular weight heparin in pediatric patients with thrombotic disease: a dose finding study. J Pediatr 1996; 128:313–318.
8. Punzalan RC, Hillery CA, Montgomery RR, Scott JP, Gill JC. Low-molecular weight heparin in thrombotic disease in children and adolescents. J Pediatr Hematol Oncol 2000; 22:137–142.
9. Massicotte MP, Adams M, Leaker M, Andrew M. A nomogram to establish therapeutic levels of the low molecular weight heparin (LMWH), clivarine in children requiring treatment for venous thromboembolism (VTE) [abstr]. Thromb Haemost 1997; (suppl):282.
10. Massicotte P, Marzinotto V, Julian J, Gent M, Shields K, Szechtman B, Chan AKC, Andrew M. Dose finding and pharmacokinetics of prophylactic doses of a low molecular weight heparin (reviparin) in pediatric patients [abstr]. Blood 1999; 94(suppl 1):27a.
11. Dix D, Andrew M, Marzinotto V, Charpentier K, Bridge S, Monagle P, deVeber G, Leaker M, Chan AKC, Massicotte P. The use of low molecular weight heparin in pediatric patients: A prospective cohort study. J Pediatr 2000; 136:439–445.
12. Broyer M, Gagnadoux MF, Sierro A, Fischer AM, Niaudet P. Preventive treatment of vascular thrombosis after kidney transplantation in children with low molecular weight heparin. Transplant Proc 1991; 23:1384–1395.
13. Andrew M, PROTEKT Investigators. A randomized control trial of low molecular weight heparin for the prevention of central venous line-related thrombotic complications in children: the PROTEKT trial [abstr]. 42nd Annual Meeting of the American Society of Hematology, San Francisco, CA, Dec 1–5, 2000.
14. Nohe N, Flemmer A, Ruemler R, Praum M, Auberger K. The low molecular weight heparin dalteparin for prophylaxis and therapy of thrombosis in childhood: a report on 48 cases. Eur J Pediatr 1999; 158(suppl 3):S134–S139.
15. Michelson AD, Bovill E, Monagle P, Andrew M. Antithrombotic therapy in children. Chest 1998; 114:748S–769S.
16. Levine MN, Gent M, Hirsh J, Leclerc J, Anderson D, Weitz J, Ginsberg J, Turpie AG, Demers C, Kovacs M. A comparison of low-molecular-weight heparin administered primarily at home with unfractionated heparin administered in the hospital for proximal deep-vein thrombosis. N Engl J Med 1996; 334:677–681.
17. Koopman MM, Prandoni P, Piovella F, Ockelford PA, Brabdjes DP, van der Meer J, Gallus AS, Simonneau G, Chesterman CH, Prins MH. Treatment of venous thrombosis with intravenous unfractionated heparin administered in the hospital as compared with subcutaneous low-molecular-weight heparin administered at home. The Tasman Study Group. N Engl J Med 1997; 334:682–687.
18. The Colombus Investigators. Low-molecular-weight heparin in the treatment of patients with venous thromboembolism. N Engl J Med 1997; 337:657–662.
19. deVeber G, Chan A, Monagle P, Marzinotto V, Armstrong D, Massicotte P, Leaker M, Andrew M. Anticoagulation therapy in pediatric patients with sinovenous thrombosis: a cohort study. Arch Neurol 1998; 55:1533–1537.
20. Massicotte MP, Dix D, Monagle P, Adams M, Andrew M. Central venous catheter related thrombosis in children: analysis of the Canadian Registry of Venous Thromboembolic Complications. J Pediatr 1998; 133:770–776.
21. Monagle P, Adams M, Mahoney M, Ali K, Barnard D, Bernstein M, Brisson L, David M, Desai S, Scully MF, Halton J, Israels S, Jardine L, Leaker M, McCusker P, Silva M, Wu J, Anderson R, Andrew M, Massicotte MP. Outcome of pediatric thromboembolic disease: a report from the Canadian Childhood Thrombophilia Registry. Pediatr Res 2000; 47:763–766.

22. Schmidt B, Andrew M. Neonatal thrombosis: report of a prospective Canadian and International registry. Pediatrics 1995; 96:939–943.

23. Dix D, Marzinotto V, Monagle P, Freedman M, Saunders EF, Doyle J, Calderwood S, Massicotte MP. Use of low molecular weight heparin (LMWH) for the management of venous thromboembolic disease (VTE) in children undergoing bone marrow transplant (BMT) [abstr]. 11th Annual Meeting of the American Society of Pediatric Hematology/Oncology, Chicago, II, Sept. 10–12, 1998.

24. Monagle P, Andrew M, Halton J, Marlar R, Jardine L, Vegh P, Johnston M, Webber C, Massicotte MP. Homozygous protein C deficiency: description of a new mutation and successful treatment with low molecular weight heparin. Thromb Haemost 1998; 79:756–761.

25. Fijnvandraat K, Nurmohamed MT, Peters M, Ploos van Amstel SLB, ten Cate JW. A cross-over dose finding study investigating a low molecular weight heparin (Fragmin) in six children on chronic hemodialysis [abstr]. Thromb Haemostas 1993; 69:649.

26. Harenberg J, Huhle G, Wang L, Hoffmann U, Bayerl C, Kerowgan M. Association of heparin-induced skin lesions, intracutaneous tests, and heparin-induced IgG. Allergy 1999; 54:473–477.

27. Fureder W, Kyrle PA, Gisslinger H, Lechner K. Low-molecular-weight heparin-induced skin necrosis. Ann Hematol 1998; 77:127–130.

28. Hottelart C, Achard JM, Moriniere P, Zoghbi F, Dieval J, Fournier A. Heparin-induced hyperkalemia in chronic hemodialysis patients: comparison of low molecular weight and unfractionated heparin. Artif Organs 1998; 22:614–617.

29. Barnes C, Deidun D, Hynes K, Monagle P. Alopecia and dalteparin: a previously unreported association [letter]. Blood 2000; 96:1618–1619.

30. Rocha E, Martinez–Gonzalez MA, Montes R, Panizo C. Do the low-molecular-weight heparins improve efficacy and safety of the treatment of deep venous thrombosis? A meta-analysis. Haematologica 2000; 85: 935–942.

31. Mismetti P, Laporte–Simitsidis S, Tardy B, Cucherat M, Buchmuller A, Juillard–Delsart D, Decousus H. Prevention of venous thromboembolism in internal medicine with unfractionated or low-molecular-weight heparins: a meta-analysis of randomized clinical trials. Thromb Haemost 2000; 83:14–19.

32. Van Ryn–McKenna J, Cai L, Ofosu FA, Hirsh J, Buchanan MR. Neutralization of enoxaparine-induced bleeding by protamine sulfate. Thromb Haemost 1990; 63:271–274.

33. Berry L, Crowther M, Pawlowski E, Chan AKC. Incomplete neutralization of low-molecular-weight heparin by protamine results from decreased binding affinity [abstr]. Thromb Haemost 1999; (suppl):451–452.

34. Melissari E, Parker CJ, Wilson NV, Monte G, Kanthou C, Pemberton KD, Nicolaides KH, Barrett JJ, Kakkar VV. Use of low-molecular-weight heparin in pregnancy. Thromb Haemost 1992; 68:652–656.

35. Shefras J, Farquharson RG. Bone density studies in pregnant women receiving heparin. Obstet Gynecol 1996; 65:171–174

36. Warkentin TE, Chong BH, Greinacher A. Heparin-induced thrombocytopenia: towards consensus. Thromb Haemost 1998; 79:1–7.

37. Warkentin TE. Heparin-induced thrombocytopenia:pathogenesis, frequency, avoidance and management. Drug Safety 1997; 17:325–341.

38. Warkentin TE, Levine MN, Hirsh J, Horsewood P, Roberts RS, Gent M, Kelton JG. Heparin-induced thrombocytopenia in patients with low-molecular-weight heparin or unfractionated heparin. N Engl J Med 1995; 332:1330–1335.

39. Neuhaus TJ, Goetschel P, Schmugge M, Leumann E. Heparin-induced thrombocytopenia type II on hemodialysis: Switch to danaparoid. Pediatr Nephrol 2000; 14:713–716.

40. Andrew M, deVeber G. Pediatric thromboembolism and stroke protocols. 2nd ed. Hamilton: BC Decker, 1999.

11

New Indications for Low-Molecular-Weight Heparins

Omer Iqbal, Debra A. Hoppensteadt, Sarfraz Ahmad, Harry L. Messmore, and
Jawed Fareed
Loyola University Medical Center, Maywood, Illinois, U.S.A.

SUMMARY

Heparin is commonly used for anticoagulation; however, its nonanticoagulant effects such as the anti-inflammatory and antiproliferative actions have been known for some time. As a polycomponent drug, heparin produces multiple effects at cellular and humoral levels. Its ability to release and modulate the generation of endogenously active substances has also been known for many years. Heparin's interactions with endogenous proteins and vascular cells are also widely appreciated. The development of low-molecular-weight heparin (LMWH) represents an improved usage of heparin-derived sulfated polymers with improved pharmacological profiles. Initially developed for the prophylaxis of deep-vein thrombosis (DVT), these drugs have found their applications in thrombotic, cardiovascular, hemodynamic, proliferative, and autoimmune disorders, to name a few indications. The clinical profiles of intravenous and subcutaneously administered LMWHs differ from unfractionated heparin (UFH) owing to their biochemical and pharmacological profiles. Because of their size, the LMWHs exhibit better vascular and cellular uptake; easy accessibility to the membrane barriers; and are capable of interacting with growth factors and other cytokines. Clinical trials designed to test the efficacy of these agents in the prophylaxis and treatment of thrombosis reveal added benefits of these drugs in patients with cancer, autoimmune diseases, sepsis, and hemodynamic disorders. Experimental investigations also demonstrated several nonanticoagulant effects of these drugs, paving their way into the management of nonthrombotic disorders. The LMWHs are now being tested in several clinical trials for such indications as thrombotic stroke, vascular dementia, inflammatory bowel disease, malignancy, autoimmune diseases, and bone–marrow-associated vascular disorders. The safety and efficacy of these drugs in the elderly, in pregnant women, the pediatric population, and weight-compromised individuals have also been established. Thus, LMWHs will provide not only an antithrombotic drug group with higher therapeutic index, but will be gradually developed in expanded indications that may include nonthrombotic diseases.

I. INTRODUCTION

Heparin was first discovered by a medical student Jay McClean in 1916 while he was studying the procoagulant actions of phospholipids [1]. Howell and Holt named this substance heparin [2]. They purified the material [3] and published a detailed report about its chemical and physiological actions [4]. It was first used clinically in 1937 by Crafoord, a Swedish surgeon who used heparin as an anticoagulant in patients suffering from postoperative pulmonary emboli [5]. Through chemical and enzymatic depolymerization of the benzylic esters of porcine mucosal heparin, a new class of antithrombotic drugs was developed in Europe in the 1980s, the *low-molecular-weight heparins* (LMWHs). These compounds have several advantages over conventionally used unfractionated heparin (UFH). LMWHs, besides inhibiting factors Xa and IIa, releasing tissue factor pathway inhibitor (TFPI), tissue plasminogen activator (t-PA), and modulating cellular adhesion molecules, also have greater than 90% bioavailability. In 1993, the first LMWH, enoxaparin, was approved by the U.S. Food and Drug Administration (FDA), solely for prophylaxis in elective hip replacement surgery.

The currently available commercial LMWHs are produced by enzymatic or chemical depolymerization of unfractionated heparin, as depicted in Figure 1.

Because of their heterogeneous nature, both the UFH and LMWHs exhibit multiple biochemical and pharmacological effects that involve cellular and humoral sites. Figure 2 depicts the polycomponent effects of these drugs. In addition to the anticoagulant effects, the LMWHs produce profibrinolytic effects by virtue of plasminogen activator inhibitor-1 (PAI-1) and thromboin activatable fibrinolytic inhibitor (TAFI) down-regulation. These agents also produce heparan-sparing effects in the regulation of cellular function. LMWHs produce endothelial modulation, and release prostacyclin, and tissue factor pathway inhibitor. Heparins also have certain effects at the regulatory level. Because of their strong anionic nature, these agents strongly interact with growth factors, modulate the expression of adhesion molecules, and inhibit heparanases. The oligosaccharide components of LMWHs also pass endogenous barriers, form complexes with macromolecules and cellular sites, and may potentially glycosylate endogenous macromolecules. This wide spectrum of activities contributes to the polypharmacological nature of heparins. Thus, the nonanticoagulant actions observed with these drugs may be related to their direct and indirect effects on various pathological processes. Because of these added actions, the LMWHs have found novel and expanded indications.

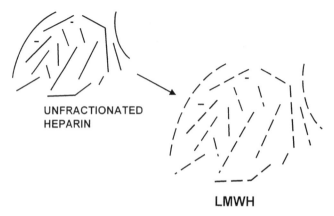

UNFRACTIONATED
HEPARIN

LMWH

Figure 1 Depolymerization of heparin to manufacture LMWHs: chemical, enzymatic, radiation, and ultrasonication methods are used to prepare these drugs, coupled with the manufacturing patent; each of the resulting LMWHs exhibits a distinct molecular and pharmacological profile.

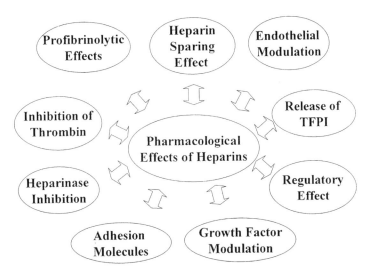

Figure 2 Pharmacological spectrum of heparins: besides producing the antithrombotic and anticoagulant effects, LMWHs produce several additional effects, which may contribute to their wide therapeutic spectrum.

1. For prevention of deep-vein thrombosis (DVT) that may lead to pulmonary embolism (PE)

    a. In patients undergoing hip-replacement surgery [6,7].
    b. For extended prophylaxis in hip replacement [8,9].
    c. In patients undergoing knee replacement surgery [10–12].
    d. In patients undergoing abdominal surgery who are at risk for thromboembolic complications [13].

2. For the treatment of acute deep-vein thrombosis (DVT), with or without pulmonary embolism (PE)

    a. For patients who can be treated at home for acute DVT without PE, in conjunction with warfarin sodium therapy [14].
    b. For hospitalized patients with acute DVT, with or without PE, in conjunction with warfarin sodium therapy [15].

3. For unstable angina and non–Q-wave myocardial infarction. For the prevention of ischemic complications of unstable angina and non–Q-wave myocardial infarction when concurrently administered with aspirin [16].

4. In geriatrics: Prophylaxis in elderly patients with venous risk factors [17].

II. THE ROLE OF LMWHs IN CARDIOLOGY AND CARDIOVASCULAR SURGERY

The LMWHs play a substantial role in the treatment of coronary arterial thrombotic disorders and may be superior to unfractionated heparin. LMWHs by inhibiting FXa, prevent the generation of thrombin. Bendetowicz et al. have shown decreased thrombin generation in platelet-rich plasma by enoxaparin [18]. It has also been reported by Melandri et al. that LMWHs can suppress thrombin activity even in the presence of activated platelets [19]. LMWHs cause less platelet activation and are less neutralized by platelet factor 4 when compared with UFH [20]. The anticoagulant activity of LMWH is not influenced by the presence of acute-phase proteins present in high concentrations following an acute thrombotic episode, such as histidine-rich glycoproteins, vitronectin, fibronectin, and von Willebrand's factor (vWF). UFH and LMWHs release TFPI that inactivates the TF-VIIa–Xa complex to promote an antithrombotic effect [21]. Furthermore, the enhanced anti-Xa/anti-IIa ratio, better bioavailability, predictable anticoagulant response, convenient dosing schedule, and potential of outpatient management of LMWHs, provide options for their therapeutic use superior to those of UFH. Five large clinical trials (FRISC, FRIC, FRAXIS, ESSENCE, TIMI 11B) have shown the efficacy and safety of three LMWHs—enoxaparin, dalteparin, and nadroparin—in the treatment of UA/NQWMI [22–26]. Enoxaparin has demonstrated superiority over UFH in preventing the composite triple endpoints of death: MI; the need for revascularization, without an increase in the risk of major bleeding events; and maintaining the clinical outcome for 1 year. ESSENCE and TIMI11B also showed equivalent clinical benefit with enoxaparin, without any increased risk of major bleeding events. There was a 20% reduction in death and serious cardiac ischemic events in a metanalysis of the data from ESSENCE and TIMI11B. Other LMWHs, such as dalteparin and nadroparin in similar trials, did not show any superiority over UFH. However, differences in trial designs and study populations may have a substantial effect over study outcome and prevent direct comparisons between different drugs.

The FRISC II trial results [27] demonstrated an initial beneficial effect of prolonged treatment with twice-daily regimen of dalteparin, in addition to aspirin, in patients with unstable angina, who were managed with a noninvasive approach. To maintain these benefits, a coronary procedure is needed in most patients [28]. Dalteparin, at a subcutaneous dosage of 120 IU/kg b.i.d. (to a maximum of 10,000 IU), and enoxaparin, at a similar dosage of 1 mg/kg are approved for use in the acute phase of unstable coronary artery disease (CAD) [29,30]. These dosages provided a median AXa level at the trough of 0.5 IU/L for dalteparin [31] and 0.6 IU/L for enoxaparin. These doses are said to be the maximum tolerated, considering the increased bleeding rates when higher doses of both of these agents are used [29,32]. Because women at body-weight-adjusted, doses had higher anti-Xa levels and a higher incidence of bleeding than men in FRISC II, the doses were not only body–weight-adjusted, but also gender-adjusted. In FRISC II, dalteparin was used for long-term treatment on an outpatient basis. In this setting the proved dose of dalteparin was 7500 IU in men of more than 70 kg and women of more than 80 kg and 5000 IU in other patients [27]. Smoking could also influence the response to LMWHs by causing lower anti-Xa levels and lower risk of bleeding [31]. As patients with renal impairment were excluded from the clinical trials, caution was necessary to adjust the dosage in older patients with renal dysfunction.

Reactivation of the acute coronary syndrome after cessation of heparin treatment has been observed in several trials of unstable CAD in which UFH, LMWHs, and direct thrombin inhibitors were used. This may be due to the waning of the protective effect, which seems to last only as long as there is adequate thrombin inhibition. Hence, there is an increased event rate after cessation of UFH, as observed in some trials [29,33,34]. In the TRIM trial [34], there was a pronounced increase of MI and refractory angina during 24 h after cessation of the 72-h FH infusion in unstable CAD patients managed noninvasively. The FRISC trial also demonstrated a similar phenomenon. However, other trials did not exhibit this phenomenon of reactivation after cessation of heparin treatment. This may be due to reactivation of the coagulation activity at the plaque rupture site with cessation of thrombin inhibition [35] and to less activation of protein C by thrombomodulin [36]. Several ongoing trials are evaluating the addition of GPIIb/IIIa inhibitors in combination with LMWH and aspirin.

Gran et al. have investigated the use of LMWHs in extracorporeal circuits, including hemodialysis and cardiopulmonary bypass [37]. In acute and chronic hemodialysis, LMWHs are generally well tolerated, with relatively few incidences of clotting within the extracorporeal circuit or of major hemorrhagic events. Dieval et al. have shown some accumulation of anti-Xa activity with some preparations [38].

III. LMWHs IN PTCA

LMWHs are increasingly being used before percutaneous (PTCA) in patients with unstable angina [39]. In a randomized pilot trial of 60 patients undergoing percutaneous coronary intervention (PCI), no difference in safety between intravenous UFH or enoxaparin (1 mg/kg) was observed [40]. This study was a pilot to the NICE-1 study that included 800 patients to test the safety of intravenous enoxaparin (1 mg/kg) in patients undergoing PCI [41]. In addition, Kereiakes et al. have published on the use of dalteparin at 40 and 60 U/kg intravenously in PCI [42]. As per the recommendations of the Sixth American College of Chest Physicians Consensus Conference on Antithrombotic Drugs, routine substitution of LMWH for UFH still cannot be recommended.

IV. LMWHs TO PREVENT RESTENOSIS FOLLOWING PTCA

In one study using a 2×2 factorial design, 814 patients were randomly assigned to treatment with omega-3 fatty acid supplementation (5.4 g daily), enoxaparin 30 mg twice daily, both, or neither [43]. No differences were observed among the four treatment groups in a 6-month angiographic assessment of minimal lumen diameters. The effects of other antithrombins, in addition to enoxaparin, were also studied [44–47]. In a randomized trial, 458 patients were randomly assigned to treatment with either enoxaparin (40-mg daily by subcutaneous injection) or placebo, for 1 month after angioplasty. There was no difference in angiographic restenosis (follow-up diameter stenosis: 43 and 45%, respectively) on clinical restenosis (e.g., freedom from death, infarction, revascularization, unstable angina, or asymptomatic angiographic narrowing), in 40% of patients in both groups [46].

V. COMBINATION OF LMWH AND GPIIb/IIIa INHIBITOR IN PCI

The National Investigators collaborating on Enoxaparin-3 (NICE-3) Trial was a prospective, nonrandomized trial designed to establish the relative bleeding safety of the concomitant use of enoxaparin with a GPIIb/IIIa inhibitor, abciximab, eptifibatide, or tirofiban, and to determine the safety of bringing the patients to the catheterization laboratory while receiving combination therapy. The results showed that the overall non-CABG major bleeding rate was 1.9%, death 0.3%, MI 3.4%, urgent target vessel revascularization 2.1%, and the composite 5.7%. In addition, NICE-4 compared the use of a reduced dose of enoxaparin (0.75 mg/kg) in combination with a standard dose of abciximab in PCI [41]. The results of this study demonstrated that enoxaparin was capable of keeping the patients anticoagulated through the PCI procedure without any bleeding or other major complications. These results, which compare favorably with those in previous studies, show that enoxaparin can be used safely as adjunctive therapy with GPIIb/IIIa inhibitors. The investigators reported that the study provided a useful experience on how to make the transition from a hospital floor or intensive care unit to the catheterization laboratory laboratory when treating with a combination of enoxaparin and GPIIb/IIIa inhibitors.

VI. LMWHs IN THROMBOTIC STROKE

Because the pathophysiology of cerebrovascular disease is similar to that of the acute coronary syndrome, it was thought that LMWHs may have a beneficial role in the management of ischemic stroke. Given this hypothesis, several trials were performed. These included the International Stroke Trial (IST) [47], the Chinese Acute Stroke Trial (CAST) [48], the TOAST Trial [49], the Hong Kong Fraxiparin in Stroke Study (FISS) Trial [50], the Fraxiparin in Stroke-2 (FISS–BISS) Trial with nadroparin [51] and the Tinzaparin in Acute Ischemic Stroke Trial (TAIST), which recently completed enrollment.

VII. LMWHs IN INFLAMMATORY BOWEL DISEASE

The pathogenesis of inflammatory bowel disease (IBD) is still not well understood. The role of heparin in IBD, particularly in ulcerative colitis has been previously reported [52]. An interplay between growth factors and cell adhesion molecules is required for tissue repair. Inflammation disturbs this normal healing process of mucosal restitution owing to loss of growth factors, cell adhesion molecules, or both. The hypothesized mechanism of action of heparin in IBD, besides its anticoagulant effects, includes the restoration of high-affinity receptor binding by basic fibroblast growth factors that act as an antiulcerogenic in the presence of coreceptors such as heparan sulfate proteoglycans, syndecan-1. In the ulcerated mucosa of patients with IBD, there is loss of syndecan-1, which leads to impaired binding of fibroblast growth factor and, as a result, impaired healing. It is hypothesized that heparin increases the rate of mucosal restitution by restoring high-affinity receptor binding of basic fibroblast growth factor [53]. Heparin has achieved clinical remission, particularly in normal stool frequency; no rectal bleeding; with a success rate of 66–90% [52,54–56]; normalization of concentrations of TNF-α [57]; decreased C-reactive protein [58]; and resolution of pyoderma gangrenosum [58] and erythema nodosum [59]. In a Russian study, a reduction in the rate of colectomy for severe colitis from 19.4 to 6.2% was reported [60].

Unfractionated heparin having anticoagulant and anti-inflammatory properties has been used earlier to treat IBD particularly ulcerative colitis (61,62). A hypercoagulable state, with histopathological findings of microthrombi and multifocal gastroenterological infarcts, exists in cases of ulcerative colitis [63,64]. There are several studies involving the use of heparin in IBD. However, in one uncontrolled study, dalteparin, a LMWH, has been used as adjuvant therapy in cases with ulcerative colitis [65,66]. Recently, an ultra-LMWH, OP2000 (Incara) is in phase II/III clinical trials for evaluation of its use in IBD. OP2000 is nearly 100% bioavailable, when administered subcutaneously, with a very wide volume of distribution. It has fewer anti-IIa effects, suggesting a decreased hemorrhagic potential, however, it retains its anti-Xa effects. OP2000, with its unique anticoagulant features, is a promising drug in the management of IBD. The results of phase II and III clinical trials are much awaited. Heparin has recently been shown to attenuate TNF-α–induced inflammatory response through a CD11b-dependent mechanism [67]. It is now understood that heparin has anti-inflammatory actions, including modulation of some of the pathophysiological effects of endotoxin and TNF-α, such as neutrophil migration, edema formation, pulmonary hypertension, and hypoxemia [68,69]. Heparin also suppresses selected neutrophil functions, such as superoxide generation [70] and chemotaxis in vitro

[71,72], to reduce eosinophil migration [73] and to diminish vascular permeability [74]. Binding of glycosaminoglycans to adhesion molecules expressed on the surface of activated endothelial cells or leukocytes are some of the proposed mechanisms of action of heparin. Heparin effectively binds to endothelial P-selectin, but not E-selectin [69,75], L-selectin, or CD11b/CD18 expressed on neutrophils [76,77]. It has been suggested in studies in rats that the anti-inflammatory action of heparin is not dependent on its anticoagulant properties. A dosage of heparin that exhibited maximum inhibition of the inflammatory response to TNF-α, did not significantly prolong the aPTT. Hence, it may be possible to administer heparin at doses capable of achieving anti-inflammatory activity, without increasing the risk of bleeding, in IBD patients [67].

VIII. LMWH IN SEPSIS

More than 40 clinical trials using multiple anti-inflammatory agents in excess of 14,000 patients with sepsis have provided convincing evidence that these anti-inflammatory agents have a beneficial effect in sepsis. Following this, a series of studies showed that inhibition of various inflammatory mediators, including interleukin (IL)-1 and platelet-activating factor (PAF), may provide better outcome in the sepsis models [78]. However, no single anti-inflammatory agent has demonstrated consistent benefit in human clinical trials [79–81]. Proinflammatory mediators, such as TNF-α and IL-1, produce a clinical picture that mimics bacterial septic shock [82–84]. Salas has recently demonstrated that heparin attenuates TNF-α–induced inflammatory response through a CD11b-dependent mechanism [67]. TNF-α also plays a pivotal role in the pathophysiology of IBD. In addition, heparins and LMWHs have the unique characteristic of releasing tissue factor pathway inhibitor (TFPI) from the endothelium. TFPI is a naturally occurring anticoagulant that also has anti-inflammatory properties. The other concept in sepsis is the release of thrombin-activatable fibrinolysis inhibitor (TAFI) which promotes fibrinolytic deficit and clotting. As the name suggests TAFI is thrombin activatable; hence, whenever there is generation of thrombin, TAFI is secreted. Heparin and LMWHs and other antithrombin agents can lower the levels of thrombin in the body so that TAFI is not released. Thus, down-regulation of thrombin may play a beneficial role in the septic process.

IX. LMWH IN BONE-MARROW TRANSPLANTATION-ASSOCIATED VENO-OCCLUSIVE DISEASE

Veno-occlusive disease (VOD) is a complication following allogeneic and autologous hematopoietic cell transplantations. The incidence varies from center to center, depending on the diagnostic criteria used. It is important to identify risk factors associated with disease progression and death in patients who develop clinical features of VOD. In one study, risk factors associated with the development of severe VOD at different times following bone marrow transplantation have been documented. Several studies have evaluated the use of recombinant tissue-type plasminogen activator t-PA and heparin based on the hypothesis of vascular endothelial damage, hypercoagulability, and clotting. These studies show a 30–40% incidence of hemorrhage and, as a result, a combination of t-PA and heparin is not advised. Defibrotide, a polydeoxyribonucleotide derived from mammalian tissue has many antithrombotic and fibrinolytic properties. Defibrotide also has a unique characteristic of releasing TFPI from the endothelium, as was found in a study of 19 patients with severe VOD and multiorgan dysfunction [85]; a larger study is in progress. Antithrombin III concentrates have also been used in ten patients with severe VOD who had antithrombin III levels of less than 88% of normal; clinical improvement was observed in all patients 1–10 days after beginning therapy [86]. In a prospective, randomized clinical trial of 161 patients who underwent allogeneic or autologous hematopoietic cell transplantation, a lower incidence of VOD, without any increase in the bleeding risk, was noted in the heparin-treated group [87,88]. LMWHs have shown a lower incidence of VOD in a pilot study of 61 patients undergoing bone marrow transplantation who were randomized to receive enoxaparin, 40 mg/day, or placebo [89].

X. LMWH IN ANTIPHOSPHOLIPID SYNDROME

The antiphospholipid (aPL) syndrome is an acquired disorder in which patients develop thrombosis with laboratory evidence of autoantibodies that recognize anionic phospholipid–protein complexes. It is considered to be secondary when this disorder is associated with systemic lupus erythematosus (SLE) or other major autoimmune disorders, and primary in their absence. Clinically, there can be vascular thrombosis or embolism and recurrent spontaneous pregnancy losses. Proposed pathogenic mechanisms include aPL antibody-mediated disruption of the annexin-V anticoagulant shield, altered eicosanoid synthesis, injury to endothelium, induction of receptors for cell adhesion molecules on endothelium, increase of endothelin, expression of tissue factor on monocytes and on endothelial cells, interference with protein C pathway, increase of plasminogen activator inhibitor 1, impairment of autoactivation of factor XII, and reduced fibrinolysis and platelet activation. Patients with spontaneous thromboembolism should be treated with long-term oral anticoagulants. Patients with catastrophic aPL may be refractory to anticoagulation alone. Women with pregnancy loss who have evidence of aPL antibodies should be treated with low-dose aspirin and UFH 5000 U given subcutaneously every 12 h [90–92]. The benefits of LMWHs include once-daily injections, a decreased rate of allergic reactions, and decreased bone loss, when compared with UFH.

XI. LMWHs IN DISSEMINATED INTRAVASCULAR COAGULATION

Thrombin is generated when procoagulants are introduced or produced in the blood, which can lead to disseminated intravascular coagulation (DIC). Patients experience multiorgan dysfunction, caused by microthrombi, and bleeding, caused by consumption of platelets, fibrinogen, factor V, factor VII, and secondary fibrinolysis. The most common trigger of DIC is tissue factor (TF) exposure to blood. Although heparin in DIC patients did not show a reduction in mortality, it has improved the levels of hemostatic factors in the treated patients [93]. Heparin may be beneficial in some categories of chronic DIC (e.g., metastatic carcinomas, purpura fulminans, dead fetus syndrome, and aortic aneurysm). However, heparin or LMWH should be used cautiously in these conditions. In chronic DIC, a continuous infusion of heparin, 500–750 U/h may be sufficient. In mismatched transfusion, amniotic fluid embolism, septic abortion, or purpura fulminans, an intravenous bolus administration of 5,000–10,000 U of heparin may be given. In some conditions a continuous infusion of 500–1000 U/h may be necessary for maintaining the beneficial response. In patients with purpura fulminans, full heparinization may be beneficial [94,95].

XII. LMWHs IN EXTRACORPOREAL CIRCUITS AND HEMODIALYSIS

Extracorporeal circulation needs anticoagulation to prevent activation of the coagulation system by the tubing system and membranes. Without anticoagulation there will be deposition of fibrin clots, eventually leading to thrombotic obstruction. The administration of UFH may occasionally cause heparin-induced thrombocytopenia (HIT), but it may also cause bleeding. LMWHs have provided convincing evidence that they are as effective as UFH [96,97]. LMWHs may be considered in patients with HIT undergoing cardiopulmonary bypass surgery. Convincing evidence exists that in hemodialysis patients LMWHs at least have efficacy and safety similar to that of UFH. Besides, there is a less frequent incidence of HIT and other adverse effects. The very important advantage of LMWHs in long-term hemodialysis patients is the efficacy of a predialysis bolus injection without the need for monitoring. Further studies to evaluate the safety of LMWHs in hemodialysis patients with a high bleeding risk are necessary.

XIII. LMWHs IN ALZHEIMER'S DISEASE

Heparin oligosaccharides are reported to pass through the blood–brain barrier and inhibit [β]-amyloid precursor protein secretion and heparin binding to [β]-amyloid peptide [98]. Heparan sulfate can promote amyloid formation under pathological conditions that are dependent on its interaction with Aβ-peptide [99–100] or with the Aβ-precursor protein (APP) [101,102]. It was thought that compounds that can cross the blood–brain barrier and inhibit the binding of heparan sulfate with the Aβ-peptide or APP may interfere with endogenous heparan sulfate, and these are likely to have a potential therapeutic advantage in Alzheimer's disease. Beatrice et al. have demonstrated that LMWH derivatives can cross the blood–brain barrier in an in vitro cell culture model, and they also have the ability to interfere with the binding of heparin to Aβ-peptide [98]. Overproduction of APP and an increase of the [β]-amyloidogenic cleavage of this protein were earlier reported to be part of the pathogenic process of amyloid formation in Alzheimer's disease [103,104]. LMWH sulfated compounds, such as heparin disaccharides, prevent the aggregation of Aβ-fibrils and can also inhibit amyloidogenesis by inhibiting the overproduction and amyloidogenic cleavage of APP [98].

XIV. LMWHs: OTHER POTENTIAL NOVEL INDICATIONS

Heparins, and possibly LMWHs, inhibit the replication and infectivity of some viruses. Viruses have been thought to contribute to the development of atherosclerosis in humans and have been identified in the atherosclerotic vascular walls. Also, inflammatory processes play a role in the development of atherosclerosis. Heparins and LMWHs could possibly exert an anti-inflammatory action based on the release of TFPI. There is as yet no convincing evidence from virus-enhanced experimental atherosclerosis.

As per the Sixth American College of Chest Physicians (ACCP) Consensus Conference on Antithrombotic Therapy, held in February 2000, for intracranial prophylaxis in neurosurgery, low-dose UFH or postoperative LMWH may be acceptable alternatives (grade 2A), and for trauma with identifiable risk factor for thromboembolism, prophylaxis with LMWH is recommended when considered safe. In acute spinal cord injury, prophylaxis with LMWH is recommended (grade 1B) and in the rehabilitation phase, continued LMWH therapy or full-dose oral anticoagulation is recommended (grade 1C). Very few cases of intraspinal hematomas that occur during prophylaxis with LMWH have been reported after a procedure of combined lumbar spinal and epidural anesthesia [105]. However, Schwander and Bachman found no complications related to intraspinal bleedings after spinal/epidural anesthesia in almost 14,000 patients who received LMWH for thromboprophylaxis [106]. Yet, in the United States, LMWHs are contraindicated during spinal/epidural anesthesia. Arterial thrombotic complications in patients with peripheral arterial occlusive disease (PAOD) can be prevented by prolonged prophylaxis with LMWHs. However, neither the group of patients who will benefit from this long-term prophylaxis, nor the adequate dose or duration have yet been determined.

The role of LMWHs in acute coronary syndrome, cancer, pregnancy, pediatrics, and venous thromboembolism has been discussed already in different chapters.

XV. CONCLUSIONS

Low-molecular-weight heparins are meeting the expectations of the physicians in the realm of their established indications. There are scores of novel indications for which LMWHs may be potentially used. Although, LMWHs are not officially approved for these indications, the preliminary data now available provide convincing evidence for their beneficial role. The role of LMWHs in the management of venous thromboembolism in cancer patients seems quite promising. The pivotal role of TNF-α in the pathophysiology of inflammatory bowel disease and the effects of heparins and LMWHs in attenuating TNF-α-induced inflammatory response through a CD11b-dependent mechanism, provides convincing evidence for the use of LMWHs in IBD and other inflammatory disorders. Low-molecular-weight sulfated compounds such as heparin disaccharides, can pass through the blood–brain barrier and have prevented the aggregation of Aβ-fibrils and can also inhibit amyloidogenesis by inhibiting the overproduction and amyloidogenic cleavage of APP. By virtue of these characteristics these compounds have a promising role in treatment of Alzheimer's disease. LMWHs may be used in conjunction with various GPIIb/IIIa inhibitors, antithrombin drugs and thrombolytic agents.

Despite several attempts to replace heparin, it has always stood the test of time. Both basic scientists and the clinicians are amazed at the enormous potential of heparins. Low-molecular-weight heparins may be used in all the indications for which unfractionated heparin is used, as well as the scores of other novel indications for which it has a promising future.

REFERENCES

1. McClean J: The discovery of heparin. Circulation 1959; 19:75–78.
2. Howell WH, Holt E. The purification of heparin and its chemical and physiologic reactions. Bull Johns Hopkins Hosp 1928; 42:199–207.
3. Howell WH, Holt E. The purification of heparin and its presence in the blood. Am J Physiol 1925; 71:533–559.
4. Howell WH, Holt E. Two new factors in blood coagulation. heparin and proantithrombin. Am J Physiol 1918; 47:328–334.
5. Crafoord C. Preliminary report on post-operative treatment with heparin as a preventive of thrombosis. Acta Chirur Scand 1937; 79:407–426.
6. Turpie AGGG, Levine MN, Hirsh J et al. A randomized controlled trial of a low molecular weight heparin (enoxaparin) to prevent deep vein thrombosis in patients undergoing elective hip surgery. N Engl J Med 1986; 315:925–929.
7. Spiro TE, Colwell CW. Efficacy and safety of enoxaparin for the prevention of deep vein thrombosis after hip replacement surgery. Orthop Rev 1994; (suppl 1):47–55.

8. Planes A, Vochelle N, Darmon JY et al. Risk of deep vein thrombosis after hospital discharge in patients having undergone total hip replacement: double-blind randomized comparison of enoxaparin versus placebo. Lancet 1996; 348:224–228.

9. Bergquist D, Benoni J, Bjorgell O, et al. Low molecular weight heparin (enoxaparin) as prophylaxis against venous thromboembolism after total hip replacement N Engl J Med 1996; 335:696–700.

10. Colwell CW Jr, Spiro TE, Trowbridge AA, et al. Efficacy and safety of enoxaparin versus unfractionated heparin for prevention of deep vein thrombosis after elective knee arthroplasty. Clin Orthop Rel Res 1995; 321:19–27.

11. Leclerc JR, Geerts WH, Desjardins L, et al. Prevention of deep vein thrombosis after major knee surgery—a randomized, double-blind trial comparing a low molecular weight heparin fragment (enoxaparin) to placebo. Thromb Haemost 1992; 67:417–423.

12. Spiro TE, Fitzgerald RH, Trowbridge AA, et al. Enoxaparin—a low molecular weight heparin and warfarin for the prevention of venous thromboembolic disease after elective knee replacement surgery. Blood 1994; 84:(10 suppl 1):246a.

13. Clagett GP, Anderson FA Jr, Heit J et al. Prevention of venous thromboembolism. Chest 1995; 108:3125–3345.

14. Levine M, Gent M, Hirsh J et al. A comparison of low-molecular-weight heparin administered primarily at home with unfractionated heparin administered in the hospital for proximal deep vein thrombosis. N Engl J Med 1996; 334:677–681.

15. Data on File. Aventis (Rhone–Poulenc–Rorer) Pharmaceuticals, Inc.

16. Cohen M, Demers C, Gurfinkel EP, et al. A comparison of low-molecular-weight heparin with unfractionated heparin for unstable coronary artery disease. N Engl J Med 1997; 337:447–452.

17. Manciet GA, Descamps A, Vergnes C, Debilly A, Trophy F, Emeriau JP, Galley P, Boisseau MR. Etude de l'efficacite et de la tolerance de Fraxiparine adminstree au long cours chez le sujet age. essai randomise en double issue (essai APTE). In: Bounameau H, Samama M, ten Cate JW, eds 2nd International Symposium on Fraxiparin. New York: Schattauer, 1989; 17.

18. Bendetowicz AV, Kai H, Knebel R, et al. The effect of subcutaneous injection of unfractionated heparin and low molecular weight heparin on thrombin generation in platelet rich plasma. A study in human volunteers. Thromb Haemost 1994; 72:705–712.

19. Melandrie G, Semprini F, Cervi V, et al. Comparison of the efficacy of low-molecular-weight heparin (parnaparin) with that of unfractionated heparin in the presence of activated platelets in healthy subjects. Am J Cardiol 1993; 72:450–454.

20. Dehmer GJ, Fisher M, Tate DA, Teo S, Bonnem EM. Reversal of heparin anticoagulation by recombinant platelet factor 4 in humans. Circulation 1995; 91:2188–2194.

21. Broze GR Jr. The tissue factor pathway of coagulation. In: Loscalzo J, Shafer AI, eds. Thrombosis and Haemorrhage. Boston, MA: Blackwell Scientific 1994; 57–86.

22. Cohen M, Demers C, Gurfinkel EP, et al. A comparison of low-molecular-weight heparin with unfractionated heparin for unstable coronary artery disease. N Engl J Med 1997; 337:447–452.

23. Antaean EM, McCabe CH, Premmereur J, et al. Enoxaparin for the acute and chronic management of unstable angina/non-Q-wave myocardial infarction: results of TIMI11B. Circulation 1998; 98(suppl):1504.

24. Wallentin L, Ohlsson J, Swahn E, et al. Low molecular weight heparin during instability in coronary artery disease. Lancet 1996; 347:561–568.

25. Klein W, Buchwald A, Hillis S, et al. Comparison of low molecular weight heparin with unfractionated heparin acutely and with placebo for 6 weeks in the management of unstable coronary artery disease. Circulation 1997; 96:61–68.

26. Leizorovicz A. FRAXIS: fraxiparine in ischemic syndromes. Presented at the European Society of Cardiology, Vienna, August 1998.

27. FISC II Investigators. Long-term low molecular mass heparin in unstable coronary artery disease. Lancet 1999; 354:701–707.

28. FRISC II Investigators. Invasive compared with noninvasive treatment in unstable coronary artery disease. Lancet 1999; 354:708–715.

29. Fragmin—During Instability in Coronary Artery Disease Study Group. Low molecular weight heparin during instability in coronary artery disease. Lancet 1996; 347:561–568.

30. Cohen M, Demers C, Gurfinkel, et al. A comparison of low molecular weight heparin with unfractionated heparin for unstable coronary artery disease. Efficacy and safety of subcutaneous enoxaparin in non–Q-wave coronary events study group. N Engl J Med 1997; 337:447–452.

31. Toss H, Wallentin L, Siegbahn A. Influences of sex and smoking habits on anticoagulation activity in low molecular weight heparin treatment of unstable coronary artery disease. Am Heart J 1999; 137:72–78.

32. The Thrombolysis in Myocardial Infarction (TIMI)11A Trial Investigators. Dose-ranging trial of enoxaparin for unstable angina: results of TIMI11A. J Am Coll Cardiol 1997; 29:1474–1482.

33. Theroux P, Waters D, Lam J, et al. Reactivation of unstable angina after the discontinuation of heparin. N Engl J Med 1992; 327:141–145.

34. The Thrombin Inhibition in Myocardial Ischemia (TRIM) Study Group. A low molecular weight, selective thrombin inhibitor, inogatran vs. heparin for unstable coronary artery disease in 1209 patients. Eur Heart J 1997; 18:1416–1425.

35. Wallentin L. Low molecular weight heparin in unstable coronary artery disease. Exp Opin Invest Drugs 2000; 9:581–592.

36. DeCristofaro R, DeCandia E, Landolfi R. Effect of high and low molecular weight heparin on thrombin–thrombomodulin interaction and protein C activation. Circulation 1998; 98:1297–1301.

37. Gran E, Siguenza E, Madnell F et al. Low molecular weight heparin (CY-216) versus unfractionated heparin in chronic hemodialysis. Nephron 1992; 62:13–17.

38. Dieval J, Moniere P, Roussel B, Bayron B, Fournier A, Delobel J. Anticoagulation in hemodialysis sessions with a low molecular weight heparin (CY-222). J Mal Vasc 1987; 12:114–118.

39. Cohen M, Bigonzi F, Le Iouver V, et al. One year follow-up of the ESSENCE Trial (enoxaparin versus heparin in unstable angina and non–Q-wave myocardial infarction) [abstr]. J Am Coll Cardiol 1998; 31:79A.

40. Rabah M, Premmereur J, Graham M, et al. Usefulness of intravenous enoxaparin for percutaneous coronary intervention in stable angina pectoris. Am J Cardiol 1999; 84:1391–1395.

41. Kerekiakes DJ, Grines C, Fry E, et al. Enoxaparin and abciximab adjunctive pharmacotherapy during percutaneous coronary intervention. J Invasive Cardiol 2001; 13:272.

42. Kereiakes DJ, Kleiman NS, Fry NS, Mwawasi G, Lengerich R, Maresh K, Burkert ML, Aquilina JW, DeLoof M, Broderick TM, Shimshak TM. Dalteparin in combination with abciximab during percutaneous coronary intervention. Am Heart J 2001; 141:348–52.

43. Cairns JA, Gill J, Morton B, et al. Fish oils and low molecular weight heparin for the reduction of restenosis after percutaneous transluminal coronary angioplasty: the AMPAR study. Circulation 1996; 94:1553–1560.

44. Ellis S, Roubin G, Wilentz J, et al. Effect of 18 to 2-hour heparin administration for prevention of restenosis after uncomplicated coronary angioplasty. Am Heart J 1989; 117:777–782.

45. Serruys P, Deckers J, Close P. A double blind randomized heparin controlled trial evaluating acute and long term efficacy of r-hirudin (CGP 39393) in patients undergoing coronary angioplasty [abstr]. Circulation 1994; 90:I–394.

46. Faxon D, Spiro T, Minor S, et al. Low molecular weight heparin in prevention of restenosis after angioplasty. results of the enoxaparin restenosis after angioplasty. results of the enoxaparin restenosis (ERA) trial. Circulation 1994; 90:908–914.

47. International Stroke Trial Collaborative Group. The International Stroke Trial (IST). A randomized trial of aspirin, subcutaneous heparin, both or neither among 19435 patients with acute ischemic stroke. Lancet 1997; 349:1569–1581.

48. CAST (Chinese Acute Stroke Trial) Collaborative Group. CAST: randomized placebo-controlled trial of early aspirin use in 20,000 patients with acute ischemic stroke. Lancet 1997; 349:1641–1649.

49. Low molecular weight heparinoid, ORG 10172 (danaparoid), and outcome after acute ischemic stroke. a randomized controlled trial. The Publications Committee for the Trial of ORG 10172 in Acute Stroke Treatment (TOAST) Investigators. JAMA 1998; 279:1265–1272.

50. Kay R, Wong K, Yu Y et al., for FISS Trial. Low molecular weight heparin for the treatment of acute ischemic stroke. N Engl. J Med 1995; 333:1588–1593.

51. Hommel M, FISS bis Investigators Group. Fraxiparine in ischemic stroke study (FISS bis) [abstr]. Cerebrovasc Dis 1998; 8(suppl 4):1–103.

52. Gaffney P, O'Leary J, Doyle, C et al. Response to heparin in patients with ulcerative colitis. Lancet 1991; 337:238–39.

53. Day R, Forbes A. Heparin cell adhesion, and pathogenesis of inflammatory bowel disease. Lancet 1999; 354:62–65.

54. Gaffney P, Doyle G, Hogan D, Annis P. Paradoxical response to heparin in 10 patients with ulcerative colitis. Am J Gastroenterol 1995; 90:220–23.

55. Evans R, Shim WV, Morris A, Rhodes J. Treatment of corticosteroid-resistant ulcerative colitis with heparin—a report of 16 cases. Alimen Pharmacol Ther 1997; 1:1037–40.

56. Brazier F, Yzet T, Boruchowicz A, Colomber J, Duchman J, Dupas J. Treatment of ulcerative colitis with heparin. Gastroenterology 1996; 110:A872.

57. Folwaczny C, Fricke H, Endres S, Jochum M, Loeschke K. Anti-inflammatory properties of unfractionated heparin in patients with highly active ulcerative colitis. a pilot study. Am J Gastroenterol 1997; 92:911–12.

58. Dwaraknath A, Yu L, Brookes C, Pryce D, Rhodes J. "Sticky" neutrophils, allergic arthritis, and response to heparin in pyoderma gangrenosum complicating ulcerative colitis. Gut 1995; 35: 585–88.

59. Brazier F, Yzet T, Cochran J, Iglicki F, Dupas J. Effect of heparin treatment on extraintestinal manifestations associated inflammatory bowel disease. Gastroenterology 1996; 110:A872.

60. Zavgorodniv L, Mustgart A. Application of anticoagulants in the complex treatment of ulcerative colitis. Clin Med 1982; 60:74–80.

61. Dobosz M, Mionskowska L, Dobrowolski S, Dymecki D, Makarewicz W, Hrabowska M, Wajda Z. Is nitric oxide and heparin treatment justified in inflammatory bowel disease? An experimental study. Scand J Clin Lab Invest 1996; 56:657–663.

62. White B, Ang YS, Mahmud N, Keeling PWN, Smith OP. Heparin and inflammatory bowel disease. Lancet 1999; 354:1122–1123.

63. Korzenik JR. IBD: a vascular disorder ? The case for heparin therapy. Inflamm Bowel Dis 1997; 3:87–94.

64. Day R, Forbes A. Heparin, cell adhesion, and pathogenesis of inflammatory bowel disease. Lancet 1999; 354:62–65.

65. Torkvist L, Loftberg R. Beneficial effects of low molecular weight heparin as adjuvant therapy in ulcerative colitis. Haemostasis 1998; 28(suppl. 3):144.

66. Torkvist L, Thoriacius H, Sjoqvist U, Bohman L, Lapidus A, Flood L, Agren B, Rauds J, Loftberg R. Low molecular weight heparin as adjuvant therapy in active ulcerative colitis. Aliment Pharmacol Ther 1999; 13:1323–1328.

67. Salas A, Sans M, Soriano A, Reverter JC, Anderson DC, Pique JM, Panes J. Heparin attenuates TNF-induced inflammatory response through a CD11b dependent mechanism. Gut 2000; 47:88–96.

68. Nelson RM, Cecconi O, Roberts WG, et al. Heparin oligosaccharides bind L- and P-selectin and inhibit acute inflammation. Blood 1993; 82:3253–8.

69. Meyer J, Cox CS, Herndon DN, et al. Heparin in experimental hyperdynamic sepsis. Crit Care Med 1993; 21:84–9.

70. Hiebert LM, Liu JM. Heparin protects cultured arterial endothelial cells from damage by toxic oxygen metabolites. Atherosclerosis 1990; 83:47–51.

71. Matzner Y, Marx G, Drexler R, et al. The inhibitory effect of heparin and related glycosaminoglycans on neutrophil chemotaxis. Thromb Haemost 1984; 52:134–7.

72. Bazzoni G, Beltran NA, Mascellani G, et al. Effect of heparin, dermatan sulfate and related oligo-derivatives on human polymorphonuclear leukocyte functions. J Lab Clin Med 1993; 121:268–75.

73. Texeira MM, Hellwell PG. Suppression by intradermal administration of heparin of eosinophil accumulation but not edema formation in inflammatory reactions in guinea pig skin. Br J Pharmacol 1993; 110:1496–500.

74. Carr J. The anti-inflammatory actions of heparin: heparin as an antagonist to histamine, bradykinin and prostaglandin E_1. Thromb Res 1979; 16:507–16.

75. Koenig A, Norgard SK, Linhardt R, et al. Differential interactions of heparin and heparan sulfate for glycosaminoglycans with the selectins. Implications for the use of unfractionated and low molecular weight heparins as therapeutic agents. J Clin Invest 1998; 101:877–89.

76. Diamond MS, Alon R, Parkos CA, et al. Heparin is an adhesive ligand for the leukocyte integrin Mac-1 (CD11b/CD18). J Cell Biol 1995; 130:1473–82.

77. Benimetskaya L, Loike JD, Khaled Z, et al. Mac-1 (CD11b/CD18) is an oligodeoxynucleotide-binding protein. Nat Med 1997; 3:414–20.

78. Ohlsson K, Bjork P, Bergenfeldt M, Hageman R, Thompson RC. Interleukin-1 receptor antagonist for interleukin-1 receptor antagonist reduces mortality from endotoxin shock. Nature 1990; 348:550–552.

79. Natanson C, Hoffman WD, Suffredini AF, Eickacker PQ, Danner RL. Selected treatment strategies for septic shock based on proposed mechanisms of pathogenesis. Ann Intern Med 1994;120:771–783.

80. Quezado ZMN, Banks SM, Natanson C. New strategies for combating sepsis: the magic bullets missed the mark. . . but the search continues. Trends Biotechnol 1995 13:56–63.

81. Freeman BD, Natanson C. Clinical trials in sepsis and septic shock. Curr Opin Crit Care 1995; 1:349–357.

82. Natanson C. Eichenholz PW, Danner RL, et al. Endotoxin and tumor necrosis factor challenges in dogs simulate the cardiovascular profile of human septic shock. J Exp Med 1989; 169:823–832.

83. Waage A, Espevik T. Interleukin-1 potentiates the lethal effects of tumor necrosis factor/cachectin in mice. J Exp Med 1988; 167:1987–1992.

84. Okusawa S, Gelfand JA, Ikejima T, Connolly RJ, Dinarello CA. Interleukin-1 induces a shock like state in rabbits: synergism with tumor necrosis factor and the effect of cyclooxygenase inhibition. J Clin Invest 1988; 81:1162–1172.

85. Richardson PG, Elias AD, Krishnan, et al. Treatment of severe veno-occlusive disease with defibrotide: compassionate use results in response without significant toxicity in a high-risk population. Blood 1998; 92:737.

86. Morris JD, Harris RE, Hashmi R, et al. Antithrombin III for the treatment of chemotherapy-induced organ dysfunction following bone marrow transplantation. Bone Marrow Transplant 1997; 20:871.

87. Attal M, Huguet F, Schlaifer D, et al. Intensive combined therapy for previously untreated aggressive myeloma. Blood 1992; 79:1130.

88. Hagglund H, Remberger M, Klaesson S, et al. Norethisterone treatment, a major risk factor for veno-occlusive disease in the liver after allogeneic bone marrow transplantation. Blood 1998; 92:4568.

89. Or R, Nagler A, Shpillberg O et al. Low molecular weight heparin for the prevention of veno-occlusive disease of the liver in bone marrow transplantation patients. Transplantation 1996; 61:1067.

90. Rai R, Cohen H, Dave M, Regan L. Randomized controlled trial of aspirin and aspirin plus heparin in pregnant women with recurrent miscarriage associated with phospholipid antibodies (or antiphospholipid antibodies) Br Med J 1997; 314:253.

91. Kutteh WH. Antiphospholipid antibody-associated recurrent pregnancy loss. treatment with heparin and low dose aspirin is superior to low dose aspirin alone. Am J Obstet Gynecol 1996; 174:1584.

92. Kutteh WH, Ermell LD. A clinical trial for the treatment of antiphospholipid antibody-associated recurrent pregnancy loss with lower dose heparin and aspirin Am J Reprod Immunol 1996; 35:402.

93. Corrigan JJ, Jordan CM. Heparin therapy in septicemia with disseminated intravascular coagulation. N Engl J Med 1970; 283:778.

94. Hjort PF, Rapaport SI, Jorgensen L. Purpura fulminans. Report of a case successfully treated with heparin and hydrocortisone. Review of 50 cases from the literature. Scand J Haematol 1964; 1:69.

95. Gerson WT, Dickerman JD, Bovill EG, Golden E. Severe acquired protein C deficiency in purpura fulminans associated with disseminated intravascular coagulation; treatment with protein C concentrate. Pediatrics 1993; 91:418.

96. Verstraete M. Pharmacotherapeutic aspects of unfractionated and low molecular weight heparins. Drugs 1990; 40:498–530.

97. Nurmohamed MT, Rosendaal FR, Buller HR, et al. Low-molecular-weight heparin versus standard heparin in general and orthopaedic surgery: a meta-analysis. Lancet 1992; 340:152.

98. Beatrice L, Wanhong D, Fenart L, Marie-Pierre D, Andrew S, Romeo C, Howard F. Heparin oligosaccharides that pass the blood brain barrier inhibit [beta]-amyloid precursor protein secretion and heparin binding to [beta]-amyloid peptide. Clin Neurochem Dis 1998; 70:736–744.

99. Snow AD, Kinsella MG, Prather PB, Nochlin D, Podlisny MB, Selkoe DJ, Kisilevsky R, Wight TN. A characteristic binding affinity between heparin and heparan sulfate proteoglycans and the A4 amyloid protein of Alzheimer's disease [abstr]. J Neuropathol Exp Neurol 1989; 48:352.

100. Buee L, Ding W, Delacourte A, Fillit H. Binding of secreted neuroblastoma proteoglycans to the Alzheimer's amyloid A4 peptide. Brain Res 1993; 601:154–163.

101. Narindrasorasak S, Lowery D, Gonzalez-DeWhitt P, Poorman RA, Greenberg BD, Kisilevsky R. High affinity interactions between the Alzheimer's [beta]-amyloid precursor proteins and the basement membrane form of heparan sulfate proteoglycans. J Biol Chem 1991; 266:12878–12883.

102. Buee l, Ding W, Anderson B, Narindrasorasak S, Kisilevsky R, Boyle NJ, Robakis N, Delacourte A, Greenberg BD, Fillit H. Vascular basement membrane heparan sulfate proteoglycan binding to the Alzheimer's amyloid precursor protein involves the N-terminal region of the A4 peptide. Brain Res 1993; 627:199–204.

103. Selkoe DJ. Normal and abnormal biology of the [beta]-amyloid precursor protein. Annu Rev Neurosci 1994; 17:489–517.

104. Maury CPJ. Molecular pathogenesis of [beta]-amyloidosis in Alzheimer's disease and other cerebral amyloidoses. Lab Invest 1995; 212:4–16.

105. Tryba M und die Teilnehmer des Workshops uber hamostaseologische Probleme bei regionalanaesthesien. Reg Anaesth 1989; 12:127.

106. Schwander D, Bachman F. Heparine et anesthesies medullaires. analyse de decision. Ann Fr Anesth Reanim 1991; 10:284.

12

Clinical Use of Argatroban

Bruce E. Lewis and Jeanine M. Walenga
Loyola University Medical Center, Maywood, Illinois, U.S.A.

SUMMARY

Argatroban is the smallest molecule of the anticoagulant class of direct thrombin inhibitors. The main attributes of this synthetic drug are its rapid onset of antithrombin action, the rapid reversibility of its anticoagulant effect, the potent inhibition of clot-bound thrombin, the absence of antibody formation, and no need for dosage adjustment in patients with renal impairment; it is eliminated by hepatic metabolism. These properties make argatroban a predictable anticoagulant with intravenous use in a routine clinical setting. Argatroban is approved in the United States for both prophylaxis and treatment of thrombosis in patients with heparin-induced thrombocytopenia (HIT). In limited trials it has also provided reliable anticoagulation during percutaneous coronary interventions on patients with HIT. Preliminary reports document the feasibility of using argatroban for anticoagulation during peripheral vascular interventions, hemodialysis, and as adjuct to thrombolysis in acute ST-elevation myocardial infarction. A consistent safety profile of argatroban has been demonstrated in all studies to date. Current recommendations for argatroban monitoring are to use the activated partial thromboplastin time (aPTT) for low doses and the activated clotting time (ACT) for high doses. Argatroban continues to be studied as an antithrombotic agent in various clinical settings.

I. INTRODUCTION

Argatroban is the smallest molecule of the anticoagulant class of direct thrombin inhibitors. This drug has been used in Japan for the management of thromboembolic disorders for several years. Despite this experience and a large number of preclinical studies on the pharmacology of argatroban, clinical trials in Europe and North America were initiated only in 1996. The main attributes of argatroban are its rapid onset of action, the rapid reversibility of its anticoagulant effect, potent inhibitioin of clot-bound thrombin, the absence of antibody formation, and no need for dosage adjustment in patients with renal impairment [1]. These characteristics of argatroban

185

make it a promising anticoagulant that is being evaluated in numerous clinical settings at this time (Table 1).

II. PHARMACOLOGY

Argatroban is a small synthetic molecule derived from L-arginine (527-Da molecular weight). The predominant mechanisn of argatroban's action is direct thrombin inhibition through a reversible interaction with the catalytic site of thrombin [2–6]. Its thrombin inhibition constant (K_i) is 3.9×10^{-8} M [4]. It is a selective thrombin inhibitor and does not inhibit other serine proteases. Argatroban differs from heparin, which requires a cofactor to inhibit thrombin. The parent compound, L-arginine, is a known nitric oxide donor. This property is retained by argatroban, thus giving it a dual mechanism of action. Nitric oxide donation induces endothelium-mediated vascular smooth-muscle relaxation and vasodilation [7].

The small molecular size of argatroban may offer a therapeutic advantage over other thrombin inhibitors for treatment of the older, more organized thrombus, in that it can penetrate and effectively inhibit thrombin despite the fibrin barrier [8,9]. Concentrations (IC_{50}) of argatroban that inhibit soluble, fibrin-bound and clot-bound thrombin, are 1.1, 2.8, and 2.4 μM [4]. Berry's work has shown that only a two-fold increase in argatroban concentration is needed to penetrate and neutralize fibrin-bound thrombin in vitro (vs. inhibition of soluble fibrin), compared with the 23-fold increase needed for hirudin and a 500-fold increase for heparin [8]. Berry's results were even more dramatic when argatroban was compared with hirudin and heparin in an in vivo clot-bound thrombin model. In this model, a two-fold increase in argatroban concentration, compared with a 4000-fold increase in hirudin and a 5000-fold increase in heparin, was required to inhibit a clot-bound thrombin.

Argatroban reaches its steady-state pharmacokinetic values, measured by its aPTT anticoagulation effect, 1–3 h after intravenous administration. After discontinuation of the drug, the aPTT returns to normal within 2–4 h. Argatroban is approximately 54% bound to plasma proteins [9]. Its volume of distribution is 0.2 L/kg, total body clearance is 0.3 L/h kg^{-1} (5 mL/min kg^{-1}) and its elimination half-life is 39–51 min [10]. Age, gender and renal function do not affect the pharmacokinetics of argatroban [10].

Argatroban is rapidly metabolised in the liver and excreted through the bile into the feces [11,12]. There are three known metabolites of argatroban (M$_1$, M$_2$, and M$_3$): M$_1$ retains a very

Table 1 Clinical Uses of Argatroban as an Anti-coagulant in HIT and Non-HIT Patients

HIT thrombosis prophylaxis[a]
HITTS thrombosis treatment[a]
Angioplasty
Peripheral vascular procedures
Cerebral vascular procedures
Adjunct therapy to thrombolysis in acute ST elevation MI
Hemodialysis

[a]FDA approved.

modest antithrombin effect, whereas M_2 and M_3 are inert. The modest antithrombin effect of M_1 requires caution with ultrahigh-argatroban–dosing strategies because M_1 can accumulate and produce a clinical anticoagulant effect [13]. The anticoagulant effect of M_1 is not clinically apparent with routine intravenous doses. However, the M_1 effect can be clinically relevant, with logarithmic dose increases in argatroban concentrations.

Volunteers with normal ($n = 12$) or impaired hepatic function ($n = 5$) showed predictable temporal pharmacokinetic profiles for a 4 h infusion of 2.5 μg/kg min^{-1} argatroban [14,15]. However, at the end of the infusion time the hepatically impaired individuals had a two-fold increase in mean argatroban plasma levels (aPTT 108 vs. 71 s), and a 2.5–4.5-fold increase in the clearance and elimination half-life of argatroban [15]; consequently, dose reduction is recommended for patients with hepatic impairment [10].

Volunteers with varying degrees of renal dysfunction ($n = 24$), ranging from normal to severe impairment, did not demonstrate any differences in clearance, steady-state plasma concentrations, steady-state volume of distribution, or elimination half-life for an intravenous infusion of 5 μg/kg min^{-1} of argatroban [16]. In contrast, hirudin and danaparoid are cleared through the kidneys and patients with renal impairment require dose reduction to avoid excess plasma concentrations.

Argatroban does not induce the formation of antibodies [17] that neutralize its anticoagulant effect, prolong its half-life, or enhance its activity, as do the antibodies generated to hirudin [18].

III. PRECLINICAL MODELS

Argatroban is an effective antithrombotic agent in several models of venous thrombosis. It produces a dose-dependent anticoagulant effect with complete inhibition of thrombosis at dosages of about 150–300 μg/kg or plasma concentrations of about 0.5–1 μg/mL (two-fold less potent than heparin gravimetrically) depending on the model. Argatroban also provides effective antithrombotic activity against thrombi formed in arterial–venous shunt models, and in models of arterial thrombosis in which thrombi contain a high degree of trapped platelets and other blood cells, as well as in modes of endothelial damage [1]. In all models, argatroban was generally as effective as heparin at relatively equal gravimetric doses.

The bleeding effect of argatroban was compared with that of heparin following intravenous administration in rabbit and rat models. It also produced dose-dependent blood loss from standarized incisions in the rabbit ear. Heparin, on the other hand, demonstrated a non–dose-dependent blood loss, with a high amount of bleeding at intravenous doses above 1 mg/kg. Only at a high dose of 5 mg/kg, however, did argatroban produce significant bleeding, equivalent to that obtained with heparin [1]. In the rat, an argatroban infusioin of 11 μg/kg min^{-1} and a heparin infusion of 2.2 μg/kg min^{-1} doubled the bleeding time from that observed in control animals [19].

Argatroban has also demonstrated effective antithrombotic activity in models of thrombolysis with t-PA, u-PA, scu-PA, urokinase, and staphylokinase [1]. Argatroban did not produce any compromise of the fibrinolytic activity by these agents and, in some cases, decreased time to lysis in the presence of the fibrinolytic agent. The results suggested that argatroban inhibits factor XIIIa generation.

Argatroban affects vascular smooth muscle in an endothelium-dependent fashion. In canine cerebral and coronary arteries, the concentration required to inhibit vasoconstriction by thrombin (ED_{50}) was approximately 0.3 μM [20,21]. Argatroban was also able to relax vessel contraction induced by thrombin. Without intact endothelium the inhibitory effect of argatroban was decreased [21]. In rat aortic smooth-muscle cells, argatroban suppressed thrombin-induced proliferation [22], and in rabbits, locally administered argatroban inhibited intimal smooth-muscle migration and proliferation [23]. Other cell culture studies suggest that argatroban may inhibit thrombin-induced induction of transforming growth factor (TGF-β) that is produced by kidney mesangial cells and leads to glomerulonephritis [24]. Additional studies have shown that argatroban may increase granulocyte–macrophage colony-stimulating factor (GM-CSF) mRNA and protein levels, suggesting a relation between cytokine production and thrombin activity [25].

The effects of argatroban on platelets appear to be limited to thrombin- and factor-induced activation [1]. Simultaneous administration of argatroban and ticlopidine did not result in additive or synergistic effects on ADP-induced platelet aggregation [26]. The activity of argatroban is not influenced by endogenous factors such platelet factor 4 (PF4) and other proteins that bind heparin [9].

IV. CLINICAL TRIALS AND STUDIES

A. Heparin-Induced Thrombocytopenia

Heparin-induced thrombocytopenia (HIT) has become recognized as one of the most devastating prothrombotic states seen in medicine. HIT is an immune-mediated process that occurs in 2–3% of patients given heparin [27]. Most of the patients who develop serological evidence of HIT will develop subclinical thrombosis, and 50% of these patients are at risk for clinical thrombosis [27,28]. The hallmark of HIT is thrombocytopenia, which requires 4–5 days of heparin exposure to initiate antibody formation, but thrombocytopenia can occur more rapidly in a patient with heparin reexposure. The immune response is usually an IgG antibody that forms in response to the heparin–PF4 complex [29]. The IgG antibody binds to the heparin–PF4 complex on the platelet membrane and activates the platelet through surface membrane Fc receptors. The activated platelet, in turn, releases highly procoagulant microparticles that perpetuate the vicious cycle of this hypercoagulable state [30]. HIT appears to impart the highest risk of thrombosis of all known hypercoagulable states. HIT patients who develop thrombosis as a result of this hypercoagulable state are at the most severe end of the HIT spectrum. This state is termed heparin-induced thrombocytopenia with thrombosis syndrome (HITTS). The heparin–PF4 antibody state generally resolves within 3 months of the heparin exposure. However, patients have had measurable antibody years after the initial heparin exposure.

The initial treatment recommendations for HIT management are the immediate discontinuation of all heparin. This recommendation is clearly necessary, but not sufficient, therapy in the setting of HIT because 50% of HIT patients will progress to clinical thrombosis, despite heparin cessation [31]. Until recently, however, alternative non–heparin-based anticoagulant compounds that could be substituted for heparin in HIT patients were not clinically approved in the United States. The heparinoid, danaparoid, and low-molecular-weight heparins (LMWHs) are less likely to induce HIT and historically have been used for HIT treatment in selected patients [32,33]. However, danaparoid and LMWHs have sufficient immunological similarity to UFH to perpetuate the hypercoagulable state of HIT, once HIT is initiated. Danaparoid and LMWHs, therefore, should be avoided once active HIT has developed. Argatroban has no immune similarity to heparin; therefore, it cannot initiate or perpetuate HIT. This distinctly different immune structure offers a therapeutic advantage for treatment of HIT.

1. Supportive Data

Multiple trials with argatroban provide data that support the use of argatroban, both in prophylaxis and treatment of HIT. The first published multicenter argatroban trial, ARG911, compared active treatment with an initial 2 μg/kg min^{-1} intravenous infusion of argatroban titrated to achieve an aPTT of 1.5–3 × baseline, for up to 14 days, in 304 HIT/HITTS patients with traditional heparin withdrawal in 193 HIT historic control patients [34]. Patients were followed for 37 days, and efficacy was clinically defined by prevention of thrombotic events, death, or amputation. The patients were further divided into a prophylactic treatment arm (HIT patients) in whom thrombocytopenia was present, but no clinical thrombus could be identified at enrollment, and a therapeutic treatment arm (HITTS patients) in whom both thrombocytopenia and clinical thrombosis were identified at enrollment. This strategy produced four distinct study arms for comparison: (1) 147 HIT historic, control patients who had no active anticoagulant therapy; (2) 160 HIT patients treated with argatroban; (3) 46 HITTS historic, control patients who had no active anticoagulant therapy; and (4) 144 HITTS patients treated with argatroban (Fig. 1).

Several important observations came from the ARG911 trial (Table 2). Control HITTS patients had a composite endpoint of death, amputation, or new thrombosis of 56.5%, which was reduced to 43.8% with argatroban treatment. Despite clinical absence of thrombus on enrollment, 39% of HIT control patients developed thrombus during the 37-day follow-up, compared with 26% of argatroban-treated patients (p = 0.014). Argatroban also showed a favorable directionality for the individual components of death and new thrombotic event rates in both HIT and HITTS patients. These data suggest that all HIT patients are at risk for the development of serious clinical thrombotic events whether thrombus is present or absent when HIT is identified. HIT patients at highest risk for new thrombotic events over the 37-day observation period are those with thrombus present (HITTS) and are clearly candidates for antithrombotic treatment. However, HIT patients without clinical thrombus also warrant consideration for prophylatic antithrombotic treatment because of high thrombotic event rates in HIT, despite absence of thrombus.

2. Mechanism of Action

The antithrombotic mechanism of action of argatroban is clearly demonstrated in Figures 2 and 3 [34]. The elimination of thrombotic death in the HIT group treated with argatroban and the near

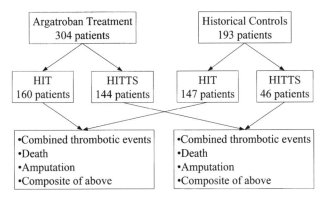

Figure 1 Trial design of the prospective ARG911 clinical investigation for the safety and efficacy of argatroban anticoagulation in patients with HIT or HITTS.

Table 2 Treatment of HIT/HITTS with Argatroban

	HIT %		HITTS %	
	Control	Arg	Control	Arg
Death	21.8	16.9	28.3	18.1
Amputation	2.0	1.9	8.7	11.1
New thrombosis	15	6.9	19.6	14.6
Composite	38.8	25.6	56.5	43.8

Results of the ARG911 trial.
*p = 0.014
Source: Ref. 34.

elimination of thrombotic death in the HITTS group treated with argatroban provide highly statistically significant support of argatroban therapy for treatment of both HIT and HITTS. These data also clearly demonstrate that argatroban is an effective antithrombotic agent.

A secondary efficacy variable in the ARG911 trial was platelet count recovery time. The reduced platelet counts seen in HIT patients, in part, reflect platelet consumption by both micro- and macrothrombotic processes. Resolution of the prothrombotic effects of HIT is indirectly reflected by platelet count increases. The platelet count recovery times were significantly reduced in argatroban-treated HIT patients compared with controls, which supports the concept of argatroban controlling propagation of the thrombus. In fact, argatroban-treated patients saw a rise in platelet counts throughout the early treatment period. The control patients had a decline in platelet counts throughout the same early observation period.

3. Ease of Use and Safety

The ease of argatroban use was highlighted in the ARG911 trial, as shown by the aPTT data. Seventy-six percent of HIT patients and 81% of HITTS patients achieved adequate antic-oagulation on the first postbolus aPTT draw. This draw was typically performed less than 5 h after the initial argatroban bolus. The daily aPTT level remained constant throughout the

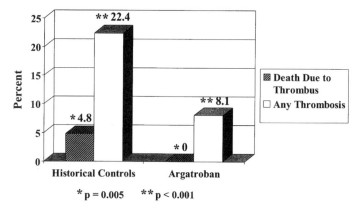

Figure 2 The antithrombotic efficacy of argatroban is demonstrated by the reduction of thrombosis/ death due to thrombosis in patients with HIT who were treated with argatroban.

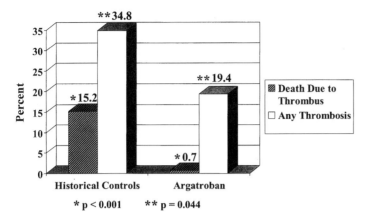

Figure 3   The antithrombotic efficacy of argatroban is demonstrated by the reduction of thrombosis/death due to thrombosis in patients with HITTS who were treated with argatroban.

remainder of the study if the drug dose remained unchanged. The laboratory data suggest that argatroban is a very predictable compound; therefore, it is easily administered in a clinical setting.

The safety of argatroban is acceptable, with an overall 6.9% incidence of major bleeding across 304 argatroban-treated patients in the ARG911 trial, which was not statistically different from the 6.7% incidence of major bleeds in the control patients who received no intravenous anticoagulants. The 6.9% argatroban major bleed rate is approximately one-half of the 13–17% major bleed rate reported in the hirudin HIT trials [35,36].

The difference in bleeding between hirudin and argatroban may be explained by two factors. First, hirudin has a nearly irreversible binding to the catalytic site on thrombin when compared with the reversible binding of argatroban with thrombin [4,37]. The resultant shorter half-life seen with argatroban compared with hirudin may permit a quicker reversal of the anticoagulant effect when bleeding is recognized. Second, hirudin itself can result in antibody production that may alter the kinetics of hirudin administration and elimination [18]. The effects of antihirudin antibody production may reduce both the predictability and the accuracy in monitoring anticoagulation levels during prolonged or repeat hirudin use.

These observations suggest that argatroban is a safe and effective anticoagulant in the setting of HIT or HITTS, despite the application to a population who manifest thrombocytopenia as part of their disease process, and it may have a safety advantage over other anticoagulants. One must acknowledge the limitations of the historic control study design as used in the ARG911 trial, however, because this may introduce bias into the study. This design was necessary, as there was no comparative treatment available and, moreover, it would have been unethical to use a placebo or withhold treatment that has been shown in preliminary studies to be effective. Knowing the limitation of the study design, in the ARG911 trial there was an attempt to minimize bias by having independent adjudication of controls and treated patients, and to minimize variability in practice each site was limited to provide only three controls per treated patient.

B.   Angioplasty in HIT and Non-HIT Patients

Frequently, patients with heparin-induced thrombocytopenia require coronary interventional procedures. Two trials (ARG215/216 and ARG310/311) have assessed the safety and efficacy of argatroban as anticoagulant therapy for percutaneous coronary interventional (PCI) procedures on HIT patients in the cardiac catheterization laboratory. Patients ($n = 91$; 112 interventions) were given a 350-μg/kg bolus followed by 25-μg/kg min^{-1} infusion of argatroban. Patients in this trial could not be randomised to heparin versus argatroban. Therefore, the safety and efficacy of argatroban administration during PCI procedures on HIT patients was compared with results obtained on non-HIT patients treated with heparin during PCI. Efficacy of anticoagulation for argatroban-treated PCI HIT patients was measured by comparison with the Cleveland Clinic PCI angioplasty registry of heparin-treated non-HIT patients during the concordant time of patient enrollment. Safety of argatroban for coronary interventional procedures was assessed by comparing the bleeding rate with argatroban with that of the heparin-only arm of the EPILOG trial, which was also conducted during the same time period as patient enrollment in the argatroban PCI trials.

The 100% acute procedural success rate with argatroban during PCI procedures on HIT patients compared favourably with the 94% procedural success rate in heparin-treated non-HIT patients (Table 3; p = not significant). Adequate anticoagulation, as measured by activated-clotting time (ACT), was achieved in 99% of argatroban-treated patients after the initial argatroban bolus. An ACT of 300–450 s was maintained throughout the interventional procedure in about 65% of the argatroban-treated patients. Fewer than 30% of patients required a repeat bolus with argatroban for the PCI procedure. When patients did require an additional bolus, 150 μg/kg generally re-established a therapeutic ACT. The safety of argatroban during PCI also appeared to be at least equivalent to the safety of heparin during PCI (1.1% major bleed rate with argatroban compared with 3.1% major bleed rate with heparin).

Argatroban has also been used for percutaneous coronary intervention in a limited number of non-HIT patients. Two studies report success in patients using a strategy of continuous infusion to maintain an aPTT of 1.5–2 times the baseline before PCI [38,39]. A third pilot study compared PCI outcomes with intravenous argatroban plus intravenous argatroban post-PCI (10 mg infused over 20 min) with conventional heparin strategies in 53 patients [1]. A reduction in the percentage of the stenosis diameter and the binary restonosis rate at a 3-month follow-up for argatroban-treated patients compared with heparin-treated patients was reported.

Although the data are promising for the use of argatroban in PCI in patients with and without HIT, there are limitations on the data interpretation of the angioplasty studies described in the foregoing. One should be aware that the registry-style data collection used for the control groups could introduce observational bias from the nonblinded nature of the study design.

The use of argatroban for peripheral vascular and cerebral vascular procedures has not been formally studied [40]. However, several case reports provide some information on the

Table 3 PCI with Argatroban Anticoagulation in Patients with HIT

Criteria	Arg HIT patients (%)	Control (heparin) non–HIT patients (%)
Procedural success rate (acute)	100[a]	94.3[c]
Major bleed rate	1.1[b]	3.1[d]

[a]*Acute procedural success* was defined as absence of death, Q-wave MI, or need for urgent revascularization.
[b]*Major bleed* was defined as > 5-gm drop in hemoglobin, need for more than two packed cell transfusions, cerebral bleed, or retroperitoneal bleed.
[c]Control arm was based on the Cleveland Clinic PCI angioplasty registry.
[d]Control arm was based on the heparin-only arm of the EPILOG trial.

feasibility of argatroban use for anticoagulation in these patients. Small-vessel interventions on tibial and peroneal arteries or intracranial vessels can probably be safely performed using coronary argatroban-dosing strategies (350-μg/kg bolus, followed by 25-μg/kg min^{-1} infusion). Larger vessels, such as iliac, and renal arteries, can probably be treated with smaller argatroban doses (250-μg/kg bolus followed by 10-μg/kg min^{-1} infusion). Further work with argatroban for anticoagulation in peripheral vascular interventional procedures is necessary to optimize dosing strategies in this setting.

C. Acute Myocardial Infarction

The investigation of argatroban as adjunct therapy to thrombolytics for patients with acute ST-elevation myocardial infarction (MI) was performed in two clinical studies. More than 1200 patients were randomised to argatroban or placebo as adjunct therapy to streptokinase, and to argatroban or heparin as adjunct therapy to t-PA. The streptokinase patients were given either a 100-μg/kg bolus of argatroban plus 1-μg/kg min^{-1} infusion, or 100-μg/kg bolus of argatroban plus 3-μg/kg min^{-1} argatroban infusion, or placebo bolus plus placebo infusion. The t-PA patients were given argatroban 1 μg/kg min^{-1}, 3-μg/kg min^{-1}, or heparin 70 μg/kg bolus plus 15 μg/kg h^{-1} infusion.

Primary efficacy outcomes were not significantly different between treatment groups with either streptokinase or t-PA. However, TIMI frame counts were improved in patients with onset of symptoms within 3 h of the procedure if treated with t-PA and argatroban confirming previous data in animal models [41,42]. TIMI grade 3 flow was also significantly more frequent in high-dose argatroban and t-PA than in t-PA and heparin patients (57 vs. 20%) in patients presenting after 3 hours. The lack of efficacy benefit in the argatroban-treated streptokinase arm, compared with placebo, was not surprising, as most coagulation experts agree that no additional benefit can be expected by adding antithrombotic therapy to streptokinase.

This study also provides important safety data on argatroban. No statistically significant differences were seen for major hemorrhage between patients treated with argatroban and streptokinase compared with placebo and streptokinase (Table 4). Similarly, no significant differences were seen in total transfusion rates between patients treated with streptokinase and argatroban when compared with patients treated with streptokinase and placebo. However, a trend toward increased bleeding and transfusion rates for patients given argatroban and streptokinase was observed. A trend toward less bleeding was observed in patients treated with argatroban and t-PA compared with heparin and t-PA (2.6% and 4.3% vs. 10.0%). Only 1% of argatroban-treated patients had a documented intracranial hemorrhage when used in combination with thrombolytics. The number of patients treated is much too small to provide statistically meaningful conclusions, but argatroban may offer such hope for improving the safety profile of combination therapy with thrombolytics and antithrombotics.

A second pilot study was conducted that compared argatroban with heparin as adjunct for alteplase during the treatment of acute MI [43]. Coronary angiography was performed at 90 min after the start of the infusion and at 5 days. The coronary angiographic results showed no statistically significant differences in patency rates between argatroban-treated patients and heparin-treated patients. Clinical outcomes were also not statistically different. However, the study did not have enough power to detect a difference in clinical outcome.

D. Hemodialysis

Argatroban has been reported as a potential alternative anticoagulant for patients who fail heparin or those who cannot be given heparin during hemodialysis. All clinical reports to date recommend maintenance of the aPTT more than 1.5 times baseline. A wide range of dosing

Table 4 Argatroban as an Adjunct to Thrombolytic Therapy in Elevated ST-segment MI Patients

(Criteria)	SK			tPA		
	+ Placebo (%)	+ Arg (1 μg/kg) (%)	+ Arg (3 μg/kg) (%)	+ Heparin (%)	+ Arg (1 μg/kg) (%)	+ Arg (3 μg/kg) (%)
Major bleed rate	3.6	5.5	5.7	10.0	2.6	4.3
Transfusion rate	3.3	5.2	5.4	17.5	10.5	6.4

Dosage adjustments were mandated by protocol for aPTT values of more than 90 s. Dosage adjustments were infrequently required in the 1-μg/kg min^{-1} argatroban-treatment group (6% for the argatroban treatment versus 3% for placebo). The 3-μg/kg argatroban-treatment group required dose adjustments in 36% of patients. The data demonstrated the ease of the use of argatroban.

strategies has been used in the hemodialysis setting. Bolus plus infusion strategies include a single 10-mg bolus of argatroban and 0.1-mg/kg h^{-1} infusion [44,45]. One report has suggested the use of 20-mg/h dosing, whereas a second report proposed 0.49-mg/kg h^{-1} dosing [46]. Both the bolus dosing and hourly dosing have had success, but the number of treated patients is very small.

V. MONITORING

Intravenous administration of argatroban has been monitored using various assays. The thrombin time has been proposed as the logical laboratory measurement for assessment of the anti-coagulation level. However, this test can be too sensitive to argatroban, thereby limiting the meaningful results it can provide across various clinical settings. In addition, the thrombin time test is not readily available in all laboratories, and methods vary from laboratory to laboratory. Therefore, thrombin times have not been useful for argatroban monitoring.

The most practical test for intravenous argatroban monitoring has been the aPTT. The slope of the dose–response curve is linear for intravenous argatroban-dosing strategies between 1 and 10 μg/kg min^{-1}. Several studies have shown that the clinical effect of argatroban correlates well with prolongation of the aPTT [1,5,14,47–51]. However, with high-dose argatroban ($> 15 \mu$g/kg min^{-1}) the aPTT response becomes nearly vertical, which is not useful.

The prothrombin time (PT) is affected by argatroban in a fairly linear fashion. This effect on the PT makes the interpretation of the warfarin (Coumadin)–argatroban interaction challenging [51]. Similarly, other coagulation tests (e.g., assays for fibrinogen, coagulation factors, and functional protein C) cannot be performed when argatroban is present, owing to argatroban's interference in the test systems [51]. This can be overcome by using chromogenic-type assays [52].

The biggest challenge yet has been the monitoring of warfarin in the face of argatroban therapy. It has been demonstrated that argatroban linearly and predictably increases the INR, the extent of which is dependent on the sensitivity of the thromboplastin used [53]. The level of anticoagulation by warfarin therefore, can be predicted during cotherapy with argatroban. A practical recommendation for warfarin titration in the background of argatroban therapy is to administer warfarin and argatroban simultaneously until an INR of 4 has been achieved [54]. Argatroban can then be withdrawn and the INR reassessed. Most experts recommend lower initial doses of warfarin in the setting of HIT because high-dose warfarin (especially in the absence of protection by a thrombin inhibitor) has been associated with paradoxical thrombosis. The paradoxical thrombosis is thought to be related to protein C depletion.

The aPTT is not accurate at high argatroban concentrations. The ACT has traditionally been used to monitor heparin for high-dose applications in angioplasty and cardiac surgery. Its dose–response curve is linear at high argatroban concentrations and it is a reasonable tool for monitoring high-dose argatroban administration. The ACT has an additional advantage of being widely available in most hospitals and is readily interpreted by clinicians. The target ACT for PCI is > 300 when argatroban is used without glycoprotein (GP) IIb/IIIa inhibitors. An ACT of 200–250 s is recommended when argatroban is used in conjunction with a GPIIb/IIIa inhibitor.

The ecarin-clotting time (ECT) is being developed as a more specific and sensitive assay for monitoring thrombin inhibitors. It has a linear dose-dependent response in the therapeutic range of argatroban. One advantage of the ECT is that heparin or clotting factor deficiencies do not influence it. A second advantage is that the ECT has been adapted to dry-chemistry test card technology and can, therefore, be applied to bedside monitoring [55]. The disadvantage of ECT monitoring at this time is the lack of clear definition of toxic and therapeutic parameters correlated to clinical outcomes.

Also available are a specific chromogenic assay for thrombin inhibition activity and a high-performance liquid chromatography (HPLC) assay for direct quantitation of argatroban and its metabolites.

VI. CONCLUSIONS AND FUTURE DIRECTIONS

Argatroban is a direct thrombin inhibitor that has a large body of data demonstrating efficacy for both prophylaxis and treatment of thrombosis in patients with HIT. Based on these studies, the U.S. FDA has granted approval for argatroban use in these clinical indications.

Argatroban also provides reliable anticoagulation during percutaneous coronary interventions on HIT patients. Preliminary reports document the feasibility of using argatroban for anticoagulation during peripheral vascular interventions and hemodialysis for HIT patients. A limited experience with argatroban as adjunct to thrombolysis in acute ST elevation myocardial infarction has not shown an efficacy advantage, but these trials suffer from underpowering and some design limitations. The improvement in TIMI frame counts with argatroban suggests more work should be done with argatroban in the setting of acute myocardial infarction.

Among all the argatroban trials a consistent safety profile has been demonstrated. The laboratory data among the various trials suggests that argatroban is a predictable anticoagulant. Current recommendations for argatroban monitoring would include the aPTT for infusions of $1–10\,\mu g/kg\,min^{-1}$ and the ACT for the high-dose argatroban administration during interventional procedures.

Clinicians must remember that the studies and trials reported suffer from design limitations, as historical controls and registry-style data collection were used, which could potentially introduce bias. Large-scale, randomized, double-blinded trials have not yet been performed.

Argatroban is of a class of drugs that differs in many respects from heparin, LMWH, and heparinoids. Many of these differences are distinct advantages of the thrombin inhibitor that make it highly beneficial for use as an anticoagulant in patients with HIT. Hirudin, similar to argatroban, is another thrombin inhibitor that shares many of the same pharmacological characteristics of argatroban. However, there are several important differences between these two thrombin inhibitors that reflect advantages of argatroban over hirudin (Table 5). Thus, as the thrombin inhibitor class of drugs becomes established as a useful clinical anticoagulant, it is

Table 5 Advantages of Argatroban Over Heparin, LMWHs, Heparinoids, and Hirudin

No cross-reaction with heparin antibody
Rapid onset of action
Rapid reversibility
Short half-life
Inhibit clot-based thrombin
Nitric oxide donor (vasodilation)
Absence of antibody formation that affects pharmacokinetics and activity
Less bleeding
Ease of intravenous administration
Effective monitoring by aPTT or ACT
No dose adjustment required in renal-impaired patients

important to identify the advantages and disadvantages, not only of the drug class itself, but also of the individual drugs within a given class.

Argatroban continues to be studied for its role as an anticoagulant in various clinical settings. Current studies are evaluating the safety and efficacy of the combined therapy of argatroban with GPIIb/IIIa inhibitor antiplatelet drugs. Argatroban is also being studied as an antithrombotic agent in models of myocardial infarction, sepsis, cerebral thrombosis, tumor colonization, disseminated intravascular coagulation, peripheral arterial occlusion, extracorporeal circulation, and glomerulonephritis [1].

REFERENCES

1. Jeske W, Walenga JM, Lewis BE, Fareed J. Pharmacology of argatroban. Exp Opin Invest Drugs 1999; 8:625–654.
2. Banner DW, Hadvary P. Inhibitor binding to thrombin with x-ray crystallographic studies. Adv Exp Med Biol 1993; 340:27–33.
3. Bauer M, Brandstetter H, Turk D, Sturzebecker J, Bode W. Crystallographic determination of thrombin complexes with small synthetic inhibitors as a starting point for the receptor-based design of antithrombotics. Semin Thromb Hemost 1993; 19:352–360.
4. Hursting MJ, Alford KL, Becker JC, Brooks RL, Joffrion JL, Knappenberger GD, Kogan PW, Kogan TP, McKinney AA, Schwarz RP. Novastan (brand of argatroban): a small-molecule, direct thrombin inhibitor. Semin Thromb Hemost 1997; 23:503–516.
5. Bush LR. Argatroban, a selective, potent thrombin inhibitor. Cardiovasc Drug Rev 1991; 9:247–263.
6. Hijikata–Okunomiya A, Okamoto S. A strategy for a rational approach to designing synthetic selective inhibitors. Semin Thromb Hemost 1992; 18:135–149.
7. Ucki Y, Matsumoto K, Kizaki Y, Yoshida K, Matsunaga Y, Yano M, Tominga Y, Eguchi K. Argatroban increases nitric oxide levels in patients with peripheral arterial occlusive disease: placebo controlled study. J Thromb Thrombolysis 1999; 8:131–137.
8. Berry CN, Girard D, Lochot S, Lecoffre C. Antithrombotic actions of argatroban in rat models of venous, mixed and arterial thrombosis, and its effects on the tail transection bleeding time. Br J Pharm 1994; 113:1209–1214.
9. Tatsuno J, Komatsu I, Iida S. [Pharmacokinetic studies of argipidine (MD-805)—protein binding and blood cell binding.] (in Japanese). Jpn Pharmacol Ther 1986; 14(suppl 5):243–249.
10. Swan SK, Hursting MJ, The pharmacokinetics and pharmacodynamics of argatroban: effects of age, gender, and hepatic or renal dysfunction. Pharmacotherapy 2000; 20:318–329.

11. Ahmad S, Ahsan A, George M, Iqbal O, Jeske WP, McKenna R, Lewis BE, Walenga JM, Fareed J. Simultaneous monitoring cf argatroban and its major metabolite using an HPLC method: potential clinical applications. Clin Appl Thromb Haemost 1999;5: 252-258.

12. Izawa O, Katsuki M, T, Iida S. [Pharmacokinetics studies of argatroban (MD-805) in human—concentrations of argatroban and its metabolites in plasma, urine and feces during and after drip intravenous infusion.] (in Japanese). Jpn PharmacoL Ther 1986; 14(suppl 5):251–263.

13. Ahmad S, Yang A, Ashan A, Fu K, Iqbal O, Hoppensteadt DA, Lewis BE, Walenga JM, Fareed J. Pharmacokinetics of argatroban in primates: evidence of endogenous uptake. Int Angiol 2000; 19:126–134.

14. Swan SK, St. PJV, Lambrecht J. Comparison of anticoagulant effects and safety of argatroban and heparin in healthy subjects. Pharmacotherapy 2000; 20:756–770. [Summary in 3 parts (Part A)].

15. Hursting MJ, Becker JC, Joffrion JL, Knappenberger GD, Schwarz RP. Effect of hepatic function on the pharmacokinetics and pharmacodynamics of argatroban [abstr]. Thromb Haemost 1997; (June):493–494.

16. Hursting MJ, Joffrion JL, Brooks RU, Swan SK. Effect of renal function on the pharmacokinetics and pharmacodynamics of argatroban (a direct thrombin inhibitor). Blood 1996; 88(suppl 1):167a.

17. Walenga JM, Ahmad S, Hoppensteadt D, Iqbal O, Ahsan A, Fareed J. Prolonged argatroban treatment does not result in the generation of neutralizing antibodies. Thromb Res 2002; in press.

18. Eichler P, Frieseri H–J, Lubenow N, Jaeger B, Greinacher A. Antihirudin antibodies in patients with heparin-induced thrombocytopenia treated with lepirudin: incidence, effects on aPTT, and clinical relevance. Blood 2000; 96:2373–2378.

19. Berry CN, Girard D, Lochot S. Lecoffre C. Antithrombotic actions of argatroban in rat models of venous, mixed and arterial thrombosis, and its effects on the tail transection bleeding time. Br J Pharm 1994; 113:1209–1214.

20. Nakamura K, Hatano Y, Mon K. Thrombin-induced vasoconstriction in isolated cerebral arteries and the influence of a synthetic thrombin inhibitor. Thromb Res 1985; 40:715–720.

21. Winn MJ, Jain K, Ku DD. Argatroban and inhibition of the vasomotor actions of thrombin. J Cardiovasc Pharmacol 1993; 22:754–760.

22. Hijikata–Okunorniya A, Nakaya Y, Inoue N, Takahashi A, Taniguchi T, Wanaka K, Tsuda Y, Okada Y, Ishikawa Y. Effects of argatroban on thrombin-induced events in cultured vascular smooth muscle cells. Thromb Res 2000; 97:257–262.

23. Imanishi T, Arita M, I-Jamada M, Tomobuchi Y, Hano T, Nishio I. Effects of local administration of argatroban using a hydrogel-coated balloon catheter on intimal thickening induced by balloon injury. Jpn Circ J 1997; 61:256–262.

24. Yamabe H, Osawa H, Inuma H, Kaizuka M, Tamura N, Tsunoda S, Baba Y, Shirato K, Onodera K. Thrombin stimulates production of transforming growth factor-beta by cultured human mesangial cells. Nephrol Dial Transpl 1997; 12:438–442.

25. Wakita H, Furukawa F, Takigawa M. Thrombin and trypsin induced granulocyte–macrophage colony-stimulating factor and interleukin-6 gene expression in cultured normal human keratinocytes. Proc Assoc Am Phys 1997; 109:190–207.

26. Kosugi T, Nakamura M, Saitoh S, Kinjoh K, Hanashiro K. Changes of rabbit platelet function following simultaneous administration of ticlopidine hydrochloride and argipidine (MD-805). Int J Tissue React 1992; 14:141–148.

27. Warkentin TE, Levine MN, Hirsh J. Induced thrombocytopenia in patients treated with low-molecular-weight heparin or unfractionated heparin. N Engl J Med 1995; 332:1330–1335.

28. Warkentin T, Kelton J. A 14-year study of heparin-induced thrombocytopenia. Am J Med 1996; 101:502–507.

29. Amiral J, Bridey F, Wolf M, Boyer–Neumann C, Fressinaud F, Vissac AM, Peynaud–Debayle E, Dreyfus M, Meyer D. Antibodies to macromolecular platelet factor 4–heparin complexes in heparin-induced thrombocytopenia: a study of 44 cases. Thromb Haemost 1995; 73:21–28.

30. Warkentin TE, Hayward CP, Boshkov LK, Santos AV, Sheppard JA, Bode AP, Kelton JG. Sera from patients with heparin-induced thrombocytopenia generate platelet-derived rnicroparticles with procoagulant activity: an explanation for the thrombotic complications of heparin-induced thrombocytopenia. Blood 1994; 84:3691–3699.

31. Wallis DE, Workman DL, Lewis BE, Steen L, Pifarre R, Moran JF. Failure of early heparin cessation as treatment for heparin-induced thrombocytopenia. Am J Med 1999; 106:629–635.

32. LeRoy J, Leclerc MH, Delahousse B, Guerois C, Foloppe P, Gruel Y, Toulemonde F. Treatment of heparin-associated thrombocytopenia and thrombosis with low molecular weight heparin (CY 216). Semin Thromb Hemost 1985; 11:326–329.

33. Magnani HN. Heparin-induced thrombocytopenia (HIT): an overview of 230 patients treated with Orgaran (Org 10172). Thromb Haemost 1993; 70:554–561.

34. Lewis BE, Wallis DE, Rerkowitz SD, Matthai WH, Fareed J, Walenga JM, Bartholomew J, Sham R, Lerner RG, Zeigler ZR, Rustagi PK, Jang IK, Rifkin SD, Moran J, Hursting MJ, Kelton JG, the ARG-911 Study Investigators. Argatroban anticoagulant therapy in patients with heparin-induced thrombocytopenia. Circulation 2001; 103:1838–1843.

35. Greinacher A, Volpel H, Janssens U, Hach–Wunderle V, Kemkes–Matthes B, Eichler P, Mueller–Velten HG, Potzsch B, the HIT Investigators Group. Recombinant hirudin (lepirudin) provides safe and effective anti-coagulation in patients with heparin-induced thrombocytopenia: prospective study. Circulation 1999: 99:73–80.

36. Greinacher A, Janssens U, Berg G, Bock M, Kwasny H, Kemkes–Matthes B, Eichler P. Volpel H, Potzsch B, Luz M, the Heparin-Associated Thrombocytopenia Study (HAT) Investigators. Lepirudin (recombinant hirudin) for parenteral anticoagulation in patients with heparin-induced thrombocytopenia. Circulation 1999; 100:587–593.

37. Stone SR, Hofsteenge J. Kinetics of inhibition of thrombin by hirudin. Biochemistry 1986; 25:4622–4628.

38. Itoh T, Nonogi H, Miyazaki S, Itoh A, Daikoko S. Local delivery of argatroban using drug delivery device "dispatch" in the prevention of restenosis following coronary angioplasty trial (40-CAT): result of the prospective randomized pilot study. Circulation 1997; 96:3635.

39. Kobayashi H, Suzuki S, Sakamoto S, Matsuo T. Argatroban, a direct thrombin inhibitor versus heparin during and after percutaneous transluminal coronary angioplasty (PTCA) [abstr]. Thromb Haemost 1997; (June):494.

40. Lewis BE, Rangel Y, Fareed J. The first report of successful carotid stent implant using argatroban anticoagulation in a patient with heparin-induced thrombocytopenia and thrombosis syndrome: a case report. Angiology 1998; 49:61–67.

41. Jang IK, Gold HK, Leinbach RC. Acceleration of reperfusion by combination of rt-PA and a selective thrombin inhibitor, argatroban. Circulation 1989; 80(Suppl II): 217.

42. Jang IK, Brown OF, Giugliano RP, Anderson HV, Losordo D, Nicolav JC, Norbady R, Liprandi A, Massey TJ, Dinsmore R, Schwarz R. A multicenter, randomized study of argatroban versus heparin as adjunct to tPA in acute MI: MI with novastan and tPA study (MINT). J Am Coll Cardiol 1999; 33:1879–1885.

43. Vermeer F, Vahanian A, Fels DW, Besse P, Radzik D, Simoons ML. Intravenous argatroban versus heparin as co-medication to alteplase in the treatment of acute myocardial infarction; preliminary results of the ARGAMI pilot study. J Am Coll Cardiol 1997; 29:195A.

44. Koide M, Yamamoto S, Matsuo M, Suzak S, Arina N, Matsuo T. Anticoagulation for heparin induced thrombocytopenia with spontaneous platelet aggregation in patients requiring haemodialysis. Nephrol Dial Transp 1955; 10:2137–2140.

45. Matsuo T, Chikahira Y, Yamada T, Nakao K. Ueshima S, Matsuo O. Effect of synthetic thrombin inhibitor (MD805) as an alternative drug on heparin-induced thrombocytopenia during hemodialysis. Thromb Res 1988; 52:165–171.

46. Matsuo T, Yamada T, Yamanashi T, Ryo R. Anticoagulant therapy with MD805 of a hemodialysis patient with heparin-induced thrombocytopenia. Thromb Res 1990; 58:663–666.

47. Bergougnan L, Moore N, Brohier S. Pharmacodynamic and pharmacokinetic profile of argatroban (1 mg/mL alcohol solution) in healthy man. J Clin Pharmacol 1998; 38:878.

48. Lewis BE, Iqbal O, Hoppensteadt D, Walenga JM, Ahsan A, Ahmad S, Schwarz RP, Fareed J. Clinical pharmacokinetic and pharmacodynamic studies on argatroban to optimize the anticoagulant dosage in interventional cardiovascular procedures [abstr]. Thromb Haemost 1997; (June):492.

49. Ahmad S, Ahsan A, Iqbal O, Hoppensteadt DA, Lewis BE, Walenga JM, Fareed J. Pharmacokinetics and pharmacodynamics of argatroban as studied by HPLC and functional methods: implications in the monitoring and dosage-optimizations in cardiovascular patients. Clin Appl Thromb Hemost 1998; 4:243–249.

50. Hursting MJ, Becker JC, Lewis BE, Iqbal O, Walenga JM, Ferguson JJ. Differential effects of argatroban and heparin on Hemochron and Hemo-Tec activated clotting times in patients undergoing coronary interventional procedures. J Am Coll Cardiol 1997; 29:500a.

51. Walenga JM, Fasanella AR, Iqbal O, Hoppensteadt DA, Ahmad S, Wallis DE, Bakhos M. Coagulation laboratory testing in patients treated with argatroban. Semin Thromb Hemost 1999; 25(suppl 1):61–66.

52. Hoppensteadt DA, Kahn S, Fareed J. Factor X values as a means to assess the extent of oral anticoagulation in patients receiving antithrombin. Clin Chem 1997; 43:1786–1788.

53. Sheth SB, DiCicco RA, Hursting MA, Montague T, Jorkasky DK. Interpreting the international normalized ratio (INR) in individuals receiving argatroban and warfarin. Thromb Haemost 2001; 85:435.

54. Hursting MJ, Zehnder JL, Joffrion IL, Becker JL, Knappenberger GD, Schwarz RP. The interventional normalization ratio during concurrent warfarin and argatroban anticoagulation: differential contributions of each agent and effects of the choice of thromboplastin used. Clin Chem 1999; 45:409–412.

55. Mize PD, Ruebsaman K. Dry chemistry ecarin clotting time for ex vivo monitoring of direct thrombin inhibitors [abstr.]. Thromb Haemost 1997; (June):436.

13

Hirudin for Acute Coronary Syndromes

John W. Eikelboom
University of Western Australia, Perth, Australia

Shamir R. Mehta and Salim Yusuf
McMaster University, Hamilton, Ontario, Canada

SUMMARY

A strong biological rationale for a therapeutic role of specific inhibitors of thrombin in the management of acute coronary syndromes has led to the development of a new class of potent antithrombotic agents that directly inhibit both fluid-phase and tissue-bound thrombin. Hirudin, the prototype direct thrombin inhibitor, has been extensively evaluated in randomized trials in unstable angina and acute myocardial infarction and, to a lesser extent, during percutaneous coronary intervention. Although hirudin is superior to unfractionated heparin in reducing early cardiac events during active treatment, it is also associated with an increased risk of major bleeding. Thus, the role of hirudin in acute coronary syndromes remains to be clearly established. The Direct Thrombin Inhibitor Trialists' Collaboration is conducting an individual patient data metanalysis of major randomized trials of direct thrombin inhibitors, which should assist in further clarifying the role of hirudin in acute coronary syndromes.

I. INTRODUCTION

Intracoronary thrombus formation is a fundamental process in the clinical evolution of the acute coronary syndromes [1]. Disruption of atherosclerotic plaque exposes thrombogenic material in the lipid-rich core of the plaque to the blood, causing platelet adhesion and activation, coagulation activation, and thrombin generation [2]. Thrombin converts fibrinogen to fibrin as well as acting as a potent platelet agonist to recruit additional platelets into the platelet-rich thrombus. The resulting intracoronary thrombus impairs coronary blood flow, which then causes myocardial ischemia and the clinical manifestations of unstable angina or acute myocardial infarction.

Aspirin and heparin are effective therapies for the prevention of myocardial infarction and death in patients with acute coronary syndromes [3,4]. Despite their widespread use, however, patients presenting with unstable angina or myocardial infarction remain at high risk of recurrent ischemic events and death during the acute and chronic phases [5]. This suggests that in a sizeable proportion of patients, the process of intracoronary thrombus formation is resistant to inhibition by aspirin and heparin. Large amounts of thrombin are generated when the coagulation mechanism is activated by tissue factor exposed at the site of arterial injury [6,7]. When bound to fibrin, soluble fibrin degradation products, or exposed subendothelial matrix proteins, thrombin is protected from inactivation by heparin, which cannot effectively inhibit bound thrombin. However, bound thrombin remains enzymatically active, amplifying its own generation through a positive-feedback loop formed by coagulation factors V and VIII, thereby promoting further clot accretion. Bound thrombin also continues to activate platelets through thromboxane A_2-independent mechanisms that cannot be blocked by aspirin [7–10].

Recognition of the importance of thrombin as a therapeutic target to prevent intracoronary thrombus formation, and its relative resistance to inhibition by aspirin and heparin has led to the development of a class of anticoagulants specifically designed to control the generation of thrombin and block its activity. These agents are known as direct thrombin inhibitors because, unlike heparin, which indirectly inhibits fluid-phase thrombin by catalyzing the naturally occurring thrombin inhibitors antithrombin III and heparin cofactor II, these newer agents bind directly to both fluid-phase and bound thrombin, preventing interaction of the enzyme with its substrate and blocking its activity. Hirudin is the prototype of direct thrombin inhibitors, and still remains the most widely studied.

This chapter outlines the biochemistry and pharmacology of hirudin and reviews the results of major randomized trials that have been performed with this agent in the setting of unstable angina, acute myocardial infarction, and during percutaneous coronary revascularization performed in patients with acute coronary syndromes.

II. HIRUDINS

Hirudins are a homologous group of naturally occurring polypeptides isolated originally from the salivary gland of the European medicinal leech *Hirudo medicinalis*, but now available through recombinant DNA technology. The anticoagulant properties of leech saliva were first described in the latter part of the 19th century, but it was not until the 1950s that Markwardt extracted hirudin from head parts of medicinal leeches, described its specific antithrombin activity and recognized its polypeptide structure [11,12]. The primary structure of hirudin was elucidated in 1976 [13].

A. Biochemistry

There are several variants of hirudin that contain either 65 or 66 amino acids. The N-terminal structure of hirudin is globular because of three disulfide bonds, whereas the C-terminal portion contains a preponderance of acidic amino acids, including a sulfated tyrosine located three amino acids from the C-terminus [14]. Native hirudin variants as well as recombinant hirudins share this common basic structure and have similar anticoagulant activities [14–16]. However recombinant hirudins lack the sulfate group on tyrosine-63 and, therefore, are known as desulfatohirudins [16].

Hirudins are highly specific inhibitors of thrombin, forming an essentially irreversible 1 : 1 stoichiometric complex with thrombin, thereby blocking the substrate-binding domain and the active center of the enzyme [10,11]. Although loss of the sulfate group on tyrosine-63 reduces the affinity of recombinant hirudin for thrombin by approximately ten fold, recombinant hirudin remains an extremely potent and selective inhibitor of thrombin [16].

The secondary and tertiary structure of hirudin is essential for its antithrombotic function [17–19]. The central core region of hirudin is tightly folded and is held together by the three disulfide bridges, whereas a six-residue N-terminus protrudes from the core region as does a longer C-terminal tail. Thrombin contains an anion-binding exosite that functions as the substrate recognition site, an active site, and an apolar-binding site adjacent to the active site that plays a role in substrate binding to the active site [16]. The N-terminal domain of hirudin binds to the active site of thrombin, whereas the C-terminal tail blocks the anion-binding exosite, thereby preventing thrombin's interaction with negatively charged substrates such as fibrinogen. The bivalent nature of the thrombin–hirudin interaction contrasts with several more recently developed low-molecular-weight thrombin inhibitors, such as argatroban, inogatran, and efegatran, which selectively block only the active site.

B. Pharmacology

The pharmacological properties of native and recombinant hirudins are similar. Although desirudin and lepirudin, the two currently available recombinant hirudins, differ slightly in their amino-terminal amino acid sequence, they have a similar overall amino acid sequence, molecular weight, potency, and antithrombotic activity [20–22].

Hirudin has many advantages over heparin (Table 1). Hirudin blocks all of the biological actions of thrombin on blood coagulation, including thrombin-mediated conversion of fibrinogen to fibrin, activation of coagulation factors XI and XIII, and positive feedback activation of coagulation factors V and VIII [11,23]. After complexing with hirudin, thrombin also loses its cellular nonhemostatic effects, such as its ability to stimulate the proliferation of fibroblasts, activate endothelial cells, or induce smooth-muscle cell contraction. In addition, hirudin prevents

Table 1 Comparison of Hirudin and Heparin

Hirudin	Heparin	
	Unfractionated	Low-molecular-weight
Specific inhibitor of thrombin	Inhibits thrombin, factors Xa, IXa, XIa	Inhibits factor Xa, thrombin
Inhibits fluid-phase and tissue-bound thrombin	Inhibits only fluid-phase thrombin	Inhibits only fluid-phase thrombin
Antithrombin III-independent	Antithrombin III-dependent	Antithrombin III-dependent
Not neutralized by plasma proteins	Neutralized by heparinase, plasma proteins, PF4	Neutralized by heparinase
Inhibits platelet function	Paradoxical activation of platelets?	Limited platelet inhibition
No effect on vascular permeability	Increases vascular permeability	No effect on vascular permeability
No thrombocytopenia	Immune and nonimmune thrombocytopenia	Thrombocytopenia rare
No hepatic toxicity	Transient rise in liver enzymes common	Can cause transient rise in liver enzymes

binding of thrombin to endothelial thrombomodulin, thus reducing protein C activation and limiting the ability of activated protein C to serve as an anticoagulant by inactivating factors Va and VIIIa [24].

Because coronary thrombi are rich in platelets, inhibition of thrombin-mediated platelet activation by hirudin is of particular relevance. Hirudin exerts an effect on platelets by several distinct mechanisms [16,25]: First, by inhibiting thrombin, hirudin blocks thrombin-mediated platelet activation [26]; second, hirudin prevents exposure of the platelet glycoprotein IIb/IIIa integrin receptor, thus preventing platelet aggregation [27]; and third, by virtue of a greater affinity for thrombin, hirudin can cause dissociation of platelet-bound thrombin [28]. Thus, hirudin inhibits activation of both blood coagulation and platelets, the two key processes involved in intracoronary thrombus formation.

The pharmacokinetic properties of hirudin were initially defined in laboratory animals, but are similar in humans [11,21,29–32]. Hirudin is not absorbed by the gastrointestinal tract and must be administered parenterally. After bolus intravenous injection, hirudin is rapidly distributed and has an elimination half-life of 20–60 min, depending on the particular form of recombinant hirudin being studied. After subcutaneous injection, peak levels are reached after 1–2 h. Hirudin is distributed in the extracellular space and is primarily renally excreted in a still active form, undergoing limited hepatic metabolism. The renal clearance of hirudin approximates that of creatinine, which suggests that it is cleared by glomerular filtration. In nephrectomized dogs, blood levels of hirudin remained virtually constant after the initial distribution phase [33], further illustrating the predominant renal route of hirudin excretion.

In plasma, hirudin produces a dose-dependent increase in the activated partial thromboplastin time (aPTT), with the half-life of this effect being 2–3 h [30,31]. However, the relation between hirudin and the aPTT is dependent on the particular aPTT reagent that is used. The aPTT reaches a plateau at higher hirudin doses [34]. More recently, the ecarin-clotting time (ECT) assay has been developed for monitoring direct thrombin inhibitors [35]. Ecarin is a snake venom that converts prothrombin to meizothrombin, which causes clotting of fibrinogen in citrated whole blood or plasma. The ECT has been used successfully to monitor hirudin therapy during coronary artery bypass surgery [36], but has not been evaluated in acute coronary syndromes.

Toxicological studies in experimental animals and tolerance studies in humans indicate that, other than its anticoagulant effects, recombinant hirudin is pharmacodynamically relatively "inert" [37]. Thus, hirudin has no direct effects on blood cells, plasma proteins, or other enzymes, and has no direct effect on platelet aggregation and release reactions induced by platelet agonists such as ADP, collagen, platelet-activating factor, or arachidonic acid. Early studies in animals and humans also demonstrated little evidence of immunogenicity or allergenicity [37,38], although more recent human studies have revealed a high incidence of antibody production against hirudin when the drug is given intravenously or subcutaneously for long periods [39,40]. However, antihirudin antibodies are not associated with the development of thrombocytopenia and appear to be of little clinical significance [39–41].

C. Preclinical Studies of the Antithrombotic Efficacy of Hirudin

The antithrombotic activity of hirudin for prevention of arterial thrombosis has been studied in numerous animal models and in settings where vascular injury has been induced with various mechanical, chemical or electrical stimuli [37,38,42–46]. In these models, hirudin is superior to heparin for the prevention of platelet-rich thrombus formation on injured carotid or coronary vessels, prevents mural thrombus formation on arterial vessels after angioplasty, and both accelerates and sustains coronary recanalization when given with streptokinase. The latter observation is of particular clinical importance because bound thrombin exposed during thrombolysis may trigger recurrent ischemic events, and is inaccessible to inhibition by heparin. Hirudin also prevents endotoxin-induced microthrombosis in models of disseminated intravascular coagulation (DIC), inhibiting the consumption of clotting factors and antithrombin III [47,48]. Similarly, hirudin prevents thrombosis on artificial surfaces, inhibits the development of occlusive thrombi in arteriovenous shunts [49], and attenuates fibrin deposition on dialysis membranes [33].

III. CLINICAL STUDIES

Hirudin has been extensively studied in patients with coronary artery disease, having been tested as a replacement for heparin in patients with unstable angina, as an adjunct to thrombolytic therapy in patients with acute myocardial infarction, and as a substitute for heparin in patients with unstable angina undergoing percutaneous coronary intervention (Table 2).

A.   Hirudin as a Replacement for Heparin in Unstable Angina

Several phase I/II studies have compared hirudin with unfractionated heparin (UFH) in patients with unstable angina or non–Q-wave myocardial infarction [50–53]. The largest of these was the Organization to Assess Strategies for Ischemic Syndromes (OASIS) pilot study [53] in which 909 patients with unstable angina or non–Q-wave myocardial infarction were randomized to a 72-h infusion of low- or medium-dose hirudin or UFH. Doses of hirudin and UFH were adjusted to achieve a target aPTT of 60–100 s. Although this study was not powered for clinical outcomes, hirudin was associated with a promising reduction in the composite primary outcome of cardiovascular death, myocardial infarction or refractory angina at 7 days (OR 0.57; 95% CI: 0.32–1.02) and a significant reduction in the composite secondary outcome of death, myocardial infarction refractory and severe ischemia requiring revascularization at 7 days (OR 0.49; 95% CI: 0.27–0.86) compared with UFH. The incidence of major bleeding was low (approximately 1% in each group) and was not significantly higher in patients treated with hirudin than in those given UFH (OR 0.86; 95% CI: 0.23–3.19). No intracranial bleeding was observed in this study.

To further compare the effects of hirudin and UFH on biochemical markers of coagulation activation in the OASIS pilot study, blood samples were collected before, during, and after study drug infusion in a subset of 395 patients for measurement of aPTT, prothrombin fragment 1.2, thrombin–antithrombin complexes, and D-dimer levels [54]. Hirudin had no effect on prothrombin fragment 1.2 levels, a marker of thrombin generation, but produced greater suppression of thrombin–antithrombin complexes and D-dimer than UFH during the study drug infusion, which is consistent with its more potent inhibition of thrombin activity. However, after cessation of study-drug, levels of D-dimer increased above baseline levels in both treatment groups, suggesting that longer-term antithrombotic strategies may be needed to passivate the culprit lesion.

In the phase III OASIS-2 trial [55], 10,141 patients with unstable angina or non–Q-wave myocardial infarction were randomized to medium-dose hirudin (0.4-mg/kg bolus, 0.15-mg/kg h^{-1} infusion) or UFH for 72 h. During treatment, there was a significant reduction in the composite outcome of death or myocardial infarction with hirudin relative to heparin (2.0 vs. 2.6%, OR 0.76; 95% CI: 0.59–0.99), but the primary outcome of death or myocardial infarction at 7 days (3.6 vs. 4.2%, OR 0.84; 95% CI: 0.69–1.02) and at 35 days (6.8 vs. 7.7%, OR 0.87 95% CI: 0.75–1.01) was not significantly different in the two groups (Table 3). However, there was no loss of benefit after cessation of the study drug, and the absolute risk reduction in death

Table 2 Design of Major Randomized Trials of Hirudin in Acute Coronary Syndromes and During Percutaneous Coronary Intervention

Study	Year	Condition	N	Design	Primary efficacy outcome
OASIS 2	1999	USA	10,141	2-arm study	Randomized heparin-controlled	CV death or MI; 7 days
HIT 3	1994	MI	302	2-arm study	Randomized heparin-controlled	Death or MI; 30 days
GUSTO 2A	1994	MI	12,142	2-arm study	Randomized heparin-controlled	Death or MI; 30 days
GUSTO 2B	1996	MI	2,564	2-arm study	Randomized heparin-controlled	Death or MI; 30 days
TIMI 9A	1994	MI	757	2-arm study	Randomized heparin-controlled	Death, MI, CCF, or shock; 30 days
TIMI 9B	1996	MI	3,002	2-arm study	Randomized heparin-controlled	Death, MI, CCF, or shock; 30 days
HELVETICA	1995	PCI	1,141	3-arm study	Randomized heparin-controlled	Death, MI, CABG, or bailout procedure; 30 weeks

CABG, coronary artery bypass graft; CCF, congestive cardiac failure; MI, myocardial infarction; PCI, percutaneous coronary intervention; USA, unstable angina.

Table 3 Death or Myocardial Infarction in Hirudin Versus Unfractionated Heparin-Treated Patients in OASIS-2

Outcome	Timing	Odds ratio	95% CI	p-Value
CV death, or MI[b]	72 hours	0.76	0.59–0.99	0.04
[a]CV death, or MI	7 days	0.84	0.69–1.02	0.08
CV death, MI, refractory angina	7 days	0.82	0.70–0.96	0.01
Death or MI	35 days	0.87	0.75–1.01	0.06

[a]Primary outcome.
[b]CV, cardiovascular; MI, myocardial infarction.

or myocardial infarction that emerged during treatment was maintained at 35 days. Compared with UFH, hirudin was associated with a significantly increased risk of major bleeding (1.2 vs. 0.7%, OR 1.73; 95% CI: 1.13–2.63), but not life-threatening bleeding (0.4 versus 0.4%, OR 0.99; 95% CI: 0.54–1.85). There were no cases of intracranial bleeding during study-drug infusion with hirudin and one case with UFH.

A pooled analysis of the OASIS pilot and OASIS-2 trials [55] indicates a statistically significant reduction in the composite outcome of death or myocardial infarction at 35 days (6.7 vs. 7.7%, OR 0.86; 95% CI: 0.74–0.99) with hirudin compared with UFH. The early treatment benefit seen in both trials was maintained for at least 35 days. The lack of rebound in clinical events after stopping hirudin seems to be inconsistent with the biochemical evidence of rebound seen in the OASIS pilot study. However, both biochemical and clinical rebound have been reported after heparin is stopped [56,57]. Because the OASIS pilot and OASIS-2 trials compared an equal duration of therapy with hirudin and UFH, any rebound in clinical events after cessation of therapy may have been "masked" by a parallel increase in clinical events in both treatment groups.

B. Hirudin as an Adjunct to Thrombolytic Therapy in Acute Myocardial Infarction

The Hirudin for Improvement of Thrombolysis (HIT) group and the Thrombolysis in Myocardial Infarction (TIMI) group conducted a series of phase II trials [58–63] evaluating hirudin as an adjunct to thrombolytic therapy with streptokinase (SK) or tissue plasminogen activator (t-PA) in acute myocardial infarction. Promising results seen with hirudin in these studies, based primarily on angiographic outcomes, prompted the initiation of several phase III randomized, heparin-controlled trials in acute coronary syndromes by the TIMI, Global Utilization of Streptokinase and Tissue Plasminogen Activator for Occluded Coronary Arteries (GUSTO), and HIT study groups. Both the TIMI-9A [64] and HIT-3 [65] trials evaluated the use of hirudin as an adjunct to thrombolysis, whereas the GUSTO-2A [66] study included patients with acute myocardial infarction receiving thrombolytic therapy as well as patients with unstable angina or myocardial infarction who were ineligible for thrombolytic therapy. However, all of these initial phase III studies were terminated prematurely because of unacceptably high rates of major hemorrhage.

The TIMI-9A trial [64] randomly assigned patients with acute myocardial infarction undergoing thrombolytic therapy to 96 h of treatment with hirudin or UFH. Patients had to be within 12 h of symptom onset, and the choice of thrombolytic therapy was left to the discretion of the investigator. Hirudin was administered as a 0.6-mg/kg intravenous bolus followed by an infusion of 0.2-mg/kg h^{-1}, the highest dose used in phase II clinical trials. As in the phase II TIMI-5 and TIMI-6 studies [62,63], the dose of hirudin in TIMI-9A was not adjusted according to the aPTT. Unfractionated heparin was given as a 5000-IU/kg bolus followed by a weight-adjusted infusion of 1000-IU/kg h^{-3} for patients weighing less than 80 kg and 1300-IU/kg for those weighing more than 80 kg. Unfractionated heparin was dose-adjusted to achieve an aPTT ratio of 2.0–3.0. The primary outcome was the composite of death or myocardial infarction at 30 days. Although the planned enrolment was 3000 patients, the trial was terminated prematurely by the Data and Safety Monitoring Board after 757 patients had been randomized because of excess hemorrhagic complications in both treatment groups, particularly with hirudin. Spontaneous major bleeding at nonintracranial sites occurred in 7.0% of hirudin-treated patients compared with 3.0% of heparin-treated patients (p = 0.02), although no difference in the incidence of intracranial bleeding was observed (1.7 vs. 1.9%, p = ns). Patients with major bleeding were older (mean age 68 vs. 61 years), had higher median aPTT values at 12 h (100 vs. 85 s), and were more likely to have a creatinine level higher than 1.5 mg/dL (15 vs. 5%) compared with patients who did not experience major bleeding.

The GUSTO-2A trial [66] randomly assigned patients presenting within 12 h of onset of symptoms of unstable angina or acute myocardial infarction to hirudin or UFH for 48–96 h, with the primary outcome being death or myocardial infarction at 30 days. The planned enrolment was 12,000 patients, with an approximately equal proportion of patients with or without ST-elevation. The doses of hirudin and unfractionated heparin were identical with those used in the TIMI-9A study, with a target aPTT of 60–90 s for UFH and no dose adjustment for hirudin. After 2564 patients had been randomized, GUSTO-2A was stopped because of an excess of intracranial bleeds in patients receiving thrombolytic therapy with 23 of the 26 intracranial bleeds occurring in this group. The overall incidence of intracranial hemorrhage was 1.8%, and there was a trend to more intracranial hemorrhage with hirudin than with heparin (1.3 vs. 0.7%, p = 0.11). Patients with intracranial hemorrhage were older (mean age 72 vs. 64 years), had a higher median aPTT at 12 h (110 vs. 87 s), and included a greater proportion of patients with body weight greater than 80 kg (58 vs. 47%) compared with patients who did not experience intracranial hemorrhage

In the HIT-3 study [65], the third study stopped prematurely because of an excess of major bleeding, patients presenting within 6 h of acute myocardial infarction who were eligible for thrombolytic therapy were randomized to 48–72 h of either hirudin or unfractionated heparin as an adjunct to t-PA. The dose of hirudin, 0.4-mg/kg bolus and 0.15-mg/kg h infusion, was lower than that used in TIMI-9A and GUSTO-2A studies, whereas the initial dose of UFH was weight-adjusted at 70-IU/kg bolus and 15-IU/kg/h^{-1} infusion. The dose of both hirudin and UFH was adjusted during infusion to a target aPTT ratio of 2.0–3.5. The frequency of dose adjustment in either direction was limited to twice and, during the first 24 h, downward dose adjustment could be performed only if there was bleeding. Although enrollment of 7000 patients was planned, the trial was terminated after 302 patients were entered because of an excess of intracranial bleeds in patients receiving hirudin (3.4 vs. 0%, p = ns). All intracranial bleeds occurred during the first 24 h of treatment. As in TIMI-9A and GUSTO-2A, the median aPTT was higher in patients who experienced major bleeding than in those, who did not (106 vs. 76 s).

There are several potential explanations for the excess of bleeding seen in the TIMI-9A, GUSTO-2A, and HIT-3 trials, particularly in patients treated with hirudin. First, a clear dose–response relation for efficacy was not seen in phase II trials evaluating hirudin as an adjunct to thrombolytic therapy, and the higher doses did not appear to confer an increased risk of bleeding. Therefore, the highest dose of hirudin evaluated in the pilot studies was used in TIMI-9A and GUSTO-2A. In retrospect, however, it is clear that the dose of hirudin used in these studies, and particularly the initial bolus dose, was inappropriately high. Second, the dose of UFH in the TIMI-9A and GUSTO-2A studies was approximately 20% higher than that used in the GUSTO-1 trial [67] in an attempt to improve on the high incidence of subtherapeutic aPTT values seen in the earlier study [68]. Levels of anticoagulation achieved with UFH in GUSTO-2A were significantly higher than those in GUSTO-1. However, the GUSTO-1 investigators subsequently showed that aPTTs of more than 70 s were associated with an excess of hemorrhagic events [69], a finding consistent with the increased bleeding seen with heparin in TIMI-9A and GUSTO-2A. Further support for the conclusion that heparin doses used in TIMI-9A and GUSTO-2A were too high comes from the finding of an excess of major bleeding in heavier patients in GUSTO-2A [66]. Third, aPTT monitoring for hirudin was not performed in TIMI-9A and GUSTO-2A and was not recommended during the first 24 h of treatment in HIT-3. However, the clear association between high aPTT and major bleeding risk, and the clustering of bleeding events during the first 24 h that was observed in all three studies, suggests that careful laboratory monitoring is essential, particularly during the first 24 h. Fourth, the association between baseline creatinine and bleeding risk in TIMI-9A suggests that the dose of hirudin needs to be reduced in patients with renal insufficiency, particularly in view of the known renal mechanism of hirudin clearance [33].

The TIMI-9B [70] and GUSTO-2B [71] trials were subsequently recommenced with lower doses of both hirudin and UFH. In both trials, the bolus dose of hirudin was reduced from 0.6 to 0.1 mg/kg and the infusion from 0.2 to $0.1 \, \text{mg/kg} \, \text{h}^{-1}$. In addition, hirudin therapy was monitored and adjusted according to the aPTT, with a target range of 55–85 s in TIMI-9B and 60-85 s in GUSTO-2B. With these modifications, planned enrolment was successfully completed in both studies.

The GUSTO-2B results showed a borderline significant reduction in the primary composite outcome of death or myocardial infarction with hirudin compared with heparin (OR 0.89; 95% CI: 0.79–1.00) at 30 days. The benefits of hirudin were similar when given as an adjunct to thrombolysis or when used for the treatment of non–ST-elevation acute coronary syndromes. During the first 24 h of treatment, there was a clear reduction in death or myocardial infarction with hirudin (1.3 vs. 2.1%, OR 0.61; 95% CI: 0.46–0.81), and a retrospective subgroup analysis suggested a favorable interaction between hirudin and streptokinase, compared with heparin and streptokinase, with a highly significant 39% reduction in death or myocardial infarction at 30 days in the hirudin-treated group (9.1 vs. 14.9%, OR 0.57; 95% CI: 0.38–0.87) [72].

In the TIMI-9B trial there was no benefit of hirudin over unfractionated heparin at 30 days, either on the primary composite outcome of death, myocardial infarction, cardiac failure, or cardiogenic shock (OR 1.09; 95% CI: 0.88–1.36) or the composite of death or myocardial infarction (OR 1.02; 95% CI: 0.80–1.31). However, there was a trend to reduction in nonfatal myocardial infarction during hospitalization (OR 0.65; 95% CI: 0.42–1.01) and at 30 days (OR 0.81; 95% CI: 0.56–1.18). Neither TIMI-9A nor GUSTO-2A demonstrated an excess of major or intracranial bleeding with hirudin.

The results of TIMI-9B and GUSTO-2B suggest that hirudin is at least as effective as UFH for the prevention of major adverse cardiovascular outcomes, including death and myocardial infarction, when used as an adjunct to thrombolytic therapy in patients with acute myocardial infarction. When the results of these two trials are pooled with results of the OASIS-2 trial, a clear benefit of hirudin over UFH is evident with a statistically significant 10% relative risk reduction in death or myocardial infarction at 30–35 days (p = 0.016) (Fig. 3) [55]. Nevertheless, the lack of a clear benefit of hirudin over UFH at 30 days in GUSTO-2B and TIMI-9B remains somewhat unexpected given the strong biological rationale for the use of direct thrombin inhibitors in the setting of thrombolytic therapy and the promising results of phase II angiographic studies. It is possible that the revised dose of hirudin employed in the TIMI-9B and GUSTO-2B trials was too low, and the duration of treatment too short, to block thrombin generated during thrombolysis. Furthermore, the timing of hirudin administration in relation to thrombolytic therapy may have been suboptimal. In TIMI-9B and GUSTO-2B, adjunctive

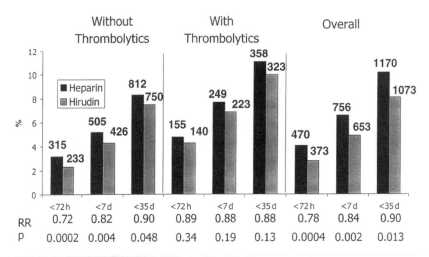

Figure 1 Pooled analysis of large trials of hirudin versus heparin in acute coronary syndromes. (From Ref. 55. Reproduced with permission from Elsevier Science.)

anticoagulant therapy was commenced a median of approximately 30–40 min after starting thrombolytic therapy [70,71]. Because exposure of thrombin may be an important trigger of recurrent ischemic events, the greatest benefit of adjunctive antithrombotic therapy during thrombolytic therapy may be realized only when treatment is started before use of thrombolytic therapy. This hypothesis is being tested in the HERO-2 study in which 20,000 patients with acute myocardial infarction will be randomized to either a direct thrombin inhibitor (bivalirudin) or UFH as an adjunct to streptokinase.

C. Hirudin During Percutaneous Coronary Intervention

The HELVETICA study [73] was a phase III randomized, double-blind trial comparing hirudin with unfractionated heparin for the prevention of restenosis after percutaneous transluminal coronary angioplasty in patients with unstable angina. This trial was conducted before the widespread use of intracoronary stents. A total of 1141 patients were randomized to either hirudin, given as a bolus and 24 h infusion followed by subcutaneous placebo or hirudin for a further 72 h, or to unfractionated heparin given as a bolus plus infusion for 24 h followed by 72 h of placebo subcutaneous injections. An additional bolus of placebo (hirudin group) or UFH (heparin group) could be administered at the discretion of the physician if the procedure lasted longer than 1 h, but no dose adjustment was allowed during the intravenous infusion. The primary outcome was event-free survival at 30 weeks, defined as the absence of death, myocardial infarction, coronary artery bypass graft surgery, or bailout angioplasty, with or without a stent at the previously dilated site. Secondary outcomes included cardiac events within the first 96 h as well as bleeding complications.

At 7 months, there were no significant differences in event-free survival in patients who received unfractionated heparin (67.3%), intravenous hirudin (63.5%), or intravenous followed by subcutaneous hirudin (68.0%). There also was no significant difference among the three groups in luminal diameter of the dilated vessel on repeat angiography at 6 months. However, hirudin was associated with a substantial, and statistically significant, reduction in the primary composite outcome at 96 h (OR 0.61; 95% CI: 0.41–0.90). Although this early benefit was preserved to 30 days, there was a subsequent divergence in the time-to-event curves, which may have been due to restenosis in both groups. No excess in minor or major bleeding was observed with hirudin.

In the context of current knowledge, the lack of benefit of hirudin in preventing restenosis at 7 months in the HELVETICA study is not surprising. Antithrombotic drugs, including glycoprotein IIb/IIIa inhibitors, heparin, and warfarin do not prevent restenosis after coronary angioplasty [74], while trials of antithrombotic therapy in acute coronary syndromes have consistently demonstrated that the benefits of therapy are achieved during active treatment, with no additional benefit after cessation of therapy [4,55,70,71,75]. This also is the pattern of benefit seen in the HELEVTICA trial, where a clear treatment effect was observed during the first few days of active therapy, with no additional benefit occurring after stopping treatment.

Emerging data from patients undergoing percutaneous coronary intervention in randomized acute coronary syndrome trials lend further support for the superiority of hirudin over UFH in this setting. In the OASIS-2 trial [55], which compared hirudin with UFH in acute coronary syndromes without ST elevation, 117 patients underwent percutaneous coronary intervention during the period of study drug infusion. At 35 days, hirudin was associated with a substantial, and highly statistically significant, reduction in death or myocardial infarction compared with UFH (6.4 vs. 22.9%, OR 0.25; 95% CI: 0.07–0.86) [76]. Similarly, in the GUSTO-2B trial [70], which compared hirudin with unfractionated heparin in acute coronary syndromes, 1404 patients received a blinded study drug during percutaneous coronary intervention and for a further 72 h thereafter. Compared with UFH, patients who received hirudin during angioplasty had a significantly reduced risk of death or myocardial infarction at 30 days (2.1 vs. 3.8%, p = 0.05) [77].

The treatment effects of hirudin during percutaneous coronary intervention appear to be analogous to the pattern of benefit seen in the glycoprotein IIb/IIIa inhibitor trials. In settings where intervention rates are low, as in the GUSTO-4 trial comparing abciximab with placebo in unstable angina, glycoprotein IIb/IIIa inhibitors are, at best, of marginal benefit [78]. By contrast, a consistent and substantial benefit of glycoprotein IIb/IIIa inhibitors was seen in percutaneous coronary intervention trials [75]. Similarly, in OASIS-2 and GUSTO-2B [55,70], the overall benefits of hirudin were modest. However, in the subset of patients undergoing percutaneous coronary intervention, the benefits of hirudin appear to be much greater. These findings emphasize the role of antithrombotic therapy at the time of vessel wall injury, and raise the possibility that monotherapy with a direct thrombin inhibitor, such as hirudin, may be comparable with combined therapy with heparin and a glycoprotein IIb/IIIa inhibitor during percutaneous coronary intervention. This concept is being explored further in trials evaluating the use of bivalirudin during percutaneous coronary intervention [79].

IV. CONCLUSIONS AND FUTURE DIRECTIONS

Randomized trials examining the usefulness of hirudin in acute coronary syndromes or during percutaneous coronary intervention indicate a clear early benefit of hirudin over unfractionated heparin, and pooled data indicate that a significant treatment effect persists at 30–35 days. Nevertheless, the role of hirudin in acute coronary syndromes remains to be defined. Several factors appear to be limiting the further development of hirudin, including the increased risk of major bleeding, and its relatively high cost. It is possible that judicious patient selection, combined with appropriate laboratory monitoring of the anticoagulant response of hirudin may lead to improvements in its safety profile.

Interpretation of early randomized experience with hirudin in acute coronary syndromes has largely focused on its relatively narrow therapeutic window. However, this feature is not unique to hirudin; it is shared by other widely accepted and effective antithrombotic agents, including UFH and warfarin. Perhaps a more important lesson from early hirudin experience is the need for adequately powered and properly monitored phase II trials to select the most appropriate dose and duration of antithrombotic agents before planning more definitive phase III trials [80].

An important unanswered question relates to the optimal duration of more potent antithrombotic agents such as hirudin. Trials examining the benefit of long-term anticoagulation using indirect thrombin inhibitors, such as low-molecular-weight heparin, have largely been disappointing [4]. Individual trials of vitamin K antagonists have been inconclusive [81], although pooled results suggest that they are beneficial [82]. However, neither low-molecular-weight heparin nor warfarin is as potent as hirudin at blocking the activity of thrombin. A polyethylene glycol-complexed long-acting hirudin derivative (PEG-hirudin) that can be given once daily by subcutaneous injection is available, and may be useful for more long-term therapy.

The Direct Thrombin Inhibitor Trialists' Collaboration is currently conducting an individual patient data-based metanalysis of major randomized trials of direct thrombin inhibitors, including hirudin, in acute coronary syndromes and during percutaneous coronary intervention [83]. This approach will provide enhanced statistical power to identify clinically important treatment effects, particularly in high-risk patients in whom the risk/benefit ratio of hirudin may be more favorable. Results of this collaborative project, which is being jointly coordinated by the Canadian Cardiovascular Collaboration, McMaster University and Duke Clinical Research Institute, will be available during 2001 and will help further clarify the role of hirudin in acute coronary syndromes.

REFERENCES

1. Fuster V, Badimon L, Badimon JJ, Chesebro J. The pathogenesis of coronary artery disease and the acute coronary syndromes. N Engl J Med 1992; 326:242–250.
2. Furie B, Furie BC. Molecular and cellular biology of blood coagulation. N Engl J Med 1992; 326:800–806.
3. Antiplatelet Trialists' Collaboration. Collaborative overview of randomised trials of antiplatelet therapy—I: prevention of death, myocardial infarction, and stroke by prolonged antiplatelet therapy in various categories of patients. Br Med J 1994; 308:81–106.
4. Eikelboom JW, Anand SS, Malmberg K, Weitz JI, Ginsberg JS, Yusuf S. Unfractionated heparin (UFH) and low-molecular-weight heparin (LMWH) in unstable angina and non–Q-wave myocardial infarction (NQMI): a meta-analysis. Lancet 2000; 355:1936–1942.
5. Mehta S, Eikelboom JW, Yusuf S. Long-term management of unstable angina and non–Q-wave myocardial infarction. Eur Heart J 2000; 2:E6–E12.
6. Chesebro JH, Zoldhelyi P, Badimon L, Fuster V. Role of thrombin in arterial thrombosis: implications for therapy. Thromb Haemost 1991; 66:1–5.
7. Weitz JI. Biologic rationale for the therapeutic role of specific antithrombins. Coronary Artery Dis 1996; 7:409–419.
8. Weitz JI, Hudoba M, Massel D, Maraganore J, Hirsh J. Clot-bound thrombin is protected from inhibition by heparin–antithrombin III but is susceptible to inactivation by antithrombin III-independent inhibitors. J Clin Invest 1990; 86:385–391.
9. Weitz JI, Leslie B, Hudoba M. Thrombin binds to soluble fibrin degradation products where it is

protected from inhibition by heparin–antithrombin but susceptible to inactivation by antithrombin-independent inhibitors. Circulation 1998; 97:544–552.

10. Bar-Shavit R, Eldor A, Vlodavsky I. Binding of thrombin to sub-endothelial extracellular matrix: protection and expression of functional properties. J Clin Invest 1989; 84:1096–1104.

11. Markwardt F. The development of hirudin as an antithrombotic drug. Thromb Res 1994; 74:1–23.

12. Markwardt F. Past, present and future of hirudin. Haemostasis 1991; 21:11–26.

13. Petersen TE, Roberts HR, Sotrup–Jensen L, Magnusson S. Primary structure of hirudin, a thrombin-specific inhibitor. In: Peeters H, ed. Protides of the Biologic Fluids. Oxford: Pergamin Press, 1976.

14. Wallis RB. Hirudins: from leeches to man. Semin Thromb Hemost 1996; 22:185–196.

15. Scharf M, Engels J, Tripier D. Primary structure of new "iso-hirudins." FEBS Lett 1989; 255:105–110.

16. Toschi V, Lettino M, Gallo R, Badimon JJ, Chesebro JH. Biochemistry and biology of hirudin. Coronary Artery Dis 1996; 7:420–428.

17. Clore GM, Sukamaran DK, Nilges M, Zabock J, Gronenborn AM. The conformations of hirudin in solutions: a study using nuclear magnetic resonance, distance geometry and restrained molecular dynamics. EMBO J 1987; 6:529–537.

18. Folkers PJM, Clore GM, Driscoll PC, Dodt J, Kohler S, Gronenborm AM. Solution structure of recombinant hirudin and the Lys-47 → Glu mutant: a nuclear magnetic resonance and hybrid distance geometry–dynamical simulated annealing study. Biochemistry 1989; 28:1601–1617.

19. Haruyama H, Wuthrich K. Conformation of recombinant desulfatohirudin in acqueous solution determined by nuclear magnetic resonance. Biochemistry 1989; 28:4301–4312.

20. Griessbach U, Sturzebecher J, Markwardt F. Assay of hirudin in plasma using a chromogenic thrombin substrate. Thromb Res 1985; 37:347–350.

21. Marbet GA, Verstraete M, Kienast J, Graf P, Hoet B, Tsakiris DA, Silling–Engelhardt G, Close P. Clinical pharmacology of intravenously administered recombinant desulfatohirudin (CGP 39393) in healthy volunteers. J Cardiovasc Pharmacol 1993; 22:364–372.

22. Longstaff C, Wong MY, Gaffney PJ. An international collaborative study to investigate standardisation of hirudin potency. Thromb Haemost 1993; 69:430–435.

23. Badimon L, Meyer BJ, Badimon JJ. Thrombin in arterial thrombosis. Haemostasis 1994; 24;69–80.

24. Hofsteenge J, Taguchi H, Stone SR. Effect of thrombomodulin on the kinetics of thrombin and inhibitors. Biochem J 1986; 237:243–247.

25. Verstraete M. Modulating platelet function with direct thrombin inhibitors. Haemostasis 1996; 26:70–77.

26. Glusa E. Hirudin and platelets. Semin Thromb Hemost 1991; 17:122–125.

27. van Willigen G, Akkerman J-WN. Regulation of glycoprotein IIbIIIa exposure on platelets stimulated with α-thrombin. Blood 1992; 79:82–90.

28. Tam SW, Fenton JW, Detwiler TC. Dissociation of thrombin from platelets by hirudin: evidence for receptor processing. J Biol Chem 1979; 254:8723–8725.

29. Meiring SM, Lotter SM, Badenhorst PN, Bucha E, Nowak G, Kotze HF. Sites of elimination and pharmacokinetics of recombinant [^{131}I] lepirudin in baboons. J Pharm Sci 1999; 88:523–529.

30. Zoldhelyi P, Webster MWI, Fuster V, Grill DE, Gaspar D, Edwards SJ, Cabot CF, Chesebro JH. Recombinant hirudin in patients with chronic, stable coronary artery disease: safety, half-life, and effects on coagulation parameters. Circulation 1993; 88:2015–2022.

31. Verstraete M, Noromohamed M, Kienast J, Siebeck M, Silling–Engelhardt G, Buller H, Hoet B, Bichler J, Close P. Biologic effects of recombinant hirudin (CGP 39393) in human volunteers. European Hirudin in Thrombosis Group. J Am Coll Cardiol 1993; 22:1080–1088.

32. Stringer KA, Lindenfeld J. Hirudins: antithrombin anticoagulants. Ann Pharmacother 1992; 26:1535–1540.

33. Markwardt F, Nowak C, Bucha E. Hirudin as an anticoagulant in experimental haemodialysis. Haemostasis 1991; 21:149–155.

34. Tripodi A, Chantarangkul V, Arbini AA, Moia M, Mannucci PM. Effects of hirudin on activated partial thromboplastin time determined with ten different reagents. Thromb Haemost 1993; 70:286–288.

35. Fareed J, Callas D, Hoppensteadt DA, Lewis BE, Bick RL, Walenga JM. Antithrombin agents as anticoagulants and antithrombotics: implications in drug development. Semin Hematol 1999; 36: 42–56.

36. Potzsch B, Madlener K, Seelig C, Riess CF, Greinacher A, Muller–Berghaus G. Monitoring of r-hirudin anticoagulation during cardiopulmonary bypass—assessment of whole blood ecarin clotting time. Thromb Haemost 1997; 77:920–925.

37. Markwardt F. Hirudin: the famous anticoagulant agent. Adv Exp Med Biol 1993; 340:191–211.

38. Markwardt F. Development of hirudin as an antithrombotic agent. Semin Thromb Haemost 1989; 15:269–282.

39. Huhle G, Hoffmann U, Song X, Wang LC, Heene DL, Harenberg J. Immunologic response to recombinant hirudin in HIT type II patients during long-term treatment. Br J Haematol 1999; 106:196–201.

40. Song X, Huhle G, Wang L, Hoffmann U, Harenberg J. Generation of anti-hirudin antibodies in heparin-induced thrombocytopenia patients treated with r-hirudin. Circulation 1999; 100:1528–1532.

41. Harenberg J, Huhle G, Wang LC, Hoffmann U, Song XH. Re-exposure to recombinant (r)-hirudin in anti-hirudin antibody positive patients with a history of heparin-induced thrombocytopenia. Br J Haematol 2000; 109:512–518.

42. Heras M, Chesebro JH, Penny WJ, Bailey KR, Badimon L, Fuster V. Effects of thrombin inhibition on the development of acute platelet-thrombus deposition during angioplasty in pigs. Heparin versus recombinant hirudin, a specific thrombin inhibitor. Circulation 1989; 79:657–665.

43. Heras M, Chesebro JH, Webster MWI, Mruk JJ, Grill DE, Penny WJ, Bowie EJ, Badimon L, Fuster V. Hirudin, heparin and placebo during deep arterial injury in the pig. The in-vivo role of thrombin in platelet-mediated thrombosis. Circulation 1990; 82:1476–1484.

44. Kelly AB, Marzec UM, Krupski W, Bass A, Cadroy Y, Hanson SR, Harker LA. Hirudin interruption of heparin-resistant arterial thrombus formation in baboons. Blood 1991; 77:1006–1012.

45. Rigel DF, Olson RW, Lappe RW. Comparison of hirudin and heparin as adjuncts to streptokinase thrombolysis in a canine model of coronary thrombolysis. Circulation 1993; 72:1091–1102.

46. Gertz SD, Fallon JT, Gallo R, Taubman MB, Banai S, Barry WL, Gimple LW, Nemerson Y, Thiruvikraman S, Naidu SS, Chesebro JH, Fuster V, Sarembock IJ, Badimon JJ. Hirudin reduces tissue factor expression in neointima after balloon injury in rabbit femoral and porcine coronary arteries. Circulation 1998; 98:589–687.

47. Nowak C, Markwardt F. Hirudin in disseminated intravascular coagulation. Haemostasis 1991; 21:142–148.

48. Pernerstorfer T, Hollenstein U, Hansen JB, Stohlawetz P, Eichler HG, Handler S, Speiser W, Jilma B. Lepirudin blunts endotoxin-induced coagulation activation. Blood 2000; 95:1729–1734.

49. Markwardt F, Kaiser S, Nowak C. Studies on the antithrombotic effects of recombinant hirudin. Thromb Res 1989; 54:377–388.

50. Fox KA. r-Hirudin in unstable angina pectoris. Rationale and preliminary data from the APT pilot study. Eur Heart J 1995; 16:28–32.

51. Topol EJ, Fuster V, Harrington RA, Califf RM, Kleiman NS, Kereiakes DJ, Cohen M, Chapekis A, Gold HK, Tannenbaum MA, Rao AK, Debowey D, Schwartz D, Henis M, Chesebro J. Recombinant hirudin for unstable angina pectoris. A multicenter, randomized angiographic trial. Circulation 1994; 89:1557–1566.

52. Rao AK, Sun L, Chesebro JH, Fuster V, Harrington RA, Schwartz D, Gallo P, Matos D, Topol EJ. Distinct effects of recombinant desulfatohirudin (Revasc) and heparin on plasma levels of fibrinopeptide A and prothrombin fragment F1.2 in unstable angina. A multicenter trial. Circulation 1996; 94:2389–2395.

53. Organisation to Assess Strategies for Ischemic Syndromes (OASIS) Investigators. Comparison of the effects of two doses of recombinant hirudin compared with heparin in patients with acute myocardial ischemia without ST elevation: a pilot study. Circulation 1997; 96:769–777.

54. Flather MD, Weitz JI, Yusuf S, Pogue J, Sussex B, Campeau J, Gill J, Schuld R, Joyner CD, Morris AL, Lai C, Theroux P, Marquis JF, Chan YK, Venkatesh G, Jessel A. Reactivation of coagulation after stopping infusions of recombinant hirudin and unfractionated heparin in unstable angina and myocardial infarction without ST elevation: results of a randomised trial. Eur Heart J 2000; 21:1473–1481.

55. Organisation to Assess Strategies for Ischemic Syndromes (OASIS-2) Investigators. Effects of recombinant hirudin (lepirudin) compared with heparin on death, myocardial infarction, refractory

angina, and revascularisation procedures in patients with acute myocardial ischaemia without ST elevation: a randomised trial. Lancet 1999; 353:429–438.

56. Theroux P, Waters D, Lam J, Juneau M, McCans J. Reactivation of unstable angina after discontinuation of heparin. N Engl J Med 1992; 327:141–145.

57. Granger CB, Miller JM, Bovill EG, Gruber A, Tracy RP, Krucoff MW, Green C, Berrios E, Harrington RA, Ohman EM. Rebound increase in thrombin generation and activity after cessation of intravenous heparin in patients with acute coronary syndromes. Circulation 1995; 91:1929–1935.

58. Molhoek GP, Laarman GJ, Lok DJ, Luz CM, Kingma JH, Van den Bos AA, Zijnen P, Bosma AH, Hertzberger DP, Takens LH. Angiographic dose-finding study with r-hirudin (HBW 023) for the improvement of thrombolytic therapy with streptokinase (HIT-SK). Interim results. Eur Heart J 1995; 16:33–37.

59. Zeymer U, von Essen R, Tebbe U, Michels HR, Jessel A, Vogt A, Roth M, Appel KF, Neuhaus KL. Recombinant hirudin and front-loaded alteplase in acute myocardial infarction: final results of a pilot study. HIT-I (hirudin for the improvement of thrombolysis). Eur Heart J 1995; 16:22–27.

60. von Essen R, Zeymer U, Tebbe U, Jessel A, Kwasny H, Mateblowski M, Niederer W, Wagner J, Maurer W, von Leitner ER, Haerten K, Roth M, Neuhaus KL. HBW 023 (recombinant hirudin) for the acceleration of thrombolysis and prevention of coronary reocclusion in acute myocardial infarction: results of a dose-finding study (HIT-II) by the Arbeitsgemeinschaft Leitender Kardiologischer Krankenhausarzte. Coronary Artery Dis 1998; 9:265–272.

61. Neuhaus KL, Molhoek GP, Zeymer U, Tebbe U, Wegscheider K, Schoder R, Camez A, Laarman GJ, Grollier GM, Lok DJA, Kuckuck H, Lazaras P. Recombinant hirudin (lepirudin) for the improvement of thrombolysis with streptokinase in patients with acute myocardial infarction. Results of the HIT-4 trial. J Am Coll Cardiol 1999; 34:966–973.

62. Cannon CP, McCabe CH, Henry TD, et al. A pilot trial of recombinant desulfatohirudin compared with heparin in conjunction with tissue-type plasminogen activator and aspirin for acute myocardial infarction: results of the Thrombolysis in Myocardial Infarction (TIMI) 5 trial. J Am Coll Cardiol 1994; 23:993–1003.

63. Lee LV. Initial experience with hirudin and streptokinase in acute myocardial infarction: results of the Thrombolysis in Myocardial Infarction (TIMI) 6 trial. Am J Cardiol 1995; 75:7–13.

64. Antman EM. Hirudin in acute myocardial infarction. Safety report from the Thrombolysis and Thrombin Inhibition in Myocardial Infarction (TIMI) 9A Trial. Circulation 1994; 90:1624–1630.

65. Neuhaus KL, von Essen R, Tebbe U, et al. Safety observations from the pilot phase of the randomized r-hirudin for Improvement of Thrombolysis (HIT-III) study. A study of the Arbeitsgemeinschaft Leitender Kardiologischer Krankenhausarzte. Circulation 1994; 90:1638–1642.

66. The Global Use of Strategies to Open Occluded Coronary Arteries (GUSTO) IIa Investigators. Randomized trial of intravenous heparin versus recombinant hirudin for acute coronary syndromes. Circulation 1994; 90:1631–1637.

67. The GUSTO-1 Investigators. An international randomized trial comparing four thrombolytic strategies for acute myocardial infarction. N Engl J Med 1993; 329:673–682.

68. Granger CB, Califf RM, Hirsh J, Woodlief LH, Topol EJ, for the GUSTO Investigators. aPTTs after thrombolysis and standard intravenous heparin are often low and correlate with body weight, age and sex: experience from the GUSTO trial [abst]. Circulation 1992; 86:I-258.

69. Granger CB, Hirsh J, Califf RM, Col J, White H, Betriu A, Woodlief LH, Lee KL, Bovill EG, Simes RJ, Topol EJ, for the GUSTO Investigators. Activated partial thromboplastin time and outcome after thrombolytic therapy for acute myocardial infarction. Results from the GUSTO-1 trial. Circulation 1996; 93:870–878.

70. The Global Use of Strategies to Open Occluded Coronary Arteries (GUSTO) IIb Investigators. A comparison of recombinant hirudin with heparin for the treatment of acute coronary syndromes. N Engl J Med 1996; 335:775–782.

71. Antman EM. Hirudin in acute myocardial infarction. Thrombolysis and Thrombin Inhibition in Myocardial Infarction (TIMI) 9B trial. Circulation 1996; 94:911–921.

72. Metz BK, White HD, Granger CB, Simes RJ, Armstrong PW, Hirsh J, Fuster V, MacAulay CM, Califf RM, Topol EJ, for the GUSTO-IIb investigators. Randomized comparison of direct thrombin inhibition

versus heparin in conjunction with fibrinolytic therapy for acute myocardial infarction: results from the GUSTO-IIb Trial. J Am Coll Cardiol 1998; 31:1493–1498.

73. Serruys PW, Herrman JP, Simon R, Rutsch W, Bode C, Laarman GJ, van Dijk R, van den Bos AA, Umans VA, Fox KA, Close P, Deckers JW. A comparison of hirudin with heparin in the prevention of restenosis after coronary angioplasty. Helvetica Investigators. N Engl J Med 1995; 333:757–763.

74. Popma JJ, Weitz J, Bittl JA, Ohman EM, Kuntz RE, Lansky AJ, King SB. Antithrombotic therapy in patients undergoing coronary angioplasty. Chest 1998; 114:728S–741S.

75. Kong DF, Califf RM, Miller DP, Moliterno DJ, White HD, Harrington RA, Tcheng JE, Lincoff AM, Hasselblad V, Topol EJ. Clinical outcomes of therapeutic agents that block the platelet glycoprotein IIb/IIIa integrin in ischemic heart disease. Circulation 1998; 98:2829–2835.

76. Mehta S, Yusuf S, Rupprecht HJ, Wittlinger T, Flather M, Pogue J, Cronin L, Hunt D, Varigos J, Keltai M, Piegas L, Lewis B, Joyner C, Anand S, Luz M. Substantial benefit of hirudin compared to heparin among unstable angina patients undergoing percutaneous coronary intervention [abstr]. J Am Coll Cardiol 2000; 35:357A.

77. Roe MT, Granger CB, Ohman EM, Califf RM, Hellkamp A, Topol EJ, White HD, Hochman J, Van der Werf F. Hirudin significantly reduces ischemic events following coronary intervention for acute coronary syndromes [abstr]. J Am Coll Cardiol 2000; 35:39A.

78. Simoons M. The GUSTO-4 study. Late Breaking Clinical Trials. European Society of Cardiology, Amsterdam, 2000.

79. Topol EJ. Evolution of improved antithrombotic and antiplatelet agents: genesis of the Comparison of Abciximab Complications with Hirulog (and back-up abciximab) Events Trial (Cachet). Am J Cardiol 1998; 82(8B):63P–68P.

80. Yusuf S. Challenges in the conduct and interpretation of phase II (pilot) randomized trials. Am Heart J 2000; 139:S136–S142.

81. Cairns JA, Theroux P, Lewis HD Jr, Ezekowitz M, Meade TW, Sutton GC. Antithrombotic agents in coronary artery disease. Chest 1998; 114:611S–633S.

82. Anand SS, Yusuf S. Oral anticoagulant therapy in patients with coronary artery disease: a meta-analysis. JAMA 1999; 282:2058–2067.

83. Direct Thrombin Inhibitor Trialists' Collaborative group. Direct thrombin inhibitors in acute coronary syndromes and during percutaneous coronary intervention: design of a meta-analysis based on individual patient data. Am Heart J 2000; in press.

14

Clinical Development of Bivalirudin

Robert A. Harrington
Duke University Medical Center, Durham, North Carolina, U.S.A.

John M. Maraganore
Millennium Pharmaceuticals, Cambridge, Massachusetts, U.S.A.

INTRODUCTION

Because of the central role of thrombosis in the complications patients may encounter when they present with acute coronary syndromes or undergo percutaneous coronary angioplasty, antithrombotic therapy has become a cornerstone of therapy for such patients. Both antiplatelet agents and indirect thrombin inhibitors, in clinical trials, have effectively reduced the ischemic complications of these disease processes. Despite these therapies, however, the morbidity and mortality associated with these syndromes remains unacceptably high.

An understanding of the pivotal role of thrombin in the thrombosis process and the limitation of currently available indirect thrombin inhibitors has lcd to a search for more potent, direct thrombin inhibitors. Thrombin plays a central role in arterial thrombogenesis. Most treatment strategies for acute coronary syndromes (ACS) target the inhibition of thrombin activity or its generation. Indirect thrombin inhibitors, such as heparin or low-molecular-weight heparin (LMWH), have several limitations that are largely overcome by direct thrombin inhibitors, such as hirudin and bivalirudin. Bivalirudin is a thrombin-specific antagonist that has recently been approved for clinical use in the United States.

Bivalirudin is a novel bivalent and reversible thrombin-specific anticoagulant. It acts initially as a non-competitive thrombin inhibitor, then as a competitive univalent inhibitor as thrombin cleaves the D-Phe-Phe-Arg-Pro moiety of bivalirudin, releasing the substrate recognition site of thrombin, but retaining a 12-amino acid carboxy-terminal bivalirudin moiety bound to the fibrinogen recognition site. This molecular reversibility of synthetic bivalirudin is in contrast with that of thrombin inhibitors such as hirudin, which is an irreversible bivalent anticoagulant isolated from leech saliva. Unlike heparin, bivalirudin is able to inhibit both free and clot-bound thrombin equally, thus preventing both the initiation and continuation of clot formation. Bivalirudin demonstrates a consistent and predictable anticoagulant effect because it does not bind to other plasma proteins. Bivalirudin's direct, reversible, specific mode of action, linear pharmacokinetics, and short half-life of approximately 25 min contribute to its predictable anticoagulant effect and may also contribute to its improved safety profile over heparin.

When treating patients with antithrombotic agents, physicians must balance the prevention of thrombotically mediated ischemic events (such as death, myocardial infarction, and recurrent ischemia) with the possible stiniulation of adverse safety events (such as thrombocytopenia and bleeding). Typically there has been a trade-off, in that potent new therapies that are more likely to suppress ischemic events may also result in an increased risk of bleeding. As our basic understanding of thrombosis continues to evolve, there may be an opportunity to develop agents that are highly specific for certain parts of the coagulation system; such agents might reduce the potential for thrombosis without markedly impairing hemostasis, therefore, they might even reduce the risk of bleeding compared with unfractionated heparin (UFH).

In a trial of more than 4000 patients treated during the era of balloon angioplasty, bivalirudin clearly reduced the ischemic complications of the angioplasty procedure while simultaneously decreasing the risk of bleeding complications compared with heparin. This was one of the first observations that one could uncouple ischemic benefit from bleeding risk, and it led to the assessment that bivalirudin provided a more stable, predictable level of anticoagulation among patients undergoing PCI, which appeared to translate into direct clinical benefit. The strength of the this data led directly to the drug application supporting the use of bivalirudin in patients undergoing balloon angioplasty and was the centerpiece of the approyal of this agent by the U.S. Food and Drug Administration (FDA).

Additionally, a systematic overview has demonstrated that bivalirudin reduces the combined incidence of death and myocardial infarction for patients with a broad array of acute coronary events. It also appears to be associated with a highly significant and consistent reduction in major hemorrhage, seen in a variety of patient settings, compared with heparin.

Finally, bivalirudin is being evaluated in every aspect of acute cardiovascular care that employs unfractionated heparin as the standard of anticoagulation. Large-scale randomized trials will be performed and reported in the next 1–3 years that will properly establish the role of this unique agent for the treatment of acute coronary dieases. Additionally, smaller trials are underway that seek to validate the use of this thrombin-specific anticoagulant in niche settings, such as heparin-induced thrombocytopenia, for which heparin is absolutely ineffective and contraindicated.

I.   IN VITRO AND IN VIVO STUDIES

A.   Advantages of Direct versus Indirect Thrombin Inhibition

Thrombin plays a central role in arterial thrombogenesis. Most treatment strategies for acute coronary syndromes (ACS) target the inhibition of thrombin activity or its generation. Indirect thrombin inhibitors, such as heparin or low-molecular-weight heparin (LMWH), have a number of limitations that are largely overcome by direct thrombin inhibitors, such as hirudin and bivalirudin.

Heparin, the most widely used indirect thrombin inhibitor, inhibits thrombin activity by binding to antithrombin III (AT III) which, in turn, binds to the active site of thrombin and forms a ternary complex [1]. This large ternary complex does not inhibit thrombin bound to fibrin [2,3], nor does it inhibit platelet-bound factor Xa. This inability to inhibit fibrin-bound thrombin and platelet-bound factor Xa may partly, contribute to heparin's variable effects in patients with ACS [4]. Furthermore, heparin binds nonspecifically to endothelium and to acute-phase plasma proteins [5] (such as platelet factor IV, a platelet protein released during clotting [6]) that are produced in patients with ACS. The resulting pharmacokinetic and pharmacodynamic characteristics of heparin are complex. Heparin dose–response is unpredictable and a variable response is observed in different disease states [7]. Therefore, heparin administered as antithrombotic therapy requires careful monitoring of anticoagulant levels to assure optimal patient management.

Direct thrombin inhibitors bind to either the active (substrate recognition) site or to both the active site and exosite-1 (fibrinogen recognition site) of thrombin without the need for a cofactor, such as antithrombin III. Bivalirudin is a novel bivalent and reversible thrombin-specific anticoagulant [1,8–10]. It initially acts as a noncompetitive thrombin inhibitor, then as a competitive univalent inhibitor as thrombin cleaves the D-Phe-Phe-Arg-Pro moiety of bivalirudin, releasing the substrate recognition site of thrombin, but retaining a 12-amino acid carboxy-terminal bivalirudin moiety bound to the fibrinogen recognition site. This molecular reversibility of synthetic bivalirudin is in contrast with that of thrombin inhibitors, such as hirudin, which is an irreversible bivalent anticoagulant isolated from leech saliva. Unlike heparin, bivalirudin is able to inhibit both free and clot-bound thrombin equally, thus preventing both the initiation and continuation of clot formation. Bivalirudin demonstrates a consistent and predictable anticoagulant effect because it does not bind to other plasma proteins. Bivalirudin's direct, reversible, specific mode of action, linear pharmacokinetics, and short half-life of approximately 25 min contribute to its predictable anticoagulant effect and may also contribute to its improved safety profile over heparin [8,10–13].

A persistent question during percutaneous coronary intervention (PCI) is the relation between the activated clotting time (ACT) and subsequent clinical outcomes. With heparin there is evidence that to achieve the maximum efficacy, there is some increase in bleeding events, whereas to minimize bleeding risk is to reduce the optimal efficacy [14]. Similarly, both the variability and the resistance of heparin may limit its optimal antithrombotic therapy in patients with ACS.

The clinical challenge of improving the therapeutic window and providing a foundation anticoagulant for modern and future care includes anticoagulation that provides maximum efficacy while reducing risks of adverse events such as bleeding. Therapeutic limitations of heparin constitute a potential advantage of direct thrombin blockade with bivalirudin. With the introduction of the reversible thrombin-specific anticoagulant, bivalirudin, progress is made toward improvements in net clinical benefit for patients undergoing coronary angioplasty.

II. DISCOVERY AND IN VITRO CHARACTERIZATION OF THE SERIES OF MOLECULES

The general class of novel synthetic peptides called *hirulogs* was designed using the protein hirudin, a natural inhibitor of thrombin, as a model [8]. Peptides from the COOH-terminus of hirudin were known to block human α-thrombin–catalyzed hydrolysis of fibrinogen. These peptides exhibit a ten-fold increase in anticoagulant activity on sulfation of the tyrosine corresponding to Tyr-63 of natural hirudin [8,15]. However, a sulfated hirudin peptide, designated S-Hir$_{53--64}$, was determined to be 50-fold less active than hirudin as an inhibitor of thrombin activity toward fibrinogen [8]. Surprisingly, S-Hir$_{53-64}$ and peptides such as those composing the COOH-terminal 21 amino acids of hirudin failed to inhibit thrombin amidolytic function. Examination of a three-dimensional model for the structure of bovine thrombin showed that the site for hirudin peptide binding is approximately 18–20 Å away from the active hydroxyl group of Ser-195 [15]. These facts provided the basis for the rational design of novel peptides, hirudin analogues, that are targeted toward both the fibrinogen recognition site or anion-binding exosite (ABE) and the catalytic site of thrombin [8].

Hirudin analogues consist of three components: 1) an active-site–specificity sequence with a restricted Arg-Pro scissle bond; (2) a polymeric linker of glycyl residues from 6 to 18 Å in length; and (3) an ABE recognition sequence such as that in the hirudin COOH-terminus (residues 53–64) [8,16]. The optimal inhibitory activity of these peptides depends on all three components of their structure. The sequence (D-Phe)-Pro-Arg-Pro was used for all the constructs because it binds tightly to the active site of thrombin. Studies on the optimal length of the oligoglycyl spacer, which forms a molecular "bridge" linking active site and ABE recognition sequences, showed that at least three to four glycines are necessary for optimal inhibitory activity [8].

III. SELECTION OF BIVALIRUDIN FROM THE RANGE OF MOLECULES CONSTRUCTED

Several analogues of hirudin were constructed. Each consisted of tetrapeptide sequence (D-Phe)-Pro-Arg-Pro, a glycine spacer of varying lengths, and the COOH-terminal dodecapeptide sequence derived from residues 53–64 of hirudin. The objective of bivalirudin design was to achieve high potency and specificity for thrombin inhibition through bivalent interactions with unique sites on thrombin. Hence, bivalirudin is a 20-amino acid peptide inhibitor of thrombin consisting of (1) the NH_2-terminal tetrapeptide sequence (D-Phe-Pro-Arg-Pro), which binds to thrombin's catalytic site; (2) the highly anionic COOH-terminal dodecapeptide sequence derived from residues 53–64 of hirudin; and (3) an intervening segment of four glycine residues. The resulting peptide, bivalirudin, is a potent and specific inhibitor of thrombin, forming a high-affinity stoichiometric complex that results in neutralization of thrombin action during blood coagulation and thrombin formation [8].

IV. MODE OF ACTION

Bivalirudin binds to thrombin's active site and exosite 1. Through this thrombin-specific bivalent binding, bivalirudin inhibits thrombin's cleavage of fibrinogen and its activation of factors V and VIII. Accordingly, bivalirudin can delay time to blood coagulation initiated by intrinsic pathway (aPTT) or extrinsic pathway (PT) activation.

Comparison of anticoagulant activities of bivalirudin, hirudin, and S-Hir$_{53-64}$ showed that bivalirudin is twofold more potent than hirudin and 100-fold more active than S-Hir$_{53-64}$ in increasing the activated partial thromboplastin time (aPTT) of normal human plasma [8].

Although the bivalirudin design was based on hirudin, there are several biochemical differences that underscore important pharmacological differences. Hirudin binds to thrombin with high affinity, forming an essentially permanent complex at both the active and anionic-binding sites, resulting in irreversible inhibition of thrombin activity. In contrast, bivalirudin's affinity for thrombin is 1000-fold lower than that of hirudin, allowing reversible binding. The reversibility of the bivalirudin–thrombin complex is facilitated by thrombin's slow cleavage of the bivalirudin Arg_3-Pro_4 bond, and results in recovery of active site functions, such as protein C activation, an important endogenous mechanism for attenuation of the coagulation cascade [8]. ABE interactions are preserved, however, maintaining bivalirudin's inhibition of fibrinogen cleavage by thrombin and its platelet thrombin receptor. Thus, the reversible binding of bivalirudin to thrombin preserves selected aspects of thrombin-mediated regulation of coagulation.

A. Serine Protease Specificity

The catalytic site of thrombin resembles that of many serine proteases. Nevertheless, the specificity of bivalirudin, examined by measuring the ability of the peptide to inhibit the activity of 15 separate serine proteases, demonstrated specificity for thrombin. Bivalirudin concentrations from 0 to 1000 μM were tested for inhibition of substrate hydrolysis by several different serine proteases. Bivalirudin concentrations more than 26,000-fold greater than those required for thrombin inhibition are required for inhibition of other serine proteases. The IC_{50} value for bivalirudin inhibition of thrombin (0.014 μM) was at least four to five orders of magnitude lower than that of other serine proteases [17]. In addition, 20 μM of bivalirudin did not inhibit in vitro fibrinolysis mediated by the serine protease plasminogen activator (t-PA) [18]. Therefore, at bivalirudin steady-state plasma concentrations employed in human clinical studies, reaching as high as 20 μg/mL (10 μM), bivalirudin activity would remain pharmacologically specific to thrombin. Specificity of bivalirudin is an important component of its pharmacological safety, as inhibition of other serine proteases can contribute to potential nonmechanism-based toxicities.

B. Lack of Binding to Red Cells and Plasma Proteins

The potential interaction of bivalirudin with plasma proteins and blood cells was investigated in various systems. The IC_{50} for bivalirudin inhibition of thrombin activity toward a chromogenic substrate was not consistently altered in the presence of increasing dilutions (0–25%) of human plasma. Over a wide range of bivalirudin concentrations, less than 10% of bivalirudin was bound with human blood cells in a nonspecific fashion [19]. Specific or nonspecific binding of bivalirudin to plasma proteins was not observed in the test systems.

C. Platelets

Thrombin is a potent agonist for platelet aggregation as are adenosine diphosphate (ADP) and collagen. In in vitro and in vivo models, bivalirudin demonstrates a dose-dependent inhibition of thrombin-induced platelet activation, and ensuing granule release, p-selectin expression, and aggregation [20]. Full inhibition of thrombin-induced platelet activation was achieved in vitro at plasma levels approximately 2.2 μg/mL. This concentration is approximately ten-fold lower than clinical steady-state plasma concentrations of 16 μg/mL reported during the first 4 h of treatment for percutaneous transluminal coronary angioplasty. Bivalirudin had no effect on platelet aggregation induced by either ADP or collagen, suggesting that platelet aggregation is still feasible, albeit reduced, in the presence of bivalirudin in vivo. Although heparin activity is neutralized in plasma samples obtained from collagen-activated platelets, bivalirudin remains a potent inhibitor of thrombin and is unaffected by platelet activation products [21].

D. Effects on Soluble and Clot-Bound Thrombin

Unlike heparin, bivalirudin inhibits both clot-bound and free-circulating thrombin. Bivalirudin inhibits the activities of clot-bound thrombin in a fashion that closely parallels its action against the soluble enzyme. In vitro studies demonstrate that bivalirudin produces a concentration-dependent inhibition of fibrinopeptide A (FPA) release mediated by free thrombin and clot-bound thrombin. After a 10-min incubation, 1.0 μM bivalirudin (2.2 μg/mL) inhibited free thrombin by 96% and clot-bound thrombin by 100%. At 60-min incubation there is a 62% inhibition of clot-bound thrombin. Less inhibition is seen at 60-min incubation as bivalirudin is slowly cleaved by thrombin. The extent of inhibition at 90 min (58%) was no different from that at 60 min [6].

E. Reversibility

The inhibition constant (K_i) for bivalirudin is 1.9 nM. Bivalirudin was slowly cleaved by thrombin at the Arg_3-Pro_4 bond with a K_{cat} value of 0.01 s^{-1}. The formation of the complex resulted in an enhancement of 44% in the intrinsic fluorescence of thrombin, and the kinetics for the increase in fluorescence were described by a double-exponential decay [11,22]. The dependence of the rate constant for the fast phase on the concentration of bivalirudin could be described by Michaelis–Menten equation with K_m and k_{max} values of 0.75±0.12 μM and 325±17 s^{-1}, respectively [11,22].

V. MANUFACTURING OF BIVALIRUDIN

The active pharmaceutical ingredient (API) bivalirudin is a medium-sized peptide comprising 20 amino acids linked by amide bonds. The molecule is synthesized using an entirely chemical process, followed by a chromatographic purification and final isolation by lyophilization. The synthetic scheme to manufacture a 20-amino–acid peptide is complex, involving over 40 individual reaction steps.

After synthesis, the final "crude" molecule is purified by reverse-phase column chromatography, a very powerful tool that is capable of removing impurities that differ from the parent molecule by as little as their chirality. A bulk lyophilization (freeze-drying) process, yielding a stable solid, isolates the final API. The use of chemical methodology allows smooth scale-up from initial small-scale research and preclinical product to a final commercial product with minimal process changes or introduction of new impurities. After testing and release the API is formulated in a manitol buffer at pH 5.0–6.0 and sterile filtered before aseptic filling into vials where the product is freeze-dried to produce a lyophile for reconstitution.

VI. PHARMACOLOGY IN ANIMAL MODELS

Animal studies with bivalirudin support the conclusions that this thrombin-specific inhibitor is superior to heparin in the prevention of thrombus formation and as adjunctive therapy with thrombolytic drugs. Furthermore, that the relation between systemic anticoagulation and antithrombotic effects for direct antithrombins differs substantially from that observed with heparin, suggesting that bivalirudin may emerge as a more potent agent for the management of thrombosis without increasing the risk for bleeding.

A. Species-Specific Anticoagulation

The anticoagulant activity of bivalirudin is apparent in various species, but exhibits a species specificity for antithrombin–anticoagulant activity. In two in vitro studies measuring activated partial thromboplastin time (aPTT), the activities in plasma from humans, cynomolgus monkey, rat, and mouse were comparable. There was slightly higher bivalirudin activity in baboon plasma, whereas the aPTT dose–response was reduced in cow, pig, dog, and rabbit. In rabbit plasma, a bivalirudin concentration of 1 μg/mL prolonged the aPTT to 138.2% of control, compared with a prolongation of aPTT in human plasma to 282.5% of control [23]. In subsequent in vivo studies, all species evaluated were pharmacologically responsive to bivalirudin with relative sensitivity of the species similar to that observed in vitro, (i.e. baboon > humans > monkeys > rats > cow > pig > dog > rabbit, with baboons being the most sensitive and rabbits being the least sensitive to bivalirudin activity) [24]. The sensitivity differences are likely related to across-species differences in the amino acid sequence of thrombin.

B. Dose-Dependent Effects

The anticoagulant activity of bivalirudin can be measured in plasma systems by aPTT following activation of the intrinsic pathway of coagulation. Anticoagulant activity can also be measured by prothrombin time (PT) following activation of extrinsic pathway of coagulation as well as by fibrin clot formation as measured by thrombin time (TT). Bivalirudin prolongs aPTT, PT, and TT measures of normal human plasma in a concentration-dependent manner [13]. In normal human plasma, the concentrations of bivalirudin required to prolong coagulation times to 300% of control values were estimated at 2600 ng/mL for PT, 820 ng/mL for aPTT, and 86 ng/mL for TT [25]. This descending order of sensitivity is likely due to the absence of prothrombinase activation in the TT assay. The curvilinear dose response of aPTT seen in vitro is consistent with that following bivalirudin administration to humans and supports the selection of this parameter as the primary pharmacodynamic marker in the nonclinical studies. Bivalirudin exhibits dose-dependent anticoagulant and antithrombotic activity that correlates with its pharmacokinetics in numerous in vivo models of venous and arterial thrombosis.

1. Porcine Carotid Artery Model

In a porcine carotid artery model of recurrent arterial thrombotic occlusion, the in vivo effects of heparin and bivalirudin on prevention of arterial thrombus formation were examined. At a bolus dose of 2.4 mg/kg followed by a 1 h infusion at 4.8 mg/kg h^{-1}, bivalirudin completely interrupted both arterial and venous thrombus formation. This dose of bivalirudin also prolonged aPTT 2.8-fold and bleeding time 2.9-fold [26].

With heparin, antithrombotic effects were observed only at a high dose (500-U/kg i.v. bolus) that markedly perturbed coagulation. At doses of 250 U/kg, heparin prolonged ex vivo blood coagulation greater than 14-fold, but failed to interrupt the frequency or severity of arterial thrombus formation. High-dose heparin significantly inhibited thrombus formation, but was associated with aPTT prolongation greater than 300 s and a fourfold prolongation in sublingual bleeding time. Thus, based on the ex vivo prolongation of aPTT, bivalirudin was a more potent inhibitor of arterial thrombosis than was heparin. Moreover, the antithrombotic effects of bivalirudin were observed at levels that provided lower systemic anticoagulant effects than with heparin.

2. Rabbit Model of Cerebral Thromboembolism

Intracarotid administration of thrombin can induce a sustained and marked accumulation of both ^{111}In-labeled platelets and ^{125}I-fibrinogen in the cerebral vasculature. Bivalirudin administered to rabbits as an ic-bolus dose at 0.05 mg/kg, 0.1 mg/kg, or 0.2 mg/kg 1 min before thrombin administration demonstrated a dose-dependent inhibition of platelet accumulation in the cranial vasculature [27]. At a dose of 0.2 mg/kg, complete inhibition of platelet accumulation was observed over the 120-min observation period. When administered after the thrombin injection, however, bivalirudin did not inhibit platelet accumulation. The effects of intracarotid injection of thrombin toward platelet activation are rapid and essentially irreversible by competitive thrombin inhibition. These data suggest a prophylactic, antithrombotic activity of bivalirudin in a rabbit model of thrombin-mediated cerebral thromboembolism.

Bivalirudin was significantly more effective than heparin at decreasing restenosis in rabbits. Focal femoral athersclerotic lesions were generated in rabbits, and balloon angioplasty performed to compare the effects of bivalirudin (5-mg/kg i.v. bolus; 5-mg/kg/h for 2 h), and heparin (150-U/kg i.v. bolus). Mean luminal diameter of the dilated vessel was quantitated by angiogram before and after angioplasty and again at 28 days. Restenosis, defined as the change in luminal diameter during the 28 days after angioplasty, was significantly lower after bivalirudin administration than after heparin administration [27]; the clinical significance of reduced restenosis rates in rabbits is unclear. In view of the complex biological phenomena associated with restenosis, it is unlikely that thrombin inhibition alone will provide a clinically meaningful reduction in restenosis.

3. Rat Model of Carotid Endarterectomy

In a rat model of microsurgical carotid endarterectomy, the antithrombotic properties of bivalirudin and heparin were compared. Bivalirudin was observed to inhibited platelet- and fibrinogen-dependent components of the thrombotic process to deep arterial injury, whereas heparin showed a trend toward reduced fibrin deposition, but was without effect on the platelet-dependent component of the thrombotic response [28].

Bivalirudin administered at a dose of 0.4-mg/kg i.v. bolus, 1-mg/kg h^{-1} i.v. infusion achieved a 68% decrease in fibrin accumulation without affecting platelet deposition on the endarterectomy surface and without inducing excessive bleeding. At a dose of 0.8-mg/kg i.v. bolus, 2.2 mg/kg h^{-1} i.v. infusion, bivalirudin resulted in a 57% inhibition of platelet deposition, but was accompanied by prolonged bleeding at the arteriotomy site [28]. Inhibition of fibrin deposition was seen at a dosage that allowed effective hemostasis microvascular anastomosis. These results suggest that bivalirudin's direct inhibitory effect on thrombin is relatively more potent toward fibrinogen cleavage than its effect on platelet activation in preventing thrombus formation.

4. Baboon Models

The effects of intravenous bivalirudin administration were examined in baboons, surgically prepared with a continuous arteriovenous (AV) shunt between the femoral artery and vein. Thrombosis formation was monitored by ^{111}In-platelet and ^{125}I-fibrin(ogen) deposition. At doses ranging from 0.12 to 24 mg/kg over a 60-min continuous infusion, bivalirudin inhibited acute platelet-dependent thrombosis following introduction of several thrombogenic surfaces (endarterectomized baboon aorta, collagen-coated Gortex, Dacron vascular graft, and a two-chamber device similar to simulated arterial and venous thrombosis). Bivalirudin had no effect on circulating platelet counts and hematocrit [29,30].

Following a single IV dose of 1 mg/kg to baboons, the aPTT was approximately 540% of control at 2 min postdose and had returned to predose levels by 3 h postdose [31]. Acute subcutaneous (s.c.) administration of 1 mg/kg resulted in aPTT values that reached 180% of baseline at approximately 60 min after bivalirudin administration. Measurable increases were still evident through 6 h postdose. The pharmacodynamic profile in baboons correlated directly with circulating levels of bivalirudin following either intravenous or subcutaneous administration. When bivalirudin was administered to rats, rabbits, and cynomolgus monkeys, pharmacodynamic and pharmacokinetic profiles and the correlation between them were similar to those observed in the baboon.

The relative rapid recovery of normal coagulation after cessation of bivalirudin administration is due to both its short half-life and the reversible nature of its binding to thrombin. These properties contribute to bivalirudin's clinical safety and negate the need for antidotal therapy to address exaggerated anticoagulant effects in patients. These observations in animals accurately predict activity of bivalirudin in patients with venous and arterial thrombotic disease.

C. Effects with t-PA

Endogenous mechanisms for fibrinolysis are involved centrally in the control and regulation of hemostasis and thrombosis. Endogenous fibrinolysis is mediated through activation of plasminogen to yield plasmin by two plasminogen activators: single-chain urokinase (UK) and tissue-type plasminogen activator (t-PA). Fibrinolysis, in turn, is regulated by endogenous antiproteases such as α_2-antiplasmin and plasminogen activator inhibitors. For the management of thrombotic disease, pharmacological fibrinolysis has been demonstrated through the use of rt-PA, various forms of UK, and streptokinase, a bacterial-derived, nonproteolytic plasminogen activator.

Fibrinolysis mediated by t-PA involves binding of t-PA to fibrin and activation of fibrin-bound plasminogen to yield plasmin. Cleavage of fibrin by plasmin requires sufficient plasminogen activation to overcome inhibition by α_2-antiplasmin, which is crosslinked to fibrin through the transglutaminase activity of factor XIIIa. Plasmin degrades fibrin to yield soluble fibrin degradation products.

The effects of bivalirudin toward t-PA–induced fibrinolysis were measured in a plasma system. At concentrations of 1 and 20 μM, bivalirudin did not modify the extent or kinetics of clot lysis mediated by 0.1 and 1.0 μg/mL of human t-PA. In the absence of bivalriudin, there was a 34.3±5.1% and 99.7±6.5% clot lysis over 120 min with 0.1 and 1.0 μg/mL t-PA, respectively. When bivalirudin was added at its highest concentration of 20 μM, there was a 25.8±4.4% and 94.5±8.0% clot lysis over 120 min with 0.1 and 1.0 μg/mL t-PA, respectively [18]. These results indicate the absence of bivalirudin interference of endogenous fibrinolytic mechanisms. However, bivalirudin may act to promote pharmacological fibrinolysis in vivo during occlusive thromboembolism by interrupting prothrombotic activities of clot-bound thrombin [6].

In a rat model of thrombolysis, bivalirudin (0.6-mg/kg i.v. bolus, 2.0-mg/kg h^{-1} infusion) potentiated recombinant tPA (rt-PA)-induced thrombolysis by decreasing the incidence of reocclusion and time to lysis, while increasing vessel patency. Compared to heparin (40-U/kg/h i.v. infusion), bivalirudin showed significant reduction in time to clot lysis (4.3±1.8 min vs. 11.8±8.1 min) and increased vessel patency (94.6±2.3% vs. 78.8±13.2%). Compared with recombinant hirudin (r-hirudin), bivalirudin showed significant reduction in time to clot lysis as evidenced by reduction in time to reperfusion (4.3±1.8 vs. 13.3±8.8 min) [31].

D. Toxicology

Bivalirudin is not associated with any clinically relevant toxicologic effects. Bivalirudin has not demonstrated any reproductive or developmental toxicity nor exhibited any mutagenic or genotoxic potential in nonclinical studies. No apparent toxic effects related to the D-Phe amino acid portion of the bivalirudin molecule have been observed. Acute and repeated dose studies in rats demonstrated no toxicity associated with the major impurities and degradation products of bivalirudin. Long-term carcinogenicity studies have not been conducted. Adverse effects of bivalirudin in nonclinical studies were limited to those resulting from exaggerated anticoagulant activity and were observed only after an extended duration of exposure.

VII. PHARMACOLOGY IN HUMANS

Following intravenous administration, bivalirudin showed immediate and rapidly reversible anticoagulant effects, with coagulation times returning to baseline between 30 and 60 min [13]. Pharmacokinetic parameters for intravenous bivalirudin show a half-life of approximately 25 min, a volume of distribution of 13.0 ± 0.7 L, and a clearance rate of approximately 419 ± 37 mL/min, or 3.4 mL/min kg^{-1} [13,22]. The short half-life of bivalirudin distinguishes it from hirudin, which has a somewhat longer half-life.

There is an excellent correlation of bivalirudin plasma levels with anticoagulant effect. Bivalirudin exhibits linear dose- and concentration-dependent anticoagulant activity for prolongation of aPTT, PT, and TT.

Subcutaneous administration of bivalirudin, however, exhibits different pharmacokinetic and pharmacodynamic profiles. Peak anticoagulant effects were observed between 1 and 2 h and this activity was sustained for several hours. Higher doses yielded prolonged elevations of aPTT [13].

A. Immunogenicity

Bivalirudin is not immunogenic and does not appear to cause platelet reactions in vitro. Plasma samples obtained 7 and 14 days following bivalirudin administration exhibited no evidence of antibivalirudin antibodies (IgG, IgM, or IgE) [13]. Heparin use is associated with two forms of heparin-induced thrombocytopenia. Heparin-associated thrombocytopenia (HAT) is typically characterized by a nonimmune-mediated, transient and mild decrease in platelet counts 1–4 days after heparin exposure [32]. The heparin-induced immune-mediated reaction, known as heparin-induced thrombocytopenia thrombosis syndrome (HITTS), is often life-threatening. Antibodies to the heparin–platelet factor 4 complex cause spontaneous platelet aggregation observed clinically as declining platelet counts and may lead to thrombotic complications [32]. Bivalirudin was tested in vitro in the presence of sera from patients with HAT/HITTS and did not cause platelet aggregation.

B. Neutralization of Heparin but not Bivalirudin by Activated Platelets

The in vitro anticoagulation activities of heparin and bivalirudin were compared in aPTT assays. Both agents showed dose-dependent prolongation of aPTT, although dose–response curves were different. For bivalirudin, a steep response of aPTT was observed at low concentrations, whereas higher concentrations showed a more shallow response in an aPTT. The opposite relation was observed for heparin.

Heparin and bivalirudin were also compared in plasma obtained from collagen-activated platelet-rich plasma (CA–PRP) to test for effects of platelet activation on the anticoagulant activities of the two agents. In CA–PRP and platelet-poor plasma, bivalirudin showed comparable anticoagulant activity. In contrast, heparin activity was reduced in CA–PRP, indicating neutralization of heparin in the presence of platelet activation. The ability of bivalirudin to escape neutralization in vitro by platelet-activation products may explain its improved in vivo antithrombotic activity, compared with heparin in certain animal models of arterial thrombus formation [16,33].

C. Activity of Bivalirudin versus Heparin in ACS Patients

The anticoagulant activities of bivalirudin and heparin were tested in plasma obtained from healthy human volunteers and from patients with stable angina, unstable angina, and acute myocardial infarction (MI). At concentrations that were determined to provide similar prolongation of aPTT to 400% of baseline, bivalirudin (1.6 μg/mL) and heparin (0.13 U/mL) were added to the healthy volunteer or patient plasma samples, and subsequent aPTT values were measured. Heparin showed greater variability than bivalirudin in prolongation of aPTT, with a standard deviation for all heparin-treated samples of 43% of the mean, whereas that for bivalirudin was 12% of the mean. No significant differences were observed in the activity of bivalirudin in plasma from volunteers or from patients with coronary artery disease. Heparin activity, however, was significantly reduced in patients with unstable angina and acute MI. The reduction of heparin activity was not correlated with plasma levels of antithrombin or platelet factor 4. Using data on the baseline characteristics of volunteers and patients from whom plasma was obtained for the study, predictors of reduced heparin activity were unstable angina ($p < 0.001$), acute MI ($p < 0.001$), and recent chest pain at rest ($p < 0.001$) [7,16]. The reduced anticoagulant effects of heparin in plasma from patients with ACS may explain the improved benefits of bivalirudin in controlled clinical studies.

VIII. CLINICAL STUDIES OF BIVALIRUDIN

From an understanding of the pathophysiology of arterial thrombosis, the mainstays of antithrombotic therapy for arterial disease appear to include both anticoagulant and antiplatelet agents. Currently, parenterally administered anticoagulants are used to treat both acute ischemic heart disease and acute cerebrovascular disease. Although there are other, less common indications for these drugs relative to arterial thrombosis, their primary indications include the treatment of acute coronary syndromes, the complications of percutaneous coronary interventions, stroke, and transient ischemic attacks.

Despite a limited body of randomised-controlled clinical trial data to support its use, unfractionated heparin has become the standard anticoagulant for the treatment of these diseases. Because heparin has emerged over a period of many decades as the standard of care, any new anticoagulant under clinical development must treat heparin as an active control, rather than using placebo as the comparator in a traditional placebo-controlled clinical trial. The introduction of a new anticoagulant into clinical practice must also take into consideration the current use of multiple antithrombotic agents, such as both oral and parentally administered antiplatelet therapy, in this group of patients, as well as that most of these therapies work in an additive way.

When treating patients with antithrombotic agents, physicians must balance the prevention of thrombotically mediated ischemic events (such as death, myocardial infarction, and recurrent ischemia) with the possible stimulation of adverse safety events (such as thrombocytopenia and bleeding). Typically there has been a trade-off, in that potent new therapies that are more likely to suppress ischemic events may also result in an increased risk of bleeding. As our basic understanding of thrombosis continues to evolve, there may be an opportunity to develop agents that are highly specific for certain parts of the coagulation system; such agents might reduce the potential for thrombosis without markedly impairing hemostasis and, therefore, might even reduce the risk of bleeding compared with unfractionated heparin.

The development of a number of antithrombotic drugs for arterial thrombosis has acknowledged pathophysiological similarities between the complications of percutaneous coronary intervention (PCI) and the adverse outcomes associated with acute coronary syndromes. Agents that prohibit thrombosis in one of these settings are often valuable and effective in the other setting.

In the past decade, percutaneous coronary intervention has commonly been the starting point for testing novel antithrombotics because the thrombotic risk can be well timed from the moment of inflation of the balloon in the coronary artery or the moment of deployment of an interventional device. There is also acknowledgment that this intense period of heightened thrombotic risk can be greatly attenuated by antithrombotic agents, which can, therefore, be measured in clinical trials. Thus, novel agents frequently begin the process of discovery among patients undergoing PCI and then proceed to the broader group of patients experiencing ACS.

The clinical development of bivalirudin followed this pathway over the last 7–10 years resulting in its approval in late 2000 for use as an anticoagulant in the setting of PCI among patients with unstable coronary syndromes. The remainder of this chapter will focus on the clinical development of bivalirudin, highlighting the experience in both PCI and ACS; it will include a discussion of the data from individual trials as well as the perspective gained from a formal systematic overview performed on all of the bivalirudin clinical data available up to that point. The chapter will close with a discussion of the plans for the continued development of bivalirudin in both percutaneous coronary intervention and acute coronary syndromes.

A.   Bivalirudin in Percutaneous Coronary Intervention

Heparin has been the basis of anticoagulation in patients undergoing PCI since Gruentzig did the first angioplasty in the 1970s. The basic technique of cardiac catheterization and percutaneous intervention carries a thrombotic risk because of the presence of sheaths, catheters, and guidewires, all of which are inherently thrombogenic. The angioplasty procedure itself necessarily involves plaque disruption, setting up the nidus for platelet activation and thrombin generation.

The early use of heparin by Gruentzig and others in the catheterization laboratory was based on empiric observations from the early days of cardiopulmonary bypass, rather than on randomized controlled data or even clearcut observational data. In the late 1980s and early 1990s, several reports emerged from the literature suggesting that there was a threshold value of anticoagulation (which could be determined by the activated-clotted time [ACT]) that needed to be achieved to minimize thrombotic ischemic events at the close of the procedure [34,35]. Although none of these data came from randomized trials, they nevertheless resulted in the acceptance in clinical practice of an ACT goal of approximately 300–350 s during the procedure. In the course of this work, investigators observed that higher levels of heparinization resulted simultaneously in fewer ischemic events and more bleeding events; in other words, the more heparin used during these procedures the fewer the ischemic events, but the greater the risk of bleeding for the patient.

Topol et al. [36] performed the first trial of bivalirudin (at that time known as hirulog) as a replacement for heparin during coronary angioplasty. The trial was designed as a dose-escalation study. It was a nonrandomized, open-label trial using ascending doses of bivalirudin in a group of patients treated with aspirin, but not heparin. There were five dosing groups: group 1—bolus of 0.15 mg/kg followed by an infusion of 0.6 mg/kg h^{-1}; group 2—0.25-mg/kg bolus followed by an infusion of 1.0 mg/kg h^{-1}; group 3—0.35-mg/kg bolus followed by an infusion of 1.4 mg/kg h^{-1}; group 4—bolus of 0.45 mg/kg followed by an infusion of 1.8 mg/kg h^{-1}; and group 5—bolus of 0.55 mg/kg followed by an infusion of 2.2 mg/kg h^{-1}. A sixth group was added later by protocol amendment—bolus of 1.0 mg/kg followed by an infusion of 2.5 mg/kg h^{-1}.

Patients underwent routine balloon angioplasty procedures at 11 participating sites between February 1991 and May 1992. The primary purpose of the trial was to examine the potential efficacy and safety of bivalirudin in patients undergoing angioplasty. The primary measure of efficacy was abrupt vessel closure occurring during or within 24 h after the procedure. Anticoagulation status was determined by measuring the ACT and the aPTT during and after the procedure. Bleeding complications were measured using definitions based on severity as determined by a drop in hemoglobin coupled with observation of the site of blood loss.

A total of 291 patients were entered into the study and 279 received the study medication; overall, they represented a typical balloon angioplasty population from the early 1990s. There was balance of baseline characteristics across all the dosing groups. Both the ACT and the aPTT demonstrated gradual increases in median values as a function of the bivalirudin dose. It was not until the higher doses of bivalirudin that a reliable increase of more than 300 s was seen in the ACT. As defined by protocol, abrupt vessel closure occurred in 18 patients (6.2%). This resulted in 6 patients with myocardial infarction and 1 death. There was a dose–response seen with abrupt closure. In a post hoc analysis based on the intention-to-treat principle, abrupt closure occurred in 12.5% of dosing groups 1–3 patients and 3.6% of groups 4–6 ($p = 0.006$). Considering only those patients who actually underwent a balloon angioplasty procedure, the occurrence of abrupt vessel closure was 10.2% in groups 1–3 and 3.8% in groups 4–6 ($p = 0.038$) [37]. Only one bleeding event occurred during the course of the trial, and there was no observation of an increased risk of bleeding with the higher doses, which were associated with the decreased risk of thrombotic episodes.

This trial suggested that bivalirudin could be used in place of heparin during coronary intervention at doses that resulted in an ACT of 300 s, or more, which did not appear to be accompanied by an increased risk of bleeding compared with lower doses. The main limitations of the trial were the lack of a heparin control group for a direct comparison and a sample size too small to determine definitive clinical outcomes. It was, however, the first report of an angioplasty procedure without adjunctive heparin anticoagulation and became the basis for a larger, definitive, clinical outcome trial as reported by Bittl [38].

The trial by Bittl et al. [38] was a comparison of bivalirudin versus heparin for patients undergoing balloon angioplasty at 121 centers in North America and Europe between March 1993 and July 1994. The trial intended to enroll a broad population of patients undergoing balloon angioplasty who had presented with either unstable angina or postinfarction angina. The original randomization plan was to stratify enrollment based on the presence of either unstable angina or postinfarction angina. Patients were to be randomized to extended therapy with unfractionated heparin at a dose of 175-U/kg bolus followed by a 24-h infusion of $15 \, U/kg \, h^{-1}$ or to treatment with bivalirudin at a dose of 1 mg/kg followed by an infusion of $2.5 \, mg/kg \, h^{-1}$ for 4 h and then 14–20 h of $0.2 \, mg/kg \, h^{-1}$.

The primary endpoint of the trial was the inhospital composite of death, myocardial infarction, abrupt vessel closure, need for repeat intervention with either coronary bypass surgery or percutaneous intervention, or placement of an intra-aorta balloon pump for ongoing ischemia. The major safety endpoint was major hemorrhage. For a variety of logistical and operational reasons, after the original reporting of the data by Bittl et al., Biogen, the manufacturer of bivalrudin, decided not to continue developing the agent.

Beginning in 1997, attempts were made to reexamine the original data from the Bittl trial to try to make the results applicable to current PCI trial standards. The data were analyzed using the primary endpoint of death, MI, and the need for revascularization at 7, 90, and 180 days. This was coupled with a safety evaluation measuring major hemorrhage, defined as overt bleeding which led to a 3 g/dL drop in hemoglobin, transfusion, intracranial hemorrhage, or retroperitoneal bleeding. The reworked analysis employed the statistical technique of logistic regression with covariates of investigative sites, post-MI angina, age, percentage stenosis, and the presence or absence of multivessel coronary disease.

A total of 4312 patients were enrolled in the trial and randomized to treatment with bivalirudin or heparin; 4098 patients actually underwent balloon angioplasty and were presented in the original Bittl et al. report. The updated final report includes the entire intention-to-treat cohort of 4312 patients. Outcome data at 180 days were available for 98% (4213) of the original cohort. Patients enrolled in the trial represented typical patients with acute coronary disease undergoing percutaneous intervention. The median age was 62–63. The majority of patients were men; approximately one in five were diabetic; approximately one-third had new-onset or accelerating angina; and 17% had had a myocardial infarction within the previous 2 weeks. Approximately 25% had undergone angioplasty at some point in the past, and approximately 10% had had previous bypass surgery. The majority of patients had single-vessel disease although 16% had three-vessel disease.

The median value of the ACT measured 5 min after treatment with bivalirudin was 345 s (25th,75th = 305,405) versus 382 s (332,450) among patients treated with heparin. Bivalirudin significantly reduced the risk of inhospital (through 7 days) death, myocardial infarction, or repeat revascularization by approximately 22%, from 7.9% among the heparintreated patients to 6.2% in the bivalirudin group (p = 0.039). The composite of death or myocardial infarction was reduced from 9.9 to 6.8% (p = 0.112) at 180 days. The reduction was consistent across all components of the primary endpoint. As had been seen in the earlier pilot trial by Topol et al. [36], the use of bivalirudin was associated with a lower incidence of hemorrhagic complications (Table 1).

Among patients with postinfarction angina as an entry criterion, the effect of bivalirudin was amplified: bivalirudin reduced the inhospital composite of death, myocardial infarction, or revascularization by more than 50% from 9.9% with heparin to 4.9% with bivalirudin (p = 0.009). The absolute difference was maintained through 180 days and remained statistically significant.

In this trial of more than 4000 patients treated during the era of balloon angioplasty, bivalirudin clearly reduced the ischemic complications, of the angioplasty procedure while simultaneously decreasing the risk of bleeding complications compared with heparin. This was one of the first observations that one could uncouple ischemic benefit from bleeding risk, and it led to the assessment that bivalirudin provided a more stable, predictable level of anticoagulation among patients undergoing PCI, which appeared to translate into direct clinical benefit. The strength of the re-examined data led directly to the drug application supporting the use of

Table 1   Bleeding Endpoints in Hospital up to Seven Days, by Treatment Group

All patients	Bivalirudin	Heparin	Odds Ratio	p
	($n = 2161$)	($n = 2151$)	(95% CI)	
Clinically significant bleeding	76 (3.5)	199 (9.3)	0.34 (0.26–0.45)	<0.001
Intracranial hemorrhage	1 (0.04)	2 (0.09)	0.50 (0.05–5.23)	0.624
Retroperitoneal bleeding	5 (0.2)	15 (0.7)	0.33 (0.13–0.87)	0.026
Red cell transfusion ≥ 2 units	43 (2.0)	123 (5.7)	0.34 (0.24–0.47)	<0.001
With >3 g/dL fall in Hb	41 (1.9)	124 (5.8)	0.33 (0.24–0.46)	<0.001
With >5 g/dL fall in Hb	14 (0.6)	47 (2.2)	0.29 (0.17–0.51)	<0.001

Hb, hemoglobin.
Source: Unpublished table, courtesy of John Bittl.

bivalirudin in patients undergoing balloon angioplasty and was the centerpiece of the approval of this agent by the U.S. Food and Drug Administration (FDA).

We will address the limitations of the bivalirudin PCI data and discuss the continued clinical development plan in the last section of this chapter.

B. Bivalirudin for Treatment of Acute Coronary Syndromes

1. ST-Segment Elevation Acute Myocardial Infarction

Large, randomized clinical trials in the 1980s demonstrated that a combination of fibrinolytic therapy with antiplatelet and antithrombin therapy could lead to preservation of left ventricular function and increased survival among patients presenting with ST-segment elevation acute myocardial infarction. As part of the GUSTO trial, Simes et al. were able to demonstrate a link between rapid and complete angiographic reperfusion and 30-day mortality [39]. In addition to the effect of reperfusion on mortality, Ohman et al. described the association between reocclusion following successful fibrinolysis and increased risk of mortality [40].

Although the data demonstrating the additive benefit of heparin when given with aspirin and fibrinolytic therapy has been somewhat weak [41], it is clear that the addition of heparin and the level of anticoagulation when using heparin in conjunction with fibrinolytic therapy add to the bleeding risk, including intracranial hemorrhage [42,43]. Therefore, it is reasonable to look toward the thrombin-specific anticoagulant bivalirudin as a potential replacement for heparin in the setting of acute myocardial infarction. Its increased thrombin specificity has led investigators to believe that it might result in a speeding of reperfusion and a lessening of reocclusion when given with fibrinolytic therapy. The hope would be that the improvement in the biology of reperfusion would translate into an improvement in clinical outcomes.

With this as a background rationale, two groups of investigators explored the feasibility of replacing heparin with bivalirudin as adjunctive therapy with streptokinase to improve early reperfusion among patients with ST-segment elevation acute myocardial infarction. The first trial, reported by Theroux et al., enrolled 70 patients at a single investigative site in a small dose-escalation and feasibility trial of bivalirudin combined with streptokinase in patients presenting with ST-segment elevation infarction [44]. All patients were to receive aspirin and then be randomized in a double-blind fashion to one of two dosages of bivalirudin or 1000 U/h of heparin for 12 h. Streptokinase was given as a dose of 1.5 million U intravenously administered over 45–60 min. The primary endpoint of the trial was TIMI flow at 90 and 120 minutes after initiation of streptokinase.

The trial was terminated for administrative reasons after 70 patients were enrolled. Two patients randomized were not included in the primary analysis because of a lack of angiographic data. The primary endpoint was ascertained at 90 min in all 68 patients who were included in the primary endpoint analysis. Ascertainment of TIMI flow at 60 min was possible in 37 patients. In the lower-dose bivalirudin group, TIMI flow grade 2 or 3 was observed in 87, 96, and 100% of patients at 60, 90, and 120 min, respectively. TIMI 3 flow was achieved in 69, 85, and 92%, respectively, at these time points. In the higher-dose bivalirudin group, TIMI 2 or 3 flow was observed in 71, 79, and 82% of patients at 60, 90, and 120 min, and TIMI 3 flow was observed in 57, 61, and 68% at the same time points. TIMI 2 or 3 flow was noted in the heparin group in 43, 46, and 62% of patients at 60, 90, and 120 min, while TIMI 3 flow was observed in 29, 31, and 46% of patients, respectively. Given the small number of patients enrolled in the trial, it is difficult to make definitive assessments of the clinical outcome events, but it should be noted that there were fewer recurrent ischemic events among the patients treated with the lower dose of bivalirudin, and less bleeding in the bivalirudin-treated patients than in the heparin-treated patients.

A larger-dose exploration trial comparing bivalirudin versus heparin in patients receiving streptokinase was led by White et al. [45] and was known as the HERO trial (hirulog versus heparin in patients receiving streptokinase and aspirin for acute myocardial infarction). HERO enrolled patients who were within 12 h of an ST-segment elevation MI. All patients received aspirin and 1.5-million U of streptokinase intravenously over 30–60 min and were then randomized in a double-blind manner to receive either heparin or bivalirudin at two different doses. Heparin was given as a bolus of 5000 U followed by an infusion for up to 60 h of 1000 U/h in patients weighing less than less than 80 kg, and 1200 U/h in patients weighing more than 80 kg. The lower dose of bivalirudin was a bolus of 0.125 mg/kg followed by an infusion of $0.25\,mg/kg\,h^{-1}$ for 12 h, then reduced by 50% for up to 60 h. The higher-dose bivalirudin group received a bolus of 0.25 mg/kg followed by an infusion of $0.5\,mg/kg\,h^{-1}$ for 12 h, followed by a 50% reduction in the infusion for up to 60 h. The primary endpoint of the trial was the assessment of angiographic patency at 90–120 min. Bleeding was monitored throughout the trial, with major bleeding defined as events that were clinically overt and associated with either a fall in hemoglobin $\geq 3\,g/dL$ or a transfusion of 2 U or more of blood.

Twenty-six participating hospitals enrolled and randomized 412 typical acute MI patients in five countries Four hundred patients underwent the early angiogram, and TIMI flow could be assessed in 393 of them. The time to angiography was 1.8 h in the three treatment groups. TIMI 3 flow was observed in 35% of the heparin-treated patients, 46% of the low-dose bivalirudin group, and 48% of the high-dose bivalirudin group. The difference between the high-dose bivalirudin group and the heparin group relative to early TIMI 3 flow was approximately a 37% relative improvement (p = 0.03). Patients treated with either dose of bivalirudin had less variability and overall lower aPTTs at both 11 and 24 h after receiving streptokinase. The combined endpoint of death or myocardial infarction at 35 days occurred in 15% of the heparin-treated patients, 11% who received low-dose bivalirudin, and 8.8% who received high-dose bivalirudin (p = 0.26). One hemorrhagic stroke occurred in the high-dose bivalirudin group. There was less major bleeding among the patients receiving bivalirudin compared with those treated with heparin (14% with low-dose, 19% with high-dose, and 27% with heparin).

These data then provided the basis for the Hirulog and Early Reperfusion/Occlusion [46] trial. In this trial, approximately 17,000 patients presenting within 6 h of acute ST-segment elevation myocardial infarction will be treated with aspirin and randomized to receive either intravenous heparin or bivalirudin along with streptokinase. The protocol recommends that the antithrombin therapy be delivered before the administration of streptokinase. The primary endpoint is 30-day mortality and, assuming a control group mortality of 7.4% at 30 days, the trial has 80% statistical power to detect a 15% reduction in 30-day mortality compared with heparin. Important secondary endpoints will include death or myocardial infarction as well as death, myocardial infarction, stroke, intracranial hemorrhage, and major bleeding.

2. Non–ST Segment Elevation Acute Coronary Syndromes

At the time the results of the Bittl angioplasty trial became known to the sponsor, Biogen, the TIMI 8 study group had just begun a randomized comparison of bivalirudin with heparin among patients with acute coronary syndromes without persistent ST-segment elevation. The TIMI 8 trial was terminated after 133 of a planned 5320 patients had been enrolled when Biogen temporarily halted further development; the sponsor did not have knowledge of the event rate and the individual treatments at the time they terminated the trial. Subsequent review of the data revealed that bivalirudin was associated with a nonsignificant decrease in the combined incidence of death or myocardial infarction at 7 days (heparin, 9.2%, bivalirudin, 2.9%). Consistent with other trials that had been performed in PCI and acute MI, bivalirudin was associated with a decreased risk of bleeding compared with heparin in the TIMI 8 trial with an inhospital major hemorrhage rate of 4.6% in the heparin group versus 0% in the bivalirudin group.

IX. BIVALIRUDIN SYSTEMATIC OVERVIEW

A systematic overview was then performed and published, using all the available bivalirudin clinical trial data from the settings of both percutaneous coronary intervention and acute coronary syndromes [47]. Because of the need for anticoagulation among this group of patients, there was felt to be a need to look at the bivalirudin data in total and to assess the effectiveness of the agent as an anticoagulant. Therefore, the methodology of the systematic overview was to divide the previously conducted bivalirudin trials into two groups. One group included the study arms that employed what was, in retrospect, felt to be a subtherapeutic dose of bivalirudin, and the second group included the study arms that were compared directly against heparin as control therapy; the particulars of the individual trials are displayed in Tables 2 and 3.

The overview considered the clinical events of death, myocardial infarction, the composite of death or MI, and the occurrence of major hemorrhage. The definition for each of the endpoints was the definition that had been specified in the individual trial. All of the outcomes were evaluated for all of the data at an early time point (7 days or during the inhospital phase). Trials that had longer follow-up had an analysis of the clinical endpoints at 30–50 days. The overview employed a random-effects model and reported the data using odds ratios and 95% confidence intervals.

Two trials involving 701 patients included subtherapeutic bivalirudin arms. Four trials using heparin as a control enrolled 4973 patients. The analyses from the systematic overview are displayed in Figs. 1 and 2.

The systematic overview demonstrated that bivalirudin reduces the combined incidence of death and myocardial infarction for patients with a broad array of acute coronary events. Perhaps even more striking was the benefit of bivalirudin for a major hemorrhage. It appears to be associated with a highly significant and consistent reduction in major hemorrhage seen in a variety of patient settings, compared with heparin. This observation may establish a new standard in the assessment of novel antithrombotic drugs. As it is now possible to dissociate the beneficial effects of antithrombotic therapy from the bleeding risks, bivalirudin produces an improvement not only in the ischemic endpoints, but also in the safety endpoints.

X. SUMMARY AND FUTURE DIRECTIONS

Given the strength of available data, bivalirudin was approved for clinical use in the United States, with an indication as an anticoagulant during percutaneous coronary intervention among patients with unstable coronary syndromes. Because the data from the pivotal trial by Bittl et al. were collected in an era predating routine coronary stent implantation and use of platelet glycoprotein IIb/IIIa inhibitors, there are questions on the applicability of these data to current coronary interventional practice. To address these questions, a large randomized clinical trial is underway (a randomized evaluation in PCI linking angiomax to reduced clinical events: REPLACE) that will enroll approximately 6000 patients in a comparison of bivalirudin, with and without glycoprotein IIb/IIIa inhibitors, versus unfractionated heparin with glycoprotein

Table 2 Subtherapeutic Bivalirudin-Controlled Trials

Ref.	n	Year	Load (mg/kg)	Infusion (mg/kg h^{-1})	Duration (h)	Bivalirudin control regimen	Primary endpoint (inhospital)	Indication
6	291	1990	0.45	1.8	4	Three dose groups:	Death, MI, bypass, abrupt closure	Angioplasty for unstable angina
			0.55	2.2		0.15 mg/kg B, then 0.6 mg/kg h^{-1} I		
			1.0	2.5		0.25 mg/kg, then 1.0 mg/kg h^{-1} I		
						0.35 mg/kg B, then 1.4 mg/kg h^{-1} I		
7	410	1992	None	0.25	72	0.02 mg/kg h^{-1}	Death, MI, ischemia, revasc	Unstable angina or non–Q-wave MI
				0.5				
				1.0				

B, bolus; I, infusion; Load, loading dose; MI, myocardial infarction; revasc, rapid clinical deterioration requiring revascularization.
Source: Ref. 47.

Table 3 Heparin-Controlled Trials

Ref.	n	Year	Load (mg/kg)	Infusion (mg/kg/h × duration)	Heparin regimen	Primary endpoint	Indication
TIMI-8	133	1993	0.1	0.25×72 h	70 U/kg B, then 15 U/kg h^{-1} I	In-hospital/14-day death or MI	Unstable angina or non-Q-wave MI
9	4312	1992	1.0	2.5×4 h, then 0.2×14–20 h	175 U/kg B, then 15 U/kg h^{-1} I	In-hospital death, MI, abrupt closure, revasc	Angioplasty for unstable angina
10	116	1991	None	0.5×12 h, then 0.1×84 h 0.1 mg/kg/h×12 h	5000 U B, then 1000 U/h I, or 1000 U/h I alone	90-min patency	Acute MI
11	412	1992	0.125 0.25	0.25×12 h, then 0.125×36–48 h 0.5×12 h, then 0.25×36–48 h	5000 U B, then 1000–1200 U/h I	90–120 min patency	Acute MI

B, bolus; I, infusion; Load, loading dose; MI, myocardial infarction; revasc, rapid clinical deterioration requiring revascularization.
Source: Ref. 47.

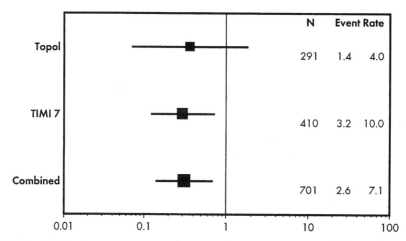

Figure 1 Odds ratios and 95% confidence intervals for the risk of death or myocardial infarction 7 days after randomization to therapeutic versus subtherapeutic bivalirudin doses. (From Ref. 47).

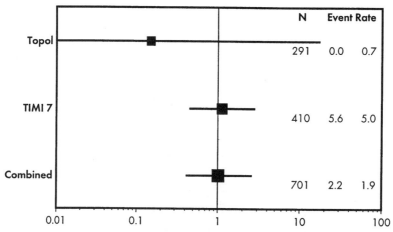

Figure 2 Odds ratios and 95% confidence intervals for the risk of in-hospital major hemorrhage after randomization to therapeutic versus subtherapeutic bivalirudin doses. (From Ref. 47).

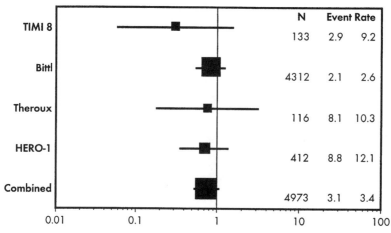

Figure 3 Odds ratios and 95% confidence intervals for the risk of death or myocardial infarction 7 days after randomization to bivalirudin versus heparin. (From Ref. 47).

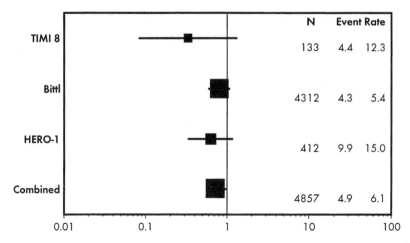

Figure 4 Odds ratios and 95% confidence intervals for the risk of death or myocardial infarction 30 to 50 days after randomization to bivalirudin versus heparin. (From Ref. 47).

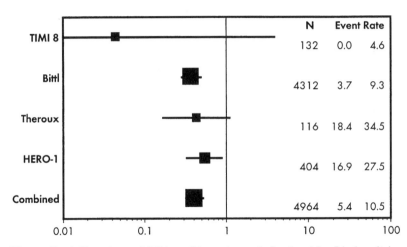

Figure 5 Odds ratios and 95% confidence intervals for the risk of in-hospital major hemorrhage after randomization to bivalirudin versus heparin. (From Ref. 47).

IIb/IIIa inhibitors. The primary endpoint of the trial (30-day composite of death, MI, urgent repeat revascularization, and major bleeding) attempts to take advantage of the unique features of bivalirudin that uncouple the ischemic and safety events.

Trials are being considered that will examine the benefit of bivalirudin compared with standard therapy of unfractionated heparin among high-risk ACS patients. The role of bivalirudin in this setting with need to be evaluated on a background of increasing glycoprotein IIb/IIIa inhibitor use and aggressive invasive management practices.

In total, bivalirudin is being evaluated in every aspect of acute cardiovascular care that employs unfractionated heparin as the standard of anticoagulation. Large-scale randomized trials will be performed and reported in the next 1–3 years that will properly establish the role of this unique agent for the treatment of acute coronary dieases. Additionally, smaller trials are underway that seek to validate the use of this thrombin-specific anticoagulant in niche settings, such as heparin-induced thrombocytopenia, for which heparin is absolutely ineffective and contraindicated.

REFERENCES

1. Bates, SM Weitz, JI, Direct thrombin inhibitors for treatment of arterial thrombosis: potential differences between bivalirudin and hirudin. Am J Cardiol 1998; 82(8B):12P–18P.
2. Weitz, J, Leslie B, Hudoba M, Thrombin binds to soluble fibrin degradation products where it is protected from inhibition by heparin and hirudin of coagulation activation during rt-PA-induced thrombolysis. Blood 1989; 74:1025–1030.
3. Hogg PJ, Jackson, CM, Fibrin monomer protects thrombin from inactivation by heparin– antithrombin III: implications for heparin efficacy. Proc Natl Acad Sci USA 1989; 86:3619–3623.
4. Hirsh J, Warkentin TE, Raschke R, et al., Heparin and low-molecular-weight heparin:mechanisms of action, pharmacokinetics, dosing considerations, monitoring, efficacy, and safety [published erratum appears in Chest 1999 Jun; 115:1760]. Chest 1998; 114(5 suppl):489S–510S.
5. Young E, Prins M, Levine MN, et al., Heparin binding to plasma proteins, an important mechanism for heparin resistance. Thromb Haemost 1992; 67:639–643.
6. Weitz JI, Hudoba M, Massel D, et al., Clot-bound thrombin is protected from inhibition by heparin– antithrombin III but is susceptible to inactivation by antithrombin III-independent inhibitors. J Clin Invest 1990; 86:385–391.
7. Maraganore J, Bourdon P, Adelman B, et al. Heparin variability and resistance: comparisons with a direct thrombin inhibitor [abstr]. Circulation 1992; 86:386.
8. Maraganore JM, Bourdon P, Jablonski J, et al. Design and characterization of hirulogs:a novel class of bivalent peptide inhibitors of thrombin. Biochemistry 1990; 29:7095–7101.
9. Ginsberg JS, Nurmohamed MT, Gent M, et al. Effects on thrombin generation of single injections of hirulog in patients with calf vein thrombosis. Thromb Haemost 1994; 72:523–525.
10. Witting JI, Bourdon P, Brezniak DV, et al. Thrombin-specific inhibition by and slow cleavage of hirulog-1 [see comments]. Biochem J 1992; 283(pt 3):737–743.
11. Parry MA, Maraganore JM, Stone SR, Kinetic mechanism for the interaction of Hirulog with thrombin. Biochemistry, 1994. 33(49):14807–14814.
12. Cannon CP, Maraganore, JM, Loscalzo, J, et al. Anticoagulant effects of hirulog, a novel thrombin inhibitor, in patients with coronary artery disease. Am J Cardiol, 1993; 71:778–782.
13. Fox I, Dawson A, Loynds P, et al. Anticoagulant activity of hirulog, a direct thrombin inhibitor, in humans. Thromb Haemost 1993; 69:157–163.
14. Chew DP, Bhatt DL, Lincoff AM, et al. Defining the optimal ACT during PCI:aggregate results from six randomized controlled trials. Circulation 2001; 103:961–966.
15. Bourdon P, Fenton JW III, Maraganore, J, Affinity labeling of lysine–149 in the anion-binding exosite of human alpha-thrombin with an N-(dinitrofluorobenzyl)hirudin C-terminal peptide. Biochemistry 1990; 29:6379–6384.
16. Maraganore JM, Hirudin and hirulog: advances in antithrombotic therapy. Perspect Drug Discov and Design 1993; 1:461–478.
17. Maraganore J, Specificity of BG8967 for human alpha-thrombin. Report TR–02 NDA Vol. 1.010, Data on File: pp. 62–95.
18. Jiang L, Chao BH, Maraganore, JM, Effects of BG8967 on tissue-type plasminogen activator (t-PA)-induced clot lysis in human plasma. Report VG–06, NDA Vol 1.010, Data on File: pp. 96–105.
19. Bourdon P, Maraganore, J, Studies on binding of BG8967 to human blood cells and plasma proteins Report TR–01 NDA Vol. 1.010, Data on File: pp. 163–189.
20. Baciu R, Fawell, S, Maraganore, J, Studies on BG8967 effect on platelet function Report TR–08 NDA Vol. 1.010, Data on File: pp. 118–125.
21. Baciu R, Fawell S, Maraganore, J, In vitro comparative studies of the anticoagulant activities of heparin and BG8967. Report TR–36a NDA Volume 1.010, Data on File: pp. 126–137.
22. Maraganore JM, Adelman BA, Hirulog:a direct thrombin inhibitor for management of acute coronary syndromes. Coron Artery Dis, 1996; 7:438–448.
23. Baciu R, Fawell S, Maraganore J, Species specific anticoagulation activity of BG8967. Report VG–01, NDA Vol. 1.010, Data on File: pp. 16–32.

24. Maraganore J, Chao BH, Joseph ML, et al. Anticoagulation activity of synthetic hirudin peptides. J Biol Chem, 1989 264:8692–8698.
25. Baciu R, Fawell S, Maraganore, J, Studies of BG8967 activity in plasma coagulation assays. Report TR–05 NDA Vol 1.010, Data on File: pp. 106–117.
26. Muller TH, Koch V, Gerster U, et al. Hirulog:a synthetic hirudin-based peptide, is superior to heparin in prevention of arterial thrombus formation. Thromb Haemost, 1991; 68:1291.
27. Page CP Maraganore J, Antithrombotic activity of BG8967 in a rabbit model of platelet embolism in the cranial vasculature. Report TR–38a, NDA Vol. 1.010, Data on File: pp. 216–226.
28. Jackson MR, Alvingm BM, Maraganore, JM, Antithrombotic activity of BG8967 in a rat model of carotid endarterectomy. Report TR–38-b, NDA Vol. 1.010, Data on File: pp. 195–215.
29. Kelly AB, Hanson SR, Chao BH, et al. Bivalent antithrombin peptide interruption of thrombus formation in vivo. Thromb Haemost, 1991; 65:735.
30. Kelly AB, Maraganore JM, Bourdon P, et al. Antithrombotic effects of synthetic peptides targeting various functional domains of thrombin Proc Natl Acad Sci USA, 1992; 89:6040–6044.
31. Klement P, Hirsh J, Maraganore J, et al. Effects of heparin and hirulog on t-PA induced thrombolysis in a rt model. Thromb Haemost 1992; 68:64.
32. Campbell AR, Mahaffey KW, Lewis BE, et al. Bivalirudin in patients with heparin-induced thrombocytopenia undergoing percutaneous coronary intervention. J Invas Cardiol 2000; 12(suppl F):14F–19F.
33. Maraganore J, Chao BH, Weitz J, et al. Comparison of antithrombin activities of heparin and hiruog 1: Basis for improved antithrombotic properties of direct thrombin inhibitors [abstr]. Thromb Haemost 1991; 65:829.
34. Bowers J, Ferguson J, The use of activated clotting times to monitor heparin therapy during and after interventional procedures. Clin Cardiol 1994; 17:357–361.
35. Narins CR, Hillegass WB Jr, Nelson CL, et al. Relation between activated clotting time during angioplasty and abrupt closure. Circulation 1996; 93:667–671.
36. Topol EJ, Bonan R, Jewitt D, et al. Use of a direct antithrombin, hirulog, in place of heparin during coronary angioplasty. Circulation 1993; 87:1622–1629.
37. Bittl JA. Bivalirudin for percutaneous coronary interventions: development perspective. J Invas Cardiol 2000; 12(suppl F):2F–6F.
38. Bittl JA, Strony J, Brinker JA, et al. Treatment with bivalirudin (hirulog) as compared with heparin during coronary angioplasty for unstable or postinfarction angina Hirulog Angioplasty Study Investigators. N Engl J Med 1995; 333:764–769.
39. Simes RJ, Topol EJ, Holmes DR, Jr, et al. Link between the angiographic substudy and mortality outcomes in a large randomized trial of myocardial reperfusion. Importance of early and complete infarct artery reperfusion GUSTO-I Investigators. Circulation, 1995; 91:1923–1928.
40. Ohman EM, Califf RM, Topol EJ, et al. Consequences of reocclusion after successful reperfusion therapy in acute myocardial infarction. Circulation 1990; 82:781–791.
41. Mahaffey KW, Granger CB, Collins R, et al. Overview of randomized trials of intravenous heparin in patients with acute myocardial infarction treated with thrombolytic therapy. Am J Cardiol 1996; 77:551–556.
42. GUSTO. Randomized trial of intravenous heparin versus recombinant hirudin for acute coronary syndromes. The Global Use of Strategies to Open Occluded Coronary Arteries (GUSTO) IIa Investigators [see comments]. Circulation, 1994; 90:1631–1637.
43. Antman EM, Hirudin in acute myocardial infarction. Safety report from the Thrombolysis and Thrombin Inhibition in Myocardial Infarction (TIMI) 9A Trial [see comments]. Circulation 1994; 90:1624–1630.
44. Theroux P, Perez–Villa F, Waters D, et al. Randomized double-blind comparison of two doses of hirulog with heparin as adjunctive therapy to streptokinase to promote early patency of the infarct-related artery in acute myocardial infarction. Circulation 1995; 91:2132–2139.

45. White HD, Aylward PE, Frey MJ, et al. Randomized, double-blind comparison of hirulog versus heparin in patients receiving streptokinase and aspirin for acute myocardial infarction (HERO) Hirulog Early Reperfusion/Occlusion (HERO) Trial Investigators [see comments]. Circulation 1997; 96:2155–2161.
46. White HD, Direct thrombin inhibition and thrombolytic therapy: rationale for the Hirulog and Early Reperfusion/Occlusion (HERO-2) trial. Am J Cardiol 1998; 82(8B):57P–62P.
47. Kong DF, Topol EJ, Bittl JA, et al. Clinical outcomes of bivalirudin for ischemic heart disease. Circulation 1999; 100:2049–2053.

15

Development of a Synthetic Heparin Pentasaccharide as an Antithrombotic Drug

Jeanine M. Walenga, Walter P. Jeske, and Jawed Fareed
Loyola University Medical Center, Maywood, Illinois, U.S.A.

M. Michel Samama
Hôtel-Dieu Hospital, Paris, France

SUMMARY

Pentasaccharide is the first of a new class of antithrombotic agents distinct from low-molecular-weight heparins and heparin. It is a totally synthetic agent that exhibits only factor (F) Xa inhibitor activity. It is dependent on binding to antithrombin III (AT) for eliciting its antithrombotic action. It has an anti-FXa activity of about 700 U/mg. The aPTT is minimally affected by pentasaccharide. It has dose-dependent antithrombotic activity in several animal models of thrombosis. The antithrombotic activity is related to the inhibition of thrombin generation through anti-FXa activity, although the maximal inhibition of thrombin generation was less than that for heparin. Plasma AT saturation occurs at high dosages and loss of anti-FXa activity occurs at AT levels of 50% or less. It does not release TFPI. No platelet interactions have been observed, even in systems positive to heparin-induced thrombocytopenia. There is no platelet factor 4 (PF4) interaction with pentasaccharide. Protamine sulfate does not neutralize the actions of pentasaccharide; however, heparinase I and heparinase II do cleave and inactivate pentasaccharide. Pharmacokinetic studies reveal nearly complete subcutaneous bioavailability, rapid onset of action, a prolonged half-life in both intravenous ($\sim$ 4 h) and subcutaneous dosing ($\sim$ 15 h) regimens and no metabolism with renal excretion. Animal studies suggest only minor bleeding at dosages far higher than required for complete protection against induced thrombosis. Phase II clinical studies have identified a dose of 2.5 mg once daily for prophylaxis of venous thrombosis. Four phase III studies (n > 8000) have demonstrated a 50% relative risk reduction of venous thromboembolic events in orthopedic surgery patients in comparison to low-molecular-weight heparin. The bleeding, as a measure of safety, however, was significantly higher statistically, in comparison with low-molecular-weight heparin. Clinical trials of pentasaccharide for treatment of established thrombosis, coronary syndromes, and adjunct to thrombolytic therapy are ongoing. At present, laboratory monitoring is not recommended. In this chapter we will discuss the development of this novel agent and the potential advantages that it may provide over other naturally derived antithrombotic agents.

I. INTRODUCTION

Heparin represents a heterogeneous drug that is composed of sulfated oligosaccharide molecules with a molecular weight range of 1,500–50,000. These oligosaccharides possess molecular and functional heterogeneity and contain consensus sequences that have different degrees of affinity with endogenous plasma and cellular ligands such as antithrombin III (AT), HCII, fibrinogen, platelet factor 4 (PF4), vitronectin, and growth factors. The main biological function of heparin is its anticoagulant effect that is mediated through AT.

Structure–activity studies of heparin have brought about the development of several low-molecular heparins (LMWH) and chemically modified heparins. Utilizing the concept that AT was of prime importance, the complete chemical synthesis of a pentasaccharide representing the consensus sequence within the heparin molecule for binding to AT was undertaken.

The original pentasaccharide sequence was isolated from natural heparin by fractionation [1,2]. This specific pentasaccharide was subsequently produced by an innovative process of glycosaminoglycan synthesis [3,4]. Its structure comprised a regular region and an irregular region of heparin. Expected spectral characteristics were shown by ^{13}C-NMR and high-affinity AT binding [5–7]. Four specific sulfate groups, critical for optimum binding to AT were present in the pentasaccharide (i.e., the 6-O sulfate on the D unit, the 3-O sulfate on the F unit, and two 2-N sulfates on the F and H units [2,8,9]. The relative positioning of the sulfated monosaccharides also proved to be of critical importance for AT binding. Pentasaccharide only partly fills the heparin-binding site on AT and does not produce a conformational change such as caused by heparin [10].

In an effort to simplify the synthetic process, and thus increase the production yield, O-sulfate and O-methyl groups were substituted for the N-sulfate and OH groups that were on the first synthetic pentasaccharide without losing activity [11]. The biological properties of both pentasaccharides (hydroxyl or methyl group on the H unit) were identical. The original pentasaccharide required 90 separate steps, today the process has been reduced to 28 steps that include 53 chemical transformations and purifications. This second-generation pentasaccharide, the α-methyl product (SR90107A/Org31540; molecular weight 1728) (Fig. 1), is being clinically developed through a cooperative effort between Sanofi–Synthélabo and Organon.

Pentasaccharide is a novel antithrombotic agent that, although based on the structure of heparin, has multiple differences from heparin and LMWH (Tables 1 and 2). The characteristics of pentasaccharide as determined from experimental data and the newly developing clinical data will be presented.

II. MECHANISM OF ACTION

Blood coagulation is inhibited when a stoichiometric complex between the serine active site of the coagulation factor and the Arg393-Ser394 bond of AT forms [12,13]. The efficient inhibition of proteases by AT requires heparin as a cofactor. The inhibition rate constant for FXa has been estimated as 3×10^3 M^{-1}min^{-1} without heparin, whereas in the presence of heparin the rate of inhibition is accelerated to 2×10^8 M^{-1}min^{-1} [14]. Pentasaccharide is a selective and reversible

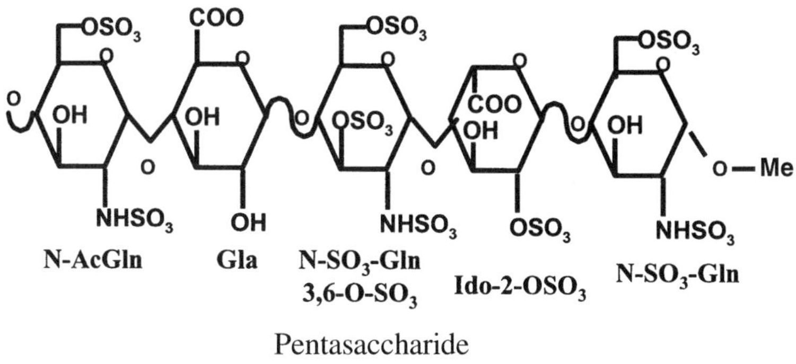

Pentasaccharide

Figure 1 Pentasaccharide Org31540/SR90107A is based on the sequence of saccharide units to which AT binds to heparin. It is composed of a regular-repeating region of heparin (trisulfated disaccharide units represented by the last two groups on the right) and an irregular region of heparin (represented by the three groups starting from the left). Within the irregular region is a 3-O sulfate group required for high-affinity binding to AT.

Table 1 Characteristics of Pentasaccharide

High affinity for AT
Activity can be expressed on a gravimetric, unit, or molar basis
Selective; single-target anti-factor Xa
No antithrombin activity
Requires AT for effect
Minimal prolongation of the aPTT
Inhibits thrombin generation
Thrombin generation is correlated with antithrombotic activity, but not completely inhibited at antithrombotic doses
Antithrombotic activity well-documented in animal models

Table 2 Differences Between Unfractionated Heparin and Pentasaccharide

Heparin has the following properties that are not associated with pentasaccharide:
    Antithrombin activity
    Inhibition of serine proteases other than FXa
    HCII interaction
    TFPI release
    Prolongation of the aPTT
    Fibrinolytic activity
    Platelet interaction
    Heparin antibody-induced platelet activation (HIT)
    PF4 interaction
    Bleeding dose–response in animal models or human volunteers
    Neutralization by protamine

inhibitor of FXa, dependent on binding to AT to elicit its activity [15]. The K_d of pentasaccharide for AT is 48 ± 11 nmol/L [16]. Pentasaccharide inhibits FXa at the same rate as heparin. It does not inhibit thrombin (FIIa), as heparin chains of more than 18 saccharide units are required for simultaneous binding to AT and thrombin to produce this inhibition [17–19].

Heparin cofactor (HC) II is another plasma serine protease inhibitor resembling AT in that it is activated by glycosaminoglycan binding [20]. HCII exhibits only weak progressive anti-FIIa activity and does not inhibit FXa. Pentasaccharide promotes only small increases in the HCII-mediated anti-FIIa activity at high concentrations [15,21,22].

III. BIOLOGICAL ACTIVITIES

A. Potency and AT Saturation

Pentasaccharide has an anti-FXa activity of about 700 anti-FXa U/mg, based on the First International Standard for low-molecular-weight heparin (for lack of a more appropriate reference standard). Thus, 1 anti-FXa U/mL is equivalent to 1.43 μg/ml or 0.83 μM of pentasaccharide. The Heptest (Haemachem; St. Louis, MO), other clot-based anti-FXa assays, and the chromogenic anti-FXa assay exhibit equal sensitivities to pentasaccharide [15].

Pentasaccharide (similar to LMWH or heparin) is dependent on equimolar amounts of AT for full expression of its anti-FXa effect. Thus, low plasma concentrations of AT are rate-limiting for the activity of pentasaccharide [23]. The normal human plasma level of AT is 2–3 μM [24]. It is estimated that clinical doses of pentasaccharide for prophylaxis will be less than 1.0 μg/mL, therapeutic doses will be 1–3 μg/mL, and doses for interventional procedures will be more than 1 μg/mL [25–28]. At concentrations of pentasaccharide higher than 3 μg/mL of plasma, no additional anticoagulant effect can be obtained with normal plasma levels of AT. More importantly, a decrease in pentasaccharide activity is observed with low AT levels (Fig. 2). For 0.5–2.0 μg/mL pentasaccharide, at AT levels of 0.5 U/mL, there is 20% loss of activity.

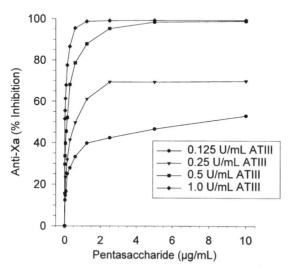

Figure 2 The in vitro anti-FXa activity of pentasaccharide is dependent on the concentration of AT. In comparison with physiologic concentrations of AT (1.0 U/mL), inhibition of FXa is reduced at lower AT concentrations. At AT concentrations less than 0.5 U/mL, the effect is marked and is observed at pentasaccharide concentrations that relate to clinical dosages (0.5–1.5 μg/mL). This loss of anti-FXa activity is translated into a loss of both thrombin generation inhibition and in vivo antithrombotic effect. (From Refs. 23,29.)

With 0.25 U/mL AT there is a 45% loss of activity, and with 0.125 U/mL AT there is a 65% loss of pentasaccharide activity in comparison with the activity obtained with 1.0 U/mL AT [29].

Saturation of AT by pentasaccharide at high doses was confirmed in a human volunteer study [30]. At doses over 17.2 mg (12,000 U), the AUC and clearance were lower than expected with an increase in the fraction excreted in the urine. It was suggested by Boneu et al. [30] that at these high doses, in which the plasma molar concentration of pentasaccharide greatly exceeds that of plasma AT, excess pentasaccharide is excreted in the urine faster than pentasaccharide bound to AT.

B. Anticoagulant Effects

Pentasaccharide has no effect on the prothrombin time (PT) or thrombin-clotting time. It has a very weak effect on the activated partial thromboplastin time (aPTT) such that prolongation is not observed with concentrations of less than 5.0 μg/mL. The aPTT cannot be prolonged by pentasaccharide even with a molar excess of AT [23,30]. Pentasaccharide does, however, show activity in the glass-activated wholeblood clotting and the nonactivated PTT (Ortho Thrombofax reagent of bovine brain cephalin) assays in which the activator is less potent.

It had been reasoned that the pentasaccharide–AT complex, owing to its large size, could not efficiently inhibit FXa bound within the prothrombinase complex [31–36]. This is probably invalid reasoning owing to the good efficacy shown in the clinical trials. The pentasaccharide–AT complex may, however, be unable to inhibit FXa at a rate equal to the rate at which FXa incorporates into the prothrombinase complex. Thus, there can be fast, efficient procoagulant activity and thrombin generation induced by the activator used in the aPTT assay versus a relatively less efficient anticoagulant activity produced by FXa inhibition within the coagulation cascade accounting for the lack of aPTT response by pentasaccharide.

Another consideration is that nearly complete inhibition of the FXa generated during clotting would be required to inhibit thrombin generation. Two mechanisms provide support for why a complete inhibition of FXa may be needed to block thrombin generation: (1) the amplification mechanism within the coagulation cascade in which a tenfold increase in activity occurs at each step; and (2) only a low level of thrombin is required to generate clot formation. Thrombin inhibitors prolong the aPTT, whereas the FXa inhibitor pentasaccharide does not. How the aPTT relates physiologically to in vivo thrombogenesis (or bleeding), however, is unknown making a comparison of the aPTT effect to the clinical efficacy (and bleeding safety) of pentasaccharide difficult.

C. Thrombin Generation

Blocking the activity of FXa inhibits the generation of thrombin. Pentasaccharide produces a dose-dependent inhibition of the amount of thrombin generated and a prolongation of the lag phase for thrombin generation by chromogenic substrate assay and F1.2 levels [15,37–40] (Fig. 3). In contrast to heparin, however, a plateau is reached in thrombin generation inhibition such that high anti-FXa activity can reduce, but not completely block, thrombin generation. There is a correlation between the inhibition of thrombin generation and antithrombotic activity in animal models [41–43]. Complete inhibition of induced in vivo thrombosis was associated with a 65% inhibition of thrombin generation measured ex vivo.

These findings were confirmed in a study utilizing plasma obtained from humans treated with pentasaccharide. After subcutaneous administration of pentasaccharide at 4,000, 8,000, and 12,000 anti-FXa IU (6, 12, 18 mg), thrombin generation was impaired up to 18 h after treatment; the time course of thrombin generation inhibition and anti-FXa activity were the same [21].

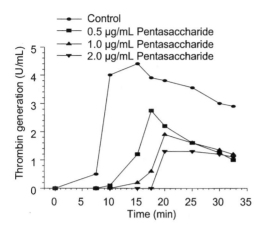

Figure 3 Pentasaccharide inhibits in vitro thrombin generation in a concentration-dependent manner. The amount of thrombin formed, as well as the time to initiate thrombin formation, is affected. This system used cephalin activation of rabbit plasma and a chromogenic substrate to quantitate thrombin; saline instead of pentasaccharide was used for control ($n = 3$). (From Refs. 15,41).

Thrombin generation following extrinsic pathway activation was more potently inhibited than intrinsic–pathway-activated thrombin generation. The weaker inhibition in the intrinsic pathway system may be due to the inability of pentasaccharide to inhibit activation by the thrombin feedback loops, such as FVIIIa formation [44].

D. Factor VII/VIIa Inhibition

Two studies have shown that heparin inactivates FVIIa bound to tissue factor [45], and that LMWH inhibits FVII consumption in surgical patients at risk of thrombosis [46]. LMWH also inhibits FVIIa generation or its activity [47]. The pentasaccharide–AT complex inhibits the coagulant activity of the tissue factor–FVIIa complex [48]. It was determined that pentasaccharide and heparin exhibit the same pseudo–first-order rate constant for the inhibition of tissue factor-bound FVIIa [48]. It is still unclear whether this mechanism is a direct effect on FVIIa by pentasaccharide or an indirect effect of FXa inhibition.

E. Tissue Factor Pathway Inhibitor

Heparin and LMWH cause an increase in plasma TFPI, and the released TFPI may significantly contribute to the antithrombotic action of heparins [49–53]. In studies with pentasaccharide, no TFPI release was detected after 100- and 200-μg/kg–intravenous injections to rabbits [54], 250- or 500-μg/kg intravenous injections to rhesus monkeys [55], or 12,000 anti-FXa IU (18-mg) subcutaneous injection to human volunteers [21]. In an in vitro system the inhibitory activity of r-TFPI against thrombin and FXa generation was more pronounced in the presence of heparin, LMWH and heparan sulfate, but not in the presence of pentasaccharide [56].

F. Facilitation of Thrombolysis

Pentasaccharide does not possess any thrombolytic activity in itself, but it may be a useful adjunct to thrombolytic therapy. In a rabbit model, pentasaccharide enhanced clot lysis induced by tissue plasminogen activator (t-PA) by 43% [57]. Pentasaccharide combined with heparin increased clot lysis to 80%. In another rabbit model, where thrombus formation was induced by vessel wall damage using a balloon catheter and 85% reduction in blood flow, pentasaccharide at 0.35 μg/kg completely prevented thrombotic reocclusion after t-PA lysis in 80% of the animals in which reocclusion occurred with t-PA alone [58]. The time to lysis was shortened from 44.8 min with t-PA alone to 25.6 min with pentasaccharide plus t-PA.

IV. EFFECT ON PLATELETS

A. Platelet and Leukocyte Interaction

Pentasaccharide from 1.5 to 100 μg/mL does not cause platelet aggregation, nor influence platelet aggregation induced by epinephrine (10 μg/mL), ADP (0.5 μM), collagen (0.8 μg/mL), or arachidonic acid (300 μg/mL) [15,59,60]. Heparin and LMWH have an intermediary effect on leukocyte aggregation, chemotaxis, phagocytosis, and burst reactions. Pentasaccharide has no effect [61].

B. Heparin-Induced Thrombocytopenia

Pentasaccharide from 1.5 to 100 μg/mL does not induce in vitro platelet aggregation or platelet activation in the [^{14}C] serotonin-release assay in the presence of heparin antibody obtained from patients with a clinical diagnosis of heparin-induced thrombocytopenia (HIT) (Fig. 4) [15,62,63]. Also, pentasaccharide with heparin antibody does not produce an increase in P-selectin expression, platelets bound to leukocytes or platelet fragment formation as determined by whole blood flow cytometry [64,65]. In contrast to pentasaccharide, comparable oversulfated ultra-LMWH and a hypersulfated lactobionic acid amide derivative produced heparin antibody-

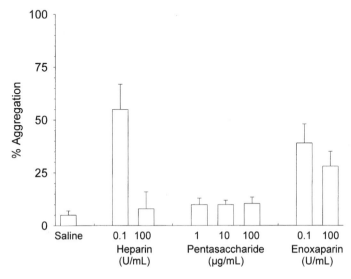

Figure 4 Pentasaccharide over a wide range of concentrations does not cause in vitro platelet aggregation in the presence of heparin antibody [heparin-induced thrombocytopenia test system (HIT) using sera from patients clinically diagnosed with HIT ($n = 30$)]. Comparative analysis with heparin and LMWH confirmed the inert nature of pentasaccharide toward preexisting heparin antibody.

mediated platelet activation [62,66]. These results are consistent with the concept that a certain degree of sulfation or size is required for a positive platelet response to heparin antibody that is not met by the ultra-LMW pentasaccharide [67].

The current understanding is that HIT is due, at least partly, to antibodies directed at a heparin–PF4 complex. There is no interaction of pentasaccharide with PF4 [15]. This supports the suggestion that pentasaccharide should not generate antibody or cause HIT, nor should it extend the disease process in patients with circulating heparin antibody.

V. PROTEIN BINDING

LMWH have a lower affinity for heparin-binding proteins than does heparin [68]. Thus, it would be expected that pentasaccharide, which is even smaller in molecular weight than the LMWH, would exhibit even less protein binding. However, the binding characteristics of oligosaccharides are also strongly influenced by charge density. Studies are needed to confirm the interactions of pentasaccharide with cells and plasma proteins.

VI. ANTITHROMBOTIC EFFECTS

A. Venous Thrombosis Models

The first study that determined that FXa inhibition alone was capable of producing an in vivo antithrombotic effect was conducted with pentasaccharide by Walenga and colleagues in 1985 [69,70]. A dose-dependent antithrombotic activity was produced by pentasaccharide in the classic Wessler stasis thrombosis rabbit model, in four modifications of the Wessler model for which different coagulation activators were used, as well as in other venous thrombosis rat and rabbit models [40,70–74]. Complete inhibition was achieved at a dose of 100 μg/kg intravenously as compared to heparin at 25 μg/kg intravenously [75]. Previous investigations using heparin oligosaccharides with lower potency than pentasaccharide did not reveal antithrombotic effects, leading to the suggestion that thrombin inhibition, not FXa inhibition, was the critical antithrombotic component of heparin [76–78]. The findings with pentasaccharide settled the question that inhibition of FXa alone was sufficient to produce an antithrombotic effect.

For subcutaneous studies, in a rat model of jugular vein clamping, the dose of pentasaccharide that doubled the baseline clamping number (thrombogenic challenge) was only 50% higher than the dose needed by intravenous administration (Fig. 5). With subcutaneous heparin, on the other hand, the dose was nearly sixfold higher than that required by intravenous administration [40,79].

The need for a higher dose of pentasaccharide than heparin to achieve complete protection against thrombosis under the same conditions in the Wessler model may be explained through the differences in mechanisms of action of the two agents. Pentasaccharide inhibits only FXa, whereas heparin has multiple points of attack on coagulation, including both anti-FXa and anti-FIIa activities. With heparin, the rate of inhibition of thrombin is tenfold more rapid than the rate of inhibition of FXa. Thus, heparin possesses not only an activity devoid in pentasaccharide, but also the anti-FIIa activity that it does possess is faster than the anti-FXa activity of pentasaccharide. In addition, the issue raised over the lack of aPTT prolongation may also be relevant to this discussion.

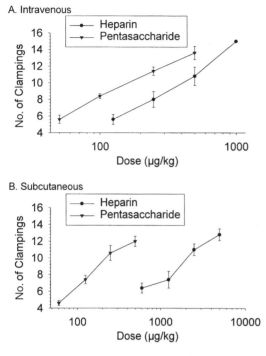

Figure 5 Pentasaccharide exhibits a dose-dependent antithrombotic effect in a rat model in which external clamping of the jugular vein to induce thrombosis and Doppler-monitored blood flow to determine the endpoint were used. Pentasaccharide was administered (A) intravenously at 100–500 μg/kg or (B) subcutaneously at 125–500 μg/kg. In comparison with heparin, pentasaccharide required lower doses to achieve the same antithrombotic activity by both routes of administration ($n = 5$) (From Ref. 40.)

B. Arterial Thrombosis Models

In a laser-induced rat thrombosis model, pentasaccharide was effective at inhibiting clot formation in the mesenteric arterioles after intravenous administration, but at a higher dose than required to suppress venous thrombosis (> 250 μg/kg) [40,80]. In a rat arteriovenous shunt model, pentasaccharide and heparin inhibited thrombus growth by 30% at an intravenous dose of 80 U/kg anti-FXa for both drugs after 15-min circulation through the shunt [74,81–83]. Platelet consumption was inhibited 48% by pentasaccharide and 63% by heparin. Thrombi formed in the presence of pentasaccharide (not heparin) became less or nonthrombogenic after a 45-min circulation period, as determined by a decrease in platelet deposition and a decrease in thrombus-induced thrombin generation ex vivo [83].

The antithrombotic effect of pentasaccharide tested in an arteriovenous shunt model in baboons showed inhibition of both arterial-type platelet-rich thrombi, measured by ^{111}In-labeled platelet deposition on a collagen-coated tubing, and venous-type fibrin-rich thrombi under static and disturbed blood flow, measured by the accumulation of ^{125}I-fibrin [35]. Higher doses were needed on the arterial side than on the venous side to achieve a comparable level of inhibition. At a relatively high concentration of 5.6 anti-FXa U/mL intravenously, and after only 40 min circulation time, did pentasaccharide significantly reduce platelet deposits in the arterial model. Thus, in animal models pentasaccharide is capable of inhibiting arterial thrombosis in a dose-dependent manner, but only at relatively high doses; it is more effective against venous thrombosis.

C. Other Models of Antithrombotic Activity

Pentasaccharide was studied in a model of hemodialysis. Compared with heparin, pentasaccharide provided equivalent anticoagulation for a 3-h period after a single intravenous dose of 1–1.5 mg/kg [84]. Based on findings for LMWH and hirudin, the small-molecular-weight pentasaccharide can be dialyzed out of the blood, depending on the type of dialysis system used (high-flow, membrane-type) (Walenga JM, personal communication, 2000). More studies are needed in this area.

Preliminary studies on the oral absorption of pentasaccharide have shown promising results. In a rat model, the anti-FXa activity for a 1-mg/kg dose of SanORG34006, a modified pentasaccharide that is hypersulfated, gave moderate anti-FXa activity 3 h after ingestion that lasted beyond 6 h (Walenga JM, personal communication, 2000).

VII. HEMORRHAGIC EFFECTS

Pentasaccharide when administered intravenously at 200 to 20,000 U/kg anti-FXa doses to rats in the tail transection model, produced only a mild increase in blood loss (twofold more than placebo). In comparison, heparin gave a fivefold increase in blood loss over placebo at an intravenous dose of 300-U/kg anti-FXa [74]. In the rabbit ear-bleeding model, pentasaccharide did not significantly increase the amount of blood loss at doses 50-fold higher than the antithrombotic dose in the stasis thrombosis model [40]. In the same animal models, heparin dose-dependently increased blood loss. At a dose tenfold higher than the dose that completely inhibited clot formation in the stasis thrombosis model, a significant increase in blood loss over placebo was observed.

By subcutaneous administration, heparin produced a hemorrhagic effect at a dose sevenfold higher than the effective antithrombotic dose. Pentasaccharide administered subcutaneously did not produce significant blood loss at a dose 40-fold higher than that which was completely effective in the stasis thrombosis model [40].

In a human volunteer study, no enhanced nor spontaneous bleeding was observed [30]. In a subgroup of this study in whom repeated injections of pentasaccharide were administered to elderly subjects, some minor hematomas at the injection or cannula site and one mild transient hematuria on day 3 occurred. With a single injection of 20,000 IU (26.6 mg) anti-FXa or 8000 IU (11.4 mg) anti-FXa daily for 7 days, rebleeding occurred following accidental removal of the scar from the template bleeding time test in a limited number of patients when plasma levels were 3.0 μg/mL (2 U/mL anti-FXa) pentasaccharide. In all patients the bleeding-time test was normal.

VIII. NEUTRALIZATION

In vitro studies performed in human plasma and in vivo studies performed in rats revealed that pentasaccharide cannot be neutralized with protamine sulfate even at a 30-fold higher gravimetric concentration of protamine to pentasaccharide [15,85]. Polybrene, however, is able to neutralize the anti-FXa activity of pentasaccharide (20.0 μg/mL polybrene/1.0 μg/mL pentasaccharide) [15].

Heparinase I (< 1.0 U/mL) is capable of splitting pentasaccharide ($<100\,\mu$g/mL) into di- and tri-saccharide components [86]. Complete neutralization of the anti-FXa, Heptest, thromboelastograph, and thrombin generation in vitro actions of pentasaccharide were demonstrated

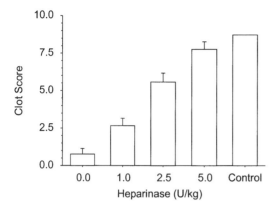

Figure 6 Heparinase I effectively neutralized the antithrombotic effect of pentasaccharide as shown in a rabbit model of stasis thrombosis using FEIBA to activate clotting ($n = 4$). The control was saline in place of pentasaccharide to demonstrate a complete clotting effect; the zero heparinase control shows the antithrombotic effect of 100 μg/kg of pentasaccharide.

with 4.0 U/mL heparinase I [87]. Heparinase I also produces a concentration-dependent inhibition of the antithrombotic activity of pentasaccharide (Fig. 6). Heparinase I and II, but not heparinase III, cleave the AT-binding site of pentasaccharide, leaving only a partially intact site as demonstrated by mass spectral analysis [88]. These data suggest a potential role for heparinase I or II as an agent for pharmacological neutralization of pentasaccharide.

IX. PHARMACOKINETICS

Early studies showed a prolonged half-life of pentasaccharide ranging from 1–4 h in rats, rabbits, and baboons, to 15–20 h in rhesus monkeys [69,89]. With its high affinity for AT, and being 98% bound to AT, the half-life of pentasaccharide was demonstrated to be similar to that of AT [90].

Human pharmacokinetics of pentasaccharide showed a subcutaneous bioavailability of nearly 100% (Table 3). Its distribution volume is consistent with the blood volume [74,91]. It has a rapid onset of action: half maximum activity is reached within 25 min after subcutaneous administration, and peak concentrations are reached in 2 h. Area under the concentration–time

Table 3 Pharmacokinetics of Pentasaccharide

Nearly 100% bioavailability by subcutaneous route
Half-life is species-dependent
Half-life is related to half-life of AT
Half-life is 15–20 h
Volume of distribution is similar to that of blood volume
Rapid onset of action
AUC and clearance are dose-dependent
Not metabolised
Excreted in urine unchanged
Steady states reached 2–3 days after repeated dosing
Elderly have increased half-life and decreased clearance

Table 4 Clinical Trials or Pentasaccharide

Trial [Ref]	Trial Phase and Penta. Dose[a]	Clinical Condition	Comparator Drug	Patients (No.)	Thrombosis (%) Penta.	Thrombosis (%) Compar.	Bleeding (%) Penta.	Bleeding (%) Compar.
Venous thrombosis								
Pentathalon [92]	IIb (No. America) 0.75, 1.5, 3, 6, or 8 mg once daily	Hip replacement	Enoxaparin 30 mg b.i.d. 1st injection >12 h post-operative	933	3 mg p < 0.001 vs. 0.75 mg and p = 0.009 (ITT) vs. enoxaparin		3 mg 4.5% vs. 3.5% enoxaparin; 6 and 8 mg discontinued owing to bleeding	
Pentatak [92]	IIb (No. America) 0.75, 1.5, 3, 6, or 8 mg once daily	Knee replacement	None	—	3 mg p = 0.013 vs. 0.75 mg		6 and 8 mg discontinued owing to bleeding	
Penthifra [25]	III (Europe) 2.5 mg once daily	Hip fracture (trauma)	Enoxaparin 40 mg preoperative (~12 h) then 40 mg once daily	1707	8.3[b]	19.0	6.3	4.4
Ephesus [26]	III (Europe) 2.5 mg once daily	Elective hip replacement	Enoxaparin 40 mg preoperative (~12 h) then 40 mg once daily	2200	4.1[b]	9.2	8.0	6.2
Pentathlon 2000 [27]	III (No. America) 2.5 mg once daily	Elective hip replacement	Enoxaparin 30 mg b.i.d. 1st injection >12 h post-operative	2200	6.2	8.3	3.2	3.0
Pentamaks [28]	III (No. America) 2.5 mg once daily	Elective major knee surgery	Enoxaparin 30 mg b.i.d. 1st injection >12 h post-operative	1000	12.5[b]	27.8	4.4	3.9

Rembrandt [93]	II 5, 7.5, or 10 mg once daily	DVT treatment	Dalteparin 100 U b.i.d.	453	No significant difference vs. dalteparin	No significant difference vs. dalteparin
Matisse DVT	III In progress	DVT treatment	Enoxaparin	2200 planned	—	—
Matisse PE	III In progress	PE treatment	Heparin	2200 planned	—	—
Cardiology						
Vuillemenot, et al. [95]	IIa Single i.v. 12-mg bolus; plus aspirin	PTCA	None	61	2 (acute vessel closure)	None
Pentua	IIb In progress	Unstable angina treatment	—	—	—	—
Pentalyse	IIb 4, 8 or 12 mg; plus tPA and aspirin	Thrombolysis for AMI	Heparin, 5000-U loading; 1000-U maintenance	326	No different from heparin	No different from heparin

[a] Fondaparinux (Arixtra)
[b] p < 0.0001 vs. enoxaparin
DVT, deep venous thrombosis; PE, pulmonary embolism; AMI, acute myocardial infarction; PTCA, percutaneous transluminal coronary angioplasty; ITT, intention to treat.

curve (AUC) and clearance correlate linearly with the dose of pentasaccharide [30]. There is no evidence of metabolism. Unbound pentasaccharide is cleared rapidly and unchanged through the kidneys, whereas pentasaccharide bound to AT is eliminated with AT [89,91]. The renal clearance rate of unbound pentasaccharide is less than 10 min, and the dissociation constant for the pentasaccharide–AT complex is $K_d = 754$ nmol/L [90]. It has been suggested that pentasaccharide may accumulate in patients with renal dysfunction. Steady-state plasma concentrations were reached 2–3 days after repeated daily administration and the clearance was 1.5–2 fold higher than that after the first injection. In elderly subjects, prolongation of the half-life (~13.5 vs. 15.8 h), larger AUC, decreased plasma clearance and reduced renal clearance were observed [30].

X. CLINICAL STUDIES

Sanofi–Synthélabo and Organon have created a joint venture for marketing, research, development, and clinical expansion. Data from several clinical trials with pentasaccharide (SR90107A/Org31540; fondaparinux; Arixtra®), targeted toward prophylaxis of venous thrombosis in total hip replacement, hip fracture, and total knee replacement in surgical patients, have recently been made public (Table 4).

A. Prophylaxis of VTE

The PENTATHLON study was the pivotal phase IIb dose-finding clinical trial for pentasaccharide that enrolled 933 hip replacement patients in North America [92]. The efficacy data for venous thromboembolic events (VTE) showed a decrease from once daily dosages of 0.75 to 8.0 mg (started 6 h after surgery) that was dose-dependent up to 3 mg, but a wide variation between centers was observed. A significant reduction in VTE was observed with 3 and 8 mg (not 6 mg) pentasaccharide in comparison with enoxaparin at 30 mg twice daily (started 12–24 h after surgery). The data for major bleeding in this trial revealed slightly higher bleeding in the 3-mg pentasaccharide group in comparison with enoxaparin, and significantly more bleeding with 6 and 8 mg. Similar data were obtained from the PENTATAK dose-finding study in knee replacement patients. From these trials it was determined that a once-daily dose of 2.5 mg of pentasaccharide would be used in the subsequent phase III trials.

Four phase III clinical trials, designated the PENTHIFRA, EPHESUS, PENTATHLON 2000, and PENTAMAKS studies, have been completed [25–28]. All trials were performed in hip replacement, hip fracture, and knee surgery patients (n > 8000) in Europe and North America. Pentasaccharide was dosed at 2.5 mg/day for a maximum of 9 days, with the first injection 6 h after surgery. Enoxaparin was dosed at 40 mg presurgery, then 40 mg once-a-day, in the European trials; and at 30 mg twice daily, with the first injection at least 12 h after surgery, in the North American trials. These trials showed that pentasaccharide is more effective than enoxaparin in preventing VTE (50% relative risk reduction for three trials and a 25% risk reduction in the PENTATHLON 2000 trial). The individual trial data showed slightly higher, but nonsignificant bleeding with pentasaccharide. However, by pooled data analysis, the bleeding was significantly higher statistically for pentasaccharide. The total bleeding event rate for the four trials was 5.6% for pentasaccharide and 4.4% for enoxaparin The total safety outcome (all severe adverse events) for the four trials was 5.9% for pentasaccharide and 5.2% for enoxaparin. The analysis of the phase II and phase III clinical trials reveals that the safety–efficacy of pentasaccharide is narrower than what was anticipated from the animal model data. Dosing of pentasaccharide in the phase IIb trial in a range of 0.75 to 8.0-mg, fixed-dose postoperative administration, revealed a steep dose–response curve. There was no enhanced efficacy with the two lower dosages, and more bleeding occurred with the two higher dosages in comparison with standard dose enoxaparin.

B. Treatment of VTE

The REMBRANDT trial was a phase II study of pentasaccharide for treatment of DVT in 334 patients, which showed that pentasaccharide was an effective and safe treatment across a dose range of 5–10 mg, once-daily administered for 6–7 days on average [93]. Based on the outcome from this trial, there are two phase III clinical trials ongoing. These are treatment studies of pentasaccharide versus enoxaparin in the MATISSE DVT trial and pentasaccharide versus heparin in the MATISSE PE trial. The MATISSE DVT is a double-blind study, whereas the MATISSE PE is an open study. Over 4000 patients will be enrolled.

C. Other Clinical Indications

The PENTALYSE phase II study of pentasaccharide as an anticoagulant adjunct to thrombolytic therapy with t-PA in acute myocardial infarction (MI), showed good efficacy and safety [94]. In 333 patients pentasaccharide and heparin had similar TIMI flow, late patency, and urgent revascularization rates. However, there was no dose–response between 4, 8, or 12 mg at the 90-min angiogram.

A pilot trial in conventional balloon angioplasty showed that a 12-mg pentasaccharide infusion, with 500 mg of intravenous aspirin, was safe and effective with only 2 of 61 (3.28%) sudden vessel closures within 24 h of the procedure [95]. There was no major bleeding. The plasma levels of pentasaccharide were $1.91 \pm 0.39 \, \mu g/mL$ at 10 min and $0.36 \pm 0.11 \, \mu g/mL$ at 23 h. During and after the procedure the ACT and aPTT remained within the normal range. This study showed that pentasaccharide was at least as effective as heparin. The PENTUA study, a phase IIb trial, is in progress during which the efficacy of pentasaccharide for the treatment of unstable angina will be determined.

Two small clinical studies were performed to determine if there were drug interactions with pentasaccharide. In a study of 12 healthy volunteers, there was no alteration of the pharmacokinetics of pentasaccharide at 4 mg subcutaneously coadministered with 10–15 mg of oral warfarin [96]. There was no effect of pentasaccharide on the PT. The second study coadministered 10-mg subcutaneous pentasaccharide with 975-mg oral aspirin to 16 healthy volunteers [97]. A small increase in the aPTT was observed, but no additional effect on the bleeding time test with pentasaccharide.

XI. LABORATORY MONITORING

In animal studies the chromogenic anti-FXa level and the Heptest clotting time correlated with antithrombotic activity for pentasaccharide ($r > 0.90$) [40]. The antithrombotic efficacy of pentasaccharide was also associated with an inhibition of thrombin generation measured by fibrinopeptide A. However, there was no prolongation of the aPTT or thrombin-clotting time assays. This has been confirmed in clinical trials [15,95,98].

Because of the dependence of pentasaccharide on AT to express its activity, there must be at least an equal-molar ratio of AT to pentasaccharide. Thus, to accurately quantitate the amount of pentasaccharide in laboratory assays, AT must be supplemented at equal- or higher-molar levels than the molar level of pentasaccharide in the test sample [29]. Supplementation should be

Table 5 Laboratory Monitoring of Pentasaccharide

Currently not recommended for prophylactic dosing
Therapeutic dosing recommendations not yet established
Considerations for the need to monitor:
    Decreased therapeutic window
    Fixed dosing
    Variation in patient weight
    Variation in AT levels
    Variation in protein levels
    Variation in renal function
    Drug interactions
Assays:
    No effect on PT, aPTT, ACT
    Use anti-FXa clot-based and chromogenic assays
    Anti-FXa assays may not provide clinically relevant information
    Should another type of assay be developed?
    Supplement AT to the assay for pharmacokinetic studies
    Should AT be supplemented to the assay for clinical monitoring?

done for pharmacokinetic studies if needed, but for pharmacodynamic studies and clinical monitoring native patient blood would provide more physiological results.

Laboratory monitoring of pentasaccharide is currently not recommended for prophylactic dosing (circulating pentasaccharide levels $< 1\,\mu g/mL$). At higher doses (0.5–$1.0\,\mu g/mL$ for treatment or more than $1\,\mu g/mL$ for procedures), however, it may be necessary to monitor the level of pentasaccharide because of the potential bleeding risk (Table 5). Also, when pentasaccharide is given in combined therapeutic modalities with thrombolytic, antiplatelet or other antithrombotic agents, laboratory monitoring may be desirable. Because the aPTT and the celite-activated clotting time (ACT) are not prolonged by pentasaccharide, the only alternative at this time is to use the anti-FXa clot-based or chromogenic assay.

There may be subpopulations of patients who will require monitoring for safety and efficacy reasons with pentasaccharide treatment. Considering the narrower-than-predicted therapeutic window of pentasaccharide (based on animal studies), the proposed fixed dosage, variations in patient weight, and variations in AT levels, monitoring may be desired. A fixed dose may be effective in patients with ideal or slightly lower body weight; however, it may not be effective in overweight and AT-compromised patients. In underweight patients, pentasaccharide may cause bleeding. Other factors that may be determinants of the safety–efficacy of pentasaccharide include hematocrit, total protein levels, and renal function.

XII. POTENTIAL ADVANTAGES OF PENTASACCHARIDE

The synthetic pentasaccharide is distinct from LMWH and heparin, with a unique therapeutic profile that has several potentially important advantages over other antithrombotic agents (Table 6). Both unfractionated and LMWH are obtained from mammalian tissues. There is an increased demand for LMWH and other glycosaminoglycans owing to their clinical efficacy [99], there are stricter agriculture controls due to the increase in bovine spongiform encephalopathy (BSE), for example, and it is projected that the supply of animal source tissue will reach a limitation. Therefore, the availability of chemically synthetic antithrombotic agents may become a timely

Table 6   Potential Advantages of Pentasaccharide

Synthetic
No viral or other animal contaminants
Well-defined pure, homogeneous molecular structure
Relatively long half-life
Superior bioavailability
Predictable dose–effect
Does not interact with PF4
No cross-reactivity with heparin antibody
At present there is no evidence that it causes HIT

source of pharmaceutical material. Because of its synthetic origin, the chemically synthesized pentasaccharide is free of viral contaminants; it can, therefore, be used universally without quarantine regulations on its production and international transportation. Furthermore, the biological–pharmacological differences among the heparins will not be seen with the pentasaccharide, owing to its defined chemical and biologic and properties [100].

Pentasaccharide possesses superior bioavailability, predictable pharmacokinetics, and because of its longer half-life, its pharmacological actions are sustained. This may be important in the long-term prophylaxis of thrombotic syndromes. Pentasaccharide should be an ideal agent for home therapy.

One main advantage of pentasaccharide is its potential use in patients with HIT. LMWH cannot be used in patients with symptomatic HIT, because these drugs continue the thrombocytopenia response. Antithrombotic alternatives in these patients need to be agents devoid of cross-reacting with the heparin antibody and devoid of extending the disease process. Pentasaccharide could be a drug of choice for thrombosis prophylaxis, and potentially for therapeutic treatment in HIT patients, for it has no known platelet activation or heparin–antibody-related reactivity. Additionally, pentasaccharide should not cause the generation of antibody.

XIII.   POTENTIAL DISADVANTAGES OF PENTASACCHARIDE

As with any new drug, there are possible disadvantages that need to be considered in the early phase for proper development of the drug (Table 7). The first clinical data on pentasaccharide indicate that this agent may have a narrower therapeutic window than predicted from animal studies. It is curious that a relatively low dose of pentasaccharide (2.5 mg [$< 40 \mu$g/kg body weight]) causes an increase in bleeding. The long half-life may, in general, have an effect on drug accumulation. Pentasaccharide exhibits interactions with antiplatelet and thrombolytic drugs. This, coupled with a long half-life, may produce additional burden on clinical bleeding with pentasaccharide. It can be speculated that because the hypercoagulable state is very high in the orthopedic patient population, pentasaccharide dosing was at the high end of the efficacy window, and thus the bleeding potential was more evident than what it may be in other patient populations. Renal impairment may also increase drug accumulation.

The mechanism of this bleeding is not understood. Endogenous interactions of pentasaccharide and the clinical manifestations of these interactions, particularly at the vascular site, are not fully known. Furthermore, the pharmacokinetic–pharmacodynamic studies of pentasaccharide are still incomplete. The bleeding potential of pentasaccharide, and the lack of understanding

Table 7 Potential Disadvantages of Pentasaccharide

Higher bleeding risk than predicated by animal models
Drug interactions
Long half-life
Traditional assays for heparin monitoring cannot be used
Lack of thrombin inhibition
Lack of TFPI release
Drug accumulation in patients with renal dysfunction
No antidote for bleeding
Price

of the mechanism of this bleeding, question the appropriateness of the fixed-dosing regimen without monitoring. It should also be considered that the traditional assays for monitoring heparin cannot be used to monitor pentasaccharide at either high or low doses. Also there is no antidote for this agent.

It has been suggested that some thrombin inhibition may be necessary for treatment of thrombosis. It is not known if the fixed dose of pentasaccharide used in the orthopedic trials is optimal for all clinical indications for thrombosis prophylaxis or treatment when thrombin generation is greater or lesser. Whether the lack of TFPI release has any clinical significance is still unknown. Endogenous variations in AT levels that can fluctuate with the disease process or with interventional procedure or surgery may influence the pharmacological response of pentasaccharide.

If the price for pentasaccharide is high its clinical acceptance will be limited. The fast development of oral heparin and oral thrombin inhibitors may also present competition for pentasaccharide.

XIV. SUMMARY

The antithrombotic action of heparin produced by its inhibition of FXa has been the focus of new drug development, as witnessed by the advent of LMWHs, and more specifically, by the heparin-derived synthetic pentasaccharide. FXa plays a pivotal role in the coagulation process being the common point between the extrinsic and intrinsic pathways. Thus, inhibition of FXa should theoretically control excessive thrombin generation and thrombosis formation by a regulated, controlled process with minimal bleeding risk because some clot formation (the good clot) should still be possible.

In the first years of development of pentasaccharide, there was doubt that anti-FXa activity alone was sufficient to produce an antithrombotic effect. Not until the pure, synthetic pentasaccharide (with its specific structure associated with high potency) became available, and after multiple investigators performed their own studies, was the concept accepted that sole anti-FXa activity is an effective means of producing antithrombotic activity. Pentasaccharide has been proved to be an effective antithrombotic agent through numerous animal model investigations and is now confirmed with the first clinical trial data.

Pentasaccharide is the first of a new class of antithrombotic agents. It is more attractive than heparin or LMWHs for several reasons. The synthetic nature of pentasaccharide provides a pure material of known chemical structure. It is characterized by complete subcutaneous bioavailability, a rapid onset of action, and no evidence of metabolism. The 15-h half-life and predictable pharmacokinetics allow for once-a-day dosing. Perhaps more importantly, pentasaccharide may potentially become the drug of choice in patients with HIT who require anti-coagulation. It also is not expected to induce antibody formation owing to its chemical structure.

Pentasaccharide is distinct from LMWH and heparin, with a unique therapeutic profile. Pentasaccharide is being evaluated as a prophylactic agent for deep-vein thrombosis, coronary indications, and as an adjunct to thrombolytic therapy. Other clinical indications such as treatment of established thrombosis, ischemic stroke, and peripheral arterial disease are also being considered for its use.

As pentasaccharide is a totally synthetic agent, it offers several additional possibilities, which include chemical derivitization, conjugated molecular forms with antithrombin and antiplatelet agents, and labeled forms that may be useful in vascular mapping when AT is bound to the lining of blood vessels. Combination therapy with pentasaccharide and such drugs as antithrombin, antiplatelet, thrombolytic agents, and recombinant forms of APC and TFPI may become useful in the management of thrombosis and vascular disorders. Pentasaccharide in mono- or polytherapeutic form may also have value in the management of nonthrombotic indications such as Alzheimer's disease, inflammation, and proliferative disorders.

Pentasaccharide and its derivatives provide unique tools for defined structure–activity relation studies related to heparin and AT. Since the original synthesis in 1983, numerous analogues and derivatives of pentasaccharide have been synthesized. Pentasaccharide can be molecularly manipulated to exhibit additional properties of heparin or to optimize half-life, potency, or others, through alteration of charge density and saccharidic chain extension [101]. Pentasaccharide conjugates with thrombin-binding domains and structures that do not interact with PF4, thereby reducing the likelihood of promoting HIT, have been produced [102,103].

The future holds promise for FXa inhibitors such as pentasaccharide. However, how and where they are used clinically, and how they will compete with LMWHs, direct thrombin inhibitors and direct FXa inhibitors remains to be determined. The role for synthetic agents is promising for the advantages they hold over naturally derived products, not the least of which is their specific chemical design to target desired biological effects.

ACKNOWLEDGMENT

This chapter is dedicated to Dr. Jean Choay, who made the pentasaccharide story possible. The expertise of Dr. Maurice Petitou in synthesizing the original and other pentasaccharides is kindly acknowledged.

REFERENCES

1. Casu B. Methods of structural analysis. In: Lane DA, Lindahl U, eds. Heparin: Chemical and Biological Properties, Clinical Applications. London: Edward Arnold, 1989;25–50.
2. Choay J, Lormeau JC, Petitou M, Sinäy P, Fareed J. Structural studies on a biologically active hexasaccharide obtained from heparin. Ann NY Acad Sci 1981; 370:644–649.
3. Sinäy P, Jaquinet JE, Petitou M, Duchaussoy P, Lederman I, Choay J, Torri G. Total synthesis of a heparin pentasaccharide fragment having high affinity for antithrombin III. Carbohydr Res 1984; 132:C5–C9.
4. Petitou M, Duchaussoy P, Lederman I, Choay J, Sinäy P, Jacquinet JC, Torri G. Synthesis of heparin fragments. A chemical synthesis of the pentasaccharide O-(2-deoxy-2-sulfamido-6-O-sulfo-α-D-glucopyranosyl)-1→4)-O-(β-D-glucopyranosyluronic acid)-(1→4)-O-(2-deoxy-2-sulfamido-3, 6-di-O-sulfo-α-D-glucopyranosyl)-(1→4)-O-(2-O-sulfo-α-L-idopyranosyluronic acid)-(1→4)-2-deoxy-2-

sulfamido-6-O-sulfo-D-glucopyranose decasodium salt, a heparin fragment having high affinity for antithrombin III. Carbohydr Res 1986; 147:221–236.

5. Atha DH, Lormeau JC, Petitou M, Rosenberg RD, Choay J. Contribution of monosaccharide residues in heparin binding to antithrombin III. Biochemistry 1985; 24:6723–6729.

6. Torri G, Casu B, Gatti G, Petitou M, Choay J, Jacquinet JC. Mono- and bidimensional 500 MHZ proton NMR spectra of a synthetic pentasaccharide corresponding to the binding sequence of heparin to antithrombin-III: evidence for conformational peculiarity of the sulfated iduronate residue. Biochem Biophys Res Commun 1985; 128:134–140.

7. Olson ST, Björk I, Sheffer R, Craig PA, Shore JD, Choay J. Role of the antithrombin-binding pentasaccharide in heparin acceleration of antithrombin-proteinase reactions. J Biol Chem 1992; 267:12528–12538.

8. Lindahl U, Bäckström G, Thunberg L. The antithrombin-binding sequence in heparin. Identification of an essential 6–0 sulfate group. J Biol Chem 1983; 258:9826–9830.

9. Riesenfeld J, Thunberg L, Höök M, Lindahl U. The antithrombin-binding sequence of heparin. Location of essential N-sulfate groups. J Biol Chem 1981; 256:2389–2394.

10. Gettins P. Examination by 1H-n.m.r. spectroscopy of the binding of a synthetic, high-affinity heparin pentasaccharide to human antithrombin III. Carbohydr Res 1989; 185:69–76.

11. Petitou M, Duchaussoy P, Lederman I, Choay J, Sinäy P, Jacquinet JC, Torri G. Synthesis of heparin fragments: a α-methyl alpha-pentaoside with high affinity for antithrombin III. Carbohydr Res 1987; 167:67–75.

12. Rosenberg RD, Damus PS. The purification and mechanism of action of human antithrombin–heparin cofactor. J Biol Chem 1973; 248:6490–6505.

13. Damus PS, Hicks M, Rosenberg RD. Anticoagulant action of heparin. Nature 1973; 246:355–357.

14. Jordan RE, Oosta GM, Gardner WT, Rosenberg RD. The kinetics of hemostatic enzyme-antithrombin interactions in the presence of low molecular weight heparin. J Biol Chem 1980; 255:10081–10090.

15. Walenga JM. Factor Xa inhibition in mediating antithrombotic actions: application of a synthetic heparin pentasaccharide. Mention tres bien. [dissertation] Universite Pierre et Marie Curie, Paris VI, Paris, France, June 1987.

16. Herbert JM, Herault JP, Bernat A, van Amsterdam RGM, Lormeau JC, Petitou M, van Boeckel C, Hoffmann P, Meuleman DG. Biochemical and pharmacological properties of SANORG 34006, a potent and long-acting synthetic pentasaccharide. Blood 1998; 91:4197–4205.

17. Holmer E, Kurachi K, Söderström G. The molecular-weight dependence of the rate-enhancing effect of heparin on the inhibition of thrombin, factor Xa, factor IXa, factor XIa, factor XIIa and kallikrein by antithrombin. Biochem J 1981; 193:395–400.

18. Laurent TC, Tengblad A, Thunberg L, Höök M, Lindahl U. The molecular weight dependence of the anticoagulant activity of heparin. Biochem J 1978; 175:691–701.

19. Oosta GM, Gardner WT, Beeler DL, Rosenberg RD. Multiple functional domains of the heparin molecule. Proc Natl Acad Sci 1981; 78:829–833.

20. Griffith MJ, Noyes LM, Church FC. Reactive site peptides structural similarity between heparin cofactor II and antithrombin III. J Biol Chem 1985; 260:2218–2225.

21. Lormeau JC, Hérault JP. The effect of the synthetic pentasaccharide SR 90107/ORG 31540 on thrombin generation ex vivo is uniquely due to AT-mediated neutralization of factor Xa. Thromb Haemost 1995; 74:1474–1477.

22. Kaiser B, Hoppensteadt D, Jeske W, Walenga JM, Fareed J, Samama M. Heparin cofactor II interactions with heparin pentasaccharide are minimal to mediate its antithrombotic actions. Thromb Haemost 1993; 69:1111.

23. Walenga JM, Bara L, Hoppensteadt D, Choay J, Fareed J, Samama M. AT III as a rate limiting factor for the measurement of pentasaccharide in laboratory assays. Thromb Haemost 1991; 65:1314.

24. Conard J, Brosstad F, Larsen ML, Samama M, Abildgaard U. Molar antithrombin concentration in normal human plasma. Haemostasis 1983; 13:363–368.

25. Eriksson B. The PENTHIFRA study: comparison of the first synthetic factor Xa inhibitor with low molecular weight heparin (LMWH) the prevention of venous thromboembolism (VTE) after hip fracture surgery. Blood 2000; 96:490A.

26. Lassen M. The EHPHESUS study: comparison of the first synthetic factor Xa inhibitor with low molecular weight heparin (LMWH) the prevention of venous thromboembolism (VTE) after elective hip replacement surgery. Blood 2000; 96:490A.

27. Turpie G. The PENTATHLON 2000 study: comparison of the first synthetic factor Xa inhibitor with low molecular weight heparin in the prevention of venous thromboembolism (VTE) after hip replacement surgery. Blood 2000; 96:491A.

28. Bauer K. The PENTAMAKS study: comparison of the first synthetic factor Xa inhibitor with low molecular weight heparin the prevention of venous thromboembolism (VTE) after elective major knee surgery. Blood 2000; 96:490A.

29. Walenga JM, Hoppensteadt D, Mayuga M, Samama MM, Fareed J. Functionality of pentasaccharide depends on endogenous antithrombin levels. Blood 2000; 96:817a.

30. Boneu B, Necciari J, Cariou R, Sié P, Gabaig AM, Kieffer G, Dickinson J, Lamond G, Moelker H, Mant T, Magnani H. Pharmacokinetics and tolerance of the natural pentasaccharide (SR90107/ORG31540) with high affinity to antithrombin III in man. Thromb Haemost 1995; 74:1468–1473.

31. Bendayan P, Boccalon H, Dupouy D, Boneu B. Dermatan sulfate is a more potent inhibitor of clot-bound thrombin than unfractionated and low molecular weight heparins. Thromb Haemost 1994; 71:576–580.

32. Bendetowicz AV, Bara L, Samama MM. The inhibition of intrinsic prothrombinase and its generation by heparin and four derivatives in prothrombin poor plasma. Thromb Res 1990; 58:445–454.

33. Hemker HC, Choay J, Béguin S. Free factor Xa is on the main pathway of thrombin generation in clotting plasma. Biochim Biophys Acta 1989; 992:409–411.

34. Eisenberg PR, Siegel JE, Abendschein DR, Miletich JP. Importance of factor Xa in determining the procoagulant activity of whole-blood clots. J Clin Invest 1993; 91:1877–1883.

35. Cadroy Y, Hanson SR, Harker LA. Antithrombotic effects of synthetic pentasaccharide with high affinity for plasma antithrombin III in non-human primates. Thromb Haemost 1993; 70:631–635.

36. Hérault JP, Pflieger AM, Savi P, Lormeau JC, Hoffman P, Bernat A, Herbert JM. Comparative effects of two factor Xa inhibitors on prothrombinase assembled in different environments. Haemostasis 1996; 26:S3.

37. Ofosu FA, Choay J, Anvari N, Smith LM, Blajchman MA. Inhibition of factor X and factor V activation by dermatan sulfate and a pentasaccharide with high affinity for antithrombin III in human plasma. Eur J Biochem 1990; 193:485–493.

38. Béguin S, Choay J, Hemker HC. The action of a synthetic pentasaccharide on thrombin generation in whole plasma. Thromb Haemost 1989; 61:397–401.

39. Lormeau JC, Hérault JP. Comparative inhibition of extrinsic and intrinsic thrombin generation by standard heparin, a low molecular weight heparin, and a synthetic AT-III binding pentasaccharide. Thromb Haemost 1993; 69:152–156.

40. Jeske W. Pharmacologic studies on synthetic analogues of heparin with selective affinity to endogenous serine protease inhibitors [dissertation]. Loyola University Chicago, Chicago, IL, May 1996.

41. Walenga JM, Bara L, Petitou M, Samama M, Fareed J, Choay J. The inhibition of the generation of thrombin and the antithrombotic effect of a pentasaccharide with sole anti-factor Xa activity. Thromb Res 1988; 51:23–33.

42. Dol F, Gaich C, Petitou M, Boneu B, Caranobe C, Bernat A, Sainte Marie M, Herbert JM. The antithrombotic activity of synthetic pentasaccharides and fraxiparine is closely correlated with their respective ability to alter thromboplastin-triggered thrombin generation ex vivo. Thromb Haemost 1993; 69:655.

43. Walenga JM, Fareed J. Relative contribution of factor Xa and factor IIa inhibition in the mediation of the antithrombotic actions of LMWHs and synthetic heparin pentasaccharides. Thromb Haemor Dis 1991; 3:53–59.

44. Ofosu FA. Modulation of the enzymatic activity of α-thrombin by polyanions: consequences on intrinsic activation of factor V and factor VIII. Haemostasis 1991; 21:240–247.

45. Rao LVM, Rapaport SI, Hoang AD. Binding of factor VIIa to tissue factor permits rapid antithrombin III/heparin inhibition of factor VIIa. Blood 1993; 81:2600–2607.

46. Ofosu FA, Leclerc J, Delorme F, Craven S, Shafai S, Frewin L, Blajchman MA. The low molecular weight heparin enoxaparin inhibits the consumption of factor VII and prothrombin activation in vivo associated with elective knee replacement surgery. Br J Haematol 1992; 83:391–399.

47. Gerotziafas GT, Bara L, Bloch MF, Makris PE, Samama MM. Treatment with LMWHs inhibits factor VIIa generation during in vitro coagulation of whole blood. Thromb Res 1996; 81:491–496.

48. Lormeau JC, Héerault JP, Herbert JM. Antithrombin mediated inhibition of factor VIIa–tissue factor complex by the synthetic pentasaccharide representing the heparin binding site to AT. Thromb Haemost 1996; 76:5–8.

49. Broze GJ, Warren LP, Novotny WF, Higuchi DA, Girard JJ, Miletich JP. Lipoprotein-associated coagulation inhibitor that inhibits the factor VII–tissue factor complex also inhibits factor Xa: insight into its possible mechanism of action. Blood 1988; 71:335–343.

50. Hoppensteadt D, Walenga JM, Fasanella A, Jeske W, Fareed J. TFPI antigen levels in normal human volunteers after IV and SC administration of heparin and a low molecular weight heparin. Thromb Res 1994; 77:175–185.

51. Bara L, Bloch MF, Zitoun D, Samama M, Collignon F, Frydman A, Uzan A, Bouthier J. Comparative effects of enoxaparin and unfractionated heparin in healthy volunteers on prothrombin consumption in whole blood during coagulation, and release of tissue factor pathway inhibitor. Thromb Res 1993; 69:443–452.

52. Lindahl AK, Sandset PM, Abildgaard U. The present status of tissue factor pathway inhibitor. Blood Coag Fibrinol 1992; 3:439–449.

53. Wun TC. Lipoprotein associated coagulation inhibitor (LACI) is a cofactor for heparin: synergistic actor between LACI and sulfated polysaccharides. Blood 1992; 79:430–438.

54. Zitoun D, Bara L, Bloch MF, Samama MM. Plasma TFPI activity after intravenous injection of pentasaccharide (PS) and unfractionated heparin in rabbits. Thromb Res 1994; 75:577–580.

55. Lojewski B, Bacher P, Jeske W, Fareed J. Molecular weight dependence on the release of tissue factor pathway inhibitor after subcutaneous and intravenous actions of heparins. Thromb Haemost 1993; 69:1174.

56. Kaiser B, Hoppensteadt DA, Jeske W, Wun TC, Fareed J. Inhibitory effects of TFPI on thrombin and factor Xa generation in vitro–modulatory action of glycosaminoglycans. Thromb Res 1994; 75:609–616.

57. Bernat A, Hoffmann P, Sainte–Marie M, Herbert JM. The synthetic pentasaccharide SR 90107A/Org 31540 enhances tissue-type plasminogen activator-induced thrombolysis in rabbits. Fibrinolysis 1996; 10:151–157.

58. Kaiser B, Fareed J. Effect of unfractionated heparin and a heparin pentasaccharide on the thrombolytic process in an experimental model in rabbits. Fibrinolysis 1996; 10(suppl 3):127.

59. Fareed J, Hoppensteadt D, Jeske W, Walenga JM. An overview of non-heparin glycosaminoglycans as antithrombotic agents. In: Poller L, ed. Recent Advances in Blood Coagulation. London: Churchill Livingstone, 1993:169–187.

60. Salzman EW, Rosenberg RD, Smith MH, Lindon JN, Favreau L. Effect of heparin and heparin fractions on platelet aggregation. J Clin Invest 1980; 65:64–73.

61. Labrouche S, Freyburger G, Belloc F, Boisseau MR. Influence of selected heparins on human neutrophil functions in vitro. Thromb Haemost 1992; 68:556–562.

62. Walenga JM, Koza MJ, Lewis BE, Pifarré R. Relative heparin-induced thrombocytopenic potential of low molecular weight heparins and new antithrombotic agents. Clin Appl Thromb/Hemost 1996; 2(suppl 1):S21–S27.

63. Elalamy I, Lecrubier C, Potevin F, Abdelouahed M, Bara L, Marie JP, Samama M. Absence of in vitro cross-reaction of pentasaccharide with the plasma heparin dependent factor of twenty-five patients with heparin associated thrombocytopenia. Thromb Haemost 1995; 74:1384–1385.

64. Ahmad S, Jeske WP, Walenga JM, Hoppensteadt DA, Wood JJ, Herbert JM, Messmore HL, Fareed J. Synthetic pentasaccharides do not cause platelet activation by antiheparin–platelet factor 4 antibodies. Clin Appl Thromb Hemost 1999; 5:259–266.

65. Jeske W, Szatkowski E, Hoppensteadt D, Walenga JM. Development of a flow cytometric assay for the detection of heparin induced thrombocytopenia. Blood 1996; 88(suppl 1):317a.

66. Jeske WP, Jay AM, Haas S, Walenga JM. Heparin-induced thrombocytopenic potential of GAG and non–GAG-based antithrombotic agents. Clin Appl Thromb Hemost 1999; 5(suppl 1):S56–S62.
67. Greinacher A, Alban S, Dummel V, Franz G, Mueller–Eckhardt C. Characterization of the structural requirements for a carbohydrate based anticoagulant with a reduced risk of inducing the immunological type of heparin-associated thrombocytopenia. Thromb Haemost 1995; 74:886–892.
68. Young E, Wells P, Holloway S, Weitz J, Hirsh J. Ex-vivo and in-vitro evidence that low molecular weight heparins exhibit less binding to plasma proteins than unfractionated heparin. Thromb Haemost 1994; 71:300–304.
69. Walenga JM, Fareed J. Preliminary biochemical and pharmacologic studies on a chemically synthesized pentasaccharide. Semin Thromb Hemost 1985; 11:89–99.
70. Wessler S, Reimer SM, Sheps MC. Biologic assay of a thrombosis-inducing activity in human serum. J Appl Physiol 1959; 14:943–946.
71. Walenga JM, Petitou M, Lormeau JC, Samama M, Fareed J, Choay J. Antithrombotic activity of a synthetic heparin pentasaccharide in a rabbit stasis thrombosis model using different thrombogenic challenges. Thromb Res 1987; 46:187–198.
72. Thomas DP, Merton RE, Gray E, Barrowcliffe TW. The relative antithrombotic effectiveness of heparin, a low molecular weight heparin, and a pentasaccharide fragment in an animal model. Thromb Haemost 1989; 61:204–207.
73. Amar J, Caranobe P, Sie P, Boneu B. Antithrombotic potencies of heparins in relation to their antifactor Xa and antithrombin activities: an experimental study in two models of thrombosis in the rabbit. Br J Haematol 1990; 76:94–100.
74. Hobbelen PMJ, Van Dinther TG, Vogel GMT, Van Boeckel CAA, Moelker HCT, Meuleman DG. Pharmacological profile of the chemically synthesized antithrombin III binding fragment of heparin (pentasaccharide) in rats. Thromb Haemost 1990; 63:265–270.
75. Walenga JM, Fareed J, Petitou M, Samama M, Lormeau JC, Choay J. Intravenous antithrombotic activity of a synthetic heparin pentasaccharide in a human serum induced stasis thrombosis model. Thromb Res 1986; 43:243–248.
76. Buchanan MR, Boneu B, Ofosu F, Hirsh J. The relative importance of thrombin inhibition and factor Xa inhibition to the antithrombotic effects of heparin. Blood 1985; 65:198–201.
77. Cade JF, Buchanan MR, Boneu B, Ockelford P, Carter CJ, Cerskus AL, Hirsh J. A comparison of the antithrombotic and haemorrhagic effects of low molecular weight heparin fractions: the influence of the method of preparation. Thromb Res 1985; 35:613–625.
78. Bergqvist D, Nilsson B, Hedner U, Pedersen PC, Ostergaard PB. The effect of heparin fragments of different molecular weights on experimental thrombosis and haemostasis. Thromb Res 1985; 38:589–601.
79. Raake W, Elling H. Rat jugular vein hemostasis–a new model for testing antithrombotic agents. Thromb Res 1989; 53:73–77.
80. Weichert W, Breddin HK. Effect of low molecular weight heparins on laser-induced thrombus formation in rat mesenteric vessels. Haemostasis 1988; 18 (suppl 3):55–63.
81. Meuleman DG, Hobbelen PMJ, Van Dinther TG, Vogel GMT, Van Boeckel CAA, Moelker HCT. Antifactor Xa activity and antithrombotic activity in rats of structural analogues of the minimum antithrombin III binding sequence: discovery of compounds with a longer duration of action than of the natural pentasaccharide. Semin Thromb Hemost 1991; 17 (suppl 1):112–117.
82. Vogel GMT, Meuleman DG, Bourgondien FGM, Hobbelen PMJ. Comparison of two experimental thrombosis models in rats, effects of four glycosaminoglycans. Thromb Res 1989; 54:399–410.
83. Vogel GMT, Van Amsterdam RGM, Kop WJ, Meuleman DG. Pentasaccharide and Orgaran arrest, whereas heparin delays thrombus formation in a rat arteriovenous shunt. Thromb Haemost 1993; 69:29–34.
84. Hoppensteadt DA, Jeske WP, Walenga JM, Fu K, Yang LH, Ing TS, Herbert JM, Fareed J. Laboratory monitoring of pentasaccharide in a dog model of hemodialysis. Thromb Res 1999; 96:115–124.
85. Bernat A, Herbert JM. Protamine sulfate inhibits pentasaccharide (SR 80027)-induced bleeding without affecting its antithrombotic and anti-factor Xa activity in the rat. Haemostasis 1996; 26:195–202.

86. Daud AN, Ahsan A, Iqbal O, Walenga JM, Silver PJ, Ahmad S, Fareed J. Synthetic heparin pentasaccharide depolymerization by heparinase I: molecular and biological implications. Clin Appl Thromb Hemost 2001; 58–64.

87. Iqbal O, Shadid H, Silver P, Walenga JM, Daud AN, Ahmad S, Fareed J. Heparinase is capable of neutralizing the anticoagulant and hemorrhagic effects of a synthetic pentasaccharide. Blood 2000; 96:52a.

88. Shriver Z, Sundaram M, Venkataraman G, Fareed J, Linhardt R, Biemann K, Sasisekharan R. Cleavage of the antithrombin III binding site in heparin by heparinases and its implication in the generation of low molecular weight heparin. Proc Natl Acad Sci USA 2000; 97:10365–10370.

89. Bacher P, Fareed J, Hoppensteadt D, Walenga JM, Iqbal O. Endogenous AT III as a limiting factor in the mediation of antiprotease actions of heparins and related oligosaccharides. Impact on the pharmaco-dynamic parameters as calculated by using functional methods. Thromb Haemost 1991; 65:932.

90. Van Amsterdam RGM, Vogel GMT, Visser A, Kop WJ, Buiting MT, Meuleman DG. Synthetic analogues of the antithrombin III-binding pentasaccharide sequence of heparin. Prediction of in vivo residence times. Arterioscler Thromb Vasc Biol 1995; 15:495–503.

91. Crépon B, Donat F, Bârzu T, Hérault JP. Pharmacokinetic (PK) parameters of AT binding pentasac-charides in three animal species: predictive value for humans. Thromb Haemost 1993; 69:654.

92. Turpie AG. A dose ranging study of a novel synthetic pentasaccharide (ORG 31540/SR90107A) in the prevention of venous thromboembolism after total hip replacement. Int J Hematol 2000; 72(suppl 1):54.

93. The Rembrandt Investigators. Treatment of proximal deep vein thrombosis with a novel synthetic compound (SR90107A/ORG31540) with pure anti-factor Xa activity. Circulation 2000; 102:2726–2731.

94. Coussement PK. SR9010A/ORG31540, a new synthetic pentasaccharide, as an adjunct to fibrinolysis in ST-elevation acute myocardial infarction: the PENTALYSE study. Presented at the Late Breaking Clinical Trials II session at the ACC 49th Annual Scientific Session, March 12–15, 2000.

95. Vuillemenot A, Schiele F, Meneveau N, Claudel S, Donat F, Fontecave S, Cariou R, Samama MM, Bassand JP. Efficacy of a synthetic pentasaccharide, a pure factor Xa inhibitor, as an antithrombotic agent—a pilot study in the setting of coronary angioplasty. Thromb Haemost 1999; 81:214–220.

96. Faaij RA, Burggraaf J, Cohen AF. Lack of pharmacokinetic (PK) and pharmacodynamic (PD) interaction between the first synthetic factor Xa inhibitor and warfarin in human volunteers. Blood 2000; 96:56a.

97. Donat F, Ollier C, Santoni A, Duvauchelle T. Safety and pharmacokinetics (PK) of co-administration of the first synthetic factor Xa inhibitor and aspirin in human volunteers. Blood 2000; 96:54a.

98. Walenga JM, Jeske WP, Bara L, Samama MM, Fareed J. State-of-the-art article. Biochemical and pharmacologic rationale for the development of a heparin pentasaccharide. Thromb Res 1997; 86:1–36.

99. Fareed J. Basic and applied pharmacology of low molecular weight heparins. Pharm Ther 1995; June:16s–24s.

100. Fareed J, Walenga JM, Hoppensteadt D, Huan XO, Nonn R. Biochemical and pharmacological inequivalence of low-molecular-weight heparins. Proc Natl Acad Sci USA 1989; 556:333–353.

101. Petitou M, van Boeckel CAA. Heparin: from the original "soup" to well-designed heparin mimetics. Pure Appl Chem 1997; 69:1839–1846.

102. Petitou M, Hérault JP, Bernat A, Driguez PA, Duchaussoy P, Lormeau JC, Herbert JM. Synthesis of thrombin-inhibiting heparin mimetics without side effects. Nature 1999; 398:417–422.

103. Petitou M, Duchaussoy P, Driguez PA, Jaurand G, Hérault JP, Lormeau JC, van Boeckel, CAA, Herbert JM. First synthetic carbohydrates with the full anticoagulant properties of heparin. Angew Chem Int Edit 1998; 37:3009–3014.

16

Oral-Direct Thrombin Inhibitors

Mark A. Crowther
McMaster University, Hamilton, Ontario, Canada

SUMMARY

Current strategies for the treatment and prevention of venous thrombosis require a mix of parenteral and oral therapies that frequently require laboratory monitoring. Oral-direct thrombin inhibitors have the potential to simplify antithrombotic therapy; these agents produce a predictable anticoagulant response so that laboratory monitoring may be unnecessary. Ximelagatran, the oral direct thrombin inhibitor in the most advanced stage of development, is a prodrug of melagatran, an active–site-directed inhibitor of thrombin. In phase II studies, ximelagatran has been evaluated as thromboprophylaxis in patients undergoing elective hip or knee replacement surgery and in patients with nonvalvular atrial fibrillation. The drug has also been studied in patients with acute venous thrombosis. In each case, ximelagatran appears to be at least as safe and effective as current antithrombotic interventions. Phase III studies with ximelagatran for these indications are currently underway. If ximelagatran lives up to its initial promise, it has the potential to revolutionize the prevention and treatment of thrombosis.

I. INTRODUCTION

Current anticoagulant practice dates to the 1940s, when oral vitamin K antagonists were first used for the prevention and treatment of thromboembolism. All currently available oral anticoagulants produce their antithrombotic effect by interfering with posttranslational processing of four vitamin K-dependent clotting proteins: factors VII, IX, X, and prothrombin [1]. Oral anticoagulants also block the posttranslational modification of two naturally occurring anticoagulants, protein C and protein S. Vitamin K antagonists act as competitive antagonists to two enzymes that catalyze the conversion of vitamin K from the epoxide to reduced form. Reduced vitamin K is required for γ-carboxylation of glutamine residues found on the amino terminals of vitamin K-dependent clotting factors [1]. γ-Carboxylation is necessary for interaction of these proteins with calcium, an essential step in the assembly of coagulation factor complexes on phospholipid surfaces.

Oral vitamin K antagonists are effective antithrombotic drugs. For example, warfarin reduces the risk of stroke in patients with atrial fibrillation by about 70% [2], and lowers the risk of recurrent deep vein thrombosis by about 90% [3]. However, oral vitamin K antagonists have four major drawbacks: (1) onset of anticoagulation is delayed because it takes several days to lower the levels of the vitamin K-dependent coagulation factors into the therapeutic range [4]; (2) multiple drug and food interactions render the anticoagulant response unpredictable so that careful laboratory monitoring is essential [5]; (3) reversal of the anticoagulant effect of vitamin K antagonists is slow unless supplemental vitamin K or fresh-frozen plasma is given [7–9] because it takes time to regenerate normal or near-normal levels of the vitamin K-dependent clotting factors; and (4) decreases in the levels of protein C or protein S on initiation of oral anticoagulant therapy can precipitate skin necrosis in individuals whose baseline levels of protein C or protein S are reduced [10].

Currently, there are no safe and effective orally available alternatives to the vitamin K antagonists. Aspirin and other orally active antiplatelet agents reduce the risk of thrombosis in a variety of patient populations, including those with atherosclerotic vascular diseases. However, antiplatelet agents are less effective than warfarin or parenteral anticoagulants in many patients at high risk of thrombosis [11,12]. Orally available heparin formulations are undergoing clinical trials, but their utility remains to be proved.

Various recombinant analogues of inhibitors of coagulation isolated from hematophagous organisms have been described. These agents produce their anticoagulant effect by binding with high-affinity to the active site of specific coagulation factors. Examples include hirudin, tick-anticoagulant peptide, and nematode anticoagulant protein, agents that target thrombin, factor Xa, and the tissue factor-bound VIIa complex, respectively. All of these anticoagulants are large molecules that must be given parenterally, a feature that limits their clinical usefulness.

Unlike heparin, which catalyzes antithrombin-mediated inactivation of thrombin, factor Xa, and other clotting enzymes, direct-acting anticoagulants do not require a plasma cofactor to express their activity. Furthermore, most of these agents target only a single clotting enzyme or coagulation factor complex. By using structure-based design, small-molecule inhibitors of coagulation enzymes have been developed. For example, once the three-dimensional structure of the hirudin–thrombin complex was elucidated, a variety of low-molecular-weight inhibitors of the active site of thrombin were produced. Subsequent chemical manipulation has led to the production of orally active direct thrombin inhibitors.

II. PHARMACOLOGY OF ORAL DIRECT THROMBIN INHIBITORS

Oral direct thrombin inhibitors have the potential to overcome many of the limitations of the vitamin K antagonists. For example, direct thrombin inhibitors have a rapid onset of action and their anticoagulant effect is dose-dependent. Because they target only a single enzyme, direct thrombin inhibitors may have a wider therapeutic window than vitamin K antagonists [13]. With short half-lives, the anticoagulant effect of oral direct thrombin inhibitors is rapidly reversible, and because these agents have no effect on the levels of protein C or protein S, there is no danger of skin necrosis.

Ximelagatran has about 20% bioavailability after oral administration, which is 100-fold better than melagatran [14–16], and the absorption of ximelagatran is unaffected by food [16]. After oral administration, ximelagatran is rapidly converted to melagatran, the levels of which peak in 1.6–1.9 h [16]. The drug has a half-life of about 3 h [15], mandating twice-daily oral administration. Melagatran is primarily eliminated via the kidneys. The half-life of ximelagatran does not vary between ethnic groups [15], but is prolonged in the elderly, reflecting their impaired renal function [17]. The pharmacokinetics and pharmacodynamics of ximelagatran are not influenced by aspirin [18] and ximelagatran does not interfere with drugs that are metabolized by the cytochrome P450 isozymes CYP2C19, CYP2C9, or CYP3A4 [19–21].

After oral absorption, ximelagatran is rapidly converted to melagatran by two intermediate metabolites, designated H 338/57 and H 415/04 [17]. Melagatran inhibits thrombin generation ex vivo and in vitro [22]. The active metabolites of ximelagatran are more effective than dalteparin for the prevention of thrombosis in rats [23].

Melagatran acts as a competitive antagonist with antithrombin for the active site of thrombin [24]. Once bound to thrombin, melagatran blocks thrombin's activity and reduces thrombin generation by blocking feedback activation of coagulation [25]. Melagatran enhances the fibrinolytic activity of tissue plasminogen activator by blocking thrombin-mediated activation of thrombin activatable fibrinolysis inhibitor [26] and blocks thrombin-mediated platelet activation [27,28].

In a phase I study in 120 healthy male subjects, 60 mg of ximelagatran administered orally produced similar suppression in the levels of prothrombin fragments F1.2, thrombin–antithrombin complexes, and β-thromboglobulin, as did 100 mg/kg of enoxaparin or a continuous infusion of hirudin [29].

A paradoxical increase in the risk of thrombosis might occur with the use of direct thrombin inhibitors because of their capacity to block protein C activation by the thrombin–antithrombin complex [30]. However, clinical results now suggest that any prothrombotic tendency is overcome by suppression of the procoagulant effects of thrombin.

The principal complication of oral direct thrombin inhibitors is likely to be hemorrhage. No specific antidotes are available for direct thrombin inhibitors. Consequently, bleeding complications must be managed symptomatically. Although not well studied, dialysis or hemoperfusion likely removes these compounds from the circulation, and the administration of activated coagulation factor complexes such as FEIBA, Autoplex, or recombinant activated factor VII (factor VIIa) may overcome their anticoagulant effect. FEIBA was effective for this indication in animal models [31], and recombinant factor VIIa reduces the anticoagulant activity of melagatran in human volunteers [32].

Because it produces a predictable anticoagulant response, routine laboratory monitoring is unlikely to be necessary for ximelagatran. If monitoring is required, enzyme-linked immunosorbent assays (ELISA) can be used to measure drug levels. Because of their cost and inconvenience, however, these assays are unlikely to be routinely available. Oral direct thrombin inhibitors do not produce predictable prolongation of the activated partial thromboplastin time (APTT) or International Normalized Ratio (INR). Consequently, these widely available tests are not useful for monitoring [33,34]. Although melagatran prolongs the APTT, the APTT declines over time despite constant plasma levels of melagatran. For example, Eriksson and colleagues [33] demonstrated that the plasma concentration of melagatran that produced a twofold prolongation of APTT was 0.4 μmol/L at the beginning of treatment and 0.9 μmol/L 8–11 days later. The INR also is prolonged in patients receiving ximelagatran, but the extent of prolongation with fixed plasma concentrations is highly dependent on the reagent used to measure the INR. For example, Mattsson and Menschik–Lundin [35] demonstrated a twofold increase in the INR with a melagatran concentration of 0.87 μmol/L if thromboplastin-S (Biopool) was used. In contrast, with SPA 50 (Stago), a less sensitive reagent, a concentration of 2.9 μmol/L was required to produce a twofold increase in the INR.

Direct thrombin inhibitors produce marked prolongation of the thrombin-clotting time, even at low plasma concentrations. The ecarin clotting time (ECT) may provide a more reliable guide to plasma levels of direct thrombin inhibitors over usual therapeutic ranges. However, the ECT has yet to be standardized and its clinical usefulness has not been established.

III. CLINICAL TRIALS WITH ORAL DIRECT THROMBIN INHIBITORS

Early-phase clinical trials have demonstrated that ximelagatran has an antithrombotic effect in humans. For example, in a phase II dose-finding study involving 1916 patients undergoing elective knee (606 patients) or hip arthroplasty, melagatran was given subcutaneously before surgery and ximelagatran was given orally in the postoperative period. When compared with dalteparin (5000 U subcutaneously once daily), the highest dose of ximelagatran reduced the incidence of venographically detected deep-vein thrombosis from 28 to 15%. The risk of proximal deep-vein thrombosis was reduced from 6.5 to 2.5% [36]. A follow-up study in 2788 patients undergoing hip or knee arthroplasty compared the effectiveness of a postoperative, subcutaneous 3-mg dose of melagatran followed by ximelagatran (24 mg orally, twice daily) with enoxaparin, 40 mg subcutaneously once daily started the evening before surgery. The rate of proximal deep-vein thrombosis and pulmonary embolism was 5.7% in those randomized to melagatran or ximelagatran and 6.2% in patients given enoxaparin, a nonsignificant difference. Bleeding and other complications were similar between the two groups [37].

In a second phase II study performed in North America, ximelagatran was compared with enoxaparin for thromboprophylaxis in 600 patients undergoing knee arthroplasty [38]. Ximelagatran, administered in twice-daily doses of 8, 12, 18, or 24 mg, was compared with enoxaparin (30 mg subcutaneously twice daily). Anticoagulants were started 12–24 h after surgery and were continued for up to 12 days until mandatory venography was performed. The results of this study are presented in Table 1. Ximelagatran appeared to be as effective as enoxaparin and, at the doses tested, did not appear to increase the risk of bleeding.

Warfarin is often used for thromboprophylaxis after knee arthroplasty in centers in North America. Warfarin was compared with ximelagatran (24-mg orally twice daily) for postoperative thromboprophylaxis in 680 patients undergoing elective knee arthroplasty [39]. The rates of total and proximal venous thrombosis were 19.2 and 3.3%, respectively, in those given ximelagatran and 25.7 and 5.0%, respectively, in those treated with warfarin. These data suggest that ximelagatran is at least as effective as warfarin for the prevention of venous thrombosis after knee arthroplasty.

Ximelagatran also has been evaluated in patients with atrial fibrillation. The SPORTIF II study randomized 257 patients with nonvalvular atrial fibrillation to receive either one of three doses of ximelagatran (20, 40, or 60 mg twice daily) or warfarin in doses sufficient to produce an INR of 2.0–3.0 [40]. Over a 12-week period, 2 of 67 (3.0%) patients allocated to warfarin had a transient ischemic attack, compare with 1 of 190 (0.5%) patients given ximelagatran who had a stroke, and 1 additional patient had a transient ischemic attack.

Table 1 Phase II Trial Comparing Ximelagatran with Enoxaparin for Thromboprophylaxis After Knee Replacement Surgery

Outcome	Ximelagatran				Enoxaparin
	8 mg	12 mg	18 mg	24 mg	30 mg
	$n = 63$	$n = 101$	$n = 87$	$n = 95$	$n = 97$
Overall VTE(%)	27.0	19.8	28.7	15.8	22.7
Proximal DVT/PE(%)	6.6	2.0	5.8	3.2	3.1
	$n = 84$	$n = 134$	$n = 124$	$n = 127$	$n = 125$
Major bleeding(%)	0.0	0.0	2.4	0.0	0.8

Oral direct thrombin inhibitors have the potential to revolutionize the treatment of acute venous thrombosis. Single-agent, nonmonitored therapy would substantially reduce the complexity and might reduce the cost of treating this common clinical problem. Ximelagatran has been evaluated in a phase II trial for initial monotherapy of deep vein thrombosis [41]. In this study, patients with objectively documented deep vein thrombosis were randomized to receive either ximelagatran (24, 36, 48, or 60 mg orally twice daily) or dalteparin, followed by warfarin. Paired venograms were compared to assess the change in thrombus size as assessed using a validated scoring system. Rates of thrombus regression and changes in clinical indicators, such as pain, edema, and leg circumference, were similar between the ximelagatran and dalteparin groups. There was a trend for increased thrombus progression in patients given ximelagatran compared with those treated with dalteparin and warfarin (8 and 3%, respectively), but this difference was not statistically significant. Based on these results Ximelagatran is currently undergoing phase III evaluation as monotherapy for acute deep vein thrombosis.

IV. SUMMARY

Oral direct thrombin inhibitors hold great promise. These agents have the potential to overcome many of the limitations of vitamin K antagonists. Even if oral direct thrombin inhibitors prove to be no more effective than vitamin K antagonists, treatment will be streamlined if the need for laboratory monitoring can be obviated.

REFERENCES

1. Furie B, Bouchard BA, Furie BC. Vitamin K-dependent biosynthesis of gamma-carboxyglutamic acid. Blood 1999; 93:1798–1808.
2. Hart RG, Sherman DG, Easton JD, Cairns JA. Prevention of stroke in patients with nonvalvular atrial fibrillation. Neurology 1998; 51:674–681.
3. Kearon C, Gent M, Hirsh J, et al. A comparison of three months of anticoagulation with extended anticoagulation for a first episode of idiopathic venous thromboembolism. N Engl J Med 1999; 340:901–907.
4. Harrison L, Johnston M, Massicotte MP, Crowther M, Moffat K, Hirsh J. Comparison of 5-mg and 10-mg loading doses in initiation of warfarin therapy. Ann Intern Med 1997; 126:133–136.
5. Ansell J, Hirsh J, Dalen J, Bussey H, Anderson D, Poller L, Jacobson AF, Deykin D, Matchar DB. Managing oral anticoagulant therapy. Chest 2001; 119:22S–38S.
6. White RH, McKittrick T, Hutchinson R, Twitchell J. Temporary discontinuation of warfarin therapy: changes in the International Normalized Ratio. Ann Intern Med 1995; 122:40–42.
7. Crowther MA, Julian J, Douketis JD, Kovacs M, Biagoni L, Schnurr T, McGinnis J, Gent M, Hirsh J, Ginsberg JS. Treatment of warfarin-associated coagulopathy with oral vitamin K: a randomized clinical trial. Lancet 2000; 356:1551–1553.
8. Shetty HG, Backhouse G, Bentley DP, Routledge PA. Effective reversal of warfarin-induced excessive anticoagulation with low dose vitamin K_1. Thromb Haemost 1992; 67:13–15.
9. Hirsh J, Dalen J, Anderson DR, Poller L, Bussey H, Ansell J, Deykin D. Oral anticoagulants: mechanism of action, clinical effectiveness, and optimal therapeutic range. Chest 2001; 119:85–215.
10. Conlan MG, Bridges A, Williams E, Marlar R. Familial type II protein C deficiency associated with warfarin-induced skin necrosis and bilateral adrenal hemorrhage. Am J Hematol 1988; 29:226–229.
11. Risk factors for stroke and efficacy of antithrombotic therapy in atrial fibrillation. Analysis of pooled data from five randomized controlled trials. Arch Intern Med 1994; 154:1449–1457.

12. Gent M, Hirsh J, Ginsberg JS, Powers PJ, Levine MN, Geerts WH, Jay RM, Leclerc J, Neemeh JA, Turpie AG. Low-molecular-weight heparinoid orgaran is more effective than aspirin in the prevention of venous thromboembolism after surgery for hip fracture. Circulation 1996; 93:80–84.
13. Elg M, Gustafsson D, Carlsson S. Antithrombotic effects and bleeding time of thrombin inhibitors and warfarin in the rat. Thromb Res 1999; 94:187–197.
14. Gustafsson D, Nystrom JE, Carlsson S, et al. Pharmacodynamic properties of H 376/95, a prodrug of the direct thrombin inhibitor melagatran, intended for oral use [abstr]. Blood 1999; 94:(10).
15. Johansson L, Eriksson UG, Frison L. et al. Pharmacokinetics and pharmacodynamics of H 376/95 after oral dosing in healthy male subjects of different ethnic origin [abstr]. Blood 2000; 96:(11).
16. Eriksson UG, Johansson L, Frison L, et al. Single and repeated oral dosing of H 736/95, a prodrug of the direct thrombin inhibitor melagatran, to young healthy male patients [abstr]. Blood 1999; 94:(10).
17. Johansson L, Eriksson UG, Frison L, et al. Pharmacokinetics of H 376/95 in young and elderly healthy subjects [abstr]. Blood 2000; 96:(11).
18. Fager G, Eriksson–Lepkowska M, Frison L, et al. Influence of acetylsalicyclic acid on the pharmacodynamics and pharmacokinetics of melagatran, the active form of the direct thrombin inhibitor H 376/95 [abstr]. Eur Heart Jl 2000; 21 (suppl):441.
19. Eriksson–Lepkowska M, Thuresson A, Bylock A, et al. The effect of the oral direct thrombin inhibitor, ximelagatran, on the pharmacokinetics of diazepam in healthy male volunteers [abstr]. Thromb Haemost 2001; 86:(1).
20. Eriksson–Lepkowska M, Thuresson A, Bylock A, et al. The effect of the oral direct thrombin inhibitor, ximelagatran, on the pharmacokinetics and pharmacodynamics of diclofenac in healthy male volunteers [abstr]. Thromb Haemost 2001; 86:(1).
21. Johansson S, Bylock A, Eriksson–Lepkowska M, et al. The effect of the oral direct thrombin inhibitor, ximelagatran, on the pharmacokinetics of nifedipine in healthy male volunteers [abstr]. Thromb Haemost 2001; 86(1).
22. Bostrom SL, Sarich TC, Wolzt M. The effects of melagatran, the active form of H 376/95, an oral, direct thrombin inhibitor, on thrombin generation [abstr]. Blood 2000; 96:(11).
23. Carlsson S, Adler G, Elg M. The oral, direct thrombin inhibitor H 376/95 reduced thrombus size in a deep venous thrombus treatment conscious rat model [abstr]. Blood 2000; 96:(11).
24. Deinum J, Elg M. The effect of melagatran on the binding of thrombin to anti-thrombin studied by plasmon resonance [abstr]. Haemostasis 2000; 30 (s1):165.
25. Bostrom SL, Sarich TC, Wolzt M. Dose-dependent reduction in endogenous thrombin potential by melagatran, the active form of the oral, direct thrombin inhibitor H 376/95 [abstr]. Haemostasis 2000; 30 (s1):167.
26. Mattsson C, Bjorkman J–A, Abrahamsson T, et al. Melagatran, the active form of the oral, direct thrombin inhibitor H 376/95, enhances the thrombolytic effects of tissue type plasminogen activator: a possible mechanism being inhibition of thrombin-mediated Pro–Cpu activation [abstr]. Blood 2000; 96:(11).
27. Nylander S, Mattsson C. Inhibition of thrombin-induced platelet activation by different anticoagulants as measured with flow cytometry [abstr] Blood 2000; 96:(11).
28. Schersten F, Wahlund G, Carlsson S, et al. Effect of melagatran, the active form of the oral direct thrombin inhibitor H 376/95, on platelet deposition and relative thrombus size in a porcine coronary artery overstretch model [abstr]. Circulation 2000; 102 (s2):130.
29. Sarich TC, Wolzt M, Eriksson UG, et al. Effect of H 376/95, an oral, direct thrombin inhibitor, versus r-hirudin and enoxaparin on markers of thrombin generation and platelet activation in shed blood from healthy male subjects [abstr]. Haemostasis 2000; 30 (s1):24–25.
30. Menschik–Lundin A, Nylander S, Mattsson C, et al. Inhibition of protein C activation by anticoagulant compounds with different modes of action [abstr]. Haemostasis 2001; 30 (s1):167–168.
31. Elg M, Borjesson I, Pehrsson S, et al. Feiba reversed bleeding times prolonged by high doses of a thrombin inhibitor and was not prothrombotic [abstr]. Blood 2000; 96:(11).
32. Ulvinge J–C, Berntsson P, Bostrom SL. Melagatran-induced inhibition of thrombin generation is reversed by Feiba [abstr]. Blood 2000; 96:(11).

33. Eriksson UG, Frison L, Gustafsson D, et al. Effect of melagatran, the active form of the oral, direct thrombin inhibitor, H 376/95, on activated partial thromboplastin time (APTT) in orthopaedic surgery patients treated to prevent deep vein thrombosis and pulmonary embolism [abstr]. Blood 2000; 96:(11).

34. Menschik–Lundin A, Mattsson C. Effects of melagatran, the active form of the oral, direct thrombin inhibitor H 376/95, on prothrombin time determined with 15 reagents of different sensitivities [abstr]. Haemostasis 2000; 30 (s1):164–165.

35. Mattsson C, Menschik–Lundin A. Prothrombin time assays are unsuitable for monitoring the effects of melagatran, the active form of the oral, direct thrombin inhibitor H 376/95 [abstr]. Blood 2000; 96:(11).

36. Eriksson BI, Lindbratt S, Kalebo P, et al. METHRO II: dose–response study of the novel oral, direct thrombin inhibitor, H 376/95 and its subcutaneous formulation, melagatran, compared with dalteparin as thromboembolic prophylaxis after total hip or total knee replacement [abstr]. Haemostasis 2000; 30 (S1):183.

37. Eriksson BI, Ogren M, Agnelli G, et al. The oral direct thrombin inhibitor ximelagatran and its subcutaneous form melagatran compared with enoxaparin as prophylaxis after total hip or knee joint replacement [abstr]. Thromb Haemos 2001; 86:(1).

38. Heit JA, Colwell CWJ, Francis CW, et al. Comparison of the oral direct thrombin inhibitor H 376/95 with enoxaparin as prophylaxis against venous thromboembolism after total knee replacement: a phase II dose-finding study [abstr]. Blood 2000; 96:(11).

39. Francis CW, Davidson BL, Berkowitz SD, et al. Randomized, double-blind, comparative study of ximelagatran, an oral direct thrombin inhibitor, and warfarin to prevent venous thromboembolism (VTE) after total knee arthroplasty (TKA) [abstr]. Thromb Haemost 2001; 86:(1).

40. Petersen P. First experience with the oral direct thrombin inhibitor H 376/95 compared with warfarin in patients with non-valvular atrial fibrillation (NVAF) [abstr]. J Gen Intern Med 2001; 16 (s1):164.

41. Eriksson H, Wahlander K, Gustafsson D, et al. Efficacy and tolerability of the novel, oral direct thrombin inhibitor, ximelagatran, compared with standard therapy for the treatment of acute deep vein thrombosis [abstr]. Thromb Haemos 2001; 86:(1).

17

Orally Active Heparin

Graham F. Pineo and Russell D. Hull
University of Calgary, Calgary, Alberta, Canada

Victor J. Marder
*David Geffen School of Medicine at UCLA and Los Angeles Orthopedic Hospital,
Los Angeles, Los Angeles, California, U.S.A.*

SUMMARY

The heparins, unfractionated heparin (UFH) and low-molecular-weight heparins (LMWH) have been used extensively in the prevention and treatment of both venous and arterial thromboembolic disorders. At present, these agents must be given by the parenteral route either subcutaneously or intravenously. The increasing use of the heparins and, in particular, LMWH in the out-of-hospital setting has stimulated interest in the development of orally absorbable antithrombotic agents, and this has renewed interest in the development of orally active heparin.

Over the years many attempts have been made to demonstrate that UFH delivered by the oral route can be absorbed in adequate quantities to produce an antithrombotic affect. Indeed although there is little effect on the plasma-activated partial thromboplastin time (APTT) or anti Xa levels, UFH or LMWH delivered by the oral route has been demonstrated to have an antithrombotic effect on thrombosis models in animals. More recently the development of simple organic compounds that when attached to either heparin or low-molecular-weight heparin increases their absorption through the gastrointestinal tract has created new interest in this approach to antithrombotic therapy. Following completion of the various phase I studies a phase II clinical trial was carried out in patients undergoing total hip replacement using two dosage regimens of oral heparin attached to sodium N-(8-(2-hydroxybenzoyl) amino) caprylate (SNAC) compared with subcutaneous UFH. This study indicated that the oral heparins were both effective and safe in this setting. A phase III multicenter international clinical trial is currently underway comparing the use of two dosage regimens of SNAC heparin for 30 days with LMWH (enoxaparin) for 10 days, followed by an oral placebo for 30 days. The main efficacy endpoint for this study is deep venous thrombosis (DVT) demonstrated by ascending bilateral venography and symptomatic venous thromboembolism confirmed by objective tests. If this phase III study proves that oral SNAC heparin is effective and safe in this indication, further studies are planned with both oral UFH and LMWH in similar settings.

I. INTRODUCTION

Unfractionated heparin is one of the most widely used pharmacological agents in hospital medicine. Administered by subcutaneous injection two to three times daily, UFH is widely used for the prevention of venous thromboembolism (VTE) (deep-vein thrombosis or pulmonary embolism) [1]. As a continuous intravenous infusion, UFH has been the agent of choice for the initial treatment of VTE; acute coronary syndromes including myocardial infarction, thrombotic stroke, and in cardiovascular surgery, using cardiopulmonary bypass and in hemodialysis [1]. The development of LMWH has simplified the regimens for the prevention and treatment of thrombotic disorders, because these agents can be administered by subcutaneous injection once or twice daily without laboratory monitoring. Thus, the LMWHs are now extensively used subcutaneously for the initial treatment of VTE both in the hospital and in the outpatient setting, and they are equivalent to UFH by intravenous infusion in the management of acute coronary syndromes [2]. In addition to their antithrombotic actions, UFH and LMWH have anti-inflammatory and antiproliferative effects that have been applied in asthma and inflammatory bowel disease, interstitial cystitis, cancer, and viral infections, including human (HIV) [3], and even in diverse conditions such as hypertension and fibromyalgia.

The increasing use of the heparins (UFH and LMWH) in the outpatient setting has stimulated interest in the development of orally absorbable antithrombotic products [4], primarily the inhibitors of thrombin or factor Xa and the heparins. For example, such agents could be of practical advantage for extended (30-day) prophylaxis following orthopedic surgery [5], for the prevention or treatment of VTE in pregnancy [6], and in patients who are refractory to coumarin therapy or for whom oral anticoagulants are not adequately controlled [2].

II. ORALLY ACTIVE HEPARIN AND LMWH WITHOUT MODIFICATIONS

Heparin is not absorbed through the gastrointestinal tract or the lower or upper respiratory system in amounts adequate to have any therapeutic effect, despite claims [7,8] for gastro-intestinal or sublingual absorption of commercial heparin or synthetic heparinoids [9]. Specifically, there has been little or no effect on tests such as the APTT or the antifactor Xa assay.

Over a number of years, Jaques, Hiebert, and their colleagues have demonstrated that UFH and more recently LMWH are indeed absorbed through the gastrointestinal tract in amounts adequate to have an antithrombotic effect on experimentally induced venous thrombosis [10–13]. Their experiments demonstrated that UFH is adequately absorbed through the stomach of animals, including mice, rats, rabbits, and pigs, but with little effect on coagulation tests, such as the APTT, Xa assay, or tissue factor pathway inhibitor (TFPI). However, with a variety of experimental approaches they have demonstrated that UFH is rapidly incorporated on endothelial cells in both the venous and arterial circulation and in a wide variety of organs, so that the ratio of UFH on endothelial cells compared with plasma is of the order of 1000:1 [11,13]. By following urinary excretion over 2–3 days, they have been able to account for excretion of much of the absorbed UFH in an unchanged form. In formalin-induced venous thrombosis in the rat jugular vein, they have demonstrated that various doses of UFH, ranging from 3.25 to 60 mg/kg administered through the stomach, were effective in a dose-dependent fashion in decreasing thrombosis when compared with a saline control [14]. These effects were seen with very little evidence of anticoagulant activity being measured by the APTT in the plasma [14]. More recently attention has been directed to the gastrointestinal absorption of LMWH in both animals and human volunteers. Earlier studies demonstrated that UFH administered either through an endobronchial tube or through a nebulizer had a beneficial effect in patients with chronic obstructive pulmonary disease (COPD), asthma, and VTE [15], but these studies were not definitive and required large amounts of heparin to affect the PTT even slightly.

III. ABSORPTION OF MODIFIED UFH AND LMWH BY THE GASTROINTESTINAL TRACT

Over the years a number of attempts have been made to improve the absorption of oral UFH through the use of adjuvants, heparin–diamine complexes, surfactants, and by producing heparin fractions of different molecular sizes [16–21]. Most of the early successes were achieved with surfactants or diamine salts of LMWH and changes could be observed in the APTT and lipoprotein lipase activity in the plasma of the experimental animals. However, none of these approaches to enhancing the oral absorption of UFH or LMWH was taken to the level of clinical trials.

IV. ORAL ABSORPTION OF HEPARIN-SNAC

UFH in combination with sodium N-[8-(2-hydroxybenzoyl)amino] caprylate (SNAC); in a 25% v/v aqueous propylene glycol solution, is absorbed through the gastrointestinal tract in amounts adequate for therapeutic purposes [22–25]. In a randomized double-blind control study in human volunteers, a series of studies was performed to demonstrate that different doses of SNAC heparin delivered by the oral route could increase the APTT antifactor Xa and antithrombin levels as well as TFPI in the plasma, whereas oral heparin alone or SNAC alone had no effect. In one of the studies aimed to taste-mask the SNAC heparin solution, tolerability of the agent as well as plasma anticoagulant changes were measured. The taste-masked preparation was well tolerated with emesis occurring only with higher doses of SNAC. As shown in Figure 1 the antifactor Xa levels and the APPT increased progressively with increasing doses of SNAC heparin. It was concluded from these studies that it was feasible to deliver anticoagulant doses of heparin when attached to SNAC. In phase I studies in human volunteers, various doses of UFH and SNAC were administered either by gastric lavage or by oral solution [26] resulting in significant elevations of the PTT, antifactor IIa, and antifactor Xa activities, and TFPI levels. This study demonstrated that oral delivery of UFH in humans can be achieved, at dosages that induce antithrombotic effects that should be effective for the prevention and treatment of thrombosis.

In the model of jugular vein thrombosis in rats [27], oral heparin–SNAC has been shown to be as equally effective as subcutaneous LMWH. Animals were assigned to one of six treatment groups for 7 days, specifically:

1. Untreated control
2. Subcutaneous UFH 300 U/kg subcutaneously t.i.d.
3. SNAC alone 300 mg/kg orally t.i.d.
4. Oral UFH 30 mg/kg orally t.i.d.
5. LMWH 5 mg/kg subcutaneously daily
6. oral UFH 30 mg/kg plus SNAC 300 mg/kg orally t.i.d. (oral heparin–SNAC)

The PTT and antifactor Xa levels were measured in plasma and after treatment, the involved vein was reexplored and the intraluminal thrombus was extracted and weighed. The incidence and weight of residual thrombus was significantly decreased in the heparin–SNAC and the LMWH groups compared with controls ($P < 0.001$) (Fig. 2). Also, the APTT values and the antifactor Xa levels were elevated at 15 min and remained significantly elevated at 4 h in the

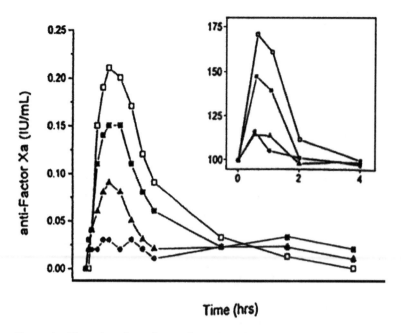

Figure 1 Mean dose-dependent prolongation of antifactor Xa activity and APTT as percent at baseline (inset) in response to taste-masked syrup containing SNAC 2.5 g and rising doses of heparin ingested per os. ● indicates 30,000 IU heparin; ▲, 60,000 IU heparin; ■, 90,000 IU heparin; and □, 150,000 IU heparin. From Ref. 26.

heparin–SNAC group as compared with SNAC alone or oral UFH alone. Figure 3 demonstrates the anti-Xa level achieved with time using oral SNAC–heparin compared with oral heparin alone or oral SNAC alone. This study indicated that oral heparin–SNAC is as effective as subcutaneous LMWH in the resolution of experimental venous thrombosis.

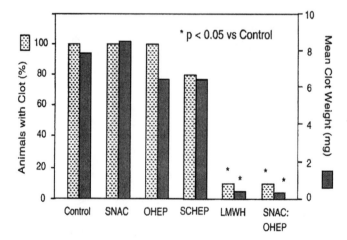

Figure 2 Administration of combination oral heparin (OHEP) and SNAC significantly reduced residual DVT and mean clot weight compared with controls: SNAC only, OHEP only, SCCCc heparin (SCHEP) only. Combination of OHEP and SNAC was as effective as LMWH. From Ref. 26.

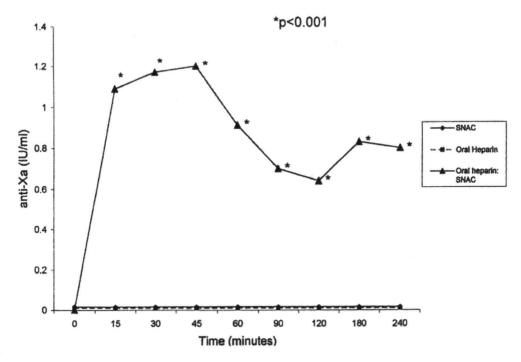

Figure 3 Administration of combination (oral heparin) OHEP and SNAC significantly increased anti-Xa levels, whereas SNAC alone or OHEP alone caused no significant change in anti-Xa levels. From Ref. 27.

In a phase II clinical trial, patients undergoing total hip replacement were randomized to receive either oral heparin–SNAC (1.5 g SNAC/60,000 U UFH or 2.25 g SNAC/90,000 U UFH), or 5000 U UFH subcutaneously every 8 h [28]. Patients received study medication for 5 days and then were observed for 35 days following surgery. Efficacy assessment was based on a 5-day bilateral full-leg venous ultrasound and patients were followed for symptomatic VTE events for 35 days. In the intention-to-treat efficacy assessment in the 123 patients, there were 6 confirmed VTE: 1 patient receiving low-dose heparin–SNAC had a proximal DVT, 3 patients receiving high-dose heparin–SNAC had a proximal DVT, and 2 patients taking subcutaneous UFH had a PE or proximal DVT. There were no deaths, two major bleeding events in the high-dose heparin–SNAC group, and minor bleeding events in 6 patients, 3 receiving low-dose heparin–SNAC, and 3 receiving subcutaneous UFH. No patients developed thrombocytopenia of less than 100×10^9/L.

A phase III multicenter clinical trial is currently underway in Canada, the United States, the United Kingdom, Australia, Poland, Czech Republic, Hungary, Spain, Denmark, and Russia to compare the efficacy and safety of two doses of heparin–SNAC with LMWH in patients undergoing total hip replacement surgery. The objectives of the study are to show superiority of either of the 30-day heparin–SNAC regimens over that of a 10-day subcutaneous LMWH regimen for the prevention of DVT, and to compare the safety of the two doses of oral heparin–SNAC with subcutaneous LMWH. Patients meeting the inclusion criteria who have signed informed consent are randomized to receive heparin–SNAC at either of the two dosages tested in the phase II trial described in the foregoing for 27–30 days beginning 4–6 h after surgery, or LMWH (enoxaparin sodium) 30 mg subcutaneously every 12 h for 10 days, beginning 12–24 h after surgery. In this double-blind, double-dummy study, the main efficacy assessment will be by bilateral ascending venography on day 27–30, but patients who experience symptomatic VTE will be investigated using objective tests. The primary safety endpoints are major and minor bleeding, wound hematoma, and thrombocytopenia. A total of 2300 patients will be studied in 120 centers.

Further studies are planned with capsule forms of oral heparin and oral LMWH.

V. CONCLUSIONS

Although UFH has been in use for several decades, early attempts to administer either UFH or LMWH by the oral route have been discouraging mainly because there was little alteration in the coagulation tests of either experimental animals or human volunteers. Subsequent studies showed that UFH and LMWH indeed can be absorbed through the stomach in sufficient amounts to achieve antithrombotic effects in animal models of venous thrombosis even though there was little effect on the plasma coagulation tests. More recently, studies have shown that the addition of a carrier (SNAC) can facilitate the absorption of UFH through the gastrointestinal tract in doses adequate for both prevention and treatment of human venous thromboembolic disorders. Initial studies have been carried out with the liquid heparin–SNAC compounds, but the technology is also available for the production of solid preparations of UFH and LMWH, permitting their use in capsules or tablets. If clinical trials are successful in demonstrating the efficacy and safety of these compounds, they will provide new impetus for the use of oral agents in a wide variety of clinical situations.

REFERENCES

1. Hirsh J, Warkentin TE, Raschke R, et al. Heparin and low-molecular-weight heparin: mechanisms of action, pharmacokinetics, dosing considerations, monitoring, efficacy, and safety. Chest 1998; 114:489S–510S.
2. Weitz JL. Low-molecular-weight heparins. N Engl J Med 1997; 337:688–698.
3. Lane DA, Adams L. Non-anti-coagulant uses of heparin. N Engl J Med 1993; 329:129–130.
4. Heit JA, Colwell CW, Francis CW, et al. Comparison of the oral direct thrombin inhibitor H 376/95 with enoxaparin as prophylaxis against venous thromboembolism after total knee replacement: a phase II dose-finding study. Arch Intern Med 2001; 161:2215–2221.
5. Hull RD, Pineo GF, Francis CW, et al. Low-molecular-weight heparin prophylaxis using dalteparin extended out-of-hospital vs in-hospital warfarin/out-of-hospital placebo in hip arthroplasty patients. Arch Intern Med 2000; 160:2208–2215.
6. Ginsberg JS, Hirsh J. Use of antithrombotic agents during pregnancy. Chest 1998; 114:524S–532S.
7. Litwins J, Vorzimer JJ, Sussman LN, Applewieg N, Etess D. Sublingual administration of heparin. Proc Soc Exp Biol Med 1951; 77:325–326.
8. Loomis TA. Absorption of heparin from the intestine. Proc Soc Exp Biol Med 1959; 101:447–449.
9. Windsor E, Freeman L. An investigation of routes of administration of heparin other than injection. Am J Med 1964; 37:408–416.
10. Sue TK, Jaques LB, Yuen E. Effects of acidity, cations and alcoholic fractionation of absorption of heparin from gastrointestinal tract. Can J Physiol Pharmacol 1976; 54:613–617.
11. Hiebert LM, Jaques LB. The observation of heparin on endothelium after injection. Thromb Res 1976; 8:195–204.
12. Jaques LB, Wice SM, Hiebert LM. Determination of absolute amounts of heparin and of dextran sulfate in plasma in microgram quantities. J Lab Clin Med 1990; 115:422–432.
13. Jaques LB, Hiebert LM, Wice SM. Evidence from endothelium of gastric absorption of heparin and of dextran sulfates 8000. J Lab Clin Med 1991; 117:122–130.

14. Hiebert LM, Wice SM, Jaques LB. Antithrombotic activity of oral unfractionated heparin. J Cardiovasc Pharmacol 1996; 28:26–29.

15. Bick RL, Ross ES. Clinical use of intrapulmonary heparin. Semin Thromb Haemost 1985; 11:213–217.

16. Tidball CS, Lipman RI. Enhancement of jejunal absorption of heparinoid sodium ethylenediaminetetraacetate in the dog. Proc Soc Exp Biol Med 1962; 111:713–715.

17. Guarani S, Ferrari W. Olive oil-provoked, bile-dependent absorption of heparin from the gastrointestinal tract in rats. Pharm Res Commun 1985; 17:685–694.

18. Engel RH, Rigg GJ. Intestinal absorption of heparin facilitated by sulphate or sulfonated surfactant. Proc Soc Exp Bio Med 1969; 13:706–710.

19. Doutremepuich C, Masse, Oca C, et al. Oral administration of low molecular weight heparin fractions in rabbits. Pathol Biol 1984; 32:45–48.

20. Lasker SE. Low molecular weight heparin-like preparations with oral activity. Semin Thromb Hemost 1985; 2:37–39.

21. Andriuoli G, Caramazza I, Galimberti G, et al. Intraduodenal absorption in the rabbit of a novel heparin solution. Haemostasis 1992; 22:113–116.

22. Leone–Bay A, Santiago N, Achan D, et al. *N*-Acylated α-amino acids as novel oral delivery agents for proteins. J Med Chem 1995; 38:4263–4269.

23. Leone–Bay A, Ho KK, Agarwal R, et al. 4-[4-(2-Hydroxybenzoyl) amino]phenylbutyric acid as a novel delivery agent for recombinant human growth hormone. J Med Chem 1996; 39:2571–2576.

24. Brayden D, Creed E, O'Connell A, Leipold H, Agarwal R, Leone–Bay A. Heparin absorption across the intestine: effects of sodium *N*-(8-(2-hydroxybenzoyl)amino)caprylate in rat in situ intestinal installations and in caco-2 monolayers. Pharma Res 1997; 14:1772–1779.

25. Rivera T, Leone–Bay A, Paton D, Leipold H, Baughman R. Oral delivery of heparin in combination with sodium *N*-(8-(2-hydroxybenzoyl)amino)caprylate: pharmacology considerations. Pharm Res 1997; 14:1830–1834.

26. Baughman RA, Kapoor SC, Agarwal RK, Kisicki J, Catella–Lawson F, FitzGerald GA. Oral delivery of anticoagulant doses of heparin: a randomized, double blind, controlled study in humans. Circulation 1998; 98:1610–1615.

27. Gonze MD, Salartash K, Sternbergh WC, Baughman RA, Leone–Bay A, Money SR. Orally administered unfractionated heparin with carrier agent is therapeutic for deep venous thrombosis. Circulation 2000; 101:2658–2661.

28. Berkowitz SD, Kosutic G, Marder VJ, Kanarek BB, Gaughman RA. Heparin administered orally via a novel carrier system (SNAC) is comparable to subcutaneous heparin when used to prevent venous thromboembolic events following elective total hip arthroplasty (THA) [abstr]. Thromb Haemost 1999; Aug (S):492.

18

Tissue Factor Pathway Inhibitor: Potential Implications in the Treatment of Cardiovascular Disorders

Debra A. Hoppensteadt and Jawed Fareed
Loyola University Medical Center, Maywood, Illinois, U.S.A.

Brigitte Kaiser
Friedrich Schiller University of Jena, Erfurt, Germany

SUMMARY

The protease inhibitor, tissue factor pathway inhibitor (TFPI), is an endogenous Kunitz-type inhibitor of the tissue factor (TF)-mediated coagulation pathway that plays an important role in hemostasis. TFPI exerts its action by first binding to factor Xa (FXa) and forming a TFPI–FXa complex, which then, in a second step, binds and effectively inhibits the tissue factor (TF)–factor VIIa (FVIIa) complex. Both full-length TFPI and chemically modified forms (e.g., truncated, glycosylated, or phosphorylated TFPI variants) exert various pharmacological effects. The anticoagulant and antiplatelet actions of TFPI, its potency in inhibiting thrombin and factor Xa generation, as well as its antithrombotic effect shown in different animal models of venous and arterial thrombosis make this inhibitor a promising agent that could be potentially useful for several clinical indications. The inhibitory action of TFPI is accelerated by both heparins and other glycosaminoglycans that are capable of releasing TFPI from the vascular endothelium, which contributes to the antithrombotic effectiveness of these drugs. The clinical relevance of TFPI continues to be explored. From the beneficial actions in animal studies and on the results obtained in the first clinical investigations, TFPI is expected to be effective in the treatment of various diseases, such as disseminated intravascular coagulation (DIC), sepsis, coronary syndromes, stroke, and acute respiratory distress syndrome (ARDS). Further clinical trials designed to clarify the role of TFPI and especially its potential usefulness as a prophylactic or therapeutic agent are ongoing.

I. INTRODUCTION

Blood coagulation and its regulation serve to maintain a balance in the clotting process as well as the integrity of the vascular system to prevent both excessive blood loss after vessel injury and the formation of intravascular thrombi after uncontrolled activation of clotting. In a cascade-like series of events, protease zymogens are converted into their active forms, which finally results in the generation of thrombin and the formation of a fibrin clot. The clotting process can be initiated by the contact system, also known as the intrinsic activation pathway, and by the tissue factor pathway, also called extrinsic activation pathway [1,2]. Tissue Factor triggers blood clotting by the binding of small amounts of available factor VIIa (FVIIa) in blood, and the TF–FVIIa complex then activates plasma factor VII to FVIIa [3,4]. The initial quantities of TF–FVIIa can also generate small amounts of factor Xa (FXa), which could then back-activate the TF-bound FVII [5,6]. In normal hemostasis the TF–FVIIa complex generates sufficient amounts of FXa, which then provides enough thrombin to induce the local aggregation of platelets, as well as the activation of the important cofactors V and VIII, thereby leading to a positive feedback with an enhancement of the generation of thrombin.

An enhanced TF expression may be important in the pathogenesis of thrombotic and vascular disorders such as disseminated intravascular coagulation or sepsis [7,8]. Tissue Factor accumulates in human atherosclerotic plaques and plays a major role in the plaque thrombogenicity. It is also readily induced in the vessel wall after acute arterial injury (e.g., by balloon angioplasty) and it accumulates in the resulting neointima [9–11].

The coagulation process is controlled by several endogenous protease inhibitors, such as antithrombin III (AT), heparin cofactor II (HC II), and protein C [12–14]. Unlike other activated coagulation proteases FVIIa is not inactivated by a direct inhibitor (i.e., it cannot be neutralized effectively unless it is bound to TF).

The only physiologically significant inhibitor of FVIIa is tissue factor pathway inhibitor (TFPI) (Fig. 1), a Kunitz-type protease inhibitor that was isolated and purified within the last

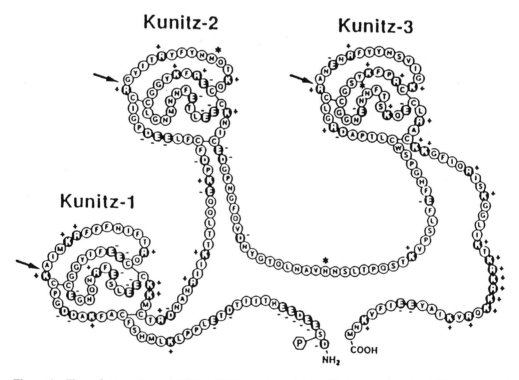

Figure 1   Tissue factor pathway inhibitor (TFPI) consists of three Kunitz-type domains. TFPI consists of 276-amino acid residues (32 kD) with 18 cysteine and 3 N-linked gylcosylation sites.

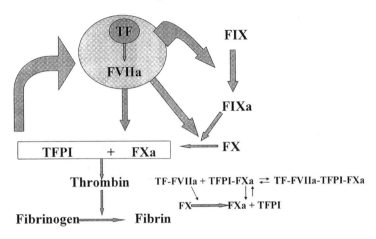

Figure 2 Activation and inhibition of the tissue factor pathway of coagulation and mechanism of action of TFPI.

several years and since then has attracted increasing attention. The properties of TFPI and its mechanism of action have led to a revised hypothesis of blood coagulation [15–17]. TFPI inhibits both FXa and the TF–FVIIa complex (Fig. 2). With the generation of FXa, the inhibitory effect of TFPI becomes apparent and prevents further production of factors Xa and IXa by TF–FVIIa. Further generation of FXa must occur through the alternative pathway involving FVIIIa and FIXa. Additional FIXa may be produced by FXIa to supplement that which is generated by TF–FVIIa, but is limited owing to the presence of TFPI. Because of the inhibition by TFPI, FXa produced by TF–FVIIa is insufficient to sustain hemostasis and must be amplified through the action of factors IXa, VIIIa, and XIa for adequate hemostasis.

II. CHEMISTRY AND MECHANISM OF ACTION

The presence of an endogenous inhibitor of tissue factor-mediated coagulation was initially demonstrated some 40 years ago. However, within the past 10 years there has been a renewed interest in this anticoagulant mechanism, leading to experimental and clinical investigations of TFPI after its purification and biochemical characterization [18,19]. Tissue factor pathway inhibitor (TFPI), previously also called lipoprotein-associated coagulation inhibitor (LACI) or extrinsic pathway inhibitor (EPI), consists, after removal of a 28-residue signal peptide, of 276-amino acid residues with 18 cysteine residues and 3 N-linked glycosylation sites. It contains an acidic N-terminal region followed by three tandemly repeated Kunitz-type serine protease inhibitory domains and a basic C-terminal region. Posttranslational modifications in the TFPI molecule include partial phosphorylation of serine-2 as well as N-linked glycosylation [18–21]. TFPI shows the typical characteristics of Kunitz-type inhibitors, such as specifically spaced cysteine residues and intramolecular disulfide bridges, which are responsible for their functional stability. Kunitz-type protease inhibitors act by a standard mechanism, producing slow, tight-binding, and competitive and reversible inhibition [18].

TFPI exerts its inhibitory action on serine proteases by a unique mechanism [22–29]. It produces a factor Xa-dependent feedback inhibition of the TF–FVIIa catalytic complex through the formation of a final, quaternary inhibitory complex consisting of TFPI–FXa–TF–FVIIa. In the first step TFPI binds and directly inhibits factor Xa via the second Kunitz-domain by hydrophobic interactions [30]. In the second step, the TFPI–FXa complex binds and inhibits FVIIa in the TF–FVIIa complex via the first Kunitz domain. Whereas Kunitz domains 1 and 2 are essential for the action of TFPI in the coagulation system, the third Kunitz domain is apparently without detectable inhibitory function [31]. However, in addition to the direct interactions between proteases and the Kunitz domains, other regions of the TFPI molecule might also be involved in its function. Secondary-site interactions are expected to enhance the inhibition of FXa [31]. Posttranslational modifications of the TFPI molecule, such as glycosylation or phosphorylation, do not seem to play a major role in its interaction with FXa; however, truncation of TFPI does affect the inhibition kinetics [23]. Full-length TFPI is a more potent inhibitor of TF–FVIIa-catalyzed activation of factor X than the C-terminally truncated TFPI that has a much lower rate constant for TFPI–FXa complex formation compared with full-length TFPI [24–26]. The C-terminus of TFPI was demonstrated to be essential for its anticoagulant activity as well as for its interaction with lipoproteins [32,33]. The degradation of this part of the molecule may result in a loss of anticoagulant potency, although it is not known whether a C-terminal fragmentation of TFPI has any physiological relevance. The first domain of TFPI also inhibits plasmin and cathepsin G, and the second domain is mainly responsible for inhibition of trypsin and chymotrypsin [31]. Another Kunitz-type serine protease inhibitor is described as TFPI-2 or placental protein 5. TFPI-2 is a potent inhibitor of trypsin, plasmin, kallikrein, and factor IXa, as well as the TF–FVIIa complex, but its function in vivo remains unclear.

III. ENDOGENOUS DISTRIBUTION OF TFPI

The TFPI mRNA has been found in a variety of cells, such as megakaryocytes, endothelial cells, and monocytes/macrophages [34,35]. The principal site of TFPI synthesis is the endothelium, which produces most of the endogenous TFPI. Endothelial-bound, heparin-releasable TFPI is the full-length protein. Thus, it has a greater anticoagulant activity than circulating TFPI, which is truncated. The average plasma concentration of TFPI in normal individuals is approximately 100 ng/mL (range: 54–142 ng/mL) corresponding to a level of about 2.5 nM [36]. In human plasma TFPI exists in several forms, and most of the circulating TFPI is associated with lipoproteins. Approximately 50% of TFPI is bound to low-density lipoproteins (LDL) and very low-density lipoproteins (VLDL): 40–45% is bound to high-density lipoproteins (HDL) and 5–10% exists in a free, non-lipoprotein-associated form [35,36]. Whereas TFPI purified from tissue cultures or released from the vasculature by heparin has a molecular weight of approximately 43 kDa, TFPI present in plasma exists in multiple molecular forms that may reflect various degrees of C-terminal truncation [37]. TFPI associated with LDL is predominantly a 34-kDa form; VLDL-associated TFPI is a mixture of 34-and 41-kDa forms, and HDL-associated TFPI is predominantly a 41-kDa form [38]. HDL-associated TFPI is covalently bound by a mixed disulfide linkage to apolipoprotein AII. It is still uncertain whether lipoprotein-associated TFPI is full-length or variably C-terminally truncated [36,37]. However, in vitro studies have demonstrated that the C-terminus of TFPI is essential for its interaction with lipoproteins [33].

Approximately 3–8% (8 ng/mL) of TFPI activity in plasma is located in the alpha-granules of platelets. TFPI is released from platelets upon their stimulation by thrombin or the calcium ionophore A-23187 [39]. TFPI is released as a stable, soluble protein from the platelet and is not associated with platelet membrane or shed vesicles [39].

Another source of TFPI is heparin-releasable TFPI. Plasma levels increase three to five fold after the infusion of heparin [40,41]. Ex vivo addition of heparin does not change the plasma TFPI level; therefore, the release of TFPI must come from intra- or extracellular stores. In cell cultures, TFPI is released from endothelial cells; it is presumed to be bound in the intima to other glycosaminoglycans on the endothelial cell surface. Heparin-releasable TFPI is structurally different from lipoprotein-associated TFPI [39].

IV. INTERACTION WITH HEPARIN AND HEPARIN DERIVATIVES

Anticoagulant and antithrombotic actions of heparin and LMWHs were considered to be mainly related to their ability to catalyze the reactions between endogenous inhibitors, such as antithrombin III (AT III) and heparin cofactor II (HC II), with serine proteases, especially thrombin and FXa; however, in addition to AT III, the heparin-dependent inactivation of FXa also requires TFPI [40]. TFPI is synthesized in vascular endothelium, and most of the intravascular pool of TFPI seems to be associated with glycosaminoglycans on vascular endothelial cells [40]. The endothelium-associated TFPI is releasable by heparin [41–44], and it is assumed that the release of TFPI from intravascular pools, as well as its direct interaction with heparin and heparin derivatives, significantly contributes to the anticoagulant and anti-thrombotic effectiveness of these drugs in vivo [45–48]. The mechanism underlying the heparin-induced release phenomenon is unknown, but may involve the displacement of TFPI from binding sites at the endothelium. New results suggest that functionally active TFPI is not released from the cell surface, and that the effect of heparin appears to be mediated by secretion of TFPI from intracellular stores [49]. In addition, heparin markedly enhances the inhibitory activity of TFPI towards TF/FVIIa [50], and exerts synergistic or even potentiating effects on the inhibition of thrombin and factor Xa generation by TFPI at concentrations that have no effect on their own [51].

Similar to unfractionated heparin, low-molecular-weight heparins (LMWHs) also release TFPI from endothelium [41]. Chemical modifications in the heparin molecule can change the physiological and biochemical properties of the heparins, resulting in a higher affinity for endothelial cells. In particular, numerous sulfate groups in the molecule and the resulting acidity may strengthen the action of LMWHs on the vascular endothelium and their TFPI-releasing capacity because the acidic character of glycosaminoglycans is important for the binding to the highly basic C-terminal region of TFPI, a likely high-affinity–binding site for heparin [52]. This view is supported by results on the influence of a supersulfated LMWH derivative on TFPI plasma concentrations after i.v. and s.c. administration in healthy volunteers [53]. After both i.v. and s.c. injection a dose-dependent increase in both total and free TFPI plasma levels was measured (Fig. 3). Maximum levels were reached 5 min after i.v. and 30 min after s.c. administration. At the highest doses used, plasma levels remained elevated at least up to 4 h (i.v.) and 8 h (s.c.), respectively.

Unfractionated as well as LMWHs are commonly used drugs for the treatment or prophylaxis of various cardiovascular disorders and, thus, it is of great interest whether the drug regimens used have any influence on TFPI plasma concentrations in patients treated with different heparins. Plasma levels of TFPI were determined in orthopedic patients who underwent total hip replacement and received either the LMWH enoxaparin (40 mg, s.c., o.d.) or placebo. In comparison with baseline levels placebo, enoxaparin caused a 1.5–2-fold increase in functional and immunological TFPI plasma levels that remained elevated throughout the 7-day treatment period (Fig. 4) [54]. This observation suggests that TFPI is released from the endothelium in its active form, which exerts inhibitory effects on the coagulation cascade. In addition to orthopedic

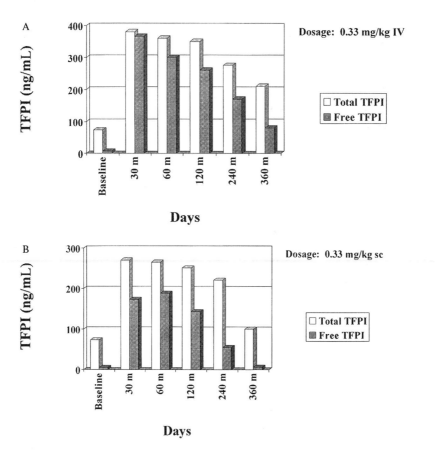

Figure 3 Plasma concentrations of free and total TFPI after (A) i.v. and (B) s.c. injection of a supersulfated low-molecular-weight heparin derivative (IK-SSH) into human volunteers (means from six determinations each).

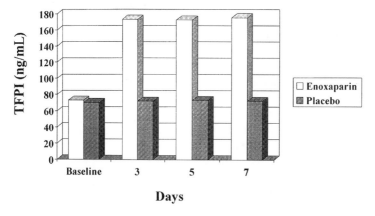

Figure 4 Immunological TFPI levels in orthopedic patients with total hip replacement after administration of enoxaparine (40 mg s.c. o.d.) or placebo.

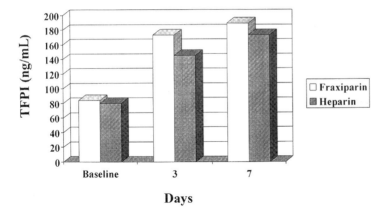

Figure 5 TFPI antigen levels after administration of unfractionated heparin (5000 IU t.i.d, $n = 100$) or fraxiparine (7500 IC AXa U/d, $n = 95$) in patients with general surgery (all results represent mean ± standard deviation).

patients, TFPI levels were also measured in patients undergoing general surgery who were treated with either UFH, calciparin (5000 IU t.i.d.), or the LMWH, fraxiparin (30 mg, s.c., o.d.). After the administration UFH and LMWH the TFPI antigen levels were increased about twofold over baseline levels 3 h after the administration of the drug on days 3 and 7 (Fig. 5). TFPI antigen was also measured during interventional cardiological procedures, such as PTCA, when a high i.v. bolus of heparin is given for the prevention of thromboembolic complications during these interventions. Changes in TFPI antigen levels after heparin in angioplasty are shown in Figure 6. After the administration of an i.v. bolus of 10,000–20,000 U of heparin, the TFPI levels increased six to eight fold above the baseline ($P < 0.001$). Approximately 2–3 h after angioplasty, the TFPI antigen levels remained elevated, indicating that large quantities of heparin-releasable TFPI were displaced from the endogenous stores.

In addition to UFH, LMWHs are now being tested as anticoagulants during PTCA. A LMWH, dalteparin was administered to patients undergoing PTCA. There was a fivefold

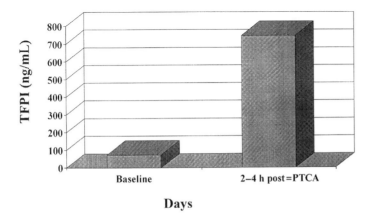

Figure 6 TFPI antigen levels after administration of UFH (10,000 to 20,000-IU i.v. bolus) in patients undergoing PTCA ($n = 30$).

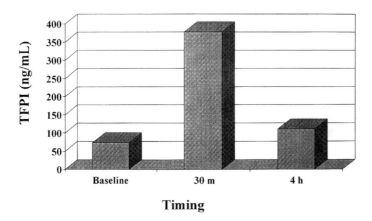

Figure 7   TFPI antigen levels in patients administered dalteparin 60 U AX/kg for anticoagulation during PTCA.

increase in the TFPI levels 30-min after the administration of 60 U AXa/kg of LMWH; as shown in Figure 7, by 4 h the TFPI levels returned to baseline levels. These results indicate that LMWHs are capable of releasing TFPI to levels similar to UFH during PTCA.

In addition to PTCA, TFPI levels were measured in patients undergoing cardiopulmonary bypass surgery (Fig. 8). TFPI antigen levels were elevated eight to tenfold from baseline 30 min after the injection of a bolus of heparin (10,000–25,000 U), and these levels remained elevated throughout bypass surgery.

The results obtained with UFH and several LMWH derivatives both in vivo and in vitro indicate that the release of TFPI from intravascular pools, as well as the direct interactions with TFPI by these drugs, may be an important factor for the mechanism and the duration of their antithrombotic action. Furthermore, TFPI seems to contribute significantly to the anticoagulant properties of the various heparins in vivo.

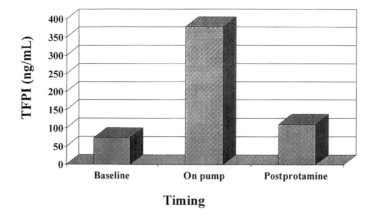

Figure 8   TFPI antigen levels in patients undergoing cardiopulmonary bypass surgery. Patients were given an intravenous bolus of unfractionated heparin (10,000–25,000 U). TFPI levels were measured at baseline, after heparin, and after surgery (postprotamine).

V. PATHOPHYSIOLOGICAL ROLE IN DISEASE STATES

Several inherited disorders that predispose to thrombosis have been identified, such as APC resistance, AT III deficiency, or deficiency of protein C or protein S [55]. However, in some patients with familial thrombophilia, the underlying defect remains unclear. Because of the major role of TF in triggering blood coagulation in normal hemostasis and the importance of TFPI as a regulator of the TF-mediated coagulation pathway, it may be assumed that a reduced level of TFPI is an important risk factor in thrombophilia; however, there are still no known clinical conditions that are related to an inherited TFPI deficiency. This may suggest that homozygous TFPI deficiency is a lethal event, a conclusion consistent with studies in mice using gene-targeting techniques. After disruption of exon 4 of the TFPI gene, which encodes Kunitz domain 1 of TFPI, 60% of mice died between embryonic days E9.5 and E11.5 with signs of yolk sac hemorrhage [56]. Animals that progress beyond E11.5 have normal organogenesis, but hemorrhage, particularly in the central nervous system and tail, seen during later gestation, none of the mice survived the neonatal period. Unregulated TF–FVIIa activity and consumptive coagulopathy accounts for the bleeding diathesis [56]. It is suggested that human TFPI-deficient embryos may suffer a similar fate and, thus, there are no thrombophilic states related to TFPI deficiency. There is, as yet only one report on low levels of TFPI in members of a family with thrombophilia [57]. Low levels of TFPI (50 and 45%), were found in two siblings exhibiting thrombotic events at an early age, whereas the parents, and especially the father, who also suffered from severe thrombosis, had normal TFPI levels. The diminished release of TFPI after heparin administration found in these patients is thought to be based on less binding of TFPI to the endothelium, compared with healthy individuals.

Various clinical studies have been performed to measure plasma concentrations of TFPI and their relevance for the pathogenesis, course, and outcome of various diseases. In samples of patients suffering from different diseases TFPI levels were normal, increased, or decreased [58–69]. Increased levels of TFPI have been observed in several illnesses. In patients with disseminated intravascular coagulation (DIC), plasma concentrations of both TF and TFPI were significantly increased compared with patients without DIC [59,60]. Furthermore, plasma levels of TF, but not of TFPI, were already increased in pre-DIC patients. During the clinical course of DIC an increase of TF antigen was followed by an increase in TFPI levels [59]. Elevated levels of TFPI were also found in DIC patients with an underlying acute nonlympho-blastic leukemia [61]. It is suggested that the release of TFPI from vascular endothelial cells reflects a DIC-related endothelial damage. TFPI might also be released from ischaemic tissues in patients with acute myocardial infarction (AMI) who showed significantly higher plasma levels of both total and free TFPI when compared with healthy volunteers and patients with pulmonary embolism or deep-vein thrombosis. TFPI levels in these AMI patients were further increased shortly after percutaneous transluminal coronary angioplasty (PTCA) and significantly reduced 24 h after PTCA [62]. Elevated TFPI levels in AMI patients could also be a sign of an up-regulated clotting system [63]; furthermore, they were closely associated with the plasma levels of LDLs [64]. A reduced TFPI activity was found in patients with ischemic stroke. TFPI activity was significantly decreased especially in the clinical subgroups of atherothrombotic and lacunar infarction, but not in cardioembolic infarction, indicating that the lower TFPI activity could be related to atherosclerotic changes in vascular cells, rather than to consumptive coagulopathy [65]. Decreased plasma levels of TFPI have also been found in patients with thrombotic thrombocytopenia purpura [66]. The adult respiratory distress syndrome (ARDS), as a complication primarily of sepsis, trauma, and shock, represents a severe pulmonary dysfunction characterized by intravascular and extravascular coagulation with fibrin deposition, an increased activity of the extrinsic coagulation pathway in the alveolar compartment of the lung, and a severe injury of the endothelium. In patients with ARDS besides a significant increase in plasma levels of von Willebrand's factor antigen there was also a significant and progressive increase of TFPI levels, indicating an increased local synthesis of TFPI in the alveolar space [67]. Other clinical studies on the relevance of increased or decreased TFPI levels included patients with chronic atherosclerotic disease treated with polyunsaturated fatty acids, which induced a small, but statistically significant, increase of TFPI plasma levels, with a down-regulation of the TF-mediated coagulation pathway [68], as well as in patients with the antiphospholipid syndrome (APS) in whom significantly elevated levels of both TF and TFPI were found, suggesting an in vivo up-regulation of TF pathway in APS patients [69].

The diagnostic significance of TFPI measurements should clearly be further elucidated. The results from the various clinical studies performed are partially contradictory, suggesting that plasma levels of TFPI do not always reflect an effective control of an increased TF–FVIIa activity and the resulting ongoing intravascular coagulation. Furthermore, it has to be taken into consideration that TFPI bound to LDLS does not inhibit TF-induced coagulation (i.e., the anticoagulant function of TFPI in human plasma is restricted to its carrier-free form [70]). In addition, no relation could be established between TFPI activity and other hemostatic parameters that indicate an activation of coagulation or fibrinolysis.

VI. ROLE OF TFPI IN CARDIOVASCULAR DISORDERS

A. Atherosclerosis and Restenosis

The most important underlying mechanism for the development of acute coronary syndromes is atherosclerotic plaque rupture. Spontaneous plaque rupture or acute interventions, such as balloon angioplasty, coronary atherectomy, or stent placement, may increase the procoagulant activity of the vessel wall and especially expose TF to circulating blood, resulting in the initiation of the clotting process, with the formation of intravascular thrombi. The effects of TF in vivo are very complex, and this membrane protein may play an important role in inflammatory processes associated with atherosclerosis and restenosis. Because TF is up-regulated after vascular injury and in atherosclerotic plaques, TFPI is expected to inhibit the development of postinjury intimal hyperplasia and thrombotic occlusion in atherosclerotic vessels.

B. Preclinical Studies

Various studies on the role of TFPI in hyperplasia of vascular smooth-muscle cells (VSMCs) have been performed using cell culture systems. In human pulmonary arteries the expression of TFPI in SMCs is up-regulated by treatment with serum or basic fibroblast growth factor (bFGF)/heparin, indicating that growth factors that can stimulate the vessel wall in vivo might locally regulate TFPI expression. The up-regulation of TFPI could be pathophysiologically important for the regulation of TF-mediated coagulation within the vessel wall; thus, for the course of hyperplasia associated with pulmonary hypertension and atherosclerosis [71]. An increased expression of TFPI after an initial expression of TF was also found in serum-stimulated cultured fibroblasts, VSMCs, and cardiac myocytes [72]. The in vitro findings suggest that TFPI not only regulates the TF-initiated clotting, but is also involved in inhibiting VSMC proliferation. Various studies have demonstrated the antiproliferative effectiveness of TFPI both in vitro and in vivo. TFPI inhibited the FVIIa–TF-induced migration of cultured VSMCs [73], the proliferation of cultured human neonatal aortic SMCs [74], as well as the growth of human umbilical vein endothelial cells [75]. Newer studies demonstrated that the antiproliferative activity of TFPI is mediated by the VLDL receptor. In addition, for the inhibition of the proliferation of bFGF-stimulated endothelial cells, that the C-terminal region of TFPI seems to be responsible because a truncated form of TFPI that contains only the first two Kunitz-type inhibitor domains is clearly ineffective [76].

In animal experiments, the effect of TFPI on the proliferation of VSMCs as well as on atherosclerotic processes was investigated. TFPI reduced angiographic restenosis and intima hyperplasia in a rabbit atherosclerotic femoral artery injury model [77]; inhibited neointima formation and stenosis in pigs after deep arterial injury of the carotid artery [78], as well as the procoagulant activity and the up-regulation of TF at injured sites [79]; and inhibited mural thrombus formation, neointima formation, and growth after repeated balloon angioplasty of the rabbit thoracic aorta [80]. Administration of TFPI attenuates arterial stenosis [81], inhibits intima hyperplasia [82], and reduces the extent of tissue ischemia and reperfusion injury [83]. Furthermore, localized delivery of TFPI intramurally at a target site within the blood vessel inhibits restenosis in recanalized vessels [84]. In a model of small autografts in the rabbit femoral artery, topically applied TFPI significantly increased the patency rates of the grafts, reduced the intimal area, as well as the percentage of stenosis, and the intima/media areas ratio [85]. Recently, published results obtained in a model of balloon-injured atherosclerotic arteries in rabbits demonstrated that an overexpression of TFPI by gene transfer markedly inhibited intimal hyperplasia without impairment of systemic hemostasis or excess bleeding [86]. In a murine model of flow cessations overexpression of TFPI by adenoviral delivery decreased vascular TF activity and inhibited neointima formation [87]. The development of atherosclerosis in mice with a homozygous apolipoprotein E (apoE) deficiency and an additional heterozygous TFPI deficiency was significantly greater than that seen in apoE knockout mice with a normal TFPI genotype, indicating that TFPI protects from atherosclerosis and is an important regulator of thrombotic events in atherosclerosis [88].

C. Studies in Human Vessels

Active TF is present in the atherosclerotic vessel wall, where it is thought to be responsible for especially acute thrombosis after plaque rupture, the major complication of primary atherosclerosis. Besides TF, TFPI is also expressed in atherosclerotic plaques [89–92]. In atherosclerotic lesions of human coronary arteries a colocalization of TF and TFPI was found in endothelial cells, macrophages, macrophage-derived foam cells, and smooth-muscle cells in intimal lesions. In type III and IV of atherosclerotic lesions the number of TF- and TFPI- positive cells is increased, accompanied by extracellular localization of TF and TFPI in the lipid core of atherosclerotic plaques [90]. In human carotid atherosclerotic plaques, biologically active TFPI was seen in endothelial cells, VSMCs, and macrophages [91]. Similar results were seen in other studies using human coronary arteries, popliteal arteries, and saphenous vein grafts. In the atherosclerotic vessels TFPI frequently colocalized with TF in endothelial cells overlying the plaque and in microvessels, as well as in the medial and neointimal SMCs, and in macrophages and T cells in areas surrounding the necrotic core [92]. TFPI was largely expressed in the normal vessel wall and enhanced in atherosclerotic vessels. It was active against the TF-dependent procoagulant activity, suggesting a significant role of the inhibitor in the regulation of TF activity. It is assumed that up-regulation of TFPI in atherosclerotic plaques may control their thrombogenicity or even prevent the complications associated with plaque rupture [92].

In the TFPI gene, three polymorphisms have recently been identified that are associated with a significant variation in plasma TFPI levels [93,94]. However, studies in patients who underwent angioplasty, with or without stent implantation, revealed that, despite significant variations in TFPI levels, there was no evidence that the polymorphism of the TFPI gene influenced the risk of angiographic restenosis after angioplasty [95].

D.   Unstable Angina and Myocardial Infarction

Several clinical studies have been performed to evaluate the significance of measuring various parameters relative to their diagnostic and prognostic value for cardiovascular disorders, especially for ischemic heart diseases such as unstable angina and acute myocardial infarction (AMI). In patients with ischemic heart diseases an excess thrombin formation was demonstrated by increased plasma concentrations of prothrombin fragment F1.2 and thrombin–antithrombin III complexes. This could be related to the elevated levels of circulating TF that was also found. In these patients plasma levels of TFPI were also increased, but not sufficiently to interrupt the TF-induced coagulation activation [96,97]. Increased plasma concentrations of both total and free TFPI measured in AMI patients may result from their release by ischemic tissues [98]. Patients with AMI show an increased procoagulant activity of monocytes that is thought to be caused by an up-regulation of TF and can be partially inhibited by surface-bound TFPI, suggesting that a direct inhibition of TF activity by a specific therapy might be particularly effective for the treatment of AMI [99]. The prognostic importance of TF and TFPI for recurrent coronary events was investigated in a long-term follow-up study over 4 years in patients after AMI [100]. There were no statistical differences in TF as well as total and free TFPI levels between patients and controls demonstrating that the TF/TFPI system is not a useful prognostic marker. By contrast, in middle-aged men without a history of coronary heart disease a significant positive correlation was found between free TFPI plasma levels and atherogenic lipids, such as total cholesterol and triglycerides, as well as factor VII and fibrinogen, which can be considered as a compensatory increase in plasma free TFPI to the occurrence of risk factors for atherothrombotic diseases in apparently healthy men [101]. A large, population study on the association between plasma levels of free and total TFPI, conventional cardiovascular risk factors, and endothelial cell markers showed that plasma levels of free TFPI correlated poorly with that of total TFPI, indicating that free and lipid-bound TFPI are regulated differently. Free TFPI strongly correlates to endothelium-derived molecules, such as thrombomodulin, von Willebrand's factor, and tissue-type plasminogen activator, whereas total TFPI is more related to conventional risk factors, such as LDL cholesterin [102].

E.   Other Cardiovascular Disorders

The endogenous, cell-associated TFPI is possibly more important for maintaining the anti-coagulant properties of the endothelium than the circulating TFPI [103]. Recombinant TFPI has been found; with only limited success, in one coronary angioplasty trial. However, the role of TFPI in the pathogenesis of acute coronary syndromes, atrial fibrillation, and heart failure is widely known. Therefore, as a mono or polytherapeutic agent, TFPI may be extremely useful. In interventional trials the role of TFPI in mediating the anticoagulant effects of heparins is well known. Therefore, pharmacological modulation or administration of TFPI may be beneficial in these patients.

VII.   SEPSIS AND DISSEMINATED INTRAVASCULAR COAGULATION

Severe sepsis is associated with the activation of various inflammatory pathways and especially with the activation of the coagulation system. Owing to endotoxin and the production of proinflammatory cytokines, TF is expressed on activated monocytes and vascular endothelial cells. TF-mediated coagulation activation can lead to microvascular thrombosis and further endothelial activation, which seems to play an important role in the development of multiple organ failure associated with severe sepsis. Given the role of TF in sepsis and DIC, it is expected that TFPI can provide a new therapeutic rationale for the treatment of sepsis. Under experimental conditions the effectiveness of TFPI in DIC and septic shock have been investigated in various animal models [104]. The results suggest that TFPI may offer benefits when used to treat severe sepsis. In various studies in humans, plasma concentrations of TF and TFPI have been determined to define the pathophysiological role of these molecules in DIC and septic shock. In patients with DIC, plasma concentrations of both TF and TFPI were significantly higher than in patients without DIC [105,106]. The increase of TF in plasma of DIC patients is followed by an increase in TFPI, which is most likely based on its release from vascular endothelium owing to endothelial cell injury [106]. In patients with DIC plasma concentrations of truncated TFPI were significantly elevated as compared with pre- and non-DIC patients. Reduced levels of the intact form of TFPI found in pre-DIC patients may suggest a hypercoagulable state in those patients with a consumption of TFPI [105,106].

In animal models of sepsis TFPI was able to completely block the coagulant response and to prevent death, as well as reduce the cytokine response. In a human model of endotoxemia, TFPI effectively and dose-dependently attenuated the endotoxin-induced coagulation activation. However, in contrast to animal experiments it did not influence leukocyte activation, chemokine release, endothelial cell activation, or the acute-phase responses. Thus, the complete prevention of coagulation activation by TFPI does not inhibit activation of inflammatory pathways during human endotoxemia [107,108]. In posttrauma patients with DIC the TF-dependent coagulation activation could not be sufficiently prevented by TFPI, which remained at normal levels. The DIC was associated with thrombotic and inflammatory responses leading to multiple organ dysfunction and a poor outcome in these patients [109].

In normal volunteers recombinant human TFPI was well tolerated without clinically significant bleeding [104]. Recently, TFPI was examined in small phase II clinical studies in patients with severe sepsis [104,110]. In the first trial, some of the patients showed an increase in the incidence of serious adverse events involving bleeding that might be caused by the relatively high doses of TFPI administered. In the two following studies lower doses of TFPI were used and then adverse events did not differ between placebo and TFPI groups [104]. A recently completed phase II study in 210 patients with sepsis showed a trend toward a relative reduction in day 28 all-cause mortality in TFPI-treated patients as compared with placebo. There was also an improvement in selected organ dysfunction scores and biochemical evidence of TFPI activity in these patients [104,110]. TFPI therapy for severe sepsis will be evaluated in a planned large, international phase III study [104].

VIII. CONCLUSIONS

Tissue Factor plays a crucial role in the pathogenesis of thrombotic, vascular, inflammatory and hemodynamic disorders. Targeting of this pathogenic mediator provides a unique therepeutic approach to the management of these disorders. The development of recombinant TFPI and its molecular variants have provided a new dimension in the management of such disorders as myocardial infraction, thrombotic stroke, microangiopathic disorders, and inflammation-associated pathogenic processes. Although the development of r-TFPI has been limited to sepsis, this polypharmacological agent and its variants will find multiple indications. Molecular manipulation of the currently available TFPI forms will provide drugs with varying degrees of pharmacokinetic and pharmacodynamic spectrums. Molecular manipulation of TFPI may also provide agents with relatively stronger affinity for endothelial or subendothelial target sites. Because TFPI is present in several forms, the identification of these forms with their differential function may lead to additional TFPI variants for specific indications. TFPI conjugates with drugs and chemicals may provide agents with a broader spectrum for the management of different diseases and desirable duration of action. During the next few years, several molecular variants of a TFPI will be developed to determine their relevant potential for different specific indications. Because of the unique nature of TFPI genomic manipulation of the vascular system will be an important consideration to enhance the endogenous release of TFPI. The TFPI gene can be readily introduced at various sites using different vectors, and it may provide an important targent to develop approaches to modulate thrombotic and vascular disorders. In addition, several oligopeptides can be mapped to mimic TFPI sites to regulate protease function.

IX. CLINICAL PERSPECTIVE

Despite the broad-spectral therapeutic nature of TFPI, this agent has found indications only in sepsis in which defined trials have been carried out. A recombinant TFPI has been administered at a dosage of $25\,\mu g/kg\,h^{-1}$ for 95 h, resulting in improved outcome in terms of surrogate markers and mortality reduction. In addition, r-TFPI has been effective in reducing abrupt closure in acute coronary syndromes, a finding that is consistent with the observation that increased TFPI levels are seen with LMWHs. Topical administration of TFPI improves capillary blood flow; thus, patients with microangiopathic disorders can benefit. This is consistent with the observation that defibrotide and other related polyelectrolytes also enhance the generation of endogenous TFPI. TFPI may be of major value in acute respiratory distress syndrome to reduce the inflammation cycle that contributes to microvascular thrombi. Recombinant-TFPI may be useful in cerebrovascular disorders, such as thrombotic and ischemic stroke. The regulatory role of TFPI in the invasiveness of glioma has been well established. In experimental animal models, r-TFPI protects vascular sites from antherosclerosis. The role of TFPI in angiogenesis is gradually emerging. Thus, r-TFPI may be of value in cancer therapy as an adjuctive drug. The anticancer effects of heparins may potentially involve the up-regulation of endogenous TFPI.

REFERENCES

1. Wachtfogel YT, Dela Cadena RA, Coleman RW. Structural biology, cellular interactions and pathophysiology of the contact system. Thromb Res 1993; 72:1–21.
2. Coleman RW, Schmaier AH. Contact system: a vascular biology modulator with anticoagulant, profibrinolytic, antiadhesive, and proinflammatory attributes. Blood 1997; 90:3819–3843.
3. Mann KG, Kalafatis M. The coagulation explosion. Cerebrovasc Dis 1995; 5:93–97.
4. Camerer E, Kolsto AB, Prydz H. Cell biology of tissue factor, the principal initiator of blood coagulation. Thromb Res 1996; 81:1–41.
5. Østerud B. Cellular interactions in tissue factor expression by blood monocytes. Blood Coag Fibrinol 1995; 6(suppl 1):S20–S25.
6. Morissey JH. Tissue factor interactions with factor VII: measurement and clinical significance of factor VIIa in plasma. Blood Coag Fibrinol 1995; 6(suppl 1):S14–S19.
7. Wada H, Wakita Y, Shiku H. Tissue factor expression in endothelial cells in health and disease. Blood Coag Fibrinol 1995; 6(suppl 1):S26–S31.
8. Francis JL, Carvalho M, Francis DA. The clinical value of tissue factor assays. Blood Coag Fibrinol 1995; 6(suppl 1):S37–S44.
9. Taubman MB, Fallon JT, Schecter AD et al. Tissue factor in the pathogenesis of atherosclerosis. Thromb Haemost 1997; 78:200–204.

10. Camerer E, Kolsto AB, Prydz H. Cell biology of tissue factor. Thromb Res 1996; 81:1–41.
11. Østerud B. Tissue factor: a complex biological role. Thromb Haemost 1997; 78:755–758.
12. Rosenberg RD, Rosenberg JS. Natural anticoagulant mechanisms. J Clin Invest 1984; 74:1–6.
13. Tollefsen DM. Insight into the mechanism of action of heparin cofactor II. Thromb Haemost 1995; 74:1209–1214.
14. Dahlback B. The protein C anticoagulant system: inherited defects as basis for venous thrombosis. Thromb Res 1995; 77:1–43.
15. Broze GJ, Jr. Tissue factor pathway inhibitor and the current concept of blood coagulation. Blood Coag Fibrinol 1995; 6(suppl 1):S7–S13.
16. Broze GJ, Jr. The role of tissue factor pathway inhibitor in a revised coagulation cascade. Semin Hematol 1992; 29:159–169.
17. Broze GJ, Jr. Tissue factor pathway inhibitor and the revised theory of coagulation. Annu Rev Med 1995; 46:103–112.
18. Broze GJ, Jr, Girard TJ, Novontny WF. Regulation of coagulation by a multivalent Kunitz-type inhibitor. Biochemistry 1990; 29:7539–7546.
19. Broze GJ, Jr. Tissue factor pathway inhibitor. Thromb Haemost 1995; 74:90–93.
20. Girard TJ, Warren LA, Novontny WF, et al. Functional significance of the Kunitz-type inhibitory domains of lipoprotein-associated coagulation inhibitor. Nature 1989; 338:518–520.
21. Girard TJ, McCourt D, Novotny WG. Endogenous phosphorylation of the lipoprotein-associated coagulation inhibitor at serine-2. Biochem J 1990; 270:621–625.
22. Broze GJ, Jr, Warren LA, Novotny WF, Higuchi DA, Girard JJ, Miletich JP. The lipoprotein-associated coagulation inhibitor that inhibits the factor VII–tissue factor complex also inhibits factor Xa: insights into its possible mechanism of action. Blood 1988; 71:335–343.
23. Huang ZF, Wun TC, Broze GJ, Jr. Kinetics of factor Xa inhibition by tissue factor pathway inhibitor. J Biol Chem 1993; 286:26950–26955.
24. Lindhout T, Franssen J, Willems G. Kinetics of the inhibition of tissue factor–factor VIIa by tissue factor pathway inhibitor. Thromb Haemost 1995; 74:910–915.
25. Lindhout T, Willems G, Blezer R, Hemker HC. Kinetics of the inhibition of human factor Xa by full-length and truncated recombinant tissue factor pathway inhibitor. Biochem J 1994; 297(pt 1):131–136.
26. Lindhout T, Salemink I, Valentin S, Willems GM. Tissue factor pathway inhibitor: regulation of its inhibitory activity by phospholipid surfaces. Haemostasis 1996; 26(suppl 4):89–97.
27. Rapaport SI. Inhibition of factor VIIa/tissue factor-induced blood coagulation: with particular emphasis upon a factor Xa-dependent inhibitory mechanism. Blood 1989; 73:359–365.
28. Warn–Cramer BJ, Rao LVM, Maki SL, Rapaport SI. Modifications of extrinsic pathway inhibitor (EPI) and factor Xa that affect their ability to interact and to inhibit factor VIIa/tissue factor: evidence for a two-step model of inhibition. Thromb Haemost 1988; 60:453–456.
29. Rapaport SI. The extrinsic pathway inhibitor: a regulator of tissue factor-dependent blood coagulation. Thromb Haemost 1991; 66:6–15.
30. Yoneda T, Komooka H, Umeyama H. A computer modeling study of the interaction between tissue factor pathway inhibitor and blood coagulation factor Xa. J Protein Chem 1997; 16:597–605.
31. Petersen LC, Bjorn SE, Olsen OH, Nordfang O, Norris F, Norris K. Inhibitory properties of separate recombinant Kunitz-type-protease inhibitor domains from tissue-factor-pathway inhibitor. Eur J Biochem 1996; 235:310–316.
32. Nordfang O, Bjorn SE, Valentin S, et al. The C-terminus of tissue factor pathway inhibitor is essential to its anticoagulant activity. Biochemistry 1991; 30:10371–10376.
33. Valentin S, Nordfang O, Bregengard C, Wildgoose P. Evidence that the C-terminus of tissue factor pathway inhibitor (TFPI) is essential for its in vitro and in vivo interaction with lipoproteins. Blood Coag Fibrinol 1993; 4:713–720.
34. Bajaj MS, Kuppuswamy MN, Saito H, Spitzer SG, Bajaj SP. Cultured normal human hepatocytes do not synthesize lipoprotein-associated coagulation inhibitor: evidence that the endothelium is the principal site of synthesis. Proc Natl Acad Sci USA 1990; 87:8869–8873.

35. Petersen LC, Valentin S, Hedner U. Regulation of the extrinsic pathway system in health and disease: The role of factor VIIa and tissue factor pathway inhibitor. Thromb Res 1995; 79:1–47.

36. Novotny WF, Girard TJ, Miletich JP, Broze GJ, Jr. Purification and characterization of lipoprotein associated coagulation inhibitor from human plasma. J Biol Chem 1989; 264:18832–18837.

37. Broze GJ, Jr, Lange GW, Duffin KL, Macphail L. Heterogeneity of plasma tissue factor pathway inhibitor. Blood Coag Fibrinol 1994; 5:551–559.

38. Glirard TJ. Tissue factor pathway inhibitor. In: Sasahara AA. Loscalzo J, eds. New Therapeutic Agents in Thrombosis and Thrombolysis. New York: Marcel Dekker, 1997; 225–260.

39. Novotny WF, Girard TG, Miletich JP, Broze GJ Jr. Platelets secrete a coagulation inhibitor functionally and antigenically similar to the lipoprotein associated coagulation inhibitor. Blood 1988; 72:2020–2025.

40. Novotny WF, Palmier M, Wun TC, Broze G, Jr, Miletich JP. Purification and properties of heparin-releasable lipoprotein-associated coagulation inhibitor. Blood 1991; 78:394–400.

41. Sandset PM, Abildgaard U, Larsen ML. Heparin induces release of extrinsic coagulation pathway inhibitor (EPI). Thromb Res 1988; 50:803–813.

42. Jesty J, Lorenz A, Rodriguez J, Wun TC. Initiation of the tissue factor pathway of coagulation in the presence of heparin: control by antithrombin III and tissue factor pathway inhibitor. Blood 1996; 87:2301–2307.

43. Hoppensteadt DA, Jeske W, Fareed J, Bermes EW, Jr. The role of tissue factor pathway inhibitor in the mediation of the antithrombotic actions of heparin and low-molecular-weight heparin. Blood Coag Fibrinol 1995; 6(suppl 1):S57–S64.

44. Hubbard AR, Weller LJ, Gray E. Measurement of tissue factor pathway inhibitor in normal and post-heparin plasma. Blood Coag Fibrinol 1994; 5:819–823.

45. Valentin S, Ostergaard P, Kristensen H, Nordfang O. Synergism between full-length TFPI and heparin: evidence for TFPI as an important factor for the antithrombotic activity of heparin. Blood Coag Fibrinol 1992; 3:221–222.

46. Wun TC. Lipoprotein-associated coagulation inhibitor (LACI) is a cofactor for heparin: synergistic anticoagulant action between LACI and sulfated polysaccharides. Blood 1992; 79:430–438.

47. Sandset PM. Tissue factor pathway inhibitor (TFPI)—an update. Haemostasis 1996; 26(suppl 4): 154–165.

48. Lindahl AK, Abildgaard U, Staalesen R. The anticoagulant effect in heparinized blood and plasma resulting from interactions with extrinsic pathway inhibitor. Thromb Res 1991; 64:155–168.

49. Tiemann C, Brinkman T, Kleesiek K. Detection of the three Kunitz-type single domains of membrane-bound tissue factor pathway inhibitor (TFPI) by flow cytometry. Eur J Clin Chem Clin Biochem 1997; 35:855–860.

50. Hamamoto T, Kisiel W. The effect of heparin on the regulation of factor VIIa–tissue factor activity by tissue factor pathway inhibitor. Blood Coag Fibrinol 1996; 7:470–476.

51. Kaiser B, Hoppensteadt DA, Jeske W, Wun TC, Fareed J. Inhibitory effects of TFPI on thrombin and factor Xa generation in vitro—modulatory action of glycosaminoglycans. Thromb Res 1994; 75:609–616.

52. Iversen N, Sandset PM, Abildgaard U, Torjesen PA. Binding of tissue factor pathway inhibitor to cultured endothelial cells—influence of glycosaminoglycans. Thromb Res 1996; 84:267–278.

53. Kaiser B, Glusa E, Hoppensteadt DA, Breddin HK, Amiral J, Fareed J. A supersulfated low molecular weight heparin (IK-SSH) increases plasma levels of free and total TFPI after i.v. and s.c. administration in man. Blood Coag Fibrinol (submitted)

54. Hoppensteadt DA. Tissue factor pathway inhibitor as a modulator of post surgical thrombogenesis. Experimental and clinical studies. PhD dissertation, University of London, 1996.

55. Bick RL, Kaplan H. Syndromes of thrombosis and hypercoagulability: congenital and acquired thrombophilias. J Appl Thromb Hemost 1998; 4:25–50.

56. Huang ZF, Higuchi D, Lasky N, Broze GJ, Jr. Tissue factor pathway inhibitor gene disruption produces intrauterine lethality in mice. Blood 1997; 90:944–951.

57. Llobet D, Falkon L, Mateo J, et al. Low levels of tissue factor pathway inhibitor (TFPI) in two out of three members of a family with thrombophilia. Thromb Res 1995; 80:413–418.

58. Novontny WF, Brown SG, Miletich JP, Rader DJ, Broze GJ, Jr. Plasma antigen levels of the lipoprotein-associated coagulation inhibitor in patient samples. Blood 1991; 78:387–393.

59. Shimura M, Wada H, Wakita Y, et al. Plasma tissue factor and tissue factor pathway inhibitor levels in patients with disseminated intravascular coagulation. Am J Hematol 1997; 55:169–174.

60. Takahashi H, Sato N, Shibata A. Plasma tissue factor pathway inhibitor in disseminated intravascular coagulation: comparison of its behavior with plasma tissue factor. Thromb Res 1995; 80:339–348.

61. Velasco F, Lopez–Pedrefa C, Borrell M, Fontcuberta J, Torres A. Elevated levels of tissue factor pathway inhibitor in acute non-lymphoblastic leukemia patients with disseminated intravascular coagulation. Blood Coag Fibrinol 1997; 8:70–72.

62. Kamikura Y, Wada H, Yamada A, et al. Increased tissue factor pathway inhibitor in patients with acute myocardial infarction. Am J Hematol 1997; 55:183–187.

63. Lorena M, Perolini S, Casazza F, Milani M, Cimminiello C. Fluvastatin and tissue factor pathway inhibitor in type IIA and IIB hyperlipidemia and in acute myocardial infarction. Thromb Res 1997; 87:397–403.

64. Moore, Hamsten A, Karpe F, Bavenholm P, Blomback M, Silveira A. Relationship of tissue factor pathway inhibitor activity to plasma lipoproteins and myocardial infarction at a young age. Thromb Haemost 1994; 71:707–712.

65. Abumiya T, Yamaguchi T, Terasaki T, Kokawa T, Kario K, Kato H. Decreased plasma tissue factor pathway inhibitor activity in ischemic stroke patients. Thromb Haemost 1995; 74:1050–1054.

66. Kobayshi M, Wada H, Wakita Y, et al. Decreased plasma tissue factor pathway inhibitor levels in patients with thrombotic thrombocytopenic purpura. Thromb Haemost 1995; 73:10–14.

67. Sabharwal AK, Bajaj SP, Ameri A, et al. Tissue factor pathway inhibitor and von Willebrand factor antigen levels in adult respiratory distress syndrome and in a primate model of sepsis. Am J Respir Crit Care Med 1995; 151:758–767.

68. Berettini M, Parise P, Ricotta S, Iorio A, Peirone C, Nenci GG. Increased plasma levels of tissue factor pathway inhibitor (TFPI) after *n*-3 polyunsaturated fatty acids supplementation in patients with chronic atherosclerotic disease. Thromb Haemost 1996; 75:395–400.

69. Amengual O, Atsumi T, Khamashta MA, Hughes GRV. The role of the tissue factor pathway in the hypercoagulable state in patients with the antiphospholipid syndrome. Thromb Haemost 1998; 79:276–281.

70. Hansen JB, Huseby KR, Huseby NE, Ezban M, Nordoy A. Tissue factor pathway inhibitor in complex with low density lipoprotein isolated from human plasma does not possess anticoagulant function in tissue factor-induced coagulation in vitro. Thromb Res 1997; 85:413–425.

71. Sato Y, Asada Y, Marutsuk AK, et al. Tissue factor pathway inhibitor inhibits aortic smooth muscle cell migration induced by tissue factor/factor VIIa complex. Thromb Haemost 1997; 78:1138–1141.

72. Kamikubo Y, Nkahara Y, Takemoto S, et al. Human recombinant tissue factor pathway inhibitor prevents the proliferation of cultured human neonatal aortic smooth muscle cells. FEBS Lett 1997; 407:116–120.

73. Hamuro T, Kamikubo Y, Nakahara Y, Miyamoto S, Funatsu A. Human recombinant tissue factor pathway inhibitor induces apoptosis in cultured human endothelial cells. FEBS Lett 1998; 421:197–202.

74. Bajaj MS, Steer S, Kuppuswamy MN, Kisiel W, Bajaj P. Synthesis and expression of tissue factor pathway inhibitor by serum-stimulated fibroblasts, vascular smooth muscle cells and cardiac myocytes. Thromb Haemost 1999; 82:1663–1672.

75. Pendurthi UR, Rao LVM, Williams JT, Idell S. Regulation of tissue factor pathway inhibitor expression in smooth muscle cells. Blood 1999; 94:579–586.

76. Hembrough TA, Ruiz JF, Papathanassiu AE, Green SJ, Strickland DK. Tissue factor pathway inhibitor inhibits endothelial cell proliferation via association with the very low density lipoprotein receptor. J Biol Chem 2001; 276:12241–12248.

77. Jang Y, Guzman LA, Lincoff AM, et al. Influence of blockade at specific levels of the coagulation cascade on restenosis in a rabbit atherosclerotic femoral artery injury model. Circulation 1995; 92:3041–3050.

78. Oltrona L, Speidel CM, Recchia D, et al. Inhibition of tissue factor-mediated coagulation markedly attenuates stenosis after balloon-induced arterial injury in minipigs. Circulation 1997; 96:646–652.

79. Asada Y, Hara S, Tsuneyoshi A, et al. Fibrin-rich and platelet-rich thrombus formation on neointima: recombinant tissue factor pathway inhibitor prevents fibrin formation and neointimal development following repeated balloon injury of rabbit aorta. Thromb Haemost 1998; 80:506–511.

80. St Pierre J, Yang LY, Tamirisa K, et al. Tissue factor pathway inhibitor attenuates procoagulant activity and upregulation of tissue factor at the site of balloon-induced arterial injury in pigs. Arterioscler Thromb Vasc Biol 1999; 19:2263–2268.

81. Abendschein DR. Method of attenuating arterial stenosis. G D. Searle & Co. U.S. Patent 5824644, 1998.

82. Brown DM, Wun TC, Khouri RK. Method of inhibiting intimal hyperplasia. Washington University, U.S. Patent 5914316, 1999.

83. Koudsi B. Wun TC. Method of inhibiting tissue ischemia and reperfusion injury. G D. Searle & Co. U.S. Patent 5648334 1997.

84. Kaplan AV. Localized intravascular delivery of TFPI for inhibition of restenosis in recanalized blood vessels. Loclamed, Inc. U.S. Patent 5772629 1998.

85. Sun LB, Utoh J, Moriyama S, Tagami H, Okamoto K, Kitamura N. Topically applied tissue factor pathway inhibitor reduced intimal thickness of small arterial autografts in rabbits. J Vasc Surg 2001; 34:151–155.

86. Zoldhelyi P, Chen ZQ, Shelat HS, McNatt JM, Willerson JT. Local gene transfer of tissue factor pathway inhibitor regulates intimal hyperplasia in atherosclerotic arteries. Proc Natl Acad Sci USA 2001; 98:4078–4083.

87. Singh R, Pan S, Mueske CS, et al. Role for tissue factor pathway in murine model of vascular remodeling. Circ Res 2001; 89:71–76.

88. Westrick RJ, Bodary PF, Xu Z, Shen YC, Broze GJ, Eitzman DT. Deficiency of tissue factor pathway inhibitor promotes atherosclerosis and thrombosis in mice. Circulation 2001; 103:3044–3046.

89. Drew AF, Davenport P, Apostolopoulos J, Tipping PG. Tissue factor pathway inhibitor expression in atherosclerosis. Lab Invest 1997; 77:291–298.

90. Caplice NM, Mueske CS, Kleppe LS, Simari RD. Presence of tissue factor pathway inhibitor in human atherosclerotic plaques is associated with reduced tissue factor activity. Circulation 1998; 98:1051–1057.

91. Kaikita K, Takeya M, Ogawa H, et al. Co-localization of tissue factor and tissue factor pathway inhibitor in coronary atherosclerosis. J Pathol 1999; 188:180–188.

92. Crawley J, Lupu F, Westmuckett AD, Severs NJ, Kakkar VV, Lupu C. Expression, localization, and activity of tissue factor pathway inhibitor in normal and atherosclerotic human vessels. Arterioscler Thromb Vasc Biol 2000; 20:1362–1373.

93. Moatti D, Haidar B, Fumeron F, et al. A new T-287C polymorphism in the 5′ regulatory region of the tissue factor pathway inhibitor gene. Association study of the T-287C and C-399T polymorphisms with coronary artery disease and plasma TFPI levels. Thromb Haemost 2000; 84:244–249.

94. Moatti D, Seknadji P, Galand C, et al. Polymorphisms of the tissue factor pathway inhibitor (TFPI) gene in patients with acute coronary syndromes and in healthy subjects: impact of the V264M substitution on plasma levels of TFPI. Arterioscler Thromb Vasc Biol 1999; 19:862–869.

95. Moatti D, Meirhaeghe A, Ollivier V, Bauters C, Amouyel P, De Prost D. Polymorphisms of the tissue factor pathway inhibitor gene and the risk of restenosis after coronary angioplasty. Blood Coag Fibrinol 2001; 12:317–323.

96. Falciani M, Gori AM, Fedi S, et al. Elevated tissue factor and tissue factor pathway inhibitor circulating levels in ischaemic heart disease patients. Thromb Haemost 1998; 79:495–499.

97. Soejima H, Ogawa H, Yasue H, et al. Heightened tissue factor associated with tissue factor pathway inhibitor and prognosis in patients with unstable angina. Circulation 1999; 99:2908–2913.

98. Kamikura Y, Wada H, Yamada A, et al. Increased tissue factor pathway inhibitor in patients with acute myocardial infarction. Am J Hematol 1997; 55:183–187.

99. Otti I, Andrassy M, Zieglgansberger D, Geith S, Schomig A, Neumann FJ. Regulation of monocyte procoagulant activity in acute myocardial infarction: role of tissue factor and tissue factor pathway inhibitor-1. Blood 2001; 97:3721–3726.

100. Roldan V, Marin F, Fernandez P, et al. Tissue factor/tissue factor pathway inhibitor system and long-term prognosis after acute myocardial infarction. Int J Cardiol 2001; 78:115–119.

101. Hansen J, Grimsgaard S, Huseby N, Sandset PM, Bonaa KH. Serum lipids and regulation of tissue factor-induced coagulation in middle-aged men. Thromb Res 2001; 102:3–13.

102. Morange PE, Renucci JF, Charles MA, et al. Plasma levels of free and total TFPI, relationship with cardiovascular risk factors and endothelial cell markers. Thromb Haemost 2001; 85:999–1003.

103. Lupu C, Poulsen E, Roquefeuil S, et al. Cellular effects of heparin on the production and release of tissue factor pathway inhibitor in human endothelial cells in culture. Arterioscler Thromb Vasc Biol 1999; 19:2251–2262.

104. Creasey AA, Reinhart K. Tissue factor pathway inhibitor activity in severe sepsis. Crit Care Med 2001; 29(7 suppl):S126–S129.

105. Yamamuro M, Wada H, Kumeda K, et al. Changes in plasma tissue factor pathway inhibitor levels during the clinical course of disseminated intravascular coagulation. Blood Coagul Fibrinol 1998; 9:491–497.

106. Shimura M, Wada H, Nakasaki T, et al. Increased truncated form of plasma tissue factor pathway inhibitor levels in patients with disseminated intravascular coagulation. Am J Hematol 1999; 60:94–98.

107. De Jonge E, Dekkers PEP, Creasey AA, et al. Tissue factor pathway inhibitor dose-dependently inhibits coagulation activation without influencing the fibrinolytic and cytokine response during human endotoxemia. Blood 2000; 95:1124–1129.

108. De Jonge E, Dekkers PEP, Creasey AA, et al. Tissue factor pathway inhibitor does not influence inflammatory pathways during human endotoxemia. J Infect Dis 2001; 183:1815–1818.

109. Gando S, Nanzaki S, Norimoto Y, Ishitani T, Kemmotsu O. Tissue factor pathway inhibitor response does not correlate with tissue factor-induced disseminated intravascular coagulation and multiple organ dysfunction syndrome in trauma patients. Crit Care Med 2001; 29:262–266.

110. Abraham E. Tissue factor inhibition and clinical trial results of tissue factor pathway inhibitor in sepsis. Crit Care Med 2000; 28(9 suppl):S31–S33.

19

Modulation of the Protein C Pathway as a Therapy for Thrombosis

Charles T. Esmon
Oklahoma Medical Research Foundation and Howard Hughes Medical Institute, Oklahoma City, Oklahoma, U.S.A.

SUMMARY

The protein C pathway plays a critical role in preventing thrombosis, particularly in the microcirculation. The pathway can be down-regulated by inflammatory mediators, oxidants, and proteases from leukocytes. The pathway also exhibits anti-inflammatory activity, probably mediated partly by preventing NFκB nuclear translocation and blocking both leukocyte adhesion and activation. The combined anticoagulant and anti-inflammatory properties of the pathway make it an attractive candidate for the treatment of acute inflammatory diseases, such as sepsis, that trigger both a hypercoaguable and hyperinflammatory state. These responses are probably heightened by the decreased levels of protein C that occur in severe sepsis. Both protein C and activated protein C supplementation have been used in severe sepsis. The results from a phase III study of activated protein C seem very promising since it was stopped approximately half way through the anticipated enrollment because of statistically significant decreases in 28-day all-cause mortality.

I. INTRODUCTION

The protein C anticoagulant pathway consists of several proteins for which the mechanisms of action are distinct from other antithrombotic agents; hence, they offer potentially novel approaches to the treatment of thrombotic diseases. A number of congenital and acquired deficiency states involving components of the pathway, however, provide potential insights into how the system might be used. There is still limited human clinical data related to the treatment of thrombosis with components of the pathway. If, however, one considers severe sepsis and disseminated intravascular coagulation (DIC) as related to thrombosis, then it appears that the protein C pathway and activated protein C (APC), in particular, may have unique therapeutic properties that have been illustrated in a wide range of animal models related to sepsis and reperfusion injury. That these results are likely to be extended into humans is supported by published abstracts of phase II results of with APC in severe sepsis [1,2]. These results appear to be applicable to humans by a recently completed randomized, double-blind, placebo-controlled trial of APC for the treatment of severe sepsis which found that APC reduced the relative risk of death 19.4% [3].

To understand the application of this pathway to thrombotic disease, it is useful to consider our current view of its mechanism of action. There are a substantial number of reviews on this area for those wishing additional information [4–6] or alternative points of view from those of the author [7–22].

The coagulation cascade is illustrated in Figure 1, with the regulatory events associated with the protein C pathway illustrated on the right side of the schematic. In this highly simplified view, coagulation is triggered by the tissue factor–factor VIIa complex. This complex can then activate either factor X or factor IX. The factor VIIIa–factor IXa complex can then activate factor X. Factor Xa generated by either mechanism can then complex with factor Va to activate prothrombin. Factor Va and VIIIa are critical to the amplification of the coagulation response. The protein C pathway is designed to block this amplification by inactivating these two critical cofactors, factors Va and VIIIa. To accomplish this, thrombin binds to thrombomodulin (TM) on the surface of the endothelium and then generates the anticoagulant, activated protein C (APC). Protein C activation is augmented by protein C binding to the endothelial cell protein C receptor (EPCR) [23]. In vivo, protein C-EPCR interaction increases protein C activation by the thrombin–TM complex at least tenfold [24]. APC complexes with protein S to inactivate factors Va and VIIIa, thus shutting down the propagation phase of the coagulation response. For simplicity the activation of factors VII, VIII, and V are not shown in this figure. It is important to realize that the precursors of the activated cofactors of the factor V and factor VIII–von Willebrand's factor complex are much more resistant to inactivation than factor Va or factor VIIIa [7–9,25,26]. This specificity may partly explain why APC administration is associated with very little bleeding in experimental animals [27]. Furthermore, in baboon models of *Escherichia coli* sepsis, administration of APC actually protects factor V and VIII from inactivation, thereby maintaining a coagulant reserve even in the presence of this potent anticoagulant [28]. Reports have indicated that factor V, but not factor Va, can serve as a cofactor to accelerate further the inactivation of the cofactors [29]. By regulating the cofactors, the protein C pathway complements the vast array of protease inhibitors the function of which is to regulate the protease components of the coagulation cascade.

A potential complication in application of this system to the treatment of thrombotic disease is that there is a common factor V variant (factor V Leiden) that is resistant to proteolytic inactivation by APC [7–13]. This trait, commonly referred to as APC resistance, is caused by a substitution of Gln at residue 506 in factor V. This corresponds to the first cleavage site in factor Va [30–32]. Factor V Leiden is also inactive as a cofactor for factor VIIIa inactivation [29]. It produces a less severe thrombogenic state, even in the homozygous form, than protein C deficiencies. The probable basis for this is that failure to cleave factor Va at Arg506 only slows the inactivation partially, and this difference is largely eliminated by protein S [32]. In addition, APC exhibits anti-inflammatory activities [33] that may further differentiate between protein C deficiency and factor V Leiden.

A schematic diagram of the components of the protein C pathway is presented in Figure 2 and a more complete schematic representation of the protein C pathway is shown in Figure 3. The protein C pathway is triggered when thrombin binds to thrombomodulin (TM). This complex exhibits altered macromolecular specificity. The complex activates protein C rapidly, but fails to promote coagulation reactions, including platelet activation [34], fibrinogen clotting [35], factor V [35], and factor XIII activation [36]. The basis for the specificity switch is illustrated in Figure 4. In addition, thrombin bound to TM is inhibited more rapidly by antithrombin [37] and the protein C inhibitor [38]. The acceleration of the inhibition by

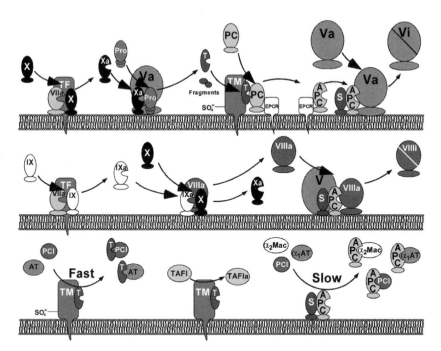

Figure 1 Coagulation is initiated when tissue factor (TF) is exposed to blood: This can occur either as the result of monocyte activation or exposure of the blood to extravascular cells. For simplicity, factor designations are not used in the figure (i.e., factor VIIa becomes VIIa). The tissue factor–VIIa complex can then activate either factor X (top row) or IX (middle row). These in turn form complexes with factor Va and VIIIa, respectively, probably on the surface of the activated platelet. The Xa–Va complex leads to explosive thrombin (T) formation. Unchecked, the thrombin would cause platelet activation, fibrin deposition, and initiate an inflammatory cascade. All steps to this point occur much better on negatively charged phospholipids. These can be made available by complement activation of the cells and by other agents that mobilize intracellular calcium. Several potent natural anticoagulant factors exist including the heparin–antithrombin mechanism responsible for the inhibition of factor Xa and thrombin and the tissue factor pathway inhibitor mechanism responsible for the control of the tissue factor–factor VIIa complex. Because the impact of inflammation on these pathways is less characterized than the protein C pathway, emphasis is placed on the latter pathway for purposes of this review. The protein C anticoagulant pathway is triggered when thrombin binds to TM on the surface of the endothelium (top row, center). This complex does not appear to need negatively charged phospholipids, especially when the endothelial cell protein C receptor (EPCR) is present. Once activated-protein C (APC) is generated, it can either remain bound to EPCR or dissociated to protein S (S). The APC–S complex can then inactivate factors Va or VIIIa. For factor VIIIa, the reaction is stimulated by factor V (V) [29].

In addition to playing a role in the regulation of the coagulation cascade per se, TM serves other functions shown on the third level of the figure. TM accelerates thrombin inhibition by antithrombin (AT) and protein C inhibitor (PCI), thus providing a mechanism for clearance of thrombin from the circulation. Thus, when TM is down-regulated by inflammatory mediators, proteolysis, and oxidation, thrombin inhibition is compromised. In addition, TM can accelerate the activation of TAFI. In its active form, this procarboxypeptidase B inhibits fibrinolysis. This loss of the fibrin stabilization resulting from TM down-regulation may compensate in part for the loss of anticoagulant functions of TM. The APC is then cleared from the circulation by α_2-macroglobulin (α_2-Mac), α_1-antitrypsin (α_1-AT), and PCI. Of importance to inflammation, α_1-AT behaves as an acute-phase reactant, and in the hemostatic balance, functions primarily as an inhibitor of APC, which, therefore, should shift the balance slightly in favor of clot formation.

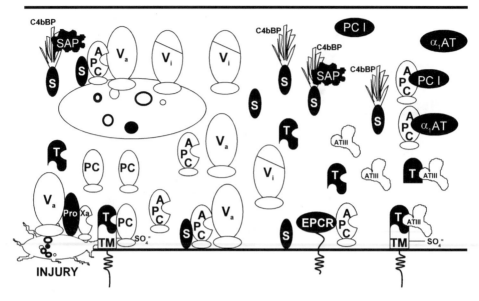

Figure 2 The protein C anticoagulant pathway under normal conditions: Vascular injury initiates prothrombin (Pro) activation that results in thrombin (T) formation. Prothrombin activation involves complex formation between factor Va (Va) and factor Xa (Xa). Thrombin then binds to thrombomodulin (TM) on the lumen of the endothelium, illustrated by the heavy line, and the thrombin-TM complex converts protein C (PC) to activated protein C (APC). Thrombin bound to TM can be inactivated very rapidly by antithrombin III (ATIII), at which time the thrombin–antithrombin III complex rapidly dissociates from TM. Activated protein C (APC) then binds to protein S (S) on cellular surfaces. The activated protein C–protein S complex then converts factor Va to an inactive complex (Vi), illustrated by the slash through the larger part of the two-subunit factor Va molecule. Protein C and APC interact with an endothelial cell protein C receptor (EPCR). This association may concentrate the zymogen and enzyme near the cell surface and facilitate the function of the pathway, but this has yet to be shown directly. Protein S circulates in complex with C4bBP, which, in turn, may bind serum amyloid P (SAP). APC is inhibited by forming complexes with either the protein C inhibitor (PCI), α_1-antitrypsin (α_1AT) or α_2-macroglobulin (not shown). See text for a more complete discussion. (From Ref. 139. Copyright © 1992 American Heart Association.)

antithrombin is dependent on the presence of a chondroitin sulfate moiety that can be covalently attached to TM [18,37,39], whereas the acceleration of the reaction with protein C inhibitor is not [38]. Thus, TM not only triggers the anticoagulant pathway, it directly blocks most of the procoagulant activities of thrombin and facilitates thrombin inactivation. Once bound to antithrombin, the complex rapidly dissociates from TM. These features create an image of a potent, multifaceted, on-demand mechanism of anticoagulant function.

This image of TM as strictly anticoagulant is clouded by some apparent contradictions. A major apparent paradox is that TM accelerates the thrombin-dependent activation of TAFI, a thrombin-dependent fibrinolytic inhibitor that is a zymogen of a procarboxypeptidase B [40]. TAFI removes Arg and Lys residues from fibrin making the lysis slower. Carboxypeptidase B activities are well known to have other effects, however. For instance, removal of the terminal Arg residue from the anaphylatoxin, complement C5a, is the major mechanism for inactivating this vasoactive toxin [41]. Thus, it may be that this carboxypeptidase has anti-inflammatory activities in addition to its antifibrinolytic properties. From the animal studies reviewed later, it would appear that the anticoagulant and anti-inflammatory properties of TM are dominant.

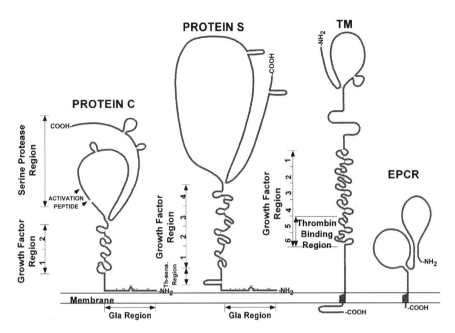

Figure 3 Schematic representation of protein C, protein S, the endothelial cell protein C receptor (EPCR), and TM. The vitamin K-dependent Gla residues of protein C and protein S are indicated by small Y-shaped symbols. Formation of these vitamin K-dependent residues is essential to full activity of protein C and protein S: Gla, γ-carboxyglutamic acid; Th.-sens., thrombin sensitive. The EPCR domain structure is based on homology to the CD1 family, and the disulfide pairing remains to be documented experimentally. (From Ref. 47; Copyright © 1989 the American Society for Biochemistry and Molecular Biology, Inc.)

Other apparently procoagulant and antifibrinolytic activities of TM have been observed. Thrombin can activate factor XI and this can be accelerated about 20-fold by TM [42]. Given that TM accelerates thrombin inactivation, the net effect of thrombin binding to TM on factor XI activation may be minimal. Furthermore, TM accelerates the inactivation of prourokinase [43,44]. This would seem to imply that the complex leads to the inhibition of fibrinolysis. This is in stark contrast with the in vivo observations that APC facilitates fibrinolysis in vivo [45–47]. Thus, the net influence of TM on the fibrinolytic system remains uncertain.

Once the thrombin–TM complex activates protein C, the resultant APC can inactivate factor Va or VIIIa. This process requires protein S. This complex functions on membrane surfaces expressing negatively charged phospholipid. The membrane specificity of the factor Va inactivation complex differs somewhat from that reported for prothrombin in that the activity of the complex is potently augmented by phosphatidylethanolamine or cardolipin in the membrane [48]. Phospholipid oxidation further enhances APC anticoagulant function while having a minimal influence on prothrombin activation in plasma [49]. It is possible that in vivo, lipid oxidation, mediated by activated leukocytes, modifies cell membrane lipids to convert them to a more anticoagulant state. In purified systems under standard conditions, protein S enhances factor Va inactivation only about twofold. Factor Xa can protect factor Va or factor IXa can protect factor VIIIa from inactivation by APC and protein S which largely eliminates this protective effect [50,51].

One of the unusual properties of APC is that it circulates with a long half-life, approximately 15 min [52]. It is also slowly inactivated in plasma [53] by the protein C inhibitor,

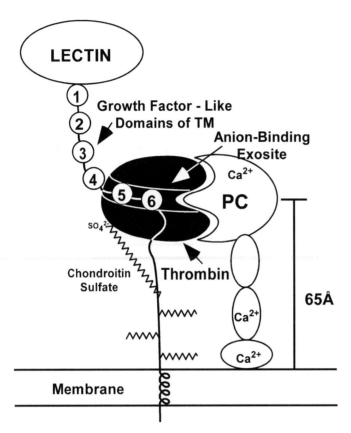

Figure 4   A model of the protein C activation complex. The small balls labeled 1–6 correspond to the EGF-like repeats in thrombomodulin, the extended structure rising from the membrane contains *O*-linked glycosylation sites (shown as zigzag lines) and is the site of attachment of the chondroitin sulfate, shown as the zigzag line with the terminal sulfate. This complex attacks protein C to release a 12-residue peptide from the amino-terminus of the heavy chain of protein C (not shown), which leads to activation. Both protein C and activated protein C interact with the activation complex [48,50]. Lectin refers to the lectin-like amino-terminal domain of thrombomodulin. (From Ref. 140; Copyright © 1993 F. K. Schattauer Verlagsgesellschaft mbH.)

α_1-antitrypsin, and in a Ca^{2+}-dependent fashion by α_2-macroglobulin and α_2-antiplasmin [53]. The slow clearance has implications about the mechanisms involved in APC function. Once generated, APC can circulate throughout the vasculature, presumably serving "sentry" duty by inactivating any cofactors on the membrane surfaces. This contrasts with the rapid clearance and inactivation by other coagulation factors, such as thrombin, that are inactivated by a single pass through the microcirculation [54].

      The ability of APC to elude the masses of plasma protease inhibitors allows one to consider the enzyme as a potential agent in therapy. There are distinct theoretical differences between considering protein C and APC as therapeutic agents. For protein C, the generation of anticoagulant activity increases with increasing thrombin challenge: this has been clearly documented in baboon studies that showed that the APC formed is approximately equivalent to the thrombin dose [55]. The thrombin is rapidly neutralized and thus additional protein C activation ceases when the thrombin generation is effectively controlled. From all of the available data, the protein C concentration in vivo is far below saturation (below K_m). Thus, the system could be augmented by infusing additional protein C. In preliminary experiments (Comp and Esmon, unpublished) this, in fact, was observed in dogs. That these animal experiments reflect the human situation is suggested by the observation that the circulating levels of APC correlate with the plasma precursor levels [56].

II. POTENTIAL THERAPEUTIC USES OF TM

The combined capacity of TM to block coagulation, activate protein C, and promote thrombin inhibition suggests that it could be useful as an antithrombotic. Limited data is available in vivo. TM has been immobilized on surfaces. As predicted based on its properties it creates nonthrombogenic surfaces in vitro [57]. I am unaware of any in vivo testing of these surfaces.

The concepts supporting the use of soluble TM as an antithrombotic are also based on these mechanisms. In cell culture, TM is down-regulated by inflammatory cytokines, raising the possibility that TM down-regulation contributes to thrombotic tendencies associated with inflammation. In vivo, down-regulation has been more difficult to document than in cell culture [58–60], but it has been observed in certain settings [61–63]. The down-regulation can be influenced by many factors, including interleukin-4 (IL4) [64] and retinoic acid (RA) [65,66], making our understanding of this potentially important phenomenon very incomplete. Nonetheless, the suggestion is attractive that TM supplementation would be useful during thrombotic complications, especially those associated with an underlying inflammatory situation. The published data on soluble TM as an antithrombotic has usually utilized models more reminiscent of DIC than thrombosis [67]. In particular, soluble TM blocks the tissue factor-induced DIC in rats [68], or endotoxin-mediated DIC [69] and the pulmonary vascular injury that ensues [70]. Most of this protective effect seems to be due to inhibition of leukocyte activation [71] probably resulting from protein C activation. Inhibition of leukocyte activation is most likely due to APC-mediated inhibition of cytokine elaboration in the tissues [72]. As is true in primates [73], active-site blocked factor Xa, which is a potent antithrombotic, failed to protect from lung injury, suggesting a protein C pathway-specific response in addition to the anticoagulant effect [70]. APC also blocked lung injury in this model [74], suggesting that the thrombomodulin effect was mediated by increased APC formation. TM, with or without the chondroitin sulfate, was effective in a tissue–factor-mediated DIC model [68]. The TM containing chondroitin sulfate was more effective on a mass basis, but was also cleared more rapidly from the circulation, 20 min versus 1 h. TM appeared to have less effect on bleeding time than heparin. When expressed as the concentration required to double the bleeding time versus the concentration required to block the decrease in platelet count 50%, TM with chondroitin was about threefold and without chondroitin twofold better than standard heparin. TM was also effective in a rat arteriovenous shunt thrombosis model. In this model, approximately 0.1 mg/kg of TM gave inhibition of thrombus mass equivalent to 10 U/kg standard heparin [75]. Thrombus formation in the injured, ligated inferior vena cava of the rat was also prevented with soluble form of TM, in this case lacking chondroitin sulfate [76,77]. These investigators found that TM blocked thrombosis at concentrations that doubled the bleeding time. Effective antithrombotic doses of hirudin or heparin resulted in bleeding times more than six times the control.

A. Protein C as an Antithrombotic and in Sepsis

Limited data are available about the use of protein C in the treatment of thrombotic disease in humans. Much of our knowledge has been gathered from the treatment of congenital deficiencies. Homozygous protein C deficiency results in life-threatening thrombotic complications in infancy. These are usually manifested as microvascular thrombosis of the skin capillaries (purpura fulminans). Replacement therapy with protein C has been shown to prevent further progression of these lesions with subsequent healing of the lesion [78,79]. These lesions are not prevented by heparinization [80]. The lesions in the homozygous infants resemble those that develop in warfarin-induced skin necrosis. In the protein C-deficient patients treated with protein C concentrate lesion progression ceases shortly after supplementation with protein C [4,81,82]. The biochemical basis for the association between protein C- and warfarin-induced skin necrosis is that protein C is vitamin K-dependent and the concentration declines more rapidly than those of prothrombin and factor IX following administration of warfarin. This temporal relation could be imagined to create a hypercoagulable window favoring procoagulant events. Consistent with this proposal, coagulation activation peptide levels have been observed to rise transiently shortly after the administration of warfarin [83]. In addition to indicating that protein C might be a logical treatment for patients with warfarin-induced skin necrosis, the data suggest that supplementation with protein C might be an effective means of safely increasing the anti-thrombotic effectiveness of warfarin with less bleeding risk than an increased intensity of oral anticoagulant treatment: this proposal remains to be tested. A universal observation, however, is that in experimental animals, even those subjected to open-chest surgery [27], APC caused relatively little bleeding complication at doses that were antithrombotic [27,84,85]. The basis for this observation is uncertain, but may be related to the fact that APC is an effective anticoagulant only at low levels of tissue factor (as might be generated within the vasculature) and that high levels of tissue factor (such as those in the extravascular space) may overcome the anticoagulant effects.

Both congenital deficiency and warfarin-induced acquired deficiency manifest themselves in microvascular thrombosis. The other situation in which microvascular thrombosis is common is inflammation-mediated DIC responses. Several lines of evidence provide a strong rationale for the use of protein C in the treatment of gram-negative septic shock, especially when purpura-like lesions are evident, as in seriously ill patients with meningococcemia. The suggestions that protein C or APC might be of use in this system comes from the observation that thrombin infusion into dogs subsequently challenged with lethal numbers of *E. coli* resulted in prevention of DIC and in improved survival [86]. With the subsequent recognition that the thrombin infusion might be functioning by activating protein C, we tested the ability of APC to prevent the lethal response to *E. coli* in baboons. APC protected the animals from death, DIC, and organ dysfunction [87]. When the protein C pathway was blocked and the animals challenged with sublethal doses of *E. coli*, all of the animals died [87,88] and the animals had much higher levels of circulating TNF-α than control animals given the same numbers of *E. coli*. Restoration of the protein C system prevented the DIC, organ damage, and elaboration of elevated cytokine levels. Taken together, these results suggest that protein C is a major regulator of microvascular thrombosis and that the system modulates the inflammatory response. In humans with meningococcemia, protein C consumption correlates better with the formation of the purpura-like lesions and death than other markers examined [89]. Protein C levels decrease significantly in patients with all forms of severe sepsis. The extent of the decrease in protein C levels is associated with an increased risk of death. In addition, the drop in protein C levels usually occurs before the diagnosis of severe sepsis or organ failure [90].

Given the link between protein C and microvascular thrombosis in congenital and acquired deficiencies, it was logical to examine protein C supplementation in the prevention of some complications of these forms of septic shock. Eleven children with severe manifestations of septic shock, usually due to meningococcemia, have been treated with protein C. Similar results were obtained in a larger study from the Smith group, bringing the total to 30 patients with only two deaths [91]. Others have argued that these uncontrolled trials are not sufficient to prove that protein C is effective [92]. In general, protein C infusion has been associated with normalization of circulating protein C levels and reversal of organ dysfunction, including a rapid regain of consciousness and kidney function [4,93]. The benefit of this treatment is not restricted to meningoccemia. One patient with a group A β-hemolytic streptococcal infection and varicella developed septic shock, DIC with consumption of protein C, and purpura [94]. His condition improved rapidly following protein C supplementation. Although these results are promising and consistent with the current basic and physiological understanding of the protein C system, a larger clinical trial is needed to verify the validity of this approach.

Potential mechanisms by which protein C might influence the septic shock process include the regulation of thrombin formation at the vessel surface or modulation of the inflammatory response. Assuming that the protein C activation mechanism is intact in the severe septic patient, one would predict that rapid protein C activation would occur in the thrombotic microvasculature where the TM and thrombin concentrations would both be high.

B.   Activated Protein C in the Treatment of Severe Sepsis

Two abstracts have been published reporting the phase II results with APC in severe sepsis (patients with one or more organ failure) [1,2]. There was a trend toward reduced mortality that failed to reach statistical significance. There was also a statistically significant decrease in IL-6 levels indicating an anti-inflammatory response. These preliminary results were confirmed and extended in a recent report of a recently completed randomized, double-blind, placebo-controlled trial of APC for the treatment of severe sepsis [3]. Treatment with APC reduced the 28-day all-cause mortality in the patients with severe sepsis from 30.8 to 24.7%. This corresponds to a 19.4% reduction in the relative risk of death.

There are several observations that provide suggestions that this system can modulate inflammation. In vitro, APC has been reported to inhibit tumor necrosis factor elaboration by monocytes [95]; to bind to these cells, probably by a specific receptor, and to prevent interferon-γ–mediated Ca^{2+} transients and cellular proliferation [96]; and to inhibit leukocyte adhesion to selectins [97]. Recently incubation of the monocytic cell line, THP 1, has been shown to block the nuclear translocation of NF-κB that normally occurs following stimulation with endotoxin [33].

An endothelial cell protein C receptor (EPCR), structurally related to the major histo-compatibility (MHC) class 1 molecules, has been identified and shown to be down-regulated by tumor necrosis factor (TNF) [98]. EPCR is released from activated endothelium by a metalloprotease [99]. Soluble EPCR binds to activated neutrophils through a complex involving Mac-1 and protease 3 [100]. Protease 3 is the primary autoantigen in Wegener's granulomatosis. It is likely that this complex modulates leukocyte adhesion, potentially contributing to the anti-inflammatory responses seen with APC. This proposal is supported by the observation that when EPCR–protein C/APC binding is blocked with monoclonal antibodies to EPCR, baboons challenged with a normally sublethal dose of *E. coli* have leukocyte extravasation, DIC, capillary leak, elevated IL-6 and IL-8, and die more rapidly than most animals given a lethal dose of the *E. coli* [101].

EPCR also appears to be involved in cell signaling. APC reduces both constitutive and phorbol-induced tissue factor expression on U937 cells, a process that is dependent on EPCR [102]. EPCR can also carry APC into the nucleus of endothelium and can elicit changes in the gene expression profile [103,104]. The exact mechanisms by which the protein C pathway modulates inflammatory responses remain obscure, but each or all of these effects may contribute to the effectiveness of this system in limiting damage caused by the host response

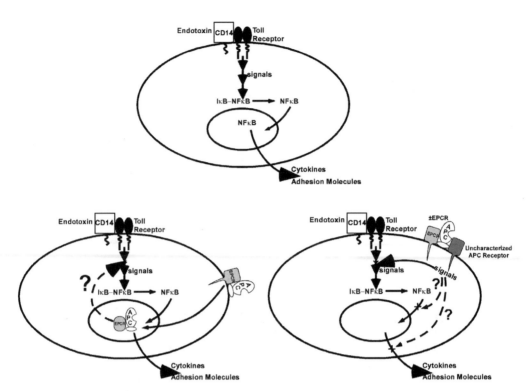

Figure 5 The role of activated protein C in modulating the inflammatory response: APC interacts with the cell surface either through EPCR or directly with a distinct APC receptor. This generates signals that block NFκB nuclear translocation. Alternatively, the EPCR–APC undergo nuclear translocation which, in turn, generates new gene products that may modulate this process. See the text for further discussion.

to infection. Potential mechanisms for APC modulation of the inflammatory response are shown in Figure 5.

In addition to being able to modulate sepsis, the system itself is sensitive to modulation by inflammatory mediators. These changes are depicted in Figure 6. In cell culture, TNF can down-regulate thrombomodulin [105] and the endothelial cell protein C receptor [98], and also can lead to protein S consumption [106–108] and increased levels of C4bBP [14,109]. Major basic protein from eosinophils can inhibit thrombomodulin function [110]. Proteolytic release of TM from the endothelium also occurs in shock and inflammatory disease [111–114]. The down-regulation of thrombomodulin mediated by inflammatory agents is less pronounced in vivo than in cell culture [58–60], although this process does seem to occur in villitis [63], over atherosclerotic plaque [115], during allograft organ rejection [62,116], and in some patients with meningococcemia [117].

III. PROTEIN S AS AN ANTITHROMBOTIC

Protein S serves as a cofactor for APC and also can block the assembly of the prothrombin activation complex by binding to factor Va and Xa [112–114,118–120]. In addition, factor Xa and IXa protect factor Va and VIIIa, respectively, and protein S largely overcomes this protection. No data is presently available to determine which of these functions is most relevant

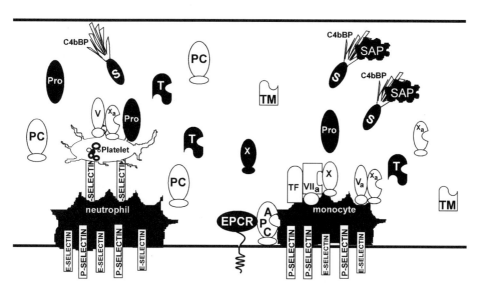

Figure 6 The protein C pathway after inflammation: In this model, inflammatory mediators lead to the disappearance of thrombomodulin from the endothelial cell surface. Endothelial cell leukocyte adhesion molecules (P-selectin) or E-selectin are synthesized or expressed on endothelial or platelet surfaces. Tissue factor (TF) is expressed on monocytes and binds factor VIIa (VIIa), and this complex converts factor X (X) to factor Xa (Xa), which forms complexes with factor Va (Va) to generate thrombin (T) from prothrombin (Pro). Because little activated protein C (APC) is formed and the little that forms does not function well because of low protein S (S), factor Va is not inactivated and prothrombin complexes are stabilized. Elevation in circulating C4bBP concentration results in little free protein S. See text for discussion: SAP, serum amyloid P. (From Ref. 139, Copyright © 1992 American Heart Association.)

physiologically. Depletion of protein S from plasma, however, has little influence on coagulation times in the absence of APC, whereas depletion of protein S decreases the anticoagulant response to APC about tenfold suggesting perhaps, that the APC-dependent activities may be more important.

Protein S as a therapeutic has not been studied extensively. Protein S deficiency has been described in patients with warfarin-induced skin necrosis [121], and patients with homozygous protein S deficiency may develop purpura fulminans [122]. Free and total protein S levels are often low in septic shock or following thrombosis [106,108,123]. Therefore, it might be reasonable to infer that protein S supplementation might be antithrombotic, especially when the levels were low due to the disease process.

Support for this concept has been obtained in a baboon model of *E. coli*-induced septic shock. Animals given 10% of the lethal numbers of *E. coli* exhibit only an acute-phase response. If free protein S is reduced by infusion of C4bBP or an antibody to protein S, infusion of the sublethal numbers of bacteria lead to death, organ failure, and either DIC or microvascular thrombosis [88]. Supplementation with sufficient protein S to return the protein S levels to normal protected the animals from death and DIC. However, the clinical experience to date with protein C infusion suggests that it is effective without simultaneous protein S supplementation. As these clinical trials continue, it will be important to determine whether patients who fail to respond to protein C infusion have unusually low protein S levels.

As yet there are no purified protein S concentrates or recombinant protein S preparations available for therapy. It is possible, however, to design forms of APC that function very effectively as anticoagulants, but no longer require protein S to do so. One such molecule is prepared as a chimera by replacing the Gla domain of protein C with the corresponding domain of prothrombin [124,125]. The resultant chimera has about four times the anticoagulant activity of APC, but no dependence on protein S. Such molecules might prove useful in treating diseases in which protein S levels are very low. One example would be patients with chickenpox who develop antiprotein S antibodies and subsequent purpura [126].

IV. PROTEIN C AND ARTERIAL THROMBOSIS

Studies from Hanson and Harker's group have shown that APC is effective in preventing platelet and fibrin accretion on vascular grafts at arterial flow rates in baboons. The concentration required to inhibit platelet accretion had little effect on bleeding time [85]. This model is highly thrombin-dependent; direct thrombin inhibitors block platelet accretion. Paradoxically, when thrombin is infused systemically, platelet accretion decreases [55]. This response is due primarily, if not exclusively, to activation of protein C, for the protective effect of thrombin in this study was eliminated by an antibody that blocks protein C activation. These studies suggest the possibility that APC might be effective in preventing arterial thrombosis. Note, however, that protein C deficiency is usually associated with venous or microvascular, rather than arterial, thrombosis. This could be due to the requirement for a development of arteriosclerosis before arterial thrombosis can occur and, therefore, protein C may not be observed as a risk factor in the heterozygous state. In the homozygous situation, the microvascular and venous thrombotic complications dominate.

V. REPERFUSION INJURY

Whenever thrombin is generated in the microvasculature, protein C activation occurs. This situation could arise in ischemia, a hypothesis supported by animal experiments. When the left anterior descending coronary artery was occluded in pigs [27] or dogs, protein C activation occurred within 2 min and activation was restricted to the region at risk. When protein C activation was blocked with a monoclonal antibody, the animal's left ventricular function did not recover as rapidly or completely from the ischemic injury. Ventricular fibrillation was often observed in the animals in which protein C activation was blocked, but not in the controls. APC infusion appeared to improve recovery of left ventricular function, although under the conditions of these experiments, this difference did not reach statistical significance. These data suggest that APC or protein C supplementation might diminish reperfusion injury. Theoretically, this would seem to be an especially attractive approach in patients with down-regulated thrombomodulin. Patients with coronary disease have been reported to have elevated TNF levels [127], possibly allowing for local thrombomodulin down-regulation. This has been suggested to occur in transplant rejection [61]. It should be emphasized that protein C activation in response to ischemia has not been documented to be due to the thrombin–TM complex. Other activators are possible. For instance, protein C can be activated and subsequently inactivated by plasmin [128,129]

In a rat model of compression-induced spinal cord injury, APC was effective in minimizing motor disturbances caused by the injury [130]. The mechanisms appear to be related to the ability to suppress tissue TNF-α levels [130] and neutrophil activation [72,131]. In contrast, active site-blocked factor Xa (a potent competitive inhibitor of the assembly of the prothrombin activation complex) failed to protect, even though it functioned as a very effective anticoagulant. From these studies the authors concluded that protection required the modulation of the inflammatory response, rather than simply providing an anticoagulant function.

VI. AMPLIFYING THE RESPONSE OF THE SYSTEM

The apparent safety and efficacy of this system observed in experimental animals suggests that supplementation with components of the system would provide safe and effective antithrombotic therapy. An alternative approach is to make the natural system better. Recently, two approaches have been extensively exploited. In the first, a protein C mutant has been designed that activates rapidly with thrombin in the absence of thrombomodulin [132]. This mutant is activated sufficiently rapidly that it anticoagulates plasma, something wild type protein C does not do in the absence of thrombomodulin.

A second approach is to modify thrombin. For this, several functions are potential aids in eliciting a selective response. In principle, one could eliminate fibrinogen-clotting activity or increase protein C activation. Enhanced protein C activation could involve either thrombo-modulin-dependent or -independent mechanisms, and several thrombin mutants with one or more of these properties have been identified [133,134]. A particularly promising thrombin mutant has been identified and studied in vivo. It has a 40-fold–decreased fibrinogen-clotting activity, is more than 50-fold less effective in activating platelets, and still retains about 50% of its protein C-activating capacity in the presence of thrombomodulin [135]. In addition, reactivity with antithrombin is reduced sevenfold. In vivo, this thrombin mutant generated the antic-oagulant response observed previously with normal thrombin, but without as much fibrinogen consumption.

VII. THROMBOMODULIN GENE THERAPY FOR PREVENTION OF THROMBOSIS AND RESTENOSIS

The properties of TM as a potent activator of protein C and the ability of APC to inhibit leukocyte infiltration have been exploited using an adenovirus delivery system in rabbit models. In arteries injured by balloon catheterization, treatment of the vessel segments with vectors capable of driving TM expression decreased thrombosis, restenosis and leukocyte infiltration into the tissues [136,137]. Even though there remain many technical difficulties with delivering genes in humans, these animal results suggest that if the technical issues of local gene therapy can be resolved, TM or possibly EPCR might be logical choices for limiting local thrombotic risk and restenosis. Others have sought to immobilize TM to make biomaterials anti-thrombotic [57,67].

Another area in which this approach might be useful is in transplant biology. In allografts, TM is down-regulated [62,116], and in xenografts there is considerable species specificity making the TM much less effective in protein C activation [138]. Therefore, modifying these transplant organs to express high levels of TM constitutively might improve transplant survival by minimizing thrombosis and inflammatory cell infiltration.

VIII. CONCLUDING REMARKS

The protein C system offers promise as a novel antithrombotic agent. The system seems to be especially important in the control of microvascular thrombosis; hence, it might provide the agents of choice in treating these diseases. All of the limited clinical data suggest that protein C supplementation is safe and effective in congenital deficiencies, warfarin-induced skin necrosis, and gram-negative sepsis. Whether protein C or APC will prove beneficial in larger, randomized clinical trials or in forms of septic shock without purpura lesions remains to be determined. If the protein C system does elicit anti-inflammatory activity, as inferred from the basic and physiological studies, modulation of this pathway may constitute a unique approach to diminish mortality and morbidity associated with septic shock. It is important to realize that studies on this system are still in their infancy. New receptors are being identified, such as the endothelial cell receptor, that can modulate APC activity [98]. As we gain a better understanding of the system, we are likely to better understand how to apply the components of the system to the treatment of thrombotic disease.

REFERENCES

1. Bernard GR, Hartman DL, Helterbrand JD, Fisher CJ. Recombinant human activated protein C (rhAPC) produces a trend toward improvement in morbidity and 28 day survival in patients with severe sepsis [abstr]. Crit Care Med 1998; 27:S4.
2. Hartman DL, Bernard GR, Helterbrand JD, Yan SB, Fisher CJ. Recombinant human activated protein C (rhAPC) improves coagulation abnormalities associated with severe sepsis [abstr]. Intensive Care Med 1998; 24:S77.
3. Bernard GR, Vincent JL, Laterre PF, LaRosa SP, Dhainaut JF, Lopez–Rodriguez A, Steingrub JS, Garber GE, Helterbrand JD, Ely EW, Fisher CJ. Efficacy and safety of recombinant human activated protein C for severe sepsis. N Engl J Med 2001; 344:699–709.
4. Esmon CT, Schwarz HP. An update on clinical and basic aspects of the protein C anticoagulant pathway. Trends Cardiovasc Med 1995; 5:141–148.
5. Esmon CT. Thrombomodulin as a model of molecular mechanisms that modulate protease specificity and function at the vessel surface. FASEB J 1995; 9:946–955.
6. Esmon CT, Fukudome K. Cellular regulation of the protein C pathway. Semin Cell Biol 1995; 6:259–268.
7. Fulcher CA, Gardiner JE, Griffin JH, Zimmerman TS. Proteolytic inactivation of human factor VIII procoagulant protein by activated protein C and its analogy with factor V. Blood 1984; 63:486–489.
8. Koedam JA, Meijers JCM, Sixma JJ, Bouma BN. Inactivation of human factor VIII by activated protein C. Cofactor activity of protein S and protective effect of von Willebrand factor. J Clin Invest 1988; 82:1236–1243.
9. Eaton D, Rodriguez H, Vehar GA. Proteolytic processing of human factor VIII. Correlation of specific cleavages by thrombin, factor Xa, and activated protein C with activation and inactivation of factor VIII coagulant activity. Biochemistry 1986; 25:505–512.
10. Griffin JH, Evatt B, Wideman C, Fernández JA. Anticoagulant protein C pathway defective in majority of thrombophilic patients. Blood 1993; 82:1989–1993.
11. Halbmayer W–M, Haushofer A, Schon R, Fischer M. The prevalence of poor anticoagulant response to activated protein C (APC resistance) among patients suffering from stroke or venous thrombosis and among healthy subjects. Blood Coagul Fibrinol 1994; 5:51–57.
12. Bertina RM, Koeleman BPC, Koster T, Rosendaal FR, Dirven RJ, de Ronde H, van der Velden PA, Reitsma PH. Mutation in blood coagulation factor V associated with resistance to activated protein C. Nature 1994; 369:64–67.
13. Dahlbäck B. Physiological anticoagulation. Resistance to activated protein C and venous thromboembolism. J Clin Invest 1994; 94:923–927.
14. Dahlbäck B. Protein S and C4b-binding protein: components involved in the regulation of the protein C anticoagulant system. Thromb Haemost 1991; 66:49–61.
15. Davie EW, Fujikawa K, Kisiel W. The coagulation cascade: initiation, maintenance and regulation. Biochemistry 1991; 30:10363–10370.

16. Walker FJ, Fay PJ. Regulation of blood coagulation by the protein C system. FASEB J 1992; 6:2561–2567.

17. Pabinger I, Brucker S, Kyrle PA, Schneider B, Korninger HC, Niessner H, Lechner K. Hereditary deficiency of antithrombin III, protein C and protein S: prevalence in patients with a history of venous thrombosis and criteria for rational patient screening. Blood Coagul Fibrinol 1992; 3:547–553.

18. Bourin MC, Lindahl U. Glycosaminoglycans and the regulation of blood coagulation. Biochem J 1993; 289:313–330.

19. Alving BM, Comp PC. Recent advances in understanding clotting and evaluating patients with recurrent thrombosis. Am J Obstet Gynecol 1992; 167:1184–1191.

20. Reitsma PH, Poort SR, Bernardi F, Gandrille S, Long GL, Sala N, Cooper DN. Protein C deficiency: a database of mutations. For the Protein C & S Subcommittee of the Scientific and Standardization Committee of the International Society on Thrombosis and Haemostasis. Thromb Haemost 1993; 69:77–84.

21. Castellino FJ. Human protein C and activated protein C. Trends Cardiovasc Med 1995; 5:55–62.

22. Reitsma PH, Bernardi F, Doig RG, Gandrille S, Greengard JS, Ireland H, Krawczak M, Lind B, Long GL, Poort SR, Saito H, Sala N, Witt I, Cooper DN. Protein C deficiency: a database of mutations, 1995 update. Thromb Haemost 1995; 73:876–879.

23. Stearns–Kurosawa DJ, Kurosawa S, Mollica JS, Ferrell GL, Esmon CT. The endothelial cell protein C receptor augments protein C activation by the thrombin–thrombomodulin complex. Proc Natl Acad Sci USA 1996; 93:10212–10216.

24. Taylor FB Jr, Peer GT, Lockhart MS, Ferrell G, Esmon CT. Endothelial cell protein C receptor plays an important role in protein C activation in vivo. Blood 2001; 97:1685–1688.

25. Walker FJ, Sexton PW, Esmon CT. Inhibition of blood coagulation by activated protein C through selective inactivation of activated factor V. Biochim Biophys Acta 1979; 571:333–342.

26. Kalafatis M, Rand MD, Mann KG. The mechanism of inactivation of human factor V and human factor Va by activated protein C. J Biol Chem 1994; 269:31869–31880.

27. Snow TR, Deal MT, Dickey DT, Esmon CT. Protein C activation following coronary artery occlusion in the in situ porcine heart. Circulation 1991; 84:293–299.

28. Taylor FB Jr, Chang A, Esmon CT, D'Angelo A, Vigano-D'Angelo S, Blick KE. Protein C prevents the coagulopathic and lethal effects of *E. coli* infusion in the baboon. J Clin Invest 1987; 79:918–925.

29. Shen L, Dahlbäck B. Factor V and protein S as synergistic cofactors to activated protein C in degradation of factor VIIIa. J Biol Chem 1994; 269:18735–18738.

30. Kalafatis M, Bertina RM, Rand MD, Mann KG. Characterization of the molecular defect in factor V^{R506Q}. J Biol Chem 1995; 270:4053–4057.

31. Billy D, Willems GM, Hemker HC, Lindhout T. Prothrombin contributes to the assembly of the factor Va–factor Xa complex at phosphatidylserine-containing phospholipid membranes. J Biol Chem 1995; 270:26883–26889.

32. Rosing J, Hoekema L, Nicolaes GAF, Thomassen MCLGD, Hemker HC, Varadi K, Schwarz HP, Tans G. Effects of protein S and factor Xa on peptide bond cleavages during inactivation of factor Va and factor Va^{R506Q} by activated protein C. J Biol Chem 1995; 270:27852–27858.

33. White B, Schmidt M, Murphy C, Livingstone W, O'Toole D, Lawler M, O'Neill L, Kelleher D, Schwarz HP, Smith OP. Activated protein C inhibits lipopolysaccharide-induced nuclear translocation of nuclear factor kappaB (NF-kappaB) and tumour necrosis factor alpha (TNF-alpha) production in the THP-1 monocytic cell line. Br J Haematol 2000; 110:130–134.

34. Esmon NL, Carroll RC, Esmon CT. Thrombomodulin blocks the ability of thrombin to activate platelets. J Biol Chem 1983; 258:12238–12242.

35. Esmon CT, Esmon NL, Harris KW. Complex formation between thrombin and thrombomodulin inhibits both thrombin-catalyzed fibrin formation and factor V activation. J Biol Chem 1982; 257:7944–7947.

36. Polgar J, Lerant I, Muszbek L, Machovich R. Thrombomodulin inhibits the activation of factor XIII by thrombin. Thromb Res 1986; 43:585–590.

37. Parkinson JF, Koyama T, Bang NU, Preissner KT. Thrombomodulin: an anticoagulant cell surface proteoglycan with physiologically relevant glycosaminoglycan moiety. Adv Exp Med Biol 1992; 313:177–188.

38. Rezaie AR, Cooper ST, Church FC, Esmon CT. Protein C inhibitor is a potent inhibitor of the thrombin–thrombomodulin complex. J Biol Chem 1995; 270:25336–25339.

39. Lin J–H, McLean K, Morser J, Young TA, Wydro RM, Andrews WH, Light DR. Modulation of glycosaminoglycan addition in naturally expressed and recombinant human thrombomodulin. J Biol Chem 1994; 269:25021–25030.

40. Bajzar L, Manuel R, Nesheim ME. Purification and characterization of TAFI, a thrombin-activable fibrinolysis inhibitor. J Biol Chem 1995; 270:14477–14484.

41. Meuer S, Hugli TE, Andeatta RH, Hadding U, Bitter–Suermann D. Comparative study on biological activities of various anaphylatoxins (C4a, C3a, C5a). Inflammation 1981; 5:263–273.

42. Gailani D, Broze GJ Jr. Factor XI activation in a revised model of blood coagulation. Science 1991; 253:909–912.

43. Molinari A, Giogetti C, Lansen J, Vaghi F, Orsini G, Faioni EM, Mannucci PM. Thrombomodulin is a cofactor for thrombin degradation of recombinant single-chain urokinase plasminogen activator in vitro and in a perfused rabbit heart model. Thromb Haemost 1992; 67:226–232.

44. de Munk GAW, Parkinson JF, Groeneveld E, Bang NU, Rijken DC. Role of the glycosaminoglycan component of thrombomodulin in its acceleration of the inactivation of single-chain urokinase-type plasminogen activator by thrombin. Biochem J 1993; 290:655–659.

45. Krishnamurti C, Young GD, Barr CF, Colleton CA, Alving BM. Enhancement of tissue plasminogen activator-induced fibrinolysis by activated protein C in endotoxin-treated rabbits. J Lab Clin Med 1991; 118:523–530.

46. Gruber A, Harker LA, Hanson SR, Kelly AB, Griffin JH. Antithrombotic effects of combining activated protein C and urokinase in nonhuman primates. Circulation 1991; 84:2454–2462.

47. Esmon CT. The roles of protein C and thrombomodulin in the regulation of blood coagulation. J Biol Chem 1989; 264:4743–4746.

48. Smirnov MD, Esmon CT. Phosphatidylethanolamine incorporation into vesicles selectively enhances factor Va inactivation by activated protein C. J Biol Chem 1994; 269:816–819.

49. Safa O, Hensley K, Smirnov MD, Merrill JT, D'Angelo A, Esmon CT, Esmon NL. Lipid oxidation enhances the function of activated protein C and anti-phospholipid antibodies. J Biol Chem 2001; 276:1829–1836.

50. Regan LM, Lamphear BJ, Huggins CF, Walker FJ, Fay PJ. Factor IXa protects factor VIIIa from activated protein C. J Biol Chem 1994; 269:9445–9452.

51. Solymoss S, Tucker MM, Tracy PB. Kinetics of inactivation of membrane-bound factor Va by activated protein C. J Biol Chem 1988; 263:14884–14890.

52. Comp PC, Esmon CT. Generation of fibrinolytic activity by infusion of activated protein C into dogs. J Clin Invest 1981; 68:1221–1228.

53. Heeb MJ, Gruber A, Griffin JH. Identification of divalent metal ion-dependent inhibition of activated protein C by alpha$_2$-macroglobulin and alpha$_2$-antiplasmin in blood and comparisons to inhibition of factor Xa, thrombin, and plasmin. J Biol Chem 1991; 266:17606–17612.

54. Lollar P, Owen W. Clearance of thrombin from the circulation in rabbits by high-affinity binding sites on endothelium. J Clin Invest 1980; 66:1222–1230.

55. Hanson SR, Griffin JH, Harker LA, Kelly AB, Esmon CT, Gruber A. Antithrombotic effects of thrombin-induced activation of endogenous protein C in primates. J Clin Invest 1993; 92:2003–2012.

56. Espana F, Zuazu I, Vicente V, Estelles A, Marco P, Aznar J. Quantification of circulating activated protein C in human plasma by immunoassays—enzyme levels are proportional to total protein C levels. Thromb Haemost 1996; 75:56–61.

57. Kishida A, Ueno Y, Maruyama I, Akashi M. Immobilization of human thrombomodulin onto biomaterials. Comparison of immobilzation methods and evaluation of antithrombogenicity. ASAIO J 1994; 40:M840–M845.

58. Laszik Z, Carson CW, Nadasdy T, Johnson LD, Lerner MR, Brackett DJ, Esmon CT, Silva FG. Lack of suppressed renal thrombomodulin expression in a septic rat model with glomerular thrombotic microangiopathy. Lab Invest 1994; 70:862–867.

59. Semeraro N, Triggiani R, Montemurro P, Cavallo LG, Colucci M. Enhanced endothelial tissue factor but normal thrombomodulin in endotoxin-treated rabbits. Thromb Res 1993; 71:479–486.

60. Drake TA, Cheng J, Chang A, Taylor FB Jr. Expression of tissue factor, thrombomodulin, and E-selectin in baboons with lethal *E. coli* sepsis. Am J Pathol 1993; 142:1458–1470.

61. Hancock WW, Tanaka K, Salem HH, Tilney NL, Atkins RC, Kupiec–Weglinski JW. TNF as a mediator of cardiac transplant rejection, including effects on the intragraft protein C/protein S/thrombomodulin pathway. Transplant Proc 1991; 23:235–237.

62. Faulk WP, Gargiulo P, Bang NU, et al. Immunopathology of hemostasis in allografted human kidneys. Blood 1987; 70(suppl. 1):371a.

63. Labarrere CA, Esmon CT, Carson SD, Faulk WP. Concordant expression of tissue factor and class II MHC antigens in human placental endothelium. Placenta 1990; 2:309–318.

64. Kapiotis S, Besemer J, Bevec D, Valent P, Bettelheim P, Lechner K, Speiser W. Interleukin-4 counteracts pyrogen-induced downregulation of thrombomodulin in cultured human vascular endothelial cells. Blood 1991; 78:410–415.

65. Dittman WA, Nelson SC, Greer PK, Horton ET, Palomba ML, McCachren SS. Characterization of thrombomodulin expression in response to retinoic acid and identification of a retinoic acid response element in the human thrombomodulin gene. J Biol Chem 1994; 269:16925–16932.

66. Koyama T, Hirosawa S, Kawamata N, Tohda S, Aoki N. All-*trans* retinoic acid upregulates thrombomodulin and down regulates tissue-factor expression in acute promyelocytic leukemia cells: distinct expression of thrombomodulin and tissue factor in human leukemic cells. Blood 1994; 84:3001–3009.

67. Maruyama I. Recombinant thrombomodulin and activated protein C in the treatment of disseminated intravascular coagulation. Thromb Haemost 1999; 82:718–721.

68. Nawa K, Itani T, Ono M, Sakano K, Marumoto Y, Iwamoto M. The glycosaminoglycan of recombinant human soluble thrombomodulin affects antithrombotic activity in a rat model of tissue factor-induced disseminated intravascular coagulation. Thromb Haemost 1992; 67:366–370.

69. Gonda Y, Hirata S, Saitoh K–I, Aoki Y, Mohri M, Gomi K, Sugihara T, Kiyota T, Yamamoto S, Ishida T, Maruyama I. Antithrombotic effect of recombinant human soluble thrombomodulin on endotoxin-induced disseminated intravascular coagulation in rats. Thromb Res 1993; 71:325–335.

70. Uchiba M, Okajima K, Murakami K, Nawa K, Okabe H, Takatsuki K. Recombinant human soluble thrombomodulin reduces endotoxin-induced pulmonary vascular injury via protein C activation in rats. Thromb Haemost 1995; 74:1265–1270.

71. Cote HCF, Bajzar L, Stevens WK, Samis JA, Morser J, MacGillivray RTA, Nesheim ME. Functional characterization of recombinant human meizothrombin and meizothrombin(desF1). Thrombomodulin-dependent activation of protein C and thrombin-activatable fibrinolysis inhibitor (TAFI), platelet aggregation, antithrombin-III inhibition. J Biol Chem 1997; 272:6194–6200.

72. Taoka Y, Okajima K, Uchiba M, Johno M. Neuroprotection by recombinant thrombomodulin. Thromb Haemost 2000; 83:462–468.

73. Taylor FB Jr, Chang ACK, Peer GT, Mather T, Blick K, Catlett R, Lockhart MS, Esmon CT. DEGR-factor Xa blocks disseminated intravascular coagulation initiated by *Escherichia coli* without preventing shock or organ damage. Blood 1991; 78:364–368.

74. Murakami K, Okajima K, Uchiba M, Johno M, Nakagaki T, Okabe H, Takatsuki K. Activated protein C attenuates endotoxin-induced pulmonary vascular injury by inhibiting activated leukocytes in rats. Blood 1996; 87:642–647.

75. Aoki Y, Takei R, Mohri M, Gonda Y, Gomi K, Sugihara T, Kiyota T, Yamamoto S, Ishida T, Maruyama I. Antithrombotic effects of recombinant human soluble thrombomodulin (rhs-TM) on arteriovenous shunt thrombosis in rats. Am J Hematol 1994; 47:162–166.

76. Solis MM, Cook C, Cook J, Glaser C, Light D, Morser J, Yu S, Fink L, Eidt JF. Intravenous recombinant soluble human thrombomodulin prevents venous thrombosis in a rat model. J Vasc Surg 1991; 14:599–604.

77. Solis MM, Vitti M, Cook J, Young D, Glaser C, Light D, Morser J, Wydro R, Yu S, Fink L, Eidt JF. Recombinant soluble human thrombomodulin: a randomized, blinded assessment of prevention of

venous thrombosis and effects on hemostatic parameters in a rat model. Thromb Res 1994; 73:385–394.

78. Dreyfus M, Masterson M, David M, Rivard GE, Muller F–M, Kreuz W, Beeg T, Minford A, Allgrove J, Cohen JD, Christoph J, Bergmann F, Mitchell VE, Haworth C, Nelson K, Schwarz HP. Replacement therapy with a monoclonal antibody purified protein C concentrate in newborns with severe congenital protein C deficiency. Sem Thromb Hemost 1995; 21:371–381.

79. Muller F–M, Ehrenthal W, Hafner G, Schranz D. Purpura fulminans in severe congenital protein C deficiency: monitoring of treatment with protein C concentrate. Eur J Pediatr 1996; 155:20–25.

80. Sills RH, Marlar RA, Montgomery RR, Desphande GN, Humbert JR. Severe homozygous protein C deficiency. J Pediatrics 1984; 105:409–413.

81. Muntean W, Finding K, Gamillscheg A, Schwarz HP. Multiple thromboses and coumarin-induced skin necrosis in a child with anticardiolipin antibodies: effects of protein C concentrate administration. Thromb Haemostas 1991; 65:2017.

82. Schramm W, Spannagl M, Bauer KA, Rosenberg RD, Birkner B, Linnau Y, Schwarz HP. Treatment of coumarin-induced skin necrosis with a monoclonal antibody purified protein C concentrate. Arch Dermatol 1993; 129:753–756.

83. Conway EM, Bauer KA, Barzegar S, Rosenberg RD. Suppression of hemostatic system activation by oral anticoagulants in the blood of patients with thrombotic diatheses. J Clin Invest 1987; 80:1535–1544.

84. Emerick SC, Murayama H, Yan SB, Long GL, Harms CS, Marks CA, et al. Preclinical pharmacology of activated protein C. In: Holcenber JS, Winkelhake JL, eds. The Pharmacology and Toxicology of Proteins, UCLA Symposia on Molecular and Cellular Biology. New York: Alan R Liss, 1987; 351–367.

85. Gruber A, Griffin JH, Harker LA, Hanson SR. Inhibition of platelet-dependent thrombus formation by human activated protein C in a primate model. Blood 1989; 73: 639–642.

86. Taylor FB Jr, Chang A, Hinshaw LB, Esmon CT, Archer LT, Beller BK. A model for thrombin protection against endotoxin. Thromb Res 1984; 36:177–185.

87. Taylor FB Jr, Stern DM, Nawroth PP, Esmon CT, Hinshaw LB, Blick KE. Activated protein C prevents E. coli induced coagulopathy and shock in the primate [abstr. 256]. Circulation 1986; 74:65.

88. Taylor F, Chang A, Ferrell G, Mather T, Catlett R, Blick K, Esmon CT. C4b-binding protein exacerbates the host response to Escherichia coli. Blood 1991; 78:357–363.

89. Powars D, Larsen R, Johnson J, Hulbert T, Sun T, Patch MJ, Francis R, Chan L. Epidemic meningococcemia and purpura fulminans with induced protein C deficiency. Clin Infect Dis 1993; 17:254–261.

90. Fisher CJ, Yan SB. Protein C levels as a prognostic indicator of outcome in sepsis and related diseases. Crit Care Med 2000; 28:S49–S56.

91. Smith OP, White B. Infectious purpura fulminans: diagnosis and treatment. Br J Haematol 1999; 104:202–207.

92. Finn A, Booy R, Levin M, Nadel S, Faust S. Infectious purpura fulminans: caution needed in the use of protein C. Br J Haematol 1999; 106:253.

93. Rivard GE, David M, Farrell C, Schwarz HP. Treatment of purpura fulminans in meningococcemia with protein C concentrate. J Pediatr 1995; 126:646–652.

94. Gerson WT, Dickerman JD, Bovill EG, Golden E. Severe acquired protein C deficiency in purpura fulminans associated with disseminated intravascular coagulation: treatment with protein C concentrate. Pediatrics 1993; 91:418–422.

95. Grey ST, Tsuchida A, Hau H, Orthner CL, Salem HH, Hancock WW. Selective inhibitory effects of the anticoagulant activated protein C on the responses of human mononuclear phagocytes to LPS, IFN-gamma, or phorbol ester. J Immunol 1994; 153:3664–3672.

96. Hancock WW, Grey ST, Hau L, Akalin E, Orthner C, Sayegh MH, Salem HH. Binding of activated protein C to a specific receptor on human mononuclear phagocytes inhibits intracellular calcium signaling and monocyte-dependent proliferative responses. Transplantation 1995; 60:1525–1532.

97. Grinnell BW, Hermann RB, Yan SB. Human protein C inhibits selectin-mediated cell adhesion: role of unique fucosylated oligosaccharide. Glycobiology 1994; 4:221–226.

98. Fukudome K, Esmon CT. Identification, cloning and regulation of a novel endothelial cell protein C/activated protein C receptor. J Biol Chem 1994; 269:26486–26491.

99. Xu J, Qu D, Esmon NL, Esmon CT. Metalloproteolytic release of endothelial cell protein C receptor. J Biol Chem 1999; 275:6038–6044.

100. Kurosawa S, Esmon CT, Stearns–Kurosawa DJ. The soluble endothelial protein C receptor binds to activated neutrophils: involvement of proteinase-3 and CDIIb/CDI8. J Immunol 2000; 165:4697–4703.

101. Taylor FB Jr, Stearns–Kurosawa DJ, Kurosawa S, Ferrell G, Chang ACK, Laszik Z, Kosanke S, Peer G, Esmon CT. The endothelial cell protein C receptor aids in host defense against *Escherichia coli* sepsis. Blood 2000; 95:1680–1686.

102. Shu F, Kobayashi H, Fukudome K, Tsuneyoshi N, Kimoto M, Terao T. Activated protein C suppresses tissue factor expression on U937 cells in the endothelial protein C receptor-dependent manner. FEBS Lett 2000; 477:208–212.

103. Xu J, Esmon CT. Endothelial cell protein C receptor (EPCR) constitutively translocates into the nucleus and also mediates activated protein C, but not protein C, nuclear translocation [abstr]. Thromb Haemostas 1999; Suppl Aug:206.

104. Esmon CT. The endothelial cell protein C receptor. Thromb Haemost 2000; 83:639–643.

105. Dittman WA. Thrombomodulin: biology and potential cardiovascular applications. Trends Cardiovasc Med 1991; 1:331–336.

106. Heeb MJ, Mosher D, Griffin JH. Activation and complexation of protein C and cleavage and decrease of protein S in plasma of patients with intravascular coagulation. Blood 1989; 73:455–461.

107. Bourin MC, Lundgren–Åkerlund E, Lindahl U. Isolation and characterization of the glycosaminoglycan component of rabbit thrombomodulin proteoglycan. J Biol Chem 1990; 265:15424–15431.

108. Fourrier F, Chopin C, Goudemand J, Hendrycx S, Caron C, Rime A, Marey A, Lestavel P. Septic shock, multiple organ failure, and disseminated intravascular coagulation. Compared patterns of antithrombin III, protein C, and protein S deficiencies. Chest 1992; 101:816–823.

109. D'Angelo A, Vigano–D'Angelo S, Esmon CT, Comp PC. Acquired deficiencies of protein S: protein S activity during oral anticoagulation, in liver disease and in disseminated intravascular coagulation. J Clin Invest 1988; 81:1445–1454.

110. Mukai HY, Ninomiya H, Ohtani K, Nagasawa T, Abe T. Major basic protein binding to thrombomodulin potentially contributes to the thrombosis in patients with eosinophilia. Br J Haematol 1995; 90:892–899.

111. Takano S, Kimura S, Ohdama S, Aoki N. Plasma thrombomodulin in health and diseases. Blood 1990; 76:2024–2029.

112. Karmochkine M, Boffa MC, Piette JC, Cacoub P, Wechsler B, Godeau P, Juhan I, Weiller PJ. Increase in plasma thrombomodulin in lupus erythematosus with antiphospholipid antibodies [Letter]. Blood 1992; 79:837–838.

113. Asakura H, Jokaji H, Saito M, Uotani C, Kumabashiri I, Morishita E, Yamazaki M, Matsuda T. Plasma levels of soluble thrombomodulin increase in cases of disseminated intravascular coagulation with organ failure. Am J Hematol 1991; 38:281–287.

114. Wada H, Ohiwa M, Kaneko T, Tamaki S, Tanigawa M, Shirakawa S, Koyama M, Hayashi T, Suzuki K. Plasma thrombomodulin as a marker of vascular disorders in thrombotic thrombocytopenic purpura and disseminated intravascular coagulation. Am J Hematol 1992; 39:20–24.

115. Laszik ZG, Ferrell G, Silva FG, Esmon CT. Endothelial protein C receptor (EPCR) and thrombomodulin (TM) are downregulated in coronary atherosclerosis. Presented at the United States Academy of Pathology (USCAP) Annual Meeting 1999, (in press).

116. Tsuchida A, Salem H, Thomson N, Hancock WW. Tumor necrosis factor production during human renal allograft rejection is associated with depression of plasma protein C and free protein S levels and decreased intragraft thrombomodulin expression. J Exp Med 1992; 175:81–90.

117. Faust SN, Heyderman RS, Harrison O, et al. Molecular mechanisms of thrombosis in meningococcal septicaemia: the role of the protein C pathway in vivo. Presented at the 2nd Annual Meeting of the British Infection Society, London, April 23, 1999.

118. Heeb MJ, Rosing J, Bakker HM, Fernandez JA, Tans G, Griffin JH. Protein S binds to and inhibits factor Xa Proc Natl Acad Sci USA 1994; 91:2728–2732.

119. Heeb MJ, Mesters RM, Tans G, Rosing J, Griffin JH. Binding of protein S to factor Va associated with inhibition of prothrombinase that is independent of activated protein C. J Biol Chem 1993; 268:2872–2877.

120. Hackeng TM, van't Veer C, Meijers JCM, Bouma BN. Human protein S inhibits prothrombinase complex activity on endothelial cells and platelets via direct interactions with factors Va and Xa. J Biol Chem 1994; 269:21051–21058.

121. Goldberg SL, Orthner CL, Yalisove BL, Elgart ML, Kessler CM. Skin necrosis following prolonged administration of coumarin in a patient with inherited protein S deficiency. Am J Hematol 1991; 38:64–66.

122. Marlar RA, Neumann A. Neonatal purpura fulminans due to homozygous protein C or protein S deficiencies. Semi Thromb Hemost 1990; 16:299–309.

123. Nguyen P, Reynaud J, Pouzol P, Munzer M, Richard O, Francois P. Varicella and thrombotic complications associated with transient protein C and protein S deficiencies in children. Eur J Pediatr 1994; 153:646–649.

124. Smirnov MD, Safa O, Regan L, Mather T, Stearns–Kurosawa DJ, Kurosawa S, Rezaie AR, Esmon NL, Esmon CT. A chimeric protein C containing the prothrombin Gla domain exhibits increased anticoagulant activity and altered phospholipid specificity. J Biol Chem 1998; 273:9031–9040.

125. Yegneswaran S, Smirnov MD, Safa O, Esmon NL, Esmon CT, Johnson AE. Relocating the active site of activated protein C eliminates the need for its protein S cofactor. A fluorescence resonance energy transfer study. J Biol Chem 1999; 274:5462–5468.

126. D'Angelo A, Valle PD, Crippa L, Pattarini E, Grimaldi LME, D'Angelo SV. Brief report: autoimmune protein S deficiency in a boy with severe thromboembolic disease. N Engl J Med 1993; 328:1753–1757.

127. Maury CPJ, Teppo A–M. Circulating tumour necrosis factor alpha (cachectin) in myocardial infarction. J Int Med Res 1989; 225:333–336.

128. Bajaj SP, Rapaport SI, Maki SL, Brown SF. A procedure for isolation of human protein C and protein S as by-products of the purification of factors VII, IX, X, and prothrombin. Prep Biochem 1983; 13:191–214.

129. Varadi K, Philapitsch A, Santa T, Schwarz HP. Activation and inactivation of human protein C by plasmin. Thromb Haemost 1994; 71:615–621.

130. Taoka Y, Okajima K, Uchiba M, Murakami K, Harada N, Johno M, Naruo M. Activated protein C reduces the severity of compression-induced spinal cord injury in rats by inhibiting activation of leukocytes. J Neurosci 1998; 18:1393–1398.

131. Hirose K, Okajima K, Taoka Y, Uchiba M, Tagami H, Nakano K–Y, Utoh J, Okabe H, Kitamura N. Activated protein C reduces the ischemia/reperfusion-induced spinal cord injury in rats by inhibiting neutrophil activation. Ann Surg 2000; 232:272–280.

132. Richardson MA, Gerlitz B, Grinnell BW. Enhancing protein C interaction with thrombin results in a clot-activated anticoagulant. Nature 1992; 360:261–264.

133. Wu Q, Sheehan JP, Tsiang M, Lentz SR, Birktoft JJ, Sadler JE. Single amino acid substitutions dissociate fibrinogen-clotting and thrombomodulin-binding activities of human thrombin. Proc Natl Acad Sci USA 1991; 88:6775–6779.

134. Le Bonniec BF, Esmon CT. Glu-192 → Gln substitution in thrombin mimics the catalytic switch induced by thrombomodulin. Proc Natl Acad Sci USA 1991; 88:7371–7375.

135. Gibbs CS, Coutré SE, Tsiang M, Li WX, Jain AK, Dunn KE, Law VS, Mao CT, Matsumura SY, Mejza SJ, Paborsky LR, Leung LLK. Conversion of thrombin into an anticoagulant by protein engineering. Nature 1995; 378:413–416.

136. Waugh JM, Yuksel E, Li J, Kuo MD, Kattash M, Saxena R, Geske R, Thung SN, Shenaq SM, Woo SL. Local overexpression of thrombomodulin for in vivo prevention of arterial thrombosis in a rabbit model. Circ Res 1999; 84:84–92.

137. Waugh JM, Li-Hawkins J, Yuksel E, Kuo MD, Cifra PN, Hilfiker PR, Geske R, Chawla M, Thomas J, Shenaq SM, Dake MD, Woo SL. Thrombomodulin overexpression to limit neointima formation. Circulation 2000; 102:332–337.

138. Kopp CW, Grey ST, Siegel JB, McShea A, Vetr H, Wrighton CJ, Schulte am Esch J, Bach FH, Robson SC. Expression of human thrombomodulin cofactor activity in porcine endothelial cells. Transplantation 1998; 66:244–251.

139. Esmon CT. The protein C anticoagulation pathway. Arterioscl Thromb © 1992; 12:135. 1992 American Heart Association.

140. Esmon CT. Molecular events that control the protein C anticoagulant pathway. Thromb Haemost 1993; 70:29.

20

Soluble Thrombomodulin

Mitsunobu Mohri

Asahi Kasei Corporation, Oh-hito, Shizuoka, Japan

SUMMARY

Soluble thrombomodulin, a soluble form of human thrombomodulin isolated from urine or produced by recombinant techniques, binds thrombin, inhibits its procoagulant activity, and promotes activation of protein C. Activated protein C inhibits thrombin generation by inactivating factors Va and VIIIa in the presence of protein S. Thus, soluble thrombomodulin attenuates thrombus growth by inhibiting thrombin generation. Intravenous soluble thrombomodulin is effective in animal models of venous thrombosis, disseminated intravascular coagulation (DIC), and arteriovenous shunt thrombosis, and it has a wider safety margin than conventional anticoagulants. The plasma half-life of soluble thrombomodulin is long, especially after subcutaneous injection. In phase II trials, soluble thrombomodulin was well tolerated in patients with DIC. Studies in venous thrombosis are planned. Thus, soluble thrombomodulin is a promising antithrombotic drug.

I. INTRODUCTION

The thrombomodulin–protein C anticoagulant pathway regulates the anticoagulant property of the vascular system [1,2]. Congenital or acquired abnormalities in this pathway are associated with venous and arterial thrombosis [3–9], reflecting the inability to inhibit thrombin activity or to control thrombin generation by activated protein C (APC).

Activated protein C, a serine protease generated when protein C is activated by the thrombin–thrombomodulin complex [1], acts as an anticoagulant by degrading factors Va and VIIIa in the presence of protein S [1,10]. In addition to its anticoagulant effects, activated protein C has anti-inflammatory activity, and suppresses endotoxin-induced tumor necrosis factor (TNF) production and CD11b down-regulation on monocytes [11,12]. Activated protein C has antithrombotic and anti-inflammatory activities in animals [13–16] and in humans [17,18].

Thrombomodulin is a membrane-bound glycoprotein found on the vascular surface of endothelial cells [19–21]. It contains 557 amino acids and is composed of an N-terminal lectin-like domain, six epidermal growth factor (EGF)-like domains, an *O*-glycosylation site-rich domain, a transmembrane domain, and a cytoplasmic domain (Fig. 1) [22]. The EGF-like domains constitute the minimum functional structure of thrombomodulin [23,24]. EGF-like domains 5 and 6 are essential for thrombin binding [25], whereas EGF-like domain 4 is required for protein C activation [26]. EGF-like domain 3 is necessary for activation of procarboxy-peptidase B, a latent carboxypeptidase B-like enzyme [27]. Thrombomodulin binds to thrombin and changes the protease's substrate specificity to protein C from fibrinogen, factors V, VIII, and XIII, and platelets [1,2].

Thrombomodulin binds the anion-binding exosite of thrombin, the site on thrombin that is critical for its interaction with its substrates [2,28,29], and induces allosteric changes in the catalytic center of thrombin that render it a potent activator of protein C [2,29]. Soluble thrombomodulin produced in mammary cells contains the various glycoforms, a high-molecular-weight form, with a chondroitin sulfate side chain, and a low-molecular-weight form, without the side chain. These two forms of thrombomodulin have different pharmacological and pharma-cokinetic properties.

Seven soluble thrombomodulin variants have been described (see Fig. 1), six are recombinant products, and one is a natural soluble form of thrombomodulin isolated from urine. Our group produced recombinant soluble thrombomodulin that comprises the extracellular domains of thrombomodulin (ART-123) in CHO cells. ART-123 is a glycoprotein consisting of 498 amino acids that has a molecular weight of approximately 62,000. ART-123 does not contain chondroitin sulfate [30]. Two groups have independently generated recombinant forms of human soluble thrombomodulin in CHO-K1 cells and U293 cells, respectively. Both contain the extracellular domains with or without chondroitin sulfate and have anticoagulant activity in vitro and in vivo [31–34].

A group developed a recombinant form of human soluble thrombomodulin composed of EGF-like domains 1–6 in insect cells [35]. This agent prevents venous thrombosis in rats, with less effect on global tests of coagulation than equally effective doses of heparin or hirudin [36,37]. Previously, we demonstrated that CHO cell-derived recombinant human soluble thrombomodulin composed of EGF-like domains 4–6 has a short half-life, but prevents

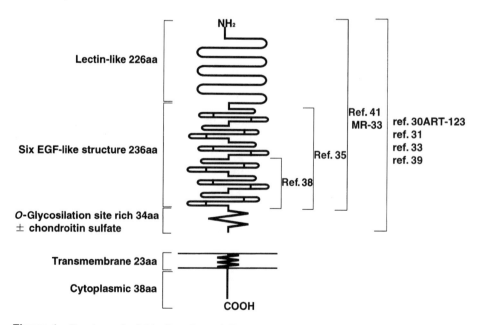

Figure 1 Structure of soluble thrombomodulins.

occlusion of an extracorporeal circuit in monkeys [38]. Chimeric recombinant soluble thrombo-modulin in which the C-terminal was modified with eight amino acids, including a glycosylation site modeled after the sequence of bovine thrombomodulin [39,40], exhibited enhanced anti-coagulant activity in vitro [39]. Soluble thrombomodulin isolated from human urine (MR-33) also exhibits anticoagulant activity in vitro and in vivo [41,42].

Although the various forms of soluble thrombomodulins have yet to be compared, all have anticoagulant activity by virtue of their ability to bind thrombin and promote protein C activation. Soluble thrombomodulin attenuates thrombin generation by inhibiting fibrin-bound thrombin-mediated thrombus growth, and have good efficacy in animals, with a wide therapeutic window. The safety of soluble thrombomodulin may reflect that its anticoagulant activity is exerted only when thrombin is generated. Consequently, soluble thrombomodulin mimics the function of cell-bound thrombomodulin.

ART-123 and MR-33 are undergoing clinical evaluation for the treatment of disseminated intravascular coagulation (DIC) and a phase II trial of ART-123 for thromboprophylaxis in orthopedic patients will soon be initiated.

II. IN VITRO PHARMACOLOGY

A. Interaction of sTM with Thrombin and Protein C

Soluble thrombomodulin (sTM) binds thrombin and alters its substrate specificity such that it prefers protein C to fibrinogen. The catalytic center of thrombin remains accessible when the enzyme is bound to soluble thrombomodulin such that thrombin retains its ability to cleave chromogenic substrates [43]. Thrombomodulin binds to exosite I on thrombin, the substrate-binding site of the enzyme, thereby inhibiting the procoagulant activities of thrombin (Fig. 2). Binding of thrombomodulin to exosite I on thrombin evokes conformational changes in the active site of the enzyme that enhance its ability to activate protein C [29]. Consequently, the anticoagulant activity of soluble thrombomodulin reflects two phenomena, direct thrombin inhibitory activity and indirect activity reflecting protein C activation. The bifunctional property of soluble thrombomodulin complicates dosing because different concentrations are needed to express these effects.

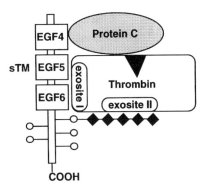

Figure 2 Hypothetical model of the interaction between thrombin and soluble thrombomodulin. EGF4 and 5 of soluble thrombomodulin cover exosite I on thrombin and alter the substrate specificity of thrombin, without affecting its enzymatic activity. EGF6 donates a binding site for protein C. The chondroitin sulfate side chain (◆) provides an additional binding site for thrombin by interacting with exosite II on the enzyme.

The activity of soluble thrombomodulin depends on its source and the extent of glycosylation. ART-123, which is produced in CHO cells, does not contain the chondroitin sulfate side chain. The IC_{50} of ART-123 for inhibition of thrombin-mediated fibrin formation in buffered fibrinogen solution is approximately 1.6 μg/mL, whereas its K_i for this reaction is 22 nM. ART-123 promotes thrombin-mediated protein C activation in a concentration-dependent manner [44] and binds thrombin with an apparent K_d of 4.0 nM in the presence of 2 nM thrombin and 10 μM protein C [44]. Kinetic parameters of the ART-123–thrombin complex-activating protein C were calculated: 5.1 μM for K_m and 48 min^{-1} for k_{cat} [44]. The catalytic efficiency of protein C activation in the presence of ART-123 is 20-fold greater than that in its absence (9.4 and 0.47 μM^{-1} min^{-1}, respectively).

The chondroitin sulfate side chain affects the affinity of thrombomodulin for thrombin and its cofactor activity for protein C activation. High-molecular-weight soluble thrombomodulin that contains the chondroitin sulfate side chain binds thrombin with fivefold higher affinity than soluble thrombomodulin without this chain (K_d values of 2.7 and 16.3 nM, respectively) and its catalytic efficiency of protein C activation is fourfold greater (378 and 84 μM^{-1} min^{-1}, respectively) [33]. Chimeric soluble thrombomodulin, which contains the bovine glycosylation sites, binds thrombin with higher affinity than intact soluble thrombomodulin (K_d values of 2.2 and 27.3 nM, respectively) but activates protein C with similar catalytic efficiency (4.3 and 5.3 μM^{-1} min^{-1}, respectively) [40]. By offering an additional binding site for thrombin, the chondroitin sulfate side chain may more efficiently alter the substrate specificity of bound thrombin (see Fig. 2) [45].

The protein–C-activating activity of soluble thrombomodulin is dependent on the calcium concentration. Calcium is thought to be necessary for the interaction of the thrombin–soluble thrombomodulin complex with the Gla domain of protein C [46]. Aspartate-349 in the fourth EGF-like domain of soluble thrombomodulin is essential for its calcium-mediated binding to protein C [47]. These findings suggest that calcium is an essential cofactor for protein C activation by thrombomodulin.

Soluble thrombomodulin binds to thrombin in a reversible fashion. Once thrombin bound to ART-123 is complexed by antithrombin, ART-123 is recycled to activate additional protein C molecules [48]. ART-123 does not affect the rate of thrombin inactivation by antithrombin [48]. In contrast, high-molecular-weight soluble thrombomodulin increases the rate of thrombin inactivation by antithrombin and heparin cofactor II [49]. This heparin-like activity is mediated by its negatively charged chondroitin sulfate chains [49].

B. Factor Va, Prothrombinase and Thrombin Generation

Prothrombin is converted to thrombin by the prothrombinase complex that comprises factor Xa, factor V, phospholipids, and calcium. Thrombin-activated factor V (factor Va) enhances the rate of thrombin generation by this complex [50]. Thus, the burst of thrombin generation evoked by prothrombinase is preceded by activation of factor V [51], an event that does not occur in factor V-deficient plasma or in plasma supplemented with an inactive form of factor V [52]. These findings suggest that thrombin-mediated factor V activation is an important positive feedback pathway. Soluble thrombomodulin attenuates this feedback pathway by activating protein C, which then inactivates factor Va [53,54].

After addition of tissue factor, calcium and phospholipid, to plasma, thrombin generation increases linearly after a lag period of 2 min and peaks at 5 min (Fig. 3). The addition of ART-123 or activated protein C produces concentration-dependent attenuation of thrombin generation. In contrast, direct thrombin inhibitors, such as hirudin or argatroban, delay the time to peak thrombin generation (see Fig. 3). These results suggest that ART-123 and activated protein C

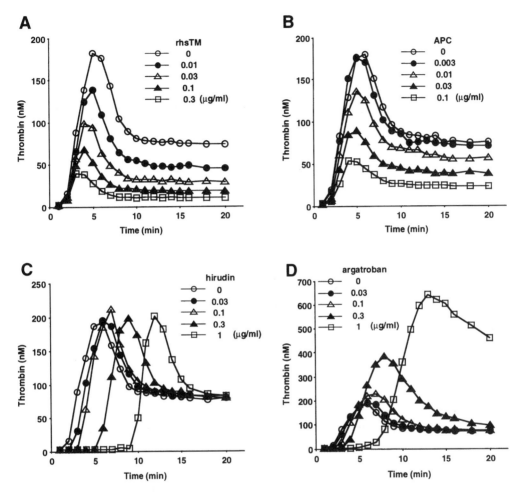

Figure 3 Effects of ART-123 and various anticoagulants on diluted tissue–factor-induced thrombin generation in plasma. The thrombin activity was determined using a chromogenic substrate. (A) ART-123 (rhsTM); (B) APC; (C) hirudin; (D) argatroban. (From Ref. 53.)

reduce the rate of thrombin generation during the propagation phase, but do not affect the initiation phase (see Fig. 3). This concept is supported by data indicating that the initial phase of thrombin generation does not require the active form of factor V [52]. Thus, small amounts of thrombin are generated by factor Xa in the presence of factor V, which is resistant to activated protein C. Once sufficient amounts of thrombin are generated to activate factor V, the propagation phase begins. Hirudin and argatroban prolong the lag phase because they inhibit factor V activation by thrombin. In contrast, soluble thrombomodulin and activated protein C affect only the propagation phase because they inactivate factor Va, but have no effect on factor V.

The IC_{50} of ART-123 in this system is 0.034 µg/mL. ART-123, which is among the most potent of the anticoagulants tested (Table 1), decreases factor Va and prothrombinase activity in plasma in a concentration-dependent manner [53]. The IC_{50} of ART-123 for factor Va and prothrombinase is 0.052 and 0.023 µg/mL, respectively. The effect of ART-123 on thrombin

Table 1 IC_{50} Values of Anticoagulants for TF-Induced Thrombin Generation in Plasma

Anticoagulants	IC_{50}	
ART-123	0.034 µg/ml	6.6×10^{-10} M
APC	0.030 µg/ml	4.9×10^{-10} M
Hirudin	0.15 µg/ml	2.1×10^{-8} M
Argatroban	0.58 µg/ml	1.1×10^{-6} M
Heparin	0.037 U/ml	2.0×10^{-8} M
Fragmin	0.065 IU/ml	8.3×10^{-8} M

Source: Ref. 46 with permission.

generation is abolished in protein C-deficient plasma [53,55] indicating that protein C is essential for its activity.

Whether soluble thrombomodulin has effects on factor VIIIa, a component of intrinsic tenase, in the same way as it does factor Va remains unclear. Activated protein C inactivates factor VIIIa [2,56], but factor Va is the preferred substrate [56]. Moreover, neither activated protein C nor thrombomodulin influences factor Xa generation or factor VIIIa degradation in the reconstituted model [57]. These results suggest that factor Va inactivation is critical for the inhibition of thrombin generation by soluble thrombomodulin.

C. Clotting Time

ART-123 produces concentration-dependent prolongation of the prothrombin time, activated partial thromboplastin time (APTT), and the factor Xa- and thrombin-clotting times, indicating a global anticoagulant effect [53]. The concentration of ART-123 required for doubling the various clotting times is 500 times higher than that needed for inhibition of thrombin generation. Prolongation of the APTT by ART-123 is somewhat dependent on plasma protein C levels [58]. The concentration of ART-123 necessary to double the thrombin-clotting time is over 500-fold lower than that required to double the APTT. In contrast, the concentrations of other anticoagulants needed to double the thrombin clotting times are only 2- to 15-fold lower than those necessary to double the APTT (Table 2). It is likely that soluble thrombomodulin has little effect on the APTT or prothrombin time because factor V activation is not necessary when clotting is

Table 2 In Vitro Safety Margin of Anticoagulants: Ratio of APTT (EC_{double}) to Thrombin Generation (IC_{50})

Anticoagulants	APTT (EC_{double})	Thrombin generation (IC_{50})	Ratio (APTT/thrombin generation)
ART-123 (µg/ml)	18	0.034	530
APC (µg/ml)	1.1	0.030	37
Hirudin (µg/ml)	0.43	0.15	2.9
Argatroban (µg/ml)	1.3	0.58	2.2
Heparin (U/ml)	0.41	0.037	11
Fragmin (U/ml)	0.94	0.065	14

Source: Ref. 46.

rapidly induced by high concentrations of initiators [52]. This concept is supported by the observation that soluble thrombomodulin is a potent anticoagulant in thromboelastography, a slow-clotting system.

High-molecular-weight soluble thrombomodulin, which contains the chondroitin sulfate side chain, has more potent anticoagulant activity than derivatives lacking this side chain [31,33]. The greater anticoagulant effect of high-molecular soluble thrombomodulin is antithrombin-mediated and is attenuated when the thrombomodulin is treated with chondroitinase [31].

D. Platelet Aggregation

Soluble thrombomodulin inhibits thrombin-mediated platelet aggregation in a concentration-dependent manner [33,59], with an IC_{50} of 1.5 µg/mL—a value 44-fold higher than the IC_{50} for inhibition of thrombin generation (Table 3), but similar to the IC_{50} for thrombin-induced fibrin formation (1.6 µg/mL). ART-123 has no effect on ADP or collagen-induced platelet aggregation. In contrast to ART-123, hirudin, argatroban, heparin, and dalteparin inhibit thrombin-induced platelet aggregation, with IC_{50} values similar to those for inhibition of thrombin generation (see Table 3).

E. Species Specificity

ART-123 and high-molecular-weight soluble thrombomodulin prolong the APTT in human, monkey, and rat plasma, but not in rabbit plasma [58]. ART-123 activates protein C and inactivates factor Va to a similar extent in human and monkey plasma, but has little activity in rat plasma [58]. Although isolated rat protein C is activated by the thrombin–thrombomodulin complex [60], its rate of activation with soluble thrombomodulin is less than that of its human counterpart [54]. *Agkistrodon* venom also fails to activate rat protein C [61], raising the possibility that rat plasma contains an inhibitor of protein C activation [58, 61].

F. Influence of Plasma Factors and Other Anticoagulants

Soluble thrombomodulin needs protein C and protein S to exert its anticoagulant activity. The effect of ART-123 on thrombin generation is influenced by the level of protein C and protein S, but not by the level of antithrombin (Fig. 4).

Factor V Leiden, a point mutation in the gene encoding for factor V [62], is the most common inherited risk factor for thrombosis in white persons [4,5,63]. Once activated, factor V Leiden is resistant to inactivation by activated protein C [62–65]. ART-123 has a normal

Table 3 In Vitro Safety Margin of Anticoagulants: Ratio of Platelet Aggregation (IC_{50}) to Thrombin Generation (IC_{50})

Anticoagulants	Platelet aggregation (IC_{50})	Thrombin generation (IC_{50})	Ratio (Platelet aggregation/ thrombin generation)
ART-123 (µg/ml)	1.5	0.034	44
Hirudin (µg/ml)	0.028	0.15	0.19
Argatroban (µg/ml)	0.054	0.58	0.093
Heparin (U/ml)	0.08	0.037	2.2
Fragmin (U/ml)	0.16	0.065	2.5

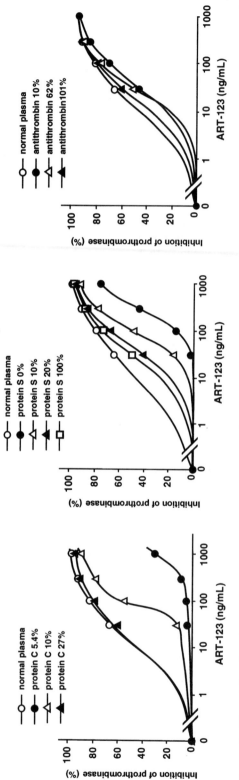

Figure 4   The activity of prothrombinase was measured in plasma containing ART-123 and various concentrations of (*left*) protein C, (*middle*) protein S, and (*right*) antithrombin. (From Ref. 44.)

inhibitory effect on prothrombinase activity in plasma from volunteers with heterozygous factor V Leiden (data not shown). However, the effect of soluble thrombomodulin on endogenous thrombin potential [66] is decreased in plasma from subjects who are heterozygous for the factor V Leiden mutation [67]. Although cleavage of factor Va at Arg^{506} is rate-limiting, it is not a critical step for factor Va inactivation by activated protein C [65]. Activated protein C eventually inactivates factor Va Leiden by cleaving at Arg^{306}, and subsequently at Arg^{679} [65]. Cleavage at Arg^{506} is no longer the rate-limiting step with high concentrations of soluble thrombomodulin [68].

The influence of heparin on the anticoagulant effect of soluble thrombomodulin is controversial. The rate of APC inactivation by protein C inhibitor increases in the presence of heparin [69]. Heparin and (LMWH) reduce the affinity of soluble thrombomodulin for thrombin, thereby decreasing the rate of protein C activation [70]. Conversely, the anticoagulant activity of activated protein C is potentiated by dermatan sulfate, LMWH heparin [71], or heparin [72].

Tissue factor pathway inhibitor (TFPI) regulates coagulation by inhibiting factor VIIa within the factor VIIa–tissue factor complex in a FXa-dependent manner [73]. Soluble thrombomodulin and TFPI act synergistically to inhibit thrombin generation [68].

Aprotinin, a broad-spectrum serine protease inhibitor, also inhibits activated protein C [74] and interferes with chromogenic substrate assays for activated protein C [75]. Consequently, aprotinin may attenuate the activity of soluble thrombomodulin.

G. Inhibitory Effect of sTM on Extension of Growing Thrombi

Fibrin-bound thrombin has the potential to promote clot growth [76]. It activates factor V, thereby amplifying thrombin generation and shortening the clotting time [77]. In addition, fibrin-bound thrombin is less sensitive to inactivation by the antithrombin–heparin complex than is fluid-phase thrombin [78,79]. Soluble thrombomodulin binds to exosite I on thrombin, the same site as that to which fibrin binds. This may explain why ART-123 binds only 2–5% of fibrin-bound thrombin and why ART-123 is unable to inhibit fibrin formation induced by fibrin-bound thrombin [43]. However, ART-123 enhances protein C activation in this system, thereby attenuating thrombin generation, fibrinopeptide A production and thrombus accretion [43]. The effect of ART-123 on fibrin-bound thrombin is abolished by the addition of antibody against protein C [43], indicating that soluble thrombomodulin inhibits thrombin in a protein C-dependent fashion.

III. IN VIVO PHARMACOLOGY

A. Effects of sTM in DIC Models

Disseminated intravascular coagulation (DIC) is a syndrome characterized by activation of coagulation, generation of intravascular fibrin and consumption of coagulation factors [80]. It is a frequent complication of sepsis or malignancy. Endotoxin down-regulates the expression of thrombomodulin on endothelial cells [81]. Moreover, protein C levels are reduced in patients with terminal sepsis [3]. These findings suggest that agents that augment the protein C anticoagulant pathway may be effective in sepsis or DIC.

Several reports suggest that soluble thrombomodulin attenuates tissue factor- or endotoxin-induced DIC in rats [32,41,42,82,83]. Soluble thrombomodulin administration blocks endotoxin-induced fibrin deposition in kidney glomeruli [42,83]. Soluble thrombomodulin also inhibits tissue factor-induced DIC in rats with decreased levels of antithrombin. In contrast, heparin is less effective when antithrombin levels are reduced [84,85].

The effects of soluble thrombomodulin in these rat models reflect primarily its ability to inhibit thrombin, rather than its capacity to activate protein C, because soluble thrombomodulin is unable to activate rat protein C [54,58]. The effective concentration of soluble thrombomodulin in rats is about $20\,\mu g/mL$, a level higher than that needed to inhibit thrombin generation (IC_{50}: $34\,ng/mL$), but sufficient to directly block thrombin activity.

To evaluate the protein C-activating activity of ART-123, the drug was given to monkeys infused with tissue factor [58]. Both ART-123 and heparin blocked the decrease in fibrinogen and platelets and the increase in levels of fibrin(ogen) degradation products (FDP) [58]. ART-123 produced a concentration-dependent decrease in the levels of thrombin–antithrombin complexes (TAT), whereas heparin did not [58]. At higher doses ($1\,mg/kg$), ART-123 prolonged the APTT more than expected based on its anticoagulant effects in vitro [58]. These findings suggest that by activating protein C, ART-123 prevents DIC by inhibiting the generation of thrombin. In contrast, heparin acts by inhibiting thrombin activity.

The dose-response with ART-123 is different from that with heparin in the monkey DIC model [58]. The dose–response with ART-123 is relatively smaller and biphasic: that with heparin is steep and linear. The effect of lower doses of ART-123 ($0.01–0.1\,mg/kg$) is mediated predominantly by its protein C-activating activity, whereas higher doses ($1\,mg/kg$) have additional thrombin inhibitory activity.

B. Effects of sTM in Thrombosis Models

Soluble thrombomodulin inhibits venous thrombosis in rats [36,37] and thrombosis in arteriovenous (AV) shunts in rats [86] and baboons [87], with a smaller effect on the bleeding time than other anticoagulants. In baboons, ART-123 prevented platelet and fibrin deposition on Dacron grafts, with less effect on the bleeding than argatroban [86]. Although activated protein C levels decreased with ART-123, the antithrombotic effect of ART-123 was abolished by administration of an antibody against protein C [86]. These findings appear at odds with the observation that ART-123 produces concentration-dependent activation of protein C in vitro [44]. However, the rate at which protein C is activated depends not only on the ART-123 concentration, but also on the thrombin concentration. Because ART-123 also inhibits thrombin generation, circulating levels of activated protein C decrease once ART-123 blocks thrombin generation. This concept is supported by the fact that ART-123 decreases TAT levels in this model [87]. These findings raise the possibility that activated protein C formed at the site of thrombin generation, reduces thrombosis.

C. Other In Vivo Effects

Soluble thrombomodulin prevents endotoxin-induced pulmonary injury [88,89], attenuates ischemia–reperfusion injury in the canine liver [90], and reduces posthepatectomy liver dysfunction in cirrhotic rats [91]. Soluble thrombomodulin also inhibits thrombin-induced neuronal cell death in vitro [92] and reduces motor disturbances caused by trauma-induced spinal cord injury [93]. An antibody against the epidermal growth factor-like structures of soluble thrombomodulin abolishes the effects of soluble thrombomodulin. The benefits of soluble thrombomodulin in these settings raises the possibility that it may have anti-inflammatory properties.

ART-123 can promote thrombin-mediated activation of procarboxypeptidase B in human or rat plasma [38]. Carboxypeptidase B is one of the exopeptidases that inactivate bradykinin [94,95] and possibly C5a, potent mediators of inflammation [94–96]. Once activated, procarboxypeptidase B also attenuates fibrinolysis by cleaving C-terminal lysine residues from fibrin, thereby reducing plasminogen–plasmin binding [97,98].

Although ART-123 inhibits plasmin-mediated fibrinolysis in vitro, inhibition of fibrinolysis has not been observed in vivo. Likely, procarboxypeptidase B is activated by thrombin bound to endothelial thrombomodulin. If this mechanism is saturated, ART-123 would not produce further activation of procarboxypeptidase B.

Activated protein C also has anti-inflammatory activity. It inhibits the responses of monocytes to inflammatory mediators by its specific receptor [11,99]. Both activated protein C and protein C inhibit endotoxin-induced and *Escherichia coli*-induced inflammatory changes in rats and baboons, respectively [15,16]. These findings suggest that soluble thrombomodulin may have anti-inflammatory activity in addition to its anticoagulant effects.

IV. PHARMACOKINETICS

The half-life of soluble thrombomodulin is dependent on not only its amino acid sequence, but also on its carbohydrate content. The half-life of low-molecular-weight soluble thrombomodulin variants (e.g., ART-123) in rats is 5–7 h [32,86]. In contrast, the high-molecular-weight form has a half-life of only 20 min [32]. If high-molecular-weight soluble thrombomodulin is treated with chondroitinase, its half-life is prolonged, suggesting that clearance is enhanced when the chondroitin sulfate side chain is present [32].

At doses of 1 or 3 mg/kg, the elimination pattern for soluble thrombomodulin is linear [86]. Its half-life in monkeys [58] and baboons [87] is similar to that in rats. A thrombomodulin variant containing the last three epidermal growth factor-like structures (E456) has an initial half-life of only 9 min in monkeys [38]. Thrombomodulin comprises 16 fewer amino acids than ART-123 has a shorter half-life than intact ART-123 [100], suggesting that the half-life of ART-123 is attributable not only to the D1 domain (N-terminal lectin-like domain) but also to the D3 domain (*O*-glycosylation site-rich domain). The half-life of MR-33 is shorter than that of ART-123 [41], likely reflecting its different carbohydrate content.

ART-123 has good bioavailability after subcutaneous injection [74–108%) and a long half-life (16–28 h) in monkeys (Fig. 5). The time to reach C_{max} is about 24 h, suggesting a slow rate of absorption from the subcutaneous injection site.

V. TOXICOLOGY

Acute and chronic toxicity studies have been performed with ART-123 in rats and monkeys. High and frequent doses of ART-123 cause bleeding in these animals. The dose that causes bleeding is lower in monkeys than in rats, reflecting species specificity. Aside from changes in hemostatic parameters, no other toxicity was observed.

ART-123 prolongs the bleeding time in rats at doses of more than 4 mg/kg (estimated plasma concentration, 70 µg/mL) [86]. This dose is higher than that required to prevent thrombosis in arteriovenous shunts [86]. Other reports suggest that soluble thrombomodulin has a wider therapeutic window in rats than heparin or hirudin [37]. At doses of 1 mg/kg (plasma concentration, 17 µg/mL 60 min after injection), ART-123 prolonged the APTT in monkeys with tissue factor-induced DIC [58]. ART-123 also prolonged the bleeding time in baboons at a dose of 1 mg/kg (plasma concentration, 14 µg/mL 60 min after injection) [87]. These results suggest that the ART-123 concentration should be maintained below 10 µg/mL to prevent bleeding. In humans, the plasma concentration of ART-123 effective for DIC was less than 2 µg/mL. No bleeding was reported.

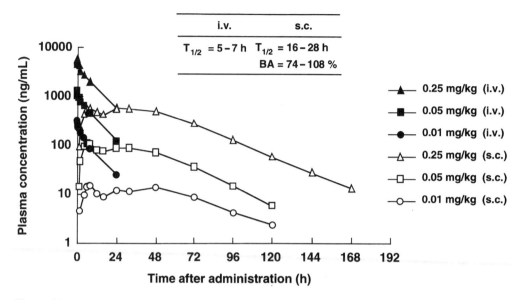

Figure 5 The elimination patterns of ART-123 after intravenous and subcutaneous injection. Monkeys were administered the indicated doses of ART-123 and the plasma concentrations were determined by ELISA. (From Ref. 44.)

VI. CLINICAL STUDIES

A. Phase I Studies

Two forms of soluble thrombomodulin (ART-123 and MR-33) have been evaluated. In a single-dose phase I study, ART-123, at doses of 0.03, 0.1, and 0.3 mg, was infused intravenously over 2 h into healthy volunteers [101]. In a multiple-dose study, 0.2 mg of ART-123 was infused intravenously over 2 h once daily for 3 days [101]. The plasma concentration of ART-123 was measured by enzyme immunoassay [86].

There was no evidence of bleeding, and ART-123 had no effect on coagulation tests or bleeding times [101]. The plasma alpha and beta half-life of ART-123 is 2.92–3.97 and 17.75–20.48 h, respectively. More than 50% is excreted into the urine within 48 h of administration [101]. In the multiple-dose study, the elimination pattern of ART-123 fitted the simulation curve calculated from the plasma concentration profile on day 1 [101]. Thus, there was no evidence of accumulation on repeated dosing.

Thrombomodulin is readily oxidized at a critical methionine residue by hydrogen peroxide or activated neutrophils. Once oxidized thrombomodulin loses its ability to activate protein C [102,103]. Consequently, plasma levels of ART-123 determined by enzyme immunoassay may overestimate the anticoagulant activity of ART-123. Clotting times, the conventional method for monitoring anticoagulant activity, were not prolonged by the doses of ART-123 used in these studies. Instead, a "prothrombinase assay" was developed. This assay is sensitive to the plasma concentration of ART-123, as well as to those of protein C and protein S [9]. Prothrombinase activity decreased by 50% after injection of 0.3 mg ART-123 and gradually increased to normal levels [104]. Inhibition of prothrombinase persisted for 48 h, and was similar to the inhibition produced by the same concentration of ART-123 in vitro [104]. These findings suggest that ART-123 has a prolonged anticoagulant effect.

In animals, ART-123 has a longer half-life after subcutaneous injection. Although the reason for the longer half-life of ART-123 in humans is unclear, this property may be advantageous for treatment or prophylaxis of thrombotic diseases.

B. Phase II Studies

The effect of soluble thrombomodulin (ART-123 and MR-33) in DIC is being evaluated in two phase II trials that are being conducted in Japan [17,105]. In an initial open-lable study, ART-123, at doses of 0.006, 0.02 and 0.06 mg/kg, produced an apparent dose–response without causing bleeding. Double-blind trials evaluating the effect of ART-123 or MR-33 in DIC are now underway [17,105]. In addition, a phase II trial evaluating the efficacy of ART-123 for thromboprophylaxis after major orthopedic surgery will soon be started.

VII. CONCLUSIONS AND FUTURE DIRECTIONS

Soluble thrombomodulin is a unique anticoagulant that acts both by activating protein C and by neutralizing thrombin. ART–123 has a long half-life after subcutaneous injection, and phase II trials with this agent in DIC are promising. The usefulness of ART-123 and other soluble thrombomodulin variants for prevention and treatment of venous thrombosis needs to be investigated. In addition to its anticoagulant activity, soluble thrombomodulin also has anti-inflammatory activity. In a phase III trial, activated protein C was well-tolerated and reduced mortality in patients with sepsis [18]. These results raise the possibility that soluble thrombo-modulin also may be effective for the treatment of sepsis.

REFERENCES

1. Esmon CT. The regulation of natural anticoagulant pathways. Science 1987; 235:1348–1352.
2. Esmon CT. The roles of protein C and thrombomodulin in the regulation of blood coagulation. J Biol Chem 1989; 264:4743–4746.
3. Esmon CT, Schwarz HP. An update on clinical and basic aspects of the protein C anticoagulant pathway. Trends Cardiovasc Med 1995; 5:141–148.
4. Koster T, Rosendaal FR, de Ronde H, Briet E, Vandenbroucke JP, Bertina RM. Venous thrombosis due to poor anticoagulant response to activated protein C: Leiden thrombophilia study. Lancet 1993; 342:1503–1506.
5. Ridker PM, Hennekens CH, Lindpainter K, Stampfer MJ, Eisenberg PR, Miletich JP. Mutation in the gene coding for coagulation factor V and the risk of myocardial infarction, stroke, and venous thrombosis in apparently healthy man. N Engl J Med 1995; 332:912–917.
6. Emmerich J, Poirier O, Evans A, Marques–Vidal P, Arveiler D, Luc G, Aiach M, Cambien F. Myocardial infarction, Arg 506 to Gln factor V mutation, and activated protein C resistance. Lancet 1995; 345:321.
7. Galli M, Duca F, Ruggeri L, Finazzi G, Negri B, Moia M. Congenital resistance to activated protein C in patients with lupus anticoagulants: evaluation of two functional assays. Thromb Haemost 1998; 80:246–249.
8. Lindoff C, Ingemarsson I, Martinsson G, Segelmark M, Thysell H, Astedt B. Preeclampsia is associated with a reduced response to activated protein C. Am J Obstet Gynecol 1997; 176:457–460.
9. Mohri M, Sata M, Gomi K, Maruyama Y, Osame M, Maruyama I. Abnormalities in the protein C anticoagulant pathway detected by a novel assay using human thrombomodulin. Lupus 1997; 6:590–596.

10. Kaiser B, Jeske W, Hoppensteadt DH, Walenga JM, Drohan W, Fareed J. In vitro studies on the effect of activated protein C on platelet activation and thrombin generation. Thromb Res 1997; 87:197–204.

11. Grey ST, Hau H, Salem HH, Hancock WW. Selective effects of protein C on activation of human monocytes by lipopolysaccharide, interferon-gamma, or PMA: modulation of effects on CD11b and CD14 but not CD25 or CD54 induction. Transplant Proc 1993; 25:2913–2914.

12. Grey ST, Tsuchida A, Hau H, Orthner CL, Salem HH, Hancock WW. Selective inhibitory effects on the anticoagulant activated protein C on the response of human mononuclear phagocytes to LPS, IFN-gamma, or phorbol ester. J Immunol 1994; 153:3664–3672.

13. Gruber A, Hanson SR, Kelly AB, Yan BS, Bang N, Griffin JH, Harker LA. Inhibition of thrombus formation by activated protein C in a primate model of arterial thrombosis. Circulation 1990; 82:578–585.

14. Hanson SR, Griffin JH, Harker LA, Kelly AB, Esmon CT, Gruber A. Antithrombotic effects of thrombin-induced activation of endogenous protein C in primates. J Clin Invest 1993; 92:2003–2012.

15. Taylor FB Jr, Chang A, Esmon CT, D'Angelo A, Vigano–D'Angelo S, Blick KE. Protein C prevents the coagulopathic and lethal effects of *E. coli* infusion in the baboon. J Clin Invest 1987; 79:918–925.

16. Murakami K, Okajima K, Uchiba M, Johno M, Nakagaki T, Okabe H, Takatsuki K. Activated protein C attenuates endotoxin-induced pulmonary vascular injury by inhibiting activated leukocytes in rats. Blood 1996; 87:642–647.

17. Maruyama I. Recombinant thrombomodulin and activated protein C in the treatment of disseminated intravascular coagulation. Thromb Haemost 1999; 82:718–721.

18. Fisher CJ, LaRosa SP, Helterbrand JD. Recombinant human activated protein C improves coagulation abnormalities, morbidity and 28 day mortality in patients with severe sepsis [abstr]. J Antimicrob Chemother 1999; 44(suppl. A):10.

19. Esmon CT, Owen WG. Identification of an endothelial cofactor for thrombin-catalyzed activation of protein C. Proc Natl Acad Sci USA 1981: 78:2249–2252.

20. Salem HH, Maruyama I, Ishii H, Majerus PW. Isolation and characterization of thrombomodulin from human placenta. J Biol Chem 1984; 259:12246–12251.

21. Maruyama I, Bell CE, Majerus PW. Thrombomodulin is found on endothelium of arteries, veins, capillaries, and lymphatics, and on syncytiophoblast of human placenta. J Biol Chem 1985; 101:363–371.

22. Suzuki K, Kusumoto H, Deyashiki Y, Nishioka J, Maruyama I, Zushi M, Kawahara S, Honda G, Yamamoto S, Horiguchi S. Structure and expression of human thrombomodulin, a thrombin receptor on endothelium acting as a cofactor for protein C activation. EMBO J 1987; 6:1891–1897.

23. Suzuki K, Hayashi T, Nishioka J, Kosaka Y, Zushi M, Honda G, Yamamoto S. A domain composed of epidermal growth factor-like structures of human thrombomodulin is essential for thrombin binding and for protein C activation. J Biol Chem 1989; 264:4872–4876.

24. Zushi M, Gomi K, Yamamoto S, Maruyama I, Hayashi T, Suzuki K. The last three consecutive epidermal growth factor-like structures of human thrombomodulin comprise the minimum functional domain for protein C-activating cofactor activity and anticoagulant activity. J Biol Chem 1989; 264:10351–10353.

25. Tolkatchev D, Ng A, Zhu B, Ni F. Identification of a thrombin-binding region in the sixth epidermal growth factor-like repeat of human thrombomodulin. Biochemistry 2000; 39:10365–10372.

26. Tsiang M, Lentz SR, Sadler JE. Functional domains of membrane-bound human thrombomodulin. EGF-like domains four to six and the serine/threonine-rich domain are required for cofactor activity. J Biol Chem 1992; 267:6164–6167.

27. Wang W, Nagashima M, Schneider M, Morser J, Nesheim M. Elements of the primary structure of thrombomodulin required for efficient thrombin-activable fibrinolysis inhibitor activation. J Biol Chem 2000; 275:22942–22947.

28. Suzuki K, Nishioka J. A thrombin-based peptide corresponding to the sequence of the thrombomodulin-binding site blocks the procoagulant activities of thrombin. J Biol Chem 1991; 266:18498–18501.

29. Fuentes–Prior P, Iwanaga Y, Huber R, Pagila R, Rumennik G, Seto M, Morser J, Light DR, Bode W. Structural basis for the anticoagulant activity of the thrombin–thrombomodulin complex. Nature 2000; 404:518–525.

30. Gomi K, Zushi M, Honda G, Kawahara S, Matsuzaki O, Kanabayashi T, Yamamoto S, Maruyama I, Suzuki K. Antithrombotic effect of recombinant human thrombomodulin on thrombin-induced thromboembolism in mice. Blood 1990; 75:1396–1399.

31. Nawa K, Sakano K, Fujisawa, Sato Y, Sugiyama N, Teruuchi T, Iwamoto M, Marumoto Y. Presence and functions of chondroitin-4-sulfate on recombinant human thrombomodulin. Biochem Biophys Res Commun 1990; 171:729–737.

32. Nawa K, Itani T, Ono M, Sakano K, Marumoto Y, Iwamoto M. The glycosaminoglycan of recombinant human soluble thrombomodulin affects antithrombotic activity in a rat model of tissue factor-induced disseminated intravascular coagulation. Thromb Haemost 1992; 67:366–370.

33. Parkinson JF, Grinnell BW, Moore RE, Hoskins J, Vlahos CJ, Bang NU. Stable expression of a secretable deletion mutant of recombinant human thrombomodulin in mammalian cells. J Biol Chem 1990; 265:12602–12610.

34. Parkinson JF, Vlahos CJ, Yan BSC, Bang NU. Recombinant human thrombomodulin. Regulation of cofactor activity and anticoagulant function by a glycosaminoglycan side chain. Biochem J 1992; 283:151–157.

35. Parkinson JF, Nagashima M, Kuhn I, Leonard J, Morser J. Structure–function studies of the epidermal growth factor domains of human thrombomodulin. Biochem Biophys Res Commun 1992; 185:567–576.

36. Solis MM, Cook C, Cook J, Glaser C, Light D, Morser J, Yu S, Fink L, Eidt JF. Intravenous recombinant soluble human thrombomodulin prevents venous thrombosis in a rat model. J Vasc Surg 1991; 14:599–604.

37. Solis MM, Vitti M, Cook J, Young D, Glaser C, Light D, Morser J, Wydro R, Yu S, Fink L, Eidt JF. Recombinant soluble human thrombomodulin: a randomized, blinded assessment of prevention of venous thrombosis and effects on hemostatic parameters in a rat model. Thromb Res 1994; 73:385–394.

38. Suzuki M, Mohri M, Yamamoto S. In vitro anticoagulant properties of a minimum functional fragment of human thrombomodulin and in vivo demonstration of its benefit as an anticoagulant in extracorporeal circulation using a monkey model. Thromb Haemost 1998; 79:417–422.

39. Edano T, Kumai N, Mizoguchi T, Ohkuchi M. The glycosylation sites and structural characteristics of oligosaccharides on recombinant human thrombomodulin. Int J Biochem Cell Biol 1998; 30:77–88.

40. Edano T, Inoue K, Yoshizaki H, Yamamoto S, Komine N, Tabunoki H, Sawada H, Koshi T, Murakami A, Wada Y, Ohkuchi M. Increased anticoagulant activity of recombinant thrombomodulin modified with glycosaminoglycan. Biol Pharm Bull 1998; 21:375–381.

41. Takahashi Y, Hosaka Y, Niina H, Nagasawa K, Naotsuka M, Sakai K, Uemura A. Soluble thrombomodulin purified from human urine exhibits a potent anticoagulant effect in vitro and in vivo. Thromb Haemost 1995; 73:805–811.

42. Takahashi Y, Hosaka Y, Imada K, Adachi T, Niina H, Watanabe M, Mochizuki H. Human urinary soluble thrombomodulin (MR-33) improves disseminated intravascular coagulation without affecting bleeding time in rats: comparison with low molecular weight heparin. Thromb Haemost 1997; 77:789–795.

43. Mohri M, Suzuki M, Sugimoto E, Sata M, Yamamoto S, Maruyama I. Effects of recombinant human soluble thrombomodulin (rhs-TM) on clot-induced coagulation in human plasma. Thromb Haemost 1998; 80:925–929.

44. Mohri M. ART-123: Recombinant human soluble thrombomodulin. Cardiovasc Drug Rev 2000; 18:312–325.

45. Parkinson JF, Koyama T, Bang NU, Preissner KT. Thrombomodulin: An anticoagulant cell surface proteoglycan with physiologically relevant glycosaminoglycan moiety. Adv Exp Med Biol 313; 177–188, 1992.

46. Kurosawa S, Galvin JB, Esmon NL, Esmon CT. Proteolytic formation and properties of functional domains of thrombomodulin. J Biol Chem 1987; 262:2206–2212.

47. Zushi M, Gomi K, Honda G, Kondo S, Yamamoto S, Hayashi T, Suzuki K. Aspartic acid 349 in the fourth epidermal growth factor-like structure of human thrombomodulin plays a role in its Ca^{2+}-mediated binding to protein C. J Biol Chem 1991; 266:19886–19889.

48. Aritomi M, Watanabe N, Ohishi R, Gomi K, Kiyota T, Yamamoto S, Ishida T, Maruyama I. Recombinant human soluble thrombomodulin delivers bounded thrombin to antithrombin III: thrombomodulin associates with free thrombin and is recycled to activate protein C. Thromb Haemost 1993; 70:418–422.

49. Koyama T, Parkinson JF, Sie P, Bang NU, Muller–Berghaus G, Preissner KT. Different glycoforms of human thrombomodulin. Their glycosaminoglycan-dependent modulatory effects on thrombin inactivation by heparin cofactor II and antithrombin III. Eur J Biochem 1991; 198:563–570.

50. Rosing J, Tans G. Coagulation factor V: an old star shines again. Thromb Haemost 1997; 78:427–433.

51. Rand MD, Lock JB, van't Veer C, Gaffney DP, Mann KG. Blood clotting in minimally altered whole blood. Blood 1996; 88:3432–3445.

52. Thorelli E, Kaufman RJ, Dahlback B. Cleavage requirements of factor V in tissue-factor induced thrombin generation. Thromb Haemost 1998; 80:92–98.

53. Mohri M, Sugimoto E, Sata M, Asano T. The inhibitory effect of recombinant human soluble thrombomodulin on initiation and extension in coagulation: a comparison with other anticoagulants. Thromb Haemost 1999; 82:1687–1693.

54. Takahashi Y, Hosaka Y, Imada K, Adachi T, Niina H, Mochizuki H. Species specificity of the anticoagulant activity of human urinary soluble thrombomodulin. Thromb Res 1988; 89:187–197

55. Ohishi R, Watanabe N, Aritomi M, Gomi K, Kiyota T, Yamamoto S, Ishida T, Maruyama I. Evidence that the protein C activation pathway amplifies the inhibition of thrombin generation by recombinant human thrombomodulin in plasma. Thromb Haemost 1993; 70:423–426.

56. Lu D, Kalafatis M, Mann KG, Long GL. Comparison of activated protein C/protein S-mediated inactivation of human factor VIII and factor V. Blood 1996; 87:4708–4717.

57. van't Veer C, Golden NJ, Kalafatis M, Mann KG. Inhibitory mechanism of the protein C pathway on tissue factor-induced thrombin generation: synergistic effect in combination with tissue factor pathway inhibitor. J Biol Chem 1997; 272:7983–7994.

58. Mohri M, Gonda Y, Oka M, Aoki Y, Gomi K, Kiyota T, Sugihara T, Yamamoto S, Ishida T, Maruyama I. The antithrombotic effects of recombinant human soluble thrombomodulin (rhsTM) on tissue factor-induced disseminated intravascular coagulation in crab-eating monkeys (*Macaca fascicularis*). Blood Coagul Fibrinol 1997; 8:274–283.

59. Esmon NL, Carroll RC, Esmon CT. Thrombomodulin blocks the ability of thrombin to activate platelets. J Biol Chem 1983; 258:12238–12242.

60. Kimura M, Kurosawa–Ohsawa K, Takahashi M, Koyama M, Tanaka S, Matsuishi T. Purification of rabbit, rat and mouse protein C with the use of monoclonal antibody to human protein C, PC01. Thromb Res 1992; 67:687–696.

61. Kogan AE, Makarov AN, Bobruskin ID, Strukova SM. Comparative study of protein C activators from the Agkistrodon snake venoms. Thromb Res 1991; 62:775–780.

62. Bertina RM, Koeleman BP, Koster T, Rosendaal FR, Dirven RJ, de Ronde H, van der Velden PA, Reitsma PH. Mutation in blood coagulation factor V associated with resistance to activated protein C. Nature 1994; 369:64–67.

63. Rees DC, Cox M, Clegg JB. World distribution of factor V Leiden. Lancet 1995; 346:1133–1134.

64. Kalafatis M, Rand MD, Mann KG. The mechanism of inactivation of human factor V and human factor Va by activated protein C. J Biol Chem 1994; 269:31869–31880.

65. Camire RM, Kalafatis M, Cushman M, Tracy RP, Mann KG, Tracy PB. The mechanism of inactivation of human platelet factor Va from normal and activated protein C-resistant individuals. J Biol Chem 1995; 270:20794–20800.

66. Hemker HC, Beguin S. Thrombin generation in plasma: its assessment via the endogenous thrombin potential. Thromb Haemost 1995; 74:134–138.

67. HC Hemker. Personal communication.

68. van't Veer C, Golden NJ, Kalafatis M, Mann KG. Inhibitory mechanism of the protein C pathway on tissue factor-induced thrombin generation. Synergistic effect in combination with tissue factor pathway inhibitor. J Biol Chem 1997; 272:7983–7994.

69. Suzuki K, Nishioka J, Kusumoto H, Hashimoto S. Mechanism of inhibition of activated protein C by protein C inhibitor. J Biochem 1984; 95:187–195.

70. De Cristofaro R, De Candia E, Landolfi R. Effect of high- and low-molecular-weight heparins on thrombin–thrombomodulin interaction and protein C activation. Circulation 1998; 98:1297–1301.

71. Fernandez JA, Petaja J, Griffin JH. Dermatan sulfate and LMW heparin enhance the anticoagulant action of activated protein C. Thromb Haemost 1999; 82:1462–1468.

72. Petaja J, Fernandez JA, Gruber A, Griffin JH. Anticoagulant synergism of heparin and activated protein C in vitro. Role of a novel anticoagulant mechanism of heparin, enhancement of inactivation of factor V by activated protein C. J Clin Invest 1997; 99:2655–2663.

73. Rapaport SI, Rao LY. The tissue factor pathway: how it has become a "prima ballerina." Thromb Haemost 1995; 74:7–17

74. Espana F, Estelles A, Griffin JH, Aznar J, Gilabert J. Aprotinin (Trasylol) is a competitive inhibitor of activated protein C. Thromb Res 1989; 56:751–756.

75. Wendel HP, Heller W, Gallimore MJ. Aprotinin in therapeutic doses inhibits chromogenic peptide substrate assays for protein C. Thromb Res 1994; 74:543–548.

76. Francis WC, Markham ER, Barlow HG, Florack MT, Dobrzynski MD, Marder JV. Thrombin activity of fibrin thrombi and soluble plasmic derivatives. J Lab Clin Med 1983; 102:220–230

77. Kumar R, Beguin S, Hemker HC. The influence of fibrinogen and fibrin on thrombin generation—evidence for feedback activation of the clotting system by clot bound thrombin. Thromb Haemost 1994; 72:713–721

78. Weitz JI, Hudoba M, Massel D, Maraganore J, Hirsh J. Clot-bound thrombin is protected from inhibition by heparin–antithrombin III but is susceptible to inactivation by antithrombin III-independent inhibitors. J Clin Invest 1990; 86:385–391.

79. Hogg PJ, Jackson CM. Fibrin monomer protects thrombin from inactivation by heparin–antithrombin III: implications for heparin efficacy. Proc Natl Acad Sci USA 1989; 86:3619–3623.

80. Muller–Berghaus G, ten Cate H, Levi M. Disseminated intravascular coagulation: clinical spectrum and established as well as new diagnostic approach. Thromb Haemost 1999; 82:706–712.

81. Moore KL, Andreoli SP, Esmon NL, Esmon CT, Bang NU. Endotoxin enhances tissue factor and suppresses thrombomodulin expression of human vascular endothelium in vitro. J Clin Invest 1987; 79:124–130.

82. Mohri M, Oka M, Aoki Y, Gonda Y, Hirata S, Gomi K, Kiyota T, Sugihara T, Yamamoto S, Ishida T, Maruyama I. Intravenous extended infusion of recombinant human soluble thrombomodulin prevented tissue factor-induced disseminated intravascular coagulation in rats. Am J Hematol 1994; 45:298–303.

83. Gonda Y, Hirata S, Saitoh K, Aoki Y, Mohri M, Gomi K, Sugihara T, Kiyota T, Yamamoto S, Ishida T, Maruyama I. Antithrombotic effect of recombinant human soluble thrombomodulin on endotoxin-induced disseminated intravascular coagulation in rats. Thromb Res 1993; 71:325–335.

84. Aoki Y, Ohishi R, Takei R, Matsuzaki O, Mohri M, Saitoh K, Gomi K, Sugihara T, Kiyota T, Yamamoto S, Ishida T, Maruyama I. Effects of recombinant human soluble thrombomodulin (rhs-TM) on disseminated intravascular coagulation model in the rats with decreased plasma antithrombin III level. Thromb Haemost 1994; 71:452–455.

85. Imada K, Takahashi Y, Hosaka Y, Adachi T, Niina H, Mochizuki H. ATIII-independence of anticoagulant effect of human urinary soluble thrombomodulin. Blood Coagul Fibrinol 1999; 10:503–511.

86. Aoki Y, Takei R, Mohri M, Gonda Y, Gomi K, Sugihara T, Kiyota T, Yamamoto S, Ishida T, Maruyama I. Antithrombotic effects of recombinant human soluble thrombomodulin (rhs-TM) on arterio-venous shunt thrombosis in rats. Am J Hematol 1994; 47:162–166.

87. Harker LA, Marzec UM, Mohri M, Fernandez JA, Kelly AB, Hanson SR, Esmon CT, Griffin JH. Antithrombotic efficacy and safety of recombinant human soluble thrombomodulin in non-human primates: inactivation of thrombin and enhanced generation of activated protein C. Circulation (submitted)

88. Uchiba M, Okajima K, Murakami K, Johno M, Mohri M, Okabe H, Takatsuki K. rhs-TM prevents ET-induced increase in pulmonary vascular permeability through protein C activation. Am J Physiol 1997; 273:889–894.

89. Uchiba M, Okajima K, Murakami K, Johno M, Okabe H, Takatsuki K. Recombinant thrombomodulin prevents endotoxin-induced lung injury in rats by inhibiting leukocyte activation. Am J Physiol 1996; 271:470–475.

90. Kaneko H, Joubara N, Yoshino M, Yamazaki K, Mitumaru A, Miki Y, Satake H, Shiba T. Protective effect of human urinary thrombomodulin on ischemia–reperfusion injury in the canine liver. Eur Surg Res 2000; 32:87–93.

91. Kaido T, Yoshikawa A, Seto S, Yamaoka S, Furuyama H, Arii S, Takahashi Y, Imamura M. Pretreatment with soluble thrombomodulin prevents intrasinusoidal coagulation and liver dysfunction following extensive hepatectomy in cirrhotic rats. Thromb Haemost 1999; 82:1302–1306.

92. Sarker KP, Abeyama K, Nishi J, Nakata M, Tokioka T, Nakajima T, Kitajima I, Maruyama I. Inhibition of thrombin-induced neuronal cell death by recombinant thrombomodulin and E5510, a synthetic thrombin receptor signaling inhibitor. Thromb Haemost 1999; 82:1071–1077.

93. Taoka Y, Okajima K, Uchiba M, Johno M. Neuroprotection by recombinant thrombomodulin. Thromb Haemost 2000; 83:462–468.

94. Babiuk C, Marceau F, St-Pierre S, Regoli D. Kininase and vascular responses to kinins. Eur J Pharmacol 1982; 78:167–174.

95. Lerner UH, Jones IL, Gustafson GT. Bradykinin, a new potential mediator of inflamation-induced bone resorption. Studies of the effects on mouse calvarial bones and articular cartilage in vitro. Arthritis Rheum 1987; 30:530–540.

96. Pellas TC, Wennogle LP. C5a receptor antagonists. Curr Pharm Discuss 1999; 5:735–755.

97. Bajzar L, Morser J, Nesheim M. TAFI, or plasma carboxypeptidase B, couples the coagulation and fibrinolytic cascades through the thrombin–thrombomodulin complex. J Biol Chem 1996; 271:16603–16608.

98. Sakharov DV, Plow EF, Rijken DC. On the mechanism of the antifibrinolytic activity of plasma carboxypeptidase B. J Biol Chem 1997; 272:14477–14482.

99. Hancock WW, Grey ST, Hau L, Akalin E, Orthner C, Sayegh MH, Salem HH. Binding of activated protein C to an aspecific receptor on human mononuclear phagocytes inhibits intracellular calcium signaling and monocyte-dependent proliferative responses. Transplantation 1995; 60:1525–1532.

100. Honda G, Masaki C, Zushi M, Tsuruta K, Sata M, Mohri M, Gomi K, Kondo S, Yamamoto S. The roles played by the D2 and D3 domains of recombinant human thrombomodulin in its function. J Biochem 1995; 118:1030–1036.

101. Nakashima M, Kanamaru M, Umemura K, Tsuruta K. Pharmacokinetics and safety of a novel recombinant soluble human thrombomodulin, ART-123, in healthy male volunteers. J Clin Pharmacol 1998; 38:40–44.

102. Conway EM, Nowakowski B, Steiner-Mosonyi M. Human neutrophils synthesize thrombomodulin that does not promote thrombin-dependent protein C activation. Blood 1992; 80:1254–1263

103. Glaser CB, Morser J, Clarke JH, Blasko E, McLean K, Kuhn I, Chang RJ, Lin JH, Vilander L, Andrews WH, Light DR. Oxidation of a specific methionine in thrombomodulin by activated neutrophils' products blocks cofactor activity. A potential rapid mechanism for modulation of coagulation. J Clin Invest 1992; 90:2565–2573.

104. Nakashima M, Uematsu T, Umemura K, Maruyama I, Tsuruta K. A novel recombinant human soluble thrombomodulin, ART-123, activates the protein C pathway in healthy male volunteers. J Clin Pharmacol 1998; 38:540–544.

105. Takahashi Y. Developmental research of human urinary soluble thrombomodulin (UTM:MR-33), a novel antithrombotic agent. BIO Clin 1999; 14:258–261.

21

Overview: Antiplatelet Therapy

Robert P. Giugliano
Harvard Medical School and Brigham and Women's Hospital, Boston, Massachusetts, U.S.A.

Shaker A. Mousa
Albany College of Pharmacy, Albany, New York, U.S.A.

James T. Willerson
University of Texas Health Science Center at Houston and Texas Heart Institute, Houston, Texas, U.S.A.

Platelet-rich thrombosis following plaque rupture plays a central role in the development of acute coronary syndromes [1,2]. Exposure of subendothelial matrix leads to platelet adhesion, predominantly mediated by the interaction between GP Ib/IX receptors and von Willebrand's factor that is magnified several hundredfold in the presence of high-shear stress [3]. Platelet adhesion at the site of endothelial injury leads to a release of adenosine diphosphate (ADP) and calcium-dependent degranulation that subsequently liberates other prothrombotic stimuli. Furthermore, calcium-mediated phospholipase A_2-dependent arachidonic acid formation provides the substrate for prostaglandin formation. Platelet activation, in turn, is augmented by a variety of mediators, including serotonin, ADP, thromboxane-A_2, collagen, and thrombin—all potential targets for antiplatelet therapies.

Indeed, many therapeutic drugs have been identified that possess clinically important antiplatelet activity (Table 1). Platelet inhibition can be achieved in numerous ways (Fig. 1), including inhibition of platelet cyclooxygenase (e.g., aspirin), inhibition of ADP receptors (e.g., clopidogrel), or inhibition of the platelet glycoprotein (GP) IIb/IIIa receptor (e.g., abciximab). Pharmacological inhibition of platelet function can also be achieved by interference with the function of the platelet glycoprotein Ib–IX receptor (monoclonal antibodies to GP1b–IX), synthetic peptides to the A_1 von Willebrand's factor domain, recombinant von Willebrand's fragments covering the A_1 domain, inhibition of thromboxane synthase, blockade of endoperoxide–thromboxane receptors, modulation of platelet adenyl or guanyl cyclase (prostacyclin analogues), and peptides that bind to but do not activate the platelet-receptor domain that interacts with thrombin.

This section focuses on new antiplatelet agents or new data with existing drugs. The section begins with a detailed review of the three currently commercially available intravenous GP IIb/IIIa inhibitors [4]. These potent antiplatelet agents block the GP IIb/IIIa receptor, the

Table 1 Classification Scheme of Antiplatelet Agents

Arachidonic acid inhibitors
  Cyclooxygenase (COX) inhibitors
    Aspirin (acetylsalicylic acid), indobufen, triflusal, nonsteroidal antiinflammatory agents (NSAIDs),
      sulfinpyrazone
  Non-COX inhibition of arachidonic acid
    Ω_3 Fatty acids, eicosanoids (prostacyclin (epoprostenol), prostaglandin analogues)
Phosphodiesterase inhibitors
  Dipyridamole, pentoxifylline, cilostazol, trapidil
Thienopyridines
  Ticlopidine, clopidogrel
Thromboxane inhibitors
  Thromboxane synthase inhibitors, thromboxane receptor blockers, combined thromboxane synthase
    inhibitors, and receptor blockers
Serotonin antagonists
Inhibitors of platelet adhesion
  von Willebrand's factor (vWF) inhibitors
    Aurintricarboxylic acid (ATA), peptide fragments derived from the human plasma vWF–GP1b–IX
      binding domain, monoclonal antibodies to vWF
  GPIb–IX inhibitors
Platelet glycoprotein IIb/IIIa receptor blockers
  Intravenous
    Abciximab, tirofiban, eptifibatide
  Oral: first-generation
    Xemilofiban, sibrafiban, orbofiban, lotrafiban
  Oral: second generation
    Roxifiban, cromofiban
Unclassified
  Multiple mechanisms
    Ditazole, anagrelide
  Other or unknown mechanisms
    Buflomedil, lexipafant, nafazatrom, carbocromen, cloricromene, ronicol
Drugs with secondary antiplatelet activity
  Direct thrombin inhibitors, heparin, nitrates, fibrates, calcium-channel antagonists and many others

final common pathway of platelet aggregation (Fig. 2). The first chapter reviews the available data with abciximab (c7E3 Fab; ReoPro®), a papain cleavage fragment of a genetically reconstructed human–mouse IgG antibody directed at the GP IIb–IIIa receptor. A pooled analysis from three landmark trials demonstrated a reduction in long-term mortality in patients undergoing percutaneous coronary intervention who received abciximab [5]. Subsequent chapters describe two "small-molecule" GP IIb/IIIa inhibitors, eptifibatide (INTEGRILIN®) and tirofiban (Aggrastat®), that have demonstrated efficacy in percutaneous coronary intervention (PCI) [6,7] and non–ST-elevation myocardial infarction [8]. Future studies with these agents are planned in ST-elevation myocardial infarction and noncoronary vascular disease.

While intravenous formulations of GP IIb/IIIa inhibitors have been quickly incorporated in clinical practice and recommended in guideline documents, experience with their oral counterparts is still largely disappointing [9]. Extension of platelet inhibition to the postacute coronary syndrome period with administration of first-generation oral GP IIb/IIIa inhibitors over the medium and long-term has met with several failures as is described in a subsequent chapter. Nonetheless, longer-acting second-generation oral agents, that more closely mimic the pharma-

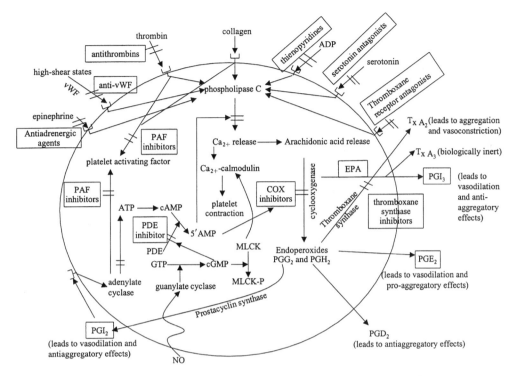

Figure 1 Mechanism of platelet activation and presumed sites of action of various platelet inhibitor agents. Platelet agonists lead to the mobilization of calcium ion (Ca^{2+}), which functions as a mediator of platelet activation through metabolic pathways dependent on epinephrine, high-shear states, thrombin, collagen, adenosine 5'diphosphate (ADP), serotonin, and thromboxane (TX) A_2. Cyclic adenosine monophosphate (cAMP) inhibits calcium mobilization from the dense tubular system. Production of guanosine 3', 5' monophosphate (cGMP) (e.g., via nitrous oxide [NO] donors) can inhibit platelet activation by inhibiting phosphodiesterase (PDE) as well as by phosphorylating myosin light-chain kinase (MLCK-P) which diminishes the affinity of MLCK for calmodulin [19]. Note that thrombin and collagen may independently activate platelets by means of platelet-activating factor. ATP, adenosine triphosphate; COX, cyclooxygenase; EPA, eicosapentaenoic acid; PAF, platelet activating factor; PG, prostaglandin; PGI_2, prostaglandin; PGI_2, prostacyclin. (From Ref. 11.)

cokinetics of intravenous preparations, are now available and undergoing evaluation. The intriguing hypothesis that GP IIb/IIIa inhibitors actually have agonist–antagonists properties [10], and that procoagulant effects may explain, at least partly, some of the failure of first general oral agents is described later this section.

In contrast, the thienopyridines (clopidogrel [Plavix®] and ticlopidine [Ticlid®]) represent an important addition to the armamentarium of oral antiplatelet agents with proved efficacy. Ticlopidine and clopidogrel are noncompetitive, irreversible, selective antagonists of ADP-induced platelet aggregation that act by specifically blocking GP IIb–IIIa activation specific for the ADP pathway (see Fig. 1). Although initial studies reported that this ADP receptor blockade led to direct inhibition of fibrinogen binding to the glycoprotein IIb/IIIa complex [12,13], more recent evidence shows that ticlopidine actually impairs the binding of von Willebrand's factor (vWF) to the GP IIb/IIIa complex [14–16]. Recent studies in patients receiving intracoronary stents and postacute coronary syndrome have demonstrated clear benefits of adding thieno-pyridine to aspirin therapy.

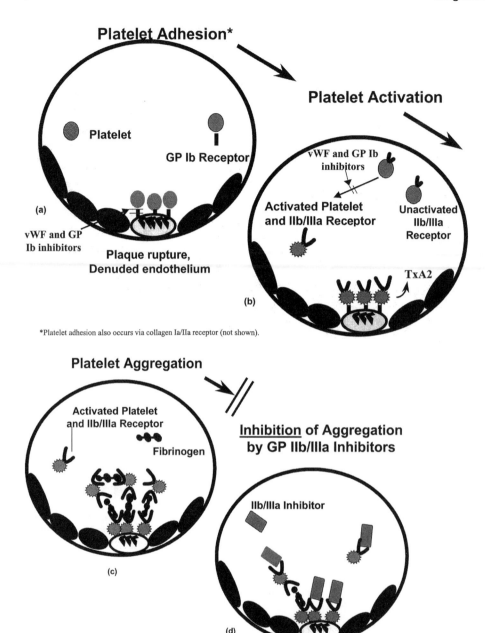

Figure 2 Three major steps in the role of platelets in thrombosis and the targets of antiplatelet therapy (2 panels) Events associated with platelet adhesion (a), activation (b), and aggregation (c–d) are shown. The initial platelet monolayer of platelet adhesion (a) is mediated by von Willebrand's factor (vWF) and the GP Ib–IX receptor, and may be inhibited by antagonists of vWF and the GP Ib–IX receptor. Activated platelets undergo a conformational change in the shape of the GP IIb/IIIa receptors, which makes them receptive to ligand binding. Fibrinogen binds to the platelet GP IIb/IIIa receptors on adjacent platelets, forming bridges between them. GP IIb/IIIa receptor inhibitors block this fibrinogen-binding receptor and, therefore, directly prevent platelets from aggregating (d). GP, glycoprotein; TxA_2, thromboxane A_2. (From Ref. 11.)

Lastly, targeting of other receptors and mediators of platelet adhesion and aggregation is ongoing. The vWF molecule has a key role in platelet adhesion, interacting with both subendothelial components and the platelet glycoprotein Ib receptor (see Fig. 2). Platelet aggregation in states associated with high-shear stress (e.g., critical arterial stenosis), is particularly mediated by the interaction between vWF and the GP1b–IX receptor [3]. Furthermore, vWF–GP1b–IX interaction leads to activation of the platelet GP IIb/IIIa receptor, resulting in fibrinogen cross-linking and platelet aggregation (see Fig. 2) [17–20]. Thus, interruption of the interaction between vWF and the GP1b–IX receptor not only may affect platelet adhesion, but also may prevent thrombus formation by blocking platelet GPIIb/IIIa activation. New agents under development that inhibit GP Ib–IX and vWF are described in the final chapter in this section.

Table 2 Choice of Antiplatelet Agents for Various Cardiovascular Indications

Indication	1st Line	2nd Line	Alternatives
Coronary artery disease			
Acute MI	Aspirin	Triflusal, ridogrel	GP IIb/IIIa inhib.[a] sulfinpyrazone
Unstable angina and non–STE-MI	Aspirin, clopidogrel	GP IIb/IIIa inhib[b]	Triflusal, ticlopidine
Chronic stable angina	Aspirin	Clopidogrel	Trapidil
2nd MI prevention	Aspirin, clopidogrel	Ticlopidine	Trapidil triflusal
Primary MI prevention	aspirin	Ω-3-FA	
PCI and Cardiac Surgery			
PCI	Aspirin clopidogrel[c] GP IIb/IIIa inhib.[c] Ticlopidine[d]	Trapidil	Cilostazol
CABG	Aspirin	Dipyridamole[c]	Indobufen, Ω-3-FA, triflusal
Cardiopulmonary bypass pump		Prostacyclin, PG analogues	
Prosthetic cardiac valves		Aspirin dipyridamole[c]	
Cerebrovascular disease			
TIA/ischemic stroke	Aspirin	Ticlopidine, clopidogrel	Dipyridamole[c]
Carotid artery disease	Aspirin		
Atrial fibrillation	Aspirin[d]		Indobufen
Peripheral vascular disease			
Peripheral arterial disease	Aspirin, clopidogrel, cilostazol, pentoxifylline	Indobufen, ticlopidine	Prostacyclin, PG analogues
Venous thromboembolism	Dextran	Aspirin	Indobufen triflusal

[a] In combination with half-dose fibrinolytic and aspirin.
[b] Eptifibatide or tirofiban; abciximab only in patients following angiography in whom a PCI is planned in the next 24 h.
[c] In combination with aspirin.
[d] In low-risk, young patients with lone atrial fibrillation.
MI, myocardial infarction; STE, ST-segment elevation; PCI, percutaneous coronary intervention; CABG, coronary artery bypass graft; TIA, transient ischemic attack; FA fatty acids; PG, prostaglandin.

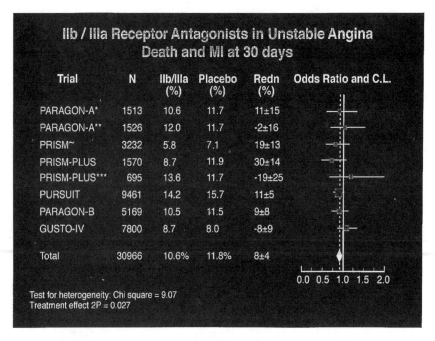

Figure 3　Metaanalysis of large GP IIb/IIIa inhibitor trials in unstable angina/non–ST elevation MI. (From Ref. 21.)

A growing number of pharmacological agents spanning multiple drug classes have been demonstrated to inhibit platelet function in humans. Recommendations for the choice of antiplatelet agent in various cardiovascular conditions, based on the available clinical data, are listed in Table 2. Aspirin remains the first-line agent for most cardiovascular diseases for which antiplatelet therapy is indicated. Newer, more potent, antiplatelet agents, such as the thienopyridines (ticlopidine, clopidogrel) and intravenous GP IIb/IIIa inhibitors (abciximab, eptifibatide, tirofiban), are promising and their role in clinical practice is likely to expand as further clinical trial data (Fig. 3) become available.

REFERENCES

1. Fuster V, Lewis A. Conner Memorial Lecture. Mechanisms leading to myocardial infarction: insights from studies of vascular biology. Circulation. 1994; 90:2126–2146.
2. Fuster V, Badimon L, Badimon JJ, Chesebro JH. The pathogenesis of coronary artery disease and the acute coronary syndromes [1]. N Engl J Med. 1992; 326:242–50.
3. Weiss HJ, Turitto VT, Baumgartner HR. Effect of shear rate on platelet interaction with subendothelium in citrated and native blood. I. Shear rate-dependent decrease of adhesion in von Willebrand's disease and the Bernard–Soulier syndrome. J Lab Clin Med 1978; 92:750–64.
4. Bhatt DL, Topol EJ. Current role of platelet glycoprotein IIb/IIIa inhibitors in acute coronary syndromes. JAMA. 2000; 284:1549–58.
5. Anderson KM, Califf RM, Stone GW, Neumann FJ, Montalescot G, Miller DP, Ferguson JJ 3rd, Willerson JT, Weisman HF, Topol EJ. Long-term mortality benefit with abciximab in patients undergoing percutaneous coronary intervention. J Am Coll Cardiol 2001; 37:2059–65.
6. O'Shea JC, Tcheng JE. Eptifibatide in percutaneous coronary intervention: the ESPRIT trial results. Curr Interv Cardiol Rep 2001; 3:62–68.

7. Kong DF, Califf RM, Miller DP, Moliterno DJ, White HD, Harrington RA, Tcheng JE, Lincoff AM, Hasselblad V, Topol EJ. Clinical outcomes of therapeutic agents that block the platelet glycoprotein IIb/IIIa integrin in ischemic heart disease [see comments]. Circulation 1998; 98:2829–35.

8. Boersma E, Akkerhuis KM, Theroux P, Califf RM, Topol EJ, Simoons ML. Platelet glycoprotein IIb/IIIa receptor inhibition in non–ST-elevation acute coronary syndromes: early benefit during medical treatment only, with additional protection during percutaneous coronary intervention. Circulation 1999; 100:2045–8.

9. Chew DP, Bhatt DL, Sapp S, Topol EJ. Increased mortality with oral platelet glycoprotein IIb/IIIa antagonists: a meta-analysis of phase III multicenter randomized trials. Circulation 2001; 103:201–206.

10. Peter K, Schwarz M, Ylanne J, Kohler B, Moser M, Nordt T, Salbach P, Kubler W, Bode C. Induction of fibrinogen binding and platelet aggregation as a potential intrinsic property of various glycoprotein IIb/IIIa (alpha IIb–beta 3) inhibitors. Blood 1998; 92:3240–9.

11. Giugliano RP, Cannon CP. Antiplatelet agents. In: Antman EM, ed. Cardiovascular therapeutics: a companion to Braunwald's heart disease. Philadelphia: WB Saunders, 2001.

12. Gachet C, Stierle A, Cazenave JP, Ohlmann P, Lanza F, Bouloux C, Maffrand JP. The thienopyridine PCR 4099 selectively inhibits ADP-induced platelet aggregation and fibrinogen binding without modifying the membrane glycoprotein IIb–IIIa complex in rat and in man. Biochem Pharmacol 1990; 40:229–38.

13. DiMinno G, Silver MJ, Cerbone AM, Riccardi G, Rivellese A, Mancini M, Thiagarajan P. Increased binding of fibrinogen to platelets in diabetes: the role of prostaglandins and thromboxane. Blood. 1985; 65:156–62.

14. Desager JP. Clinical pharmacokinetics of ticlopidine. Clin Pharmacokinet. 1994; 26:347–55.

15. Meyer D, Pietu G, Fressinaud E, Girma JP. von Willebrand factor: structure and function. Mayo Clin Proc 1991; 66:516–23.

16. Di Minno G, Cerbone AM, Mattioli PL, Turco S, Iovine C, Mancini M. Functionally thrombasthenic state in normal platelets following the administration of ticlopidine. J Clin Invest 1985; 75:328–38.

17. Grainick HR, Williams SB, Coller BS. Asialo von Willebrand factor interactions with platelets. Interdependence of glycoproteins Ib and IIb/IIIa for binding and aggregation. J Clin Invest 1985; 75:19–25.

18. De Marco L, Girolami A, Russell S, Ruggeri ZM. Interaction of asialo von Willebrand factor with glycoprotein Ib induces fibrinogen binding to the glycoprotein IIb/IIIa complex and mediates platelet aggregation. J Clin Invest. 1985; 75:1198–203.

19. De Marco L, Mazzuccato M, Grazia Del Ben M, Budde U, Federici AB, Girolami A, Ruggeri ZM. Type IIB von Willebrand factor with normal sialic acid content induces platelet aggregation in the absence of ristocetin. Role of platelet activation, fibrinogen, and two distinct membrane receptors. J Clin Invest 1987; 80:475–82.

20. Loscalzo J, Welch G. Nitric oxide and its role in the cardiovascular system. Prog Cardiovasc Dis 1995; 38:87–104.

21. White HD. Unstable angina: ischemic syndromes. In: Topol EJ, ed. Text book of Cardiovascular Medicine. Philadelphia: Lippincott Williams & Wilkins, 2001.

22

Abciximab

Deepak L. Bhatt and A. Michael Lincoff
Cleveland Clinic Foundation, Cleveland, Ohio, U.S.A.

SUMMARY

Abciximab, a monoclonal antibody, is a potent intravenous blocker of the platelet glycoprotein IIb/IIIa receptor. In addition to its antiplatelet effects, abciximab acts on other receptors, although the clinical significance of these effects is unclear. It has reduced ischemic events after percutaneous coronary intervention (PCI), and its benefit applies to all interventional modalities and all lesion types. It has decreased 1-year mortality, resulting in a high degree of cost-effectiveness. The reduction in periprocedural ischemic events, as well as intermediate-term mortality, is particularly robust in diabetic patients. Abciximab has been studied in the medical management of non–ST-elevation acute coronary syndromes, with disappointing results and no clear evidence of benefit. However, patients with acute coronary syndromes, when treated by early revascularization, benefit greatly from abciximab. Abciximab, as an adjunct to balloon angioplasty or stenting for acute ST-elevation myocardial infarction, improves outcomes. Abciximab, in combination with fibrinolytic therapy, is being studied for acute myocardial infarction; phase II studies have been promising, but phase III data are awaited. The study of abciximab for acute stroke and limb ischemia, as well as an adjunct to carotid and peripheral intervention, is in its infancy.

I. BIOLOGY

Abciximab (c7E3 Fab) is a monoclonal antibody that consists of a half-human, half-murine chimeric Fab fragment, in which the heavy- and light-chain variable regions from the murine antibody are attached to the constant regions of the human IgG_1 and κ-chains [1]. It is a powerful antiplatelet agent, likely to decrease clinical thrombosis. Abciximab binds with high affinity to the glycoprotein (GP) IIb/IIIa receptor, although with low specificity [2]. These properties differentiate it from the other intravenous GP IIb/IIIa inhibitors that have been studied. The prolonged platelet inhibition produced by abciximab is another differentiating feature [3]. At 8 days after abciximab bolus and infusion, there is still 29% blockade of the GP IIb/IIIa receptor, owing to reequilibration of abciximab among the circulating platelets. At 15 days, there remains 13% blockade of the GP IIb/IIIa receptor. This prolonged duration of platelet inhibition, with a

349

gradual recovery, may account for some of the long-term benefit of abciximab that has been noted in clinical practice.

In addition to its antiplatelet effects, mediated by binding to the GP IIb/IIIa receptor, abciximab has other biological actions that may be important in reducing thrombosis or inflammation [4,5]. Abciximab binds to the $\alpha_v\beta_3$ receptor as well as the Mac-1 receptor [6]. These effects of abciximab may influence platelet–leukocyte interactions [7]. The $\alpha_v\beta_3$ receptor, as well as the GP IIb/IIIa receptor, appears to play a role in attenuating thrombin generation in response to tissue factor [4]. This effect on thrombin generation may be particularly relevant in conditions such as acute myocardial infarction (MI) [8]. In one study of patients with acute MI, abciximab decreased platelet attachment to monocytes, whereas heparin alone did not [8]. Much about the biology of GP IIb/IIIa inhibitors, however, is not well understood. For example, the contribution of the internal pool of GP IIb/IIIa receptors to platelet aggregation has perhaps been underappreciated [9]. Although abciximab does become internalized, its inhibition of the internal GP IIb/IIIa receptor pool is incomplete, but circulating drug binds externalized receptors.

II. PERCUTANEOUS CORONARY INTERVENTION

The U.S. Food and Drug Administration (FDA)-approved indications for abciximab use are as an adjunct to percutaneous coronary intervention (PCI) for the prevention of cardiac ischemic complications in patients undergoing PCI or in patients with unstable angina not responding to conventional medical therapy when PCI is planned within 24 h. The so-called EPI trials have laid the foundation for the use for GP IIb/IIIa inhibitors during PCI (Table 1): Evaluation of Platelet IIb/IIIa Inhibition for Prevention of Ischemic Complication (EPIC), Evaluation in PTCA to Improve Long-term Outcome with Abciximab GP IIb/IIIa Blockade (EPILOG), and Evaluation of Platelet IIb/IIIa Inhibitor for Stenting (EPISTENT) were randomized clinical trials evaluating abciximab versus placebo in a broad range of patients undergoing PCI [10–12].

A. EPIC

The EPIC study enrolled 2099 high-risk patients undergoing angioplasty [10]. All patients had unstable angina, evolving acute MI, or complex angiographic lesion morphology combined with advanced age, female gender, or diabetes mellitus. Patients were treated with aspirin and heparin and were randomized to placebo, abciximab bolus, or abciximab bolus and 12-h infusion. Compared with placebo, the rates of death, nonfatal MI, unplanned surgical revascularization, or repeat percutaneous procedure, unplanned stent implantation, or insertion of an intra-aortic balloon pump for refractory ischemia were reduced with abciximab bolus plus infusion from 12.8 to 8.3%, p = 0.008. The composite event rate for the group randomized to bolus-only was 11.5%, which was not significantly different from the placebo rate. Bleeding complications were significantly increased in the bolus and infusion group compared with the other two groups.

The three-year follow-up from EPIC showed that the initial benefit seen with periprocedural abciximab was sustained [13]. The rate of death, MI, or revascularization was reduced from 47.2 to 41.1% for the bolus and infusion group, compared with placebo, p = 0.009; the rate in the bolus-only group was 47.4%. The individual components of the composite endpoint were all affected favorably by the bolus and infusion of abciximab. Additionally, the EPIC 3-year follow-up confirmed that periprocedural creatine kinase elevations were linked to long-term mortality [13].

Table 1 Randomized, Clinical Trials of Abciximab in Cardiology

Trial	N	Population	Endpoint	Results Placebo	Results Abciximab
EPIC	2099	PCI for unstable angina, evolving MI, high-risk lesion morphology	30-day death, MI, unplanned TVR, unplanned stenting, IABP	12.8%	8.3%
EPILOG	2792	PCI, urgent or elective	30-day death, MI, urgent TVR	11.7%	5.2%
EPISTENT	2399	PCI, urgent or elective	30-day death, MI, urgent TVR	10.8%[a]	5.3%[a]
CAPTURE	1265	PCI for refractory unstable angina	30-day death, MI, urgent TVR	15.9%	11.3%
GUSTO IV	7800	ACS	30-day death, MI	8.0%	8.2%, 9.1%[b]
RAPPORT	483	MI	30-day death, MI, urgent TVR	11.2%	5.8%
ADMIRAL	300	MI	30-day death, MI, urgent TVR	14.7%	7.3%
CADILLAC	2082	MI	30-day death, stroke, MI, ischemic TVR	6.7%	4.3%
STOP–AMI	140	MI, primary PCI vs. t-PA	6-month death, reinfarction, stroke	23.2%	8.5%

PCI, percutaneous coronary intervention days; IABP, intra-aortic balloon pump; ACS, acute coronary syndromes.
[a] stented patients.
[b] 24- and 48-h infusions of abciximab.

B. EPILOG

EPILOG broadened the inclusion criteria of EPIC to include patients undergoing either urgent or elective intervention [11]. Moreover, EPILOG evaluated the safety and efficacy of weight-adjusted, reduced-dose heparin as a means of decreasing the excess bleeding risk observed with abciximab in the prior EPIC trial. While the study had initially planned to enroll 4800 patients, an interim analysis revealed positive results and the trial was terminated after 2792 patients. The rate of death, MI or urgent revascularization by 30 days was 11.7% in the placebo group, 5.4% in the arm that received abciximab and standard-dose, weight-adjusted heparin, and 5.2% in the abciximab plus low-dose, weight-adjusted heparin group, p = 0.001 (Fig. 1). Rates of major bleeding were similar among all three groups. Minor bleeding, however, was more frequent in the abciximab plus standard-dose heparin group. Thus, the EPILOG trial demonstrated that the increased rates of bleeding seen with abciximab in the EPIC trial could be reduced to the level of placebo, if adjunctive low-dose, weight-adjusted heparin were used. Furthermore, EPILOG showed that even patients undergoing elective intervention derive clinical benefit from abciximab. Also, of note, the EPILOG trial protocol emphasized conservative femoral access site management, by discouraging routine placement of venous sheaths and minimizing sheath dwell time, as well as discontinuation of heparin at the conclusion of the interventional procedure. This strategy is now the standard of care, both with and without abciximab. Vascular hemostasis devices also appear to be safe and effective with abciximab [14].

C. EPISTENT

Although EPIC and EPILOG clearly demonstrated that abciximab was beneficial with either balloon angioplasty or directional atherectomy, it was not known if the benefits of this agent would be additive to those of stenting [12]. The EPISTENT trial, therefore, randomized 2399 patients to angioplasty and abciximab, stent plus placebo, or stent plus abciximab. The primary composite endpoint consisted of death, MI, or urgent revascularization by 30 days. In the 809 patients randomized to stenting and placebo, the composite event rate was 10.8%; in the 794

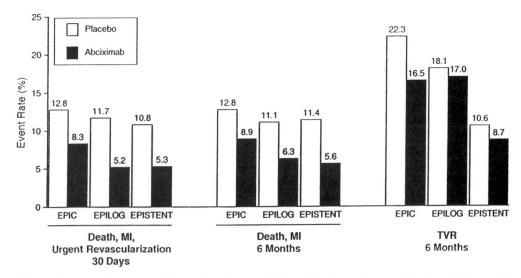

Figure 1 The 30-day rates of death, MI, and urgent TVR and the 6-month rates of death and MI, as well as TVR, from EPIC, EPILOG, and EPISTENT.

patients randomized to stent plus abciximab, the rate was reduced to 5.3%, p = 0.001; in the 796 patients randomized to balloon angioplasty and abciximab, the rate was 6.9%, p = 0.007 compared with stent–placebo. Most of abciximab's benefit was due to reductions in large MI and death. There were no significant differences among the rates of major bleeding: 2.2% with stent–placebo, 1.5% with stent–abciximab, and 1.4% with balloon–abciximab.

At 6 months follow-up in EPISTENT, there was preservation of the benefit of abciximab in reducing the rates of death and MI [15]. By 1 year, a mortality benefit was seen with the combination of abciximab and stenting: 2.4% in the stent–placebo group, 2.1% in the balloon–abciximab group, and 1.0% in the stent–abciximab group (p = 0.037) [16].

Thus, in aggregate, the EPIC, EPILOG, and EPISTENT trials show that abciximab decreases the risk of death, MI, and urgent revascularization in patients undergoing PCI for either urgent or elective indications. This benefit is durable over time. Pooled data show a significant reduction in 1-year mortality, with particular benefit and complementarity with stenting (Fig. 2).

D. Restenosis

The 6-month results of EPIC showed a significant 26% reduction in the rate of target vessel revascularization (TVR) with the bolus and infusion of abciximab, suggesting that this agent may reduce clinical restenosis [17]. Subsequent studies have failed to confirm this finding in the general population of patients undergoing PCI. In EPILOG, rates of TVR were not significantly different in the three treatment groups. In a mechanistic study, the ERASER trial of 215 patients who received stents and were randomized to placebo or abciximab infusion, restenosis was assessed both by intravascular ultrasound and quantitative coronary angiography; there was no observed difference in 6-month restenosis with abciximab given as either a 12- or 24-h infusion [18]. In another study involving stenting for acute myocardial infarction, there was no effect of abciximab on TVR or angiographic restenosis rates [19]. Likewise, EPISTENT did not find a statistically significant reduction in TVR in the overall enrolled population treated with

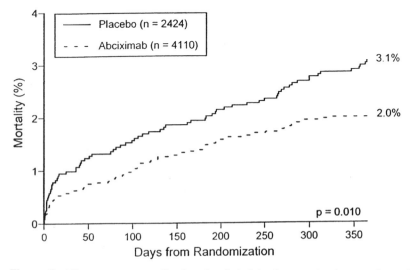

Figure 2   The one-year mortality benefit of abciximab over placebo seen in pooled data from EPIC, EPILOG, and EPISTENT. (From Ref. 44).

abciximab. However, in a subgroup of patients with diabetes, there was a reduction in TVR and angiographic restenosis (see Sec. II.I on diabetes) [15,20].

E. Lesion Types

Abciximab has provided clinical benefit during coronary revascularization of all lesion subtypes [21]. It provides similar relative risk reduction in both simple and complex lesions, although the absolute benefit is larger in complex lesions, given their higher baseline event rates [22]. Similarly, therapy with abciximab is beneficial with intervention in both large- and small-caliber vessels [22].

Abciximab infused locally into saphenous vein grafts appeared to reduce thrombus burden significantly in a pilot study [23]. Potentially, this strategy may apply to other lesion types at high risk of containing thrombus, such as in culprit lesions during acute MI. Anecdotally, angiographically visible thrombus has been dissolved by abciximab when other methods were unsuccessful [24]. Another potential approach may be to pretreat with abciximab for a period of several hours before attempting intervention of a thrombus-laden vein graft [25].

F. Devices

Whether balloon angioplasty, directional atherectomy, elective stenting or bailout stenting is used, abciximab reduces the rate of death or MI, both at 30 days and 6 months (Fig. 3) [26,27]. In a strategy of balloon angioplasty, the prophylactic use of abciximab decreases the need for unplanned stenting [28]. When bailout stenting does occur, abciximab improves the outcome [26,29].

The benefits of abciximab are also seen with rotational atherectomy [30]. Rotational atherectomy is an excellent in vivo model for embolization, with obligatory particulate debris created by the procedure, leading to transient (or permanent) perfusion defects on myocardial imaging, which abciximab can prevent [31]. Abciximab decreases the platelet activation that occurs with high-speed rotational atherectomy, and this may be one mode of benefit [32].

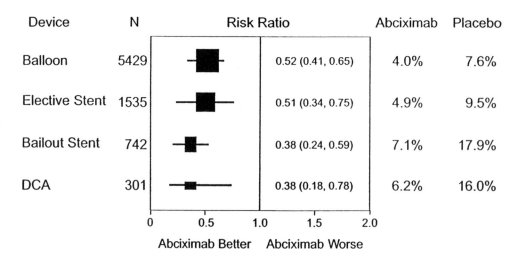

Figure 3   The benefit of abciximab is seen regardless of the interventional device that is used. (From Ref. 26).

Additionally, abciximab may lessen the impact of embolization on the microvasculature by blunting any thrombotic response to particulate debris or interrupting any inflammatory cascade an embolic shower may produce, thereby decreasing periprocedural MI [33–36].

G. Provisional Use

Despite a lack of prospective, randomized data validating provisional "bailout" use of abciximab, some catheterization laboratories utilize this strategy in an attempt to reduce costs. A retrospective analysis has been performed of 63 patients undergoing angioplasty who developed threatened or abrupt vessel closure and were treated with provisional abciximab [37]. Following abciximab administration, thrombus burden was seen to decrease and coronary flow improved. Another observational study of 29 patients undergoing PTCA also showed a decrease in thrombus score and an increase in TIMI flow with abciximab administration at the time of the complication [38]. A larger study of 298 consecutive patients treated with "rescue" abciximab showed relatively low rates of in-hospital complications [39].

H. Cost-Effectiveness

Abciximab is expensive, costing approximately 1450 dollars/dose, which discourages its use. In EPIC, excess bleeding nearly cancelled out any cost savings, although this did not occur in EPILOG or EPISTENT [40,41]. In EPISTENT, the cost effectiveness of abciximab was similar to that of stent deployment and in the range of coronary artery bypass grafting for left main disease (approximately 6000 dollars/life-year saved). This falls within the bounds of therapies generally accepted as cost effective in the United States (that is, less than 50,000 dollars/life-year saved). Among other benefits, abciximab led to shorter hospital stays for angioplasty patients [42]. In a single-center analysis of 1472 coronary interventions, in addition to a survival advantage at 6 months, abciximab therapy resulted in considerable cost savings [43]. With propensity scoring to adjust for nonrandomization, the average adjusted cost per life-year gained in this study was 1243 dollars.

I. Diabetes

One-year mortality is significantly reduced by the use of abciximab at the time of PCI in diabetic patients. In fact, the mortality of diabetic patients treated with abciximab is reduced to that of nondiabetics treated with placebo (Fig. 4) [44]. Furthermore, an angiographic analysis of diabetics undergoing stenting in EPISTENT found that rates of repeat TVR by 6 months after stenting were reduced from 16.6 to 8.1% in diabetics, $p = 0.02$, while no effect on TVR post-stenting was seen in non-diabetics [15,20]. This combination of reduction in mortality and restenosis with abciximab use in diabetics is particularly relevant to the treatment of multivessel disease [45]. Although bypass surgery is generally considered the preferred mode of revascularization for diabetics with multivessel coronary artery disease, the use of abciximab may reduce or eliminate the disparity in outcomes between percutaneous and surgical revascularization in these patients.

J. Thrombocytopenia

Abciximab increases the rate of thrombocytopenia when compared with placebo [46]. Of particular concern, abciximab may also cause a sudden, profound thrombocytopenia to less than 20–50 thousand/μL. This occurs in about 1% of patients receiving abciximab for the first time,

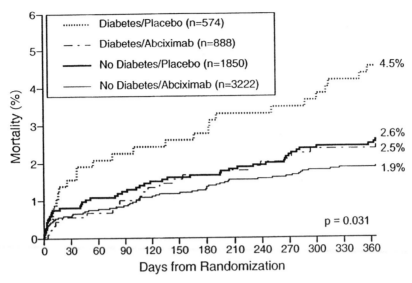

Figure 4 Diabetics derive enhanced benefit from abciximab at the time of PCI. (From Ref. 44).

usually within a few hours, and can be associated with bleeding [46a]. There is no evidence of ongoing platelet clearance if the thrombocytopenia is recognized and abciximab is stopped. Platelet transfusions are durable and protective for profound thrombocytopenia. Thus, it is important to check platelet counts at 2 and 12 h in all patients receiving this drug. Additionally, it is necessary to distinguish abciximab-induced thrombocytopenia from pseudothrombocytopenia, which is a laboratory artifact that is meaningless from a clinical standpoint [47].

K. Readministration

Abciximab can be readministered safely in patients undergoing PCI, although human anti-chimeric antibodies (HACA) develop in approximately 5% of patients within 1 month of receiving abciximab [48,49]. Allergic and anaphylactic reactions do not appear to occur, and HACA does not appear related to bleeding or ischemic complications. Among 500 patients in a readministration registry of abciximab, rates of profound thrombocytopenia were higher (4%) than expected for first-time administration, emphasizing the importance of platelet monitoring following readministration [50].

L. Emergency Coronary Artery Bypass Grafting for Failed PCI

The need for emergency coronary artery bypass grafting (CABG) in the modern era is unusual as a complication of PCI, yet one concern has been that abciximab administered at the time of PCI could create a prohibitive bleeding risk if emergent CABG were required. Reassuringly, pooled data from EPILOG and EPISTENT found that patients treated with abciximab had an 88% rate of major bleeding, versus 79% in the placebo arm, p = 0.27 [51]. Blood cell transfusions were utilized in 80% of the abciximab-treated patients versus 74% of placebo-treated patients (p = 0.53), although platelet transfusions were more frequently administered in the abciximab-treated patients to reverse antiplatelet effect (52% versus 32%, p = 0.059). Death and myocardial infarction tended to occur less frequently after failed PCI if abciximab had been used.

M. Comparisons with Other GP IIb/IIIa Inhibitors

The Do Tirofiban and ReoPro Give Similar Efficacy Outcomes Trial (TARGET) is the first randomized comparison of GP IIb/IIIa inhibitors [52]. A total of 4812 patients undergoing PCI with the intent to stent all lesions were randomized to either abciximab or tirofiban. Clopidogrel and aspirin were administered before the procedure. Abciximab was superior to tirofiban in reducing the primary endpoint of 30-day death, MI, or urgent revascularization (7.55% in the tirofiban-treated patients and 6.01% in the abciximab-treated patients, p = 0.037). No randomized comparisons of abciximab versus eptifibatide have been performed.

III. COMBINATION THERAPY

The effect of thienopyridines on thrombus inhibition may be additive to that of abciximab [53]. In whole-blood samples in a cone-and-plate viscometer at shear rates meant to simulate arterial flow, the combination of abciximab and ticlopidine produced a more sustained effect on mural thrombus formation than either agent alone [54]. Additionally, ticlopidine effectively continues the platelet inhibition that is initiated by abciximab [55]. These effects likely also apply to the combination of clopidogrel and abciximab.

Abciximab appears to have an antithrombin effect, and this may account for its ability to increase the activated clotting time (ACT) beyond that of heparin [56]. Abciximab also raises the ACT in the presence of hirudin [57]. The effect of abciximab in increasing the ACT may not be apparent until 10 min after its administration [58].

There has been some experience combining low-molecular-weight heparins (LMWHs) with abciximab. Enoxaparin and abciximab have been successfully used during percutaneous intervention [59,60]. In the National Investigators Collaborating on Enoxaparin (NICE)-4 registry, a 0.75-mg/kg bolus of intravenous enoxaparin was used with abciximab. This resulted in levels of bleeding that were no higher than historic controls, and no apparent diminished efficacy compared with unfractionated heparin. Another low-molecular-weight heparin, dalteparin, was used in a subset of patients in Global Use of Strategies to Open Occluded Coronary Arteries (GUSTO) IV trial, and the combination with abciximab appeared to be safe, with no suggestion of excess bleeding [61]. The NICE-3 registry included 147 patients taking enoxaparin for acute coronary syndromes who also received abciximab [61a]. Clinical outcomes and rates of major bleeding were similar to historic controls in this study as well.

Direct thrombin inhibitors, such as bivalirudin, are promising adjuncts to abciximab [62]. The CACHET pilot compared a strategy of planned abciximab and unfractionated heparin against bivalirudin plus provisional abciximab; the rate of death, MI, revascularization, or major hemorrhage was 14.1% in the heparin arm and 3.5% in the bivalirudin arm. The REPLACE trial will test combination therapy with bivalirudin and abciximab in a large population of patients undergoing PCI, as well as test the hypothesis that bivalirudin may obviate the need for abciximab in some patients.

IV. ACUTE CORONARY SYNDROMES

A. Abciximab During PCI

The benefit of abciximab during PCI appeared to be strongest among those with acute coronary syndromes (ACS) [63]. In EPIC, those patients with unstable angina had a 62% reduction in 30-day death, MI, or urgent revascularization with abciximab versus placebo, from 12.8 to 4.8%, p = 0.012 [63]. In those patients from EPIC who were specifically enrolled owing to unstable angina or evolving MI, the rate of death at 3 years was decreased from 12.7 to 5.1%, p = 0.01. A pooled analysis of EPIC, EPILOG, and EPISTENT confirmed that those patients with acute coronary syndromes derived greater benefit from abciximab [64].

The c7E3 Fab Antiplatelet Therapy in Unstable Refractory Angina (CAPTURE) trial enrolled 1265 patients with unstable angina refractory to conventional medical therapy including heparin and nitroglycerin and a coronary lesion suitable for angioplasty [65]. After diagnostic angiography, patients were randomized to either placebo or an 18 to 24-h infusion of abciximab before angioplasty and continued for 1 h after the angioplasty. The rate of death, MI, or urgent intervention by 30 days was reduced with abciximab from 15.9 to 11.3%, p = 0.029. The benefit of abciximab in reducing MI in CAPTURE was seen both before and after PCI. Abciximab also diminishes ischemia as measured by continuous ST-segment monitoring [66], and promotes angiographic resolution of thrombus [67]. Retrospective analysis identified those patients who were enrolled into CAPTURE with an elevated troponin as a group of patients particularly likely to benefit from abciximab [68].

B. Abciximab as Medical Therapy: GUSTO IV

The role of abciximab among patients treated medically for non–ST-elevation ACS was evaluated in the GUSTO IV trial. A total of 7800 patients with chest pain of at least 5-min duration and either ST-depression or troponin elevation were enrolled and were randomized to placebo, a 24-h infusion of abciximab, or a 48-h infusion of abciximab [61]. PCI during the drug infusion was discouraged and was performed on only 1.6% of patients. No reduction in the endpoint of death or MI was seen in either abciximab arm relative to placebo at 30 days (8.0% for placebo, 8.2% for 24-h abciximab, 9.1% for 48-h abciximab). High-risk subgroups of patients defined by troponin positivity did not exhibit benefit from abciximab either. Possible explanations for this negative result include too low an infusion dose, particularly for 48 h, whereby the level of platelet inhibition may have decreased further if agonist-induced activation of an internal pool of GP IIb/IIIa receptors occurred [69]. Potentially, a fall in abciximab levels below the therapeutic range may have even led to a prothrombotic state, as has been hypothesized to occur with the oral GP IIb/IIIa inhibitors [70]. Perhaps monitoring of the degree of platelet inhibition with adjustment of the dose to maintain at least 80% inhibition would have led to a better outcome in this trial. However, one important issue concerning the apparent lack of efficacy of abciximab in this trial is likely related to the very low rates of early revascularization. Other potential explanations include the possibility of enrollment of a low-risk population and the use of troponin for risk stratification.

Although other ACS trials have suggested benefit of GP IIb/IIIa blockade during the medical management phase of ACS, event reduction has been substantially less in magnitude and durability than among patients who undergo early revascularization by either percutaneous or surgical means. Thus, the results of GUSTO IV in no way diminish the proved benefit of abciximab in conjunction with PCI [71].

V. USE OF ABCIXIMAB FOR ACUTE ST-ELEVATION MI

There are four potential roles for GP IIb/IIIa inhibition with abciximab in acute ST-segment elevation MI. Administration at the time of either primary balloon angioplasty or stenting may be expected to enhance outcomes. There may be a role as stand-alone "lysis." Abciximab could be given after full-dose fibrinolytics or, alternatively, concomitant with partial-dose fibrinolytics. All these strategies have been tested to some degree. Additionally, the possibility of combining reduced-dose fibrinolysis, abciximab, and PCI exists.

A. Abciximab During Primary PCI for Acute ST-Elevation MI

The ReoPro and Primary PTCA Organization and Randomized Trials (RAPPORT) first established that abciximab during primary balloon angioplasty decreased the risk of death, MI, or urgent revascularization at 7 days, 30 days, and 6 months [72]. Abciximab also accelerated the rate of reperfusion, as reflected by a reduced time for the creatine kinase to peak (10.5 h for abciximab vs. 13.5 h for placebo, p = 0.015). [73].

Although stents reduce rates of target vessel revascularization compared with balloon angioplasty, they do not decrease mortality in acute MI. Rather, stenting has been associated with a degradation in coronary flow and trends toward increased mortality [74]. The Abciximab Before Direct Angioplasty and Stenting in Myocardial Infarction Regarding Acute and Long-Term follow-up (ADMIRAL) trial extended the benefit of abciximab during primary angioplasty seen in RAPPORT to primary stent deployment [75]. Abciximab provided an almost 50% reduction in the risk of death, MI, or urgent revascularization by 30 days.

The Stent versus Thrombolysis for Occluded Coronary Arteries in Patients with Acute Myocardial Infarction (STOP–AMI) trial randomized 140 patients to stent plus abciximab or to an accelerated infusion of alteplase [76]. The primary endpoint, a serial scintigraphic assessment of myocardial salvage, revealed a significantly greater preservation of myocardium at risk in those patients randomized to stenting plus abciximab. The secondary endpoint, death, reinfarction, or stroke by 6 months, was 8.5% in the stent–abciximab group versus 23.2% in the accelerated alteplase group, p = 0.02.

A study of patients with acute MI undergoing stenting by Neumann et al. provided mechanistic insight into the actions of abciximab [77]. Although nearly all patients had thrombolysis in myocardial infarction (TIMI) 3 epicardial vessel flow established by stenting, improvements in coronary flow velocity, as determined by Doppler wire measurements, were observed in the group of patients with acute MI randomized to abciximab versus conventional therapy at the time of PCI. There was also a corresponding improvement in infarct zone regional wall motion and ejection fraction in those patients treated with abciximab (ejection fraction of 62 vs. 56%, p = 0.003). Thus, part of the benefit abciximab appears to be mediated by improvements in microvascular flow and function, with associated preservation of left ventricular function.

The Controlled Abciximab and Device Investigation to Lower Late Angioplasty Complications (CADILLAC) trial randomized 2082 acute MI patients to four groups: angioplasty alone, angioplasty plus abciximab, stenting alone, and stenting plus abciximab [77a]. The primary endpoint of death, reinfarction, disabling stroke, or target vessel revascularization (TVR), owing to ischemia at 6 months, occurred in 18.4% of the angioplasty group, 14.2% of the angioplasty plus abciximab group, 10.4% of the stent group, and 9.5% of the stent plus abciximab group. Ischemic TVR at 30 days was reduced in patients receiving abciximab, from 4.2 to 2.4%, p = 0.02 [78]. Additionally, there were no increases in bleeding, stroke, or thrombocytopenia owing to abciximab. Of note, CADILLAC randomized patients after angiography, perhaps leading to exclusion of the highest-risk patients.

B. Abciximab as Monotherapy for Acute ST-Elevation MI

In the Glycoprotein Receptor Antagonist Patency Evaluation (GRAPE) pilot study, about 20% of patients awaiting primary angioplasty who received abciximab in the emergency department achieved TIMI 3 flow by 45 min [79]. In TIMI 14, the rate of TIMI 3 flow with abciximab alone at 90 min was 32% and in Strategies for Patency Enhancement in the Emergency Department (SPEED), the rate was 27% at 60–90 min. Therefore, as stand-alone therapy, abciximab provides patency rates equivalent to streptokinase and is not an improvement over current fibrinolytics. However, these data imply a complementarity with fibrinolysis. Furthermore, it may be reasonable to initiate abciximab while mobilizing a team that performs primary angioplasty.

C. Abciximab with Fibrinolysis for Acute ST-Elevation MI

Fibrinolytic therapy, while highly effective, itself creates a prothrombotic state by promotion of thrombin generation [80]. This occurs despite treatment with heparin, which itself has been associated with platelet activation [81]. However, combination of fibrinolytic agents with GP IIb/IIIa inhibitors may be a promising therapy to suppress platelet activation and enhance the speed and quality of fibrinolytic reperfusion [82]. Supporting this concept are data showing that platelet activation, as assessed by P-selectin expression, was stimulated by either alteplase or reteplase therapy for acute MI [83]. However, concomitant abciximab therapy reduced ADP-induced platelet aggregation despite an enhanced level of platelet activation with fibrinolytic therapy.

Abciximab has been studied after conventional full-dose fibrinolysis. The Thrombolysis and Angioplasty in Myocardial Infarction (TAMI)-8 pilot study first tested the concept of cautiously administering abciximab after full-dose alteplase [84]. There was a suggestion that abciximab improved the rate of angiographic TIMI 3 flow at 5 days. However, concerns about bleeding risks have limited this approach.

Partial-dose fibrinolytics combined with abciximab as a reperfusion strategy has been tested in three phase II studies. The TIMI 14 trial combined various regimens of fibrinolytics and abciximab [85]. The rate of TIMI 3 flow at 90 min for abciximab alone was 32%, for accelerated t-PA alone it was 62%, and for a 15-mg bolus of t-PA followed by a 35-mg infusion over 60 min plus abciximab was 77%. There was no significant increase in bleeding with the combination of half-dose t-PA and abciximab. The TIMI 14 trial also demonstrated that the combination of abciximab and reduced dose t-PA improved tissue level perfusion, as measured by electrocardiographic ST resolution [86]. The r-PA phase of TIMI 14 found that complete ($\geq$70%) ST-segment resolution at 90 min occurred in 56% of patients receiving a reduced dose of reteplase in combination with abciximab, when compared with 48% of patients receiving reteplase alone [87]. The SPEED trial showed that a double-bolus of low-dose r-PA plus abciximab and 60 U/kg of unfractionated heparin produced TIMI 3 flow in 61% of patients at 60 min [88]. Thus, both TIMI 14 and SPEED suggested that half-dose fibrinolysis with alteplase or reteplase plus abciximab resulted in better patency than full-dose fibrinolysis alone. The potential for improved safety (less bleeding) and greater efficacy (patency and mortality) is being evaluated in the large-scale GUSTO V trial that is examining abciximab plus low-dose double-bolus r-PA versus full-dose r-PA in a cohort of 16,600 patients.

The ENTIRE trial (TIMI 23) is examining combinations of abciximab, tenecteplase (TNK), and either unfractionated heparin or enoxaparin to determine which regimen produces the highest rates of TIMI 3 flow at 60 min in patients with acute MI. There are four treatment arms: half-dose TNK plus abciximab with unfractionated heparin, half-dose TNK plus abciximab with enoxaparin, full-dose TNK plus unfractionated heparin, and full-dose TNK plus enoxaparin. The ASSENT-3 trial is comparing full-dose TNK plus full-dose unfractionated heparin, half-dose TNK plus abciximab with low-dose unfractionated heparin, and full-dose TNK plus enoxaparin. The ENTIRE and ASSENT-3 trials will help determine the appropriate roles of abciximab and enoxaparin in the treatment of acute MI.

D. Facilitated PCI with Abciximab

In a subset analysis of patients who failed fibrinolysis in the GUSTO III trial and subsequently underwent rescue PCI with abciximab, there was a tendency toward a lower 30-day mortality in the 83 patients receiving abciximab than in those not treated with abciximab [89]. Patients receiving abciximab did have more episodes of severe bleeding (3.6% vs. 1.0%, p = 0.08), but there were no intracranial hemorrhages. An analysis of the patients in SPEED who underwent PCI within 60–90 min of receiving abciximab and low-dose rPA revealed a 5.7% rate of 30-day death, MI, or urgent revascularization [90]. Additional reports also demonstrate that facilitated PCI after low-dose fibrinolytics plus abciximab appears to be effective as well as safe, quite different from prior reports of early PCI after failed fibrinolysis, although the physician must still be cautious about increased bleeding risks [91,91a–d]. This concept will be more extensively tested in the FINESSE trial, comparing primary PCI with abciximab and stenting versus facilitated PCI after fibrinolytic therapy and abciximab. A total of 2700 patients will be randomized either to primary PCI plus abciximab or half-dose reteplase plus abciximab, followed by PCI in an open-label trial for patients presenting within 6 h of ST-segment elevation MI onset.

VI. STROKE

Animal data from a murine model support the value of abciximab in improving microvascular perfusion of ischemic brain tissue [92]. The Abciximab in Acute Ischemic Stroke investigators conducted a pilot study of 74 patients within 24 h of an acute ischemic stroke [93]. In the 54 patients who received various doses of abciximab, there were no cases of symptomatic intracranial hemorrhage. There was a trend toward less disability at 3 months in patients who received abciximab instead of placebo. The Abciximab for Emergency Stroke Treatment (AbESTT) trial is enrolling patients within 6 h of acute ischemic stroke and randomizing them to treatment with either abciximab or placebo. The primary endpoint is neurological outcome at 3 months. The major safety endpoint is fatal or nonfatal symptomatic intracranial hemorrhage. Just as with the treatment of acute MI, the possibility of using reduced-dose fibrinolytic therapy with abciximab also exists in the setting of stroke [94].

VII. CAROTID STENTING

As is true with PCI, embolization occurs during carotid stenting [34]. This creates a logical basis for use of abciximab during percutaneous interventions in the carotid artery. The initial experiences with use of abciximab in a population at greater risk for cerebral hemorrhage than in the PCI trials are encouraging, with no clear increase in intracranial hemorrhage rate [95–97]. The benefits of abciximab may also extend to vertebrobasilar intervention [98,99]. As yet, there have been no randomized comparisons of abciximab versus placebo for carotid intervention. Whether the advent of emboli protection devices will diminish the perceived need for abciximab remains to be seen.

VIII. PERIPHERAL ARTERIAL DISEASE

Peripheral arterial ischemia provides a possible role for intravenous antiplatelet therapy. Tepe et al. [100] studied 14 patients with acute or subacute iliofemoral or popliteal occlusions who were treated with urokinase, abciximab, heparin, and aspirin, as well as angioplasty of the residual stenosis. There was only 1 case of distal embolization and no episodes of major bleeding. Schweizer et al. randomized 84 patients with femoral or popliteal artery occlusion to intravenous abciximab or aspirin. All patients received alteplase and heparin, as well as mechanical thrombectomy [101]. The time to lysis was significantly decreased in the abciximab-treated patients, and the patency rate at 3 months was significantly increased. The rate of rehospitalization, reintervention, or amputation was also decreased in the abciximab group, from 73.1 to 52.4%, $p < 0.05$. The Platelet Receptor Antibodies in Order to Manage Peripheral Artery Thrombosis (PROMPT) study was the first randomized trial of GP IIb/IIIa inhibition in peripheral arterial occlusion [102]. Abciximab was combined with urokinase delivered intra-arterially. Three-month follow-up revealed that 4% of the group who received both abciximab and urokinase underwent amputation, versus 20% of the group who received urokinase alone. Therefore, abciximab appears to have a substantial potential in the treatment of peripheral arterial occlusion as an adjunct to fibrinolysis or percutaneous intervention.

IX. CONCLUSION

Abciximab has had a substantial influence on decreasing periprocedural ischemic events and long-term mortality after PCI. The benefit of abciximab is present in both urgent and elective intervention, and amplified in acute coronary syndromes. The ability of abciximab to reduce death, MI, and urgent revascularization is present across the spectrum of interventional devices utilized, and is complementary to the benefits of stenting in reducing target vessel revascularization. Diabetic patients especially derive marked benefit from abciximab, with reduction of mortality to the level of placebo-treated nondiabetics. Additionally, abciximab appears to reduce angiographic restenosis in diabetic patients with stents. Despite its expense, abciximab is cost-effective in the broad range of patients undergoing PCI. The role, if any, of abciximab for the medical management of acute coronary syndromes without the performance of PCI has not been defined. The usefulness of abciximab in conjunction with primary percutaneous revascularization for acute ST-elevation MI is well established. Large-scale evaluation is now underway to define the efficacy of combination therapy with abciximab and reduced dose fibrinolytics for acute MI. The use of abciximab outside of cardiology is likely to grow, particularly for the treatment of cerebrovascular and peripheral arterial diseases.

REFERENCES

1. Coller BS. Glycoprotein IIb/IIIa antagonists: development of abciximab and pharmacology of select agents. In: Lincoff AM, Topol EJ, eds. Platelet Glycoprotein IIb/IIIa Inhibitors in Cardiovascular Disease. Totowa, NJ: Humana Press, 1999; 67–89.
2. Topol EJ, Byzova TV, Plow EF. Platelet GPIIb–IIIa blockers. Lancet 1999; 353:227–231.
3. Mascelli MA, Lance ET, Damaraju L, Wagner CL, Weisman HF, Jordan RE. Pharmacodynamic profile of short-term abciximab treatment demonstrates prolonged platelet inhibition with gradual recovery from GP IIb/IIIa receptor blockade. Circulation 1998; 97:1680–1688.
4. Reverter JC, Beguin S, Kessels H, Kumar R, Hemker HC, Coller BS. Inhibition of platelet-mediated, tissue factor-induced thrombin generation by the mouse/human chimeric 7E3 antibody. Potential implications for the effect of c7E3 Fab treatment on acute thrombosis and "clinical restenosis." J Clin Invest 1996; 98:863–874.
5. Coller BS. Potential non-glycoprotein IIb/IIIa effects of abciximab. Am Heart J 1999; 138:S1–S5.
6. Coller BS. Binding of abciximab to alpha V beta 3 and activated alpha M beta 2 receptors: with a review of platelet-leukocyte interactions. Thromb Haemost 1999; 82:326–336.

7. Mickelson JK, Ali MN, Kleiman NS, Lakkis NM, Chow TW, Hughes BJ, Smith CW. Chimeric 7E3 Fab (ReoPro) decreases detectable CD11b on neutrophils from patients undergoing coronary angioplasty. J Am Coll Cardiol 1999; 33:97–106.

8. Neumann FJ, Zohlnhofer D, Fakhoury L, Ott I, Gawaz M, Schomig A. Effect of glycoprotein IIb/IIIa receptor blockade on platelet–leukocyte interaction and surface expression of the leukocyte integrin Mac-1 in acute myocardial infarction. J Am Coll Cardiol 1999; 34:1420–1426.

9. Gawaz M, Ruf A, Pogatsa-Murray G, Dickfeld T, Rudiger S, Taubitz W, Fischer J, Muller I, Meier D, Patscheke H, Schomig A. Incomplete inhibition of platelet aggregation and glycoprotein IIb–IIIa receptor blockade by abciximab: importance of internal pool of glycoprotein IIb–IIIa receptors. Thromb Haemost 2000; 83:915–922.

10. The EPIC Investigators. Use of a monoclonal antibody directed against the platelet glycoprotein IIb/IIIa receptor in high-risk coronary angioplasty. The EPIC investigation. N Engl J Med 1994; 330:956–961.

11. The EPILOG Investigators. Platelet glycoprotein IIb/IIIa receptor blockade and low-dose heparin during percutaneous coronary revascularization. N Engl J Med 1997; 336:1689–1696.

12. The EPISTENT Investigators. Randomised placebo-controlled and balloon–angioplasty-controlled trial to assess safety of coronary stenting with use of platelet glycoprotein-IIb/IIIa blockade. Evaluation of Platelet IIb/IIIa Inhibitor for Stenting. Lancet 1998; 352:87–92.

13. Topol EJ, Ferguson JJ, Weisman HF, Tcheng JE, Ellis SG, Kleiman NS, Ivanhoe RJ, Wang AL, Miller DP, Anderson KM, Califf RM. Long-term protection from myocardial ischemic events in a randomized trial of brief integrin beta-3 blockade with percutaneous coronary intervention. EPIC Investigator Group. Evaluation of Platelet IIb/IIIa Inhibition for Prevention of Ischemic Complication. JAMA 1997; 278:479–484.

14. Chamberlin JR, Lardi AB, McKeever LS, Wang MH, Ramadurai G, Grunenwald P, Towne WP, Grassman ED, Leya FS, Lewis BE, Stein LH. Use of vascular sealing devices (VasoSeal and Perclose) versus assisted manual compression (Femostop) in transcatheter coronary interventions requiring abciximab (ReoPro). Catheter Cardiovasc Interv 1999; 47:143–147 [discussion 148].

15. Lincoff AM, Califf RM, Moliterno DJ, Ellis SG, Ducas J, Kramer JH, Kleiman NS, Cohen EA, Booth JE, Sapp SK, Cabot CF, Topol EJ. Complementary clinical benefits of coronary-artery stenting and blockade of platelet glycoprotein IIb/IIIa receptors. Evaluation of Platelet IIb/IIIa Inhibition in Stenting investigators. N Engl J Med 1999; 341:319–327.

16. Lincoff AM, Tcheng JE, Califf RM, Kereiakes DJ, Kelly TA, Timmis GC, Kleiman NS, Booth JE, Balog C, Cabot CF, Anderson KM, Weisman HF, Topol EJ. Sustained suppression of ischemic complications of coronary intervention by platelet GP IIb/IIIa blockade with abciximab: one-year outcome in the EPILOG trial. Evaluation in PTCA to Improve Long-term Outcome with abciximab GP IIb/IIIa blockade. Circulation 1999; 99:1951–1958.

17. Topol EJ, Califf RM, Weisman HF, et al. Randomised trial of coronary intervention with antibody against platelet IIb/IIIa integrin for reduction of clinical restenosis: results at six months. The EPIC Investigators. Lancet 1994; 343:881–886.

18. The ERASER Investigators. Acute platelet inhibition with abciximab does not reduce in-stent restenosis (ERASER study). Circulation 1999; 100:799–806.

19. Neumann FJ, Kastrati A, Schmitt C, Blasini R, Hadamitzky M, Mehilli J, Gawaz M, Schleef M, Seyfarth M, Dirschinger J, Schomig A. Effect of glycoprotein IIb/IIIa receptor blockade with abciximab on clinical and angiographic restenosis rate after the placement of coronary stents following acute myocardial infarction. J Am Coll Cardiol 2000; 35:915–921.

20. Marso SP, Lincoff AM, Ellis SG, Bhatt DL, Tanguay JF, Kleiman NS, Hammoud T, Booth JE, Sapp SK, Topol EJ. Optimizing the percutaneous interventional outcomes for patients with diabetes mellitus: results of the EPISTENT (Evaluation of Platelet IIb/IIIa Inhibitor for Stenting trial) diabetic substudy. Circulation 1999; 100:2477–2484.

21. Ellis SG, Lincoff AM, Miller D, Tcheng JE, Kleiman NS, Kereiakes D, Califf R, Topol EJ. Reduction in complications of angioplasty with abciximab occurs largely independently of baseline lesion morphology. EPIC and EPILOG investigators. Evaluation of 7E3 for the Prevention of Ischemic Complications. Evaluation of PTCA to Improve Long-term Outcome with Abciximab GPIIb/IIIa Receptor Blockade. J Am Coll Cardiol 1998; 32:1619–1623.

22. Bhatt DL, Patel VB, Robbins MA, Wolski KE, Moliterno DJ, Ellis SG. Effect of Coronary Morphology and Vessel Size on the Benefit of Abciximab with Stenting. Circulation 1999; 100:I-857.

23. Barsness GW, Buller C, Ohman EM, Schechter E, Pucillo A, Taylor MA, Miller MJ, Reiner JS, Churchill D, Chandler AB, Gonzalez M, Smith J, Tommaso C, Berdan LG, Wildermann NM, Hasdai D, Holmes DR Jr. Reduced thrombus burden with abciximab delivered locally before percutaneous intervention in saphenous vein grafts. Am Heart J 2000; 139:824–829.

24. Bartorelli AL, Trabattoni D, Galli S, Grancini L, Cozzi S, Ravagnani P. Successful dissolution of occlusive coronary thrombus with local administration of abciximab during PTCA. Catheter Cardiovasc Interv 1999; 48:211–213.

25. Robinson N, Barakat K, Dymond D. Platelet IIb/IIIa antagonists followed by delayed stent implantation. A new treatment for vein graft lesions containing massive thrombus. Heart 1999; 81:434–437.

26. Bhatt DL, Lincoff AM, Califf RM, Simoons ML, Tcheng JE, Brener SJ, Wolski KE, Topol EJ. The benefit of abciximab in percutaneous coronary revascularization is not device-specific. Am J Cardiol 2000; 85:1060–1064.

27. Ghaffari S, Kereiakes DJ, Lincoff AM, Kelly TA, Timmis GC, Kleiman NS, Ferguson JJ, Miller DP, Califf RA, Topol EJ. Platelet glycoprotein IIb/IIIa receptor blockade with abciximab reduces ischemic complications in patients undergoing directional coronary atherectomy. EPILOG investigators. Evaluation of PTCA to Improve Long-term Outcome by c7E3 GP IIb/IIIa Receptor Blockade. Am J Cardiol 1998; 82:7–12.

28. Bhatt DL, Lincoff AM, Kereiakes DJ, Tcheng JE, Simoons ML, van der Wieken LR, Godfrey N, Califf RM, Topol EJ. Reduction in the need for unplanned stenting with the use of platelet glycoprotein IIb/IIIa blockade in percutaneous coronary intervention. Am J Cardiol 1998; 82:1105–6, A6.

29. Kereiakes DJ, Lincoff AM, Miller DP, Tcheng JE, Cabot CF, Anderson KM, Weisman HF, Califf RM, Topol EJ. Abciximab therapy and unplanned coronary stent deployment: favorable effects on stent use, clinical outcomes, and bleeding complications. EPILOG trial investigators. Circulation 1998; 97:857–864.

30. Braden GA, Applegate RJ, Young TM, Love WW, Sane DC. Abciximab decreases both the incidence and magnitude of creatine kinase elevation during rotational atherectomy. J Am Coll Cardiol 1997; 29:499A.

31. Koch KC, vom Dahl J, Kleinhans E, Klues HG, Radke PW, Ninnemann S, Schulz G, Buell U, Hanrath P. Influence of a platelet GPIIb/IIIa receptor antagonist on myocardial hypoperfusion during rotational atherectomy as assessed by myocardial Tc-99m sestamibi scintigraphy. J Am Coll Cardiol 1999; 33:998–1004.

32. Williams MS, Coller BS, Vaananen HJ, Scudder LE, Sharma SK, Marmur JD. Activation of platelets in platelet-rich plasma by rotablation is speed-dependent and can be inhibited by abciximab (c7E3 Fab; ReoPro). Circulation 1998; 98:742–748.

33. Bhatt DL, Topol EJ. Embolization as a pathological mechanism. In: Topol EJ, ed. Acute Coronary Syndromes. 2nd ed. New York: Marcel Dekker, 2000; 79–110.

34. Topol EJ, Yadav JS. Recognition of the importance of embolization in atherosclerotic vascular disease. Circulation 2000; 101:570–580.

35. Mak KH, Challapalli R, Eisenberg MJ, Anderson KM, Califf RM, Topol EJ. Effect of platelet glycoprotein IIb/IIIa receptor inhibition on distal embolization during percutaneous revascularization of aortocoronary saphenous vein grafts. EPIC investigators. Evaluation of IIb/IIIa Platelet Receptor Antagonist 7E3 in Preventing Ischemic Complications. Am J Cardiol 1997; 80:985–988.

36. Lefkovits J, Blankenship JC, Anderson KM, Stoner GL, Talley JD, Worley SJ, Weisman HF, Califf RM, Topol EJ. Increased risk of non-Q wave myocardial infarction after directional atherectomy is platelet dependent: evidence from the EPIC trial. Evaluation of c7E3 for the Prevention of Ischemic Complications. J Am Coll Cardiol 1996; 28:849–855.

37. Haase KK, Mahrholdt H, Schroder S, Baumbach A, Oberhoff M, Herdeg C, Karsch KR. Frequency and efficacy of glycoprotein IIb/IIIa therapy for treatment of threatened or acute vessel closure in

     1332 patients undergoing percutaneous transluminal coronary angioplasty. Am Heart J 1999; 137:234–240.

38. Muhlestein JB, Karagounis LA, Treehan S, Anderson JL. "Rescue" utilization of abciximab for the dissolution of coronary thrombus developing as a complication of coronary angioplasty. J Am Coll Cardiol 1997; 30:1729–1734.

39. Fuchs S, Kornowski R, Mehran R, Gruberg L, Satler LF, Pichard AD, Kent KM, Stone GW, Leon MB. Clinical outcomes following "rescue" administration of abciximab in patients undergoing percutaneous coronary angioplasty. J Invas Cardiol 2000; 12:497–501.

40. van Hout BA, Bowman L, Zelinger DJ, Simoons ML. Costs and effects in therapy for acute coronary syndromes: the case of abciximab in high-risk patients undergoing percutaneous transluminal coronary angioplasty in the EPIC study. Evaluation of 7E3 for the Prevention of Ischemic Complications. Eur Heart J 1998; 19 (suppl D):D59–66.

41. Topol EJ, Mark DB, Lincoff AM, Cohen E, Burton J, Kleiman N, Talley D, Sapp S, Booth J, Cabot CF, Anderson KM, Califf RM. Outcomes at 1 year and economic implications of platelet glycoprotein IIb/IIIa blockade in patients undergoing coronary stenting: results from a multicentre randomised trial. EPISTENT investigators. Evaluation of Platelet IIb/IIIa Inhibitor for Stenting [published erratum appears in Lancet 2000 Mar 25; 355:1104]. Lancet 1999; 354:2019–2024.

42. Lage MJ, Barber BL, Bowman L, Ball DE, Bala M. Shorter hospital stays for angioplasty patients who receive abciximab. J Invasive Cardiol 2000; 12:179–186.

43. Kereiakes DJ, Obenchain RL, Barber BL, Smith A, McDonald M, Broderick TM, Runyon JP, Shimshak TM, Schneider JF, Hattemer CR, Roth EM, Whang DD, Cocks D, Abbottsmith CW. Abciximab provides cost-effective survival advantage in high-volume interventional practice. Am Heart J 2000; 140:603–610.

44. Bhatt DL, Marso SP, Lincoff AM, Wolski KE, Ellis SG, Topol EJ. Abciximab reduces mortality in diabetics following percutaneous coronary intervention. J Am Coll Cardiol 2000; 35:922–928.

45. Bhatt DL, Chew DP, Topol EJ. The importance of intravenous antiplatelet therapy with abciximab during percutaneous coronary intervention in diabetic patients. Cardiovasc Rev Rep 2001; 21:161–164.

46. Giugliano RP, Hyatt RR. Thrombocytopenia with GP IIb/IIIa inhibitors: a meta-analysis. J Am Coll Cardiol 1998; 31:185A.

46a. Dasgupta H, Blankenship JC, Wood GC, Frey CM, Demko SL, Menapace FJ. Thrombocytopenia complicating treatment with intravenous glycoprotein IIb/IIIa receptor inhibitors: a pooled analysis. Am Heart J 2000; 140:206–211.

47. Sane DC, Damaraju LV, Topol EJ, Cabot CF, Mascelli MA, Harrington RA, Simoons ML, Califf RM. Occurrence and clinical significance of pseudothrombocytopenia during abciximab therapy. J Am Coll Cardiol 2000; 36:75–83.

48. Madan M, Kereiakes DJ, Hermiller JB, Rund MM, Tudor G, Anderson L, McDonald MB, Berkowitz SD, Sketch MH, Jr, Phillips HR 3rd, Tcheng JE. Efficacy of abciximab readministration in coronary intervention. Am J Cardiol 2000; 85:435–440.

49. Tcheng JE, Kereiakes DJ, Braden GA, Jordan RE, Mascelli MA, Langrall MA, Effron MB. Readministration of abciximab: interim report of the ReoPro Readministration Registry. Am Heart J 1999; 138:S33–38.

50. Tcheng JE. Clinical challenges of platelet glycoprotein IIb/IIIa receptor inhibitor therapy: bleeding, reversal, thrombocytopenia, and retreatment. Am Heart J 2000; 139:S38–S45.

51. Lincoff AM, LeNarz LA, Despotis GJ, Smith PK, Booth JE, Raymond RE, Sapp SK, Cabot CF, Tcheng JE, Califf RM, Effron MB, Topol EJ. Abciximab and bleeding during coronary surgery: results from the EPILOG and EPISTENT trials. Improve long-term outcome with abciximab GP IIb/IIIa blockade. Evaluation of platelet IIb/IIIa inhibition in STENTing. Ann Thorac Surg 2000; 70:516–526.

52. Topol EJ, Moliterno DJ, Herrmann HC, Powers ER, Grines CL, Cohen DJ, Yakubov SJ, Cohen EA, Bertrand M, Neumann F–J, Stone GW, DiBattiste PM, Demopoulos L, for the TARGET investigators. Comparison of two platelet glycoprotein IIb/IIIa inhibitors, tirofiban and abciximab, for the prevention of ischemic events with percutaneous coronary intervention. N Engl J Med 2001; 344:1888–1894.

53. Kleiman NS, Grazeiadei N, Maresh K, Taylor RJ, Frederick B, Lance ET, Effron MB, Jordan RE, Mascelli MA. Abciximab, ticlopidine, and concomitant abciximab–ticlopidine therapy: ex vivo platelet aggregation inhibition profiles in patients undergoing percutaneous coronary interventions. Am Heart J 2000; 140:492–503.

54. Fredrickson BJ, Turner NA, Kleiman NS, Graziadei N, Maresh K, Mascelli MA, Effron MB, McIntire LV. Effects of abciximab, ticlopidine, and combined abciximab/ticlopidine therapy on platelet and leukocyte function in patients undergoing coronary angioplasty. Circulation 2000; 101:1122–1129.

55. Peter K, Kohler B, Straub A, Ruef J, Moser M, Nordt T, Olschewski M, Ohman ME, Kubler W, Bode C. Flow cytometric monitoring of glycoprotein IIb/IIIa blockade and platelet function in patients with acute myocardial infarction receiving reteplase, abciximab, and ticlopidine: continuous platelet inhibition by the combination of abciximab and ticlopidine. Circulation 2000; 102:1490–1496.

56. Dangas G, Badimon JJ, Coller BS, Fallon JT, Sharma SK, Hayes RM, Meraj P, Ambrose JA, Marmur JD. Administration of abciximab during percutaneous coronary intervention reduces both ex vivo platelet thrombus formation and fibrin deposition: implications for a potential anticoagulant effect of abciximab. Arterioscler Thromb Vasc Biol 1998; 18:1342–1349.

57. Ammar T, Scudder LE, Coller BS. In vitro effects of the platelet glycoprotein IIb/IIIa receptor antagonist c7E3 Fab on the activated clotting time. Circulation 1997; 95:614–617.

58. Ambrose JA, Hawkey M, Badimon JJ, Coppola J, Geagea J, Rentrop KP, Domiguez A, Duvvuri S, Elmquist T, Arias J, Doss R, Dangas G. In vivo demonstration of an antithrombin effect of abciximab. Am J Cardiol 2000; 86:150–152.

59. Kereiakes DJ, Fry E, Matthai W, Niederman A, Barr L, Brodie B, Zidar J, Casale P, Christy G, Moliterno D, Lengerich R, Broderick T, Shimshak T, Cohen M. Combination enoxaparin and abciximab therapy during percutaneous coronary intervention: "NICE guys finish first." J Invasive Cardiol 2000; 12 (suppl A):1A–5A.

60. Tramuta DA, Kereiakes DJ, Dippel EJ, Lengerich R, Broderick TM, Abbottsmith CW, Whang DD, Roth EM, Schneider JF, Howard W, Shimshak TM. Combination enoxaparin–abciximab therapy during coronary intervention: the next standard of care? J Invasive Cardiol 2000; 12 (suppl C):3C–6C.

61. Simoons ML. GUSTO IV ACS. Presented at the European Society of Cardiology, Amsterdam, Netherlands, 2000.

61a. Ferguson JJ. NICE-3. Presented at the European Society of Cardiology, Amsterdam, Netherlands, 2000.

62. Kleiman NS, Lincoff AM, Sapp SK, Maresh KJ, Topol EJ. Pharmacodynamics of a direct thrombin inhibitor combined with a GP IIb–IIIa antagonist: first experience in humans. Circulation 1999; 100: I-328.

63. Lincoff AM, Califf RM, Anderson KM, Weisman HF, Aguirre FV, Kleiman NS, Harrington RA, Topol EJ. Evidence for prevention of death and myocardial infarction with platelet membrane glycoprotein IIb/IIIa receptor blockade by abciximab (c7E3 Fab) among patients with unstable angina undergoing percutaneous coronary revascularization. EPIC investigators. Evaluation of 7E3 in Preventing Ischemic Complications. J Am Coll Cardiol 1997; 30:149–156.

64. Roe MT, Gum PA, Booth JE, Jia G, Damaraju L, Fitzpatrick SE, Kereiakes DJ, Tcheng JE. Consistent and durable reduction in death and myocardial infarction with abciximab during coronary intervention in acute coronary syndromes and stable angina: a pooled analysis from EPIC, EPILOG, and EPISTENT. Circulation 1999; 100:I-187.

65. The CAPTURE Investigators. Randomised placebo-controlled trial of abciximab before and during coronary intervention in refractory unstable angina: the CAPTURE study. Lancet 1997; 349:1429–1435.

66. Klootwijk P, Meij S, Melkert R, Lenderink T, Simoons ML. Reduction of recurrent ischemia with abciximab during continuous ECG–ischemia monitoring in patients with unstable angina refractory to standard treatment (CAPTURE). Circulation 1998; 98:1358–1364.

67. van den Brand M, Laarman GJ, Steg PG, De Scheerder I, Heyndrickx G, Beatt K, Kootstra J, Simoons ML. Assessment of coronary angiograms prior to and after treatment with abciximab, and the outcome of angioplasty in refractory unstable angina patients. Angiographic results from the CAPTURE trial. Eur Heart J 1999; 20:1572–1578.

68. Hamm CW, Heeschen C, Goldmann B, Vahanian A, Adgey J, Miguel CM, Rutsch W, Berger J, Kootstra J, Simoons ML. Benefit of abciximab in patients with refractory unstable angina in relation to serum troponin T levels. c7E3 Fab Antiplatelet Therapy in Unstable Refractory Angina (CAPTURE) study investigators. N Engl J Med 1999; 340:1623–1629.

69. Kleiman NS, Raizner AE, Jordan R, Wang AL, Norton D, Mace KF, Joshi A, Coller BS, Weisman HF. Differential inhibition of platelet aggregation induced by adenosine diphosphate or a thrombin receptor-activating peptide in patients treated with bolus chimeric 7E3 Fab: implications for inhibition of the internal pool of GPIIb/IIIa receptors. J Am Coll Cardiol 1995; 26:1665–1671.

70. Chew DP, Bhatt DL, Sapp S, Topol EJ. Increased mortality with oral platelet glycoprotein IIb/IIIa antagonists: a meta-analysis of the phase III multicenter randomized controlled trials. Circulation 2001; 103:201–206.

71. Bhatt DL, Topol EJ. Current role of platelet glycoprotein IIb/IIIa inhibitors in acute coronary syndromes. JAMA 2000; 284:1549–1558.

72. Brener SJ, Barr LA, Burchenal JE, Katz S, George BS, Jones AA, Cohen ED, Gainey PC, White HJ, Cheek HB, Moses JW, Moliterno DJ, Effron MB, Topol EJ. Randomized, placebo-controlled trial of platelet glycoprotein IIb/IIIa blockade with primary angioplasty for acute myocardial infarction. ReoPro and Primary PTCA Organization and Randomized Trial (RAPPORT) investigators. Circulation 1998; 98:734–741.

73. Brener SJ, Barr LA, Burchenal JE, Wolski KE, Effron MB, Topol EJ. Effect of abciximab on the pattern of reperfusion in patients with acute myocardial infarction treated with primary angioplasty. RAPPORT investigators. ReoPro and Primary PTCA Organization and Randomized Trial. Am J Cardiol 1999; 84:728–730, A8.

74. Grines CL, Cox DA, Stone GW, Garcia E, Mattos LA, Giambartolomei A, Brodie BR, Madonna O, Eijgelshoven M, Lansky AJ, O'Neill WW, Morice MC. Coronary angioplasty with or without stent implantation for acute myocardial infarction. Stent Primary Angioplasty in Myocardial Infarction Study Group. N Engl J Med 1999; 341:1949–1956.

75. Montalescot G, et al. ADMIRAL study. N Engl J Med, 2001; 344:1895–1903.

76. Schomig A, Kastrati A, Dirschinger J, Mehilli J, Schricke U, Pache J, Martinoff S, Neumann FJ, Schwaiger M. Coronary stenting plus platelet glycoprotein IIb/IIIa blockade compared with tissue plasminogen activator in acute myocardial infarction. Stent versus thrombolysis for occluded coronary arteries in patients with acute myocardial infarction study investigators. N Engl J Med 2000; 343:385–391.

77. Neumann FJ, Blasini R, Schmitt C, Alt E, Dirschinger J, Gawaz M, Kastrati A, Schomig A. Effect of glycoprotein IIb/IIIa receptor blockade on recovery of coronary flow and left ventricular function after the placement of coronary-artery stents in acute myocardial infarction. Circulation 1998; 98:2695–2701.

77a. Stone GW, Grines CL, Cox DA, Garcia E, Tcheng JE, Griffin JJ, Guagliumi G, Stuckey T, Turco M, Carroll JD, Rutherford BD, Lansky AJ. Comparison of angioplasty with stenting, with or without abciximab, in acute myocardial infarction. N Engl J Med 2002; 346:957–966.

78. Tcheng JE, Effron M, Grines CL, Garcia E, Cox D, Stuckey T, Carroll J, Guagliumi G, Rutherford B, Lansky AJ, Esente P, Griffin J, Stone GW. Abciximab use during percutaneous intervention in patients with acute myocardial infarction improves early and late clinical outcomes: final results of the CADILLAC trial. J Am Coll Cardiol 2001; 37:343A.

79. van den Merkhof LF, Zijlstra F, Olsson H, Grip L, Veen G, Bar FW, van den Brand MJ, Simoons ML, Verheugt FW. Abciximab in the treatment of acute myocardial infarction eligible for primary percutaneous transluminal coronary angioplasty. Results of the Glycoprotein Receptor Antagonist Patency Evaluation (GRAPE) pilot study. J Am Coll Cardiol 1999; 33:1528–1532.

80. Owen J, Friedman KD, Grossman BA, Wilkins C, Berke AD, Powers ER. Thrombolytic therapy with tissue plasminogen activator or streptokinase induces transient thrombin activity. Blood 1988; 72:616–620.

81. Xiao Z, Theroux P. Platelet activation with unfractionated heparin at therapeutic concentrations and comparisons with a low-molecular-weight heparin and with a direct thrombin inhibitor. Circulation 1998; 97:251–256.

82. Hudson MP, Greenbaum AB, Harrington RA, Ohman EM. Use of glycoprotein IIb/IIIa inhibition plus fibrinolysis in acute myocardial infarction. J Thromb Thrombolysis 1999; 7:241–245.

83. Coulter SA, Cannon CP, Ault KA, Antman EM, Van de Werf F, Adgey AA, Gibson CM, Giugliano RP, Mascelli MA, Scherer J, Barnathan ES, Braunwald E, Kleiman NS. High levels of platelet inhibition with abciximab despite heightened platelet activation and aggregation during thrombolysis for acute myocardial infarction: results from TIMI (thrombolysis in myocardial infarction) 14. Circulation 2000; 101:2690–2695.

84. Kleiman NS, Ohman EM, Califf RM, George BS, Kereiakes D, Aguirre FV, Weisman H, Schaible T, Topol EJ. Profound inhibition of platelet aggregation with monoclonal antibody 7E3 Fab after thrombolytic therapy. Results of the Thrombolysis and Angioplasty in Myocardial Infarction (TAMI) 8 pilot study. J Am Coll Cardiol 1993; 22:381–389.

85. Antman EM, Giugliano RP, Gibson CM, McCabe CH, Coussement P, Kleiman NS, Vahanian A, Adgey AA, Menown I, Rupprecht HJ, Van der Wieken R, Ducas J, Scherer J, Anderson K, Van de Werf F, Braunwald E. Abciximab facilitates the rate and extent of thrombolysis: results of the thrombolysis in myocardial infarction (TIMI) 14 trial. The TIMI 14 investigators. Circulation 1999; 99:2720–2732.

86. de Lemos JA, Antman EM, Gibson CM, McCabe CH, Giugliano RP, Murphy SA, Coulter SA, Anderson K, Scherer J, Frey MJ, Van Der Wieken R, Van De Werf F, Braunwald E. Abciximab improves both epicardial flow and myocardial reperfusion in ST-elevation myocardial infarction: observations from the TIMI 14 trial. Circulation 2000; 101:239–243.

87. Antman EM, Gibson CM, de Lemos JA, Giugliano RP, McCabe CH, Coussement P, Menown I, Nienaber CA, Rehders TC, Frey MJ, Van der Wieken R, Andresen D, Scherer J, Anderson K, Van de Werf F, Braunwald E. Combination reperfusion therapy with abciximab and reduced dose reteplase: results from TIMI 14. The Thrombolysis in Myocardial Infarction (TIMI) 14 Investigators. Eur Heart J 2000; 21:1944–1953.

88. The SPEED Group. Trial of abciximab with and without low-dose reteplase for acute myocardial infarction. Strategies for Patency Enhancement in the Emergency Department (SPEED) group. Circulation 2000; 101:2788–2794.

89. Miller JM, Smalling R, Ohman EM, Bode C, Betriu A, Kleiman NS, Schildcrout JS, Bastos E, Topol EJ, Califf RM. Effectiveness of early coronary angioplasty and abciximab for failed thrombolysis (reteplase or alteplase) during acute myocardial infarction (results from the GUSTO-III trial). Global Use of Strategies To Open occluded coronary arteries. Am J Cardiol 1999; 84:779–784.

90. Herrmann HC, Moliterno DJ, Bode C, Betriu A, Lincoff AM, Ohman EM. Combination abciximab and reduced-dose reteplase facilitates early PCI in acute MI: results from the SPEED trial. J Am Coll Cardiol 2000; 36:1489–1496.

91. Gibson CM. Primary angioplasty compared with thrombolysis: new issues in the era of glycoprotein IIb/IIIa inhibition and intracoronary stenting. Ann Intern Med 1999; 130:841–847.

91a. Sundlof DW, Rerkpattanapitat P, Wongpraparut N, Pathi P, Kotler MN, Jacobs LE, Ledley GS, Yazdanfar S. Incidence of bleeding complications associated with abciximab use in conjunction with thrombolytic therapy in patients requiring percutaneous transluminal coronary angioplasty. Am J Cardiol 1999; 83:1569–1571, A7.

91b. Cantor WJ, Kaplan AL, Velianou JL, Sketch MH Jr, Barsness GW, Berger PB, Ohman EM. Effectiveness and safety of abciximab after failed thrombolytic therapy. Am J Cardiol 2001; 87:439–442, A4.

91c. Schweiger MJ, Antman EM, Piana RN, Giugliano RP, Burkott B, Van de Werf F. Effect of abciximab (ReoPro) on early rescue angioplasty in TIMI 14. Circulation 1998; 98:I-17.

91d. Ronner E, van Domburg RT, van de Brand MJBM, de Feyter PJ, Foley DP, van der Giessen WJ, Serrus PW, Simoons ML. Platelet glycoprotein IIb/IIIa receptor blockade after failed thrombolysis is associated with risk of bleeding. J Am Coll Cardiol 2000; 35:371A.

92. Choudhri TF, Hoh BL, Zerwes HG, Prestigiacomo CJ, Kim SC, Connolly ES Jr, Kottirsch G, Pinsky DJ. Reduced microvascular thrombosis and improved outcome in acute murine stroke by inhibiting GP IIb/IIIa receptor-mediated platelet aggregation. J Clin Invest 1998; 102:1301–1310.

93. The Abciximab in Ischemic Stroke Investigators. Abciximab in acute ischemic stroke: a randomized, double-blind, placebo-controlled, dose-escalation study. Stroke 2000; 31:601–609.
94. Winkley JM, Adams HP Jr. Potential role of abciximab in ischemic cerebrovascular disease. Am J Cardiol 2000; 85:47C–451C.
95. Kapadia SR, Bajzer CT, Ziada KM, Bhatt DL, Wazni OM, Silver MJ, Beven EG, Ouriel K, Yadav JS. Initial experience of platelet glycoprotein IIb/IIIa inhibition with abciximab during carotid stenting: a safe and effective adjunctive therapy. Stroke 2001; 32:2328–2332.
96. Cecena FA, Hoelzinger DH, Miller JA, Abu–Shakra S. The platelet IIb/IIIa inhibitor abciximab as adjunctive therapy in carotid stenting of potential thrombotic lesions. J Intervent Cardiol 1999; 12:355–362.
97. Schneiderman J, Morag B, Gerniak A, Rimon U, Varon D, Seligsohn U, Shotan A, Adar R. Abciximab in carotid stenting for postsurgical carotid restenosis: intermediate results. J Endovasc Ther 2000; 7:263–272.
98. Qureshi AI, Suri MF, Khan J, Fessler RD, Guterman LR, Hopkins LN. Abciximab as an adjunct to high-risk carotid or vertebrobasilar angioplasty: preliminary experience. Neurosurgery 2000; 46:1316–1324 [discussion 1324–1325].
99. Rasmussen PA, Perl J 2nd, Barr JD, Markarian GZ, Katzan I, Sila C, Krieger D, Furlan AJ, Masaryk TJ. Stent-assisted angioplasty of intracranial vertebrobasilar atherosclerosis: an initial experience. J Neurosurg 2000; 92:771–778.
100. Tepe G, Schott U, Erley CM, Albes J, Claussen CD, Duda SH. Platelet glycoprotein IIb/IIIa receptor antagonist used in conjunction with thrombolysis for peripheral arterial thrombosis. Am J Roentgenol 1999; 172:1343–1346.
101. Schweizer J. Short- and long-term results of abciximab versus aspirin in conjunction with thrombolysis for patients with peripheral obstructive arterial disease. Angiology 2000; 51:913–923.
102. Tepe G, Schott U, Erley C, Albes J, Claussen CD, Duda SH. Conjunctive platelet glycoprotein IIb/IIIa receptor antagonism and thrombolysis for peripheral arterial thrombosis: results of the pilot trial platelet receptor antibodies in order to manage peripheral arterial thrombosis (PROMPT). Radiology 1998; 209:303.

23

Eptifibatide: A Potent Inhibitor of the Platelet Receptor Integrin, Glycoprotein IIb/IIIa

J. Conor O'Shea, James E. Tcheng, Robert A. Harrington, and Robert M. Califf
Duke University Medical Center, Durham, North Carolina, U.S.A.

SUMMARY

Elucidation of the pivotal role of the platelet glycoprotein (GP) IIb/IIIa integrin as the receptor that mediates platelet aggregation has provided the framework for investigating the GP IIb/IIIa receptor antagonists. Among the most specific inhibitors is eptifibatide (Integrilin, COR Therapeutics, S. San Francisco, CA), a cyclic heptapeptide based on a peptide recognition sequence found in the venom of the Southeastern Pygmy rattlesnake *Sistrurus m. barbouri*. Peptide inhibitors such as eptifibatide bind competitively to GP IIb/IIIa and have a short half-life, allowing the effect to be relatively rapidly reversible and providing a favorable overall safety profile, although there is a slightly increased incidence of major and minor bleeding.

Eptifibatide has reduced acute ischemic complications in percutaneous coronary intervention, ST-segment and non–ST-segment acute myocardial infarction (MI), and unstable angina. In the Enhanced Suppression of the Platelet IIb/IIIa Receptor with Integrilin Therapy (ESPRIT) trial, two 180-μg/kg boluses of eptifibatide 10 min apart, followed by an 18- to 24-h infusion at 2 μg/kg min^{-1}, given as adjunctive therapy in nonurgent percutaneous coronary stent implantation reduced the 30-day composite of death, MI, and need for urgent target vessel revascularization from 10.4 to 6.8%, compared with placebo.

Among the patients with acute coronary syndromes in the Platelet Glycoprotein IIb/IIIa in Unstable Angina: Receptor Suppression Using Integrilin Therapy (PURSUIT) trial, eptifibatide given as a 180-μg/kg single bolus, followed by a 72-h infusion at 2 μg/kg min^{-1} produced a significant (1.5%) absolute reduction in the 30-day composite of death and nonfatal MI. The Integrelin to Manage Platelet Aggregation to Prevent Coronary Thrombosis in Acute Myocardial Infarction (IMPACT–AMI) study was the first trial to evaluate GP IIb/IIIa inhibition concurrent with thrombolytic therapy. This randomized, blinded, dose-ranging trial of eptifibatide with full-dose, accelerated regimen t-PA suggested that GP IIb/IIIa inhibition would improve both the proportion of patients achieving reperfusion as well as the kinetics of reperfusion.

I. INTRODUCTION

Platelet activation, adhesion, and aggregation are central in the pathogenesis of acute coronary syndromes. Platelet deposition and subsequent thrombus formation result in unstable angina, myocardial infarction, and abrupt vessel closure after percutaneous coronary interventions (PCI). Inhibition of platelet aggregation has, therefore, become a prime therapeutic target in the management of acute coronary syndromes and the ischemic complications of coronary intervention [1]. The primary membrane glycoprotein mediating platelet aggregation is glycoprotein GP IIb/IIIa ($\alpha_{IIb}\beta_3$) (2–6). The GP IIb/IIIa receptor is thought to be the final common pathway of platelet aggregation that binds adhesive macromolecules, which can then allow cross-linking of platelets and, ultimately platelet aggregation [7,8]. The cyclic heptapeptide, eptifibatide binds competitively to the GP IIb/IIIa receptor and inhibits platelet aggregation.

II. INTEGRINS AND THE IIb/IIIa RECEPTOR

The platelet glycoproteins have been identified and classified as members of one of five gene families, the most abundant of which is the integrins. Integrins are a widely dispersed, heterodimeric family of cell adhesion molecules found on many cell types, including leukocytes and platelets, and mediate a large number of cell and adhesive protein interactions [4,5,7,9]. The glycoprotein GP IIIb/IIIa receptor is the only integrin for which expression is limited to platelets [6]. GP IIb/IIIa is a calcium-dependent heterodimer consisting of two transmembrane proteins: a 136-kDa α-subunit, consisting of a heavy and a light chain, and a 92-kDa β-subunit. The surface of a typical platelet contains 50,000–80,000 GP IIb/IIIa receptors [10]. The binding of adhesive proteins to $\alpha_{IIb}\beta_3$ occurs through two peptide sequences: RGD (Arg–Gly–Asp) and KQAGDV (Lys–Gln–Ala–Gly–Asp–Val) (Fig. 1) [3,11–14]. The RGD sequence is found on fibrinogen, fibronectin, von Willebrand's factor (vWF), vitronectin, thrombospondin, and type I collagen [3,7,15–17]. The KQAGDV peptide-binding sequence is located at 400–411 on the Y chain of fibrinogen and consists of the dodecapeptide sequence HHLGGAKQAGDV (see Fig. 1)

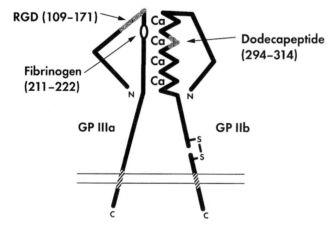

Figure 1 Structure of the GP IIIb/IIIa complex and binding sites: The dodecapeptide from the γ-chain of fibrinogen crosslinks to GPIIb. RGD peptides have been crosslinked to GPIIIa. The α and β subunits are dependent on calcium. Chelation of calcium will dissociate the heterodimer and cause loss of function. (From Ref. 6.)

[18–23]. Of these adhesive molecules, fibrinogen appears to be the most important ligand in thrombosis because it exists in high concentrations in the blood and, as it is divalent, it can simultaneously bind to glycoprotein IIb/IIIa receptors on separate platelets resulting in platelet aggregation [24].

III. EPTIFIBATIDE

The path leading to the synthesis of eptifibatide (Integrilin, COR Therapeutics, South San Francisco, CA) has its roots in the search for GP IIb/IIIa inhibitors among naturally occurring proteins. RGD sequences similar to that of fibrinogen are present in snake venom proteins and reversibly bind GP IIb/IIIa in vitro and in vivo and inhibit platelet aggregation [25–29]. These peptides, termed *disintegrins*, reversibly block the adhesive interactions of multiple RGD-dependent integrins and thereby inhibit binding of a variety of ligands [13,16,30–34]. Scarborough et al. screened 62 snake venoms [31] and found an isolate from the Southeastern Pygmy rattlesnake *Sistrurus m. barbouri*, called barbourin, that selectively inhibited fibrinogen binding to the IIb/IIIa receptor without inhibiting binding to the other RGD-dependent receptors [31]. The reason for the increased specificity of barbourin was that it differed by a single conservative amino acid substitution of lysine (K) for arginine (R) [32]. Eptifibatide was created based on the KGD sequence found in barbourin and was engineered with a ring structure to impart resistance to proteolysis (Fig. 2). The potential benefits of KGD cyclic peptide inhibitors of GP IIb/IIIa, such as eptifibatide, include the ability of the peptide to bind to the GP IIb/IIIa receptor with high specificity and affinity, blocking the binding of ligands fibrinogen and vWF without affecting the binding properties of other integrins. In addition, it is nonimmunogenic, potent, and has effects that are rapidly reversible.

A. Clinical Pharmacology

When administered intravenously, eptifibatide inhibits ex vivo platelet aggregation in a concentration-dependent manner. Platelet aggregation inhibition reverses after cessation of an eptifibatide infusion, with clearance of the drug from the plasma compartment. In preclinical studies performed in baboons and dogs, inhibition of ex vivo ADP-induced platelet aggregation

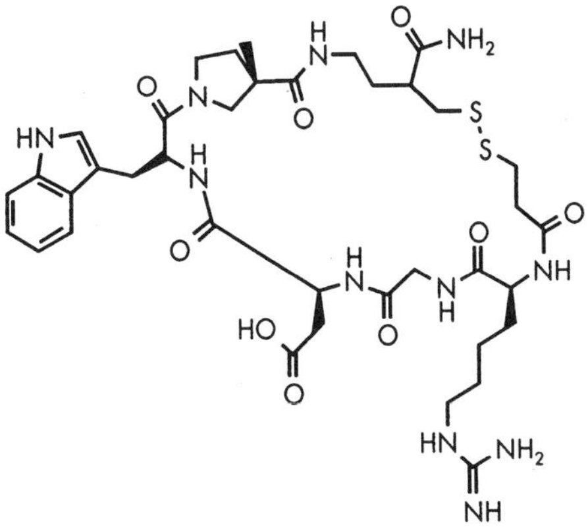

Figure 2   The chemical structure of eptifibatide.

in citrate-anticoagulated blood was obtained shortly after the initiation of an eptifibatide infusion [35,36]. Bleeding times were modestly elevated in baboons, but not elevated in dogs. In three early studies of pharmacodynamics in humans, platelet aggregation was inhibited in blood that was anticoagulated in citrate, and bleeding times were prolonged, but returned to near baseline within an hour after cessation of treatment [37–39]. The pharmacokinetics of eptifibatide are linear and dose-proportional for bolus doses ranging from 90 to 250 µg/kg and infusion rates from 0.2 to 1.5 µg/kg min^{-1}, with a half-life of 50–60 min [40]. The recommended regimens of a bolus followed by infusion produce an early peak level, followed by a small decline, with attainment of steady state within 4–6 h.

B. Toxicology

No long-term studies in animals have been performed to evaluate the carcinogenic potential of eptifibatide. Eptifibatide was not genotoxic in the Ames test, the mouse lymphoma forward mutation test, the human lymphocyte chromosomal aberration test, or the mouse micronucleus test [41]. When administered by continuous infusion at total daily doses up to 72 mg day^{-1} (about four times the recommended maximum daily human dose on a body surface area basis), eptifibatide had no effect on fertility and reproductive performance of male and female rats [41].

C. Efficacy Studies

A list of phase II and III cardiovascular trials of eptifibatide is shown in Table 1.

1. Trials in Percutaneous Coronary Intervention

During percutaneous transluminal coronary intervention, the treatment device causes serious vascular injury, resulting in the ideal milieu for coronary thrombosis [42–44]. Clinical trials of the monoclonal antibody abciximab (c7E3 Fab; ReoPro; Eli Lilly and Company/Centocor) have documented inhibition of the GP IIb/IIIa receptor (see Chap. 22). Two phase II trials of eptifibatide as an adjunct to PCI were conducted in the early 1990s to establish the pharmacodynamic and (preliminary) safety profiles of the agent. The first, the Integrelin to Minimize Platelet Aggregation and Coronary Thrombosis (IMPACT) study, was a randomized, placebo-controlled trial of 150 patients undergoing elective PCI [38]. Patients were allocated to one of three treatment approaches: placebo, a 90 µg/kg bolus before the initiation of the coronary intervention, followed by a 1.0-µg/kg min^{-1} infusion of eptifibatide for 4 h after the bolus, or the same 90-µg/kg bolus followed by a 1.0-µg/kg min^{-1} infusion of eptifibatide for 12 h. In blood collected in citrate, the 90-µg/kg bolus produced an 86% inhibition of platelet aggregation to stimulation with 20-µM ADP. There was a trend toward lower composite adverse clinical event rates with the longer infusions (12.2% for placebo, 9.6% for the 4-h infusion (p = 0.67), and 4.1% for the 12-h infusion (p = 0.13). Major bleeding event rates were 5% with either eptifibatide treatment, compared with 8% with placebo. Minor bleeding, primarily at the vascular access site, occurred in 40% versus 14%, respectively. Although the bleeding profile appeared acceptable, higher dosing of eptifibatide (and potentially better clinical efficacy) appeared to be possible. This led to the second phase II study in PCI, the IMPACT High/Low Low trial.

The IMPACT High/Low study was a placebo-controlled, randomized, dose-escalation trial that measured ex vivo platelet aggregation, bleeding time, and plasma eptifibatide concentration in 73 patients [39]. As with the IMPACT study, all patients also received aspirin and heparin sufficient to maintain the ACT at more than 300 s. Four different bolus-plus-infusion combina-

Table 1 Cardiovascular Trials of Eptifibatide

Study (Ref.)	Patients Number indication	Dose(s) Bolus infusion	Major clinical endpoints Phase 3 studies only
Percutaneous coronary intervention			
IMPACT (38)	150 Elective	90 μg/kg $1\ \mu g/kg\ min^{-1}$ for 4 or 12 h	
IMPACT II (45)	4010 All-comers	135 μg/kg 0.5 or $0.75\ \mu g/kg\ min^{-1}$ for 20–24 h	22% reduction in 30-day death, MI, UTVR, abrupt closure requiring stent; 11.6 vs. 9.1%; p = 0.035
ESPRIT (49)	2064	2×180 μg/kg boluses	37% relative reduction in 48 h composite of death, MI, UTVR; 10.5 vs. 6.6%; p = 0.0015
Acute coronary syndromes			
IMPACT USA (50)	157 "Unstable angina"	90 μg/kg 0.5 or $1.0\ \mu g/kg\ min^{-1}$ for 24 h	
PURSUIT (53)	10,948 ACS with ECG and/or +ve CKMB	180 μg/kg $2\ \mu g/kg\ min^{-1}$ for 72 h	10% reduction in 30-day composite of all-cause mortality and MI; 15.7 vs. 14.2%; p = 0.042
ST-elevation MI			
IMPACT-AMI (57)	180 Acute MI with t-PA	35–180 μg/kg 0.2–$0.75\ \mu g/kg\ min^{-1}$ for 24 h	
Integrilin and SK (58)	181 Acute MI with streptokinase for 24 h	180 μg/kg 0.75–$2.0\ \mu g/kg\ min^{-1}$	

tions were evaluated. The highest-dosing regimen tested was a 180-µg/kg bolus followed by a 1.0-µg/kg min^{-1} infusion. This regimen produced almost complete inhibition (>95%) of platelet aggregation (in whole blood anticoagulated with citrate). However, increasing rates of both minor and major bleeding were observed with increasing doses of eptifibatide. Given the available pharmacodynamic profiles coupled with concerns about bleeding, dosing regimens lower than the maximal doses tested in the IMPACT High/Low trial were ultimately selected for testing in the pivotal phase III study of eptifibatide, the IMPACT II study.

2. Phase III Trials in Percutaneous Coronary Intervention

a. IMPACT II. IMPACT II was a multicenter, parallel-group, double-blind, randomized, controlled clinical trial that recruited 4010 patients undergoing percutaneous revascularization [45]. Patients were assigned one of three treatment regimens: 135-µg/kg bolus of eptifibatide followed by a 0.5-µg/kg min^{-1} infusion for 20–24 h; a 135-µg/kg bolus, followed by a 0.75 µ/kg min^{-1} infusion for 20–24 h; or placebo bolus and placebo infusion. The bolus was administered and the infusion begun just before the PCI procedure. All patients received aspirin (325 mg) and heparin (100 U/kg), with addition heparin as needed to maintain an ACT of 300–350 s. The primary clinical endpoint was the 30-day composite of death, myocardial infarction (periprocedural MB-CK three times or more the upper limit of normal), urgent or emergency repeat coronary intervention, urgent or emergency coronary artery bypass surgery, or placement of an intracoronary stent during the index procedure for the management of true abrupt closure.

In IMPACT II, the "treated-as-randomized" analysis of the 3871 (96.5%) of patients who received any study drug (whether or not they underwent PCI) demonstrated a statistically significant 22% reduction in the primary composite clinical endpoint at 30 days, with the 135/0.5 treatment approach compared with placebo (9.1 vs 11.6%, p = 0.035; odds ratio 0.76 [0.5–0.98]). A trend toward improved outcomes was observed with the 135/0.75 dosing approach (10.0 vs. 11.6%, p = 0.18). An "all-randomized" analysis that included all patients enrolled in the study whether or not the patient received any study drug or underwent coronary intervention, showed only strong trends favoring a treatment effect. The composite primary endpoint occurred in 151 (11.4%) patients in the placebo group, compared with 124 (9.2%) in the 135/0.5-treatment group (p = 0.063) and 132 (9.9%) in the 135/0.75 treatment group (p = 0.22). In absolute terms, treatment with the 135/0.5 regimen prevented 25 events per 1000 patients in the first 30 days. A consistent, similar degree of benefit was imparted to all patients, regardless of baseline demographic characteristics, medical history, procedures performed, angiographic features, or risk strata.

In the context of the very impressive efficacy results in trials of abciximab in PCI, the results of IMPACT II were somewhat disappointing. Studies performed after IMPACT II suggested that this might have been due to underdosing of eptifibatide in the study. In the original phase-II dose-finding studies for eptifibatide, platelet aggregometry was conducted using blood anticoagulated with sodium citrate (Fig. 3). In retrospect, this overestimated the pharmacodynamic effects of eptifibatide, because citrate chelates calcium, and because calcium normally occupies the ligand-binding site within GP IIb/IIIa. Thus ex vivo ADP-induced platelet aggregation was artificially enhanced compared with the in vivo clinical effect. The best current estimate is that the eptifibatide doses used in IMPACT-II achieved only 30–50% of maximal platelet GP IIb/IIIa integrin blockade [46]. The early clinical trials with abciximab suggested that 80% receptor occupancy by a GP IIb/IIIa inhibitor would be required to maintain optimal continuous arterial perfusion [47]. The Platelet Aggregation and Receptor Occupancy with Integrilin—Dynamic Evaluation (PRIDE) study coupled with further pharmacodynamic modeling identified a "180/2.0/180" double-bolus regimen (a 180-µg/kg bolus followed 10 min later

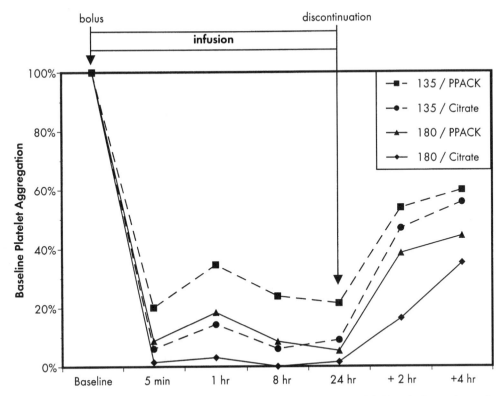

Figure 3 Inhibition of platelet aggregation by eptifibatide—the PRIDE trial: Two dosing regimens from the PRIDE trial are shown: 135-μg/kg bolus plus 0.75-μg/kg min^{-1} infusion and 180-μg/kg bolus plus 2.0-μg/kg min^{-1} infusion. Blood samples were suspended in either sodium citrate anticoagulant or PPACK anticoagulant. Assays of blood in citrate reported higher degrees of platelet inhibition than blood in PPACK at the same concentration of eptifibatide. The higher-dose (180/2.0) regimen suppressed platelet aggregation below 20% of baseline, whereas the lower-dose (135/0.75) regimen did not. Data are normalized to 100% aggregation at baseline. PPACK D–Phe–Pro–Arg–CH$_2$Cl.

by a second 180-μg/kg bolus of eptifibatide combined with a 2.0-μg/kg min^{-1} infusion) as a dosing approach that replicates or exceeds (in terms of inhibition of platelet aggregation) the pharmacodynamic profile of abciximab [48].

    b. ESPRIT. The latest trial of eptifibatide therapy is the Enhanced Suppression of the Platelet IIb/IIIa Receptor with Integrilin Therapy (ESPRIT) trial [49]. This randomized trial of a high-dose, double-bolus regimen of eptifibatide as adjunctive therapy in coronary stenting focused on three main areas: the underdosing of eptifibatide in previous clinical trials, the rapid changes in PCI since IMPACT II (including the use of lower procedural heparin dosing and the increased use of thienopyridines), and the increasing use of GP IIb/IIIa inhibition as a bailout therapy in PCI. Patients with coronary artery disease who were scheduled to undergo PCI with stent implantation in a native coronary artery, and who, in the opinion of the treating physician, would not routinely be treated with a GP IIb/IIIa inhibitor during PCI were considered for enrollment. Study drug was started immediately before the initiation of the PCI procedure, which was performed per local standards. The dosing of eptifibatide was a first bolus of 180 μg/kg immediately followed by the initiation of a 2.0-μg/kg min^{-1} (or 1.0 μg/kg min^{-1} in patients with serum creatinine > 2 mg/dL) continuous infusion. A second bolus of 180 μg/kg of eptifibatide was given 10 min after the first. The infusion was continued until hospital discharge or up to 18–24 h, whichever occurred first. A weight-adjusted heparin regimen was recommended (initial bolus of 60 U/kg, not to exceed 6000 U) to target an activated clotting time between 200 and 300 s.

With 2064 patients randomized, enrollment was terminated prematurely for efficacy on the recommendation of an independent data and safety monitoring board. The primary composite clinical endpoint of death, MI, urgent target vessel revascularization, or crossover bailout therapy for thrombotic complications at 48 h occurred in 108 of the 1024 placebo-treated patients and in 69 of the 1040 eptifibatide-treated patients, a relative risk reduction of 37% (p = 0.0015). All components and combinations of components of the primary endpoint were reduced in incidence to approximately the same relative degree as the primary composite endpoint. Benefit was realized irrespective of baseline characteristics, including age, weight, gender, diabetes, and disease presentation.

The key secondary composite endpoint of death, MI, and urgent target vessel revascularization at 30 days occurred in 6.8% of patients treated with eptifibatide and 10.5% of those treated with placebo (p = 0.0034), a relative risk reduction of 35%. Figure 4 shows Kaplan–Meier plots of events to 30 days. After the first 48 h, curves for both death and MI (see Fig. 4a) and for death, MI, and urgent target vessel revascularization (see Fig. 4b) were fairly flat. Over 88% of all events occurred in the first 48 h. The degree of heparin anticoagulation as measured by the activated-clotting time did not predict efficacy events. In the placebo group, the incidence of the primary composite endpoint was similar among patients when divided into tertiles of maximum-activated clotting time (10.0% in the lowest tertile, 11.5% in the middle tertile, and 10.3% in the highest tertile; Fig. 5). The relative benefit of treatment with eptifibatide was also similar across the tertiles of activated-clotting time, with the lowest overall event rate of the primary composite endpoint occurring in patients receiving eptifibatide who were in the lowest tertile of activated-clotting time. In contrast, rates of bleeding increased as the activated-clotting time increased, with bleeding being enhanced by treatment with eptifibatide.

There were three patients who sustained an intracerebral hemorrhage, one in the placebo group and two in the treatment group (Table 2). There were also two cases of acute profound thrombocytopenia in the eptifibatide group (a decrease in the platelet count to less than 20×10^9/L within 24 h of the initiation of treatment). Both were managed conservatively without platelet transfusion; thrombocytopenia began to resolve within hours of discontinuation of eptifibatide, and there were no clinical sequelae. Finally, rates of red blood cell transfusion were low overall, with slightly more than 1% of patients receiving a transfusion during the course of the trial.

3. Trials in Acute Coronary Syndromes

a. IMPACT: United States. The first comparative safety and efficacy evaluation of eptifibatide in unstable angina was a randomized, double-blind, placebo-controlled trial at 17 centers. Patients with unstable angina (>24 h from their last episode of angina) were randomized to placebo ($n = 51$) or one of two doses of eptifibatide [90-μg/kg bolus then 0.5-μg/kg min^{-1} ($n = 50$) or 90-μg/kg bolus then 1.0-μg/kg min^{-1} ($n = 56$)]. Infusions were continued for 24 h. Patients who received placebo also received aspirin, and all patients received heparin. Patients who received the higher-dose eptifibatide had fewer ischemic episodes and shorter mean duration of ischemia as measured by Holter monitor (p < 0.05) [50].

A second phase II dose-finding study of eptifibatide in unstable angina (IMPACT—USA) was designed to further examine the pharmacodynamics, pharmacokinetics, and safety of eptifibatide in this patient population [51]. Sixty-one patients were enrolled at five sites and received one of three open-label–dosing regimens. Platelet aggregation was suppressed 70–80%

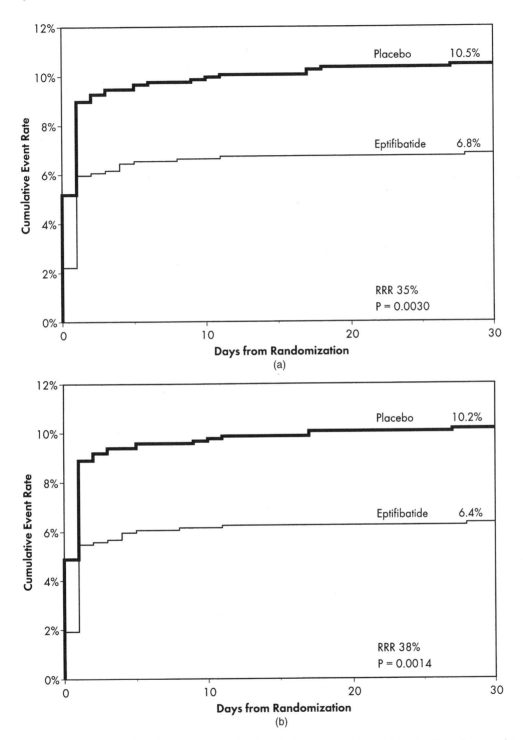

Figure 4 Kaplan–Meier plots of events to 30 days in the ESPRIT trial: (a) Probability of composite endpoint of death and MI to 30 days. (b) Probability of composite endpoint of death, MI, and urgent target vessel revascularization to 30 days. RRR, relative risk reduction.

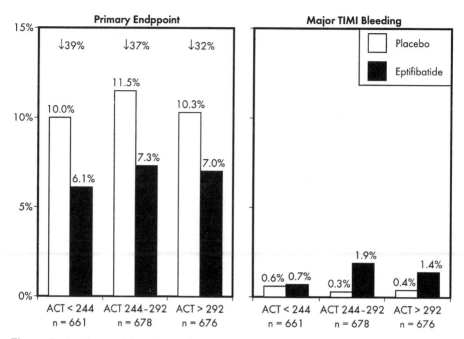

Figure 5 Incidence of the primary efficacy endpoint and major TIMI bleeding by tertiles of ACT in the ESPRIT trial.

from baseline values in the majority of patients receiving bolus doses of 135 and 150 µg/kg, and suppression was maintained with infusion of 1.0 and 1.25 µg/kg min^{-1}. Dosages required for 70–80% reduction in platelet aggregation indices were higher in patients with unstable angina than for normal patients or patients with stable angina [52].

4. Phase III Trials in Acute Coronary Syndromes

a. PURSUIT The largest randomized clinical trial in unstable angina/non-ST-segment elevation myocardial infarction ever performed was the Platelet Glycoprotein IIb/IIIa in Unstable Angina: Receptor Suppression Using Integrilin Therapy (PURSUIT) trial [53]. Eligible patients were those who presented with more than 10 min of chest pain of suspected ischemic origin within the past 24 h. In addition, patients must have had either specific electrocardiographic changes (ST-segment elevation between 0.6 and 1 mm, ST-segment depression > 0.5 mm, or T-wave inversion > 1 mm) or positive creatine kinase–myocardial band assay results. All patients randomized to eptifibatide received a 180 µg/kg bolus and either a 1.3-µg/kg min^{-1} infusion or 2.0-µg/kg min^{-1} infusion for 72 h. After 1487 patients were randomized into the 1.3-µg/kg min^{-1} approach, this arm was discontinued following a prespecified review by the data and safety monitoring board, for the safety profile observed in the 2.0-µg/kg min^{-1} arm. It was recommended, though not required, that all study patients receive aspirin and weight-adjusted heparin. Other than study drug treatment, all other decisions were left to the discretion of the treating physician.

The primary endpoint was a composite of all-cause mortality and nonfatal MI (or reinfarction) at 30 days. Secondary endpoints included death and (re)MI at 30 days, the composite at 96 h and 7 days, and safety and efficacy outcomes in patients undergoing PCI. Coronary angiography was performed in 60% of patients, and PCI was performed in 24%.

Table 2 Bleeding Events and Transfusions in the ESPRIT, PURSUIT, and IMPACT II Studies

PURSUIT	Placebo n (%)	Eptifibatide 180/1.3[a] n (%)	Eptifibatide 180/2.0 n (%)
Patients	4696	1472	4679
Major bleeding[b]	425(9.3)	152(10.5)	498(10.8)
Minor bleeding[a]	347(7.6)	152(10.5)	604(13.1)
Requiring transfusions[a]	490(10.4)	188(12.8)	601(12.8)

IMPACT II	Placebo n (%)	Eptifibatide 1350/0.5 n (%)	Eptifibatide 135/0.75 n (%)
Patients	1285	1300	1286
Major bleeding[b]	55(4.5)	55(4.4)	58(4.7)
Minor bleeding[b]	115(9.3)	146(11.7)	177(14.2)
Requiring transfusions[a]	66(5.1)	71(5.5)	74(5.8)

ESPRIT	Placebo n (%)	Eptifibatide 180/2.0/180 n (%)
Patients	1024	1040
Major bleeding[b]	4(0.4)	13(1.3)
Minor bleeding[b]	18(2)	29(3)
Requiring transfusions[c]	10(1)	15(1.4)

Note: the denominator is based for whom data are available.
[a]Administered only until the first interim analysis.
[b]For major and minor bleeding, patients are counted only once according to the most severe classification.
[c]Includes transfusions of whole blood, packed red blood cells, fresh-frozen plasma, cryoprecipitate, platelets, and autotransfusion during the initial hospitalization.

Roughly half of these (12.7% or 1228 patients) underwent intervention within 72 h of randomization while receiving the study drug.

Patients receiving eptifibatide experienced a 16.5% relative risk reduction in death or nonfatal MI at 96 h (7.6 vs. 9.1%; p = 0.011) and a 12.9% reduction at 7 days (10.1 vs. 11.6%; p = 0.016) (Table 3). At 30 days, a 9.6% relative, and 1.5% absolute, reduction in the primary endpoint of death or nonfatal MI remained in patients who received eptifibatide compared with placebo (14.2 vs. 15.7%; p = 0.042) (see Table 3). This reduction was maintained up to 6 months, with an 8% relative risk (RR) reduction (17.8 vs. 19%; p = 0.03). The benefit of eptifibatide was apparent across the spectrum of patient subgroups, although regional and gender variations were observed.

A significant reduction in composite events before the procedure was also evident (5.5 vs. 1.8%; p = 0.001) suggesting that eptifibatide may stabilize patients and thus minimize the risk of intervention. Reduction in the composite events with eptifibatide was also observed among the 8211 patients who did not undergo percutaneous interventions within 72 h (5.4 vs. 6.5% in the placebo group at 72 h, p = 0.038, and 14.6 vs 15.6% in the placebo group at 30 days, p = 0.226). Finally, patients who underwent early surgical revascularization derived particular benefit from eptifibatide therapy with a greater than 14% absolute reduction in death and nonfatal MI at both 72 h (16.3 vs. 30.8% in the placebo group, p = 0.001) and 30 days (18.4 vs. 33.5% in the placebo group, p = 0.001).

Table 3 The PURSUIT Study: Components of the Composite Endpoint, According to Study Group[a]

Time and event	Eptifibatide group (n = 4722) (%)	Placebo group (n = 4739) (%)	p-value
96 h			
Death	0.9	1.2	0.11
MI	7.1	8.3	0.03
Death or nonfatal MI	7.6	9.1	0.01
7 days			
Death	1.5	2.0	0.05
MI	9.3	10.4	0.08
Death or nonfatal MI	10.1	11.6	0.02
30 days			
Death	3.5	3.7	0.53
MI	12.6	13.5	0.14
Death or nonfatal MI	14.2	15.7	0.04

[a]All patients randomly assigned to receive the higher dose of eptifibatide or placebo are included.

Rates of major bleeding were 9.3% with placebo and 10.8% with eptifibatide (see Table 2). Most of the major bleeding complications occurred in patients undergoing bypass surgery, and treatment with eptifibatide did not increase the risk of these complications. Among patients who did not undergo CABG, major bleeding occurred in 1.1% of patients in the placebo group and 2.6% of those in the eptifibatide group, primarily at femoral artery access sites in patients undergoing percutaneous procedures.

The incidence of thrombocytopenia (platelet count less than $100,000/mm^3$) was similar in both PURSUIT treatment groups: 6.9% of eptifibatide-treated patients and 7.0% of placebo-treated patients, with a median time to onset of 4 days [61]. In addition. the incidence of stroke was similar in the eptifibatide- and the placebo-treated patients (0.7 vs. 0.8%, respectively, $p = 0.41$); most strokes were nonhemorrhagic (0.6 vs. 0.7%) [54]. Examination of the timing of eptifibatide administration in PURSUIT found an increased benefit associated with early use in these patients [55]. Compared with the overall absolute benefit of 1.5%, patients receiving eptifibatide within 6 h of presentation had a 2.8% absolute reduction in death and MI at 30 days compared with placebo; absolute reductions of 2.3 and 1.7% were achieved with eptifibatide given within 6–12 h and 12–24 h of presentation, respectively. There was no benefit from eptifibatide in the late (>24-h) treatment group. While the results of multivariable adjustment for differences in baseline risk are awaited with interest (it may be that the sickest patients were randomized earlier), these results suggest that GP IIb/IIIa inhibitor therapy should be administered as soon as possible to patients presenting with an acute coronary syndrome.

5. Trials in Acute ST-Segment Elevation Myocardial Infarction

Platelet adhesion and aggregation play an important role in the success or failure of thrombolytic and antithrombotic therapy. Aspirin, a weak platelet inhibitor, has established benefit in the management of acute MI [56]. Therefore, there is substantial interest in the more potent GP IIb/IIIa platelet inhibitors as primary antithrombotic treatments.

   a. IMPACT—AMI.   The safety and benefit of t-PA with heparin, aspirin, and eptifibatide in patients with acute myocardial infarction was addressed as part of the IMPACT—AMI trial [57]. A total of 180 patients were randomized to placebo or to eptifibatide in conjunction with accelerated alteplase. The first phase of the trial examined escalating doses of eptifibatide (bolus 35, 72, 108, 135, or 180 µg/kg, followed by an infusion at 0.2, 0.4, 0.6, 0.75, 0.75 µg/kg min^{-1}, respectively) administered in conjunction with t-PA. All patients had 90-min angiograms, and 30 patients had ADP-induced platelet aggregation studies performed in citrate. All tested doses showed increased antiplatelet effects and increased patency rates compared with placebo, and higher doses resulted in improved 24- and 6-h inhibition of aggregation. Results of the early phase of this trial, when compared with other patient populations [52], suggest that platelets are markedly activated during acute MI and that larger doses of eptifibatide may be needed to inhibit platelets fully in patients with ACS.

   The highest dose, 180-µg/kg bolus followed by infusion of 0.75 µg/kg min^{-1} was studied in 51 patients (with patients from the dose-escalation phase being pooled with those in the randomized dose-confirmation phase). Clinical outcomes in these patients were compared with 55 patients receiving placebo. Angiograms at 90 min were available for all patients, and 87 patients had 24-h continuous ST-segment monitoring. Patients treated with eptifibatide had improved patency at 90 min (TIMI 3 66 vs. 39%, p = 0.006) and decreased time to steady state as quantified by continuous ST-segment monitoring (65 vs. 116 min, p = 0.05). Eptifibatide-treated patients also had less recurrent ischemia (31% vs. 50%) and area under the ST curve during the first 6 h (2868 vs. 6670), but these differences were not statistically significant in this small size sample.

6.   Integrilin and Streptokinase Trial

Ronner and colleagues reported the results of a study using a combination of eptifibatide as a 180-µg/kg bolus followed by an infusion of 0 75- 1.33-, or 2.0-µg/kg min^{-1} with 1.5-million U of streptokinase in 181 patients with acute myocardial infarction [58]. The combined therapy yielded a modest increase in early (90-min) TIMI grade 3 flow (53% integrilin 180/0.75) compared with streptokinase with placebo (38%). The highest-dose arm was discontinued when an increased bleeding rate was observed. Coupled with the results of the Platelet Aggregation Receptor Antagonist Dose Investigation for Reperfusion Gain in Myocardial Infarction (PARA-DIGM) trial of lamifiban in combination with streptokinase or t-PA 59, these findings are disappointing, particularly relative to the potentiation of thrombolysis by streptokinase. These data would suggest an intrinsic difference in the ability of GP IIb/IIIa blockade to enhance thrombolytic potency with streptokinase in contrast with the more selective thrombolytic agents such as t-PA and r-PA.

IV.   OPINION

The GP IIb/IIIa inhibitors represent a new class of therapeutic compounds that are revolutionizing the way we treat patients with atherosclerotic coronary artery disease. Eptifibatide, a highly specific and rapidly reversible inhibitor of GP IIb/IIIa, has been extensively investigated in the setting of both PCI and acute coronary syndromes.

   The results of PURSUIT clearly establish a role for eptifibatide as front-line therapy for patients with high-risk acute coronary syndromes. This includes patients with characteristic chest pain, positive cardiac markers (including elevated troponin), or ST segment shifts on the elcctrocardiogram.

In the setting of percutaneous coronary intervention, the less-than-expected treatment effect seen with eptifibatide in IMPACT II compared with that seen with abciximab in EPIC and EPILOG may have been a result of underdosing of eptifibatide. The ESPRIT trial, which tested an eptifibatide dosing regimen shown to achieve more than 80% platelet inhibition, produced highly and statistically significant and clinically relevant reductions in the ischemic clinical complications of this procedure. These benefits were achieved despite the exclusion of subjectively higher-risk patients; patients enrolled in ESPRIT were believed by their physicians not to warrant GP IIb/IIIa receptor blockade as a pretreatment. In addition, the results were achieved against the background of aspirin, heparin, and thienopyridine treatment. Given the relatively low procurement costs of eptifibatide, these findings, particularly if they are maintained over a 6- to 12-month period, could have substantial economic and therapeutic implications; with a reduced economic barrier to entry, treatment benefit can be provided to the greatest number of patients. The caveat remains, however, that longer-term follow-up will be required to define the mortality benefit, if any, of eptifibatide in PCI.

All of the pilot trials of eptifibatide used in conjunction with thrombolytic therapy for ST–segment elevation MI have demonstrated trends consistent with improved restoration of coronary perfusion; large-scale phase III trials are ongoing to determine if these angiographic findings correlate with reduced mortality. Finally, the role of eptifibatide as an adjunct to direct coronary intervention is still undefined. The hope is that adjunctive therapy will improve procedural outcomes, reduce subacute closure, and permit the earlier discharge home of patients than is practiced today.

REFERENCES

1. Fuster V, Adams PC Badimon JJ, Chesebro JH. The pathogenesis of coronary artery disease and the acute coronary syndromes. N Engl J Med 1992; 326:242–250.
2. Hynes RO. Integrins: family of cell surface receptor. Cell 1987; 48:549–554.
3. Hynes RO. Integrins: versatility, modulation, and signaling in cell adhesion. Cell 1992; 69:1 1–25.
4. Jang U, Lincoff AM, Plow EF, Topol EJ. Cell adhesion molecules in coronary artery disease. J Am Coll Cardiol 1994; 24:1591–1601.
5. Phillips DR, Charo IF, Parise LV, Fitzgerald LA. The platelet membrane glycoprotein IIb/IIIa complex. Blood 1988; 71:831–843.
6. Phillips DR, Charo IF, Scarborough RM. GPIIb–IIIa: the responsive integrin. Cell 1991; 65:359–362.
7. Charo IF, Kieffer N, Phillips DR. Platelet membrane glycoproteins. In: Colman RW, ed. Hemostasis and Thrombosis: Basic Principles and Clinical Practice. Philadelphia: JB Lippincott, 1994; 489–507.
8. Lefkovits J, Plow EF, Topoi EJ. Platelet glycoprotein IIb/IIIa receptors in cardiovascular medicine. N Engl J Med 1995; 332:1553–1559.
9. Ginsberg J, Kearon C, Hirsh J. Critical decisions in thrombosis and hemostasis. Malden, MA: Decker, 1998.
10. Gold HK, Gimple LW, Yasuda T, et al. Pharmacodynamic study of $F(ab')_2$ fragments of murine monoclonal antibody 7E3 directed against human platelet glycoprotein IIb/IIIa in patients with unstable angina pectoris. J Clin Invest 1990; 86:651–659.
11. Ginsberg M, Pierschbacher MD, Ruoslahti E, Marguerie G, Plow E. Inhibition of fibronectin binding to platelets by proteolytic fragments and synthetic peptides which support fibroblast adhesion. J Biol Chem 1985; 260:3931–3936.
12. Pierschbacher M, Hayman EG, Ruoslahti E. Synthetic peptide within cell attachment activity of fibronectin. Proc Natl Acad Sci USA 1983; 80:1224–1227.
13. Pierschbacher MD, Ruoslahti E. Variants of the cell recognition site of fibronectin that retain attachment-promoting activity. Proc Natl Acad Sci USA 1984; 81:5985–5988.
14. Plow EF, Pierschbacher MD, Ruoslahti E, Marguerie GA, Ginsberg MH. The effect of Arg–Gly–Asp–

containing peptides on fibrinogen and von Willebrand factor binding to platelets. Proc Natl Acad Sci USA 1985; 82:8057–8061.

15. Ruoslahti E, Pierschbacher MD. New perspectives in cell adhesion: RGD and integrins. Science 1987; 238:491–497.

16. Pierschbacher MD, Ruoslahti E. Cell attachment activity of fibronectin can be duplicated by small synthetic fragments of the molecule. Nature 1984; 309:30–33.

17. Plow EF, Pierschbacher MD, Ruoslahti E, Marguerie G, Ginsberg MH. Arginyl–glycyl–aspartic acid sequences and fibrinogen binding to activated platelets. Blood 1987; 70:110–115.

18. Dolittle RF, Watt KW, Cottrell BA, Strong DD, Riley M. The amino acid sequence of the alpha-chain of human fibrinogen. Nature 1979; 280:464–468.

19. Hawiger J, Timmons S, Kloczewiak M, Strong DD, Doolittle RF. Gamma- and alpha-chains of human fibrinogen possess sites reactive with human platelet receptors. Proc Natl Acad Sci USA 1982; 79: 2068–2071.

20. Harker LA. Maraganore JM, Hirsh J. Novel antithrombotic agents. In: Colman RW, ed, Hemostasis and Thrombosis: Basic Principles and Clinical Practice. Philadelphia: JB Lippincott, 1994; 1638–1660.

21. Plow EF, Ginsberg MH. Cellular adhesion: GPIIb–IIIa as a prototypic adhesion receptor. Prog Hemost Thromb 1989; 9:117–156.

22. D'Souza SE, Ginsberg MU, Burke TA, Plow EF. The ligand binding site of the platelet integrin receptor GPIIb–IIIa is proximal to the second calcium binding domain of its alpha subunit. J Biol Chem 1990; 265:3440–3446.

23. D'Souza SE, Ginsberg MU, Burke TA, Lam SC, Plow EF. Localization of an Arg–Gly–Asp recognition site within an integrin adhesion receptor. Science 1988; 242:91–93.

24. Charo IF, Nannizzi L, Phillips DR, Hsu MA, Scarborough RM. Inhibition of fibrinogen binding to GP IIb–IIIa by a GP IIIa peptide. J Biol Chem 1991; 266:1415–1421.

25. Huang TF, Holt JC, Lukasiewicz H, Niewiarowski S. Trigramin: a low molecular weight peptide inhibiting fbrinogen integration with platelet receptors expressed on glycoprotein IIb–IIIa complex. J Biol Chem 1987; 262:16157–16163.

26. Dennis MS, Henzel WJ, Pitti RM, Lipari MT, Napier MA, Deisher TA, Bunting S, Lazarus RA. Platelet glycoprotein IIb–IIIa protein antagonists from snake venoms: evidence for a family of platelet-aggregation inhibitors. Proc Natl Acad Sci USA 1990; 87:2471–2475.

27. Gan ZR, Gould RJ, Jacobs JW, Freidman PA, Polokoff MA. Echistatin. A potent platelet aggregation inhibitor from the venom of the viper, Echis carinatus. J Biol Chem 1988; 263:19827–19832.

28. Cook JJ, Huang TF, Rucinski B, Strzyzewski M, Tuma RF. Williams JA, Niewiarowski S. Inhibition of platelet hemostatic plug formation by trigramin, a novel RGD-peptide. Am J Physiol 1989; 256:H1038–H1043.

29. Gould RJ, Polokoff MA, Friedman PA, Huang TF, Holt JC, Cook JJ, Niewiarowski S. Disintegrins: a family of integrin inhibitory proteins from viper venoms. Proc Soc Exp Biol Med 1990; 195:168–171.

30. Scarborough RM, Rose JW, Naughton MA, Phillips DR, Nannizzi L, Arfsten A, Campbell AM, Charo IF. Characterization of the integrin specificities of disintegrins isolated from American pit viper venoms. J Biol Chem 1993; 268: 1058–1065.

31. Scarborough RM, Rose JW, Hsu MA, Phillips DR, Fried VA, Campbell AM, Nannizzi L. Charo IF. Barbourin: GPIIb–IIIa-specific integrin antagonist from the venom of Sistrurus m. barbouri. J Biol Chem 1991; 266:9359–9362.

32. Scarborough RM, Naughton MA, Teng W, Rose JW, Phillips DR, NannizziL, Arfsten A, Campbell AM, Charo IF. Design of potent and specific integrin antagonists. Peptide antagonists with high specificity for glycoprotein IIb–IIIa. J Biol Chem 1993; 268:1066–1073.

33. Savage B, Marzec UM, Chao BH, Harker LA, Maraganore JM, Ruggeri ZM. Binding of the snake venom-derived proteins applaggin and echistatin to the arginine–glycine–aspartic acid recognition sites(s) on platelet glycoprotein IIb–IIIa complex inhibits receptor function. J Biol Chem 1990; 265:11766–11772.

34. Knudsen KA, Tuszynski GP, Huang TF, Niewiarowski S. Trigramin, an RGD-containing peptide from snake venom, inhibits cell-substratum adhesion of human melanoma cells. Exp Cell Res 1988; 179:42–49.

35. Hanson SR, Kotze HF, Savage B, et al. Platelet interactions with Dacron grafts: a model of acute thrombosis baboons. Arteriosclerosis 1985; 5:595–603.

36. Uthoff K, Zehr KJ, Geerling R, et al. Inhibition of platelet adhesion during cardiopulmonary by-pass reduces postoperative bleeding. Circulation 1994; 90:269–274.

37. Charo IF, Scarborough RM, Du Mee CP, et al. Therapeutics I: pharmacodynamics of the glycoprotein IIb/IIIa antagonist integrelin: phase 1 clinical studies in normal healthy volunteers. Circulation 1992; 86(suppl I): I-260.

38. Tcheng JE, Harrington RA, Kottke–Marchant K, et al. Multicenter, randomized, double blind, placebo-controlled trial of the platelet integrin glycoprotein IIb/IIIa blocker integrelin in elective coronary intervention. Circulation 1995; 91:2151–2157.

39. Harrington RA, Klieman NS, Kottke–Marchant K, et al. Immediate and reversible platelet inhibition after intravenous administration of a peptide glycoprote in IIb/IIIa inhibitor during percutaneous coronary intervention. Am J Cardiol 1995: 76:1222–1227.

40. Philips DR, Scarborough RM. Clinical pharmacology of eptifibatide. Am J Cardiol 1997; 80(4A): 11B–20B.

41. Medical Economics. The Physicians Desk Reference. Oradell, NJ, 1999.

42. Neuhaus KL, Zeymer U. Prevention and management of thrombotic complications during coronary interventions. Eur Heart J 1995; 16(suppl L):L63–67.

43. Wilentz JR, Sanborn TA, Haudenschild CC, et al. Platelet accumulation in experimental angioplasty: time-course and relation to vascular injury. Circulation 1987; 76:1225–1234.

44. Steele PM, Chesebro JH, Stanson AW, Holmes DR, Jr, Dewanjee MK, Badimon L, Fuster V. Balloon angioplasty: natural history of the pathophysiological response to injury in a pig model. Circ Res 1985; 57:105–112.

45. The IMPACT II Investigators. Randomised placebo-controlled trial of effect of eptifibatide on complications of percutaneous coronary intervention. Lancet 1997; 349:1422–1428.

46. Phillips DR, Teng W, Arfsten A, et al. Effect of Ca^{2+} on GP IIb–IIIa interactions with integrilin: enhanced GP IIb–IIIa binding and inhibition of platelet aggregation by reductions in the concentration of ionised calcium in plasma anticoagulated with citrate. Circulation 1997; 96:1488–1494.

47. Tcheng JE. Glycoprotein IIb/IIIa receptor inhibitors: putting the EPIC, IMPACT II, RESTORE, and EPILOG trials into perspective. Am J Cardiol 1996; 78:35–40.

48. Tcheng JE, Thel MC, Jennings L. Platelet glycoprotein IIb/IIIa receptor blockade with high dose integrilin in coronary intervention. Results of the PRIDE study. Eur Heart J 1997; 18:P3615.

49. The ESPRIT investigators. Novel dosing regimen of eptifibatide in planned coronary stent implantation (ESPRIT): a randomised, placebo-controlled trial. Lancet 2000; 356:2037–2044.

50. Schulman SP, Goldschmidt–Clermont PJ, Topol EJ, et al. Effects of integrelin, a platelet glycoprotein IIb/IIIa receptor antagonist, in unstable angina. Circulation 1996; 94:2083–2089.

51. Harrington RA, Schulman SP, Kleiman NS, et al. Profound, sustained and reversible platelet inhibition following administration of a glycoprotein IIb/IIIa inhibitor with and without heparin in patients with unstable angina [abstr]. Circulation 1994; 90(suppl I):I-232.

52. Harrington RA, Ohman EM, Sigmon KN, et al. Intensity of inhibition of the platelet glycoprotein IIb/IIIa receptor differs among disease states. [abstr.]. Circulation 1995; 92(suppl I):I-488–489.

53. PURSUIT Trial Investigators. Inhibition of platelet glycoprotein IIb/IIIa with eptifibatide in patients with acute coronary syndromes. N Engl J Med 1998; 339:436–443.

54. Mahaffey KW, Harrington RA, Simoons ML, et al. for the PURSUIT Investigators. Stroke in patients with acute coronary syndromes: incidence and outcomes in the PURSUIT trial, Circulation 1999; 99:2371–2377.

55. Bhatt D, Marso S, Houghtaling P. Labinaz M, Lauer M. Does earlier administration of eptifibatide reduce death and MI in patients with acute coronary syndromes? [abstr] Circulation 1998; 98: I-560.

56. The ISIS-2 Investigators. Randomised trial of intravenous streptokinase, oral aspirin, both, or neither among 17,187 cases of suspected acute myocardial infarction. Lancet 1988; 2:349–360.

57. Ohman EM, Kleiman NS, Gacioch G, et al. for the IMPACT–AMI Investigators. Combined accelerated tissue plasminogen activator and platelet glycoprotein IIb/IIIa integrin blockade with integrilin in acute

myocardial infarction: results from a randomized, placebo-controlled, dose-ranging trial. Circulation 1997; 95:846–854.

58. Ronner E, van Kesteren HA, Zijnen P, et al. Safety and efficacy of eptifibatide vs. placebo in patients receiving thrombolytic therapy with streptokinase for acute myocardial infarction; a phase II dose escalation, randomized, double-blind study. Eur Heart J 2000; 21:1530–1536.

59. Militerno DJ, Harrington RA, Krucoff MW, et al. for the PARADIGM Investigators. Randomized, placebo-controlled study of lamifiban with thrombolytic therapy for the treatment of acute myocardial infarction: rationale and design for the PARADIGM study. J Thromb Thrombol 1995; 2:165–169.

24

Tirofiban: A Paradigm for "Small-Molecule" Glycoprotein IIb/IIIa Receptor Antagonists?

John K. French and Harvey D. White
Green Lane Hospital, Auckland, New Zealand

SUMMARY

Tirofiban is a nonpeptide GP IIb/IIIa antagonist that binds reversibly to IIb/IIIa receptors. Its efficacy has been evaluated in many clinical scenarios, including acute coronary syndromes with and without ST elevation, PCl, and as treatment prior to early revascularization. In the PRISM-Plus study, which enrolled patients with acute coronary syndromes without persistent ST-segment elevation who were treated with intravenous heparin, those randomized to receive tirofiban had a lower incidence of death or nonfatal myocardial infarction (MI) at 30 d than those randomized to receive a placebo (8.7 vs. 11.9%, p = 0.03). In the PRISM study, which also enrolled patients with non-ST-elevation acute coronary syndromes, the 30-day incidence of death or MI was 5.8% in patients randomized to tirofiban, compared with 7.1% in those randomized to heparin (p = 0.12), but in patients who had elevated troponin T levels (≥ 0.1 µg/L) 6–8 h after presentation, the comparative rates were 13.7 and 3.5%, respectively (p < 0.01). In the RESTORE trial in high-risk patients who underwent angioplasty, tirofiban reduced the combined 30-day incidence of death, MI, or urgent revascularization from 10.5 to 8.0% (p = 0.052).

In the TACTICS-TIMI-18 trial, 4–48 h of tirofiban treatment followed by early revascularization was compared with an early conservative strategy in patients with non–ST-elevation acute coronary syndromes and reduced the 6-month incidence of death, MI, or severe angina requiring hospitalisation from 26.3 to 16.4% (p = 0.006) in patients with ≥ 0.5 mm of ST-segment depression and from 24.2 to 14.3% (p < 0.001) in patients with elevated troponin levels.

The TARGET trial compared tirofiban with abciximab in patients undergoing percutaneous coronary intervention for an acute coronary syndrome or stable angina. The primary endpoint of death, MI, or urgent target-vessel revascularization within 30 d occurred in 7.5% of those who received tirofiban versus 6% of those who received abciximab (p = 0.037).

Clinical trials using angiographic assessment have also been performed to evaluate the efficacy and safety of tirofiban in conjunction with low-molecular-weight heparin, and in patients receiving fibrinolytic agents for ST-elevation acute coronary syndromes. It is now established that tirofiban is effective and safe for patients presenting with non–ST-elevation acute coronary

Table 1 Abbreviations and Acronyms

ACE	Angiotensin-converting enzyme
ACUTE	Antithrombotic Combination Using Tirofiban and Enoxaparin
ADP	Adenosine diphosphate
CI	Confidence interval
EPISTENT	Evaluation of Platelet IIb/IIIa Inhibition in Stenting
FASTER	Fibrinolytic and Aggrastat ST-Elevation Resolution
FRISC	Fragmin During Instability in Coronary Artery Disease
GP	Glycoprotein
ISIS	International Studies of Infarct Survival
KQAGDV	Lysine–glutamine–alanine–glycine–aspartate–valine
MI	Myocardial infarction
M_r	Relative molecular mass
OR	Odds ratio
PCI	Percutaneous coronary intervention
PRISM	Platelet Receptor Inhibition in Ischemic Syndrome Management
PRISM-Plus	Platelet Receptor Inhibition in Ischemic Syndrome Management in Patients Limited by Unstable Signs and Symptoms
RESTORE	Randomized Efficacy Study of Tirofiban for Outcomes and Restenosis
RGD	Arginine–glycine–aspartate
RR	Relative risk
TACTICS-TIMI-18	Treat Angina with Aggrastat and Determine Cost of Therapy with an Invasive or Conservative Strategy
TARGET	Do Tirofiban and ReoPro Give Similar Efficacy
TIMI	Thrombolysis in Myocardial Infarction

syndromes, whether it is used as part of a conservative medical strategy or as treatment before revascularization procedures.

Table 1 defines the abbreviations and acronyms used in this chapter.

I. INTRODUCTION

GP IIb/IIIa receptor antagonists have a wide variety of structures, but they have as a common feature a positive and negative charge 1–2 nm apart [1], similar to the charge separation on peptide sequence RGD and, probably, KQAGDV [2]. Synthetic IIb/IIIa antagonists bind to the RGD- or KQAGDV-binding site(s) and are competitive inhibitors of fibrinogen binding.

II. TIROFIBAN

Tirofiban (MK-383 or Aggrastat) is a nonpeptide tyrosine derivative (N-(butylsulfonyl)-O-[4-(4-piperidinyl)butyl]-L-tyrosine monohydrochloride monohydrate) and is highly selective for the IIb/IIIa receptor. The molecular structure of tirofiban is shown in Figure 1 [3]. Tirofiban inhibits aggregation of gel-filtered platelets induced by 10 μM of ADP, with an IC_{50} of 9 nM. Infusion of tirofiban in a canine coronary thrombosis model causes dose-dependent inhibition of (5 μM) ADP-induced platelet aggregation, as measured by the maximal rate of change in light transmission (i.e., the slope). Infusion of 3 μg/kg min^{-1} for 6 h causes 80% inhibition, and 10 μg/kg min^{-1} causes more than 95% inhibition. Platelet aggregation returns to 70% of normal

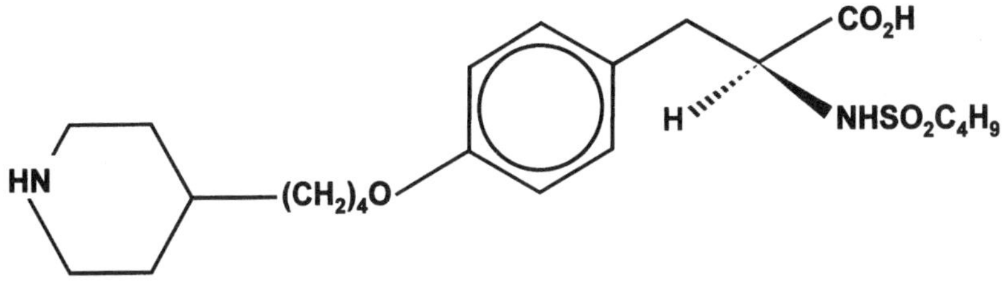

Figure 1 The structure of tirofiban.

within 30 min of ending the infusion [4]. In in vitro [3] assays of platelet function, tirofiban may be affected by anticoagulants in the tube into which the blood is aspirated, including citrate.

Tirofiban has an approximate volume of distribution of 22–42 L and a plasma half-life of 30 min. Its major excretion route in humans is in the urine, whereas dogs and rats excrete the majority of tirofiban in the bowel, through the biliary system. Following administration of an intravenous bolus, the drug is concentrated in the blood, kidneys, and biliary system. Approximately 35% of tirofiban is bound to plasma proteins in the blood.

The plasma clearance of tirofiban is, on average, 175–200 mL min^{-1}, but this is reduced by at least 50% in patients with renal failure and a creatinine clearance of less than 30 mL min^{-1} [5]. In these patients the loading and maintenance doses of tirofiban should be reduced by 50%, as uremia modifies both binding of ligands to IIb/IIIa receptors and the volume of distribution of tirofiban.

The blood levels of tirofiban are not significantly altered by coadministration of aspirin or heparin [5]. Patients in the PRISM study [6] who received other usual cardiac medications, such as β-blockers, calcium-channel antagonists, vasodilators, angiotension-converting enzyme (ACE) inhibitors, diuretics or digoxin, did not have significant changes in their plasma clearance of tirofiban.

Regardless of concomitant medications, tirofiban achieves 85–90% inhibition or more than 95% inhibition of (5 μM) ADP-induced platelet aggregation in humans when administered as a loading dose of 0.4 or 0.6 mg/kg min^{-1}, respectively [7]. These levels of inhibition are maintained at infusion rates of 0.1 or 0.5 mg min^{-1}, respectively. A plasma concentration of approximately 40 ng/mL is required to achieve more than 85% ADP-induced platelet inhibition. This concentration is almost invariably achieved by the 0.6-mg/kg bolus plus 0.15-mg/kg min^{-1} infusion regimen, but is not always achieved by the 0.4-mg/kg bolus plus 0.10-mg/kg min^{-1} regimen. Six hours after stopping either regimen, plasma levels are less than 3 ng/mL [7].

Although coadministration of heparin does not alter tirofiban concentrations, it does prolong bleeding times slightly (from 2.5- to 3-fold to approximately 4-fold) in patients with acute coronary syndromes. In this setting, a tirofiban infusion of 0.15 μg/kg min^{-1} for 4 h produced a 2.5- ±1.1-fold increase in the bleeding time and 97±5% inhibition of (3.4 μM) ADP-induced platelet aggregation [8]. The plasma clearance rate was 329 mL/min and the plasma half-life was 1.6 h. The bleeding time returned to normal and platelet aggregation returned to over 80% of the pretreatment value 4 h after stopping the infusion of tirofiban. Coadministration of aspirin caused an approximate fourfold prolongation of the bleeding time, which was not moderated by an increase in tirofiban plasma levels. The plasma concentration of tirofiban required to inhibit platelet aggregation by 50% decreased from 12 to 9 ng/mL when the patients were also given aspirin.

In patients undergoing angioplasty and receiving aspirin and heparin, a pilot dose-ranging study [7] showed that a tirofiban bolus of 10 μg/kg inhibited (5 μM) ADP-induced platelet aggregation by 93% or more within 5 min (Fig. 2), although data on platelet aggregation sooner

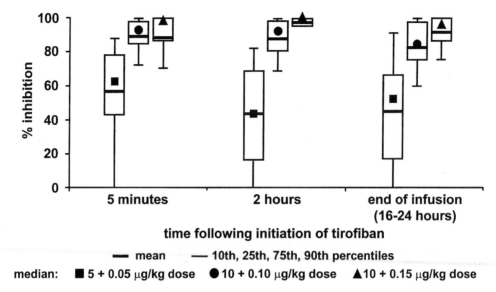

Figure 2 Effects of three different tirofiban-dosing regimens on inhibition of (5 μM) ADP-induced platelet aggregation ex vivo, measured at 5 min, at 2 h and at the end of the infusion. The doses are shown as bolus + infusion. (From Ref. 7.)

than 2 h after this initial bolus are not available. In patients undergoing angioplasty and receiving high-dose heparin (>100 U/kg), the bleeding time was more prolonged than with heparin alone. The bleeding time at 2 h was more than 30 min when a 10-μg/kg bolus was followed by either a 0.1 or 0.15 μg/kg min^{-1} infusion for 16–24 h, at which time ADP-induced platelet aggregation was inhibited by 87 and 95%, respectively. Four hours after terminating the infusions, platelet aggregation had returned to more than 50% of normal [9].

When the combination of tirofiban plus enoxaparin was compared with tirofiban plus heparin in patients with non–ST-elevation acute coronary syndromes, the adjusted bleeding times were 19.6 min versus 24.9 min (p = 0.02) [10,11]. Subsequently, in the ACUTE-II trial [12], the frequency of bleeding was examined in 525 patients with nonpersistent ST-elevation acute coronary syndromes who were treated with tirofiban and randomized in a 3 : 2 fashion to receive either enoxaparin or unfractionated heparin. In patients treated with enoxaparin, the major and minor bleeding rates (classified according to the TIMI criteria) [13] were 0.3 and 2.5%, respectively, as opposed to 1.0 and 4.3% in patients with unfractionated heparin (p = 0.57 and p = 0.11, respectively). There were no differences in clinical events (which is not surprising in a study of this size), except for an increase in the rate of rehospitalization for unstable angina in patients randomized to receive unfractionated heparin (7.1 vs. 1.6%, p = 0.002). The influence of enoxaparin and tirofiban on clinical outcomes is being evaluated in ongoing larger clinical trials. The phase III trials are outlined in Table 2.

A. Randomized Trials of Tirofiban in Acute Coronary Syndromes Without Persistent ST-Segment Elevation

In the PRISM study [6] the rate of the primary endpoint (death, new MI or refractory ischemia at 48 h) was 37% lower in patients who received tirofiban than in those who received intravenous heparin (3.8 vs. 5.6%, p<0.01). At 30 days the mortality rate was 39% lower in the tirofiban group (2.3 vs. 3.6%, p = 0.02). The benefit of tirofiban was observed almost entirely in patients

Table 2 Completed Phase III Trials of Tirofiban

Trial	Population	Dose (bolus + infusion)	N	Primary endpoint	Relative risk reduction (%)
PRISM [6]	ACS	0.6 µg/kg+ 0.15 µg/kg min^{-1}	3232	Death, new myocardial infarction or refractory ischemia within 48 h	33 (p = 0.01)
PRISM-Plus [14]	ACS	0.6 µg/kg+ 0.15 µg/kg min^{-1}	1560	Death, new myocardial infarction or refractory ischemia within 7 days	34 (p = 0.004)
RESTORE [22]	High-risk PCI	10 µg/kg+ 0.15 µg/kg min^{-1}	2212	Death, MI, CABG, repeat target vessel PCI or stent insertion for abrupt closure within 30 days	16 (p = 0.160)[a]
TARGET[b] [26]	PCI	10 µg/kg+ 0.15 µg/kg min^{-1}	4812	Death, MI, or urgent revascularization	20 (p = 0.037)

[a]p = 0.052 when the endpoint included urgent target vessel PCI according to the same criteria as those used in other trials of GP IIb/IIIa antagonists during PCI.
[b]TARGET randomized patients undergoing PCI (61% for ACS) to receive either tirofiban or abciximab (0.25-µg/kg bolus followed by a 12-h infusion of 0.125 µg/kg min^{-1}).
ACS, acute coronary syndromes.

with elevated troponin T ($>0.1\,\mu g/L$) or troponin I ($\geq 1.0\,\mu g/L$) levels 6–8 h after presentation, and in those with elevated troponin T levels the 30-d incidence of death or MI was reduced from 13.7 to 3.5% ($p < 0.01$) (Fig. 3) [12]. In the tirofiban group overall there was a trend toward a reduction in death or MI at 30 days (from 7.1 to 5.8%; RR 0.80; 95% CI 0.60–1.05; $p = 0.11$). In the subgroup of 629 patients with troponin I levels of 1 µg/L or higher, the effect of tirofiban in reducing the 30-day incidence of death, MI, or recurrent ischemia was independent of revascularization (revascularization OR 0.37; 95% CI 0.15–0.93; $p = 0.02$; no revascularization OR 0.30; 95% CI 0.10–0.84; $p = 0.004$) (Fig. 4) [12]. Similar results were observed in patients with elevated troponin T levels.

The PRISM-Plus study [14] enrolled clinically higher-risk patients, 59% of whom had ST-segment depression (compared with 32% in the PRISM study). All patients received aspirin. PRISM-Plus was initially designed to compare tirofiban, heparin, and the combination of the two, but the tirofiban-alone limb of the study was stopped early, after recruiting 345 patients, owing to an excessive mortality rate at 7 days (4.6 vs. 1.1% in the heparin group and 1.5% in the combination treatment group). The most likely explanation for this finding is chance, although heparin-rebound may also have been a contributing factor because 70% of the patients in PRISM-Plus were already receiving unfractionated heparin at randomization. At 7 days the combined incidence of death, MI, or refractory ischemia was 34% lower in the patients who received tirofiban and heparin than in those who received heparin alone (12.9 vs. 17.9%, $p = 0.004$). At 30 days the rates of death or MI were 8.7 and 11.9%, respectively ($p = 0.03$).

Combined analysis of the data from PRISM and PRISM-Plus shows that tirofiban treatment was associated with significant reductions in primary endpoint events, reducing the overall incidence of death or MI by 22% (from 8.6 to 6.7%, $p < 0.01$) at 30 days. A cost-effectiveness analysis of PRISM-Plus showed that tirofiban treatment reduced health costs [15]. In PRISM-Plus tirofiban improved outcomes in all patient subgroups, particularly those at higher risk such as diabetics [16], patients already taking aspirin therapy, and patients who had previously undergone coronary bypass surgery (Fig. 5) [14].

In the PRISM Study the rates of TIMI major bleeding [13], transfusion, and intracranial hemorrhage were 0.4, 1.9, and 0.1, respectively. There was no difference in bleeding between the treatment groups, except for the rates of transfusion, which were 1.4% in the heparin group and

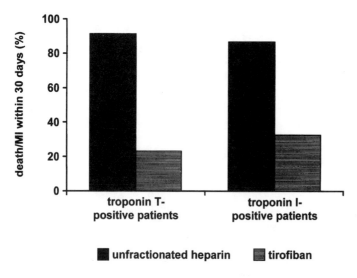

Figure 3 Effects of tirofiban on the 30-day endpoint of death/MI in patients in the PRISM study with elevated troponin T or I levels 6–8 h after presentation. (From Ref. 17.)

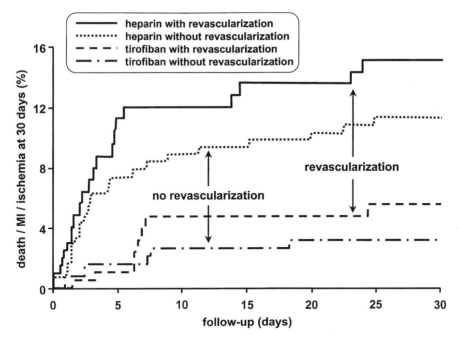

Figure 4 Thirty-day rates of death, MI, and recurrent ischemia in patients with elevated troponin I levels who received heparin or tirofiban and did or did not undergo revascularization procedures in the PRISM study. (From Ref. 12.)

2.4% in the tirofiban group (p = NS). Thrombocytopenia (platelet count <50,000/mm^3) occurred in 0.4% of the heparin group and 0.1% of the tirofiban group (p = 0.04). In patients randomized to receive heparin and tirofiban in the PRISM-Plus study, the rates of major bleeding, transfusion and thrombocytopenia were 4.0, 4.0, and 0.5%, vs. 3.0, 2.8, and 0.3% in

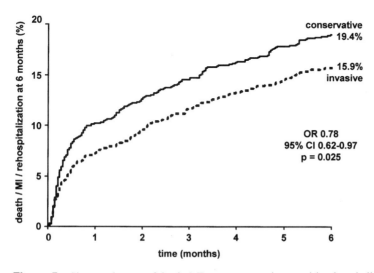

Figure 5 Six-month rates of death, MI, or severe angina requiring hospitalization in patients randomized to early invasive or early conservative treatment in the TACTICS-TIMI-18 trial. The discrimination level for ST-segment depression was ≥0.5 mV, and the discrimination level for troponin T was 0.01 μg/L. (From Ref. 18.)

patients randomized to heparin alone (comparison p values = 0.34, 0.21, and 0.44, respectively). No intracranial hemorrhages were reported in the PRISM-Plus study.

In the TACTICS-TIMI-18 trial [18], patients with non–ST-elevation acute coronary syndromes were given aspirin, heparin, and tirofiban for a median of 24 h, and randomized to undergo either early invasive or early conservative treatment. Early revascularization was performed surgically in 19% of the invasive treatment group and percutaneously in 41%. Thirty-six percent of the conservative treatment group also had revascularization procedures owing to recurrence of symptoms or inducible ischemia. At 6 months there was no difference in mortality between the groups, but the primary endpoint of death, MI, or rehospitalization for angina was reduced by 18% in the invasive treatment group [15.9 vs. 19.4% in the conservative treatment group (p = 0.025)]. Early revascularization was particularly beneficial in patients with $\geq$0.5 mm of ST-segment depression [19] or elevated troponin T levels ($>$0.1 µg/L), reducing their primary endpoint rates from 26.3 to 16.4% (p = 0.006) and from 24.2 to 14.3% (p $<$ 0.001), respectively (see Fig. 4). Major bleeding occurred in 5.5% of the invasive treatment group and in 3.3% of the conservative treatment group (p = NS). Patients in the invasive treatment group spent on average 1 day less in hospital (5 days vs. 6 days, p $<$ 0.05) than did those in the conservative treatment group.

TACTICS-TIMI-18 was the first trial to show that interventions improve clinical outcomes if performed within 48 h. The study design differed from that of the FRISC-II study [20], in which the invasive treatment group underwent percutaneous coronary intervention (PCI) at a median of 4 days or coronary artery bypass surgery at a median of 7 days. In FRISC-II the rate of periprocedural MI was higher in the invasive treatment group despite pretreatment with dalteparin, whereas this was not so in TACTICS-TIMI-18, in which patients were pretreated with tirofiban. Among the 15% of patients in TACTICS-TIMI-18 with a TIMI risk stratification score of higher than 4, those randomized to early revascularization had a risk reduction of 45% [21]. Economic analysis of this study showed that at 6 months the costs were similar in both trial limbs for patients with ST depression and those with elevated troponin levels.

B. Percutaneous Coronary Intervention

The RESTORE trial [22] compared tirofiban (10 µg/kg over 3 min followed by 0.15-µg/kg min^{-1} for 36 h) with a placebo in patients undergoing PCI (without elective stent deployment) within 72 h after presenting with an acute coronary syndrome. Six percent of patients underwent primary PCI. Although there appeared to be some early benefit of tirofiban within the first 2 days, there was no difference in the primary 30-day endpoint of death, MI or target vessel revascularization (10.3% with tirofiban vs. 12.2% with placebo, p = 0.16). However, when the RESTORE trial data were reanalyzed using the same definition for the revascularization component of the primary composite endpoint as was used in the abciximab trials [23–25], tirofiban was found to reduce the incidence of the primary composite endpoint from 10.5 to 8.0% (p = 0.052) at 30 days, an effect similar to those seen in trials of other IIb/IIIa antagonists.

The TARGET trial [26] compared tirofiban with abciximab in patients undergoing PCI for an acute coronary syndrome or stable angina, using the RESTORE Trial [22] dosing regimen for tirofiban and the EPISTENT trial [23] dosing regimen for abciximab. All patients received aspirin, clopidogrel, and heparin (70 IU/kg) targeted to an activated clotting time of 250 s. The primary endpoint of death, MI, or urgent revascularization occurred in 6.0% of the tirofiban group versus 4.8% of the abciximab group within 72 h, and in 7.5% of the tirofiban group versus 6.0% of the abciximab group within 30 days (interaction p = 0.037). In patients undergoing PCI for acute coronary syndromes, the rates of the primary endpoint at 30 days were 8.3% with tirofiban versus 6.2% with abciximab, whereas in those undergoing elective PCI the rates were 4.7 versus 6.3%, respectively (p = 0.038). These outcomes indicate that there was an interaction between treatment randomization and clinical indications for PCI. There was no difference between the groups in the incidence of major bleeding, which occurred in 1.17% of the tirofiban group and 0.95% of the abciximab group (p = 0.47), but there was an increase in minor bleeding with abciximab (3.3% with tirofiban vs. 5.6% with abciximab, p = 0.002), suggesting that the tirofiban dose could possibly be increased without incurring an unacceptable bleeding rate. At 12 months the mortality rates were 1.9% in the tirofiban group vs. 1.7% in the abciximab group overall (p = 0.66), and 2.1% vs. 2.9%, respectively, in diabetics (p = 0.44).

Possible explanations for these findings include the dosing regimens used in the trial and the duration of platelet inhibition achieved. Because abciximab also has binding affinity for other integrin receptors, including the vitronectin receptor (αv-β3) expressed on other cell types, such as macrophages [27], it may have other therapeutic effects in addition to its antiplatelet properties. The combined results of TACTICS-TIMI-18, TARGET, and PRISM-Plus indicate that tirofiban should be used early in the initial treatment of patients with acute coronary syndromes without persistent ST-segment elevation [28], and abciximab should be used when indicated in the cardiac catheterization laboratory. Epitifibatide, another small-molecule IIb/IIIa antagonist which reduces events following percutaneous intervention [29], has not been evaluated in similar comparative efficacy trials.

C. ST-Elevation Myocardial Infarction

Fibrinolytic agents reduce mortality and preserve left ventricular function when administered within 12 h of the onset of symptoms of acute MI with ST-segment elevation or new left bundle-branch block on the presenting electrocardiogram [30]. The importance of platelet inhibition in acute MI was first demonstrated in the large, randomized ISIS-2 study [31], which reported that aspirin and streptokinase reduced mortality, both individually and synergistically. Conventional fibrinolytic regimens achieve TIMI grade 3 (i.e., "normal") flow in the infarct-related artery in less than 60% of patients at 90 min [32].

Fibrinolytic agents are relatively ineffective at dissolving platelet-rich thrombi, and cause further thrombin generation, which activates platelets locally. The FASTER trial tested various bolus doses of tirofiban (between 10 and 15 μg/kg followed by 0.15 μg/kg min^{-1} for 24 h) in combination with half or two-thirds doses of tenecteplase (0.27 or 0.36 mg/kg, respectively). A control group received full-dose tenecteplase alone (0.53 mg/kg). The patients receiving the half and two-thirds doses of tenecteplase were given a 40 IU/kg heparin bolus (maximum 3,000 IU) and 7 IU/kg h^{-1} infusion (maximum 800 IU h^{-1}) to maintain an APTT of 50–70 s, while those receiving full-dose tenecteplase (the control group) were given a 60 IU/kg heparin bolus (maximum 4,000 IU) and a 12 IU/kg h^{-1} infusion (maximum 1,000 IU). The endpoints of the trial were TIMI grade 3 flow in the infarct artery at 60 min, the corrected TIMI frame count at 60 min, and ST-segment resolution at 60 and 180 min. TIMI grade 3 flow was acheived by 60 min in 59% of the tirofiban groups overall vs. 58% of the control group, and there were no differences in their corrected TIMI frame counts. Complete ST-segment resolution was achieved by 60 min in 41% of the tirofiban groups overall vs. 29% of the control group (p = 0.07), and by 180 min in 76% vs. 65%, respectively (p = 0.10). TIMI major bleeding [13] occurred within the first 48 h in 2.3% of the tirofiban groups overall vs. 4.7% of the control group. There were no episodes of intercranial hemorrhage [personal communication from Dr. EM Ohman].

III. CONCLUSION

In large, randomized clinical trials, tirofiban has been efficacious in patients with acute coronary syndromes and in those undergoing PCI, without an associated increase in hemorrhagic risk. The uses of tirofiban in acute MI, either with modified fibrinolytic regimens or before primary angioplasty in conjunction with aspirin, clopidogrel, and unfractionated or low-molecular-weight heparins, require further definition. Further research is needed to define the limits of its therapeutic efficacy and safety, the ideal levels of platelet inhibition, the need for individualization of dosage based on bedside measures of platelet function, the optimal combination of adjunctive pharmacotherapy, and the most effective duration of treatment.

REFERENCES

1. Hartman GD, Egbertson MS, Halczenko, et al. Non-peptide fibrinogen receptor antagonists. 1. Discovery and design of exosite inhibitors. J Med Chem 1992; 35:4640–4642.
2. Mayo KH, Fan F, Beavers MP, Eckardt A, Keane P, Hoekstra WJ, Andrade–Gordon P. RGD induces conformational transition in purified platelet integrin GPIIb/IIIa–SDS system, yielding multiple binding states for fibrinogen gamma-chain C-terminal peptide. FEBS Lett 1996; 378:82.
3. Eide BL, Turck CW, Escobedo JA. Identification of yr-397 as the primary site of tyrosine phosphorylation and pp6osrc association in the focal adhesion kinase, pp125FAK. Mol Cell Biol 1995; 15:2819–2827.
4. Lynch JJ Jr, Cook JJ, Sitko GR, Holahan MA, Ramjit DR, Mellott MJ, Stranieri MI, Stabilito II, Zhang G, Lynch RJ, et al. Nonpepfide glycoprotein IIb/IIIa inhibitors. 5. Antithrombotic effects of MK-0383. J Pharmacol Exp Ther 1995; 272:20–32.
5. Merck & Co, Inc. Tirofiban hydrochloride: worldwide clinical summary. West Point, PA: Merck & Co, Inc, 1997.
6. The Platelet Receptor Inhibition in Ischemic Syndrome Management (PRISM) Study Investigators. A comparison of aspirin plus tirofiban with aspirin plus heparin for unstable angina. N Engl J Med 1998; 338:1498–1505.
7. Kereiakes D, Kleiman NS, Ambrose J, Cohen M, Rodriguez S, Palabrica C, Herrmann HC, Sutton JM, Weaver WDD, McKee DB, Fitzpatrick V, Sax F. Randomized, double-blind, placebo-controlled dose-ranging study of tirofiban (MK-383) platelet IIb/IIIa blockade in high risk patients undergoing coronary angioplasty. J Am Coll Cardiol 1996; 27:536–542.
8. Zhang J, Zhang J, Shattil SJ, Cunningham MC, Rittenhouse SE. Phosphoinositide 3-kinase gamma and p85/phosphoinositide 3-kinase in platelets: relative activation by thrombin receptor or betaphorbol rnyristate acetate and roles in promoting the ligand-binding function of alphaIIb beta3 integrin. J Biol Chem 1996; 271:6265–6272.
9. Guinebault C, Payrastre B, Racaud–Sultan C, Mazarguil H, Breton M, Mauco G, Plantavid M, Chap H. Integrin-dependent translocation of phosphoinositide 3-kinase to the cytoskeleton of thrombin-activated platelets involves specific interactions of p85 alpha with actin filaments and focal adhesion kinase. J Cell Biol 1995; 129:831–842.
10. Cohen M, Théroux P, Weber S, Laramée P, Huynh T, Borzak S, Diodati JG, Squire IB. Deckelbaum LI, Thornton AR, Harris KE, Sax FL, Lo M–W, White HD. Combination therapy with tirofiban and exoxaparin in acute coronary syndromes. Int J Cardiol 1999; 71:273–281.
11. Cohen M. Initial experience with the low-molecular-weight heparin, enoxaparin, in combination with the platelet glycoprotein IIb/IIIa blocker, tirofiban, in patients with non–ST-segment elevation acute coronary syndromes. J Invasive Cardiol 2000; 12(suppl E):E5–E28.
12. Heeschen C, Hamm CW, Goldmann B, Deu A, Langenbrink L, White HD, for the PRISM Study Investigators. Troponin concentrations for stratification of patients with acute coronary syndromes in relation to therapeutic efficacy of tirofiban. Lancet 1999; 354:1757–1762.
13. Rao AK, Pratt C, Berke A, Jaffe A, Ockene I, Schreiber TL, Bell WR, Knatterud G, Robertson TL,

Terrin ML. Thrombolysis in Myocardial Infarction (TIMI) Trial—phase I: hemorrhagic manifestations and changes in plasma fibrinogen and the fibrinolytic system in patients treated with recombinant tissue plasminogen activator and streptokinase. J Am Coll Cardiol 1988; 11:1–11.

14. The Platelet Receptor Inhibition in Ischemic Syndrome Management in Patients Limited by Unstable Signs and Symptoms (PRISM-Plus) Study Investigators. Inhibition of the platelet glycoprotein IIb/IIIa receptor with tirofiban in unstable angina and non–Q-wave myocardial infarction. N Engl J Med 1998; 338:1488–1497.

15. Szucs TD, Meyer BJ, Kiowski W. Economic assessment of tirofiban in the management of acute coronary syndromes in the hospital setting: an analysis based on the PRISM PLUS Trial. Eur Heart J 1999; 20:1253–1260.

16. Theroux P, Alexander J Jr, Pharand C, Barr E, Snapinn S, Ghannam AF, Sax FL. Glycoprotein IIb/IIIa receptor blockade improves outcomes in diabetic patients presenting with unstable angina/non-ST-elevation myocardial infarction: results from the Platelet Receptor Inhibition in Ischemic Syndrome Management in Patients Limited by Unstable Signs and Symptoms (PRISM-PLUS) study. Circulation 2000; 102:2466–2472.

17. White HD. Non–ST-elevation acute coronary syndromes. New Ethic J 2000; Nov:65–72.

18. Cannon CP, Weintraub WS, Demopoulos LA, Vicari R, Frey MJ, Lakkis N, Neumann F-J, Robertson DH, DeLucca PT, DiBattiste PM, Gibson CM, Braunwald E, the TACTICS–Thrombolysis in Myocardial Infarction 18 Investigators. Comparison of early invasive and conservative strategies in patients with unstable coronary sundromes treated with the glycoprotein IIb/IIIa inhibitor tirofiban. N Engl J Med 2001; 344:1879–1887.

19. Hyde TA, French JK, Wong C–K, Straznicky IT, Whitlock RML, White HD. Four-year survival of patients with acute coronary syndromes without ST-segment elevation and prognostic significance of 0.5-mm ST-segment depression. Am J Cardiol 1999; 84:379–385.

20. Wallentin L, Lagerqvist B, Husted S, Kontny F, Ståhle F, Swahn E, for the FRISC II Investigators. Outcome at 1 year after an invasive compared with a non-invasive strategy in unstable coronary-artery disease: the FRISC II invasive randomised trial. Lancet 2000; 356:9–16.

21. Antman EM, Cohen M, Bernink PJ, McCabe CH, Horacek T, Papuchis C, Mautner B, Corbalan R, Radley D, Braunwald E. The TIMI risk score for unstable angina/non–ST elevation MI: a method for prognostication and therapeutic decision making. JAMA 2000; 284:835–842.

22. The RESTORE Investigators. Effects of platelet gycoprotein IIb/IIIa blockade with tirofiban on adverse cardiac events in patients with unstable angina or acute myocardial infarction undergoing coronary angioplasty. Circulation 1997; 96:1445–1453.

23. Lincoff AM, Califf RM, Anderson KM, Weisman HF, Aguirre FV, Kleiman NS, Harrington RA, Topol EJ, for the EPIC Investigators. Evidence for prevention of death and myocardial infarction with platelet membrane glycoprotein IIb/IIIa receptor blockade by abciximab (c7E3 Fab) among patients with unstable angina undergoing percutaneous coronary revascularization. J Am Coll Cardiol 1997; 30:149–156.

24. The EPILOG Investigators. Platelet glycoprotein IIb/IIIa receptor blockade and low-dose heparin during percutaneous coronary revascularization. N Engl J Med 1997; 336:1689–1696.

25. The EPISTENT Investigators. Randomised placebo-controlled and balloon–angioplasty-controlled trial to assess safety of coronary stenting with use of platelet glycoprotein-IIb/IIIa blockade. Lancet 1998; 352:87–92.

26. Topol EJ, Moliterno DJ, Herrmann HC, Powers ER, Grines CL, Cohen DJ, Cohen EA, Bertrand M, Neumann F-J, Stone GW, DiBattiste PM, Yakubov SJ, DeLucca PT, Demopoulos L, the TARGET Investigators. Comparison of two platelet glycoprotein IIb/IIIa inhibitors, tirofiban and abciximab, for the prevention of ischemic events with percutaneous coronary revascularization. N Engl J Med 2001; 344:1888–1894.

27. Topol EJ, Byzova TV, Plow EF. Platelet GPIIb–IIIa blockers. Lancet 1999; 353:227–231.

28. Theroux P, Alexander J Jr, Dupuis J, Pesant Y, Gervais P, Grandmont D, Kouz S, Laramee P, Huynh T, Barr E, Sax FL. PRISM–PLUS I. Upstream use of tirofiban in patients admitted for an acute coronary syndrome in hospitals with or without facilities for invasive management. PRISM–PLUS Investigators. Am J Cardiol 2001; 87:375–380.

29. The ESPRIT Investigators. Novel dosing regimen of eptifibatide in planned coronary stent implantation (ESPRIT): a randomised, placebo-controlled trial. Lancet 2000; 356:2037–2044.

30. Fibrinolytic Therapy Trialists' (FTT) Collaborative Group. Indications for fibrinolytic therapy in suspected acute myocardial infarction: collaborative overview of early mortality and major morbidity results from all randomised trials of more than 1000 patients. Lancet 1994; 343:311–322.

31. ISIS-2 (Second International Study of Infarct Survival) Collaborative Group. Randomised trial of intravenous streptokinase, oral aspirin, both, or neither among 17,187 cases of suspected acute myocardial infarction: ISIS-2. Lancet 1988; 2:349–360.

32. The GUSTO Angiographic Investigators. The effects of tissue plasminogen activator, streptokinase, or both on coronary-artery patency, ventricular function, and survival after acute myocardial infarction [published erratum appears in N Engl J Med 1994; 330:516]. N Engl J Med 1993; 329:1615–1622.

25

Procoagulant Activities of Glycoprotein IIb/IIIa Receptor Blockers

Karlheinz Peter and Christoph Bode
University of Freiburg, Freiburg, Germany

SUMMARY

Potential procoagulant effects of GP IIb/IIIa blockers are probably the most controversially discussed issues for this class of drugs, especially because clinical trials with oral GP IIb/IIIa blockers revealed disappointing results. The following chapter first reviews structural and functional data on the integrin receptor $\alpha_{IIb}\beta_3$. Second, based on the finding that currently clinically used GP IIb/IIIa blockers are ligand mimetics, experimental data is shown, demonstrating an intrinsic activating effect of ligand mimetic GP IIb/IIIa blockers that potentially results in fibrinogen binding to $\alpha_{IIb}\beta_3$ and in platelet aggregation. At the same time, data are discussed describing nonligand mimetic GP IIb/IIIa blockers as pharmacological alternatives without any intrinsic-activating property. Furthermore, the inhibitory effect of aspirin on GP IIb/IIIa blocker-induced platelet aggregation is discussed as a clinically relevant finding. And finally, the potential association of GP IIb/IIIa blocker-induced thrombocytopenia with procoagulant effects is described.

I. INTRODUCTION

The development of GP IIb/IIIa blockers is one of the most fascinating stories in cardiovascular medicine within the recent years. The technology for the production of monoclonal antibodies, the technique to "humanize" these antibodies, and the advances of molecular biology allowing identification of Arg–Gly–Asp the (RGD) sequence within fibrinogen as the "binding sequence" were the basis for the development of drugs that block the binding of fibrinogen to the platelet integrin $\alpha_{IIb}\beta_3$ (GP IIb/IIIa). [1–4]. The clinical use of GP IIb/IIIa blockers as intravenous drugs has been very beneficial in numerous large studies and has become an important part of the daily practice in cardiology within a few years [1–4]. The enormous commercial success of these drugs has fostered the fast development of many orally applicable GP IIb/IIIa blockers. The results of initial clinical trials were disappointing and may even be the cause of a premature end in the development of orally available GP IIb/IIIa blocking drugs [5–7]. Thus, success and failure of GP IIb/IIIa blockers are as close together as is rarely seen in drug development.

For the understanding of the blocking function, but especially for the understanding of potential adverse effects of GP IIb/IIIa blockers, the knowledge of the structure of GP IIb/IIIa and the ligand-binding function of this integrin is essential. The following chapter first describes the structural knowledge on GP IIb/IIIa, the pharmacological properties of the GP IIb/IIIa blockers, and then discusses data on recently revealed adverse effects of GP IIb/IIIa blockers that may participate in the limitations of these drugs in clinical trials.

II. THE STRUCTURE OF $\alpha_{IIb}\beta_3$ (GP IIb/IIIa)

The term *GP IIb/IIIa* originates from platelet protein gel electrophoresis describing initially band number II and III and, later on, with better spatial separation, IIb and IIIa [8]. GP IIb consists of two chains (105-kDa heavy chain and 25-kDa light chain) that are linked by a disulfide bond [9,10]. GP IIIa is a 95-kDa single-chain protein [9,10]. Cloning the genes was achieved in the late 1980s, and GP IIb and GP IIIa were both located on chromosome 17 [11,12]. GP IIb/IIIa is the most abundant platelet membrane receptor with 50,000 to 80,000 glycoproteins per platelet, thereby constituting up to 2% of the amount of total platelet protein [13]. The genetic defect of Glanzmann disease helped to identify the role of this glycoprotein for fibrinogen binding and for platelet aggregation [14–16]. Later on, the two glycoprotein bands were shown to be identical to the antibody epitopes CD41 and CD61. Finally, it was recognized that GP IIb/IIIa is a member of the adhesion molecule family called *integrins*, describing their integrative function between extracellular ligands and the cytoskeleton [17]. According to the original term GP IIb/IIIa, $\alpha_{IIb}\beta_3$ was chosen as a term within the integrin nomenclature [17–19]. More than 20 different integrins are known, and all of them consist of two subunits (α- and β-subunits) that are noncovalently linked to each other [18,19]. With the exception of α_4, all integrin subunits have a short cytoplasmic tail, one transmembraneous region, and a large extracellular domain [17–19]. For several of these integrins, different conformational states could be demonstrated [17–19]. During cell stimulation, integrins can change their conformation from a low- to a high-affinity state relative to their ligand-binding properties. Integrins overall have two major functions: First, they mechanically couple the cytoskeleton to the extracellular matrix or to surface receptors of other cells; second, they transmit signals from the inside of the cell to the outside of the cell and vice versa [18,19].

The platelet receptor $\alpha_{IIb}\beta_3$ is probably the most intensively studied integrin. Nevertheless, the conformational changes of $\alpha_{IIb}\beta_3$ that are necessary for ligand binding are not well understood. It is known neither how many conformational states do exist for $\alpha_{IIb}\beta_3$, nor whether this receptor can switch between these states without restriction. Unstimulated platelets express a default state of $\alpha_{IIb}\beta_3$ that does not allow binding of soluble fibrinogen. Stimulation of platelets causes a conformational change of $\alpha_{IIb}\beta_3$, allowing a high–affinity-binding of fibrinogen [20,21]. This conformational change results in the exposure of new epitopes on $\alpha_{IIb}\beta_3$, which are named ligand-induced binding sites (LIBS) [22–24]. In addition, a conformational change of $\alpha_{IIb}\beta_3$ has been described after binding of RGD peptides [25]. These peptides are ligand mimetics, as they represent one of the sites within fibrinogen that bind to $\alpha_{IIb}\beta_3$. The small size of RGD peptides allows binding to $\alpha_{IIb}\beta_3$ without prior platelet stimulation and, thereby, results in a conformational change of $\alpha_{IIb}\beta_3$ [25,26]. Because the commercially available GP IIb/IIIa blockers are either derivatives of the RGD/KGD peptides (e.g., eptifibatide), or are modeled after the RGD structure (e.g., tirofiban), or are antibody fragments that probably bind at or close to the fibrinogen-binding pocket (e.g., abciximab), GP IIb/IIIa blockers are ligand mimetics. Indeed, GP IIb/IIIa blockers induce binding of various antibodies directed against LIBS epitopes [26–30]. Interestingly, the pattern of anti-LIBS antibodies varies with each GP IIb/IIIa blocker

[27–29]. This implies that different GP IIb/IIIa blockers induce different conformational changes of $\alpha_{IIb}\beta_3$. As described later, because the GP IIb/IIIa blocker-induced conformational change may be the basis of an intrinsic-activating property, GP IIb/IIIa blockers may vary in their procoagulant activity.

The integrin $\alpha_{IIb}\beta_3$ transduces mechanical force between the cytoskeleton and the extracellular environment of the platelet, which is either composed of extracellular matrix or the cell membrane of neighboring cells [31]. For a strong force transduction, $\alpha_{IIb}\beta_3$, as do other integrins, uses a natural "trick" of mechanics. By the mechanical coupling through cytoskeletal anchorage of many integrin receptors, the mechanical force is potentiated. Without coupling, a cell can be disengaged by a kind of peeling effect. Integrin–ligand pairs are disengaged one after the other, and the mechanical force of a single integrin–ligand pair is low. If integrins are coupled by the cytoskeleton, a peeling is no longer possible, for all of the coupled integrin–ligand pairs have to be disengaged simultaneously [32–34]. Also in signal transduction, ligand binding to $\alpha_{IIb}\beta_3$ on the one side and cytoskeletal anchorage and coupling on the other side are two distinguishable phenomena. For outside-in signaling, the binding of a monovalent ligand compared with the binding of a multivalent ligand, that allows clustering of $\alpha_{IIb}\beta_3$, causes different signaling responses [35]. GP IIb/IIIa blocker used in clinical practice are monovalent. This is important in the context of outside-in signal transduction, as will be discussed later on.

III. INTRINSIC ACTIVATING PROPERTY OF GP IIb/IIIa BLOCKER

The binding of the natural ligand fibrinogen and the ligand mimetic RGD peptide induces a conformational change of $\alpha_{IIb}\beta_3$ that can be detected by anti-LIBS antibodies [22,25–27,36–39]. Pharmaceuticals that are either cyclic peptides, derived from the RGD or KGD sequence, or chemical compounds that are modeled after the RGD structure, competitively bind to the fibrinogen-binding pocket within $\alpha_{IIb}\beta_3$ and, therefore, are ligand mimetics. Additionally, these agents are able to bind to the nonactivated $\alpha_{IIb}\beta_3$ on unstimulated platelets and, thereby, cause a conformational change of $\alpha_{IIb}\beta_3$ without prior platelet activation [25,26,36–38]. Indeed, these GP IIb/IIIa blockers cause LIBS epitope expression as a reflection of a conformational change induced by these agents [39]. From these findings, we hypothesized that at the moment a ligand mimetic dissociates from GP IIb/IIIa this receptor is left in a conformation that is active and thus enables the receptor to bind fibrinogen. This hypothesis is schematically shown in Figure 1. To prove this hypothesis, platelets were incubated with ligand mimetics (RGD-peptides, abciximab [c7E3], the original IgG 7E3, and low-molecular-weight GP IIb/IIIa blockers). In a following experimental step, these ligand mimetics were washed out, and afterward fibrinogen binding was determined in flow cytometry. Indeed, after dissociation of the ligand mimetics, the receptor was left in an active, fibrinogen-binding conformation (Fig. 2) [26]. To exclude platelet-specific artifacts similar experiments were performed with an $\alpha_{IIb}\beta_3$-expressing CHO cell line. The isolated $\alpha_{IIb}\beta_3$ receptor, which cannot be activated by inside–out signaling in CHO cells, was also switched to an active, fibrinogen-binding receptor by ligand mimetics [26]. Thus, ligand mimetics have the intrinsic property of activating the $\alpha_{IIb}\beta_3$ receptor both on platelets and on a model cell line expressed as a recombinant receptor.

Interestingly, abciximab (c7E3), a human–mouse chimeric Fab antibody fragment, also reacted as a ligand mimetic [26,40]. This finding can be explained if abciximab binds at or close to the fibrinogen-binding pocket of GP IIb/IIIa. Indeed, the original publications of the IgG monoclonal antibody describe 7E3 as an activation-dependent antibody [41], which would be in agreement with a binding of abciximab at or close to the fibrinogen-binding pocket.

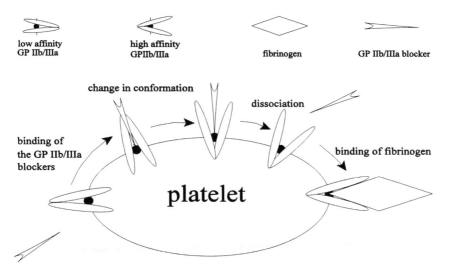

low affinity
GP IIb/IIIa

high affinity
GPIIb/IIIa

fibrinogen

GP IIb/IIIa blocker

change in conformation

dissociation

binding of
the GP IIb/IIIa
blockers

binding of fibrinogen

platelet

Figure 1 Schematic drawing of the proposed mechanism of the intrinsic-activating property of GP IIb/IIIa blockers.

Although the washout experiments are primarily an artificial, experimental setup, they possess pharmacological relevance. During start and end of intravenous therapy low plasma concentrations of the GP IIb/IIIa blockers are present. But even more relevant, low plasma concentrations may be repeatedly present with oral GP IIb/IIIa blocker therapy. At high concentrations, if a GP IIb/IIIa blocker dissociates, $\alpha_{IIb}\beta_3$ will immediately be blocked by another GP IIb/IIIa blocker. Thus, at high concentrations the intrinsic activating effect of GP IIb/IIIa blockers is masked. In contrast, at low concentrations, if a GP IIb/IIIa blocker dissociates, the probability that another blocker occupies the receptor is again low, and thus the activated $\alpha_{IIb}\beta_3$ receptor may be able to bind fibrinogen. Indeed, if platelets are incubated with increasing concentrations of the GP IIb/IIIa blocker abciximab, fibrinogen binding can be demonstrated at low concentrations (Fig. 3) [26]. The consequence of this fibrinogen binding at low concentrations of GP IIb/IIIa blockers, the formation of platelet aggregates can be seen directly in light microscopy (Fig. 4) [26]. Interestingly, abciximab-induced platelet aggregates are smaller and seem less stable compared with ADP-induced platelet aggregates (see Fig. 4), a finding that may partly explain why clinically apparent thrombi or the induction of myocardial infarction have not been reported as adverse effects of intraveneous or oral GP IIb/IIIa blocker therapy, even in patients without concomitant aspirin therapy [42].

Interestingly, monoclonal antibodies (P2, 2G12) that block fibrinogen binding to $\alpha_{IIb}\beta_3$ probably by steric hindrance but not by direct binding to the fibrinogen-binding pocket, do not induce fibrinogen binding to $\alpha_{IIb}\beta_3$ (see Fig. 2) [26]. These antibodies do not reveal ligand mimetic properties; therefore, they do not exert an intrinsic-activating effect. Antibodies with these properties may be the basis for the development of alternative GP IIb/IIIa blockers without intrinsic-activating properties. Other interesting alternatives are activation-specific antibodies such as PAC-1. These antibodies cannot bind to $\alpha_{IIb}\beta_3$ on unstimulated platelets; thus, they cannot cause a conformational change from a "resting" $\alpha_{IIb}\beta_3$ to an "activated" $\alpha_{IIb}\beta_3$ [26]. Furthermore, activation-specific antibodies as therapeutic agents may have the advantage that they may not inhibit adhesion of platelets on immobilized fibrinogen (e.g., during vessel injury). Because this may result in fewer bleeding complications, the safety profile of activation-specific antibodies may be more favorable. Also the total amount of antibodies needed and, consequently,

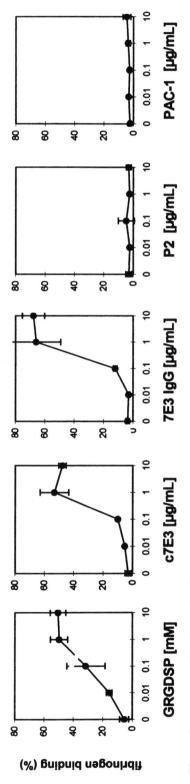

Figure 2 Induction of fibrinogen binding to platelets by ligand mimetics (GRGDSP, c7E3, 7E3): Nonligand mimetics do not induce fibrinogen binding to platelets. Platelets were incubated with the listed ligand mimetics and nonligand mimetics and after washout of these agents fibrinogen binding was determined as percentage of platelets binding fibrinogen with a fluorescence-labeled antibody in flow cytometry.

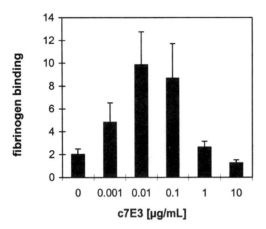

Figure 3 Induction of fibrinogen binding to platelets by low concentrations of abciximab (c7E3): Platelets were incubated with various concentrations of abciximab, and without washout, fibrinogen binding was determined in flow cytometry as the percentage of platelets binding fibrinogen.

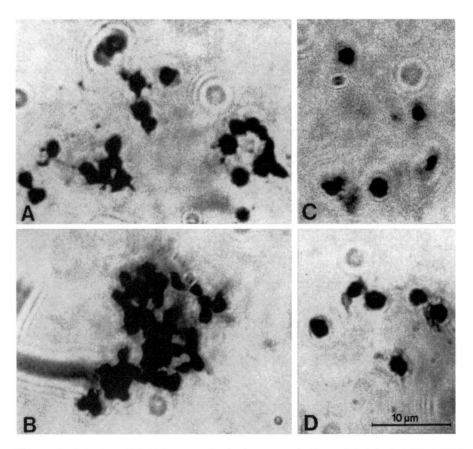

Figure 4 Induction of platelet aggregation by low concentrations of abciximab (c7E3): (A) Incubation with a low concentration (0.1 μg/mL; (B) incubation with 20 μM ADP as a positive control; (C) no addition; (D) incubation with 10 μg/mL abciximab (c7E3).

the costs, are expected to be low, because only the relatively few activated $\alpha_{IIb}\beta_3$ receptors must be occupied.

GP IIb/IIIa blocker therapy is most often accompanied by the coadministration of aspirin, heparin, ADP receptor antagonists, and most recently by fibrinolytics [1–3,43–45]; but, with the exception of aspirin, none of these drugs have an effect on the intrinsic-activating property of GP IIb/IIIa blockers [26]. The effect of aspirin was suprising. The conformational change of $\alpha_{IIb}\beta_3$ induced by GP IIb/IIIa blockers was not inhibited [26]; nevertheless, GP IIb/IIIa blocker-induced platelet aggregation was inhibited by aspirin [26]. This effect may be explained by postreceptor mechanisms, such as decreased cytoskeletal anchorage. Indeed, aspirin reduces tyrosin phosphorylation of proteins in the cytoskeleton, resulting in a decrease of actin polymerization and, thereby, aspirin may affect the anchorage of GP IIb/IIIa in the cytoskeleton [46]. Thus, usually when GP IIb/IIIa blockers are used, the intrinsic-activating effect of these drugs may be masked because of the aggregation-inhibiting effect of aspirin. Nevertheless, occasionally aspirin coadministration is contraindicated or is missed during intravenous application of GP IIb/IIIa blockers. This may be even more relevant during studies of oral GP IIb/IIIa blocker therapy without concomitant aspirin (e.g., Symphony I) [7,42].

One of the most interesting issues of GP IIb/IIIa blocker pharmacology is the question of whether binding of GP IIb/IIIa blocker induces outside-in–signal transduction. Because GP IIb/IIIa blockers are monovalent, it is not expected that they induce integrin clustering, which may be a precondition for outside-in–signal transduction. Indeed, binding of the GP IIb/IIIa blocker abciximab did not result in outside-in–signaling, as platelet shape and granularity was unchanged. P selectin surface expression was not increased, and no secretion of platelet factor 4 or β-thromboglobulin was detected on unstimulated platelets [unpublished results 26]. Nevertheless, if platelets were preactivated by thrombin, outside-in–signaling by GP IIb/IIIa blockers was detected as determined by platelet Ca^{2+} concentration measurements [47]. Interestingly, only GP IIb/IIIa blockers that reveal a conformational change, as detected by a certain set of anti-LIBS antibodies, induce Ca^{2+} signalling [47]. In acute coronary syndromes and percutaneous coronary interventions, it can be expected that platelet stimulatory conditions are present; therefore, platelets may well be preactivated. This process may be locally restricted at a stenosis or at a developing clot and may be locally relevant even if we cannot detect this platelet activation by examining the peripheral blood. Furthermore, with the oral GP IIb/IIIa blocker orbofiban, platelet activation could be directly demonstrated in ex vivo blood of treated patients [48,49]. In addition, thromboxane formation could be induced when orbofiban was incubated with platelets together with a GP IIb/IIIa receptor-crosslinking antibody [49]. Also, for other GP IIb/IIIa blockers a paradoxical platelet activation has been demonstrated [50]. Overall, there is emerging evidence for outside-in–signal transduction induced by GP IIb/IIIa blocker, whereby the different GP IIb/IIIa blockers may differ in their potential to induce this signal transduction pathway.

IV. GP IIb/IIIa BLOCKER-INDUCED THROMBOCYTOPENIA IS POTENTIALLY ASSOCIATED WITH A PROCOAGULANT EFFECT

Profound thrombocytopenia has been repeatedly described as an adverse effect in patients treated with GP IIb/IIIa blockers, but its mechanism has not yet been elucidated [51–53]. The generally preferred explanation is essentially based on the finding that binding of GP IIb/IIIa blocker to the receptor induces a conformational change and thereby exposes LIBS epitopes on $\alpha_{IIb}\beta_3$. It is then postulated that patients who develop thrombocytopenia during GP IIb/IIIa blocker therapy have preformed anti-LIBS antibodies that react with the GP IIb/IIIa blocker-occupied $\alpha_{IIb}\beta_3$ and cause a clearance of platelets [54]. Also the complex between GP IIb/IIIa blocker and $\alpha_{IIb}\beta_3$ may constitute an antigenic site for preformed antibodies. Binding of anti-LIBS antibody may crosslink the $\alpha_{IIb}\beta_3$ receptors that are additionally occupied with GP IIb/IIIa blockers, and the combination of both may well cause outside-in–signal transduction resulting in platelet activation.

In one patient treated with the GP IIb/IIIa blocker abciximab a procoagulant effect was reported [55]. Abciximab caused platelet activation, as seen by an increase in binding of fibrinogen and PAC-1 (an activation-specific monoclonal antibody) and an increase of P selectin surface expression [55]. Furthermore, a direct formation of platelet aggregates could be seen [55]. These effects could be repeated later on by in vitro addition of abciximab to the patients' blood [55]. The patient survived the abciximab-induced thrombocytopenia without an obvious thrombotic or bleeding event. An initial screening for autoantibodies potentially bound to the platelet surface was negative [55]. Nevertheless, undetected preformed anti-LIBS antibodies may have caused platelet activation. Alternatively, this patient may have a genetically determined abnormal signal transduction that causes platelet activation by the binding of a GP IIb/IIIa blocker to $\alpha_{IIb}\beta_3$. Overall, patients with GP IIb/IIIa blocker-induced thrombocytopenia should be carefully monitored for bleeding and also thrombotic complications.

V. CONCLUSIONS

The "activation" of $\alpha_{IIb}\beta_3$ (GP IIb/IIIa) based on a conformational change of the receptor, and thereby, the induced fibrinogen binding to $\alpha_{IIb}\beta_3$, is the final common response of various platelet stimulatory pathways. Therefore, the blockade of $\alpha_{IIb}\beta_3$ is an effective approach to inhibit platelet aggregation. The pharmacological strategy for the development of GP IIb/IIIa blocker has been focused on agents that are ligand mimetics. But this strategy is accompanied by two major disadvantages: (1) Ligand binding to integrins results in outside-inside signal transduction. Thus, if ligand-mimetic GP IIb/IIIa blockers bind to the integrin $\alpha_{IIb}\beta_3$, platelet activation can be the direct consequence. (2) Ligand-mimetic GP IIb/IIIa blockers possess an intrinsic-activating property that can result in fibrinogen binding to $\alpha_{IIb}\beta_3$, and this can thereby induce platelet aggregation. Both mechanisms may be involved in GP IIb/IIIa blocker-induced thrombocytopenia. Furthermore, the unfavorable results of the large trials with oral GP IIb/IIIa blockers may partly be explained by the ligand–mimetic properties of the investigated agents. Overall, a provocative conclusion may be drawn: The blockade of $\alpha_{IIb}\beta_3$ by ligand–mimetic GP IIb/IIIa blockers may be only the first step that has indeed proved the concept of $\alpha_{IIb}\beta_3$ blockade, but has also shown its limitations. The next step may have to be the development of GP IIb/IIIa blockers that are either activation-specific or that are not ligand–mimetics.

REFERENCES

1. Topol EJ, Byzova TV, Plow EF. Platelet GPIIb-IIIa blockers. Lancet. 1999; 353:227–231.
2. Lefkovits J, Plow EF, Topol E. Platelet glycoprotein IIb/IIIa receptors in cardiovascular medicine. N Engl J Med 1995; 23:1553–1559.
3. Coller BS. Platelet GPIIb/IIIa antagonists: the first anti-integrin receptor therapeutics. J Clin Invest 1997; 99:1467–1471.
4. Pow EF, Pierschbacher MB, Ruoslathi E, Marguerie GA, Ginsberg MH. The effect of Arg–Gly–Asp-containing peptides on fibrinogen and von Willebrand factor binding to platelets. Proc Natl Acad Sci USA 1985; 82:8057–8061.

5. O'Neill WW, Serruys P, Knudtson M, van Es GA, Timmis GC, van der Zwaan C, Kleiman J, Gong J, Roecker EB, Dreiling R, Alexander J, Anders R. Long-term treatment with a platelet glycoprotein-receptor antagonist after percutaneous coronary revascularization. EXCITE Trial Investigators. Evaluation of Oral Xemilofiban in Controlling Thrombotic Events. N Engl J Med. 2000; 342:1316–1324.

6. Cannon CP, McCabe CH, Wilcox RG, Langer A, Caspi A, Berink P, Lopez–Sendon J, Toman J, Charlesworth A, Anders RJ, Alexander JC, Skene A, Braunwald E. Oral glycoprotein IIb/IIIa inhibition with orbofiban in patients with unstable coronary syndromes (OPUS–TIMI 16) trial. Circulation 2000; 102:149–156.

7. The SYMPHONY investigators. Comparison of sibrafiban with aspirin for prevention of cardiovascular events after acute coronary syndromes: a randomised trial. Sibrafiban versus Aspirin to Yield Maximum Protection from Ischemic Heart Events Post-acute Coronary Syndromes. Lancet 2000; 355:337–345.

8. Phillips DR, Jennings LK, Edwards HH. Identification of membrane proteins mediating the interaction of human platelets. J Cell Biol 1980; 86:77–86.

9. Phillips DR, Charo IF, Parise LV, Fitzgerald LA. The platelet membrane glycoprotein IIb–IIIa complex. Blood 1988;71:831–843.

10. Calvete JJ. Platelet integrin GPIIb/IIIa: structure–function correlations. An update and lessons from other integrins. Proc Soc Exp Biol Med 1999; 222:29–38.

11. Bray PF, Rosa JP, Johnston GI, Shiu DT, Cook RG, Lau C, Kan YW, McEver RP, Shuman MA. Platelet glycoprotein IIb. Chromosomal localization and tissue expression. J Clin Invest 1987; 80:1812–1817.

12. Rosa JP, Bray PF, Gayet O, Johnston GI, Cook RG, Jackson KW, Shuman MA, McEver RP. Cloning of glycoprotein IIIa cDNA from human erythroleukemia cells and localization of the gene to chromosome 17. Blood 1988; 72:593–600.

13. Wagner CL, Mascelli MA, Neblock DS, Weisman HF, Coller BS, Jordan RE. Analysis of GPIIb/IIIa receptor number by quantification of 7E3 binding to human platelets. Blood 1996; 88:907–914.

14. Glanzmann E. Herditaere haemorrhagische Thrombasthenie: ein Beitrag zur Pathologie der Blutplaettchen. Jahrb Kinderheilk 1918; 88:113–114.

15. Nurden AT, Caen JP. Specific roles for platelet surface glycoproteins in platelet function. Nature 1975; 255:720–722.

16. Phillips DR, Agin PP. Platelet membrane defects in Glanzmann's thrombasthenia. Evidence for decreased amounts of two major glycoproteins. J Clin Invest 1977; 60:535–545.

17. Hynes RO. Integrins: a family of cell surface receptors. Cell 1987; 48:549–554.

18. Springer TA. Adhesion receptors of the immune system. Nature 1990; 346:425–434.

19. Hynes RO. Integrins: versatility, modulation, and signalling in cell adhesion. Cell 1992; 69:11–25.

20. Marguerie GA, Plow EF, Edgington TS. Human platelets possess an inducible and saturable receptor specific for fibrinogen. J Biol Chem 1979; 254:5357–5363.

21. Bennett JS, Vilaire G. Exposure of platelet fibrinogen receptors by ADP and epinephrine. J Clin Invest 1979; 64:1393–1401.

22. Frelinger AL III, Lam SCT, Plow EF, Smith MA, Loftus JC, Ginsberg MH. Occupancy of an adhesive glycoprotein receptor modulates expression of an antigenic site involved in cell adhesion. J Biol Chem 1988; 263:12397–12402.

23. Frelinger AL III, Cohen I, Plow EF, Smith MA, Roberts J, Lam SCT, Ginsberg MH. Selective inhibition of integrin function by antibodies specific for ligand-occupied receptor conformers. J Biol Chem 1990; 265:6346–6352.

24. Frelinger AL III, Du X, Plow EF, Ginsberg MH. Monoclonal antibodies to ligand-occupied conformers of integrin $\alpha IIb\beta_3$ (glycoprotein IIb-IIIa) alters receptor affinity, specificity, and function. J Biol Chem 1991; 266: 6346–6352.

25. Du X, Plow EF, Freelinger AL III, O'Toole TE, Loftus JC, Ginsberg MH. Ligands "activate" integrin $\alpha_{IIb}\beta_3$ (platelet GP IIb–IIIa). Cell 1991; 65:409–416.

26. Peter K, Schwarz M, Ylänne I, Kohler B, Moser M, Nordt T, Salbach P, Kübler W, Bode C. Induction of fibrinogen binding and platelet aggregation as a potential intrinsic property of various glycoprotein IIb/IIIa ($\alpha_{IIb}\beta_3$) inhibitors. Blood. 1998; 92:3240–3249.

27. Gawaz M, Neumann FJ, Schömig A. Evaluation of platelet membrane glycoproteins in coronary artery disease: consequences for diagnosis and therapy. Circulation 1999; 92:e1–e11.

28. Quinn M, Deering A, Stewart M, Cox D, Foley B, Fitzgerald D. Quantifying GPIIb/IIIa receptor binding using 2 monoclonal antibodies: discriminating abciximab and small molecular weight antagonists. Circulation 1999; 99:2231–2238.

29. Honda S, Tomiyama Y, Pelletier AJ, Annis D, Honda Y, Orchekowski R, Ruggeri Z, Kunicki TJ. Topography of ligand-induced binding sites, including a novel cation-sensitive epitope (AP5) at the amino terminus, of the human integrin beta$_3$ subunit. J Biol Chem. 1995; 270:11947–11954.

30. Mondoro TH, Wall CD, White MM, Jennings LK. Selective induction of a glycoprotein IIIa ligand-induced binding site by fibrinogen and von Willebrand factor. Blood 1996; 88:3824–3830.

31. Sastry SK, Burridge K. Focal adhesions: a nexus for intracellular signaling and cytoskeletal dynamics. Exp Cell Res 2000; 261:25–36.

32. Peter K, O'Toole TE. Modulation of cell adhesion by changes in $\alpha_L\beta_2$ (LFA-1, CD11a/CD18) cytoplasmic domain/cytoskeleton interaction. J Exp Med 1995; 181:315–326.

33. Lotz M, Burdsal C, Erickson H, and McClay D. Cell adhesion to fibronectin and tenascin: quantitative measurements of initial binding and subsequent strengthening response. J Cell Biol 1989; 109:1795–1805.

34. Tözeren A, Mackie L, Lawrence M, Chan P, Dustin M, and Springer T. Micromanipulation of adhesion of phorbol 12-myristate-13-acetate-stimulated T lymphocytes to planar membranes containing intercellular adhesion molecule-1. Biophys J 1992; 63:247–258.

35. Miyamoto S, Katz BZ, Lafrenie RM, Yamada KM. Fibronectin and integrins in cell adhesion, signaling, and morphogenesis. Ann NY Acad Sci 1998; 857:119–129.

36. Mondoro TH, Wall CD, White MM, Jennings LK. Selective induction of a glycoprotein IIIa ligand-induced binding site by fibrinogen and von Willebrand factor. Blood 1996; 88:3824–3830.

37. Murphy NP, Pratico D, Fitzgerald DJ. Functional relevance of the expression of ligand-induced binding sites in the response to platelet GP IIb/IIIa antagonists in vivo. J Pharmacol Exp Ther 1998; 86:945–951.

38. Scarborough RM, Kleiman NS, Phillips DR. Platelet glycoprotein IIb/IIIa antagonists. What are the relevant issues concerning their pharmacology and clinical use? Circulation 1999; 100:437–444.

39. Leisner TM, Wencel–Drake JD, Wang W, Lam SC. Bidirectional transmembrane modulation of integrin alphaIIbbeta3 conformations. J Biol Chem 1999; 274: 12945–12949.

40. Gawaz M, Ruf A, Neumann FJ, Pogatsa–Murray G, Dickfeld T, Zohlnhofer D, Schömig A. Effect of glycoprotein IIb–IIIa receptor antagonism on platelet membrane glycoproteins after coronary stent placement. Thromb Haemost 1998; 80:994–1001.

41. Coller BS. A new murine monoclonal antibody reports an activation-dependent change in the conformation and/or microenvironment of the platelet glycoprotein IIb/IIIa complex. J Clin Invest 1985; 76:101–108.

42. Derek PC, Deepak LB, Shelly S, Topol EJ. Increased mortality with oral platelet glycoprotein IIb/IIIa antagonists. A meta-analysis of phase III multicenter randomized trials. Circulation 2000; 103:201–206.

43. Verstraete M. Synthetic inhibitors of platelet glycoprotein IIb/IIIa in clinical development. Circulation 2000; 101:E76–E80.

44. Herrmann HC, Molitern DJ, Ohman EM, Stebbins AL, Bode C, Betriu A, Forycki F, Miklin JS, Bachinsky WB, Lincoff AM, Califf RM, Topol EJ. Facilitation of early percutaneous coronary intervention after reteplase with or without abciximab in acute myocardial infarction: results from the SPEED (GUSTO-4 Pilot) trial. J Am Coll Cardiol 2000; 36:1489–1496.

45. Antman EM, Giugliano RP, Gibson CM, McCabe CH, Coussement P, Kleiman NS, Vahanian A, Adgey AA, Menown I, Rupprecht HJ, Van der Wieken R, Ducas J, Scherer J, Anderson K, Van de Werf F, Braunwald E. Abciximab facilitates the rate and extent of thrombolysis: results of the thrombolysis in myocardial infarction (TIMI) 14 trial. The TIMI 14 Investigators. Circulation 1999; 99:2720–2732.

46. Santos MT, Moscardó A, Vallés J, Martinez M, Piñón M, Aznar J, Broekman MJ, Marcus AJ. Participation of tyrosine phosphorylation in cytoskeletal reorganization, $\alpha_{IIb}\beta_3$ integrin receptor activation, and aspirin-insensitive mechanisms of thrombin-stimulated human platelets. Circulation 2000; 102:1924–1930.

47. Honda S, Tomiyama Y, Aoki T, Shiraga M, Kurata Y, Seki J, Matsuzawa Y. Association between ligand-induced conformational changes of integrin $\alpha_{IIb}\beta_3$ and $\alpha_{IIb}\beta_3$-mediated intracellular Ca^{2+} signaling. Blood 1998; 92:3675–3683.

48. Holmes MB, Sobel BE, Cannon CP, Schneider DJ. Increased platelet reactivity in patients given orbofiban after an acute coronary syndrome: an OPUS–TIMI 16 substudy. Orbofiban in patients with unstable coronary syndromes. Thrombolysis in myocardial infarction. Am J Cardiol 1999; 84:203–207.

49. Cox D, Smith R, Quinn M, Theroux P, Crean P, Fitzgerald DJ. Evidence of platelet activation during treatment with a GPIIb/IIIa antagonist in patients presenting with acute coronary syndromes. J Am Coil Cardiol 2000; 36:1514–1519.

50. Schneider DJ, Taatjes DJ, Sobel BE. Paradoxical inhibition of fibrinogen binding and potentiation of alpha-granule release by specific types of inhibitors of glycoprotein IIb-IIIa. Cardiovasc Res 2000; 45:437–446.

51. Kereiakes DJ, Essell JH, Abbotsmith CW, Broderick TM, Runyon JP. Abciximab-associated profound thrombocytopenia: therapy with immunoglobulin and platelet transfusion. Am J Cardiol 1996; 78:1161–1163.

52. Berkowitz SD, Harrington RA, Rund MM, Tcheng JE. Acute profound thrombocytopenia after c7E3 Fab (abciximab) therapy. Circulation 1997; 95:809–813.

53. Giugliano RP. Drug-induced thrombocytopenia: is it a serious concern for glycoprotein IIb/IIIa receptor inhibitors? J Thromb Thrombolysis 1998; 5:191–202.

54. Bednar B, Cook JJ, Holahan MA, Cunningham ME, Jumes PA, Bednar RA, Hartman GD, Gould RJ. Fibrinogen receptor antagonist-induced thrombocytopenia in chimpanzee and rhesus monkey associated with preexisting drug-dependent antibodies to platelet glycoprotein IIb/IIIa. Blood 1999; 94:587–599.

55. Peter K, Straub A, Kohler B, Volkmann M, Schwarz M, Kübler W, Bode C. Platelet activation as a potential mechanism of GP IIb/IIIa inhibitor-induced thrombocytopenia. Am J Cardiol 1999; 84:519–524.

26

Inhibitors of von Willebrand Factor Binding to Platelet Glycoprotein Ib

Joel L. Moake
Baylor College of Medicine and Rice University, Houston, Texas, U.S.A.

James T. Willerson
University of Texas Health Science Center at Houston and Texas Heart Institute, Houston, Texas, U.S.A.

SUMMARY

In this chapter we review the mechanisms of platelet thrombus formation on injured and exposed vascular subendothelium. The chapter reviews the biology of von Willebrand factor (vWF) multimer binding to a primary vWF receptor on platelet membranes. This vWF receptor is the GP Ibα component of the GP Ibα/Ibβ–IX–V complex, often referred to as "GP Ib" and abbreviated "GP Ibα" in the manuscript. Within the Weibel–Palade bodies of human endothelial cells and the α-granules of megakaryocytes and platelets, vWF monomers of molecular mass 280,000 Da form disulfide bonds and polymerize into vWF multimers. The largest vWF multimers may contain more than 40 subunits, with a molecular mass in excess of 20 million Da. These large and biologically active vWF multimers are released from the endothelial cells both forward into the bloodstream and backward into the subendothelium. The large subendothelial vWF multimers mediate the adhesion of platelets from the blood at sites of vascular damage. Each platelet contains approximately 25,000 copies of the GP Ibα/Ibβ–IX–V complex. Under arterial flowing conditions, the normal adhesion of platelets from whole blood onto exposed subendothelial vascular surfaces after endothelial cell injury depends on large vWF multimers immobilized with collagen in the subendothelium. Platelets adhere, tether, and roll on exposed subendothelium through the reversible binding of platelet GP Ibα components to regions within the A1 domain of the vWF monomeric subunits that comprise the large vWF multimers. Fluid shear stress in rapidly flowing arterial blood may enhance this adhesive interaction by altering the conformation of the vWF-binding site in the GP Ibα molecules. Large vWF multimers composed of these monomers are entangled with collagen in the subendothelium. Interactions between activated GP IIb/IIIa receptors and subendothelial large vWF multimers strengthen the initial platelet GP Ibα–vWF bonds responsible for platelet tethering and rolling on an exposed subendothelial surface. The platelets are arrested on the exposed subendothelium to complete the adhesion process. The subsequent aggregation of platelets from flowing blood onto the platelets initially adherent to the subendothelium is dependent predominantly on the bridging of activated GP IIb/IIIa receptors on contiguous platelets by fibrinogen, fibronectin, and large vWF multimers from the plasma. The attachment of GP Ibα molecules on adherent platelets to vWF multimers on the surface of platelets flowing past may also contribute to the aggregation process. Inhibitors of the GP IIb/IIIa receptors have been successful in reducing thrombosis after atherosclerotic plaque fissuring, or ulceration and vascular injury following interventional procedures, including angioplasty and stenting. However, complete protection has not been provided and a significant number of individuals experiencing these clinical events continue to have arterial thrombosis and consequent myocardial infarction or death. Therefore, it is important to evaluate whether inhibitors of platelet adhesion alone and in combination with inhibitors of GP IIb/IIIa receptors might provide added benefit in individuals with vascular injury and high risk of thrombosis.

GP Ibα–vWF interactions are inhibited by synthetic polycationic peptides that have the general formula $(Arg-Lys)_n$, $(Arg)_n$, or $(Lys)_n$. This includes the arginine-rich cationic polypeptide, protamine sulfate. The glycopeptide antibiotic, ristocetin, induces the binding of large vWF multimers to platelet GP Ibα molecules. Commercially available aurin tricarboxylic acid (ATA) is a heterogeneous mixture of polycarboxylic (polyanionic) and polyphenolic polymers derived from the acid-catalyzed polymerization of salicylic acid, methylene disalicylic acid, and formaldehyde. Ristocetin-induced platelet clumping mediated by large vWF multimers is inhibited in a concentration-dependent fashion by unfractionated ATA. There is also a direct relation between the concentration of unfractionated ATA and inhibition of shear-induced, vWF-mediated platelet aggregation.

In this chapter, we review potential beneficial effects of polycarboxylic and polyphenolic polymers derived from acid-derived polymerization of salicylic acid, methylene disalicylic acid and formaldehyde (e.g., ATA) and recombinant vWF fragments that interfere with in vivo platelet adhesion and aggregation by blocking large vWF multimer binding to GP Ibα. Results in experimental animals using these approaches, as well as the results of murine monoclonal antibodies directed against GP Ibα and the effects of a variety of purified snake venom proteins, are also discussed.

I. INTRODUCTION

Interference with platelet aggregation by the blockade of fibrinogen and von Willebrand's factor (vWF) binding to platelet glycoprotein (GP) IIb/IIIa receptors has improved prophylaxis and therapy in arterial thrombotic disorders. Several GP IIb/IIIa inhibitors are now in clinical use. This chapter will review agents presently available, or under development, that are capable of blocking the attachment of large vWF multimers to the primary vWF receptor on platelet membranes. This vWF receptor is the GP Ibα component of the GP Ibα/Ibβ–IX–V complex (often referred to as "GP Ib"; abbreviated as "GP Ibα" in the discussion to follow).

II. MECHANISMS OF PLATELET THROMBUS FORMATION

In small arteries partially obstructed by atherosclerosis or vasospasm, fluid shear stresses increase manyfold above the normal time–average level of about $20\,dynes/cm^2$. These abnormally elevated shear stresses may cause or contribute to platelet thrombosis. Among the most likely mechanisms to explain platelet thrombosis in diseased arteries are: (1) adhesion of blood platelets onto the exposed subendothelium of injured or atherosclerotic arteries containing vWF and collagen, with subsequent platelet aggregation; or (2) direct vWF-mediated, shear stress-induced aggregation of platelets in constricted areas of the arterial circulation (even in the presence of an intact endothelial cell lining) [1,2].

A. Platelet Adhesion and Aggregation on Injured, Exposed Vascular Subendothelium

Within the Weibel–Palade bodies of human endothelial cells and the α-granules of megakaryocytes and platelets, vWF monomers of molecular mass 280,000 Da (280 kDa), form disulfide bonds and polymerize into vWF multimers. The largest vWF multimers may contain more than 40 subunits, with a molecular mass in excess of 20 million Da. These largest and most biologically active vWF multimers are released from endothelial cells both forward into the bloodstream and backward into the subendothelium [7–15].

Large subendothelial vWF multimers mediate the adhesion of platelets from the blood at sites of vascular damage. Each mature vWF monomeric subunit that is polymerized to form vWF multimers contains a sequence of structural domains [6–8]. These include the A1 domain (amino acids 497–716) that includes a cysteine 509–cysteine 695 disulfide loop. The A1 domain contains separate binding sites for platelet GP Ibα, collagen, heparin, and sulfatides; the A3 domain contains an additional binding site for collagen; and the C1 domain contains a binding site for platelet GP IIb/IIIa ($\alpha_{IIb}\beta_3$) receptors. This latter binding site in each vWF monomeric subunit comprises the sequence arginine–glycine–aspartate (RGD) at amino acids 1744–1746. The RGD triple amino acid sequence is also found in fibrinogen and fibronectin, and these proteins are also capable of binding to platelet GP IIb/IIIa receptors.

Each platelet contains approximately 25,000 copies of the GP Ibα/Ibβ–IX–V complex. These transmembrane proteins have molecular mass values of about 150 kDa (GP Ibα), 25 kDa (GP Ibβ), 19 kDa (GP IX), and 83 kDa (GP V), and are characterized by leucine-rich repeat sequences. Each complex is assembled in platelet membranes as two copies of covalently linked GP Ibα/GP Ibβ molecules, two GP IX molecules, and one molecule of GP V. The vWF-binding site is within extracellular N-terminal amino acids 1–282 of GP Ibα. Amino acids 271–279 of GP Ibα may be especially important for vWF attachment [8].

Under arterial flowing conditions, the normal adhesion of platelets from whole blood onto exposed subendothelial vascular surfaces after endothelial cell injury or removal depends upon large vWF multimers immobilized with collagen in the subendothelium. Platelets adhere, tether, and roll on exposed subendothelium through the reversible binding of platelet GP Ibα components to regions within the A1 domain of the vWF monomeric subunits that compose the large vWF multimers. Fluid shear stresses in rapidly flowing arterial blood enhance this adhesive interaction by altering the conformation of the vWF binding site in GP Ibα molecules [9–11], and possibly also the GP Ibα-binding sites within the A1 domains of vWF monomeric subunits [12]. Large vWF multimers composed of these monomers are entangled with collagen in the subendothelium.

In association with the adherence of extracellular platelet GP Ibα to exposed subendothelial vWF multimers, GP Ibα cytoplasmic tails interact with actin-binding proteins and stimulate actin polymerization [13,14]. As a consequence, platelets change from flat disks to spiny spheres. This alteration in shape allows the platelets to attach to subendothelial collagen fibrils intertwined with the subendothelial vWF multimers [1,15–17]. Collagen attachment to specific collagen receptors on platelets (including platelet $\alpha_2\beta_1$ molecules) initiates internal Ca^{2+} mobilization, the secretion of P selectin and large vWF multimers onto the platelet surface from platelet α-granules, and activation of platelet surface GP/IIb-IIIa receptors into a ligand-receptive conformation.

Interactions between activated platelet GP IIb/IIIa receptors and subendothelial large vWF multimers strengthen the initial platelet GP Ibα–vWF bonds responsible for platelet tethering and rolling on an exposed subendothelial surface. The platelets are, thereby, arrested on the exposed subendothelium to complete the adhesion process. The subsequent cohesion (aggregation) of platelets from flowing blood onto the platelets initially adherent to the subendothelium is dependent predominantly on the bridging of activated GP IIb/IIIa receptors on contiguous platelets by fibrinogen, fibronectin, and large vWF multimers from the plasma. The attachment of GP Ibα molecules on adherent platelets to vWF multimers on the surface of platelets flowing past may also contribute to the aggregation process [18].

Arterial thrombus formation under conditions of elevated fluid shear stresses, as a result of the adhesion and excessive aggregation of platelets from rapidly flowing blood onto the exposed subendothelium of injured or atherosclerotic arteries, can be simulated in real-time in a model system. A parallel-plate flow chamber, fibrillar collagen-coated slides, and mepacrine-labeled (fluorescent) platelets in whole blood at various flow rates are used [1]. Blood anticoagulated with citrate, hirudin, unfractionated porcine heparin, or low-molecular-weight heparin flows over the collagen-coated slides for 1–2 min at wall shear rates of 100–3000 s (about 4–120 dynes/cm^2). The precise sequence of interactions among vWF, GPIbα and GPIIb/IIIa during platelet adhesion and subsequent aggregation has been resolved for this model system from real-time observations using computerized epifluorescence video microscopy [1]. Adhesion at high shear rates is the result of the rapid adsorption of large vWF multimers from the normal blood onto collagen, followed by the binding of platelet GPIbα to the insolubilized vWF [1]. Platelet GP IIb/IIIa binding to insolubilized vWF contributes to platelet adhesion. Collagen then activates the adherent platelets, and aggregation occurs subsequently [1]. Aggregation requires the binding of fibrinogen, fibronectin, or vWF to platelet GPIIb/IIIa complexes by their RGD binding regions. [1,19].

B. Direct Shear Stress-Induced Platelet Aggregation

A rotational cone and plate viscometer in which platelet surface interactions are minimal has been a useful model for studying direct shear-induced platelet aggregation in vitro [20–22]. Platelets aggregate from platelet-rich plasma (PRP) or whole blood under conditions of abnormally elevated fluid shear stresses in the presence of large vWF multimers, adenosine diphosphate (ADP), and Ca^{2+}. These components may either be in the fluid exogenous to the platelets [20,21] or, alternatively, derived from the α granules of the sheared platelets themselves [21]. Shear-induced, vWF-mediated platelet aggregation requires both functional GPIbα receptors and intact GP IIb/IIIa complexes [20–22], and does not require ristocetin, other exogenous agents, or chemical modification of vWF. Although GPIX and GPV are noncovalently associated with the disulfide-linked GP Ibα/Ibβ molecules in the platelet membrane [23], their precise role in shear-induced platelet signal transduction or aggregation has not been established.

Very high shear stresses in turbulent flowing blood may produce intense, sustained conformational changes in platelet GP Ibα, and possibly also in the vWF A1 domain of fluid-phase large vWF multimers [2,12]. The resulting vWF–GP Ibα binding sends cytoplasmic signals via GP Ibα that are sufficient to initiate the secretion of ADP from platelet-dense granules, and to activate the ligand-receptive conformational change in GP IIb/IIIa complexes. Among these chemical signals is the dimeric 14-3-3 zeta protein [24], which dissociates from the cytoplasmic tail of platelet GP Ibα in association with the attachment of large vWF multimers to extracellular GP Ibα receptors [25].

III. AGENTS THAT INHIBIT GP Ib–vWF INTERACTIONS IN CURRENT USE

A. Protamine Sulfate

Interactions of GP Ibα-vWF are inhibited by synthetic polycationic peptides that have the general formulae $(Arg-Lys)_n$, $(Arg)_n$, or $(Lys)_n$. This includes the arginine-rich cationic polypeptide, protamine sulfate [26]. Protamine is used to neutralize the anticoagulant effect of the negatively charged sulfated mucopolysaccharide, heparin, following cardiopulmonary bypass procedures.

The glycopeptide antibiotic, ristocetin, induces the binding of large vWF multimers to platelet GP Ibα molecules [27,28]. Protamine sulfate, in excess of heparin, inhibits ristocetin-induced, vWF-mediated platelet agglutination in human PRP. Furthermore, at a concentration of 200 µg/mL, protamine sulfate suppresses the platelet GP Ibα–vWF attachments required to initiate platelet adherence from human blood onto insolubilized vWF/collagen in a parallel plate flow chamber at elevated arterial-like levels of shear stress (approximately 26–104 dynes/cm^2) [26]. These observation may explain why protamine sulfate in the circulation in excess of heparin may occasionally cause bleeding.

B. Fibrinolytic Agents

Plasmin is generated from plasminogen by tissue plasminogen activator (t-PA)-mediated proteolysis of plasminogen, or by streptokinase–plasminogen binding. Plasmin produced by t-PA addition to PRP proteolyzes large vWF multimers and inhibits direct platelet aggregation in the presence of elevated shear stress (120 dynes/cm^2) in the cone-and-plate viscometer [29]. This activity may contribute, along with fibrinolysis, to the therapeutic effect of t-PA (or streptokinase) in arteries occluded by thrombi. Proteolysis of large vWF multimers may also be responsible for some of the bleeding complications that accompany the use of t-PA or streptokinase.

IV. INVESTIGATIONAL AGENTS THAT INHIBIT GP Ib–vWF INTERACTIONS

A. Aurin Tricarboxylic Acid

Commercial ATA is a heterogeneous mixture of polycarboxylic (polyanionic) and polyphenolic polymers derived from the acid-catalyzed polymerization of salicylic acid, methylene disalicylic acid, and formaldehyde (Fig. 1) [30,31].

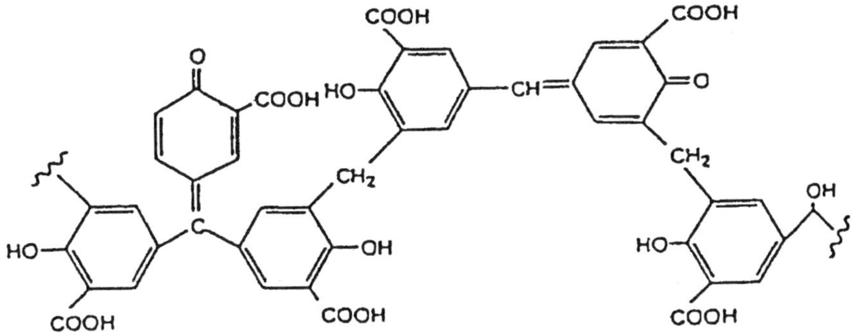

Figure 1 Commercial aurin tricarboxylic acid (ATA) is a heterogenous mixture of polymers composed of several different protomeric components (see text). (From Ref. 31).

In the aggregometer, ristocetin-induced platelet clumping mediated by large vWF multi-mers is inhibited in a concentration-dependent fashion by unfractionated ATA [32]. There is also a direct relation between the concentration of unfractionated ATA and inhibition of shear-induced, vWF-mediated platelet aggregation [31,32].

ADP-mediated platelet aggregation in fresh human PRP is usually unaffected by the addition of ATA [32]. Because fibrinogen is a cofactor for ADP-induced platelet aggregation [33,34], this is indirect evidence that ATA does not impair the function of ADP receptors, fibrinogen or the GP IIb/IIIa complex.

After the trisodium salt of ATA (obtained from Aldrich Chemical, Milwaukee, WI) is dissolved in phosphate-buffered saline, pH 7.4, relatively larger ATA polymers can be separated from smaller forms by a 50-kDa cutoff dialysis membrane [1]. A filter-sterilized stock solution of polymeric ATA with molecular mass values greater than 2500 ($A_{280}^{1\%} = 80$) can be prepared using these simple techniques, and then stored for weeks to months at room temperature. This polymeric form of ATA produces dose-dependent inhibition of shear aggregation [1] (Fig. 2A). The effect of different fluid shear stresses on the capacity of polymeric ATA, at $80\,\mu g/mL$, to inhibit shear aggregation in normal citrated PRP samples is shown in Figure 2B.

In perfusion studies [1], citrated normal whole blood was preincubated for 5 min with polymeric ATA at 28.5, 57, or $114\,\mu g/mL$, or buffer alone as control, and then perfused at $1500\,s^{-1}$ (about 60 dynes/cm^2 wall shear stress) for 1 min (Fig. 3). There was concentration-dependent inhibition by ATA of total platelet accumulation onto vWF/collagen, which was about 85–90% at $114\,g/mL$ of polymeric ATA. Inhibition was caused by ATA suppression of platelet adhesion by GP Ibα to vWF multimers insolubilized onto collagen. Subsequent studies [35] confirmed that ATA inhibits platelet adhesion to human vWF/collagen at a high wall-shear rate ($2600\,s^{-1}$), but not at lower rates ($650\,s^{-1}$ and $100\,s^{-1}$).

Polymers of ATA are likely to bind to one or more positively charged region(s) between amino acids 509 and 695 of the A1 domain disulfide loop of the vWF monomeric subunits that comprise large vWF multimers [35]. This interaction between ATA and vWF A1 domains may sterically hinder the attachment of vWF multimers to platelet GP Ibα.

The polymeric ATA structure must contain a minimum number of protomers to bind optimally to the A1 domain of vWF monomers and alter the vWF binding site for GP Ibα [31]. The molecular mass of ATA that optimally inhibits shear-induced, vWF-mediated platelet aggregation is about 2500 Da. This corresponds to an ATA polymer composed of 16 residues of methyl salicylic acid, a probable protomeric subunit of ATA, with a molecular mass of 2560 Da. Polymers larger than this would not be expected to be more inhibitory on a molar basis and, indeed, they are not. Negative charges on the aromatic residues of ATA are also required for inhibition of the interactions between vWF and GP Ibα. Aurin, which lacks carboxyl groups, is without effect [31].

1. Animal Studies

In a model system developed by Folts et al. [36–38] and adapted for use in different animals, vWF-mediated [39] cyclic reductions in arterial blood flow occur as a result of the intermittent formation of platelet thrombi in a stenotic, high-shear region created by the placement of an external constrictor on the vessel.

Strony, et al. [40] studied the effect of ATA on platelet-dependent cyclic flow reductions in a canine coronary stenosis model (>80% stenosis; 350 dynes/cm^2 estimated local average shear stress). In dose–response experiments, six animals received 4 mg/kg of unfractionated, filter-sterilized ATA by bolus infusion, followed by 1 mg/kg every 10 min. Total inhibition of cyclic flow reductions was observed in all animals after 6.7 mg/kg of ATA. A bolus intravenous

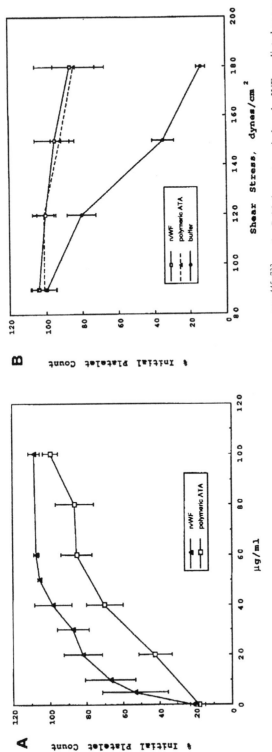

Figure 2 Effects of preincubation for 5 min at room temperature with polymeric ATA or rvWF[445-733] on the fluid shear stress-induced, vWF-mediated aggregation of platelets from citrated normal PRP in a cone-and-plate viscometer (1). Shear stresses, applied at room temperature, were (A) 180 dynes/cm² and (B) were varied over a range. Preshear platelet counts in the PRP samples were 233,000–340,000/μL.

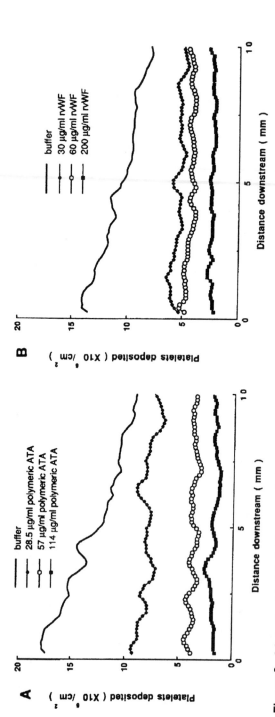

Figure 3 Mepacrine-labeled platelet accumulation along vWF–collagen type I surfaces from normal citrated whole blood perfused for 1 min at 37°C at a wall shear rate of $1500 \, s^{-1}$ (about 60 dynes/cm²) (A) after preincubation with ATA or (B) with rvWF[445–733]. (From Ref. 1.)

injection of 10 mg/kg of ATA in another 4 dogs and in rats [40a] also caused total inhibition of cyclic flow reductions. ATA did not alter hemodynamics, thrombin time, platelet count, or ADP–epinephrine-induced platelet aggregation ex vivo [40]. ATA also reduced platelet deposition in high-shear areas of injured, stenotic rabbit carotid arteries [41], and inhibited cyclic flow reductions in a laser-induced guinea pig arterial injury model [40b]. These observations indicate that vWF interactions with platelet GP Ibα in a region of high-shear stress are important during coronary artery occlusion in animals, and demonstrate that ATA prevents arterial thrombosis in vivo under these conditions.

The effects of unfractionated ATA on rat carotid and dog femoral artery models of rethrombosis following the infusion of streptokinase or t-PA have been studied [40a,40b]. Intravenous ATA at 10 mg/kg prevented rethrombosis after fibrinolytic therapy in these animal models. In the rat [40a], in contrast to the dog [40,42], values for the prothrombin time, partial thromboplastin time, thrombin time, and bleeding time were all prolonged in vivo by ATA. Platelet counts were not affected in either animal by the administration of 10 mg/kg or less ATA [40,40a,42].

2. Other Effects

ATA and its various fractions have biological activities in addition to those already discussed. A fraction of ATA with an average molecular mass of 2500 Da inhibits thrombin-induced platelet aggregation [43]. Negatively charged ATA may interact with positively charged areas on the outer surface of thrombin molecules. This inhibitory effect on thrombin may contribute to the suppression of tissue–factor-induced venous thrombosis and thromboembolism in rats and mice [44] by unfractionated intravenous ATA (10–40 mg/kg).

It has been reported [43,45] that ATA, especially at low concentrations and in solutions with low protein concentrations, may have paradoxical platelet-stimulatory effects in vitro. Whether or not these effects influence platelet thrombus formation in vivo is doubtful.

3. Toxicity

The medium lethal dose (LD_{50}) of ATA has been reported to be 340 mg/kg in mice [43]. This is about two orders of magnitude greater than an effective antithrombotic dose in dogs. No overt, acute toxicity has been observed in the animal studies discussed in the foregoing [40,40b,42,45a,45b]. Chronic toxicity studies have not been reported in any animal model. No efficacy or toxicity studies have yet been described in humans using ATA or any ATA derivative.

B. Recombinant vWF Fragments

1. rvWF 445–733

A recombinant vWF fragment that contains amino acids 445–733 was prepared 10 years ago by Sugimoto et al. [46]. This rvWF$^{445-733}$ fragment contains the A1 domain-binding sites for GP Ibα, collagen, and unfractionated heparin. The fragment also includes the carboxyl-terminal portion of the D3 domain that precedes A1 in vWF monomers. The rvWF$^{445-733}$ fragment, after reduction and alkylation, attaches to platelet GP Ibα in the absence of any modulator and blocks the binding of large vWF multimers. At concentrations between 30 and 200 μg/ml, rvWF$^{445-733}$ progressively inhibits shear stress-induced, vWF-mediated platelet aggregation using PRP in the viscometer (see Fig. 2). The fragment also suppresses platelet adhesion from whole blood onto vWF/collagen under arterial-like flowing conditions in a perfusion chamber [1] (see Fig. 3). In these in vitro experiments, the inhibitory effects of $rvWF^{445-733}$ were demonstrable in PRP or whole blood anticoagulated with citrate or hirudin. Unfractionated heparin, but not low-molecular weight heparin, binds to $rvWF^{445-733}$ and counteracts its inhibitory effect. The $rvWF^{445-733}$ fragment suppresses in vivo platelet aggregation in a Folts monkey model of constrictive coronary thrombosis [47].

2. VCL

A second recombinant vWF fragment has been produced that consists of amino acids 504–728 of the A1 domain.

VCL (Bio-Technology General, Inc.) is a recombinant fragment of vWF, Leu^{504}–Lys^{728}, with a single intrachain disulfide bond that links residues Cys^{509} and Cys^{695}. A canine model has been used to determine the effect of VCL on (1) the formation of intracoronary thrombosis and (2) reocclusion of coronary arteries after thrombolysis with t-PA [48]. In mongrel dogs after electrical stimulation, all animals developed total occlusion of the affected coronary arteries. The elapsed time from electrical stimulation to total occlusion of the coronary arteries was significantly longer in dogs pretreated with VCL ($p < 0.001$) or aspirin ($p < 0.05$) than in dogs pretreated with saline (see Fig. 4). Three hours after the occlusion of coronary arteries, only t-PA was given to the animals. The administration of t-PA resulted in thrombolysis in 4 of 12 saline-treated dogs (33%), 5 of 7 VCL-treated dogs (71%), and 4 of 8 aspirin-treated dogs

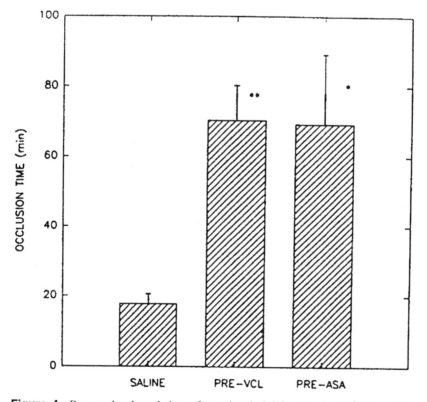

Figure 4 Bar graph: elapsed times from electrical injury to the formation of occlusive thrombi in coronary arteries of animals pretreated (PRE) with saline, VCL, and aspirin (ASA) intravenously (protocol 1). Compared with saline, *p < 0.05; **p < 0.001.

(50%). The average elapsed time from t-PA treatment to thrombolysis (thrombolysis time) was significantly shorter in VCL-treated than in saline-treated dogs (47 ± 12 vs. 81 ± 4 min; $p<0.05$) (Fig. 5).

Dogs that were not pretreated before their coronary arteries were occluded received thrombolytic treatments 3 h after coronary artery occlusion: t-PA and heparin induced thrombolysis in 5 of 7 dogs (71%); t-PA, heparin, and VCL induced thrombolysis in 6 of 7 dogs (86%); t-PA, heparin, and aspirin induced thrombolysis in 7 of 8 dogs (85%); and t-PA, heparin, VCL, and aspirin induced thrombolysis in 8 of 8 dogs (100%). The average thrombolysis time in dogs treated with t-PA, heparin, VCL, and aspirin was about half that in dogs treated only with t-PA and heparin (23.5 ± 4 vs 45 ± 12 min).

After thrombolysis, many animals developed reocclusion of the coronary arteries during the 3-hour–monitoring period. In animals pretreated with VCL, the frequency of reocclusion was not significantly different among dogs pretreated with saline (4 of 4), aspirin (4 of 4), or VCL (4 of 5). However, the average time from thrombolysis to reocclusion (reocclusion time) was significantly longer in dogs pretreated with VCL (114 ± 18 min) than in dogs pretreated with saline (42 ± 4 min) or aspirin (55 ± 14 min) ($p<0.05$). In animals that were not pretreated, coronary artery reocclusion developed in 5 of 5 dogs treated with TPA and heparin, and the addition of aspirin did not change the frequency of reocclusion (7 of 7). The addition of VCL to TPA and heparin significantly reduced the frequency of reocclusion in the reperfused coronary arteries of dogs (2 of 6; $p<0.05$ compared with the t-PA and heparin group). The addition of

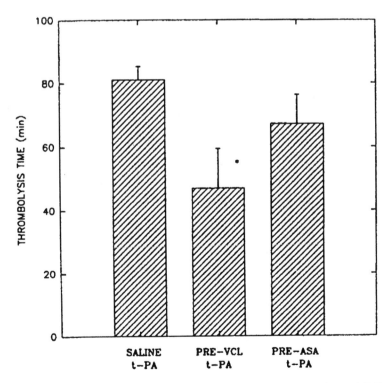

Figure 5 Bar graph: elapsed times from tissue plasminogen activator (t-PA) administration to thrombolysis in coronary arteries of animals pretreated (PRE) with saline, VCL, or aspirin (ASA) intravenously (protocol 1). Compared with saline, *p < 0.05.

VCL and aspirin also significantly reduced the frequency of reocclusion (1 of 8; p<0.01). The average reocclusion time was also significantly longer in VCL-treated dogs than in dogs who did not receive VCL (Fig. 6).

C. Monoclonal Antibodies

A murine monoclonal antibody ("Mo 6B4") Fab fragment directed against human platelet GP Ibα was injected into baboons. The anti-GP Ibα Fab fragments blocked ex vivo ristocetin–vWF-attachment to GP Ibα on baboon platelets. Platelet GP Ibα–vWF/collagen adhesion, using baboon blood in a perfusion chamber at 28–40 dynes/cm², was inhibited. Baboon platelet adherence onto an implanted collagen-rich thrombogenic surface by platelet GP Ibα–vWF/collagen interaction was also impaired [49].

A monoclonal antibody against human vWF inhibited ristocetin–vWF binding to human platelet GP Ibα, platelet GP Ibα–vWF–collagen adhesion in a perfusion system, and direct high shear stress-induced platelet aggregation in a cone-and-plate viscometer [50,50a]. This antibody, AJvW-2, also suppressed arterial thrombosis (without prolonging bleeding times) in guinea pigs [50]. Another monoclonal antibody ("antibody 712") directed against the vWF A1 domain that

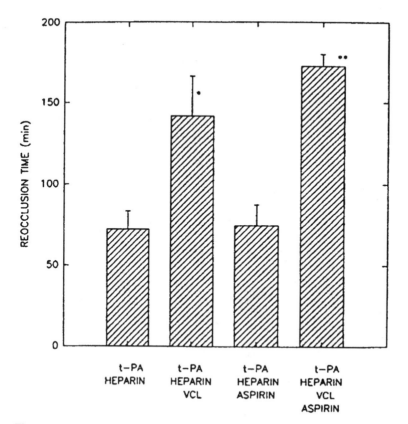

Figure 6 Bar graph: elapsed times from thrombolysis to reocclusion of coronary arteries of animals treated with tissue plasminogen activator (t-PA), heparin, VCL, and aspirin (protocol 2) when compared with t-PA plus heparin and t-PA plus heparin plus aspirin, *p < 0.05, **p < 0.001.

binds to platelet GP Ibα also suppressed injury-induced arterial thrombosis in guinea pigs, without inducing thrombocytopenia or prolonging bleeding times [51].

D. Snake Venom Proteins

A variety of purified snake venom proteins attach to, or near, the N-terminal vWF-binding region on platelet GP Ibα and block GP Ibα–vWF interactions. These proteins include: echicetin (from *Echis carinatus*) [52]; crotalin (from *Crotalus atrox*) [53]; agkistin (from *Deinagkistrodon acutus*) [54,55]; tokaracetin (from *Trimeresurus tokarensis*) [56]; and flavocetin-A (from the habu snake) [57,58]. Most of these are small-molecular-mass proteins (about 30 kDa).

Crotalin both suppressed platelet-rich thrombus formation in injured mice mesenteric vessels and prolonged bleeding times [53]. Tokaracetin suppressed direct-shear stress-induced, vWF-mediated platelet aggregation [56].

Agkistin, by binding to endothelial cell GP Ib, had the unexpected (and potentially unwelcome) property of disrupting angiogenesis ex vivo in chick embryo chorioallantoic membranes [55].

Flavocetin, with its greater molecular mass (149 kDa), may have the paradoxical (and possibly unacceptable) effect of cross-linking platelets and inducing the formation of small platelet aggregates [57].

V. ASSOCIATION BETWEEN INFLAMMATION AND PLATELET THROMBOSIS

Neutrophils and monocytes accumulate in the media of arteries occluded by platelet thrombi as a consequence of atherosclerosis, neointimal thickening after angioplasty or implantation of an endovascular stent, or injury from ischemia and reperfusion [59,60]. Leukocytes tether and roll on platelet thrombi through the binding of P-selectin glycoprotein ligand-1 (PSGL-1) on neutrophil and monocyte membranes to P selectin molecules released from platelet α-granules onto the surfaces of activated platelets in nascent thrombi. These initial leukocyte–platelet attachments are followed by the formation of even stronger adhesive bonds and the migration of leukocytes into the arterial wall.

The stronger leukocyte–platelet binding occurs by the attachment of activated Mac-1 integrin molecules ($\alpha_M\beta_2$, or CD11b/CD18) on leukocytes to GP Ibα receptors on platelets in the thrombi. More specifically, this interaction is mediated by the I (inserted) domains of the α_M (CD11b) subunits of leukocyte Mac-1 molecules that are structurally similar to the A1 (GP Ibα-binding) domain of vWF monomers [59,60]. These I-domains in Mac-1 α_M molecules are predominantly responsible for the strong adhesion of leukocytes onto platelet thrombi, and for their subsequent migration into the media of the arterial wall.

Suppression of leukocyte–platelet binding using any agent under development capable of inhibiting GP Ibα–vWF binding may also be useful in reducing the inflammation of the arterial wall and, possibly, the extent of tissue infarction associated with thrombosis.

VI. CONCLUSION

This chapter has reviewed the role of von Willebrand's factor binding to platelet glycoprotein Ib receptors, and it has emphasized the importance of vWF binding to platelet glycoprotein Ib receptors in platelet adherence and the development of a platelet-initiated thrombus. Furthermore, evidence has been presented that various inhibitors of the binding of vWF to platelet glycoprotein Ib receptors may prevent thrombosis in experimental animal arteries that have been injured and in which the subendothelium has been exposed. Aurin tricarboxylic acid, recombinant vWF fragments, and monoclonal antibodies directed against human platelet GP Ib receptor protect against arterial thrombosis in experimental animal models with arterial injury. The clinical benefit of using similar inhibitors of vWF binding to platelet glycoprotein Ib receptors in humans with acute coronary syndromes and interventional procedures remains to be established. However, there is a potential for such agents to exert a beneficial effect in protecting against arterial thrombosis and one that may be additive to other platelet inhibitors. The safety, as well as the efficacy, of such interventions will have to be carefully evaluated.

REFERENCES

1. Alevriadou BR, Moake JL, Turner NA, Ruggeri ZM, Folie BJ, Phillips MD, Schreiber AB, Hrinda ME, McIntire LV. Real-time analysis of shear-dependent thrombus formation and its blockade by inhibitors of von Willebrand factor binding to platelets. Blood 1993; 81:1263–76.
2. Kroll MH, Hellums JD, McIntire LV, Schafer AI, Moake JL. Platelets and shear stress. Blood 1996; 88:1525–1541.
3. Ruggeri ZM. Developing basic and clinical research on von Willebrand factor and von Willebrand disease. Thromb Haemost 2000; 84:147–149.
4. Ruggeri ZM. Old concepts and new developments in the study of platelet aggregation. J Clin Invest. 2000; 105:699–701.
5. Sadler JE, Mannucci PM, Berntorp E, Bochkov N, Boulyjenkov V, Ginsburg D, Meyer D, Peake I, Rodeghiero F, Srivastava A. Impact, diagnosis and treatment of von Willebrand disease. Thromb Haemost 2000; 84:160–174.
6. Cruz MA, Diacovo TG, Emsley J, Liddington R, Handin RI. Mapping the glycoprotein Ib-binding site in the von Willebrand factor A1 domain. J Biol Chem 2000; 275:19098–19105.
7. Miura S, Li CQ, Cao Z, Wang H, Wardell MR, Sadler JE. Interaction of von Willebrand factor domain A1 with platelet glycoprotein Ibalpha-(1–289). Slow intrinsic binding kinetics mediate rapid platelet adhesion. J Biol Chem 2000; 275:7539–7546.
8. Vasudevan S, Roberts JR, McClintock RA, Dent JA, Celikel R, Ware J, Vaurghese KI, Ruggeri ZM. Modeling and functional analysis of the interaction between von Willebrand factor A1 domain and glycoprotein Ibalpha. J Biol Chem 2000; 275:12763–127688.
9. Fredrickson BJ, Dong JF, McIntire LV, Lopez JA. Shear-dependent rolling on von Willebrand factor of mammalian cells expressing the platelet glycoprotein Ib–IX–V complex. Blood 1998; 92:3684–3693.
10. Dong JF, Berndt MC, Schade A, McIntire LV, Andrews RK, Lopez JA. Ristocetin-dependent, but not botrocetin-dependent, binding of von Willebrand factor to the platelet glycoprotein Ib–IX–V complex correlates with shear-dependent interactions. Blood 2001; 97:162–168.
11. Afshar–Kharghan V, Gineys G, Schade AJ, Sun L, Li CQ, McIntire LV, Dong JF, Lopez JA. Necessity of conserved asparagine residues in the leucine-rich repeats of platelet glycoprotein Ib alpha for the proper conformation and function of the ligand-binding region. Biochemistry 2000; 39:3384–3391.
12. Miyata S, Ruggeri Z. Distinct structural attributes regulating von Willebrand factor A1 domain interaction with platelet glycoprotein Ib alpha under flow. J Biol Chem 1999; 274:6586–6593.
13. Cranmer SL, Ulsemer P, Cooke BM, Salem HH, de la Salle C, Lanza F, Jackson SP. Glycoprotein (GP) Ib–IX–transfected cells roll on a von Willebrand factor matrix under flow. Importance of the GPIb/actin-binding protein (ABP-280) interaction in maintaining adhesion under high shear. J Biol Chem. 1999; 274:6097–6106.
14. Yuan Y, Kulkarni S, Ulsemer P, Cranmer SL, Yap CL, Nesbitt WS, Harper I, Mistry N, Dopheide SM, Hughan SC, Williamson D, de la Salle C, Salem HH, Lanza F, Jackson SP. The von Willebrand factor–glycoprotein Ib/V/IX interaction induced actin polymerization and cytoskeletal reorganization in rolling platelets and glycoprotein Ib/V/IX-transfected cells. J Biol Chem 1999; 274:36241–36251.

15. Moroi M, Jung SM, Nomura S, Sekiguchi S, Ordinas A, Diaz–Ricart M. Analysis of the involvement of the von Willebrand factor–glycoprotein Ib interaction in platelet adhesion to a collagen-coated surface under flow conditions. Blood 1997; 90:4413–4424.

16. Di Paola J, Federici AB, Mannucci PM, Canciani MT, Kritzik M, Kunicki TJ, Nugent D. Low platelet alpha2beta1 levels in type I von Willebrand disease correlate with impaired platelet function in a high shear stress system. Blood 1999; 93:3578–3582.

17. Jung SM, Moroi M. Signal-transducing mechanisms involved in activation of platelet collagen receptor integrin alpha(2)beta(1). J Biol Chem 2000; 275:8016–8026.

18. Kulkarni S, Dopheide SM, Yap CL, Ravanat C, Freund M, Mangin P, Heel KA, Street A, Harper IS, Lanza F, Jackson SP. A revised model of platelet aggregation. J Clin Invest 2000; 105:783–791.

19. Wu YP, Vink T, Schiphorst M, van Zanten GH, Ijsseldijk MJ, de Groot PG, Sixma JJ. Platelet thrombus formation on collagen at shear rates is mediated by von Willebrand factor-glycoprotein Ib interaction and inhibited by von Willebrand factor–glycoprotein IIb/IIIa interaction. Arterioscler Thromb Vasc Biol 2000; 20:1161–1667.

20. Moake JL, Turner NA, Stathopoulos NA, Nolasco LH, Hellums JD. Involvement of large plasma von Willebrand factor (vWF) multimers and unusually large vWF forms derived from endothelial cells in shear stress-induced platelet aggregation. J Clin Invest 1986; 78:1456–1461.

21. Moake JL, Turner NA, Stathopoulos NA, Nolasco L, Hellums JD. Shear-induced platelet aggregation can be mediated by vWF released from platelets, as well as by exogenous large or unusually large vWF multimers, requires adenosine diphosphate, and is resistant to aspirin. Blood 1988; 71:1366–1374.

22. Peterson DM, Stathopoulos NA, Giorgio TD, Hellums JD, Moake JL. Shear-induced platelet aggregation requires von Willebrand factor and platelet membrane glycoproteins Ib and IIb–IIIa. Blood 1987; 69:625–628.

23. Modderman PW, Admiraal LG, Sonnenberg A, von dem Borne AE. Glycoproteins V and Ib–IX form a noncovalent complex in the platelet membrane. J Biol Chem 1992; 267:364–369.

24. Gu M, Xi X, Englulnd GD, Berndt MC, Du X. Analysis of the roles of 14-3-3 in the platelet glycoprotein Ib–IX-mediated activation of integrin alpha(IIb)beta(3) using a reconstituted mammalian cell expression model. J Cell Biol 1999; 147:1085–1096.

25. Feng S, Christodoulides N, Resendiz JC, Berndt MC, Kroll MH. Cytoplasmic domains of GpIb alpha and GpIb beta regulates 14-3-3zeta binding to GpIb/IX/V. Blood 2000; 95:551–557.

26. Barstad RM, Stephens RW, Hamers MJ, Sakariassen KS. Protaimine sulphate inhibits platelet membrane glycoprotein Ib–von Willebrand factor activity. Thromb Haemost 2000; 83:334–337.

27. Moake JL, Olson JD, Troll JH, Weinger RS, Peterson DM, Cimo PL. Interaction of platelets, von Willebrand factor, and ristocetin during platelet agglutination J Lab Clin Med 1980; 96:168–184.

28. Moake JL, Olson JD, Troll JH, Tang SS, Funicella T, Peterson DM. Binding of radioiodinated human von Willebrand factor to Bernard–Soulier, thrombasthenic and von Willebrand's disease platelets. Thromb Res 1980; 19:21–27.

29. Kamat SG, Michelson AD, Benoit SE, Moake JL, Rajasekhar D, Hellums JD, Kroll MH, Schafer AI. Fibrinolysis inhibits shear stress-induced platelet aggregation. Circulation 1995; 92:1399–1407.

30. Gonzalez RG, Blackburn BJ, Schleich T. Fractionation and structural elucidation of the active components of aurintricarboxylic, a potent inhibitor of protein nucleic acid interactions. Biochim Biophys Acta 1979; 562:534–545.

31. Weinstein M, Vosburgh E, Phillips M, Turner N, Chute–Rose L, Moake J. Isolation from commercial aurintricarboxylic acid (ATA) of the most effective polymeric inhibitors of von Willebrand factor interaction with platelet glycoprotein Ib. Blood 1991; 78:2291.

32. Phillips MD, Moake JL, Nolasco L, Turner N. Aurin tricarboxylic acid: a novel inhibitor of the association of von Willebrand factor and platelets. Blood 1988; 72:1898–1903.

33. Nachman RL, Leung LLK. Complex formation of platelet membrane glycoproteins IIb and IIIa with fibrinogen. J Clin Invest 1982; 69:263–269.

34. Mustard JF, Packham MA, Kinlough–Rathbone RL, Perry DW, Regoeczi E. Fibrinogen and ADP-induced platelet aggregation. Blood 1978; 52:453–466.

35. Girma JP, Fressinaud E, Christophe O. Aurin tricarboxylic acid inhibits platelet adhesion to collagen by

binding to the 509–695 disulphide loop on von Willebrand factor and competing with glycoprotein Ib. Thromb Haemost 1992; 68:707–713.

36. Folts JD, Crowell EB, Rowe GG. Platelet aggregation in partially obstructed vessels and its elimination with aspirin. Circulation 1976; 54:365–370.

37. Folts JD. Drugs for the prevention of coronary thrombosis: from animal model to clinical trials. J Cardiovasc Drugs Ther 1995; 9:31–43.

38. Maalej N, Folts JD. Increased shear stress overcomes the antithrombotic platelet inhibitory effect of aspirin in stenosed dog coronary arteries. Circulation 1996; 93:1201–1205.

39. Bellinger DA, Nichols TC, Read MS. Prevention of occlusive coronary artery thrombosis by a murine monoclonal antibody to porcine von Willebrand factor. Proc Natl Acad Sci USA 1987; 84:8100–8104.

40. Strony J, Phillips M, Brands D, Moake J, Adelman B. Aurintricarboxylic acid in a canine model of coronary artery thrombosis Circulation 1990; 81:1106–1114.

40a. Kawasake T, Kaku S, Kohinata T. Inhibition by aurintricarboxylic acid of von Willebrand factor binding to platelet GP Ib, platelet retention, and thrombus formation in vivo. Am J Hematol 1994; 47:6–15.

40b. Assam K, Cisse–Thiam M, Drouet L. The antithrombotic effect of aurintricarboxylic acid in the guinea pig is not solely due to its interaction with the von Willebrand factor–GP Ib axis. Thromb Haemost 1996; 75:203–210.

41. Golino P, Ragni M, Cirillo P. Aurintricarboxylic acid reduces platelet deposition in stenosed and endothelially injured rabbit carotid arteries more effectively than other antiplatelet interventions. Thromb Haemost 1995; 74:974–979.

42. Strony J, Song A, Rusterholtz L, Adelman B. Aurintricarboxylic acid prevents rethrombosis in a canine model of arterial thrombosis. Thromb Vasc Biol. 1995; 15:359–366.

43. Guo Z, Weinstein MJ, Phillips MD, Kroll MH. Mr 6400 aurin tricarboxylic acid directly activates platelets. Thromb Res 1993; 71:77–78.

44. Bernat A, Lale A, Herbert J–M. Aurin tricarboxylic acid inhibits experimental venous thrombosis. Thromb Res. 1994; 74:617–627.

45. Kinlough–Rathbone RL, Packham MA. Unexpected effects of aurin tricarboxylic acid on human platelets. Thromb Haemost 1992; 68:189–193.

45a. Golino P, Ragni M, Cirillo P. Aurintricarboxylic acid reduces platelet deposition in stenosed and endothelially injured rabbit carotid arteries more effectively than other antiplatelet interventions. Thromb Haemost 1995; 74:974–979.

45b. Skidmore AF, Beebee TJC. Characterization and use of the potent ribonuclease inhibitor aurintricar- boxylic acid for the isolation of RNA from animal tissues. Biochem J 1989; 263:73–80.

46. Sugimoto M, Ricca G, Hrinda ME, Schreiber AB, Searfoss GH, Bottini E, Ruggeri ZM. Functional modulation of the islated glycoprotein Ib-binding domain of von Willebrand factor expressed in *Escherichia coli.* Biochemistry 1991; 30:5202.

47. Kasiewski C, Crook J, Hrinda M, Newman J, Perrone M. Inhibition of thrombus formation in monkeys by RG 12986, a recombinant von Willebrand factor fragment. Circulation 1991; 84(suppl II):II-247.

48. Yao SK, Ober JC, Garfinkel LI, Hagay Y, Ezov N, Ferguson JJ, Anderson HV, Panet A, Gorecki M, Buja LM, Willerson JT. Blockade of platelet membrane glycoprotein Ib receptors delays intracoronary thrombogenesis, enhances thrombolysis, and delays coronary artery reocclusion in dogs. Circulation 1994; 89:2822–2828.

49. Cauwenberghs N, Meiring M, Vauterin S, van Wyk V, Lamprecht S, Roodt JP, Novak L, Hartrijk J, Deckmyn H, Kotze HF. Antithrombotic effect of platelet glycoprotein Ib-blocking monoclonal antibody Fab fragments in nonhuman primates. Arterioscler Thromb Vasc Biol 2000; 20:1347–1353.

50. Kageyama S, Yamamoto H, Nagano M, Arisaka H, Kayahara T, Yoshimoto R. Anti-thrombotic effects and bleeding risk of AJvW-2, a monoclonal antibody against human von Willebrand factor. Br J Pharmacol 1997; 122:165–171.

50a. Eto K, Isshiki T, Yamamoto H, Takeshita S. Ochiai M, Yokoyama N, Yoshimoto R, Ikeda Y, Sato T. AJvW-2, an anti-vWF monoclonal antibody, inhibits enhanced platelet aggregation induced by high shear stress in platelet-rich plasma from patients with acute coronary syndromes. Arterioscler Thromb Vasc Biol 1999; 19:877–882.

51. Cisse–Thiam M, Girma JP, Meyer D, Drouet L. Inhibition of thrombus formation by anti-Willebrand monoclonal antibodies in the guinea pig. Dakar Med 1999; 44:45–48.

52. Peng M, Lu W, Beviglia L, Niewiarowski S, Kirby EP. Eichicetin: a snake venom protein that inhibits binding of von Willebrand factor and alboaggregins to platelet glycoprotein Ib. Blood 1993; 81:2321–2328.

53. Chang MC, Lin HK, Peng HC, Huang TF. Antithrombotic effect of crotalin, a platelet membrane glycoprotein Ib antagonist from venom of *Crotalus atrox*. Blood 1998; 91:1582–1589.

54. Chen YL, Tsai KW, Chang T, Hong TM, Tsai IH. Glycoprotein Ib-binding protein from the venom of *Deinagkistrodon acutus*—cDNA sequence, functional characterization, and three-dimensional modeling. Thromb Haemost 2000; 83:119–126.

55. Yeh CH, Wang WC, Hsieh TT, Huang TF. Agkistin, a snake venom-derived glycoprotein Ib antagonist, disrupts von Willebrand factor–endothelial cell interaction and inhibits angiogenesis. J Biol Chem 2000; 275:18615–18618.

56. Kawasaki T, Taniuchi Y, Hisamichi N, Fujimura Y, Suzuki M, Titani K, Kaku S, Satoh N, Takenaka T. Takaracetin, a new platelet antagonist that binds to platelet glycoprotein Ib and inhibits von Willebrand factor-dependent shear-induced platelet aggregation. Biochem J. 1995; 308:947–953.

57. Taniuchi Y, Kawasaki T, Fujimura Y. The high molecular mass, glycoprotein Ib-binding protein flavocetin-A induces only small platelet aggregates in vitro. Thromb Res 2000; 97:69–75.

58. Fukuda K, Mizuno H, Atoda H, Morita T. Crystal structure of flavocetin-A, a platelet glycoprotein Ib-binding protein, reveals a novel cyclic tetramer of C-type lectin-like heterodimers. Biochemistry 2000; 39:1915–1923.

59. Simon DI, Chen Z, Xu H, Li CQ, Dong J, McIntire LV, Ballantyne CM, Zhang L, Furman MI, Berndt MC, Lopez JA. Platelet glycoprotein Ibα is a counterreceptor for the leukocyte integrin Mac-1 (DC11b/CD18). J Exp Med 2000; 192:193–204.

60. Simon DI, Chen Z, Seifert P, Edelman ER, Ballantyne CM, Rogers C. Decreased neointiamal formation in Mac-1 −/− mice reveals a role for inflammation in vascular repair after angioplasty. J Clin Invest 2000; 105:293–300.

27

Thienopyridines: Ticlopidine and Clopidogrel

Peter J. Sharis
Beth Israel Deaconess Medical Center, Boston, Massachusetts, U.S.A.

Joseph Loscalzo
Whitaker Cardiovascular Institute, Boston University School of Medicine, Boston, Massachusetts, U.S.A.

I. INTRODUCTION

Antiplatelet agents are used widely to prevent and treat arterial thrombosis. Aspirin is a relatively weak platelet inhibitor that has shown significant benefits in patients with acute coronary syndromes [1,2]. The newer glycoprotein IIb/IIIa inhibitors have demonstrated promise in several studies to date, although additional data and follow-up are needed to define their precise indications and long-term effects [3,4].

Thienopyridines are a third class of antiplatelet agents that result in intermediate levels of platelet inhibition. Ticlopidine has been available for several years, but its use has been limited by the risk of neutropenia ($\sim$1%). Clopidogrel is a newer agent of this class that has a more favorable side effect profile. Clopidogrel was initially approved for the treatment of symptomatic atherosclerosis. Subsequent studies have resulted in its supplanting ticlopidine as the preferred agent for prevention of coronary stent thrombosis. A recent, large, randomized study found long-term administration of ticlopidine in patients with unstable angina or non–ST-elevation myocardial infarction (MI) resulted in an approximately 20% reduction in cardiovascular death, stroke, and nonfatal MI. Ongoing studies have been designed to study its efficacy in additional settings, such as acute myocardial infarction.

II. Mechanism of Action and Pharmacology

Ticlopidine and clopidogrel are thienopyridine derivatives that inhibit platelet aggregation. Clopidogrel differs structurally from ticlopidine by the presence of one additional carboxymethyl side group (Fig. 1). Both agents are inactive in vitro, requiring activation in the liver by the hepatic cytochrome P450-1A enzyme system [5,6]. The active metabolites have yet to be identified and appear to be excreted renally [7,8]. Ticlopidine is rapidly absorbed after ingestion;

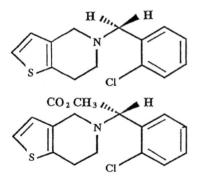

Figure 1 Chemical structure of ticlopidine (top) and clopidogrel (bottom).

maximal bioavailability occurs when it is taken after meals and is impaired by concomitant antacid use. Clopidogrel is also rapidly metabolized; however, its bioavailability appears unaffected by food intake.

Ticlopidine and clopidogrel appear to achieve their antiplatelet action by inhibiting the binding of adenosine 5′-diphosphate (ADP) to its receptors on platelets (Fig. 2) [9–11]. Recent studies suggest the existence of at least two types of ADP receptors [9,12]. The first is a low-affinity type-2 purinergic receptor (P2$_{AC}$) that is G–protein-coupled and results in mobilization

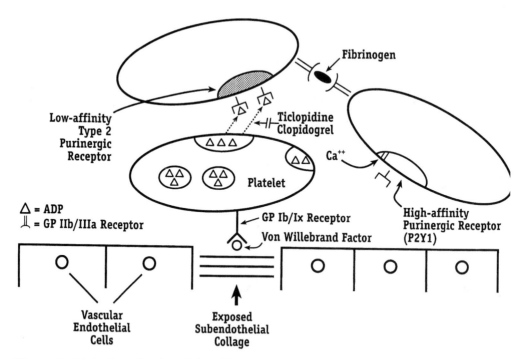

Figure 2 Mechanism of action of ticlopidine and clopidogrel. Damage to vascular endothelial cells exposes collagen. Platelets then bind to the collagen by glycoprotein (GP) Ib/Ix receptors complexed to von Willebrand factor. The bound platelets undergo degranulation, releasing adenosine 5′-diphosphate (ADP). The released ADP binds to two types of receptors, a low-affinity type-2 purinergic receptor (recently cloned; see text) and a high-affinity purinergic receptor (P2Y1). Ticlopidine and clopidogrel exert their antiplatelet effect by blocking the binding of ADP to the type-2 purinergic receptor and preventing the activation of the GP IIb/IIIa receptor complex and subsequent platelet activation.

of calcium from internal stores [13,14]. This results in a conformational change in and activation of the glycoprotein (GP) IIb/IIIa receptor complex, fibrinogen binding, and platelet aggregation. The second type of ADP receptor is a membrane protein (P2Y1) with high affinity that is responsible for rapid calcium influx and platelet shape change [13,14]. A second type of P2 receptor (P2X1), which appears to be a voltage-dependent receptor, has been cloned; however, its functional significance is unclear. Ticlopidine and clopidogrel appear to achieve their effect by interacting with the type 2 purinergic ADP receptor, but do not affect shape change or calcium influx [11,12,14,15]. Importantly, Hollopeter and colleagues recently reported cloning this purinergic receptor (P2Y12), asserting that it is both the ADP receptor as well as the thienopyridine target [16].

The inhibition of platelet aggregation by ticlopidine and clopidogrel is concentration-dependent. Standard dosing of ticlopidine (250 mg twice daily) results in maximal platelet inhibition within 4–7 days [17]. The reasons for this observed delay are poorly understood, although it has been postulated that impaired megakaryocytopoiesis in the bone marrow plays a role in addition to the direct effect of the agent on circulating platelets [18]. Actual clinical responses have been observed to occur earlier than those predicted solely based on the time course of the metabolism of ticlopidine. The fastest responses have been demonstrated with the administration of a loading dose of clopidogrel (300 mg) [19–21]: in one study, an antithrombotic effect was measurable within 90 min of the loading dose, and by 6 h the effect was equivalent to that seen at 10 days [19]. Although both ticlopidine and clopidogrel also prevent the platelet aggregation elicited by shear stress [22–24], studies suggest clopidogrel is more potent than either aspirin or ticlopidine in preventing high-shear stress-mediated coronary stent thrombosis.

Ticlopidine administration results in moderate platelet inhibition: 20–30% when measured using 20 μmol/L ADP [25]. In comparison, standard doses of GP IIb/IIIa inhibitors result in much greater platelet inhibition, usually 80–90% [26]. The antiplatelet activity of ticlopidine and clopidogrel persists for 7–10 days after the drugs are discontinued. This time interval corresponds to a circulating platelet's lifespan, suggesting the platelet inhibition is irreversible.

Studies have shown that the concomitant use of aspirin with ticlopidine or clopidogrel results in synergistic inhibition of platelet aggregation [27,28]. This effect appears to be a consequence of the potentiation of aspirin's effect on collagen-induced platelet aggregation [29,30]. A recent study found that ticlopidine also enhances the antiplatelet effects of tirofiban, a GP IIb/IIIa receptor antagonist [31].

Ticlopidine and clopidogrel prolong bleeding time approximately twofold [8,11], with maximal prolongation occurring after 5–6 days [11,32]. Normalization of the bleeding time occurs approximately 10 days after cessation of the drug's administration, a time interval that, again, corresponds to a platelet's lifespan. There are conflicting data on whether ticlopidine reduces erythrocyte aggregability [33], blood viscosity [34,35], or fibrinogen levels [33,36]. Finally, neither ticlopidine nor clopidogrel have an effect on the cyclooxygenase pathway; thereby indicating that these agents act independently of aspirin.

III. CLINICAL APPLICATIONS

A. Secondary Prevention of Stroke and Transient Ischemic Attacks

Two studies examined the effects of ticlopidine in populations with prior cerebrovascular events. The Canadian American Ticlopidine Study (CATS) compared ticlopidine, 250 mg twice daily, with placebo in a randomized, double-blind fashion in 1072 patients with a recent thromboembolic stroke [37]. The ticlopidine group had a significant 23.3% reduction in the combined endpoint of stroke, myocardial infarction, or vascular death compared with the placebo group

(11.3 vs. 14.8%/year, p = 0.02). The lack of a comparison between ticlopidine and aspirin was a major weakness of this study.

The Ticlopidine Aspirin Stroke Study (TASS) addressed the question of comparability of aspirin, enrolling 3069 patients with recent transient ischemic attacks, amaurosis fugax, or minor strokes. Patients were randomized to receive ticlopidine, 250 mg twice daily, or high-dose aspirin, 625 mg twice daily [38]. At 3 years, the ticlopidine group had a 12% reduction in the primary endpoint, consisting of nonfatal stroke or death from any cause, compared with the aspirin group (17 vs. 19%; p = 0.048). The observed benefit of ticlopidine use was primarily driven by a 21% reduction in all strokes with ticlopidine compared with aspirin (10 vs. 13%, p = 0.024). A subsequent analysis also found ticlopidine use associated with a lower incidence of recurrent transient ischemic attacks (TIAs) (30 vs. 43%; p = 0.007) [39]. Of note, ticlopidine was most efficacious during the first year of treatment, reducing the risk of death and stroke by 42%.

From the CATS and TASS data, ticlopidine received U.S. Food and Drug Administration (FDA) approval for use in persons who fail to respond to, or do not tolerate, aspirin [40]. However, because of the substantial risk of neutropenia with ticlopidine, aspirin remains the agent of choice for those with a history of stroke or transient ischemic attack.

A subsequent overview by the Antiplatelet Trialists' Collaboration (ATC) included a meta-analysis of trials that directly compared ticlopidine and aspirin [2]. Although TASS provided nearly 90% of the 3471 patients, the analysis found that ticlopidine use was associated with a statistically *insignificant* 10% reduction in myocardial infarction, stroke, or vascular death. However, it is important to note that this endpoint differs from the primary endpoint of TASS by including nonfatal myocardial infarctions and excluding nonvascular deaths.

An additional study completed since the ATC overview was the Ticlopidine Indobufen Stroke Study (TISS), which enrolled 1632 patients with a recent transient ischemic attack, amaurosis fugax, or minor stroke. Patients were randomized in an open-label fashion to ticlopidine, 250 mg/day, or indobufen (a nonsteroidal anti-inflammatory drug), 200 mg/day. The ticlopidine group had a highly statistically significant 50% lower incidence of death, myocardial infarction, or stroke compared with the indobufen group (absolute event rates of 2.9 vs. 5.8%, p = 0.004) [41].

Table 1 summarizes the finding in various studies.

B. Peripheral Arterial Occlusive Disease

Before the large Clopidogrel vs. Aspirin in Patients at Risk for Ischemic Events (CAPRIE) trial, there were only a few small trials of ticlopidine in patients with peripheral vascular disease, and these studies had heterogeneous inclusion criteria and clinical endpoints. In the Swedish Ticlopidine Multicenter Study (STIMS), 687 patients with intermittent claudication were randomized to ticlopidine, 250 mg twice daily, or placebo [42]. The intention-to-treat analysis found no significant difference between the groups in the incidence of myocardial infarction, stroke, or transient ischemic attack (25.7% [ticlopidine group] vs. 29.0% [placebo]; p = 0.24). However, among patients actually receiving treatment, the ticlopidine group had a lower incidence of primary events (13.8 vs. 22.4%; p = 0.017), including 29% fewer deaths (18.7 vs. 26.1%, p = 0.015). The mortality reduction was primarily driven by fewer deaths from ischemic heart disease (26% reduction, p < 0.01). A STIMS substudy found no significant improvement in leg flow variables among ticlopidine-treated patients, as demonstrated by venous occlusion plethysmography, ankle/brachial index, and maximum walking distance before claudication [43]. However, other smaller, double-blind studies of intermittent claudication

Table 1 Randomized Trials of Ticlopidine and Clopidogrel

Study	Population	No. pts	Regimen	Endpoint	Event rate	Event rate	p value
Stroke and TIA							
CATS	Recent thromboembolic stroke	1,072	T 250 b.i.d. or placebo	Stroke, MI, vascular death	11.3%/yr	14.8%/yr	0.02
TASS	Recent TIA or minor stroke	3,069	T 250 b.i.d. or A 625 b.i.d.	Nonfatal stroke or death	17%	19%	0.048
TISS	Recent TIA, amaurosis fugax, or minor stroke	1,632	T or indubofen (median doses 250 and 200 mg/d)	Death, stroke + MI at 1 yr	2.9%	5.8%	0.004
Peripheral Arterial Occlusive Disease							
STIMS	Intermittent claudication	687	T 250 b.i.d. or placebo	MI, stroke, and TIA	25.7%	29.0%	>0.2
Arcan et al.	Chronic intermittent claudication	169	T 250 b.i.d. or placebo	CVA, TIA + peripheral ischemia requiring surgery at 6 mo	2.4%	10.5%	0.03
EMATAP	Intermittent claudication	615	T 250 b.i.d. or placebo × 24 wks	Death, MI, stroke, and CV intervention due to clinical deterioration	1.0%	6.4%	0.002
Unstable Angina and Myocardial Infarction							
Balsano et al.	Unstable angina	652	Conventional therapy with or without T 250 b.i.d.	Vascular death and nonfatal MI at 6 mo	7.3%	13.6%	0.009
CURE	Unstable angina, non-STEMI	12,652	ASA or ASA + C 75 q.d. (300-mg loading dose)	CV death + stroke + MI	9.3%	11.3%	<0.001
STAMI	ST elevation MI treated with thrombolytic therapy	1,470	A 160/d or T 500/d	Death, stroke, recurrent MI, angina with objective evidence of ischemia	8.0%	8.0%	NS
Symptomatic atherosclerosis							
CAPRIE	Ischemic stroke, MI, or documented PAD	19,185	C 75 q.d. or ASA 325 q.d.	Ischemic stroke+ MI + vascular death	5.32%/yr	5.83%/yr	0.043
Coronary stent thrombosis							
ISAR	Coronary stenting	517	A200 + T500 × 1 mo or PH	Cardiac death, MI, PTCA, and coronary bypass surgery			

(continued over)

Table 1 (Continued)

Study	Population	No. pts	Regimen	Endpoint	Event rate	Event rate	p value
1.6%	6.2%	0.01					
STARS	Coronary stenting	1,653	A325 and T 500 × 28 d, A325 + warfarin, or A325 alone	Death, MI, PTCA, and coronary bypass surgery	0.5%	2.7%	0.007
CLASSIC S	Coronary stenting	700	T 250 b.i.d. or C 75 q.d.; all received ASA 100 q.d.	Discontinuation of medication, noncardiac death, stroke, severe PVD or bleeding events	4.5%	9.6%	0.01
TOPPS	Coronary stenting	1,016	T 250 b.i.d. (50-mg load) or C 75 q.d. (300-mg load) × 1 mo	Major cardiac events	3.8%	4.6%	NS
Herz–Zentrum	Coronary stenting	800	C 75 q.d. or T 250 b.i.d. (500-mg load)	Major cardiac events	1.7%	3.1%	NS
Saphenous vein graft patency							
Chevigne et al.	Coronary bypass surgery	77	T 250 b.i.d. (started before surgery) or placebo	Graft occlusion at 3 mo angiography	10.1%	20.3%	<0.1
Limet et al.	Coronary bypass surgery	173	T 250 b.i.d. (first dose on day 2) or placebo	Graft occlusion at 30 days	15.9%	26.1%	<0.01
Becquemin et al.	Femoropopliteal or femorofemoral bypass surgery	243	T 250 b.i.d. or placebo	Femoropopliteal or femorofemoral graft patency	82%	63%	0.002

CATS, Canadian American Ticlopidine Study; TASS, Ticlopidine Aspirin Stroke Study; TISS, Ticlopidine Indobufen Stroke Study; STIMS, Swedish Ticlopidine Multicenter Study; EMATAP, Estudio Multicentrico Argentino de la Ticlopidine en las Arteriopatias Peifericas; CURE, Clopidogrel versus Aspirin in Patients at Risk for Ischemic Events; ISAR, Intracoronary Stenting and Antithrombotic Regimen study; STARS, Stent Antithrombotic Regimen Study; TOPPS, Ticlopidine or Plavix post stent. A, aspirin; C, clopicogrel; CABG, coronary artery bypass surgery; CV, cardiovascular; CVA, cardiovascular accident; MI, myocardial infarction; PAD, peripheral arterial disease; PH, phenprocoumon; PTCA, percutaneous transluminal coronary angioplasty; STEMI, ST elevation myocardial infarction; T, ticlopidine; TIA, transient ischemic attack; W, warfarin.

patients have found significant benefits in outcome measures of unclear clinical significance, such as ankle : brachial index [44], walking ability [45,46], cutaneous microcirculation [46], and ischemic ulcer diameter [47].

A smaller, randomized, double-blind trial of 169 patients with chronic intermittent claudication also compared ticlopidine, 250 mg twice daily, with placebo [45]. At 6 months follow-up, the ticlopidine group had a 77% lower incidence of transient ischemic attack, cerebrovascular accident, and peripheral ischemic episodes requiring vascular surgical intervention (2.4 vs. 10.5%, p = 0.03). A recent trial of 615 patients with a similar design (ticlopidine 250 mg, compared with placebo) confirmed these findings [48]: at 6 months, the ticlopidine group had a 75% lower incidence in the combined endpoint of death, myocardial infarction, stroke, or cardiovascular intervention related to clinical deterioration (1.6 vs. 6.4%, p = 0.002).

C. Symptomatic Atherosclerosis

The Clopidogrel vs. Aspirin in Patients at Risk for Ischemic Events (CAPRIE) trial enrolled over 19,000 patients with symptomatic atherosclerosis, defined as recent ischemic stroke (1 week to 6 months), myocardial infarction (within 35 days), or documented peripheral arterial disease [49]. Patients were randomized to clopidogrel, 75 mg once daily, or aspirin, 325 mg once daily. At a mean follow-up of 1.9 years, clopidogrel was associated with an overall significant 8.7% reduction in the primary endpoint, consisting of ischemic stroke, myocardial infarction, or vascular death (5.32/yr vs. 5.83%/yr; p = 0.043).

Of note, there was significant heterogeneity among the three patient entry criteria groups. Among patients with documented peripheral arterial disease as the qualifying event, there was a significant 23.8% reduction in the combined primary endpoint (3.71%/yr compared with 4.86%/yr; p = 0.0028) [49]. This reduction was primarily due to fewer myocardial infarctions (1.2 vs. 1.9%/yr) and vascular deaths (1.1 vs. 1.5%/yr), as the stroke rates were similar (1.4%/yr). Among patients with a recent ischemic stroke as the qualifying event, there was a statistically insignificant 7.3% reduction in the primary endpoint among clopidogrel-treated patients compared with aspirin-treated patients (7.15 vs. 7.71%/yr; p = 0.26). Among the patients enrolled based on a myocardial infarction within 35 days of randomization, there was a statistically insignificant 3.7% increase in the combined endpoint of myocardial infarction, stroke, and vascular death (p = 0.66; see following, Sec. IV, D for further discussion). It is unclear what the mechanism of action is to explain the apparent preferential benefit of clopidogrel in patients with documented peripheral arterial disease.

Several preliminary secondary analyses of the CAPRIE data have generated interesting findings. Among patients with diabetes mellitus, there appears to be an amplification of the benefit of clopidogrel over aspirin (21 and 38% reduction in the primary endpoint in all diabetics and insulin-dependent diabetics, respectively) [50]. Patients with a prior history of coronary artery bypass graft surgery also benefited more from clopidogrel therapy with 36% fewer primary events compared with the aspirin group (15.9 vs. 22.3%, p = 0.001) [51].

The CAPRIE data led to FDA approval of clopidogrel for the secondary prevention of vascular events in patients with symptomatic atherosclerosis. Ongoing and planned studies will help evaluate the efficacy of aspirin and clopidogrel, a combination not studied in CAPRIE.

D. Acute Coronary Syndromes

Only one randomized trial has studied the effects of ticlopidine in unstable angina patients. A total of 652 patients were randomized, in an open-label fashion, to conventional therapy, consisting of calcium channel antagonists, β-blockers, or nitrates, or to conventional therapy plus ticlopidine, 250 mg twice daily [52]. Aspirin was not considered part of conventional therapy, for at the time of protocol design it was not routinely used to treat unstable angina. The ticlopidine group had a significant 46% reduction in the primary combined endpoint of vascular death and nonfatal myocardial infarction at 6 months (7.3 vs. 13.6%; p = 0.009). The number of events in the two groups was similar until after 10 days, which is consistent with ticlopidine's delayed antiplatelet effect.

In the CAPRIE trial, the subgroup of 6302 patients enrolled based on myocardial infarction within 35 days had a statistically insignificant 3.7% increase in the combined endpoint of myocardial infarction, stroke, and vascular death (p = 0.66) [49]. However, among patients enrolled based on documented peripheral vascular disease or a recent stroke, there were an additional 2144 patients with a history of myocardial infarction occurring months or years before the qualifying event. In a posthoc secondary analysis of all 8446 patients with any history of myocardial infarction, clopidogrel use was associated with a statistically insignificant 7.4% decrease in the combined endpoint. Interestingly, another analysis of all 19,185 enrolled patients found a statistically significant 19.2% reduction in the myocardial infarction event rate [53]. Based on these data, the use of clopidogrel in all patients with recent myocardial infarction, stroke, or documented peripheral arterial disease appears to result in a reduced risk of subsequent myocardial infarction.

The Clopidogrel in Unstable Angina to Prevent Recurrent Ischemic Events (CURE) trial, whose preliminary results were announced at the 2001 American College of Cardiology Annual Scientific Session, examined the efficacy of clopidogrel in addition to current background therapy in patients with unstable angina or non–Q-wave MI. A total of 12,562 patients were randomized to aspirin (75–325 mg/day) plus clopidogrel (300 mg loading dose then 75 mg/day) or aspirin alone. The aspirin and clopidogrel group had a highly statistically significant 20% reduction in the composite primary endpoint, consisting of cardiovascular death, myocardial infarction, and stroke (9.3 vs. 11.3% [aspirin alone]; p < 0.001). Of note, most of the benefit was observed within the first 48 h of treatment, suggesting that the loading dose of clopidogrel results in rapid and effective platelet inhibition.

One randomized trial has examined the use of a thienopyridine in patients with acute ST-elevation MI. The Ticlopidine vs. Aspirin After MI (STAMI) trial enrolled 1470 such patients, all of whom received thrombolysis therapy [54]. Patients were randomized in double-blind fashion to aspirin 160 mg/day or ticlopidine 500 mg/day. There was no difference between the two groups in the incidence of the primary endpoint, consisting of death, recurrent MI, stroke, or angina with objective evidence of ischemia (8.0% [at 6 months] in both groups). Another large, ongoing study will focus on the use of clopidogrel in acute myocardial infarction patients. The Clopidogrel and Metoprolol in Myocardial Infarction Trial/Second Chinese Cardiac Study (COMMIT/CCS-2) trial will evaluate the addition of clopidogrel to aspirin in the chronic phase of secondary prevention after an acute MI.

E. Prevention of Coronary Artery Stent Thrombosis

Early experience with coronary stenting was hindered by high rates of subacute stent thrombosis, a serious complication that frequently results in myocardial infarction or even death [54–56]. Antithrombotic regimens consisting of several agents, including aspirin, dipyridamole, dextran, heparin, and warfarin [57,58], were associated with stent thrombosis in 5–20% of cases [56,59–61]. Not surprisingly, these aggressive regimens led to frequent bleeding complications and prolonged hospital stays [62–64].

The major breakthrough in this area occurred when the focus shifted to the use of more aggressive antiplatelet regimens. Initial nonrandomized studies added ticlopidine (250 mg twice daily) to aspirin and heparin or low-molecular-weight heparin. The French Multicenter Group reported their experience with a total of 1251 patients who received a 1-month postprocedural regimen of ticlopidine, aspirin (100 mg once-daily), and heparin (1–2 weeks) or low-molecular-weight heparin (1 month). The addition of ticlopidine resulted in much lower stent thrombosis rates of 1.3–1.8% [65]. After removal of low-molecular-weight heparin from the regimen, the thrombosis rate remained low (1.1%). This simplified regimen was also associated with nearly 70% fewer bleeding complications.

Another group of investigators in Milan soon reported their experience with a regimen consisting of only antiplatelet agents [66]. A total of 321 patients with adequate stent expansion after high-pressure balloon inflation (average 15 atm), which was verified by intravascular ultrasound, were treated with either ticlopidine, 250 mg twice daily, for 1 month and aspirin, 325 mg once daily, for 5 days, or with aspirin alone for 1 month. At 6 months, the stent thrombosis rate was 0.8% for the group treated with aspirin and ticlopidine and 1.4% for the group treated with aspirin alone (p = NS). Because this was not a randomized study, the lower thrombosis rate could have been a reflection of the new high-pressure balloon technique [67] and other uncontrolled variables, such as increasing operator experience.

A randomized trial of 517 patients, the Intracoronary Stenting and Antithrombotic Regimen (ISAR) study, soon confirmed the advantage of an antiplatelet regimen over an anticoagulant regimen [68]. Patients were randomized to intravenous heparin for 12 hours, ticlopidine, 250 mg twice daily, and aspirin, 100 mg twice daily, for one month; or intravenous heparin for 5–10 days, aspirin, 100 mg twice daily, and phenprocoumon (target international normalized ratio [INR] 3.5–4.5) for 1 month. The antiplatelet group had 75% fewer cardiac endpoints at 30 days, consisting of cardiac death, myocardial infarction, coronary artery bypass graft surgery, or repeat coronary angioplasty. Of note, the incidence of stent thrombosis was an impressive 86% lower in the antiplatelet group (Table 2). These reductions remained significant at 6 and 12 months of follow-up [69].

Table 2 Bleeding Complications and Subacute Stent Thrombosis in Coronary Stenting Regimens

Study	Regimen (doses in mg/d)	Stent thrombosis	Bleeding
Ticlopidine-containing regimens			
French Registry	A 100, IVH, LMWH, T 500 × 1 mo	0.8%	2.2%
French Registry	A 100, IVH, T 500 × 2 d, 250 × 28 d	1.1%	1.1%
Colombo et al.	A 325 and T 500 × 1 mo or A 325 alone	0%/1.4%	0.6%
ISAR	A 200 and T 500 × 1 mo	0%	0%
STARS	A 325 and T 500 × 28 d	0.6%	2.0%
Other regimens			
French Registry	A 25 and D 225[a] × 6 mo, iD × 24 h, IVH × 5 d, W × 2 mo	6.5%	6.9%
BENESTENT	A 250–500, D 225[a] × 1 mo, iD[b], IVH × 36 h, W × 3 mo	3.5%	13.5%
STRESS	A 325, D 75 × 3, iD[b], IVH × 3 d, W × 1 mo	3.4%	7.3%
ISAR	A 200/d, IVH × 5–10 d, Ph × 1 mo		

STARS, Stent Antithrombotic Regimen Study; BENESTENT, Belgium and Netherlands Stent Study Group; STRESS, Stent Restenosis Study; ISAR, Intracoronary Stenting and Antithrombotic Regimen.
A, Aspirin; D, dipyridamole; iD, intravenous dextran; h, hours; IVH, intravenous heparin; LMWH, low molecular weight heparin; mo, months; Ph, phenprocoumon; SST, subacute stent thrombosis; T, ticlopidine; W, warfarin.
[a]75 mg three times daily.
[b]Periprocedure infusion.

A larger randomized trial, the Stent Antithrombotic Regimen Study (STARS), subsequently demonstrated a clear benefit of a ticlopidine-containing regimen over both anticoagulation and aspirin-only regimens [70]. A total of 1653 patients were randomized to either aspirin, 325 mg once daily, plus warfarin (target INR 2.0–2.5); aspirin plus ticlopidine, 250 mg twice daily; or aspirin alone for 1 month. At 30 days, the aspirin plus ticlopidine group had an 80% reduction in the combined endpoint of death, Q-wave myocardial infarction, emergency surgery, target vessel revascularization, and angiographic thrombus/restenosis (0.5 vs. 2.7% [aspirin plus warfarin; $p = 0.007$] and 3.6% [aspirin only; $p < 0.001$]).

Importantly, the increasing utilization of thienopyridines and subsequent elimination of oral anticoagulants from antithrombotic regimens led to shorter average lengths of hospital stay. In addition, post-procedural intravenous heparin is no longer routinely utilized, which has also led to a reduction in length of stay.

After the publication of the CAPRIE trial results and subsequent FDA approval of clopidogrel, many centers began to use clopidogrel instead of ticlopidine after stent implantation. Several centers soon reported their experience with this off-label approved use of clopidogrel. A single-center prospective analysis of 875 consecutive stent patients found a similar incidence at 30 days of death, nonfatal MI, and need for target vessel revascularization among 514 patients receiving clopidogrel and 361 ticlopidine patients (2.1 vs. 1.4%; $p = NS$) [71]. Another single-center experience of 500 patients that utilized loading doses of clopidogrel (300 mg followed by 75 once-daily for 14 days) and ticlopidine (500 mg then 250 mg twice-daily for 14 days) showed a similar incidence of major adverse events [72]. A third report from two centers of 1689 patients (ticlopidine: 1406; clopidogrel: 283), again, found a similar 30-day incidence of stent thrombosis (1.5 vs. 1.4%) and major adverse events (3.1 vs. 2.4%). The ticlopidine group, however, had a significantly higher incidence of side effects (10.6 vs. 5.3%; $p = 0.006$), primarily due to more frequent diarrhea and rash [73].

The first randomized study to compare the two agents, CLASSICS, was designed to determine if clopidogrel was, indeed, better tolerated and had a lower incidence of neutropenia than ticlopidine [74]. CLASSICS was not powered to detect a difference in the incidence of major cardiac events between the two groups. A total of 700 patients who underwent successful stenting were randomized to ticlopidine, 500 mg/day, or clopidogrel, 75 mg/day; all received aspirin, 100 mg/day. The clopidogrel group had a 50% lower incidence of the primary composite endpoint (4.5 vs. 9.6%; $p = 0.01$), which consisted of any adverse effect resulting in the discontinuation of study medication, as well as noncardiac death, stroke, and severe peripheral vascular or hemorrhagic events. The difference between the groups was driven by a higher intolerance of ticlopidine (e.g., allergic exanthema, diarrhea, nausea, hepatic enzyme elevation). Of note, neutropenia did not occur in any clopidogrel-treated patient, but did occur in three ticlopidine-treated patients ($p = 0.07$). The clopidogrel group also had a nonsignificant reduction in cardiac events at 30 days (1.7 vs. 3.1%, $p = 0.24$), consisting of cardiac death, urgent target vessel revascularization, angiographically documented thrombotic stent occlusion, or nonfatal MI. One concerning finding was a higher incidence of thrombotic stent occlusion associated with clopidogrel use (2.0 vs. 0.6%; $p = 0.10$).

Findings from two additional randomized trials have confirmed the better tolerability of clopidogrel compared with ticlopidine. The Ticlopidine Or Plavix [clopidogrel] poststent (TOPPS) study was a randomized, nonblinded study of 1016 patients who received ticlopidine (including 500-mg–loading dose) or clopidogrel (300-mg–loading dose) for 1 month [75]. Clopidogrel was better tolerated (intolerability in 1.6 vs. 3.6%; $p = 0.04$), and its use was associated with nonsignificant reductions in major cardiac events (3.8 vs. 4.6%) and death (0.6 vs. 1.5%) (presented at TCT 2000). The Herz–Zentrum study was a single-center, nonblinded study of 800 patients who underwent successful stenting; patients were randomized to clopidogrel, 75 mg/day, or ticlopidine, 500 mg/day (including a 500-mg–loading dose) [75]. The clopidogrel group had a significantly lower incidence of noncardiac events (4.5 vs. 9.6%; $p = 0.01$) and a nonsignificant reduction in cardiac events (1.7 vs. 3.1%).

A metanalysis was recently performed that combines data on the 2661 patients from these three randomized studies with an additional 11,166 patients from seven registries [76]. The incidence of major adverse effects was nearly 50% lower in clopidogrel-treated patients compared with ticlopidine-treated patients (2 vs. 3.9%, $p = 0.001$). The findings of this metanalysis are limited by the heterogeneity in the definition of major adverse events and drug dosage levels. Additionally, the significant difference between the clopidogrel and ticlopidine groups was primarily driven by data from the registries (odds ratio 0.45 [$p = 0.01$] vs. 0.93 [$p = NS$] in three clinical trials).

Two additional, important issues associated with the administration of thienopyridines in coronary stent patients are "pretreatment" dosing (initiation of drug therapy before stenting) and the use of loading doses. Both of these methods aim to achieve an earlier adequate level of platelet inhibition, as peak platelet activation occurs within 48–72 h of stent implantation and the majority of stent thromboses also occurs early (mean 0.7 days in the large STARS trial [70]). An analysis of the FANTASTIC trial data, in which there was no ticlopidine pretreatment, found a higher acute (< 24-h) occlusion rate in the ticlopidine group (2.4 vs. 0.9%; $p = 0.06$) [77]. The ISAR trial had a similar design, and an analysis of its data showed no influence on stent thrombosis rates until after 3 days of ticlopidine therapy [68]. A nonrandomized study of coronary stent patients, most of whom did receive ticlopidine pretreatment, found the duration of use before stenting correlated significantly with the incidence of postprocedural non–Q-wave MI [78]. Another study of 116 patients in which ticlopidine was given for 1 or more days before stenting showed subacute stent thrombosis occurring in only 1 patient (0.9%) [79]. Of note, analysis of data from the EPISTENT study found no additive benefit of ticlopidine pretreatment among patients who received a GP IIb/IIIa inhibitor; additional studies of this interaction are needed. In many patients, especially those with acute coronary syndromes, it is not possible to provide the patient with pretreatment, and loading doses are utilized to achieve rapid platelet inhibition (typically 300 mg of clopidogrel and 500 mg of ticlopidine).

F. Future Stenting Studies

The benefits of ticlopidine and clopidogrel in the expanding number of clinical settings for which stents are utilized, such as chronic total coronary occlusions [80–82], saphenous vein graft disease [83,84], and more recently, acute myocardial infarction [85–86], require additional study. However, several studies have thus far suggested a beneficial role of ticlopidine for all of these indications [87,88]. In addition, poststenting radiotherapy has recently received FDA approval for treatment of in-stent restenosis [89–91]. Reports of late stent thrombosis in these radiation-treated patients have led some investigators to prescribe clopidogrel for 6 months or more [92]; formal studies of this prolonged treatment regimen have yet to be performed. The use of clopidogrel in conjunction with newer antithrombotic agents, particularly GP IIb/IIIa inhibitors, also requires further study.

G. Other Uses

The effect of ticlopidine on the patency of saphenous vein grafts and restenosis has been examined in several studies. One study randomized 77 patients 3 days before coronary artery bypass surgery to ticlopidine, 250 mg twice-daily, or placebo [93]. At three months, saphenous vein graft patency was assessed by both coronary angiography and thallium imaging. There was a statistically insignificant 50% reduction in graft occlusion among ticlopidine-treated patients compared with placebo (10.1 vs. 20.3%); however, on-treatment analysis showed a significant 67% reduction in occlusion rates (7.1 vs. 21.8%; p < 0.02). A similar study randomized 173 patients 2 days after coronary artery bypass graft surgery to ticlopidine, 250 mg twice daily, or placebo. The ticlopidine group had a significant reduction in graft occlusion rates at post-operative days 10, 180, and 360 (p all < 0.05) [94]. Another study demonstrated the effectiveness of ticlopidine in patients with femoropopliteal or femorotibial saphenous vein grafts for effects on graft patency. Patients were randomized to ticlopidine 250 mg twice daily, or placebo [95]. The ticlopidine group had better graft patency at the 2-year follow-up (82 vs. 63%; p = 0.002).

The Ticlopidine Microangiopathy of Diabetes study (TIMAD) is the only major study to evaluate the efficacy of ticlopidine in patients with diabetic retinopathy [96]. A total of 435 patients with nonproliferative diabetic retinopathy were randomized to ticlopidine, 250 mg twice-daily, or placebo [109]. The ticlopidine group had significant reductions at 3 years in overall disease progression (p = 0.04) and microaneurysm progression (p = 0.03).

IV. SIDE EFFECTS

The use of ticlopidine and clopidogrel in stent trials is associated with very low rates of major hemorrhage. With the elimination of dextran, warfarin, prolonged infusions of intravenous heparin, and low-molecular-weight heparin from poststenting regimens, the incidence of bleeding decreased substantially (from >5% to <2%). Longer-term use of ticlopidine is also associated with low bleeding rates, as demonstrated in the secondary-stroke prevention trials. In the TASS trial, major hemorrhage occurred in only 0.5% of ticlopidine-treated patients compared with 1.4% of aspirin-treated patients (p < 0.05) [38,39]. The incidence of minor bleeding was similar with the two treatments (9 vs. 10%). In the CATS trial, major bleeding rates were similar in the ticlopidine and placebo groups (0.2 vs. 0.4%); however, the ticlopidine group had more frequent minor bleeding episodes (6.5 vs. 3.0%; p not reported) [37].

Clopidogrel use is also associated with a low incidence of major bleeding. In the CAPRIE trial, the clopidogrel group had a 1.4% incidence of major hemorrhage, compared with 1.6% in the aspirin group [49]. Of note, the clopidogrel group did have a lower incidence of gastrointestinal bleeding (1.99 vs. 2.66%).

Ticlopidine use is associated with an approximate 1% incidence of severe neutropenia, a potentially fatal side effect [112]. In the TASS trial, the incidence of neutropenia (absolute neutrophil count [ANC] <1200/mm^3) was 2.4%, whereas severe neutropenia (ANC <450/mm^3) occurred in 0.9% (vs. 0% with aspirin) [38]. In the CATS trial, severe neutropenia (<450/mm^3) occurred in 0.8% of patients [37]. In the ISAR and STARS trials [68,70], two large coronary stenting trials, the incidence of neutropenia was similar to the control groups (0.5 vs. 0.2%; 0 vs. 0%), a finding likely due to the short, 1-month duration of therapy. In most cases, neutropenia occurs in the first few months after initiation of therapy, and usually does not occur in the first 2–3 weeks of therapy. Blood counts should be obtained every 2 weeks for at least the first 3 months of therapy. Neutropenia resolves with discontinuation of ticlopidine in most patients [97]. In contrast, clopidogrel does not appear to be associated with an increased risk of neutropenia. In the CAPRIE trial, severe neutropenia occurred in only 0.1% of clopidogrel-treated patients, compared with 0.17% of aspirin-treated patients [49]. Another hematological complication associated with ticlopidine use is thrombotic thrombocytopenic purpura [98–102]. This serious complication was associated with a 33% mortality in one review of 60 cases [101]. The incidence of thrombotic thrombocytopenic purpura has been reported to be between 1:1600 and 1:5000. Shorter duration of use is associated with a lower likelihood of occurrence, although 2 of 60 cases in the largest review occurred during the initial 2 weeks of therapy. Clopidogrel appears to be associated with a lower risk of thrombotic thrombocytopenic purpura. A recent report estimated an incidence of 1:15,000 among persons taking clopidogrel [103,104]; this calculation is based on the assumption that only 10% of cases are detected by current surveillance techniques. However, some investigators argue that most cases are known and the actual incidence is much closer to the background incidence of thrombotic thrombocytopenic purpura in the general population (1:270,000).

The most common side effects associated with ticlopidine use are gastrointestinal symptoms. Diarrhea, nausea, vomiting, and anorexia occur in 20–50% of patients [11,37,38]. In the TASS trial, more ticlopidine-treated patients stopped therapy because of diarrhea (6 vs. 2% for aspirin) or rash (3 vs. 1% for aspirin) than for any other reason [38]. These gastrointestinal side effects usually occur during the first 2–3 weeks of ticlopidine administration. Modestly higher total serum cholesterol levels (+9%) were associated with ticlopidine use in the TASS trial [38], whereas in the CAPRIE trial, clopidogrel had no significant effect on cholesterol levels [49].

Other less common adverse effects of these two agents include pruritus, urticaria, ecchymosis, and epistaxis. These adverse effects appear to occur less often with clopidogrel than with ticlopidine. Most of these reactions are mild and resolve when the drug is stopped. Additional uncommon adverse events associated with ticlopidine use include thrombocytopenia [105], aplastic anemia [106], severe cholestasis [107,108], and acute interstitial nephritis [109]. Elderly women (>75 years old) have the highest incidence of hematological side effects [110].

Several medications have interactions with ticlopidine and clopidogrel. For example, the clearance of ticlopidine is decreased by 50% with concomitant cimetidine therapy [111]. Ticlopidine, in turn, affects the metabolism of certain medications. Cyclosporin doses need to be increased with concomitant ticlopidine administration [112], whereas phenytoin, carbamazepine, and theophylline doses often need to be decreased [113–115]. Clopidogrel does not appear to affect the pharmacokinetics of theophylline [116].

V. CONCLUSIONS

Ticlopidine has shown benefit in the secondary prevention of stroke, peripheral vascular disease, and unstable angina. However, the risk of severe neutropenia has limited its use to those who are aspirin-intolerant or considered aspirin "failures." The large CAPRIE trial demonstrated the efficacy of clopidogrel in symptomatic atherosclerosis patients, with no increased risk of neutropenia compared with aspirin. The large CURE trial found the use of clopidogrel in addition to aspirin in patients with unstable angina or non-ST–elevation MI results in a 20% reduction in major cardiovascular events. The use of clopidogrel in patients with acute ST-elevation MI is currently being evaluated in ongoing studies.

The use of thienopyridine in conjunction with aspirin in coronary stent patients results in a significant reduction in the incidence of stent thrombosis and major cardiac complications. Recent data have demonstrated an improved safety profile and similar (or better) efficacy of clopidogrel compared with ticlopidine in this setting. As a result, most centers now use this agent in stent patients. Ongoing studies will help better define the role of pretreatment and loading doses, and determine if longer courses of therapy (>1 month) are indicated for certain high-risk patients.

REFERENCES

1. Awtry EH, Loscalzo J. Aspirin. Circulation 2000; 101:1206–1218.
2. Antiplatelet Trialists' Collaboration. Collaborative overview of randomised trials of antiplatelet therapy—I: prevention of death, myocardial infarction, and stroke by prolonged antiplatelet therapy in various categories of patients. Br Med J 1994; 308:81–106.
3. Moliterno DJ, Topol EJ. Meta-analysis of platelet GP IIb/IIIa antagonist randomized clinical trials in ischemic heart disease: consistent, durable salutary effects [abstr]. Circulation 1997; 96(suppl I):I-475.
4. Chew DP, Moliterno DJ. A critical appraisal of platelet glycoprotein IIb/IIIa inhibition. J Am Coll Cardiol 2000; 36:2028–2035.
5. Desager JP. Clinical pharmacokinetics of ticlopidine. Clin Pharmacokinet 1994; 26:347–355.
6. Savi P, Combalbert J, Gaich C, Rouchon MC, Maffrand JP, Berger Y, Herbert JM. The antiaggregating activity of clopidogrel is due to a metabolic activation by the hepatic cytochrome P450–1A. Thromb Haemost 1994; 72:313–317.
7. Teitelbaum P. Pharmodynamics and pharmacokinetics of ticlopidine. In: Haas WK, Easton JD, eds. Ticlopidine, Platelets, and Vascular Disease. New York: Springer-Verlag, 1993:27–40.
8. Harbison JW. Ticlopidine hydrochloride. In: Messerli FH. Cardiovascular Drug Therapy. Philadelphia: W. B. Saunders, 1996; 1465–1473.
9. Mills DC, Puri R, Hu CJ, Minniti C, Grana G, Freedman MD, Colman RF, Colman RW. Clopidogrel inhibits the binding of ADP analogues to the receptor mediating inhibition of platelet adenylate cyclase. Arterioscler Thromb 1992; 12:430–436.
10. Schafer AI. Antiplatelet therapy. Am J Med 1996; 101:199–209.
11. Quinn MJ, Fitzgerald DJ. Ticlopidine and clopidogrel. Circulation 1999; 100:1667–1672.
12. Gachet C, Cattaneo M, Ohlmann P, Hechler B, Lecchi A, Chevalier J, Cassel D, Mannucci PM, Cazenave JP. Purinoceptors on blood platelets: further pharmacological and clinical evidence to suggest the presence of two ADP receptors. Br J Haemotol 1995; 91:434–444.
13. Hourani SM, Hall DA. Receptors for ADP on human blood platelets. Trends Pharmacol Sci 1994; 15:103–108.
14. Geiger J, Brich J, Honig–Liedl P, Eigenthaler M, Schanzenbacher P, Herbert JM, Walter U. Specific impairment of human platelet P2Y(AC) ADP receptor-mediated signaling by the antiplatelet drug clopidogrel. Arterioscler Thromb Vasc Biol 1999; 19: 2007–2011.
15. Hechler B, Eckly A, Ohlmann P, Cazenave JP, Gachet C. The P2Y1 receptor, necessary but not sufficient to support full ADP-induced platelet aggregation, is not the target of the drug clopidogrel. Br J Haemotol 1998; 103: 858–866.
16. Hollopeter G, Jantzen HM, Vincent D, Li G, England L, Ramakrishnan V, Yang RB, Nurden P, Nurden A, Julius D, Conley PB. Identification of the platelet ADP receptor targeted by antithrombotic drugs. Nature 2001; 409:202–207.
17. Coukell AJ, Markham A. Clopidogrel. Drugs 1997; 54:745–750.
18. Harker LA, Bruno JJ. Ticlopidine's mechanism of action on platelets. In: Hass WK, Easton JD, eds. Ticlopidine, Platelets, and Vascular Disease. New York: Springer-Verlag, 1993:41–59.
19. Cadroy Y, Bossavy JP, Thalamas C, Sagnard L, Sakariassen K, Boneu B. Early potent antithrombotic effect with combined aspirin and a loading dose of clopidogrel on experimental arterial thrombogenesis in humans. Circulation 2000; 101:2823–2838.
20. Savcic M, Hauert J, Bachmann F, Wyld PJ, Geudelin B, Cariou R. Clopidogrel loading dose regimens: kinetic profile of pharmacodynamic response in healthy subjects. Semin Thromb Hemost 1999; 25:15–19.
21. Helft G, Osende JI, Worthley SG, Zaman AG, Rodriguez OJ, Lev EI, Farkouh ME, Fuster V, Badimon JJ, Chesebro JH. Acute antithrombotic effect of a front-loaded regimen of clopidogrel in patients with atherosclerosis on aspirin. Arterioscler Thromb Vasc Biol 2000; 20:2316–2321.
22. Gawaz M, Neumann FJ, Ott I, May A, Rudinger S, Schomig A. Platelet activation and coronary stent implantation. Effect of antithrombotic therapy. Circulation 1996; 94:279–285.
23. Roald HE, Barstad RM, Kierulf P, Skjorten F, Dickinson JP, Kieffer G, Sakariassen KS. Clopido-

grel—a platelet inhibitor which inhibits thrombogenesis in non-anticoagulated human blood independently of the blood flow conditions. Thromb Haemost 1994;71:655–662.

24. Makkar RR, Eigler NL, Kaul S, Frimerman A, Nakamura M, Shah PK, Forrester JS, Herbert JM, Litvack F. Effects of clopidogrel, aspirin and combined therapy in a porcine ex vivo model of high-shear induced stent thrombosis. Eur Heart J 1998; 19:1538–1546.

25. Kereiakes DJ, Kleiman N, Ferguson JJ, Runyon JP, Broderick TM, Higby NA, Martin LH, Hantsbarger G, McDonald S, Anders RJ. Sustained platelet glycoprotein IIb/IIIa blockade with oral xemilofiban in 170 patients after coronary stent deployment. Circulation 1997; 96:1117–1121.

26. Kereiakes DJ, Kleiman N, Ambrose J, Cohen M, Rodriguez S, Palabrica T, Herrmann HC, Sutton JM, Weaver WD, McKee DB, Fitzpatrick V, Sax FL. Randomized, double–blind, placebo-controlled dose-ranging study of tirofiban (MK-383) platelet IIb/IIIa blockade in high risk patients undergoing coronary angioplasty. J Am Coll Cardiol 1996; 27:536–542.

27. Rupprecht HJ, Darius H, Borkowski U, Voigtlander T, Nowak B, Genth S, Meyer J. Comparison of antiplatelet effects of aspirin, ticlopidine, or their combination after stent implantation. Circulation 1998; 97:1046–1052.

28. Herbert J, Dol F, Bernat A, Falotico R, Lale A, Savi P. The antiaggregating and antithrombotic activity of clopidogrel is potentiated by aspirin in several experimental models in the rabbit. Thromb Haemost 1998; 80:512–518.

29. Uchiyama S, Sone R, Nagayama T, Shibagaki Y, Kobayashi I, Maruyama S, Kusakabe K. Combination therapy with low-dose aspirin and ticlopidine in cerebral ischemia. Stroke 1989; 20:1643–1647.

30. Darius H, Veit K, Rupprecht HJ. Synergistic inhibition of platelet aggregation by ticlopidine plus aspirin following intracoronary stent placement [abstr]. Circulation 1996; 94 (suppl I):I-257.

31. Umemura K, Kondo K, Ikeda Y, Nakashima M. Enhancement by ticlopidine of the inhibitory effect on in vitro platelet aggregation of the glycoprotein IIb/IIIa inhibitor tirofiban. Thromb Haemost 1997; 78:1381–1384.

32. Verstraete M, Zoldhelyi P. Novel antithrombotic drugs in development. Drugs 1995; 49:856–884.

33. Tanahashi N, Fukuuchi Y, Tomita M, Matsuoka S, Takeda H. Ticlopidine improves the enhanced erythrocyte aggregability in patients with cerebral infarction. Stroke 1993; 24:1083–1086.

34. Fagher B, Peterson S, Persson G, Larsson H. Blood viscosity during long-term treatment with ticlopidine in patients with intermittent claudication. A double-blind study. Angiology 1993; 44:300–306.

35. Randi ML, Fabris F, Crociani ME, Battocchio F, Girolami A. Effects of ticlopidine on blood fibrinogen and blood viscosity in peripheral atherosclerotic disease. Arzneimittelforschung 1985; 35:1847–1849.

36. Tohgi H, Takahashi H, Kashiwaya M, Watanabe K. Effect of plasma fibrinogen concentration on the inhibition of platelet aggregation after ticlopidine compared with aspirin. Stroke 1994; 25:2017–2021.

37. Gent M, Blakely JA, Easton JD, Ellis DJ, Hachinski VC, Harbison JW, Panak E, Roberts RS, Sicunella J, Turpie AG. The Canadian American Ticlopidine Study (CATS) in thromboembolic stroke. Lancet 1989; 1:1215–1230.

38. Hass WK, Easton JD, Adams HP Jr, Pryse–Phillips W, Molony BA, Anderson S, Kamm B. A randomized trial comparing ticlopidine hydrochloride with aspirin for the prevention of stroke in high-risk patients. Ticlopidine Aspirin Stroke Study Group. N Engl J Med 1989; 321:501–507.

39. Bellavance A. Efficacy of ticlopidine and aspirin for prevention of reversible cerebrovascular ischemic events. Ticlopidine Aspirin Stroke Study Group. Stroke 1993; 24:1452–1457.

40. Guidelines for treatment for stroke prevention. American College of Physicians. Ann Intern Med 1994; 121:54–55.

41. Bergamasco B, Benna P, Carolei A, Rasura M, Rudelli G, Fieschi C. A randomized trial comparing ticlopidine hydrochloride with indobufen for the prevention of stroke in high-risk patients (TISS study). Ticlopidine Indobufen Stroke Study. Funct Neurol 1997; 12:33–43.

42. Janzon L, Bergqvist D, Boberg J, Boberg M, Eriksson I, Lindgarde F, Persson G, Almgren B, Fagher B, Kjellstrom T. Prevention of myocardial infarction and stroke in patients with intermittent

claudication; effects of ticlopidine. Results from STIMS, the Swedish Ticlopidine Multicentre Study. J Intern Med 1990; 227:301–308.

43. Fagher B. Long-term effects of ticlopidine on lower limb blood flow, ankle/brachial index and symptoms in peripheral arteriosclerosis. A double–blind study. The STIMS Group in Lund. Swedish Ticloipdine Multicenter Study. Angiology 1994; 45:777–788.

44. Balsano F, Coccheri S, Libretti A, Nenci GG, Catalano M, Fortunato G, Grasselli S, Violi F, Hellemans H, Vanhove P. Ticlopidine in the treatment of intermittent claudication: a 21-month double-blind trial. J Lab Clin Med 1989; 114:84–91.

45. Arcan JC, Blanchard J, Boissel JP, Destors JM, Panak E. Multicenter double-blind study of ticlopidine in the treatment of intermittent claudication and the prevention of its complications. Angiology 1988; 39:802–811.

46. Qian S, Iwai T. Effect of ticlopidine on the cutaneous circulation in peripheral vascular disease. Angiology 1993; 44:627–631.

47. Katsumura T, Mishima Y, Kamiya K, Sakaguchi S, Tanabe T, Sakuma A. Therapeutic effect of ticlopidine, a new inhibitor of platelet aggregation, on chronic arterial occlusive diseases, a double-blind study versus placebo. Angiology 1982; 33:357–367.

48. Blanchard J, Carreras LO, Kindermans M, the EMATAP Group. Results of EMATAP: a double-blind placebo-controlled multicentre trial of ticlopidine in patients with peripheral arterial disease. Nouv Rev Fr Hematol 1993; 35:523–528.

49. CAPRIE Steering Committee. A randomized, blinded trial of clopidogrel versus aspirin in patients at risk of ischaemic events (CAPRIE). Lancet 1996; 348:1329–1339.

50. Bhatt DL, Marso SP, Hirsch AT, Ringleb P, Hacke W, Topol EJ. Superiority of clopidogrel versus aspirin in patients with a history of diabetes mellitus [abstr]. J Am Coll Cardiol. 2000; 35:409A.

51. Bhatt DL, Hirsch AT, Chew DP, Ringleb P, Hacke W, Topol EJ. Marked superiority of clopidogrel versus aspirin in patients with a history of previous cardiac surgery [abstr]. J Am Coll Cardiol 2000; 35:383A.

52. Balsano F, Rizzon P, Violi F, Scrutinio D, Cimminiello C, Aguglia F, Pasotti C, Rudelli G. Antiplatelet treatment with ticlopidine in unstable angina. A controlled multicenter trial. The Studio della Ticlopidina nell'Angina Instabile Group. Circulation 1990; 82:17–26; 53.

53. Gent M. Benefit of clopidogrel in patients with coronary artery disease. [abstr]. Circulation. 1997; 96(suppl I):I-467.

54. Moussa I, DiMario C, Reimers B, Akiyama T, Tobis J, Colombo A. Subacute stent thrombosis in the era of intravascular ultrasound-guided coronary stenting without anticoagulation: frequency, predictors and outcome. J Am Coll Cardiol 1997; 29:6–12.

55. Hasadi D, Garratt KN, Holmes DR Jr, Berger PB, Schwartz RS, Bell MR. Coronary angioplasty and intracoronary lysis are of limited efficacy in resolving early intracoronary stent thrombosis. J Am Coll Cardiol 1996; 28:361–367.

56. Mak KH, Belli G, Ellis SG, Moliterno DJ. Subacute stent thrombosis: evolving issues and current concepts. J Am Coll Cardiol 1996; 27: 494–503.

57. Sigwart U, Puel J, Mirkovitch V, Joffre F, Kappenberger L. Intravascular stenting to prevent occlusion and restenosis after transluminal angioplasty. N Engl J Med. 1987; 316:701–706.

58. Wong SC, Baim DS, Schatz RA, Teirstein PS, King SB 3rd, Curry RC Jr, Heuser RR, Ellis SG, Cleman MW, Overlie P. Immediate results and late outcomes after stent implantation in saphenous vein graft lesions: the multicenter US. Palmaz–Schatz stent experience. The Palmaz–Schatz Stent Study Group. J Am Coll Cardiol 1995; 26:704–712.

59. Eeckhout E, Kappenberger L, Goy JL. Stents for intracoronary placement: current status and future directions. J Am Coll Cardiol 1996; 27:757–765.

60. Bittl JA. Advances in coronary angioplasty. N Engl J Med 1996; 335:1290–1302.

61. Serruys PW, Strauss BH, Beatt KJ, Bertrand ME, Puel J, Rickards AF, Meier B, Goy JJ, Vogt P, Kappenberger L. Angiographic follow-up after placement of a self-expanding coronary-artery stent. N Engl J Med 1991; 324:13–17.

62. Serruys PW, de Jaegere P, Kiemeneij F, Macaya C, Rutsch W, Heyndrickx G, Emmanuelson H, Marco J, Legrand V, Materne P. A comparison of balloon-expandable stent implantation with balloon

angioplasty in patients with coronary artery disease. Benestent Study Group. N Engl J Med 1994; 331:489–495.

63. Fischman DL, Leon MB, Baim DS, Schatz RA, Savage MP, Penn I, Detre K, Veltri L, Ricci D, Nobuyoshi M. A randomized comparison of coronary-stent placement and balloon angioplasty in the treatment of coronary artery disease. Stent Restenosis Study Investigators. N Engl J Med 1994; 331:496–501.

64. More RS, Chauhan A. Antiplatelet rather than anticoagulant therapy with coronary stenting. Lancet 1997; 349:146–147.

65. Karrillon GJ, Morice MC, Benveniste E, Benouf P, Aubry, Cattan S, Chevalier B, Commeau P, Cribier A, Eiferman C, Grollier G, Guerin Y, Henry M, Lefevre T, Livarek B, Louvard Y, Marco J, Makowski S, Monassier JP, Pernes JM, Rioux P, Spaulding C, Zemour G. Intracoronary stent implantation without ultrasound guidance and with replacement of conventional anticoagulation by antiplatelet therapy. Circulation 1996; 94:1519–1527.

66. Colombo A, Hall P, Nakamura S, Almagor Y, Maiello L, Martini G, Gaglione A, Goldberg SC, Tobis JM. Intracoronary stenting without anticoagulation accomplished with intravascular ultrasound guidance. Circulation 1995; 91:1676–1788.

67. Nakamura S, Hall P, Gaglione A, Tiecco F, Di Maggio M, Maiello L, Martini G, Columbo A. High pressure assisted coronary stent implantation accomplished without intravascular ultrasound guidance and subsequent anticoagulation. J Am Coll Cardiol 1997; 29:21–27.

68. Schomig A, Neumann FJ, Kastrati A, Schuhlen H, Blasini R, Hadamitzky M, Walter H, Zitzmann–Roth EM, Richardt G, Alt E, Schmitt C, Ulm K. A randomized comparison of antiplatelet and anticoagulant therapy after the placement of coronary artery stents. N Engl J Med 1996; 334:1084–1089.

69. Dirschinger J, Schuhlen H, Walter H, Hadamitzky M, Zitzmann EM, Wehinger A. Intracoronary stenting and antithrombotic regimen trial: 1-year clinical follow-up [abstr]. Circulation 1997; 94(suppl I):I-257.

70. Leon MB, Baim DS, Popma JJ, Gordon PC, Cutlip DE, Ho KK, Giambartolomei A, Diver DJ, Lasorda DM, Williams DO, Pocock SJ, Kuntz RE. A clinical trial comparing three antithrombotic-drug regimens after coronary-artery stenting. Stent Anticoagulation Restenosis Study Investigators. N Engl J Med 1998; 339:1665–1671.

71. Mishkel GJ, Aguirre FV, Ligon RW, Rocha–Singh KJ, Lucore CL. Clopidogrel as adjunctive antiplatelet therapy during coronary stenting. J Am Coll Cardiol. 1999; 34:1884–1890.

72. Berger PB, Bell MR, Rihal CS, Ting H, Barsness G, Garratt K, Bellot V, Mathew V, Melby S, Hammes L, Grill D, Holmes DR Jr. Clopidogrel versus ticlopidine after intracoronary stent placement. J Am Coll Cardiol 1999; 34:1891–1894.

73. Moussa I, Oetgen M, Roubin G, Colombo A, Wang X, Iyer S, Maida R, Collins M, Kreps E, Moses JW. Effectiveness of clopidogrel and aspirin versus ticlopidine and aspirin in preventing stent thrombosis after coronary stent implantation. Circulation 1999; 99:2364–2366.

74. Müller C, Büttner HJ, Petersen J, Roskamm H. A randomized comparison of clopidogrel and aspirin versus ticlopidine and aspirin after the placement of coronary-artery stents. Circulation 2000; 101:590–593.

75. Ticlopidine Or Plavix Post Stent (TOPPS) study. Presented at Transcatheter Cardiovascular Therapeutics Conference, 2000.

76. Bhatt DL, Bertrand ME, Berger PB, L'Allier PL, Moussa I, Moses JW. Reduction in major adverse cardiac events, including mortality, after stenting using clopidogrel instead of ticlopidine [abstr]. Circulation 2000; 102;II-565.

77. Bertrand ME, Legrand V, Boland J, Fleck E, Bonnier J, Emmanuelson H, Vrolix M, Missault L, Chierchia S, Casaccia M, Niccoli L, Oto A, White C, Webb–Peploe M, Van belle E, McFadden EP. Randomized multicenter comparison of conventional anticoagulation versus antiplatelet therapy in unplanned and elective coronary stenting. The full anticoagulation versus aspirin and ticlopidine (FANTASTIC) study. Circulation 1998; 98:1597–1603.

78. Steinhubl S, Lauer M, Mukherjee D, Moliterno D, Lincoff A, Ellis S, Topol E. The duration of pretreatment with ticlopidine prior to stenting is associated with the risk of procedure-related non–Q-wave myocardial infarctions. J Am Coll Cardiol 1998; 32:1366–1370.

79. vom Dahl J, Klues HG, Reffelamann T, Hendricks F, Hanrath P. Combined antiplatelet pretreatment with aspirin and ticlopidine reduces in-hospital cardiac events following elective coronary angioplasty [abstr]. J Am Coll Cardiol 1997; 29(suppl A):98A.

80. Goldberg SL, Colombo A, Maiello L, Borrione M, Finci L, Almagor Y. Intracoronary stent insertion after balloon angioplasty of chronic total occlusions. J Am Coll Cardiol 1995; 26:713–719.

81. Sirnes PA, Golf S, Myreng Y, Molstad P, Emmanuelson H, Albertsson P, Brekke M, Mangschau A, Endresen K, Kjekshus J. Stenting in Chronic Coronary Occlusion (SICCO): a randomized, controlled trial of adding stent implantation after successful angioplasty. J Am Coll Cardiol 1996; 28:1444–1451.

82. Savage MP, Douglas JS Jr, Fischman DL, Pepine CJ, King SB 3rd, Werner JA, Bailey SR, Overlie PA, Fenton SH, Brinker JA, Leon MB, Goldberg S. Stent placement compared with balloon angioplasty for obstructed coronary bypass grafts. Saphenous Vein De Novo Trial Investigators. N Engl J Med 1997; 337:740–747.

83. de Jaegere PP, van Domburg RT, Feyter PJ, Ruygrok PN, van der Giessen WJ, van den Brand MJ, Serruys PW. Long-term clinical outcome after stent implantation in saphenous vein grafts. J Am Coll Cardiol 1996; 28:89–96.

84. Schomig A, Neumann FJ, Walter H, Schuhlen H, Hadamitzsky M, Zitzmann–Roth EM, Dirschinger J, Hausleiter J, Blasini R, Schmitt C, Alt E, Kastrati A. Coronary stent placement in patients with acute myocardial infarction: comparison of clinical angiographic outcome after randomization to antiplatelet or anticoagulation therapy. J Am Coll Cardiol 1997; 29:28–34.

85. Stone GW, Brodie BR, Griffin JJ, Morice MC, Costantini C, St. Goar FG, Overlie PA, Popoma JJ, McDonell JJ, Jones D, O'Neill WW, Grines CL. Prospective, multicenter study of the safety and feasibility of primary stenting in acute myocardial infarction: in-hospital and 30-day results of the PAMI Stent Pilot Trial. Primary Angioplasty in Myocardial Infarction (PAMI) Stent Pilot Trial Investigators. J Am Coll Cardiol 1998; 31:23–30.

86. Grines CL, Cox DA, Stone GW, Garcia E, Mattos LA,Giambartolomei A, Brodie BR, Madonna O, Eijgelshoven M, Lansky AJ, O'Neill WW, Morice MC. Coronary angioplasty with or without stent implantation for acute myocardial infarction. Stent Primary Angioplasty in Myocardial Infarction Study Group. N Engl J Med 1999; 341:1949–1956.

87. Leon MB, Ellis SG, Moses J, King SB 3rd, Heuser R, Kent KM. Interim report from the Reduced Anticoagulation Vein Graft Stent (RAVES) study [abstr]. J Am Coll Cardiol 1997; 29(suppl A):683A.

88. Itoh A, Hall P, Maiello L, Di Mario C, Moussa I, Blengino S, Ferraro M, Martinin G, Di Francesco L, Finci L, Colombo A. Intracoronary stent implantation in native coronary arteries and saphenous vein grafts: a consecutive experience with six types of stents without prolonged anticoagulation. Mayo Clin Proc 1997; 72:101–111.

89. Teirstein PS, Massullo V, Jani S, Popma JJ, Mintz GS, Russo RJ. Catheter-based radiotherapy to inhibit restenosis after coronary stenting. N Engl J Med 1997; 336:1697–1703.

90. Raizner AE, Oesterle SN, Waksman R, Serruys PW, Colombo A, Lim YL, Yeung AC, van der Giessen WJ, Vandertie L, Chiu JK, White LR, Fitzgerald PJ, Kaluza GL, Ali NM. Inhibition of restenosis with beta-emitting radiotherapy: report of the Proliferation Reduction with Vascular Energy Trial (PREVENT). Circulation 2000; 102:951–958.

91. Leon MB, Teirstein PS, Moses JW, Tripuraneni P, Lansky AJ, Jani S, Wong SC, Fish D, Ellis S, Holmes DR, Kerieakes D, Kuntz RE. Localized intracoronary gamma-radiation therapy to inhibit the recurrence of restenosis after stenting. N Engl J Med 2001; 344:250–256.

92. Costa MA, Sabaté M, van der Giessen et al. Late coronary occlusion after intracoronary brachytherapy. Circulation 1999; 100:789–792.

93. Chevigne M, David JL, Rigo P, Limet R. Effect of ticlopidine on saphenous vein bypass patency rates: a double-blind study. Ann Thorac Surg 1984; 37:371–378.

94. Limet R, David JL, Magotteaux P, Larock MP, Rigo P. Prevention of aorta–coronary bypass graft occlusion. Beneficial effect of ticlopidine on early and late patency rates of venous coronary bypass grafts: a double–blind study. J Thorac Cardiovasc Surg. 1987; 94:773–783.

95. Becquemin JP. Effect of ticlopidine on the long-term patency of saphenous-vein grafts in the legs. Etude de la Ticlopidine Apres Pontage Femore–Poplite and the Assocaition Universitaire de Recherche en Chirurgie. N Engl J Med 1997; 337:1726–1731.

96. TIMAD Study Group. Ticlopidine treatment reduces the progression of nonproliferative diabetic retinopathy. Arch Ophthalmol 1990; 108:1577–1583.
97. Shear NH, Appel C. Prevention of ischemic stroke. N Engl J Med 1995; 333:460.
98. Page Y, Tardy B, Zeni F, Comtet C, Terrana R, Bertrand JC. Thrombotic thrombocytopenic purpura related to ticlopidine. Lancet 1991; 337:774–776.
99. Ellie E, Durrieu C, Besse P, Julien J, Gbipki–Benissan G. Thrombotic thrombocytopenic purpura associated with ticlopidine. Stroke 1992; 23:922–923.
100. Kovacs MJ, Soong PY, Chin–Yee IH. Thrombotic thrombocytopenic purpura associated with ticlopidine. Ann Pharmacother 1993; 27:1060–1061.
101. Bennett CL, Weinberg PD, Rozenberg–Ben–Dror K, Yarnold PR, Kwaan HC, Green D. Thrombotic thrombocytopenic purpura associated with ticlopidine. A review of 60 cases. Ann Intern Med 1998; 128:541–544.
102. Bennett CL, Davidson CJ, Raisch DW, Weinberg PD, Bennett PD, Feldman MD. Thrombotic thrombotycopenic purpura associated with ticlopidine in the setting of coronary stroke prevention. Arch Intern Med 1999; 159:2524–2528.
103. Bennett CL, Connors JM, Carwile JM, Moake JL, Bell WR, Tarantolo SR, McCarthy LJ, Sarode R, Hatfield AJ, Feldman MD, Davidson CJ, Tsai HM. Thrombotic thrombocytopenic purpura associated with clopidogrel. N Engl J Med 2000; 342:1773–1777.
104. Bennett CL, Connors JM, Moake JL. Clopidogrel and thrombocytopenic purpura [reply to Letters to Editor]. N Engl J Med 2000; 343:1193–1194.
105. Takashita S, Kawazoe N, Yoshida T, Fukiyama K. Ticlopidine and thrombocytopenia [letter]. N Engl J Med 1990; 323:1487–1488.
106. Yeh SP, Hsueh EJ, Wu H, Wang YC. Ticlopidine-associated aplastic anemia. A case report and review of the literature. Ann Hematol 1998; 76:87–90.
107. Grimm IS, Litynski JJ. Severe cholestasis associated with ticlopidine. Am J Gastroenterol 1994; 89:279–280.
108. Naschitz JE, Khamessi R, Elias N, Yeshurun D. Ticlopidine-induced prolonged cholestasis. J Toxicol Clin Toxicol 1995; 33:379–380.
109. Rosen H, el-Hennawy AS, Greenberg S, Chen CK, Nicastri AD. Acute interstitial nephritis associated with ticlopidine. Am J Kidney Dis 1995; 25:934–936.
110. Wysowski DK, Bacsanyi J. Blood dyscrasias and hematologic reactions in ticlopidine users. JAMA 1996; 276:952.
111. Shah J, Fratis A, Ellis D, Murakami S, Teitelbaum P. Effect of food and antacid on absorption of orally administered ticlopidine hydrochloride. J Clin Pharmacol 1990; 30:733–736.
112. Boissonnat P, de Lorgeril M, Perroux V, Salen P, Batt AM, Barthelemy JC, Brourard P, Serres E, Delaye J. A drug interaction study between ticlopidine and cyclosporin in heart transplant recipients. Eur J Clin Pharmacol 1997; 53:39–45.
113. Riva R, Cerullo A, Albani F, Baruzzi A. Ticlopidine impairs phenytoin clearance: a case report. Neurology 1996; 46:1172–1173.
114. Brown RI, Cooper TG. Ticlopidine–carbamazepine interaction in a coronary stent patient. Can J Cardiol 1997; 13:853–854.
115. Colli A, Buccino G, Cocciolo M, Parravicini R, Elli GM, Scaltrini G. Ticlopidine–theophylline interaction. Clin Pharmacol Ther 1987; 41:358–362.
116. Calpain H, Thebault JJ, Necciari J. Clopidogrel does not affect the pharmacokinetics of theophylline. Semin Thromb Hemost 1999; 25(suppl 2):65–68.

28

Oral Antiplatelet Therapies Beyond Aspirin and Thienopyridines

Shaker A. Mousa
Albany College of Pharmacy, Albany, New York, U.S.A.

Konstantinos Konstantopoulos
John Hopkins University, Baltimore, Maryland, U.S.A.

Robert P. Giugliano
Harvard Medical School and Brigham and Women's Hospital, Boston, Massachussets, U.S.A.

I. INTRODUCTION

Intravascular thrombosis is one of the most frequent pathological events affecting mankind and a major cause of morbidity and mortality in developed countries. There is abundant evidence suggesting that platelets play a pivotal role in the pathogenesis of arterial thrombotic disorders, including unstable angina (UA), myocardial infarction (MI), and stroke [1–3]. The underlying pathophysiological mechanism of these processes has been recognized as the disruption or erosion of a vulnerable atherosclerotic plaque leading to local platelet adhesion, activation, and subsequent formation of partially or completely occlusive platelet thrombi. Moreover, large-scale clinical trials have documented the benefit of antiplatelet therapy in acute coronary syndromes [1,4,5]. Aspirin is the prototypical platelet inhibitor that blocks thromboxane A_2-dependent platelet aggregation, and represents the standard reference compound for the management of acute MI, UA, and secondary prevention of MI [1]. Newer-generation antiplatelet drugs, such as ticlopidine and clopidogrel, which are adenosine diphosphate (ADP) receptor antagonists, have also been introduced in clinical practice [4]. Although all of the aforementioned agents have demonstrated clinical benefit, significant mortality still occurs, presumably because they are not effective against platelet aggregation in response to all agonists. The final common step in homotypic platelet aggregate formation, regardless of the stimulus, involves the interaction of the adhesive proteins such as fibrinogen and von Willebrand's factor (vWF) with the platelet GP IIb/IIIa receptor [6,7]. Hence, this platelet integrin receptor has emerged as a rational therapeutic target in the management of acute coronary syndromes.

This chapter highlights the benefits and limitations of various antiplatelet therapies, ranging from aspirin and clopidogrel to platelet GP IIb/IIIa antagonists and beyond in thrombotic disorders, and presents future directions in the antithrombotics.

II. DIFFERENTIAL RESPONSES OF THE VARIOUS GP IIb/IIIa ANTAGONISTS

Platelet GP IIb/IIIa antagonists can be distinguished on the basis of their chemical nature (i.e., monoclonal antibody, linear peptide, cyclic peptide, peptidomimetic, or nonpeptide); route of administration (intravenous or oral), binding kinetics profiles (K_d) to activated versus unactivated platelet GP IIb/IIIa, and differences in the platelet dissociation rate constants (K_{off}). For instance, abciximab binds to both resting and activated platelet GP IIb/IIIa receptors with comparable K_d values, and exhibits relatively slow platelet dissociation rates [8–10]. Limited GP IIb/IIIa receptor occupancy by abciximab can be detected even 7–14 days after drug administration, presumably because abciximab is redistributed on the surface of newly released platelets [11]. Consequently, abciximab exhibits prolonged inhibitory effects [11], and restoration of normal platelet function requires synthesis of new platelets. In distinct contrast, eptifibatide, and tirofiban display relatively higher affinity for the activated, rather than the resting, form of GP IIb/IIIa along with relatively fast platelet dissociation rates [9]. Their inhibitory effects on platelet function usually resolve within 4–8 h of discontinuation of drug administration [12].

Accumulating evidence suggests that relatively short infusions (24–36 h) of rapidly reversible GP IIb/IIIa inhibitors such as eptifibatide and tirofiban result in early reduction in recurrent ischemic complications after percutaneous coronary intervention (PCI), with a loss of significance of the reduction at the later time points [13,14]. One notable difference between abciximab and eptifibatide or tirofiban is that the former exhibits a long receptor-bound lifetime with antiplatelet efficacy detected even 7 days after administration [11,12]. This finding along with the beneficial effects of relatively long infusions (2–4 days) of eptifibatide and tirofiban [15,16] suggest that the prolonged antiplatelet efficacy of the GP IIb/IIIa antagonists might be responsible for their sustained clinical benefit.

Sustained antiplatelet efficacy can be achieved with intravenous bolus and infusion regimens. However, ex vivo monitoring has to reflect the actual in vivo antiplatelet efficacy to optimize therapeutic dose-regimens and thus achieve clinical benefit. Citrated platelet-rich plasma (cPRP) aggregation using light transmittance aggregometry has been the most commonly used method for assessing the pharmacodynamic effects of the various GP IIb/IIIa antagonists in clinical trials. Unfortunately, the anticoagulant citrate partially chelates calcium that is necessary for maintaining the integrity of the GP IIb/IIIa receptor complex, which is a calcium-dependent association of the GP IIb and GP IIIa subunits, and for optimal receptor–ligand binding. Consequently, the ex vivo potency of certain GP IIb/IIIa antagonists can be artificially enhanced in the presence of citrate as opposed to a non–calcium-chelating anticoagulant such as heparin [9,17]. Evidence suggests that the platelet dissociation rate constant (K_{off}) appears to be the major determinant affecting the antiplatelet efficacy of a GP IIb/IIIa antagonist in response to changes in plasma calcium levels [9]. Antiplatelet efficacy of GP IIb/IIIa antagonists with relatively slow platelet dissociation rates, such as abciximab is not affected by changes in plasma calcium concentrations. In contrast, antiplatelet efficacy of agents with relatively fast dissociation rates, such as eptifibatide and others is significantly affected by changes in plasma calcium levels. Consequently, several studies have recommended the use of non–calcium-chelating anticoagulants along with a whole blood, rather than PRP platelet functional assay to determine the true antiplatelet efficacy of GP IIb/IIIa antagonists [9,17].

Small-molecule nonpeptide GP IIb/IIIa antagonists exhibiting high affinity for both resting and activated forms of GP IIb/IIIa, along with relatively slow platelet dissociation rates, have also been developed (e.g., XV454, roxifiban; DuPont Pharmaceuticals, Co.) [8,18,19]. A key feature among all nonpeptide GP IIb/IIIa receptor antagonists is the presence of an anionic carboxy acid terminal (COO−) separated by a spatial chemical moiety and certain distance from the cationic basic amine terminal (benzamidine, piperidine, guanidine). The distance between the anionic and cationic terminals is very critical for optimal affinity binding and specificity to the platelet GP IIb/IIIa receptors with minimal to no cross-reactivity with other closely related RGD-dependent integrins such as $\alpha_v\beta_3$, $\alpha_v\beta_5$, and $\alpha_5\beta_1$. The potential clinical advantages or disadvantages of class I (e.g., abciximab, XV454, roxifiban) versus class II (e.g., eptifibatide, tirofiban, and others) GP IIb/IIIa antagonists remain to be defined in clinical trials.

III. PROLONGED THERAPY WITH PLATELET GP IIb/IIIa ANTAGONISTS: INSIGHTS FROM CLINICAL TRIALS

The new class of intravenous GP IIb/IIIa antagonists combined with aspirin and heparin decrease the incidence of death and ischemic events in patients undergoing PCI, as well as in patients with acute coronary syndrome. Several lines of evidence suggest that complex or ulcerated plaques that may promote further thrombotic events persist for up to, or more than, 1 month after the acute event. Consequently, it has been hypothesized that long-term administration of oral GP IIb/IIIa antagonists might stabilize intravascular plaque and prevent additional ischemic events. Of note, oral GP IIb/IIIa inhibitors are typically prodrugs, requiring liver transformation to yield active antagonism.

Recent clinical experiences with the oral platelet GP IIb/IIIa antagonists xemilofiban, orbofiban, and sibrafiban were disappointing. The evaluation of Oral Xemilofiban in Controlling Thrombotic Events (EXCITE) clinical trial with 7232 patients scheduled for elective PCI did not show a benefit in combined endpoints (death, nonfatal MI, or urgent revascularization) at 30 days and 6 months [20]. The Orbofiban in Patients with Unstable Coronary Syndromes (OPUS-TIMI 16) trial, which included 10,302 patients who had had an acute coronary syndrome within the previous 72 h, also failed to show a benefit in the primary composite endpoint (death, MI, recurrent ischemia requiring rehospitalization, urgent revascularization, or stroke) [21]. This study was also stopped prematurely because of excess mortality in the orbofiban-treated group. However, it is noteworthy that the increased mortality rate occurred in patients with creatinine clearance of less than 90 mL/min, suggesting that the dose may need to be individualized.

In EXCITE and OPUS-TIMI 16, the oral GP IIb/IIIa inhibitor was added to background aspirin treatment, whereas in the Sibrafiban versus Aspirin to Yield Maximum Protection from Ischemic Heart Events Postacute Coronary Syndromes (SYMPHONY) trial low and high doses of sibrafiban were directly compared with the standard aspirin therapy [22]. The SYMPHONY trial and previous dose-ranging studies [22,23] showed clear correlation between the dose of sibrafiban administered with the extent of ex vivo inhibition of platelet aggregation and the rate of bleeding complications. However, the frequency of the primary endpoint (death, nonfatal MI, or severe recurrent ischemia) did not differ between sibrafiban and aspirin groups at 90-days. Furthermore, sibrafiban administration was associated with a higher frequency of hemorrhage.

The lack of clinical benefit for the oral GP IIb/IIIa antagonists as compared with the well-documented benefit with the intravenous agents is puzzling. A likely explanation might be the paucity of a significant and sustained in vivo platelet GP IIb/IIIa blockade owing to a possible overestimation of the ex vivo antiplatelet efficacy of the aforementioned inhibitors (class II GP IIb/IIIa antagonists displaying fast K_{off} rates) as determined in citrated PRP specimens [9]. Along these lines, pharmacokinetic characteristics such as the uptake or elimination of the oral inhibitors might have also led to variable and possibly insufficient plasma concentrations between doses. Furthermore, a substantial proportion of patients in the OPUS-TIMI 16 and SYMPHONY trials might not have been at risk of thrombotic events after stabilization of the acute coronary syndrome. The results of the CAPTURE and PARAGON-B clinical trials indicate that intravenous GP IIb/IIIa inhibitors were most effective in patients with raised serum troponin T levels [24,25]. Perhaps, high-risk patients such as those with high troponin T levels might also benefit from lengthy treatment with oral GP IIb/IIIa inhibitors. This hypothesis is further supported by results from a subgroup analysis in the FROST trial in which the oral GP IIb/IIIa inhibitor lefradafiban was evaluated for clinical use in patients with acute coronary syndromes without persistent ST elevation [26]. The results indicate that lefradafiban displayed a favorable trend toward a reduction in cardiac events that was particularly evident in patients with raised troponin levels [26]. We hope that other ongoing clinical trials will hopefully yield more critical information on the clinical usefulness of oral GP IIb/IIIa inhibitors.

IV.   ISSUES IN THE CLINICAL USE OF GP IIb/IIIa ANTAGONISTS

A.   Thrombocytopenia with GP IIb/IIIa Inhibitors

Thrombocytopenia is a potential, but rather infrequent, complication of GP IIb/IIIa antagonists that may contribute to hemorrhagic risk. Abciximab administration has been shown to induce thrombocytopenia (platelet count fewer than 100,000 μL) in about 2.4% of patients [27]. Thrombocytopenia also occurs, albeit less frequently, in patients administered small-molecule GP IIb/IIIa antagonists, such as eptifibatide, tirofiban, or lamifiban. The exact mechanisms of thrombocytopenia induced by GP IIb/IIIa antagonists are unknown. It has been postulated that ligand-induced binding site (LIBS) expression in vivo may facilitate the production of antibodies against GP IIb/IIIa and cause subsequent immune thrombocytopenia. However, the association between LIBS expression and the potential to induce thrombocytopenia has yet to be studied in more detail [28].

Development of thrombocytopenia with abciximab is not necessarily a contraindication to subsequent use of GP IIb/IIIa antagonists. Most notably, recent studies have shown that patients who developed severe reversible thrombocytopenia after treatment with abciximab, did not exhibit this adverse side effect when treated with eptifibatide or tirofiban at a later time point [29,30].

B.   Bleeding Risk

All GP IIb/IIIa antagonists (intravenous or oral), because of their steep dose–response relation, have a narrow therapeutic window for antiplatelet efficacy versus bleeding risk. Several studies have documented correlation between the drug dose, the degree of inhibition of platelet function and the frequency of bleeding complications. The bleeding risk associated with the use of GP IIb/IIIa inhibitors in the clinical trials reported here ranges from 0 to 3%.

C.   Monitoring and Dosing of GP IIb/IIIa Antagonists

Ex vivo monitoring has to reflect the actual in vivo platelet responses to determine the optimal therapeutic dose regimens of the various GP IIb/IIIa antagonists. Assuming the existence of a bedside assay to rapidly and accurately assess platelet function, one might be able to titrate the drug dose to a target degree of platelet inhibition; thereby adjusting the dose on the basis of patient platelet state [23]. However, one could initially use fixed-dosing, but lower the dose if repeated bleeding complications were encountered [23]. Such strategies could potentially improve the overall safety of these potent antiplatelet agents and provide optimal benefit.

V. FUTURE CONSIDERATIONS IN THE DEVELOPMENT OF GP IIb/IIIa ANTAGONISTS

GP IIb/IIIa antagonists are one of the most exciting and promising pharmacological advances in the treatment and prevention of various thromboembolic disorders. However, the clinical evolution of these inhibitors has reached a crossroads. Despite the well-documented benefit of intravenous use of GP IIb/IIIa antagonists, the oral agents of this class are facing tremendous challenges owing to the lack of superior benefit over aspirin. Clinical experiences (efficacy/safety ratio) gained with injectable GP IIb/IIIa antagonists will provide valuable insights into the potential of long-term chronic usage of oral GP IIb/IIIa antagonists. However, testing oral agents in long-term indications, such as in secondary prevention of ischemic events after MI or stroke, is considerably more complex. The risk of hemorrhage in these settings might dictate lower levels of inhibition of platelet aggregation than those targeted for short-term indications, such as PCI and in acute coronary syndromes [23,28]. Perhaps, the most challenging question to be addressed with oral GP IIb/IIIa inhibitors is what degree of inhibition of platelet function is needed to yield a clear therapeutic benefit in the absence of serious and less clinically serious bleeding events. Moreover, will these agents be used alone or in combination with other antiplatelet therapies?

It is noteworthy that the oral GP IIb/IIIa inhibitors examined in various clinical investigations exhibited relatively faster dissociation rates than abciximab [10]. In contrast, XV454 and roxifiban are potent GP IIb/IIIa antagonists with long receptor-bound lifetimes, and thus extended antiplatelet effects [10,18]. This prolonged antiplatelet efficacy would avoid the possibility of "on-off" proaggregatory effects of GP IIb/IIIa antagonists that could potentially be observed with oral agents such as orbofiban between doses [28,31]. Consequently, we are tempted to speculate that an oral version of a high-affinity antagonist with slow platelet dissociation rates, such as roxifiban or XV454, might have higher chances for success rather than the short-acting GP IIb/IIIa antagonists, although this aspect still lies in the future. As we gain experience with this new class of agents, the benefits and pitfalls associated with their use will become clearer. Furthermore, newer compounds under consideration for prolonged administration as platelet inhibitors and antithrombotic drugs include among others GP Ib antagonists, inhibitors of thrombin, tissue factor/FVIIa, and FXa.

A. Other Potential GP IIb/IIIa Antagonists Applications

Ample evidence supports the notion that platelets facilitate the hematogenous dissemination of tumor cells. The most convincing evidence is the inhibition of metastasis by experimental thrombocytopenia, and the reconstitution of metastatic potential after platelet repletion [32,33]. However, the mechanisms by which platelets assist metastatic spread are not clearly understood. It has been suggested that platelets, by adhering to tumor cells, provide a protective shield that masks them from the cytotoxic activity of the immune cells [34]. Moreover, platelets may facilitate the escape of tumor cells from the harsh environment of the circulatory system by potentiating tumor cell adhesive interactions with the vessel wall [35]. Alternatively, activated

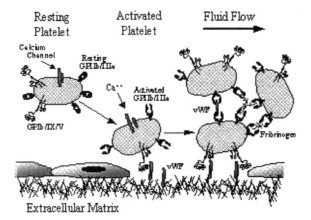

Figure 1 Schematic representation of platelet adhesion to subendothelial matrix and subsequent arterial thrombus formation under high-shear conditions.

platelets may contribute to tumor-induced angiogenesis by releasing potent angiogenesis stimulators [36]. Therefore, blockade of tumor cell–platelet adhesive interactions might provide a potential antimetastatic benefit. We have recently demonstrated that platelet P-selectin and GP IIb/IIIa cooperate to mediate optimal colon carcinoma cell adhesion to immobilized, activated platelets under dynamic flow conditions [37]. Specifically, platelet P-selectin is required for the efficient tethering/rolling of free-flowing colon carcinoma cells in shear flow, whereas subsequent platelet GP IIb/IIIa involvement converts these transient tethering interactions into stable adhesion (Fig. 2) [37,38]. The firm adhesion step is at least partially mediated by vWF which acts to bridge platelet GP IIb/IIIa with a yet unidentified receptor on the colon cancer cell surface (see Fig. 2). GP IIb/IIIa has also been implicated in the interactions of platelets with a variety of melanoma, breast and colon cancer cells [33,39]. Consequently, use of GP IIb/IIIa antagonists, such as XV454 that can effectively interfere with tumor cell–platelet adhesive interactions in vitro [37], might prove to be a promising therapeutic strategy to combat blood-borne metastasis.

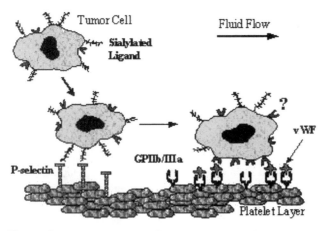

Figure 2 Proposed model of human colon carcinoma cell adhesion to surface-bound immobilized platelets under dynamic flow conditions.

V. OTHER ORAL ANTIPLATELET AGENTS

Several additional oral antiplatelet agents have been developed, studied, and are approved for clinical use. Four of the most promising oral drugs include cilostazol, indobufen, triflusal, and trapadil. Each of these drugs is discussed in detail in the following.

A. Cilostazol

Cilostazol is a quinolinone derivative that inhibits cellular phosphodiesterase (more specific for phosphodiesterase type III) with reversible antiplatelet activity. Initially developed in Japan [40], cilostazol was approved by the Ministry of Health and Welfare in Japan in 1988 for the treatment of intermittent claudication and over 725,000 patients have been treated [41]. In 1999 cilostazol was approved by the U.S. Food and Drug Administration (FDA) [42] following three trials performed in the United States [2,4,5] with an indication for the reduction of symptoms of intermittent claudication, as indicated by an increased walking distance [42,45–48]. Several in-depth reviews of cilostazol have been published [49–53].

The mechanism of the effects of cilostazol on the symptoms of intermittent claudication is not fully understood [48,54–57]. Cilostazol and several of its active metabolites are cyclic AMP (cAMP) phosphodiesterase III inhibitors that inhibit phosphodiesterase activity and suppress cAMP degradation by blocking its hydrolysis, with a resultant increase in cAMP in platelets and blood vessels leading to inhibition of platelet aggregation and vasodilation, respectively [58–64]. In studies comparing inhibition of platelet aggregation, cilostazol has a more potent antiplatelet effect than aspirin (by a factor of 10–30) [58] or even ticlopidine [65,66]. Unlike aspirin, cilostazol does not inhibit prostacyclin I_g (prostacyclin PGI_2) synthesis, which may be important since endothelium-derived PGI_2 potentiates the effects of the inhibition of platelet aggregation by cilostazol [67] and inhibits both primary and secondary aggregation [68].

In addition to its antiplatelet effects, cilostazol is an arterial vasodilator, producing nonhomogeneous dilation of vascular beds, with greater dilation in the femoral bed than in vertebral, carotid, or superior mesenteric arterial beds, probably by its direct action on vascular smooth muscle [54,69–72]. However, the importance of the role of vasodilation in the beneficial effects observed with cilostazol in intermittent claudication is unclear. Cilostazol also produces a reduction in triglycerides and an increase in high-density lipopolysaccharide (HDL)–cholesterol (predominantly HDL-2) of approximately 15 and 10%, respectively [43,73–76], and reduces carotid intima media thickness in diabetics [77]. Cilostazol inhibits smooth-muscle cell proliferation, which may be mediated through increased levels of intracellular cAMP in smooth-muscle cells [78], and is the leading hypothesis explaining its mechanism of action in preventing restenosis [79–82]. Lastly, cilostazol has positive chronotropic activity and also increases levels of brain naturetic peptide [83].

Noncardiovascular effects of cilostazol include bronchodilation [84,85], improved nerve conduction [62,86–88], and increased insulin sensitivity [89] in diabetics, and antiproliferative effect on tumor cells [90,91].

The recommended dose of cilostazol is 100-mg bi.d., which should be taken at least 30 min before or 2 h after meals [92]. Because cilostazol is metabolized extensively by cytochrome P-450 isoenzymes (primarily 3A4, but also 2C19), if concomitant use of inhibitors of this system such as ketoconazole, itraconazole, erythromycin [93], lovastatin [94], diltiazem, or omeprazole [95] are administered, the dose of cilostazol should be decreased to 50 mg b.i.d. [92]. Patients should refrain from drinking grapefruit juice as it also inhibits CPY3A4 and the interaction of grapefruit juice with cilostazol has not been well-characterized. No dose adjustment is required with quinidine [96], aspirin [97], or warfarin [98], as cilostazol does not cause any additional changes on coagulation parameters or pharmacokinetics compared with use of these agents individually.

The dose of cilostazol does not require adjustment in patients with renal [99] or mild liver dysfunction [100], although caution should be exercised in patients with moderate–severe hepatic impairment [100].

1. Clinical Uses

a. Peripheral Arterial Disease. Consistent symptom reduction manifested by increased walking distance and speed were observed in eight randomized placebo-controlled, double-blind trials of twice daily cilostazol (Fig. 3) [92]. The range of improvement reported across the eight clinical trials in patients treated with the 100-mg twice-daily dose, expressed as the median change from baseline, was 17–72%, with intermediate benefit observed for the 50-mg twice-daily dose. Improvements in walking distance were observed within 2–4 weeks after initiating therapy. These results are corroborated by improvements in subjective quality-of-life assessments, functional status, and global evaluations [41]. A randomized, double-blind, placebo-controlled trial [46] compared cilostazol and pentoxifylline, the only two drugs approved by the FDA for intermittent claudication. Mean maximal walking distance was significantly greater for patients receiving cilostazol at every postbaseline visit, whereas results with pentoxifylline were intermediate and not statistically different from placebo. Death, serious adverse advents and withdrawals from treatment were similar in each group, although cilostazol was associated with a higher frequency of minor side effects.

Cilostazol may be especially beneficial in patients with diabetes and atherosclerosis [76,101]. Current evidence suggests cilostazol improves lipid, uric acid, and glucose metabolism in patients with impaired glucose tolerance or type 2 diabetes [74,76], inhibits vascular damage caused by platelet-derived microparticles in diabetics [102], and also increases insulin sensitivity [89]. Cilastozol's favorable, albeit modest, effects on plasma lipoproteins may also contribute to

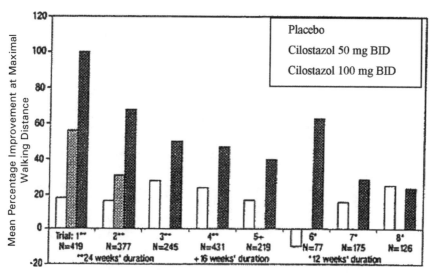

Figure 3 Mean percentage improvement in maximal walking distance at study end for the eight randomized, double-blind, placebo-controlled clinical trials. (From Ref. 53.)

the beneficial effects through improvement in the underlying peripheral arterial disease or coexisting atherosclerotic vascular disease [43,56,73,77], and deserves further investigation.

No large studies comparing cilostazol with thienopyridines (e.g., clopidogrel) for intermittent claudication have been published. In light of the marked benefit of the subgroup of patients with peripheral arterial disease in the CAPRIE trial [103] with clopidogrel, this comparison is necessary to assess the relative efficacy and safety of these potent oral platelet inhibitors.

b. Percutaneous Coronary Intervention. Several studies have demonstrated the usefulness of cilostazol in patients undergoing PCI, with or without stent implantation [79,82,104,105]. Cilostazol significantly reduced restenosis (17.9 vs. 39.5%, p < 0.001) and urgent target lesion revascularization (11.4 vs. 28.7%, p < 0.001) in patients with successful PCI compared with aspirin monotherapy [106]. In another study [107], cilostazol 200 mg/day plus aspirin 81 mg/day reduced restenosis compared with aspirin 81 mg monotherapy in patients undergoing balloon angioplasty (12.5 vs. 43.8%). In this same trial, cilostazol plus aspirin had a lower rate of restenosis compared to ticlopidine 200 mg plus aspirin 243 mg among patients undergoing intracoronary stent implantation (14.3 vs. 32.7%). A second larger study [108] comparing cilostazol versus ticlopidine as add-on therapy to aspirin in patients undergoing stent placement demonstrated no difference in angiographic restenosis (27.0 vs. 22.9%). Cilostazol and ticlopidine, each in combination with aspirin, achieved similar degrees of inhibition of sheer stress-induced platelet inhibition among patients with acute ST-elevation MI undergoing primary PCI [61]. Comparisons of cilostazol with clopidogrel in patients receiving aspirin post-PCI are awaited.

2. Other Uses

Cilostazol may be useful in patients with chronic cerebral ischemia [70–72], and also has been studied in patients with sick-sinus syndrome and other bradyarrhthymias [83,109,110]. However, definitive large-scale trials have not been completed for either indication.

3. Safety

An analysis of the cilostazol safety database summarizing safety data from eight cilostazol phase III controlled clinical trials in 2702 patients (1374 of whom received cilostazol) has been published [111]. There were a total of 475 patient-exposure years in the cilostazol group. Headache, diarrhea, and other gastrointestinal symptoms were observed more frequently in patients receiving cilostazol than those receiving placebo and pentoxifylline. The only adverse event in clinical studies that resulted in discontinuation of therapy in more than 3% of patients was headache (3.5–3.7%) [92–111], and this has been associated with increased flow in the external carotid arteries [112]. Discontinuation of therapy due to headache was dose-related with cilostazol (1.3% for 50 mg b.i.d. vs. 3.7% for 100 mg b.i.d.), and more frequent than with placebo (0.3%).

Because several other phosphodiesterase inhibitors have caused decreased survival compared with placebo in patients with class III–IV heart failure [113,114], cilostazol is contraindicated in patients with congestive heart failure of any severity. Available survival data in nearly 2000 patients studied with cilostazol suggests no increase in the risk of death (RR = 1.2, 95% CI 0.5–3.1); however, there are no longer-term data or studies in patients with more severe underlying heart disease [42]. Postmarketing surveillance in the United States including over 70,000 patient-years of cilostazol exposure has shown minimal accounts of myocardial infarction, stroke, or death. Thus, the safety profile of cilostazol in doses up to

200 mg/p day appears to offer an acceptable risk–benefit ratio in patients with intermittent claudication [111].

B. Indobufen

Indobufen is an isoindolinyl phenylbutyric acid derivative that reversibly inhibits platelet cyclooxygenase [115], resulting in a decreased production of thromboxane B_2 [116,117]. Indobufen inhibits the second wave of platelet aggregation induced by ADP, epinephrine, and platelet-activating factor, and exhibits a dose-dependent inhibitory effect on collagen- and arachidonic acid-induced aggregation [118,119]. Other effects include a reduction in platelet levels of ATP [118], serotonin [120], platelet factor 3 [121–123], platelet factor 4 [122–125], thromboglobulin [124,125], neutrophil activation [126], and impaired platelet adhesion [124,127]. Bleeding times are prolonged slightly, but remain within the upper limits of normal [128–130].

1. Clinical Uses

Two manuscripts review the clinical uses of indobufen in detail [116,131].

a. Peripheral Arterial Disease. Clinical trials in patients with intermittent claudication have consistently demonstrated an increase in pain-free walking and total walking distance with indobufen compared with placebo [132–135]. Two studies comparing indobufen to active control demonstrated that indobufen is superior to aspirin [136], and marginally better than aspirin plus dipyridamole [137], in increasing pain-free and total walking distances.

Indobufen is also effective in maintaining peripheral arterial graft patency following surgical bypass. Patency rates at 1 month and 1 year were similar in patients randomized to indobufen 200 mg b.i.d.–t.i.d. versus the combination of aspirin plus dipyridamole [138]. No large trials have been published comparing indobufen to more potent oral antiplatelet regimens (e.g. aspirin plus clopidogrel, cilostazol) currently in use for treatment of peripheral arterial disease.

b. Cardiogenic Embolism. Indobufen, 100–200 mg b.i.d. was compared with warfarin (INR 2.0–3.5) for 12 months in 916 patients with nonrheumatic atrial fibrillation and a recent cerebral ischemic episode in a randomized equivalence trial [139]. No significant differences in the primary endpoint (composite of nonfatal stroke, pulmonary or systemic embolism, non-fatal MI, and vascular death) were observed between the two treatments, while patients treated with warfarin had more noncerebral bleeding (5.1 vs. 0.6%, $p < 0.01$), and tended to have more cerebral and major gastrointestinal hemorrhage.

Indobufen was superior to placebo in preventing thromboembolic complications in 196 patients with heart disease at high risk for cardiogenic embolism (90 with atrial fibrillation) that were followed for a median of 34.5 months [140]. In a study of indobufen versus aspirin in patients with cerebrovascular disease, no significant differences in new cerebrovascular events were found [141]. Two additional nonrandomized studies suggested that indobufen was effective in secondary prevention of TIA and stroke [142,143]. In a double-blind, placebo-controlled pilot trial [144] of patients undergoing carotid endarterectomy, indobufen, 400-mg daily, was associated with a reduction in platelet accumulation using postoperative scintigraphy, and better ultrasonic tomographic and angiographic outcomes at a minimum of 6 months following surgery.

A metanalysis [145] of five randomized, controlled trials in patients with nonrheumatic atrial fibrillation published between 1989 and 1999 comparing warfarin versus indobufen plus aspirin demonstrated no significant difference in stroke deaths (OR 0.74; 95% CI 0.39–1.40) or vascular deaths (OR 0.86; 95% CI 0.63–1.17). There was a borderline significant reduction in nonfatal stroke with warfarin; however, there was a 45% increase in the odds of major bleeding with warfarin. Limitations of this metanalysis include marked heterogeneity between trials and limited data.

2. Cerebrovascular Disease

Indobufen was inferior to ticlopidine in the Ticlopidine Indobufen Stroke Study (TISS) that randomized 1632 patients with a recent transient ischemic attack, amaurosis fugax, or minor stroke to ticlopidine or indobufen [146]. Treatment with ticlopidine resulted in a 50% reduction in death, MI, or stroke compared with indobufen (2.9 vs. 5.8%; p = 0.004) [146].

    a. Coronary Revascularization. Following several small trials that demonstrated promising results with indobufen following CABG [147,148], two large prospective, randomized, double-blind, 12-month clinical trials, the Studio Indobufene nel Bypass Aortocoronarico [149] (SINBA) and the United Kingdom (UK) study [150], compared indobufen 200 mg twice daily to aspirin plus dipyridamole in patients after CABG surgery. In a combined analyses of these two studies [151], there were no significant differences between the two treatment groups relative to occlusion of the bypass graft or distal anastomoses (Fig. 4). Likewise there was no difference in the rate of major postoperative cardiovascular events (2.7 vs. 3.7%). Fewer adverse events and less gastrointestinal bleeding were seen with indobufen in both trials.

    Indobufen, 400 mg twice daily, and aspirin, 325 mg t.i.d. were compared in 323 patients undergoing PCI. At 6 months, patients receiving indobufen experienced a marginally lower incidence of restenosis (31 vs. 38%) that did not achieve statistical significance [152].

    b. Venous Thromboembolism. In a 3-year study of indobufen (200 mg) compared with placebo, the rate of recurrent DVT was reduced from 46 to 5% with indobufen therapy [153,154]. Among 224 patients with a recent episode of DVT followed for 3 years, rates of recurrent DVT were lowest with indobufen plus graduated compression stockings (2.1%),

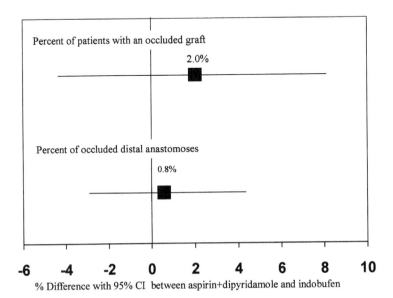

Figure 4 Combined analysis of difference in occlusion of coronary artery bypass graft occlusions at 1-year in a combined analysis [124] comparing aspirin + dipyridamole vs. indobufen. A number greater than 0 indicates fewer occlusions with indobufen.

intermediate if either alone was used (indobufen 5.0%, stockings 9.4%), and highest if neither was used (46%) [153,154]. In a direct comparison with oral acenocoumarol, no significant difference was found in the incidence of DVT as documented by I^{125} fibrinogen scanning in 150 patients with acute MI [155].

   c. Other.   Indobufen may also be useful in preventing platelet aggregation on hemodialysis membranes [156,157] and in the treatment of migraine headaches [158].

3. Safety

Few large studies comparing indobufen with other antiplatelet agents are available to assess the relative safety of indobufen. Lower incidences of adverse effects and drug discontinuation have been reported in patients receiving indobufen compared with high-doses of aspirin (≥ 900 mg) [116]. However, a comparison of the incidence of hemorrhagic events following indobufen versus lower doses (75–325 mg) of aspirin is needed.

C. Triflusal

Triflusal is a 4-trifluoromethyl benzoate derivative of salicylate, structurally similar to aspirin, but exhibiting different pharmacodynamic properties [159–163]. Triflusal has been widely studied for a variety of cardiovascular indications in Europe and Latin America, and appears most promising as a potentially safer alternative to aspirin.

   Triflusal irreversibly inhibits platelet cyclooxygenase, but, unlike aspirin, has only minimal inhibition of endothelial cyclooxygenase, thus having the desirable effect of maintaining prostacyclin synthesis. Triflusal also inhibits platelet phosphodiesterase, with a resulting increase in platelet cAMP levels, which can inhibit platelet activation, whereas this effect is negligible with aspirin [159–161,164–167]. Other actions of triflusal include stimulation of nitric oxide production in neutrophils (to a greater extent than that of aspirin [163,168]); inhibition of superoxide anion release in human neutrophils (an indirect vasodilatory effect); inhibition of transcription factors NF-κB and NF-κB-induced inflammatory mediators, such as the vascular cell adhesion molecule 1 (VCAM-1) [169–171] and other endothelial cell adhesion molecules [163,165]; and a reduction in subendothelial platelets [172]. Most importantly, an active deacetylated metabolite of triflusal [159] potentiates the effect of triflusal on platelet cyclooxygenase, and itself is an inhibitor of platelet cyclooxygenase, increasing the levels of cAMP (greater than the parent compound) [161,172]. This secondary antiplatelet effect of the active metabolite, following initial inhibition by the parent compound, may confer additional efficacy beyond that seen with aspirin.

1. Clinical Studies

   a. Myocardial Infarction.   Triflusal appears to have efficacy similar to aspirin in reducing mortality and cardiovascular events when administered postinfarction with a potential to lower the risk of intracranial hemorrhage in combination with fibrinolytic therapy based on the results of the Triflusal in Myocardial Infarction (TIM) study (Fig. 5) [173]. In this double-blind equivalence trial of triflusal 600 mg daily versus aspirin 300 mg once-daily for 35 days in 2275 patients with recent (<24 h) myocardial infarction (70% treated with fibrinolysis), the null hypothesis of no difference between treatments in the primary composite endpoint of death, nonfatal MI, or nonfatal CVA, was accepted after the fifth data inspection when the lower bound of the 95% confidence limit for superiority was crossed (i.e., p-value for equivalence < 0.05). The frequency of the primary composite were slightly, but not significantly, lower with triflusal (triflusal 9.1 vs. aspirin 10.2%; OR = 0.88; 95% CI 0.63 to 1.23; p-value for super-

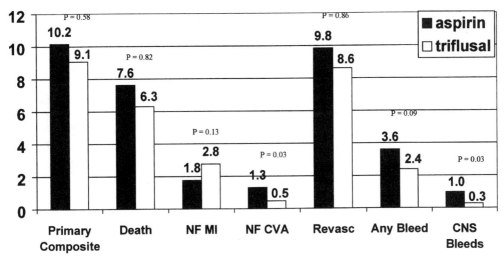

Figure 5 Rates of the primary composite endpoint (death, nonfatal MI, or nonfatal CVA) and other clinically important endpoints in the Triflusal in Myocardial Infarction (TIM) study comparing triflusal with aspirin for 35 days following AMI. p-Values shown are for superiority. The equivalence p-value for the primary composite was < 0.05 (see text for details). NF, non-fatal; MI, myocardial infarction; CVA, stroke; Revasc, revascularization; CNS, central nervous system.

iority $= 0.58$). Rates of death (6.3 vs. 7.6%; $p = 0.28$), nonfatal CVA (0.48 vs. 1.31%; $p = 0.03$), and revascularization (8.6 vs. 9.8%; $p = 0.33$) were all lower with triflusal whereas there was a nonsignificant increase in the rate of nonfatal MI with triflusal (2.8 vs. 1.8%, $p = 0.13$). Of particular interest, triflusal was associated with a significant reduction in CNS bleeding (0.27 vs. 0.97; $p = 0.03$) and a trend toward a reduction in all organ-related bleeding (2.4 vs. 3.6%; $p = 0.09$). If confirmed in other large studies, this latter finding of lower hemorrhagic rates may allow a safer antiplatelet agent (i.e., triflusal) to be substituted for aspirin in patients with increased risk of bleeding. Further studies comparing triflusal with other antiplatelet agents (e.g., clopidogrel) and additional data on its safety and cost-effectiveness are needed [174].

    b. Unstable Angina.   Triflusal 300 mg t.i.d. in a double-blind, placebo-controlled trial of 281 patients with unstable angina reduced the incidence of nonfatal MI from 12 to 4% after 6 months of treatment [175].

    c. Coronary Artery Revascularization.   Triflusal appears moderately effective in preventing vein graft occlusion following CABG [176] and reducing complications after PCI in a retrospective study [177], probably by reducing platelet activation caused by the bypass pump [178]. Triflusal 300 mg daily plus dipyridamole 75 mg t.i.d. reduced graft occlusion at 6 months compared with placebo, and was as effective as the combination of low-dose (50 mg) aspirin plus dipyridamole 75 mg t.i.d. [176].

    d. Peripheral Vascular Disease.   Triflusal, 300 mg twice daily, increased total and pain-free walking distance in a placebo-controlled trial of patients with chronic obliterative peripheral arteriopathy [179]; however, larger confirmatory studies are awaited.

    e. Thrombotic Stroke.   In two small studies [166,180] evaluating triflusal in patients with cerebrovascular disease, favorable trends for clinical benefit with triflusal 900 mg compared with aspirin 330 mg daily were observed in patients treated for 4 years. Preliminary results from larger randomized, double-blind, multicenter trials presented at the International Stroke Conference in February 2001 suggest that triflusal is at least equivalent to aspirin for the prevention of a second stroke, and offers the additional benefit of significantly fewer bleeding complications [181]. Both trials, the Triflusal, Aspirin, Cerebral Infarction Prevention (TACIP) Study [182] and the Triflusal Versus Aspirin for the Prevention of Infarction: A Randomized Stroke Study (TAPIRSS) [183], enrolled patients with recent TIA or stroke and compared the efficacy of triflusal and aspirin administered for 2–3 years in the secondary prevention of cerebral infarction.

   f. Venous Thromboembolism. Triflusal 300 mg was ineffective in reducing thromboembolic complications in studies of patients undergoing hip surgery [184,185]. The observed rates of DVT and PE were similar in a trial comparing triflusal plus heparin with heparin alone [184], and in a latter study [185], there was no difference between patients assigned postoperative triflusal, aspirin, or placebo.

2. Safety

The most common adverse effects of triflusal are nausea, vomiting, epigastric pain, and heartburn, and may occur in up to 15% of patients [164,175,176,179,184,186]. In the largest study to date with triflusal [173], there was no increase in the rate of gastrointestinal hemorrhage compared with aspirin (triflusal 0.9, aspirin 1.5%); however, smaller studies [176,184] have suggested a slightly higher rate of gastric intolerance compared with aspirin. Other reported side effects of triflusal include headache and vertigo [176,179], skin rash [164,175,176,179,184], and photosensitivity [187–190].

D. Trapidil

Trapidil is a potent antiplatelet agent with multiple modes of action. It can be administered either orally or intravenously, has been widely used as an antianginal drug (typical dose 200-mg orally b.i.d. or t.i.d.) in Japan and some European countries for two decades [191], and has been studied in various other conditions, as well [192,193].

   Trapidil has a complex mechanism of action including inhibition of phosphodiesterase types I–IV, thromboxane and its synthesis; antagonism of platelet-derived growth factor by receptor blockade; and stimulation of PGI_2 [191–195]. Trapidil, in vitro, inhibits ADP-, arachidonic acid-, thrombin-, and thromboxane A_2-induced platelet aggregation [196]. In addition to its antiplatelet effects, trapidil is also a coronary vasodilator, with positive inotropic, lusitropic, and chronotropic effects [197]; it is a peripheral arterial dilator that tends to lower diastolic pressure; it is an inhibitor of histamine; is a smooth muscle relaxant; and may have antihyperlipidemic and antiatherosclerotic effects [192,198,199]. Recent studies have shown that trapidil possesses antiproliferative activity in vascular smooth-muscle cells [200,201].

1. Clinical Uses

   a. Percutaneous Coronary Intervention. Trapidil appears to prevent restenosis [198,202–204] perhaps owing to its antagonism of platelet-derived growth factor [202] or inhibition of smooth-muscle cell proliferation [205]. Trapidil may be superior to aspirin alone [198] or the combination of aspirin plus dipyridamole [202]. The largest study to date with trapidil in PCI was the Studio Trapidil versus Aspirin nella Restenosi Coronarica (STARC) trial [198]. This multicenter, randomized, double-blind trial assessed the effects of trapidil in angiographic restenosis prevention of PCI, and found that the restenosis rate in 254 patients undergoing repeat angiography at 6 months was reduced in patients who received trapidil, 100 mg t.i.d. compared with aspirin (24.2 vs. 39.7%; p < 0.01). Clinical events at follow-up were similar in the two groups, except that recurrent angina was significantly more frequent in the aspirin group, 43.7 vs. 25.8% in the trapidil group (p < 0.01). Trapidil was well tolerated, with the same number of patients discontinuing trapidil as in the aspirin group (3%).

A metanalysis [206] concluded that trapidil reduced restenosis after PCI by 40–53% compared with control patients. The rate of per-patient restenosis in the patients receiving trapidil was more than halved compared with controls (OR 0.44; 95% CI 0.29–0.66). Tolerability with trapidil was good, and rare adverse events (gastrointestinal intolerance, thrombocytopenia, headache, increased liver function enzymes) were transient or resolved after therapy was discontinued.

   b.   *Post Myocardial Infarction.*   Limited experience with trapidil in patients following myocardial infarction has been reported. In the Japanese Antiplatelet Myocardial Infarction Study (JAMIS) [207], a multicenter, open-label, randomized controlled trial of aspirin 81 mg/day, trapidil 300 mg/day, or no antiplatelet therapy, 723 patients with a recent (<1 month) myocardial infarction were studied. After a mean follow-up of 475 days, long-term use of aspirin reduced the incidence of recurrent MI compared with no antiplatelet therapy (RR = 0.27; 95% CI 0.10–0.72; p = 0.0045), while the effect of trapidil was borderline (RR = 0.51; 95% CI 0.23–1.10; p = 0.08). The composite incidence of cardiovascular events (cardiovascular death, recurrent MI, unstable angina requiring readmission, ischemic stroke) was reduced by trapidil compared with no antiplatelet therapy (RR = 0.50; 95% CI 0.31–0.80; p = 0.0039), but only a modest effect (RR = 0.79; 95% CI 0.53–1.19; p = 0.20) was seen for aspirin compared with no antiplatelet agent.

   c.   *Angina.*   In several small studies of patients with coronary artery disease, trapidil reduced anginal attacks and use of nitroglycerin [208], increased exercise tolerance [209], delayed the onset of ST segment depression [209], and had beneficial effects on preload and afterload [210,211]. Observations with 4014 patients treated for 12 weeks with trapidil in a medical practice confirmed these clinical benefits, with a low rate of side effects (< 4%), mainly limited to gastrointestinal complaints or headache [212].

2.   Safety

In a Japanese study of 12,227 patients [213], trapidil infrequently caused nausea and vomiting (0.70%), anorexia (0.57%), epigastric discomfort (0.38%), a feeling of abdominal fullness (0.21%), or headaches (0.20%). Rarely, trapidil may cause flushing, orthostatic hypotension, and chest pressure; these may be associated with an excessively rapid intravenous infusion [214]. Allergic dermatological reactions have rarely been observed [214].

VI.   FUTURE CONSIDERATIONS FOR ORAL ANTIPLATELET AGENTS BEYOND GP IIB/IIIA ANTAGONISTS

Antiplatelet agents with anti-inflammatory efficacy as well as other desirable pharmacological effects such as vasodilation or vasorelaxation could be suited for various thromboembolic disorders. Additionally, oral antiplatelet agents could represent a useful adjunct therapy of tumor-associated thrombocytopenia and tumor metastasis. However, additional clinical trials are needed to document those added benefits for an antiplatelet agent.

REFERENCES

1.   Antiplatelet Trialist Collaboration. Collaborative overview of randomized trials of antiplatelet therapy—I: prevention of death, myocardial infarction and stroke by prolonged antiplatelet therapy in various categories of patients. Br Med J 1994; 308:81–106.

2. Fitzgerald DJ, Roy L, Catella F, Fitzgerald GA. Platelet activation in unstable coronary disease. N Engl J Med 1986; 315:983–989.

3. Fuster V. Mechanisms leading to myocardial infarction: insights from studies of vascular biology. Circulation 1994; 90:2126–2146.

4. CAPRIE Steering Committee. A randomised, blinded, trial of clopidogrel versus aspirin in patients at risk of ischaemic events (CAPRIE). Lancet 1996; 348:1329–1339.

5. The CAPTURE Investigators: Randomised placebo-controlled trial of abciximab before and during coronary intervention in refractory unstable angina: the CAPTURE study. Lancet 1997; 349:1429–1435.

6. Konstantopoulos K, Kukreti S, McIntire LV: Biomechanics of cell interactions in shear fields. Adv Drug Deliv Rev 1998; 33:141–164.

7. Pytela R, Pierschbacher MS, Ginsberg MH, Plow EF, Ruoslahti E. Platelet membrane glycoprotein IIb/IIIa: member of a family of RGD specific adhesion receptors. Science 1986; 231:1559–1562.

8. Mousa SA, Bozarth, JM, Lorelli W, Forsythe M., Thoolen M, Slee A, Reilly TM, Friedman PA. Antiplatelet efficacy of XV459, a novel nonpeptide platelet GP IIb/IIIa antagonist: comparative platelet binding profiles with c7E3. J Pharmacol Exp Therap 1998; 286:1277–1284.

9. Mousa SA, Bozarth J, Forsythe MS, Slee A. Differential antiplatelet efficacy for various GP IIb/IIIa antagonists: role of plasma calcium levels. Cardiovasc Res (2000; 47:819–826.

10. Mousa SA, Khurana S, Forsythe MS. Comparative in vitro efficacy of different platelet glycoprotein IIb/IIIa antagonists on platelet-mediated clot strength induced by tissue factor with the use of thromboelastography. Differentiation among glycoprotein IIb/IIIa antagonists. Arterioscler Thromb Vasc Biol 2000; 20:1162–1167.

11. Konstantopoulos K, Kamat SG, Schafer AI, Bañez EI, Jordan R, Kleiman NS, Hellums JD. Shear-induced platelet aggregation is inhibited by in vivo infusion of an anti-glycoprotien IIb/IIIa antibody fragment, c7e3 fab, in patients undergoing coronary angioplasty. Circulation 1995; 91:1427–1431.

12. Kamat SG, Turner NA, Konstantopoulos K, Hellums JD, McIntire LV, Kleiman NS, Moake JL. Effects of integrilin on platelet function in flow models of arterial thrombosis. J Cardiovasc Pharmacol 1997; 29:156–163.

13. The IMPACT II Investigators. Randomised placebo-controlled trial of effect of eptifibatide on complications of percutaneous coronary intervention: IMPACT-II. Integrilin to minimise platelet aggregation and coronary thrombosis–II. Lancet 1997; 349:1422–1428.

14. The RESTORE Investigators. Effects of platelet glycoprotein IIb/IIIa blockade with tirofiban on adverse cardiac events in patients with unstable angina or acute myocardial infarction undergoing coronary angioplasty. Circulation 1997; 96:1445–1453.

15. The PURSUIT Investigators: Inhibition of platelet glycoprotein IIb/IIIa with eptifibatide in patients with acute coronary syndromes. The PURSUIT Trial Investigators. Platelet glycoprotein IIb/IIIa in unstable angina: receptor suppression using integrilin therapy. N Engl J Med 1998; 339:436–443.

16. PRISM-PLUS Study Investigators: Inhibition of the platelet glycoprotein IIb/IIIa receptor with tirofiban in unstable angina and non–Q-wave myocardial infarction. Platelet receptor inhibition in ischemic syndrome management in patients limited by unstable signs and symptoms. N Engl J Med 1998; 338:1488–1497.

17. Phillips DR, Teng W, Arfsten A, et al. Effect of Ca^{2+} on GP IIb/IIIa interactions with integrilin: enhanced GP IIb/IIIa binding and inhibition of platelet aggregation by reduction in the concentration of ionized calcium in plasma anticoagulated with citrate. Circulation 1997; 96:1488–1494.

18. Abulencia JP, Tien N, McCarty OJT, Plymire D, Mousa SA, Konstantopoulos K. Comparative antiplatelet efficacy of a novel, nonpeptide GP IIb/IIIa antagonist (XV454; and abciximab (c7E3; in flow models of thrombosis. Arterioscler Thromb Vasc Biol 2001; 27:149–156.

19. Mousa SA, Forsythe M, Bozarth JM, Youssef A, Wityak J, Olson R, Sielecki T. XV454, a novel nonpeptide small-molecule platelet GP IIb/IIIa antagonist with comparable platelet $\alpha IIb\beta 3$-binding kinetics to c7E3. J Cardiovasc Pharmacol 1998; 32:736–744.

20. O'Neill WW, Serruys P, Knudtson M, et al. Long-term treatment with a platelet glycoprotein-receptor antagonist after percutaneous coronary revascularization. EXCITE Trial Investigators. Evaluation of Oral Xemilofiban in Controlling Thrombotic Events. N Engl J Med (2000; 342:1316–1324.

21. Cannon CP, McCabe CH, Wilcox RG, et al. Oral glycoprotein IIb/IIIa inhibition with orbofiban in patients with unstable coronary syndromes (OPUS–TIMI 16; trial. Circulation (2000; 102:149–156.

22. The SYMPHONY Investigators. Comparison of sibrafiban with aspirin for prevention of cardiovascular events after acute coronary syndromes: a randomised trial. The SYMPHONY Investigators. Sibrafiban versus aspirin to yield maximum protection from ischemic heart events post-acute coronary syndromes. Lancet 2000; 355:337–345.

23. Cannon CP, McCabe CH, Borzak S, et al. Randomized trial of an oral platelet glycoprotein IIb/IIIa antagonist, sibrafiban, in patients after an acute coronary syndrome: results of the TIMI 12 trial. Thrombolysis in Myocardial Infarction. Circulation 1998; 97:340–349.

24. Newby LK, Ohman EM, Christenson RH, et al. Benefit of glycoprotein IIb/IIIa inhibition in patients with acute coronary syndromes and troponin T-positive status: the PARAGON-B troponin T substudy. Circulation 2001; 103:2891–2896.

25. Hamm CW, Heeschen C, Goldmann B, Vahanian A, Adgey J, Miguel CM, Rutsch W, Berger J, Kootstra J, Simoons ML. Benefit of abciximab in patients with refractory unstable angina in relation to serum troponin T levels. c7E3 Fab Antiplatelet Therapy in Unstable Refractory Angina (CAPTURE) study investigators. N Engl J Med 1999; 340:1623–1629.

26. Akkerhuis KM, Neuhaus KL, Wilcox RG, et al. Safety and preliminary efficacy of one month glycoprotein IIb/IIIa inhibition with lefradafiban in patients with acute coronary syndromes without ST-elevation; a phase II study. Eur Heart J 2000; 21:2042–2055.

27. Kereiakes DJ, Berkowitz SD, Lincoff AM, Tcheng JE, Wolski K, Achenbach R, Melsheimer R, Anderson K, Califf RM, Topol EJ. Clinical correlates and course of thrombocytopenia during percutaneous coronary intervention in the era of abciximab platelet glycoprotein IIb/IIIa blockade. Am Heart J 2000; 140:74–80.

28. Scarborough RM, Kleiman NS, Phillips DR. Platelet glycoprotein IIb/IIIa antagonists. What are the relevant issues concerning their pharmacology and clinical use? Circulation 1999; 100:437–444.

29. Desai M, Lucore CL. Uneventful use of tirofiban as an adjunct to coronary stenting in a patient with a history of abciximab-associated thrombocytopenia 10 months earlier. J Invas Cardiol 2000; 12:109–112.

30. Rao JR, Mascarenhas DA. Successful use of eptifibitide as an adjunct to coronary stenting in a patient with abciximab-associated acute profound thrombocytopenia. J Invas Cardiol 2001; 13:471–473.

31. Holmes MB, Sobel BE, Cannon CP, Schneider DJ. Increased platelet reactivity in patients given orbofiban after an acute coronary syndrome. An OPUS–TIMI 16 substudy. Am J Cardiol 2000; 85:491–493.

32. Gasic GJ, Gasic TB, Stewart CC. Antimetastatic effects associated with platelet reduction. Proc Natl Acad Sci USA 1968; 61:46–52.

33. Karpatkin S, Pearlstein E, Ambrogio C, Coller BS. Role of adhesive proteins in platelet tumor interaction in vitro and metastasis formation in vivo. J Clin Invest 1988; 81:1012–1019.

34. Nieswandt B, Hafner M, Echtenacher B, Mannel DN. Lysis of tumor cells by natural killer cells in mice is impeded by platelets. Cancer Res 1999; 59:1295–1300.

35. Felding–Habermann B, Habermann R, Salvidar E, Ruggeri ZM. Role of β_3 integrins in melanoma cell adhesion to activated platelets under flow. J Biol Chem 1996; 271:5892–5900.

36. Pinedo HM, Verheul HMW, D'Amato RJ, Folkman J. Involvement of platelets in tumor angiogenesis? Lancet 1998; 352:37 1775–1777.

37. McCarty OJT, Mousa SA, Bray PF, Konstantopoulos K. Immobilized platelets support human colon carcinoma cell tethering, rolling, and firm adhesion under dynamic flow conditions. Blood 2000; 96:1789–1797.

38. Burdick MM, McCarty OJT, Jadhav S, Konstantopoulos K. Cell–cell interactions in inflammation and cancer metastasis. IEEE Eng Med Biol 2001; 20:86–91.

39. Honn KV, Tang DG, Crissman JD. Platelets and cancer metastasis. Cancer Metast Rev 1992; 11:325–351.

40. Nishi T, Kimura Y, Nakagawa K. [Research and development of cilostazol: an antiplatelet agent]. Yakugaku Zasshi 2000; 120:1247–1260.

41. Beebe HG, Dawson DL, Cutler BS, Herd JA, Strandness DE Jr, Bortey EB, Forbes WP. A new pharmacological treatment for intermittent claudication: results of a randomized, multicenter trial. Arch Intern Med 1999; 159:2041–2050.
42. Miller JL. Cilostazol approved for use in intermittent claudication [news]. Am J Health Syst Pharm 1999; 56:404.
43. Dawson DL, Cutler BS, Meissner MH, Strandness DE Jr. Cilostazol has beneficial effects in treatment of intermittent claudication: results from a multicenter, randomized, prospective, double-blind trial. Circulation 1998; 98:678–686.
44. Money SR, Herd JA, Isaacsohn JL, Davidson M, Cutler B, Heckman J, Forbes WP. Effect of cilostazol on walking distances in patients with intermittent claudication caused by peripheral vascular disease. J Vasc Surg 1998; 27:267–274; discussion 274–275.
45. Dawson DL. Comparative effects of cilostazol and other therapies for intermittent claudication. Am J Cardiol 2001; 87:19D–27D.
46. Dawson DL, Cutler BS, Hiatt WR, Hobson RW 2nd, Martin JD, Bortey EB, Forbes WP, Strandness DE Jr. A comparison of cilostazol and pentoxifylline for treating intermittent claudication. Am J Med 2000; 109:523–530.
47. Weismantel D. Is cilostazol more effective than pentoxifylline in the treatment of symptoms of intermittent claudication? J Fam Pract 2001; 50:181.
48. Liu Y, Fong M, Cone J, Wang S, Yoshitake M, Kambayashi J. Inhibition of adenosine uptake and augmentation of ischemia-induced increase of interstitial adenosine by cilostazol, an agent to treat intermittent claudication. J Cardiovasc Pharmacol 2000; 36:351–360.
49. Tjon JA, Riemann LE. Treatment of intermittent claudication with pentoxifylline and cilostazol. Am J Health Syst Pharm 2001; 58:485–493; quiz 494–496.
50. Cariski AT. Cilostazol: a novel treatment option in intermittent claudication. Int J Clin Pract Suppl 2001:11–18.
51. Cada D, Baker D, Leiven T. Cilostazol. Hosp Pharm 1999; 34:859–866.
52. Ikeda Y. Antiplatelet therapy using cilostazol, a specific PDE3 inhibitor. Thromb Haemost 1999; 82:435–438.
53. Reilly MP, Mohler ER 3rd. Cilostazol: treatment of intermittent claudication. Ann Pharmacother 2001; 35:48–56.
54. Cone J, Wang S, Tandon N, Fong M, Sun B, Sakurai K, Yoshitake M, Kambayashi J, Liu Y. Comparison of the effects of cilostazol and milrinone on intracellular cAMP levels and cellular function in platelets and cardiac cells. J Cardiovasc Pharmacol 1999; 34:497–504.
55. Lee TM, Su SF, Tsai CH, Lee YT, Wang SS. Differential effects of cilostazol and pentoxifylline on vascular endothelial growth factor in patients with intermittent claudication. Clin Sci (Lond) 2001; 101:305–311.
56. Otsuki M, Saito H, Xu X, Sumitani S, Kouhara H, Kurabayashi M, Kasayama S. Cilostazol represses vascular cell adhesion molecule-1 gene transcription via inhibiting NF-kappaB binding to its recognition sequence. Atherosclerosis 2001; 158:121–128.
57. Hirose T, Kurebayashi S, Kasayama S. Antiplatelet agent cilostazol potentiates adipocyte differentiation of 3T3-L1 cells. Atherosclerosis 2001; 158:19–22.
58. Kimura Y, Tani T, Kanbe T, Watanabe K. Effect of cilostazol on platelet aggregation and experimental thrombosis. Arzneimittelforschung 1985; 35:1144–1149.
59. Uehara S, Hirayama A. Effects of cilostazol on platelet function. Arzneimittelforschung 1989; 39:1531–1534.
60. Tanaka K, Gotoh F, Fukuuchi Y, Amano T, Uematsu D, Kawamura J, Yamawaki T, Itoh N, Obara K, Muramatsu K. Effects of a selective inhibitor of cyclic AMP phosphodiesterase on the pial microcirculation in feline cerebral ischemia. Stroke 1989; 20:668–673.
61. Tanigawa T, Nishikawa M, Kitai T, Ueda Y, Okinaka T, Makino K, Ito M, Isaka N, Ikeda Y, Shiku H, Nakano T. Increased platelet aggregability in response to shear stress in acute myocardial infarction and its inhibition by combined therapy with aspirin and cilostazol after coronary intervention. Am J Cardiol 2000; 85:1054–1059.
62. Inada H, Shindo H, Tawata M, Onaya T. Cilostazol, a cyclic AMP phosphodiesterase inhibitor,

stimulates nitric oxide production and sodium potassium adenosine triphosphatase activity in SH-SY5Y human neuroblastoma cells. Life Sci 1999; 65:1413–1422.

63. Kariyazono H, Nakamura K, Shinkawa T, Yamaguchi T, Sakata R, Yamada K. Inhibition of platelet aggregation and the release of P-selectin from platelets by cilostazol. Thromb Res 2001; 101:445–453.

64. Inoue T, Sohma R, Morooka S. Cilostazol inhibits the expression of activation-dependent membrane surface glycoprotein on the surface of platelets stimulated in vitro. Thromb Res 1999; 93:137–143.

65. Momo K, Someya K, Tachiiri T, Mitsuoka Y, Nakamura K, Imai S, Ino T, Ohkubo H. Effects of the new antiplatelet agent 2-methyl-3-1,4,5,6-tetrahydronicotinoyl)pyrazolo[1,5-a]pyridine on platelet aggregation and thrombosis in experimental animals. Arzneimittelforschung 1992; 42:32–39.

66. Ikeda Y, Kikuchi M, Murakami H, Satoh K, Murata M, Watanabe K, Ando Y. Comparison of the inhibitory effects of cilostazol, acetylsalicylic acid and ticlopidine on platelet functions ex vivo. Randomized, double-blind cross-over study. Arzneimittelforschung 1987; 37:563–566.

67. Igawa T, Tani T, Chijiwa T, Shiragiku T, Shimidzu S, Kawamura K, Kato S, Unemi F, Kimura Y. Potentiation of anti-platelet aggregating activity of cilostazol with vascular endothelial cells. Thromb Res 1990; 57:617–623.

68. Sorkin EM, Markham A. Cilostazol. Drugs Aging 1999; 14:63–71; [discussion 72, 73].

69. Tanaka T, Muneyuki T, Oka Y, Sada T, Kira Y. [Effect of long-term cilostazol administration on coronary flow velocity and coronary flow reserve]. J Cardiol 1999; 34:183–188.

70. Oishi M, Mochizuki Y, Shikata E, Satoh Y. Effect of cilostazol on cerebral blood flows in chronic stage of cerebral circulation. Keio J Med 2000; 49 Suppl 1:A145–A147.

71. Torigoe R, Hayashi T, Anegawa S, Furukawa Y, Tomokiyo M, Katsuragi M. [Effects of long-term administration of cilostazol on chronic cerebral circulatory insufficiency—with special reference to cerebral blood flow and clinical symptoms]. No To Shinkei 1998; 50:829–839.

72. Torigoe R, Hayashi T, Anegawa S, Harada K, Toda K, Maeda K, Katsuragi M. Effect of propentofylline and pentoxifylline on cerebral blood flow using ^{123}I-IMP SPECT in patients with cerebral arteriosclerosis. Clin Ther 1994; 16:65–73.

73. Elam MB, Heckman J, Crouse JR, Hunninghake DB, Herd JA, Davidson M, Gordon IL, Bortey EB, Forbes WP. Effect of the novel antiplatelet agent cilostazol on plasma lipoproteins in patients with intermittent claudication. Arterioscler Thromb Vasc Biol 1998; 18:1942–1947.

74. Cilostzol: beneficial lipid effects in IGT/type 2 diabetes mellitus. Inpharma Wly 2001; 1293:15.

75. Tani T, Uehara K, Sudo T, Marukawa K, Yasuda Y, Kimura Y. Cilostazol, a selective type III phosphodiesterase inhibitor, decreases triglyceride and increases HDL cholesterol levels by increasing lipoprotein lipase activity in rats. Atherosclerosis 2000; 152:299–305.

76. Toyota T, Oikawa S, Abe R, Sano R, Suzuki N, Hisamichi S, Fukai A, Group CDDMLS. Effect of cilostazol on lipid, uric acid, and glucose metabolism in Patients with Impaired Glucose Tolerance or Type 2 Diabetes Mellitus: A Double-blind, placebo-controlled study. Clin Drug Invest 2001; 21:325–335.

77. Ahn CW, Lee HC, Park SW, Song YD, Huh KB, Oh SJ, Kim YS, Choi YK, Kim JM, Lee TH. Decrease in carotid intima media thickness after 1 year of cilostazol treatment in patients with type 2 diabetes mellitus. Diabetes Res Clin Pract 2001; 52:45–53.

78. Takahashi S, Oida K, Fujiwara R, Maeda H, Hayashi S, Takai H, Tamai T, Nakai T, Miyabo S. Effect of cilostazol, a cyclic AMP phosphodiesterase inhibitor, on the proliferation of rat aortic smooth muscle cells in culture. J Cardiovasc Pharmacol 1992; 20:900–906.

79. Tsuchikane E, Katoh O, Sumitsuji S, Fukuhara A, Funamoto M, Otsuji S, Tateyama H, Awata N, Kobayashi T. Impact of cilostazol on intimal proliferation after directional coronary atherectomy. Am Heart J 1998; 135:495–502.

80. Takai S, Jin D, Nishimoto M, Sakaguchi M, Kirimura K, Yuda A, Miyazaki M. Cilostazol suppresses intimal formation in dog grafted veins with reduction of angiotensin II-forming enzymes. Eur J Pharmacol 2001; 411:301–304.

81. Ishizaka N, Taguchi J, Kimura Y, Ikari Y, Aizawa T, Togo M, Miki K, Kurokawa K, Ohno M. Effects of a single local administration of cilostazol on neointimal formation in balloon-injured rat carotid artery. Atherosclerosis 1999; 142:41–46.

82. Kozuma K, Hara K, Yamasaki M, Morino Y, Ayabe S, Kuroda Y, Tanabe K, Ikari Y, Tamura T. Effects of cilostazol on late lumen loss and repeat revascularization after Palmaz–Schatz coronary stent implantation. Am Heart J 2001; 141:124–130.

83. Kishida M, Watanabe K, Tsuruoka T. [Effects of cilostazol in patients with bradycardiac atrial fibrillation]. J Cardiol 2001; 37:27–33.

84. Fujimura M, Tachibana H, Myou S, Kita T, Matsuda T. Bronchoprotective effect of an intrabronchial administration of cilostazol powder and a nebulized PDE1 and PDE4 inhibitor KF19514 in guinea pigs. Int Arch Allergy Immunol 1998; 116:220–227.

85. Fujimura M, Kamio Y, Saito M, Hashimoto T, Matsuda T. Bronchodilator and bronchoprotective effects of cilostazol in humans in vivo. Am J Respir Crit Care Med 1995; 151:222–225.

86. Yamamoto Y, Yasuda Y, Kimura Y, Komiya Y. Effects of cilostazol, an antiplatelet agent, on axonal regeneration following nerve injury in diabetic rats. Eur J Pharmacol 1998; 352:171–178.

87. Yamamoto Y, Yasuda Y, Komiya Y. Cilostazol prevents impairment of slow axonal transport in streptozotocin-diabetic rats. Eur J Pharmacol 2000; 409:1–7.

88. Suh KS, Oh SJ, Woo JT, Kim SW, Yang IM, Kim JW, Kim YS, Choi YK, Park IK. Effect of cilostazol on the neuropathies of streptozotocin-induced diabetic rats. Korean J Intern Med 1999; 14:34–40.

89. Nakaya Y, Minami A, Sakamoto S, Niwa Y, Ohnaka M, Harada N, Nakamura T. Cilostazol, a phosphodiesterase inhibitor, improves insulin sensitivity in the Otsuka Long–Evans Tokushima Fatty Rat, a model of spontaneous NIDDM. Diabetes Obes Metab 1999; 1:37–41.

90. Murata K, Kameyama M, Fukui F, Ohigashi H, Hiratsuka M, Sasaki Y, Kabuto T, Mukai M, Mammoto T, Akedo H, Ishikawa O, Imaoka S. Phosphodiesterase type III inhibitor, cilostazol, inhibits colon cancer cell motility. Clin Exp Metast 1999; 17:525–530.

91. Ikeda Y, Matsumata T, Takenaka K, Yamagata M, Sugimachi K. Effects of doxorubicin and/or cilostazol on cancer cells during liver regeneration after two-thirds hepatectomy in rats. Oncology 1998; 55:354–356.

92. Product-Information. Pletal(r), cilostazol. In: Otsuka America Pharmaceutical, Rockville, MD. 1999.

93. Suri A, Forbes WP, Bramer SL. Effects of CYP3A inhibition on the metabolism of cilostazol. Clin Pharmacokinet 1999; 37:61–68.

94. Bramer SL, Brisson J, Corey AE, Mallikaarjun S. Effect of multiple cilostazol doses on single dose lovastatin pharmacokinetics in healthy volunteers. Clin Pharmacokinet 1999; 37:69–77.

95. Suri A, Bramer SL. Effect of omeprazole on the metabolism of cilostazol. Clin Pharmacokinet 1999; 37:53–59.

96. Bramer SL, Suri A. Inhibition of CYP2D6 by quinidine and its effects on the metabolism of cilostazol. Clin Pharmacokinet 1999; 37:41–51.

97. Mallikaarjun S, Forbes WP, Bramer SL. Interaction potential and tolerability of the coadministration of cilostazol and aspirin. Clin Pharmacokinet 1999; 37:87–93.

98. Mallikaarjun S, Bramer SL. Effect of cilostazol on the pharmacokinetics and pharmacodynamics of warfarin. Clin Pharmacokinet 1999; 37:79–86.

99. Mallikaarjun S, Forbes WP, Bramer SL. Effect of renal impairment on the pharmacokinetics of cilostazol and its metabolites. Clin Pharmacokinet 1999; 37:33–40.

100. Bramer SL, Forbes WP. Effect of hepatic impairment on the pharmacokinetics of a single dose of cilostazol. Clin Pharmacokinet 1999; 37:25–32.

101. Hayakawa T, Shouzu A, Nishikawa M, Miyake Y, Shimizu H, Omoto S, Inada M. Effects of beraprost and cilostazol and renal function on serum thrombomodulin levels in diabetic patients. Arzneimittelforschung 2000; 50:535–538.

102. Nomura S, Shouzu A, Omoto S, Hayakawa T, Kagawa H, Nishikawa M, Inada M, Fujimura Y, Ikeda Y, Fukuhara S. Effect of cilostazol on soluble adhesion molecules and platelet-derived microparticles in patients with diabetes. Thromb Haemost 1998; 80:388–392.

103. A randomised, blinded, trial of clopidogrel versus aspirin in patients at risk of ischaemic events (CAPRIE). CAPRIE Steering Committee [see comments]. Lancet 1996; 348:1329–1339.

104. Take S, Matsutani M, Ueda H, Hamaguchi H, Konishi H, Baba Y, Kawaratani H, Sugiura T, Iwasaka T, Inada M. Effect of cilostazol in preventing restenosis after percutaneous transluminal coronary angioplasty. Am J Cardiol 1997; 79:1097–1099.

105. Tsutsui M, Shimokawa H, Higuchi S, Yoshihara S, Hayashida K, Sobashima A, Kuga T, Matsuguchi T, Okamatsu S. Effect of cilostazol, a novel anti-platelet drug, on restenosis after percutaneous transluminal coronary angioplasty. Jpn Circ J 1996; 60:207–215.

106. Tsuchikane E, Fukuhara A, Kobayashi T, Kirino M, Yamasaki K, Izumi M, Otsuji S, Tateyama H, Sakurai M, Awata N. Impact of cilostazol on restenosis after percutaneous coronary balloon angioplasty. Circulation 1999; 100:21–26.

107. Tanabe Y, Ito E, Nakagawa I, Suzuki K. Effect of cilostazol on restenosis after coronary angioplasty and stenting in comparison to conventional coronary artery stenting with ticlopidine. Int J Cardiol 2001; 78:285–291.

108. Park SW, Lee CW, Kim HS, Lee HJ, Park HK, Hong MK, Kim JJ, Park SJ. Comparison of cilostazol versus ticlopidine therapy after stent implantation. Am J Cardiol 1999; 84:511–514.

109. Toyonaga S, Nakatsu T, Murakami T, Kusachi S, Mashima K, Tominaga Y, Yamane S, Uesugi T, Kanai H, Tsuji T. Effects of cilostazol on heart rate and its variation in patients with atrial fibrillation associated with bradycardia. J Cardiovasc Pharmacol Ther 2000; 5:183–191.

110. Atarashi H, Endoh Y, Saitoh H, Kishida H, Hayakawa H. Chronotropic effects of cilostazol, a new antithrombotic agent, in patients with bradyarrhythmias. J Cardiovasc Pharmacol 1998; 31:534–539.

111. Pratt CM. Analysis of the cilostazol safety database. Am J Cardiol 2001; 87:28D–33D.

112. Yamashita K, Kobayashi S, Okada K, Tsunematsu T. Increased external carotid artery blood flow in headache patients induced by cilostazol. Preliminary communication. Arzneimittelforschung 1990; 40:587–588.

113. Packer M, Carver JR, Rodeheffer RJ, et al. Effect of oral milrinone on mortality in severe chronic heart failure. The PROMISE Study Research Group [see comments]. N Engl J Med 1991; 325:1468–1475.

114. Cohn JN, Goldstein SO, Greenberg BH, Lorell BH, Bourge RC, Jaski BE, Gottlieb SO, McGrew F 3rd, DeMets DL, White BG. A dose-dependent increase in mortality with vesnarinone among patients with severe heart failure. Vesnarinone Trial Investigators [see comments]. N Engl J Med 1998; 339:1810–1816.

115. Fuccella LM, Corvi G, Moro E, Pogliani E, Tamassia V, Tosolini G. Pharmacokinetic, bioavailability and pharmacodynamic study of indobufen (K 3920), an inhibitor of platelet aggregation, after a single dose in man. Eur J Clin Pharmacol 1979; 15:323–327.

116. Wiseman LR, Fitton A, Buckley MM. Indobufen. A review of its pharmacodynamic and pharmacokinetic properties, and therapeutic efficacy in cerebral, peripheral and coronary vascular disease. Drugs 1992; 44:445–464.

117. Cipollone F, Patrignani P, Greco A, Panara MR, Padovano R, Cuccurullo F, Patrono C, Rebuzzi AG, Liuzzo G, Quaranta G, Maseri A. Differential suppression of thromboxane biosynthesis by indobufen and aspirin in patients with unstable angina. Circulation 1997; 96:1109–1116.

118. Cattaneo M, Bevilacqua C, Lecchi A, Mannucci PM. In vitro and ex vivo effects of indobufen on human platelet aggregation, the release reaction and thromboxane B_2 production. Haemostasis 1987; 17:293–300.

119. Davi G, Francavilla G, Mattini A, Catalano I, Licata G. Indobufen treatment in angina pectoris: effects on platelet function and thromboxanc synthcsis. Curr Ther Res 1988; 43:1031–1037.

120. Pogliani E, Corvi G, Mandelli V, Fuccella LM. Preliminary human pharmacology studies on the inhibition of platelet aggregation by indobufen (K 3920). Haematologica 1981; 66:160–170.

121. Crow MJ, Salter MC, Donaldson DR, Rajah SM. Inhibition of platelet function with indobufen: correlation with plasma drug level. Thromb Res 1985; 38:303–306.

122. Ciavarella N, Corvi G, Coviello M, Parato M, Pilolli Dea. The effect of indobufen (K 3920) on platelet aggregation, platelet factors 3, 4 and some coagulation parameters in patients with venous thrombosis. Curr Ther Res 1981; 29:503–508.

123. Vinazzer H, Fuccella LM. Clinical pharmacology studies with indobufen (K 3920): inhibitor of platelet aggregation. J Clin Pharmacol 1980; 20:316–325.

124. Carrieri P, Oferfice G. Study of platelet function in vitro and in vivo in patients with transient cerebral ischaemia: effects of short-term treatment with a new platelet antiaggregant drug, indobufen. Curr Ther Res 1984; 36:681–686.

125. Orefice G, Carrieri P, Indaco A, Iorillo L, Fioretti A. A comparative study between indobufen and acetylsalicylic acid on β-thromboglobulin, platelet factor 4 and platelet aggregation in patients with transient ischemic attacks. Acta Neurologica 1984; 6:97–102.

126. Chello M, Mastroroberto P, Celi V, Romano F, Marchese AR, Colonna A. Reduction by indobufen of neutrophil activation in peripheral arterial occlusive disease. J Cardiovasc Pharmacol 1996; 27:417–423.

127. Moia M, Della Valle P, Castellana P, Cattaneo M, Mannucci PM. Indobufen inhibits thrombus formation and platelet adhesion to subendothelium both in vitro and ex vivo. In: 10th International Conference on Thrombosis. Athens, Greece. 1988.

128. Nenci GG, Berrettini M, Iadevaia V, Parise P, Ballatori E. Inhibition of spontaneous platelet aggregation and adhesion by indobufen (K 3920). A randomized, double-blind crossover study on platelet, coagulation and fibrinolysis function tests. Pharmatherapeutica 1982; 3:188–194.

129. Pogliani EM, Fantasia R, Perini C, Corvi G. Prevention of in vivo platelet aggregation by indobufen in angina patients during exercise. J Int Med Res 1981; 9:113–119.

130. Italian Multicenter Study Group. Long-term antiplatelet activity and safety of indobufen in patients with cardiovascular disease. Int J Clin Pharmacol Ther Toxicol 1985; 23:439–446.

131. Bhana N, McClellan KJ. Indobufen: an updated review of its use in the management of athero-thrombosis. Drugs Aging 2001; 18:369–388.

132. Belcaro G. Vasospasm in patients with intermittent claudication: the role of indobufen. Curr Ther Res 1990; 47:795–801.

133. Belcaro G. Vasospasm in intermittent claudication. Curr Ther Res 1990; 48:667–675.

134. Signorini GP, Salmistraro G, Maraglino G. Efficacy of indobufen in the treatment of intermittent claudication. Angiology 1988; 39:742–746.

135. Tonnesen KH, Albuquerque P, Baitsch G, Gomez Alonso A, Ibanez F, Kester RC, Leveson S, Poredos P. Double-blind, controlled, multicenter study of indobufen versus placebo in patients with intermittent claudication. Int Angiol 1993; 12:371–377.

136. Belcaro G, De Simone P. Long-term evaluation of indobufen in peripheral vascular disease. Angiology 1991; 42:8–14.

137. Fabris F, Steffan A, Randi ML, Avruscio GP, Cordiano I, Girolami A. Indobufen versus dipyridamole plus aspirin in the treatment of patients with peripheral atherosclerotic disease. J Med 1992; 23:81–92.

138. D'Addato M, Curti T, Bertini D, Donini I, Ferrero R, Fiorani P, Pellegrino F, Vecchioni R, Visconti W, Zinicola N. Indobufen vs. acetylsalicylic acid plus dipyridamole in long-term patency after femoro-popliteal bypass. Int Angiol 1992; 11:106–112.

139. Morocutti C, Amabile G, Fattapposta F, Nicolosi A, Matteoli S, Trappolini M, Cataldo G, Milanesi G, Lavezzari M, Pamparana F, Coccheri S. Indobufen versus warfarin in the secondary prevention of major vascular events in nonrheumatic atrial fibrillation. SIFA (Studio Italiano Fibrillazione Atriale) Investigators. Stroke 1997; 28:1015–1021.

140. Fornaro G, Rossi P, Mantica PG, Caccia ME, Aralda D, Lavezzari M, Pamparana F, Milanesi G. Indobufen in the prevention of thromboembolic complications in patients with heart disease. A randomized, placebo-controlled, double-blind study. Circulation 1993; 87:162–164.

141. Amabile G, Matteoli S, Fattapposta F, Lavezzari M, Trappolini M, Heiman F, Morocutti C. [Italian Study on Atrial Fibrillation (SIFA): status report]. Cardiologia 1993; 38:327–332.

142. Rogan J. Indobufen in secondary prevention of transient ischaemic attack. Multicentre Ischaemic Attack Study Group. J Int Med Res 1990; 18:240–244.

143. Belcaro G, Pierangeli A, Piolli DS. Long-term evaluation of the safety and efficacy of indobufen in cerebrovascular disease. Curr Ther Res 1990; 47:444–451.

144. Pratesi C, Pulli R, Milanesi G, Lavezzari M, Pamparana F, Bertini D. Indobufen versus placebo in the prevention of restenosis after carotid endarterectomy: a double-blind pilot study. J Int Med Res 1991; 19:202–209.

145. Taylor FC, Cohen H, Ebrahim S. Systematic review of long term anticoagulation or antiplatelet treatment in patients with non-rheumatic atrial fibrillation. BMJ 2001; 322:321–326.

146. Bergamasco B, Benna P, Carolei A, Rasura M, Rudelli G, Fieschi C. A randomized trial comparing ticlopidine hydrochloride with indobufen for the prevention of stroke in high-risk patients (TISS study). Ticlopidine Indobufen Stroke Study. Funct Neurol 1997; 12:33–43.

147. Rohn V, Pirk J, Mach T. [The effect of indobufen on aortocoronary bypass patency after 1 week and after 1 year] Cor Vasa 1993; 35:162–164.

148. Pirk J, Rohn V, Peregrin J. The effect of ibustrin on early aortocoronary bypass patency. Cor Vasa 1990; 32:258–262.

149. Group TS. Indobufen versus aspirin plus dipyridamole after coronary artery bypass surgery. Coronary Artery Dis 1991; 2:897–906.

150. Rajah SM, Nair U, Rees M, et al. Effects of antiplatelet therapy with indobufen or aspirin–dipyridamole on graft patency one year after coronary artery bypass grafting. J Thorac Cardiovasc Surg 1994; 107:1146–1153.

151. Cataldo G, Heiman F, Lavezzari M, Marubini E. Indobufen compared with aspirin and dipyridamole on graft patency after coronary artery bypass surgery: results of a combined analysis. Coronary Artery Dis 1998; 9:217–222.

152. Dalla Volta S, Coronarica. oboSSIsA. Antiplatelet treatment in the prevention of restenosis after PTCA: an Italian multicenter study. Blood 1989; 74:176A.

153. Belcaro G, Errichi BM, De Simone P. Prevention of recurrent deep venous thrombosis with indobufen. A 3-year follow-up study using color duplex scanning. Angiology 1993; 44:328–331.

154. Belcaro G, Laurora G, Cesarone MR, De Sanctis MT. Prophylaxis of recurrent deep venous thrombosis. A randomized, prospective study using indobufen and graduated elastic compression stockings. Angiology 1993; 44:695–699.

155. Peters SH, Jonker JJ, de Boer AC, den Ottolander GJ. The incidence of deep venous thrombosis in patients with an acute myocardial infarction treated with acenocoumarol or indobufen. Thromb Haemost 1982; 48:222–225.

156. Salter MC, Mayor P, Crow MJ, Rajah SM, Davison AM. Microthrombus formation on hemodialysis membranes: a placebo controlled randomized trail of two doses of indobufen. Clin Nephrol 1985; 24:31–36.

157. Pogliani EM, Colombi M, Cristoforetti G, Valenti G, Miradoli et al. beta-Thromboglobulin and platelet factor 4 plasma levels during haemodialysis: effect of indobufen. Pharmatherapeutica 1982; 3:127–132.

158. Carrieri PB, Orefice G, Sorge F. A double-blind placebo-controlled trial of indobufen in the prophylaxis of migraine. Acta Neurol Scand 1988; 77:433–436.

159. de la Cruz JP, Mata JM, Sanchez de la Cuesta F. Triflusal vs aspirin on the inhibition of human platelet and vascular cyclooxygenase. Gen Pharmacol 1992; 23:297–300.

160. De la Cruz JP, Pavia J, Garcia–Arnes J, Sanchez de la Cuesta F. Effects of triflusal and acetylsalicylic acid on platelet aggregation in whole blood of diabetic patients. Eur J Haematol 1988; 40:232–236.

161. Dalla–Volta S. Pharmacological basis of antiplatelet drugs in acute myocardial infarction: focus on triflusal. Eur Heart J 1999; 1(suppl F):7F–11F.

162. Theroux P. Antiplatelet drugs in the acute phase of myocardial infarction. Eur Heart J 1999; 1(suppl F):29F–33F.

163. Sanchez de Miguel L, Casado S, Farre J, Garcia–Duran M, Rico LA, Monton M, Romcro J, Bellver T, Sierra MP, Guerra JI, Mata P, Esteban A, Lopez–Farre A. Comparison of in vitro effects of triflusal and acetylsalicylic acid on nitric oxide synthesis by human neutrophils. Eur J Pharmacol 1998; 343:57–65.

164. Dominguez MJ, Vacas M, Saez Y, Olabarria I, Velasco A, Iriarte JA, Forn J. Effects of triflusal in patients with prosthetic heart valves. Clin Ther 1985; 7:357–360.

165. Cruz Fernandez JM, Lopez G, Aranda V, Marfil Montoya F, et al. Managing acute myocardial infarction: clinical implications of the TIM study. Eur Heart J 1999; 1(suppl F):12F–18F.

166. McNeely W, Goa KL. Triflusal. Drugs 1998; 55:823–33 [discussion 834–835].

167. Messa GL, Franchi M, Auteri A, Di Perri T. Action of 2-acetoxy-trifluoromethylbenzoic acid (triflusal) on platelet function after repeated oral administration in man: a pharmacological clinical study. Int J Clin Pharmacol Res 1993; 13:263–273.

168. De Miguel LS, Jimenez A, Monton M, Farre J, Del Mar Arriero M, Rodriguez–JA, Garcia-Canete J, Rico L, Gomez J, Nunez A, Casado S, Farre AL. A 4-trifluoromethyl derivative of salicylate, triflusal,

stimulates nitric oxide production by human neutrophils: role in platelet function. Eur J Clin Invest 2000; 30:811–817.

169. Fernandez de Arriba A, Cavalcanti F, Miralles A, Bayon Y, Alonso A, Merlos M, Garcia–Rafanell J, Forn J. Inhibition of cyclooxygenase-2 expression by 4-trifluoromethyl derivatives of salicylate, triflusal, and its deacetylated metabolite, 2-hydroxy–4-trifluoromethylbenzoic acid. Mol Pharmacol 1999; 55:753–760.

170. Bayon Y, Alonso A, Sanchez Crespo M. 4-trifluoromethyl derivatives of salicylate, triflusal and its main metabolite 2-hydroxy–4-trifluoromethylbenzoic acid, are potent inhibitors of nuclear factor kappaB activation. Br J Pharmacol 1999; 126:1359–1366.

171. Hernandez M, de Arriba AF, Merlos M, Fuentes L, Crespo MS, Nieto ML. Effect of 4-trifluoromethyl derivatives of salicylate on nuclear factor kappaB-dependent transcription in human astrocytoma cells. Br J Pharmacol 2001; 132:547–555.

172. De La Cruz JP, Villalobos MA, Garcia PJ, Smith–Agreda JM, Sanchez de la Cuesta F. Effects of triflusal and its main metabolite HTB on platelet interaction with subendothelium in healthy volunteers. Eur J Clin Pharmacol 1995; 47:497–502.

173. Cruz–Fernandez JM, Lopez–Bescos L, Garcia–Dorado D, Lopez Garcia–Aranda V, Cabades A, Martin–Jadraque L, Velasco JA, Castro–Beiras A, Torres F, Marfil F, Navarro E. Randomized comparative trial of triflusal and aspirin following acute myocardial infarction [in process citation]. Eur Heart J 2000; 21:457–465.

174. Bayes de Luna A. May aspirin be replaced in the treatment of myocardial infarction? [in process citation]. Eur Heart J 2000; 21:430–432.

175. Plaza L, Lopez–Bescos L, Martin–Jadraque L, et al. Protective effect of triflusal against acute myocardial infarction in patients with unstable angina: results of a Spanish multicenter trial. Grupo de Estudio del Triflusal en la Angina Inestable. Cardiology 1993; 82:388–398.

176. Guiteras P, Altimiras J, Aris A, et al. Prevention of aortocoronary vein-graft attrition with low-dose aspirin and triflusal, both associated with dipyridamole: a randomized, double-blind, placebo-controlled trial. Eur Heart J 1989; 10:159–167.

177. Masotti M, Tura A, Crexells C, Oriol A. Antiplatelet agents and their effect on complications during or soon after percutaneous transluminal coronary angioplasty. J Int Med Res 1991; 19:414–418.

178. Prieto MA, De La Cruz JP, Del Prado MF, Sanchez de la Cuesta F. Influence of triflusal on platelet activation after coronary artery bypass graft. Blood Coagul Fibrinolysis 2000; 11:191–197.

179. Auteri A, Angaroni A, Borgatti E, et al. Triflusal in the treatment of patients with chronic peripheral arteriopathy: multicentre double-blind clinical study vs. placebo. Int J Clin Pharmacol Res 1995; 15:57–63.

180. Matias–Guiu J, Alvarez–Sabin J, Codina A. [Comparative study of the effect of low-dosage acetylsalicylic acid and triflusal in the prevention of cardiovascular events among young adults with ischemic cerebrovascular disease]. Rev Neurol 1997; 25:1669–1672.

181. Bankhead C. Triflusal safer than aspirin in stroke? Inpharma Wk 2001; 1280:19–20.

182. Triflusal Versus Acetysalicylic Acid in Secondary Prevention of Cerebral Infarction: TACIP study (Triflusal, Aspirin, Cerebral Infarction Prevention). Stroke 1999; 30:1305.

183. Triflusal Versus Aspirin for the Prevention of Infarction: a Randomized Stroke Study (TAPIRSS). Stroke 1998; 29:553.

184. Monreal M, Lafoz E, Roca J, Granero X, Soler J, Salazar X, Olazabal A, Bergqvist D. Platelet count, antiplatelet therapy and pulmonary embolism—a prospective study in patients with hip surgery. Thromb Haemost 1995; 73:380–385.

185. Putz P, Buyse H, Delvaux D, Kutnowski M, Demulder A, Dumont N, Lavenne E, Claes R, Rosillon D. Triflusal versus acetysalicylic acid: a double-blind study for the prophylaxis of deep vein thrombosis after hip surgery. Acta Chir Belg 1991; 91:269–276.

186. Kwon SU, Ahn JY, Yun BW, et al. A clinical trial on the safety and the inhibitory effect of platelet aggregation by triflusal (Disgren) in the patients with cerebral thrombosis. Kor J Clin Pharmacol Ther 1996; 4:20–28.

187. Lee AY, Yoo SH, Lee KH. A case of photoallergic drug eruption caused by triflusal (Disgren). Photodermatol Photoimmunol Photomed 1999; 15:85–86.

188. Serrano G, Aliaga A, Planells I. Photosensitivity associated with triflusal (Disgren). Photodermatology 1987; 4:103–105.

189. Bosca F, Cuquerella MC, Marin ML, Miranda MA. Photochemistry of 2-hydroxy-4-trifluoromethylbenzoic acid, major metabolite of the photosensitizing platelet antiaggregant drug triflusal. Photochem Photobiol 2001; 73:463–468.

190. Nagore E, Perez–Ferriols A, Sanchez–Motilla JM, Serrano G, Aliaga A. Photosensitivity associated with treatment with triflusal. J Eur Acad Dermatol Venereol 2000; 14:219–221.

191. Mest HJ, Thomas E. [Is there a renaissance for trapidil?]. Z Ges Inn Med 1986; 41:217–220.

192. Mest K. Trapidil: a potent inhibitor of platelet aggregation. J Drug Dev 1990; 3:143–149.

193. Ohnishi H, Yamaguchi K, Shimada S, Suzuki Y, Kumagai A. A new approach to the treatment of atherosclerosis and trapidil as an antagonist to platelet-derived growth factor. Life Sci 1981; 28:1641–1646.

194. Ohnishi H, Kosuzume H, Hayashi Y, Yamaguchi K, Suzuki Y, Itoh R. Effects of trapidil on thromboxane A_2-induced aggregation of platelets, ischemic changes in heart and biosynthesis of thromboxane A_2. Prostaglandins Med 1981; 6:269–281.

195. Harder S, Thurmann PA, Hellstern A, Benjaminov A. Pharmacokinetics of trapidil, an antagonist of platelet derived growth factor, in healthy subjects and in patients with liver cirrhosis. Br J Clin Pharmacol 1996; 42:443–449.

196. Suzuki Y, Yamaguchi K, Shimada S, Kitamura Y, Ohnishi H. Antithrombotic activity and the mechanism of action of trapidil (Rocornal). Prostaglandins Leukotiene Med 1982; 9:685–695.

197. Raubach KH, Vlahov V, Wolter K, Bussmann WD. Double-blind randomized multicenter study on the efficacy of trapidil versus isosorbide dinitrate in stable angina pectoris. Clin Cardiol 1997; 20:483–488.

198. Maresta A, Balducelli M, Cantini L, et al. Trapidil (triazolopyrimidine), a platelet-derived growth factor antagonist, reduces restenosis after percutaneous transluminal coronary angioplasty. Results of the randomized, double-blind STARC study. Studio Trapidil versus Aspirin nella Restenosi Coronarica. Circulation 1994; 90:2710–2715.

199. Fachinformation: Rocornal, trapidil. Laupheim. Dr Rentschler Arzneimittel GmbH & Co, 1996.

200. Cheng Y, Liu P, Chen H, Zeng F. Antiproliferative effects of trapidil in vascular smooth muscle cells are associated by inhibition of MAPK and P34(cdc2) activity. J Cardiovasc Pharmacol 2000; 35:1–6.

201. Cercek B, Ebrahimi R, dimayuga P, Khorsandi M, Forrester JS. Trapidil prevents rat smooth muscle cell proliferation in vitro and in vivo [abstr]. J Am Coll Cardiol 1991; 17(suppl):72A.

202. Okamoto S, Inden M, Setsuda M, Konishi T, Nakano T. Effects of trapidil (triazolopyrimidine), a platelet-derived growth factor antagonist, in preventing restenosis after percutaneous transluminal coronary angioplasty. Am Heart J 1992; 123:1439–1444.

203. Liu MW, Roubin GS, Robinson KA, Black AJ, Hearn JA, Siegel RJ, King SBd. Trapidil in preventing restenosis after balloon angioplasty in the atherosclerotic rabbit. Circulation 1990; 81:1089–1093.

204. Nishikawa H, Ono N, Motoyasu M, Aoki T, Shimizu Y. Preventive effects of trapidil on restenosis after PTCA [abstr]. Circulation 1992; 86(suppl I):I–53.

205. Tiell ML, Sussman, II, Gordon PB, Saunders RN. Suppression of fibroblast proliferation in vitro and of myointimal hyperplasia in vivo by the triazolopyrimidine, trapidil. Artery 1983; 12:33–50.

206. Serruys PW, Banz K, Darcis T, Mignot A, van Es GA, Schwicker D. Results of a meta-analysis of trapidil, a PDGF inhibitor N. A sufficient reason for a second look to the pharmacological approach to restenosis. J Invas Cardiol 1997; 9:505–512.

207. Yasue H, Ogawa H, Tanaka H, Miyazaki S, Hattori R, Saito M, Ishikawa K, Masuda Y, Yamaguchi T, Motomiya T, Tamura Y. Effects of aspirin and trapidil on cardiovascular events after acute myocardial infarction. Japanese Antiplatelets Myocardial Infarction Study (JAMIS) investigators. Am J Cardiol 1999; 83:1308–1313.

208. Circo A LgP, chiaranda G et al. Studio clinico sull'attivita antianginosa e antiaggregante piastrinica e sulla tollerabilita del trapidil in pazienti affetti da angina pectoris. Clin Eur 1991; I:33–43.

209. Metra M, Danesi, R, Guaini, T, et al. Il trapidil net trattemento acuto e cronica dell'angina da sforzo: studio dose-riposta. Clin Ter Cardiovasc 1988; 7:37–45.

210. Di Donato M, Dabizzi RP, Maioli Mea. Acute haemodynamic effects of intravenous administration of trapidil in man. Arzneimittelforschung 1985; 35:1295–1298.
211. Kurita A, Satomura K, Kawaguchi S, Takase B, Shibuya T, Arakawa K, Mizuno K, Sugawara H, Isojima K. The effects of trapidil on left ventricular function and platelet aggregation in patients with coronary artery disease subjected to pacing. Jpn Heart J 1991; 32:287–296.
212. Lohr E. [Therapy of ischemic heart disease with trapidil. Observations with 4,014 patients in medical practice]. Fortschr Med 1994; 112:446–450.
213. Vertraeglichkeit: "Sehr gut." Erfahrungen aus Japan. Fortschr Med 1992; 110:14–15.
214. Trapidil, in Mikropharm 2, electronic version, In: Webe-und Vetriebsgesellschaft Deutscher Apotheker (W + V). Frankfurt/Main, Germany: ABDA-Datenbank International, 1993.

29

Overview of New Therapeutic Agents

Marc Verstraete
University of Leuven, Leuven, Belgium

The use of thrombolytic drugs has revolutionized the treatment of patients with acute myocardial infarction. If used within the first 6 h after the onset of symptoms, streptokinase and urokinase, plus aspirin and heparin, reduce in-hospital mortality by more than half and considerably improve long-term survival. Although these first-generation fibrinolytic agents (streptokinase, urokinase) are effective at thrombolysis, they are not fibrin-specific; they also convert circulating plasminogen to plasmin. Because plasminogen in the thrombus and in the plasma are in equilibrium, the plasminogen within the thrombus is also gradually depleted. This "plasminogen steal" reduces clot lysis. Furthermore, streptokinase is immunogenic, resulting in drug resistance, fever, and allergic reactions. To address some of these problems, a complex of streptokinase and acylated human plasminogen, termed anisoylated streptokinase activator complex (APSAC) or anistreplase, was developed. This molecule can be administered as a bolus owing to its longer plasma half-life than that of streptokinase. The hope for a higher fibrin (thrombus) affinity and fibrinolytic efficacy compared with streptokinase was not fulfilled in clinical trials. Moreover, the compound still elicits antigenic responses in patients; pyrexia and hypotension are infrequent adverse reactions.

The second-generation agents (tissue-plasminogen activator [t-PA] or alteplase; single-chain urokinase-type plasminogen activator [scu-PA], or prourokinase) are fibrin-selective. They were developed to avoid the systemic thrombolytic state that causes depletion of circulating fibrinogen and plasminogen. However, the high doses of these agents that are required for the treatment of myocardial infarction do produce a mild to moderate decrease in levels of circulating fibrinogen and plasminogen. Moreover, the risk of intracranial hemorrhage with t-PA is slightly greater than with streptokinase (0.7 vs. 0.5%). These limitations of second-generation thrombolytic agents (Table 1) explain the quest for better agents as discussed in this section of the book.

Table 1. Shortcomings of Second-Generation Thrombolytic Drugs in Patients with Myocardial Infarction

Procoagulant effects
Resistance to recanalization in 15 to 40% of patients
Only about half of patients reach TIMI[a] perfusion grade 3
Angiographically documented reocclusion rates of 5–10% at 7 days and 25% at 3 months
Time to reperfusion > 45 min
Intracranial bleeding in 0.3–0.7% of patients

[a] TIMI, Thrombolysis in Myocardial Infarction trial.

Clinical and Preclinical Profile of the Novel Recombinant Plasminogen Activator Reteplase

Michael Waller and Steven Mack
Centocor, Inc., Malvern, Pennsylvania, U.S.A.

Ulrich Martin
Seil Biomedicals GmbH, Martinsried, Germany

Paul A. Minella
University of Florida, Gainesville, Florida, and Centocor, Inc., Malvern, Pennsylvania, U.S.A.

Reteplase is a novel recombinant plasminogen activator consisting of the kringle 2 and protease domains of tissue-type plasminogen activator (t-PA). Because of its production in *Escherichia coli* cells, reteplase is not glycosylated. As shown experimentally, consequences of the structural changes are a virtual lack of functional fibrin binding and a lower affinity to endothelial cells and liver cells, resulting in a longer half-life. The longer half-life of reteplase compared with t-PA has an influence on pharmacodynamic characteristics: It contributes to the higher thrombolytic potency, allowing dose reduction, and it enables intravenous-bolus injection, which is associated with more rapid reperfusion than after administration of reference thrombolytic agents. The double-bolus regimen of reteplase stabilizes coronary artery blood flow after successful reperfusion. At equieffective doses, the degree of systemic lytic state after reteplase is comparable with that after t-PA.

The clinical evaluation of reteplase has shown that 10 plus 10 U of reteplase restores blood flow to the heart more rapidly than alteplase. Furthermore, the restored blood flow is more complete and stable after injected double-bolus reteplase than after alteplase. As a consequence, reteplase-treated patients required fewer coronary interventions and had higher myocardial salvage than alteplase-treated patients, as evidenced by improved global and regional left ventricular function.

Reteplase is effective in improving survival after acute myocardial infarction. The INJECT trial demonstrated that double-bolus reteplase was at least as effective as streptokinase in reducing 35-day mortality after acute myocardial infarction. At 6 months, mortality in the reteplase group was 1% lower than in the streptokinase group, which constitutes a nonsignificant, but favorable, trend for reteplase. In the INJECT trial, patients treated with reteplase had a significantly lower incidence of heart failure than those treated with streptokinase, suggesting a better quality of life for survivors of acute myocardial infarction. The GUSTO III trial showed no significant differences between therapy with reteplase and accelerated alteplase in 30-day mortality, stroke, and noncerebral bleeding events. Overall, reteplase has a safety profile similar to that of other thrombolytic agents.

Emerging data from preclinical studies and phase II trials of fibrinolytic therapy, combined with the glycoprotein (GP) IIb/IIIa inhibitor abciximab, suggest that concomitant use of these agents may further improve clinical outcomes. Promising results of using combination therapy with reteplase and abciximab demonstrated that fibrinolysis occurs more rapidly and more completely when compared with using either agent alone. Furthermore, electrocardiographic results indicate that combination treatment may be beneficial in terms of restoring myocardial microcirculation. The clinical benefit of a combination of reduced-dose reteplase with abciximab over standard thrombolytic therapy with reteplase alone is currently being investigated in GUSTO V, a large-scale mortality trial.

I. INTRODUCTION

Thrombolytic treatment of patients with acute myocardial infarction (AMI) has become an established therapy [1]. The most widely used thrombolytic agents are streptokinase and tissue-type plasminogen activator (t-PA). Analyses of large clinical studies have shown not only a significant decrease in mortality from acute myocardial infarction by thrombolysis, but also the beneficial effects of early myocardial reperfusion [2]. Early and complete reperfusion is associated with reduced in-hospital mortality, whereas incomplete reperfusion resulted in a short-term prognosis similar to that of persistent occlusion of the coronary artery [3]. Therefore, coronary artery recanalization should be accomplished as rapidly and as completely as possible. Furthermore, restored blood flow should be maintained and stable, because reocclusion is associated with substantial morbidity and mortality [4]. The currently available thrombolytic agents include urokinase, APSAC, streptokinase, alteplase, reteplase, and tenecteplase. Mortality rates of trials studying thrombolytic therapy have ranged between 6 and 8%. In an attempt to achieve faster, increased TIMI 3 flow rates, lower mortality, and improve long-term outcomes, much research has focused on the combination of reduced-dose thrombolytic therapy and glycoprotein (GP) IIb/IIIa receptor inhibition.

II. PRECLINICAL PROFILE OF RETEPLASE

A. Mechanism of Action and Biochemistry

Plasminogen activators catalyze the cleavage of endogenous plasminogen to generate plasmin, a relatively nonspecific protease that degrades the fibrin matrix of a thrombus. Therefore, plasminogen activators are defined as thrombolytic agents. First-generation thrombolytic agents (e.g., streptokinase and urokinase) are "non-fibrin–selective" and catalyze the activation of both fibrin-bound and free plasminogen. Second-generation thrombolytic agents (e.g., tissue-type plasminogen activator [t-PA; e.g., alteplase]) are "fibrin-selective" because they preferentially activate fibrin-bound, but not fluid-phase plasminogen. The fibrin selectivity can be explained by the marked stimulation of t-PA activity in the presence of fibrin [5]. The fibrin selectivity of t-PA is due to its high-affinity binding to fibrin, mainly through the finger domain but also through the kringle 2 domain [6], and by enhancement of its plasminogenolytic activity by fibrin at the kringle 2 domain [7,8].

The third-generation thrombolytic agent reteplase is a recombinant plasminogen activator derived from t-PA. Reteplase differs structurally from t-PA and consists of the kringle 2 and

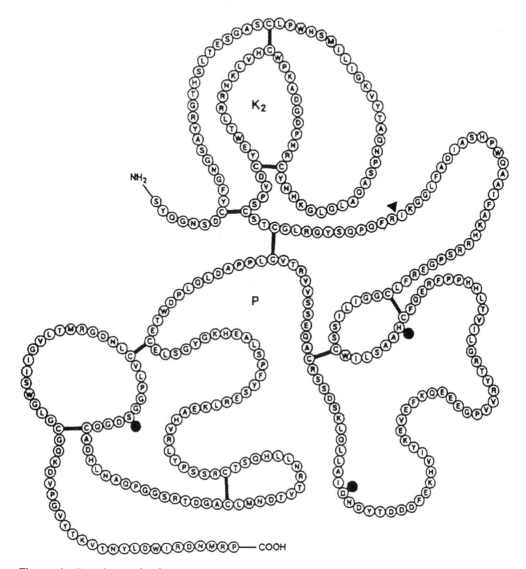

Figure 1 Reteplase molecule.

protease domains, but lacks carbohydrate side chains owing to production in *E. coli* cells. The completely single-chain reteplase molecule consists of 355 amino acids and has a molecular weight of 39 kDa (Fig. 1) [9].

Functional analysis revealed that fibrin binding of reteplase at therapeutic concentrations in vitro (10–2000 ng/mL) is about that of urokinase, which is 30% of that of t-PA [9]. This low fibrin binding of reteplase might have an effect on reduction of severe-bleeding complications, as discussed later. The low-affinity fibrin binding compared with t-PA did not affect the amidolytic activity [9,10]. Kinetic analysis showed similar values for reteplase and t-PA in the single-chain (sc) and two-chain (tc) forms for K_m and K_{cat}. Amidolytic activity merely reflects the protease function, which appears to be unaltered for reteplase when compared with t-PA. This assumption is supported by kinetic analysis of the plasminogenolytic activity (i.e., formation of plasmin), which demonstrated the same low-catalytic efficiency of reteplase and t-PA in the absence of a stimulator [9]. However, the plasminogenolytic activity of reteplase in the presence of fragments of fibrinogen as stimulator was lower by a factor of 3.8 in comparison with t-PA on a molar basis [9]. If soluble fibrin monomers were used as stimulator for the tc forms of either enzyme, the catalytic efficiency K_{cat}/K_m of reteplase was half than that of t-PA [11].

Use of fibrin monomers and of the two-chain forms probably simulates the in vivo situation of a fibrin-containing clot better than use of fragments of fibrinogen. Reteplase was rapidly and completely converted from the single-chain to the two-chain form at therapeutic concentrations (peak: 5–10 µg/mL) in a human plasma milieu in vitro [12]. This was caused by cleavage of the Arg_{275}–Ile_{276} bond. The cleavage rate by plasmin was the same for reteplase and t-PA [9]. The catalytic efficiency of reteplase was enhanced by a factor of 311 in the presence of fibrin monomers, compared with that in the absence of fibrin monomers [11]. The relevance of this in vitro comparison may be negligible, because in vivo peak concentration of reteplase after bolus injection is higher than the steady-state concentration during alteplase infusion in patients [13,14].

The lower catalytic efficiency and the lower fibrin affinity of reteplase might be explained by the lack of the finger domain in the reteplase molecule. Reteplase appears to interact with fibrin by the lysine-binding site in the kringle 2 domain because binding of reteplase to fibrin could be completely suppressed by addition of the lysine analogue ε-amino caproic acid [9]. Reteplase was susceptible to inactivation by plasminogen activator inhibitor type I (PAI-I) in a manner similar to t-PA [15,16], and might be explained by the missing finger and epidermal growth factor domains, which seem to be responsible for the interaction with endothelial cells [17,18]. The low affinity to cellular surfaces might also contribute to reduce the bleeding tendency, as discussed later.

B. In Vitro Clot Lysis

Reteplase achieved concentration- and time-dependent lysis of human plasma clots [19]. The maximal efficacy (E_{max}) of reteplase in lysis of fresh, platelet-poor plasma clots was virtually identical with that of alteplase. However, the effective molar concentration of reteplase to achieve 50% clot lysis in vitro (EC_{50}) was 6.4-fold higher than that of alteplase. This difference was more marked than for catalytic efficiency in the buffer milieu of the plasminogenolytic assay (6.4-fold vs. 1.8-fold). An explanation might be the greater susceptibility of reteplase to inactivation in plasma by protease inhibitors in comparison with alteplase [12], whereas the plasminogenolytic activity of reteplase and alteplase was equally stable over time in Tris buffer [20]. The relevance of the low in vitro potency of reteplase will be discussed later in view of in vivo pharmaco-dynamic and pharmacokinetic data.

Variation of clot composition and clot age revealed that reteplase was less effective than alteplase in lysis of cell-rich and aged clots [19]. This diminished thrombolytic efficacy toward old thrombi might lower lysis of hemostatic plugs and thereby lower excess bleeding following administration of reteplase. Hemostatic plugs are believed to be older clots that physiologically seal small vessel wall injuries [21].

"Carryover" experiments functionally confirmed the lower fibrin binding of reteplase by the absence of further lysis after transfer of the clot preincubated with the activator to fresh plasma with no activator added [19]. This implies that lysis by reteplase is coupled to its presence in plasma and that after "washout" of reteplase from plasma, extended lytic action is not to be expected because reteplase is only marginally bound to the fibrin of the clot. The more limited fibrinolytic action of reteplase might also contribute to reducing bleeding rates without affecting the thrombolytic action. In contrast, t-PA showed sustained lysis in vivo after clearance from the circulation [22].

The ability of reteplase and alteplase to penetrate and lyse a clot under physiological conditions was investigated in a "dynamic plasma clot lysis model" [23]. In this model, a constant pressure gradient is applied to a clot that has been placed in a tube system filled with saline, mimicking the in vivo situation of an occluded coronary artery in the body. In a series of experiments, various concentrations of the thrombolytic agent are added to the saline on the "upstream" end of the clot. The pressure gradient promotes migration of the saline and the thrombolytic agent through the clot. In this experiment, t-PA remained trapped at the upstream surface of the clot, whereas reteplase penetrated the clot quickly and thoroughly. The difference can be explained by high-affinity fibrin binding of t-PA, which is not present in reteplase owing to the absence of the finger domain, the fibrinonectin-like portion of t-PA that promotes high-affinity fibrin binding. The results of angiographic clinical trials in patients with acute myocardial infarction (compare Sec. III.B) suggest that this difference between reteplase and t-PA may actually translate into faster and more complete thrombolysis and reperfusion of the infarct-related artery.

C. In Vivo Thrombolysis

In the rabbit model of jugular vein thrombosis, reteplase dose-dependently increased thrombolysis, correlating to the area under the plasma concentration–time curve (AUC) [24]. The maximal efficacy of reteplase was comparable with that of alteplase. Reteplase was more potent in thrombolysis than alteplase, as evidenced by a 5.3-fold lower effective dose of 50% thrombolysis (ED_{50}). Even on a molar basis, reteplase was 2.2-fold more potent than alteplase. This is in contrast to the 6.4-fold lower in vitro clot lysis potency and 2-fold lower catalytic efficiency. The discrepancy between in vitro and in vivo potency of reteplase can be explained by its lower clearance rate and its longer half-life compared with alteplase.

A canine model of coronary artery thrombosis was used to characterize reteplase in the lead indication (i.e., acute myocardial infarction). A systematic dose–response study with intravenous-bolus injection confirmed the higher in vivo thrombolytic potency of reteplase compared with alteplase by a factor of 4.3 on a molar basis [25]. A single intravenous-bolus injection of 0.14 U/kg = 0.24 mg/kg) was equieffective (66% reperfusion rate) to a 90-min intravenous infusion of 1 mg/kg alteplase.

A comparative study revealed the predominant characteristic of reteplase is rapid induction of reperfusion. The time to reperfusion was significantly shorter than for alteplase, streptokinase, urokinase, and APSAC at clinically relevant doses and regimens [26]. The property of rapid thrombolysis appears to be influenced by the pharmacokinetic profile after intravenous-bolus injection, because such infusion of reteplase as well as of alteplase was not associated with rapid thrombolysis [25]. The rapid onset of action after reteplase-bolus injection was also found in a canine model of pulmonary hypertension induced by thromboembolism [27].

The aforementioned studies in the canine model of coronary thrombolysis revealed the occurrence of reocclusion shortly after successful thrombolysis by reteplase as well as by alteplase, despite the concomitant use of intravenous heparin. However, this phenomenon is model-related and is known from t-PA studies, where it represents the subpopulation of thrombolytically treated patients with reocclusion [28,29]. In dogs, an intravenous-double–bolus administration regimen of reteplase was superior to single-intravenous–bolus administration in stabilizing the coronary artery blood flow and reducing reocclusion, whereas doubling the single-bolus dose did not [30]. It appeared that the longer half-life of reteplase compared with alteplase favored the double-bolus regimen because it combines the advantages of high peak concentrations after bolus injection followed by an infusion-like plasma level of the drug. In contrast, double-bolus alteplase would require higher bolus doses owing to the shorter half-life, but followed by a steep decline of the plasma concentration. This pharmacokinetic profile of double-bolus alteplase would imply a higher bleeding risk owing to the very high peak concentrations, without the benefit of sustained plasma levels required for effective thrombolysis.

Another strategy to prevent deterioration of coronary blood flow might be the use of hirudin, a novel direct thrombin inhibitor, as an adjunct to reteplase. Hirudin in addition to single-bolus or double-bolus reteplase significantly improved coronary blood flow after reperfusion, whereas aspirin did not [31,32]. However, hirudin is an investigational drug and is not available for adjunctive use with reteplase.

Results of animal experiments in the aforementioned model suggest that intravenous heparin is required as an adjunct to reteplase to maintain coronary blood flow after reperfusion in the absence of a systemic lytic state [33]. On the basis of these data, it is recommended that intravenous heparin be used, because it cannot be predicted in the individual patients whether nonspecific fibrinogenolysis by reteplase generates enough fibrinogen degradation products with anticoagulant properties [34].

D. In Vivo Interaction of Reteplase with Platelets and the Hemostatic System

A pharmacologically effective dose of 0.2 U/kg reteplase induced only a slight reduction of plasma fibrinogen in rabbits and in dogs [24,25]. Systematic investigation with pharmacological doses in anesthetized rabbits revealed a dose-dependent reduction of the hemostasis proteins—fibrinogen, plasminogen, and α_2-antiplasmin [24]. At equieffective doses of 50% thrombolysis, the degree of in vivo fibrin selectivity of reteplase, was virtually identical with that of alteplase. It can be concluded that in vivo reteplase has a relative (i.e., a dose-dependent) fibrin selectivity similar to that of alteplase. The exact extent of fibrinogen reduction depends on the dose. The relevance of a marked fibrinogen reduction for the occurrence of bleeding is questioned because there are only weak relations between markers of systemic lysis and bleeding [35].

Alteration of platelet function by reteplase could be relevant for a bleeding tendency if platelet function or count were reduced [36], or to a reocclusion tendency if platelet activity were increased [37]. Ex vivo platelet aggregation measurements in rabbits and dogs at pharmacological doses showed a tendency to slight reduction, rather than an increase in platelet aggregation [26,31,38]. In vitro experiments with citrated human platelet-rich plasma revealed a concentration- and time-dependent inhibitory effect of reteplase on platelet aggregation, which appeared to be plasmin-dependent. There was no evidence of a proaggregatory effect [39].

E. Bleeding Risk

In general, bleeding after treatment with plasminogen activators is caused by lysis of physiologically formed "hemostatic plugs," which may either be young and fresh, especially when induced by invasive procedures (e.g., by catheterization), or old (e.g., after trauma, surgery, or after endogenous sealing of vascular leakages). Intracerebral, retroperitoneal, and gastrointestinal bleedings are of major concern because they may be life-threatening. The results of the GUSTO I trial showed that the fibrin-selective plasminogen activator alteplase actually caused significantly more intracerebral (i.c.) bleedings than the nonfibrin-selective plasminogen activator streptokinase [40], indicating that extensive reduction in fibrinogen by streptokinase is of little importance for the induction of i.c. bleeding.

There is a hypothesis that major bleeding (e.g., intracerebral) may be caused by prolonged and effective fibrinolysis of old clots [41]. This might explain why alteplase caused more i.c.

bleeds. Since alteplase is infused over 90 min to 3 h, it effectively lyses old, platelet-rich clots, and strongly binds to the fibrin surface of clots and endothelial cells, thereby extending its fibrinolytic action beyond its presence in plasma [22]. Because of genetic variation, reteplase has low-affinity fibrin binding [9], low-affinity endothelial cell binding [15,16], low-efficacy lysis of old, platelet-rich clots [19], low-fibrinolytic activity at low concentrations [19], and a short presence in plasma after bolus injection [26]. These properties do not affect the desired pharmacodymaic effect on pathological, acute thrombi (e.g., in the coronary artery), and they may contribute to a reduction in the incidence of major bleeding.

F. Pharmacokinetics

The short half-life of human t-PA is explained mainly by its rapid clearance in the liver by receptor-medicated mechanisms [42]. The structures in t-PA responsible for hepatic uptake appear to be carbohydrate moieties [43] and parts of the polypeptide sequence encoding the finger or growth factor domains [44]. These domains and the carbohydrate moieties are lacking in reteplase. Recent experiments suggest that two independent receptor systems (i.e., the mannose receptor on liver endothelial cells and the low-density lipoprotein receptor-related protein (LFP) on liver parenchymal cells, are involved in the hepatic clearance of t-PA [45].

As a result of genetic engineering, the pharmacokinetic profile of reteplase was changed compared with that of t-PA. Alteplase-controlled studies in rats, rabbits, dogs, and nonhuman primates with reteplase consistently confirmed a 4.5- to 12.3-fold prolongation of the half-life and a 3.2- to 8.5-fold lowering of the total plasma clearance rate. Analysis of plasma concentration of reteplase activity after a single-intravenous–bolus injection revealed predominantly first-order kinetics, with a best-fit in most individuals to single-phase elimination in contrast to alteplase [46,47]. Dose–response evaluation of reteplase after intravenous-bolus injection of pharmacological doses in rabbit and dog models of thrombolysis revealed a linear increase in the plasma concentration–time curves, resulting in a dose-independent pharmaco-kinetic profile [24,25]. The longer half-life of reteplase makes it more suitable for bolus administration than alteplase. This difference in half-life may explain the high incidence of bleeding and hemorrhagic stroke after administration of double-bolus alteplase in clinical trials.

G. Metabolism

The rapid clearance of $[^{125}I]$-t-PA in rats is mainly mediated (80%) by its uptake in the liver [48], whereas only 14% of $[^{125}I]$-reteplase was dose-independently taken up in the liver [49]. Even use of the $[^{125}I]$-tyramine cellobiose label, which accumulates in the lysosomes, showed the limit of hepatic uptake to be 37% of a pharmacological dose of reteplase. Twenty percent of the injected dose was actively taken up and degraded in the kidneys. However, only 4% of the injected dose was recovered in the bladder and urine. Use of the ^{125}I-label may be misleading because degradation products artificially accumulate (e.g., in the intestine and the skin).

The liver and kidneys are the main organs of active uptake and lysosomal degradation. In the liver, parenchymal cells contributed more (65%) to the metabolism by a receptor-mediated uptake mechanism and subsequent lysosomal degradation. The type of kidney cell responsible for active uptake was not identified. Binding of reteplase to liver parenchymal cells could be displaced by t-PA, indicating that LRP might be involved in the binding of reteplase. In in vivo investigations, GST-RAP (fusion protein of glutathione S-transferase and the 39-kDa protein or receptor-associated protein), which is an inhibitor of LRP, significantly inhibited the uptake of reteplase in the liver in vivo [49]. The contribution of endothelial cells to the liver metabolism of reteplase was low, owing to the lack of carbohydrates in contrast to t-PA [48].

Organ failure studies were conducted to elucidate the metabolic capacity of the liver and kidneys. Bilateral nephrectomy in rats resulted in a longer half-life, an increase in liver uptake, and a reduced clearance rate compared with t-PA [20]. Nevertheless, plasma activity concentration decreased over time, indicating that there are compensatory mechanisms. In addition to the liver, blood or plasma was identified as contributing to inactivation of reteplase by inhibitors (e.g., C1-inactivator, α_2-antiplasmin, and α_1-antitrypsin) [12]. In the healthy rat, the relative contribution of this inhibition pathway to total clearance of reteplase was calculated to be 32.3%. Results of functional studies suggest that the catabolic role of the kidneys might be higher than proposed by the uptake studies (20%), potentially by filtration, as has been shown for other mutants of t-PA [44]. Further studies with varying degrees of renal dysfunction indicated that slight impairment of renal function does not significantly influence the pharmacokinetic properties of reteplase [50]. Chemically induced hepatic failure reduced the clearance rate only marginally (by 14%), indicating that liver failure can be compensated better than kidney failure. In studies with renal and hepatic failure in rats, reteplase was still inactivated in plasma [20].

III. CLINICAL PROFILE OF RETEPLASE

A. Clinical Pharmacology in Healthy Volunteers

The first human experience with reteplase was gained in healthy male volunteers [51]. The study was performed in a stepwise dose-escalating manner to examine tolerability, pharmacokinetics, and effects on the hemostatic and fibrinolytic systems. The systemic effects of reteplase on the hemostatic and fibrinolytic systems do not reflect the principal pharmacodynamic effect, which is restoring patency of the previously thrombosed coronary artery. However, they do reflect the dose–response characteristics and provide insight into the fibrinolytic action and fibrin selectivity of reteplase.

At the doses studied (up to 5.5 U) of reteplase, there was no reduction in plasma fibrinogen or prolongation of the clotting times (thrombin time, prothrombin time, activated partial thromboplastin time). Measurement of plasminogen and α_2-antiplasmin, which are the main components of the fibrinolytic system, revealed a reduction in plasminogen to a nadir of 86% of baseline and consumption of α_2-antiplasmin up to 70% of baseline at the higher doses. α_2-macroglobulin and antithrombin III remained unchanged. The decreases most probably reflected nonspecific systemic formation of plasmin by reteplase. Indirect evidence of the fibrinolytic action of reteplase was obtained by a dose-dependent increase in fibrin D-dimers up to 1147 ± 380 ng/mL and in fibrin degradation products. The reduction in plasminogen activator inhibitor (PAI)-1 activity indicated normal interaction of reteplase with PAI-1.

Bleeding time, platelet count, and platelet aggregation were in the normal range after administration of reteplase. Evaluation of hemodynamic, clinicochemical, and urinalysis parameters of safety did not reveal relevant changes after 2-min intravenous bolus injection of reteplase. Formation of antibodies to reteplase was not found in samples taken up to 1-year postadministration. The AUC values of reteplase activity showed a dose-dependent linear increase beginning at doses of 2.2 U reteplase. At the highest dose studied (5.5 U), the total plasma clearance for reteplase activity was 306 ± 40 mL/min and the half-life was 14.4 ± 1.1 min.

Following the first human experience with reteplase in the foregoing dose-escalating study, reteplase was evaluated in a single-dose, randomized, placebo-controlled crossover phase I study in seven male volunteers [52]. The dose of 6 U in this study was based on pharmacokinetic calculations from the first study, which suggested that 6 U would represent about half the expected effective dose in the human.

As expected, 6 U did not decrease plasma fibrinogen, but significantly reduced plasminogen and α_2-antiplasmin to 83 and 64% of baseline, respectively, again indicating systemic activation of the fibrinolytic system. This assumption was supported by a significant increase in fibrin D-dimers to a maximum of 1016 ± 216 ng/mL. Fibrinogen degradation products were elevated only marginally, to 555 ± 152 ng/mL (normal range: 125–425 ng/mL). In the control group, these parameters remained unchanged. Measurement of bleeding time and platelet count did not reveal abnormalities. Safety parameters including analysis of antibody formation to reteplase measured in samples taken up to 1 year postadministration failed to show any abnormalities. Pharmacokinetic analysis of reteplase plasma concentrations of activity and antigen revealed a dominant half-life of 11.2 ± 0.4 min and 13.9 ± 0.7 min, respectively, and a total plasma clearance of 371 ± 13 mL/min and 183 ± 15 mL/min.

B. Patency Trials with Reteplase in Patients with Acute Myocardial Infarction

Reteplase was evaluated in four different patency trials in patients with acute myocardial infarction.

1. GRECO (German Recombinant Plasminogen Activator) Study

The GRECO study was the first study conducted in patients with acute myocardial infarction [53]. This open-label sequential trial enrolled 142 patients. Principal entry criteria were an age of 18–75 years, typical symptoms of acute myocardial infarction with duration of more than a half-hour, but less than 6 h, and ST-segment elevation in at least two standard leads. The primary efficacy parameter was patency of the infarct-related coronary artery (Thrombolysis in Myocardial Infarction Trial [TIMI] grade 2 or 3), assessed from angiograms obtained 90 min after administration of reteplase. A sequential design was used to ensure that study of doses with 90-min patency of less than 70% was terminated early. Concomitant therapy consisted of heparin (5000 IU as a bolus and 1000 IU/h for 48 h) and acetylsalicylic acid (200 mg daily).

Forty-two patients received 10 U of reteplase as a single-intravenous bolus injection over 2 min. The 90-min TIMI grade 2 or 3 patency rate after the 10-U dose was 66%. Because this patency rate was less than 70%, the dose was increased to 15 U of reteplase. A total of 100 patients were treated at that dose. The 90-min patency rate (TIMI 2 or 3) and TIMI 3 rate after the 15-U dose were 76 and 69%, respectively. Angiographically confirmed reocclusions at 24–48 h after reperfusion were found in two patients, both in the 15-U dose group.

During the hospital stay, five deaths occurred among the 142 patients (3.5%). One nonfatal intracranial hemorrhage was encountered, and eight patients had a reinfarction. There was no evidence of antibody formation to reteplase. Angiography at 30 and 60 min after the bolus injection revealed a patent (TIMI 2 or 3) infarct-related artery in 66 and 74%, respectively, of patients treated with 15 U of reteplase. Very early reocclusion, defined as TIMI grade 0 or 1 at 90 min, that had been patent (TIMI grade 2 or 3) at 30 or 60 min angiography, occurred in 10 of 78 (13%) patients.

2. Double-Bolus (GRECO DB) Study

GRECO DB was an extension of the first GRECO study to evaluate the concept of the double-bolus regimen. This concept was effective in maintaining coronary artery blood flow in animals reperfused with reteplase [30]. The double-bolus was expected to stabilize the very early reperfused coronary artery and avoid fluctuations in the patency of the infarct-related artery, thereby encouraging complete and stable coronary thrombolysis. Therefore, patients with acute myocardial infarction were treated with a double-bolus regimen of 10 U reteplase, followed by 5 U reteplase 30 min later. The primary objective of the trial was to determine the effect of double-bolus administration on coronary artery patency. This study was conducted by the same group of investigators who carried out the GRECO study and used the same protocol [54].

Fifty patients underwent 90-min angiography. The TIMI 2 or 3 patency rate and the TIMI 3 rate at this time were 78 and 58%, respectively. The incidence of reocclusion was very low, with only one patient having angiographically confirmed reocclusion between the 90-min angiogram and the 24- to 48-h angiogram. Very early cycling of the patency status was seen in some patients. Five patients with an open vessel at 30 or 60 min had a closed vessel at 90 min (very early reocclusion rate of 10%), while 16 patients with a closed vessel at 30 or 60 min showed a patent artery at 90 min. There were no deaths and no strokes in the study.

3. Recombinant Plasminogen Activator Angiographic Phase II International Dose-Finding (RAPID) Study

RAPID was a randomized, open-label, dose-response study comparing reteplase at doses of 15 U, 10 + 5 U, and 10 + 10 U and the conventional 3-h infusion of alteplase (100 mg) in patients with acute myocardial infarction [55]. The primary objective of the study was to assess the effects of the three reteplase regimens in comparison with the 3-h infusion of alteplase on coronary artery patency (TIMI grade 2 or 3) and TIMI grade 3 flow at 90 min after the initiation of thrombolytic therapy. Although this was an open-label study, all angiograms were read blinded by a central core laboratory. Patients were eligible if they had ST-segment elevation and if the interval between the onset of the ischemic pain and the treatment was less than 6 h. Patients must have been 18–75 years of age. All patients were scheduled to receive acetylsalicylic acid at a dose of 200–350 mg/day before thrombolytic therapy and until hospital discharge. The heparin regimen consisted of an intravenous 5000-IU bolus that was administered before thrombolytic therapy and an infusion of 1000 IU/h for at least 24 h, also initiated before thrombolytic therapy.

Six hundred and six patients were randomized to one of four treatment groups. The 10 + 10 U regimen of reteplase produced higher 30-, 60-, 90-min, and follow-up patency and TIMI 3 rates more than either the 15-U and 10 + 5-U reteplase regimens. Based on these results, which were supported by other efficacy and safety results, the 10 + 10-U regimen was selected for evaluation in further studies. As a result, all further discussions of the RAPID study focus on comparison of the 10 + 10-U regimen with the alteplase control.

The 10 + 10-U reteplase group achieved significantly higher 60-, 90-, and 5- to 14-day TIMI 3 flow than the alteplase group (51 vs. 49%), suggesting a 30-min advantage with reteplase in achieving complete reperfusion of coronary arteries. TIMI 2 or 3 patency rates were significantly higher for the 10 + 10-U reteplase regimen relative to the alteplase control at the follow-up evaluation. Patients who had a patent (TIMI 2 or 3) infarct-related artery at the 90-min angiogram and a nonpatent artery (TIMI 0 or 1) at any follow-up assessment were classified as having had a reocclusion. The difference in reocclusion rates between reteplase and alteplase was not statistically significant (2.9 vs. 7.8%).

The global ejection fraction and regional wall motion in the 10 + 10-U reteplase group were significantly superior to those of the alteplase group at hospital discharge (53 ± 1.3% vs. 49 ± 1.3% and −2.19 ± 0.12 vs. −2.61 ± 0.13 SD per chord, respectively). The 30-day mortality rate in the 10 + 10-U reteplase group was 1.9, compared with 3.9% in the alteplase group. There was only one stroke (15-U group) in all reteplase groups (1 of 452 patients), compared with 6 in the alteplase group (6 of 154 patients). The incidence of stroke in the 10 + 10-U reteplase group was significantly less than in the alteplase group. Bleeding complications were similar between the groups.

4.   Recombinant Plasminogen Activator Angiographic Phase II International
     Dose-Finding (RAPID-2) Study

The RAPID-2 study was a randomized, open-label, angiographic study in 324 patients with acute
myocardial infarction [56]. It was designed to compare the effect of $10 + 10\,$U reteplase with
that of accelerated-dose alteplase ($100\,$mg over $90\,$min) on the TIMI grade of the infarct-related
coronary artery $90\,$min after the initiation of thrombolytic therapy. All angiograms were read
blinded by a central core laboratory. There was no age limit, and patients were recruited up to
$12\,$h after symptom onset. All patients were scheduled to receive acetylsalicylic acid at a dose of
$160–350\,$mg/day before thrombolytic therapy and until hospital discharge. The heparin regimen
consisted of a 5000-IU–intravenous bolus that was administered before thrombolytic therapy and
an infusion of $1000\,$IU/h for at least $24\,$h, also initiated before thrombolytic therapy.

In this study, reteplase achieved earlier and more complete reperfusion than accelerated-
dose alteplase. TIMI grade 2 or 3 patency and TIMI grade 3 flow rates of the infarct-related
artery at $90\,$min were significantly higher for reteplase relative to the alteplase control (83.4 vs.
73.3% and 59.5 vs. 45.2%, respectively). At $60\,$min, both the TIMI grade 2 or 3 patency and the
TIMI grade 3 flow rates were significantly higher for reteplase than with alteplase. Reteplase-
treated patients required significantly fewer additional coronary interventions within the first $6\,$h
of treatment (13.3 vs. 26.5%). There were no significant differences between the reteplase and
alteplase groups relative to 35-day mortality (4.1 vs. 8.4%) and hemorrhagic stroke (1.2 vs.
1.8%).

C.   Hemostatic and Pharmacokinetic Parameters of Reteplase in Patients
with Acute Myocardial Infarction

Reteplase induced a decrease in median fibrinogen from 2.79 to $1.69\,$g/L after $10\,$U and from
2.54 to $0.92\,$g/L after $15\,$U in the GRECO study [53]. More detailed analysis of a subgroup of
the GRECO study receiving $15\,$U of reteplase showed residual concentrations of plasminogen
and of α_2-antiplasmin at $2\,$h after onset of thrombolysis of 43 and 22%, respectively, after $10\,$U,
and of 39 and 21%, respectively [57]. The double-bolus of $10 + 5\,$U in the GRECO DB study
induced a decrease in median fibrinogen from $2.86\,$g/L to 37% of baseline at $2\,$h [54]. In the
RAPID study, median plasma fibrinogen concentrations were significantly lower in all reteplase
dose groups than in the alteplase group. However, the bleeding complications did not seem to
parallel the reduction in fibrinogen [55].

Analysis of plasma antigen concentrations in the subgroup of the GRECO study
demonstrated a dominant half-life of $19.2\,$min after $10\,$U of reteplase and of $18.8\,$min after
$15\,$U of reteplase in patients with acute myocardial infarction [57]. The dominant half-life for
alteplase antigen after accelerated dosing of $100\,$mg over $90\,$min was reported to be $3.5\,$min [14].
Therefore, the antigen half-life of reteplase is about 5.4-fold longer than that of alteplase, making
reteplase more suitable for bolus administration than alteplase. Plasma clearance of reteplase
antigen [58] was $104\,$mL/min ($10\,$U) and $139\,$mL/min ($15\,$U) and thus about 4.6-fold lower than
alteplase antigen clearance ($572\,$mL/min) [14].

D.   Mortality Trials with Reteplase in Patients with Acute Myocardial
Infarction

1.   International Joint Efficacy Comparison of Thrombolysis (INJECT) Study

The INJECT study was the first study to evaluate the effects of reteplase in reducing mortality
following acute myocardial infarction [59]. The study was designed to determine whether the

reteplase was at least as effective in mortality reduction (within 1% of fatality rate) as a standard streptokinase regimen. In this double-blind study, 3004 patients were randomized to a double bolus of 10 + 10 U of reteplase, 30 min apart, and 3006 patients were randomized to 1.5 MU of streptokinase over 60 min. Patients with symptoms and electrocardiographic criteria consistent with acute myocardial infarction were recruited. Treatment could be started up to 12 h from onset of symptoms. There was no upper age limit for enrollment into the study. All patients received intravenous heparin for at least 24 h. Patients were given 250–325 mg acetylsalicylic acid initially, then 75–150 mg daily. The primary event was 35-day outcome.

Among treated patients, the mortality rate was 8.9% in the reteplase group and 9.53% in the streptokinase group. The difference in 35-day mortality (reteplase–streptokinase) was −0.53, indicating a beneficial trend in favor of reteplase. The 95% confidence interval for this difference ranged from −1.98 to 0.94%. Because the upper limit of the 90% confidence interval (CI) for this difference is 0.71%, this result shows that reteplase is at least as effective as streptokinase. At 6 months, mortality rates were 11.02% for reteplase and 12.05% for streptokinase, a difference of −1.03% (95% CI: −2.65–0.59%). Thus, the trend in favor of reteplase was stronger at 6 months than at 35 days. These results provide further evidence that reteplase is effective in reducing mortality after acute myocardial infarction.

Bleeding events were similar in the two groups (0.7% for reteplase and 1.0% for streptokinase). The in-hospital stroke rates were 1.23% for reteplase and 1.0% for streptokinase. The incidence of recurrent myocardial infarction was similar in the two groups. There were significantly fewer cases of atrial fibrillation, asystole, cardiac shock, heart failure, allergic reactions, and hypotension in the reteplase group relative to the streptokinase group. There was no evidence of antibody formation to reteplase.

In a subgroup study of the INJECT trial, the prognostic power of early ST-segment elevation resolution was assessed to test the value of differences in ST resolution as a surrogate endpoint [60]. The results showed that the 35-day mortality in patients with infarct age less than 6 h for complete, partial, or no ST resolution was 2.5, 4.3, and 17.5%. The percentage of patients with complete ST resolution was larger, and with no ST resolution smaller, with reteplase compared with streptokinase (p = 0.006). Mortality rates among all evaluated patients in the substudy were 5.2% for reteplase-treated patients and 7.2% for streptokinase-treated patients (not significant).

2. Global Use of Strategies to Open Occluded Coronary Arteries (GUSTO III) Study

The GUSTO III trial was a multinational study designed to compare 30-day mortality rates between reteplase and accelerated alteplase therapy [61]. A total of 15,059 patients were enrolled at 807 sites worldwide. Patients were randomized in a 2:1 fashion to receive therapy with either 10 + 10 U reteplase (n = 10,138) or accelerated alteplase (100 mg over 90 min, n = 4921). Patients who presented within 6 h of the onset of signs or symptoms consistent with acute myocardial infarction were enrolled. All patients were treated concomitantly with heparin and aspirin. The concomitant use of antiarrhythmics, calcium channel blockers, nitrates, angiotensin-converting enzyme (ACE) inhibitors, and other cardiovascular medications was left to the discretion of the investigator.

The primary endpoint of 30-day mortality was realized in 7.47% of reteplase- and 7.24% of alteplase-treated patients. The 95% confidence interval was −1.11–0.66. The net clinical benefit, combined endpoint of death and nonfatal disabling stroke, was a nonsignificant difference of 7.89% in reteplase-treated patients and 7.91% in alteplase-treated patients (95% CI: 0.88–1.13).

Rates of hemorrhagic stroke were 0.91% for reteplase and 0.93% for alteplase. Rates of severe or life-threatening bleeds as well as moderate bleeds for reteplase and alteplase were 0.95 versus 1.20% and 6.9 versus 6.8%, respectively. All comparisons for bleeding events revealed nonsignificant differences between the two treatment arms. Rates of reinfarction, recurrent ischemia, and cardiac arrhythmias revealed no significant differences between reteplase and alteplase.

A subgroup analysis was conducted involving 392 patients from GUSTO III who underwent percutaneous transluminal coronary angioplasty (PTCA) of the infarct-related artery within 24 h of thrombolytic therapy [62]. In this group, 83 patients received abciximab in conjunction with PTCA while 309 did not. There was a significant improvement in the mortality at 30 days in patients given abciximab in conjunction with PTCA versus those treated with PTCA alone (3.6 vs. 9.7%, p = 0.042). The combined incidence of mortality, myocardial infarction, and stroke was reduced among abciximab patients initially randomized to reteplase (n = 55) versus alteplase (n = 28) (7 vs. 21%, p = 0.08). Although severe bleeding was increased among abciximab-treated patients (3.6 vs. 1.0%, p = 0.08), no intracranial hemorrhages occurred with abciximab.

One-year follow-up information for 97.4% of the 15,059 patients enrolled into the GUSTO III trial is available [63]. Overall, the mortality rates for alteplase and reteplase were not significantly different, 11.06 and 11.20% (p = 0.77), respectively. The absolute mortality difference at 1 year between the two groups was 0.14% (95% CI: −1.21–0.93%. The absolute mortality difference narrowed over time from 0.31 at 24 h to 0.14% at 1 year. The Kaplan Meier curve (Fig. 2) for the 1-year mortality results reveal no clear separation between the two therapies. In fact, the curves converge and even cross over one another at several time-points.

One-year mortality rates in the prospectively defined subgroups of advanced age (>75 years), infarct location, and time to treatment were compared and showed no statistically significant differences between reteplase and alteplase. For patients receiving treatment with alteplase or reteplase within 0–2 h after symptoms onset, 1-year mortality rates were 8.33 and 8.04% (p = 0.25); for 2–4 h the rates were 11.05 and 11.37% (p = 0.67); and for more than 4 h the rates were 12.70 and 14.34% (p = 0.18), respectively. Mortality rates for reteplase patients aged over 75 years were 29.6 versus 30.9% in alteplase-treated patients (p = 0.46). Inferior infarction patients had mortality rates of 7.92 and 7.95% (p = 0.95) for reteplase and alteplase patients. Anterior infarction patients had 1-year mortality rates of 14.39 and 14.18% (p = 0.74), respectively.

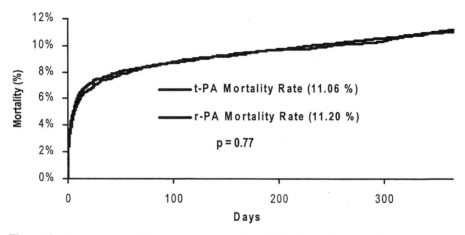

Figure 2 One-year mortality (Kaplan-Meier estimate) for the GUSTO III trial.

E. Angiographic Trials Using the Combination of Reduced-Dose Reteplase and Abciximab in Patients with Acute Myocardial Infarction

1. Thrombolysis in Myocardial Infarction (TIMI 14) Trial

The TIMI 14 trial was designed to study the effect of the combination of abciximab and reteplase, alteplase, or streptokinase on angiographic evidence of infarct-related coronary artery reperfusion [64]. TIMI 14 was an international phase II dose-finding, dose-confirmation, and safety trial comparing different fibrinolytic and fibrinolytic–antiplatelet regimens in 1187 patients with acute myocardial infarction. Patients aged between 18 and 75 years presenting within 12 h of the onset of AMI symptoms were enrolled. Patients were to receive one of several regimens consisting of abciximab (0.25- or 0.30-mg/kg–intravenous bolus, followed by 0.125 µg/kg min^{-1}-intravenous infusion for 12 h) in combination with streptokinase, alteplase, or reteplase at various dosing regimens, or to control regimens of standard fibrinolytic therapy with alteplase or reteplase alone.

The reteplase arm of TIMI 14 enrolled 299 patients. These patients were randomized to abciximab (0.25 mg/kg–intravenous bolus, followed by 0.125-µg/kg min^{-1}–intravenous infusion for 12 h) plus reduced-dose reteplase 5 + 5 U or 10 + 5 U and low-dose or very low-dose heparin, or a control regimen of full-dose reteplase 10 + 10 U and standard-dose heparin. The primary efficacy endpoint was angiographic TIMI grade 3 flow at 90 min after the onset of therapy. Secondary endpoints included TIMI flow grade at 60 min, TIMI frame count at 60 and 90 min, and safety endpoints such as major hemorrhage and intracranial hemorrhage [65].

Standard-dose heparin consisted of an initial bolus of 70 U/kg followed by an initial intravenous infusion rate of 15 U/kg h^{-1}. The low-dose heparin regimen comprised an initial bolus of 60 U/kg followed by an initial infusion rate of 7 U/kg h^{-1}, whereas the very low-dose heparin regimen consisted of an initial bolus of 30 U/kg followed by an initial infusion rate of 4 U/kg h^{-1}. The infusion was adjusted to maintain an activated partial thromboplastin time (aPTT) of 50–70 s.

The rates of complete infarct-related artery reperfusion observed in the reduced dose (5 + 5 U) reteplase + abciximab group compared with the reteplase-alone control group were 70 versus 73%, respectively (Fig. 3). TIMI Myocardial Perfusion Grade (TMPG) 2/3 was obtained in 42% of reteplase–only-treated patients versus 60 of reteplase–abciximab-treated patients (Fig. 4). A subset of the TIMI 14 trial examined the rates of complete ST-segment resolution, defined as ≥ 70% resolution. Complete ST-segment resolution was achieved in 48% of reteplase treated patients compared with 56% of patients receiving combination therapy with reteplase and abciximab.

The incidence of major bleeding events, intracranial hemorrhage, and death was similar in patients treated with reteplase only and in patients receiving 5 + 5 U of reteplase and abciximab. In the patients treated with 10 + 5 U reteplase and abciximab, higher rates of major bleeding and an adverse trend in terms of death and intracranial hemorrhage were noted. However, the treatment groups in this trial were too small to enable dependable statistical comparisons of clinical events occurring with low-frequency, such as death and intracranial hemorrhage.

2. Strategies for Patency Enhancement in the Emergency Department (SPEED) Trial

Enrollment in the SPEED trial, or GUSTO V pilot trial, included 528 patients with acute myocardial infarction diagnosed by electrocardiographic ST-segment elevation. Inclusion and exclusion criteria were similar to the TIMI 14 trial; however, SPEED had no upper age limit for enrollment, and patients could be enrolled up to 12 h after chest pain onset. In the dose-finding

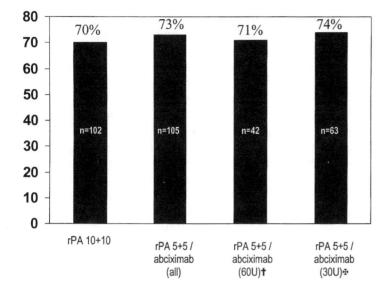

† All patients received heparin 60 U/kg-IV bolus, followed by a 7 U/kg h^{-1} infusion
⌖ All patients received heparin 30 U/kg-IV bolus, followed by a 4 U/kg h^{-1} infusion
All patients received abciximab at a dose of 0.252 mg/kg IV bolus, followed by a
0.125 μcg/kg min^{-1} infusion (10 μcg/min max) for 12 h

Figure 3 TIMI 14 angiographic results.

stage (phase A, $n = 304$) of the SPEED trial, patients were randomized in a 4 : 1 ratio to receive experimental single-bolus (5, 7.5, 10 U) and double-bolus (5 + 2.5 U, 5 + 5 U) reteplase doses in combination with standard-dose abciximab and low-dose heparin. This group was compared with a control regimen of standard-dose abciximab plus low-dose heparin. In the dose-

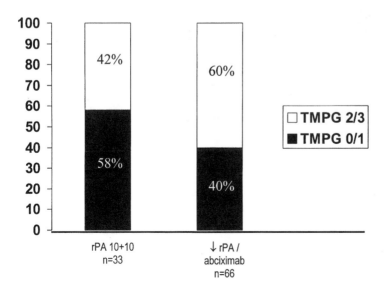

Figure 4 TIMI 14 TMPG results.

confirmation stage (phase B, $n = 224$), the combination regimens of reteplase $5 + 5$ U, standard-dose abciximab, and low-dose heparin were compared with control regimens of $10 + 10$-U double-bolus reteplase plus standard-dose heparin. The primary efficacy endpoint was TIMI grade 3 flow in the infarct-related artery at 60–90 min following initiation of the reperfusion regimen. Following the 60–90-min angiogram, PTCA was performed at the investigators' discretion [67].

Heparin regimens utilized in SPEED also differed from TIMI 14. In the dose-finding stage (phase A) and in the beginning of the dose-confirmation stage (phase B), patients randomized to combination treatment with reteplase and abciximab were treated with an initial intravenous heparin bolus of 60 U/kg, with additional heparin given to maintain an activated clotting time of 200 s, or more, during cardiac catheterization or intervention. During the dose-confirmation stage (phase B) and after release of the TIMI 14 results, the heparin-bolus dose for patients randomized to combination therapy was reduced to 40 U/kg (maximum 4000 U). Patients in the reteplase-only group received a 70-U/kg bolus (maximum 5000 U).

Angiographic results from the dose-finding and dose-confirmation phases are shown in Figure 5. The combination of reteplase $5 + 5$ U plus standard-dose abciximab was associated with the greatest percentage of TIMI grade 3 and TIMI grade $2 + 3$ flow. Note that these data represent angiographic findings at an average of 62 min after initiation of therapy. Overall patency (TIMI $2 + 3$ flow) rates observed in phase B patients were 77% in the reteplase-alone group and 77% in the combination of abciximab and half-dose reteplase.

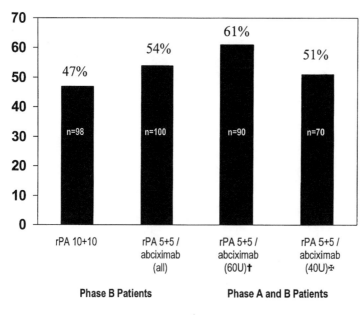

† All patients received heparin 60 U/kg^{-1} IV bolus
✠ All patients received heparin 40 U/kg^{-1} IV bolus
All patients received abciximab at a dose of 0.252 mg/kg^{-1} IV bolus, followed by a
0.125 μcg/kg min^{-1} infusion (10 μcg/min max) for 12 h
Data represented at a 62 min mean time to angiography

Figure 5   SPEED angiographic results, phase A and B.

Corrected TIMI frame count (cTFC) is a more dynamic measure of coronary flow than TIMI flow grades. Values below 27 are considered normal. In the reteplase-only and the combination group cTFC were 44 and 34, respectively.

There were no statistical differences between the groups receiving reteplase only and combination treatment relative to death, intracranial hemorrhage, major and minor bleeding, and thrombocytopenia. However, the treatment groups were too small to rule out small, but still clinically relevant, differences.

Overall, the results of SPEED confirmed those of the TIMI 14 trial. Combination therapy with reteplase $5 + 5$ U plus standard-dose abciximab produced higher TIMI grade 3 flow rates compared with standard-dose reteplase (Fig. 6). In comparison with lower heparin doses, use of adjunctive heparin at a dose of 60 U/kg with combination therapy appeared to improve TIMI grade 3 flow rates without a substantial increase in major bleeding. The trend toward lower cTFC [67] and a greater percentage of patients with complete ST-segment resolution [65] in the combination arm supports the hypothesis that combination therapy may lead to superior microvascular reperfusion than would therapy with reteplase alone.

F. Mortality Trial Utilizing the Combination of Reduced-Dose Reteplase and Abciximab in Patients with Acute Myocardial Infarction

1. Global Use of Strategies to Open Occluded Coronary Arteries (GUSTO V) Trial

The GUSTO V study is a global, prospective, randomized comparison of reteplase 5 + 5-U–double-bolus, standard-dose abciximab, and low-dose heparin (experimental regimen) versus reteplase 10 + 10-U–double-bolus (control regimen). Subsequent to the experience in SPEED and TIMI 14 summarized earlier, the experimental low-dose heparin regimen will consist of a 60-U/kg bolus (not to exceed 5000 U) followed by infusion at an initial rate of $7\,U/kg\,h^{-1}$.

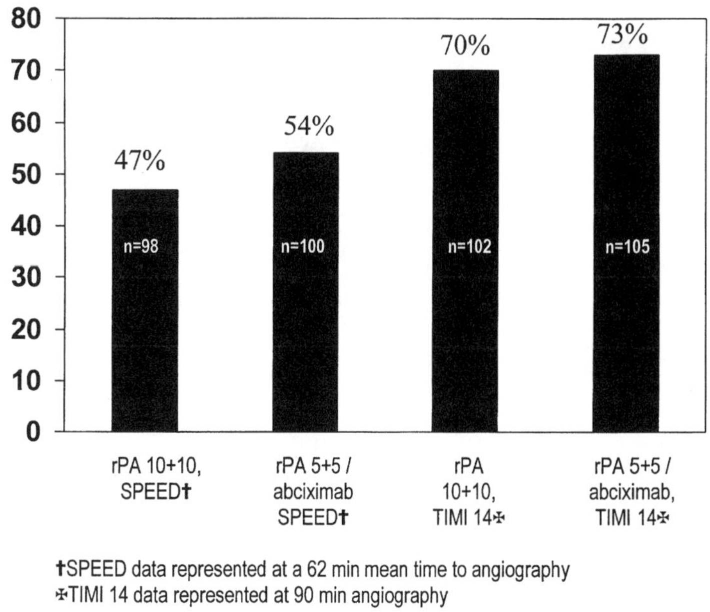
80
70
60
50
40
30
20
10
0
47%
n=98
54%
n=100
70%
n=102
73%
n=105
rPA 10+10, SPEED†
rPA 5+5 / abciximab SPEED†
rPA 10+10, TIMI 14✠
rPA 5+5 / abciximab, TIMI 14✠
†SPEED data represented at a 62 min mean time to angiography
✠TIMI 14 data represented at 90 min angiography

Figure 6 SPEED and TIMI 14 angiographic results.

Enrollment is planned to include approximately 16,600 patients. The primary endpoint will be mortality at 30 days.

IV. SUMMARY AND CONCLUSION

Reteplase is a novel recombinant plasminogen activator consisting of the kringle 2 and protease domains of t-PA. Owing to its production in *E. coli*, reteplase is not glycosylated. As shown experimentally, consequences of the structural changes are a virtual lack of functional fibrin binding and a lower affinity for endothelial cells and liver cells, resulting in a longer half-life and a higher thrombolytic potency compared with t-PA. The longer half-life enables administration as bolus injection, which is associated with more rapid reperfusion than after administration of standard thrombolytic agents.

In the clinical evaluation of reteplase $10 + 10\,\text{U}$ restores blood flow to the heart more rapidly than alteplase. Furthermore, the restored blood flow is more complete and stable after double-bolus reteplase than after alteplase. As a consequence, reteplase-treated patients require fewer coronary interventions and have higher myocardial salvage than do alteplase-treated patients, as evidenced by improved global and regional left ventricular function.

Reteplase is effective in improving survival after acute myocardial infarction. The INJECT trial demonstrates that double-bolus reteplase is at least as effective as streptokinase in reducing 35-day mortality after acute myocardial infarction. At 6 months, mortality in the reteplase group was 1% lower than in the streptokinase group, which constitutes a nonsignificant but favorable trend for reteplase. In the INJECT trial, patients treated with reteplase had a significantly lower incidence of heart failure than patients treated with streptokinase, suggesting a better quality of life for survivors of acute myocardial infarction. In GUSTO III, direct comparison of double-bolus reteplase with an accelerated infusion of alteplase in patients with acute myocardial infarction showed very similar efficacy and safety profiles of the two agents, with no statistically significant or clinically relevant differences in mortality, nonfatal stroke, death, hemorrhagic stroke, intracranial hemorrhage, and noncerebral bleeding.

Angiographic phase II trials combining reduced doses of reteplase with the GP IIb/IIIa receptor antagonist abciximab in ST-elevation acute myocardial infarction indicate a potential benefit of combination therapy over treatment with reteplase alone. The actual clinical value of this combination is currently investigated in a large-scale mortality trial, GUSTO V.

REFERENCES

1. Granger CB, Califf RM, Topol EJ. Thrombolytic therapy for acute myocardial infarction—a review. Drugs 1992; 44:293–325.
2. Task Force on Myocardial Reperfusion. Reperfusion in acute myocardial infarction. Circulation 1994; 90:2091–2102.
3. Vogt A, von Essen R, Tebbe U, Feuerer W, Appel KF, Neuhaus KL. Impact of early perfusion status of the infarct-related artery on short-term mortality after thrombolysis for acute myocardial infarction: retrospective analysis of four German multicenter studies. J Am Coll Cardiol 1993; 21:1391–1395.
4. Ohman EM, Califf RM, Topol EJ, et al. and the TAMI Study Group. Consequences of reocclusion after successful reperfusion therapy in acute myocardial infarction. Circulation 1990; 82:781–791.
5. Holylaerts M, Rijken DC, Lijnen HR, Collen D. Kinetics of the activation of plasminogen by human tissue plasminogen activator. J Biol Chem 1982; 257:2912–2919.
6. van Zonnefeld AJ, Veerman H, Pannekoek H. On the interaction of the finger and the kirngle-2 domain of tissue-type plasminogen activator with fibrin. J Biol Chem 1986; 261:14214–14218.

7. van Zonnefeld AJ, Veerman H, Pannekoek H. Antonomous functions of structural domains on human tissue-type plasminogen activator. Proc Natl Acad Sci USA 1986; 83:4670–4674.

8. Verheijen JH, Caspers MPM, Chang GTG, de Munk GAW, Pouwels PH, Enger–Valk BE, Involvement of finger domain and kringle 2 domain of tissue-type plasminogen activator in fibrin binding and stimulation of activity by fibrin. EMBO J 1986; 5:3525–3530.

9. Kohnert U, Rudolph R, Verheijen JH, et al. Biochemical properties of the kringle 2 and protease domains are maintained in the refolded t-PA deletion variant BM 06.022. Protein Eng 1992; 5:93–100.

10. Sturzebecher J, Neumann U, Kohnert U, Kresse GB, Fischer S. Mapping of the catalytic site of CHO-t-PA and the t-PA variant BM 06.022 by synthetic inhibitors and substrates. Protein Sci 1992; 1:1007–1013.

11. Kohnert U, Horsch B, Fischer S. A variant of tissue plasminogen activator (t-PA) comprised of the kringle 2 and the protease domain shows a significant difference in the in vitro rate of plasmin formation as compared to the recombinant human t-PA from transformed Chinese hamster ovary cells. Fibrinolysis 1993; 7:365–372.

12. Rijken DC, Groeneveld E, Barrett–Bergshoeff MM. In vitro stability of a tissue-type plasminogen activator mutant BM 06.022, in human plasma. Thromb Haemost 1994; 72:906–911.

13. Grunewald M, Ellbruck D, Mohren M, et al. Single vs. double bolus thrombolysis with the recombinant plasminogen activator BM 06.022 in patients with acute myocardial infarction—pharmacokinetics and hemostatic changes [abstr]. Thromb Haemost 1995; 73:1328.

14. Tanswell P, Tebbe U, Neuhaus KL, Glasle–Schwarz L, Wojcik J, Seifried E. Pharmacokinetics and fibrin specificity of alteplase during accelerated infusions in acute myocardial infarction. J Am Coll Cardiol 1992; 19:1071–1075.

15. Mulder M, Kohnert U, Fischer S, Verheijen JH. Comparison of the interaction of tissue type plasminogen activator and recombinant plasminogen activator (rpa/BM 06.022) with human umbilical vein endothelial cells [abstr]. Fibrinolysis 1944; 48(suppl. 1):12.

16. Stockinger H, Kubbies M, Rudolph R, Stern A, Kohnert U, Fischer S. Binding of recombinant variants of human tissue-type plasminogen activator (t-PA) to human umbilical vein endothelial cells. Thromb Res 1992; 67:589–599.

17. Beebe DB, Miles LA, Plow EF. A linear amino acid sequence involved in the interaction of t-PA with its endothelial cell receptor. Blood 1988; 74:2034–2037.

18. Hajjar KA. The endothelial cell tissue plasminogen activator receptor. J Biol Chem 1991; 266:21962–21970.

19. Martin U, Sponer G, Strein K. Differential fibrinolytic properties of the recombinant plasminogen activator BM 06.022 in human plasma and blood clot systems in vitro. Blood Coagul Fibrinol 1993; 4:235–242.

20. Martin U, Sponer G, Strein K. Influence of hepatic and renal failure on pharmacokinetic properties of the novel recombinant plasminogen activator BM 06.022 in rats. Drug Metab Dispos 1993; 21:236–241.

21. Kanamasa K, Watanabe I, Cereck B, Yano J, Fishbein MC, Ganz W. Selective decrease in lysis of old thrombi after rapid administration of tissue-type plasminogen activator. J Am Coll Cardiol 1989; 14:1359–1364.

22. Agnelli G, Buchanan MR, Fernandez F, Van Ryn J, Hirsh J. Sustained thrombolysis with DNA–recombinant tissue-type plasminogen activator in rabbits. Blood 1985; 66:399–401.

23. Fischer S, Kohnert U. Major mechanistic differences explain the higher clot lysis potency of reteplase over alteplase: lack of fibrin binding is an advantage for bolus application of fibrin-specific thrombolytics. Fibrinolysis Proteolysis 1997; 11:129–135.

24. Martin U, Fischer S, Kohnert U, et al. Thrombolysis with an *Escherichia coli*-produced recombinant plasminogen activator (BM 06.022) in the rabbit model of jugular vein thrombosis. Thromb Haemost 1991; 65:560–564.

25. Martin U, Fischer S. Kohnert U, et al. Coronary thrombolytic properties of a novel recombinant plasminogen activator (BM 06.022) in a canine model. J Cardiovasc Pharmacol 1991; 18:111–119.

26. Martin U, Sponer G, Strein K. Evaluation of thrombolytic and systemic effects of the novel recombinant plasminogen activator BM 06.022 compared with alteplase, anistreplase, streptokinase and urokinase in a canine model of coronary artery thrombosis. J Am Coll Cardiol 1992; 19:433–440.

27. Martin U, Sponer G, Strein K. Rapid reversal of canine thromboembolic pulmonary hypertension by bolus injection of the novel recombinant plasminogen activator BM 06.022. J Cardiovasc Pharmacol 1993; 21:455–461.

28. Shebuski RJ, Sitko GR, Claremon DA, Baldwin J, Remy DC, Stern AM. Inhibition of factor XIIa in a canine model of coronary artery thrombosis: effect on reperfusion and acute reocclusion after recombinant tissue type plasminogen activator. Blood 1990; 75:1455–1459.

29. Shebuski RJ, Stabilito IJ, Sitko GR, Polokoff MH. Acceleration of recombinant tissue-type plasminogen activator-induced thrombolysis and prevention of reocclusion by the combination of heparin, and the Arg–Gly–Asp-containing peptide bitistatin in a canine model of coronary thrombosis. Circulation 1990; 82:169–177.

30. Martin U, Sponer G, Konig R, Smolarz A, Meyer–Sabellek W, Strein K. Double bolus administration of the novel recombinant plasminogen activator BM 06.022 improves coronary blood flow after reperfusion in a canine model of coronary thrombosis. Blood Coagul Fibrinol 1992; 3:139–147.

31. Martin U, Sponer G, Strein K. Hirudin and sulotroban improve coronary blood flow after reperfusion induced by the novel recombinant plasminogen activator BM 06.022 in a canine model of coronary artery thrombosis. Int J Hematol 1992; 56:143–153.

32. Martin U, Doerge L, Fischer S. Comparison of desulfatohirudin (REVASC) and heparin as adjuncts to thrombolytic therapy with reteplase in a canine model of coronary thrombosis. Br J Pharmacol 1996; 118:271–276.

33. Martin U, Fischer S, Sponer G. Influence of heparin and systemic lysis on coronary blood flow after reperfusion induced by the novel recombinant plasminogen activator BM 06.022 in a canine model of coronary thrombosis. J Am Coll Cardiol 1993; 22:914–920.

34. Marder VJ, Shulman NR. High molecular weight derivatives of human fibrinogen produced by plasmin. J Biol Chem 1969; 244:2120–2124.

35. Stump DC, Califf RM, Topol EJ, et al., TAMI Study Group. Pharmacodynamics of thrombolysis with recombinant tissue-type plasminogen activator: correlation with characteristics of and clinical outcomes in patients with acute myocardial infarction. Circulation 1989; 80:122–1230.

36. Harrington RA, Sane DC, Califf RM, et al. Clinical importance of thrombocytopenia occurring in the hospital phase after administration of thrombolytic therapy for acute myocardial infarction. J Am Coll Cardiol 1994; 23:891–898.

37. Paris P, Agnelli, G. Thrombus resistance to lysis and reocclusion after thrombolysis: the role of platelets. Blood Coagul Fibrinol 1991; 2:749–758.

38. Martin U, Dalchau H, Sponer H. Effects of the novel recombinant plasminogen activator BM 06.022 on platelets and bleeding time in rabbits. Platelets 1992; 3:247–253.

39. Martin U, Sponer G, Strein K. Effects of the novel recombinant plasminogen activator BM 06.022 on human platelet aggregation in vitro. Fibrinolysis 1993; 7:203–210.

40. The GUSTO Investigators. An international randomized trial comparing four thrombolytic strategies for acute myocardial infarction. N Engl J Med 1993; 329:673–682.

41. Sherry S. Unresolved clinical pharmacologic questions in thrombolytic therapy for acute myocardial infarction. J Am Coll Cardiol 1988; 12:519–525.

42. Rijken DC, Otter M, Kuiper J, van Berkel TJC. Receptor-mediated endocytosis of tissue-type plasminogen activator (t-PA) by liver cells. Thromb Res 1990; suppl X:63–71.

43. Hotchkiss A, Refino CJ, Leonard CK, et al. The influence of carbohydrate structure on the clearance of recombinant tissue-type plasminogen activator. Thromb Haemost 1988; 60:255–261.

44. Larsen GR, Metzger M, Henson K, Blue Y, Horgan P. Pharmacokinetic and distribution analysis of variant forms of tissue-type plasminogen activator with prolonged clearance in rat. Blood 1983; 73:1842–1850.

45. Narita M, Bu G, Herz J, Schwartz AL. Two receptor systems are involved in the plasma clearance of tissue-type plasminogen activator (t-PA) in vivo. J Clin Invest 1995; 96:1164–1168.

46. Martin U, Fischer S, Kohnert U, et al. Pharmacokinetic properties of an *Escherichia-coli*-produced recombinant plasminogen activator (BM 06.022) in rabbits. Thromb Res 1991; 62:137–146.

47. Martin U, Kohler J, Sponer G, Strein G. Pharmacokinetics of the novel recombinant plasminogen activator BM 06.022 in rats, dogs, and non-human primates. Fibrinolysis 1992; 6:39–43.

48. Kuiper J, Otter M, Rijken DC, van Berkel TJC. Characterization of the interaction in vivo of tissue-type plasminogen activator with liver cells. J Biol Chem 1988; 263:18220–18224.

49. Kuiper J, van de Bilt H, Martin U, van Berkel TJC. Uptake, internalization and degradation of the novel plasminogen activator reteplase (BM 06.022) in the rat. Thromb Haemost 1995; 74:1501–1510.

50. Martin U, Doerge L, Stegmeier KH, Muller–Beckmann B. Influence of the degree of renal dysfunction on the pharmacokinetic properties of the novel plasminogen activator reteplase in rats. Drug Metab Disp 1996; 24:288–291.

51. Martin U, von Mollendorff E, Akpan W, Keintsch–Engel R, Kaufmann B, Neugebauer G. Dose-ranging study of the novel recombinant plasminogen activator BM 06.022 in healthy volunteers. Clin Pharmacol Ther 1991; 50:429–436.

52. Martin U, von Mollendorff E, Akpan W, Keintsch–Engel R, Kaufmann B, Neugebauer G. Pharmacokinetic and hemostatic properties of the recombinant plasminogen activator BM 06.022 in healthy volunteers. Thromb Haemost 1991; 66:569–574.

53. Neuhaus KL, von Essen R, Vogt A, et al. Dose finding with a novel recombinant plasminogen activator (BM 06.022) in patients with acute myocardial infarction: results of the German Recombinant Plasminogen Activator Study. J Am Coll Cardiol 1994; 24:55–60.

54. Tebbe U, von Essen R, Smolarz A, et al. Open, noncontrolled dose-finding study with a novel recombinant plasminogen activator (BM 06.022) given as a double bolus in patients with acute myocardial infarction. Am J Cardiol 1993; 72:518–524.

55. Smalling RW, Bode C, Kalbfleisch J, et al., the RAPID Investigators. More rapid, complete, and stable coronary thrombolysis with bolus administration of reteplase compared with alteplase infusion in acute myocardial infarction. Circulation 1995; 91:2725–2732.

56. Bode C, Smalling RW, Kalbfleisch J, et al., the RAPID Investigators. Randomized comparison of double bolus reteplase (r-PA) and front-loaded alteplase (rt-PA) in patients with acute myocardial infarction (RAPID II) [abstr]. Eur Heart J 1995; 16(suppl):11.

57. Seifried E, Mueller MM, Martin U, Koenig R, Hombach V. Bolus application of a novel recombinant plasminogen activator in acute myocardial infarction patients: pharmacokinetic and effects on the hemostatic system. Ann NY Acad Sci 1992; 667:417–420.

58. Seifried E, Mueller MM, Eggeling T, Martin U, Koenig R, Hombach V. Bolus application of a mutant of tissue plasminogen activator in acute myocardial infarction patients—pharmacokinetics and hemostatic effects [abstr]. Ann Hematol 1993; 66:A40.

59. International Joint Efficacy Comparison of Thrombolytics Trialists. Randomised, double-blind comparison of reteplase double-bolus administration with streptokinase in acute myocardial infarction (INJECT): trial to investigate equivalence. Lancet 1995; 346:329–336.

60. Schroeder R, Wegscheider K, Schroeder K, Dissmann R, Meyer–Sabellek W. Extent of early ST segment elevation resolution: a strong predictor of outcome in patients with acute myocardial infarction and a sensitive measure to compare thrombolytic regimens. A substudy of the International Joint Efficacy Comparison of Thrombolytics (INJECT). J Am Coll Cardiol 1995; 26:1657–1664.

61. GUSTO III Investigators. A comparison of reteplase and alteplase for acute myocardial infarction. N Engl J Med 1997; 337:1118–1123.

62. Miller JM, Smalling R, Ohman EM, et al. Effectiveness of early coronary angioplasty and abciximab for failed thrombolysis (reteplase or alteplase) during acute myocardial infarction (results from the GUSTO III trial). Am J Cardiol 1999; 84:779–784.

63. Topol EJ, Ohman EM, Armstrong PW, et al. Survival outcomes 1 year after reperfusion therapy with either alteplase or reteplase for acute myocardial infarction; results from the global utilization of streptokinase and t-PA for occluded coronary arteries (GUSTO) III trial. Circulation 2000; 102:1761–1765.

64. Antman EM, Giugliano RP, Gibson CM, et al. Abciximab facilitates the rate and extent of thrombolysis; results from the thrombolysis in myocardial infarction (TIMI) 14 trial. Circulation 1999; 99:2720–2732.

65. Antman EM, Gibson CM, de Lemos JA, et al. Combination reperfusion therapy with abciximab and reduced dose reteplase: results from TIMI 14. Eur Heart J 2000; 21:1944–1953.

66. de Lemos JA, Antman EM, Gibson CM, et al. Abciximab improves both epicardial flow and myocardial reperfusion in ST-elevation myocardial infarction; observations from the TIMI 14 trial. Circulation 2000; 101:239–243.
67. SPEED Investigators. Trial of abciximab with and without low-dose reteplase for acute myocardial infarction; strategies for patency enhancement in the emergency department (SPEED) group. Circulation 2000; 101:2788–2794.

31

Tenectaplase: Biochemistry, Pharmacology, and Clinical Experience

Edward R. McCluskey, Canio J. Refino, and Thomas F. Zioncheck
Genentech, Inc., South San Francisco, California, U.S.A.

Richard Y. Chin
Genentech, Inc., South San Francisco, and Stanford University Medical School, Palo Alto, California, U.S.A.

SUMMARY

Extensive experience in clinical trials has shown the superiority of recombinant tissue plasminogen activator (t-PA) over streptokinase and has led to the concept that the ideal thrombolytic should be easy and rapid to administer, be fibrin-specific (so as not to induce a systemic lytic state), not be inhibited by endogenous inhibitors (e.g., PAI-1), and have a more favorable safety profile (i.e., less intracranial hemorrhage) than tissue plasminogen activator.

Tenectaplase (TNK–t-PA) is a bioengineered form of t-PA that has been modified at three sites [T103N, N117Q, KHRR(296–299)AAAA] to create a new molecule that has decreased clearance (allowing bolus administration), more fibrin specificity (thus causing less fibrinogen depletion), and less inhibition by PAI-1 in in vitro and in vivo models of fibrinolysis. Four clinical trials, with a total of 21,183 patients, have characterized the biochemical and pharmacological properties of TNK and demonstrated its clinical safety and efficacy for the treatment of acute myocardial infarction. TNK is easy to administer, effective in decreasing mortality following myocardial infarction with equivalent ICH rates and decreased major and minor hemorrhage rates, compared with t-PA. Additional trials are now underway to study the combination of different doses of TNK with glycoprotein (GP) IIb/IIIa inhibitors and with alternate heparinization regimens.

I. INTRODUCTION

In the early 1980s tissue plasminogen activator (t-PA) was recognized as a potent and fibrin-specific plasminogen activator [1]. Since that time, t-PA has been extensively investigated and is used as a therapeutic agent in the treatment of acute thrombotic disorders, such as acute myocardial infarction (AMI) [2,3], pulmonary embolism, and ischemic stroke [4]. The Global Utilization of Streptokines and t-PA for Occluded Coronary Arteries (GUSTO) I trial demonstrated the superiority of an accelerated infusion regimen of t-PA for reperfusion and mortality reduction, compared with other available thrombolytic regimens [5,6]. At the same time, GUSTO also provided a rationale to develop new thrombolytic agents with advantages beyond those of t-PA.

The GUSTO angiographic trial [5] demonstrated that t-PA results in coronary reperfusion (TIMI 2 and 3 flow) in 81% of patients with AMI. Only 54% of patients, however, achieved TIMI-3 flow by 90 min following treatment. The increased patency profile of t-PA correlated with lower mortality and a lower major adverse event rate (30-day mortality plus in-hospital nonfatal stroke) compared with streptokinase. Intracerebral hemorrhage is a rare, but severe-side effect, of t-PA, which occurred in approximately 0.7% of t-PA-treated patients. Although t-PA is fibrin-specific, therapeutic doses induce a systemic lytic state in a significant minority of patients, with resulting depletion of clotting factors [7]. Reocclusion of recanalized coronary arteries occurs in approximately 5% of patients [6]. Finally, because t-PA is rapidly cleared from the circulation it must be administered primarily as an intravenous (IV) infusion. Thus, the ideal thrombolytic agent would induce rapid, sustained, and complete reperfusion (TIMI-3 flow grade), have little or no risk of intracranial hemorrhage or severe bleeding, and can be rapidly administered as a single bolus.

Several strategies have been employed to develop a safer, more effective, and easier-to-administer thrombolytic agent. The use of other thrombolytic molecules (staphylokinase, bat PA, u-PA, and others) and the use of truncated (and less active) forms of the t-PA molecule (r-PA, n-PA) are discussed in other chapters. This chapter will focus on the use of molecular biological and pharmacological techniques to determine where in the t-PA molecule the amino acid residues responsible for the clinical and biochemical properties are located, how they are altered to produce the current TNK–t-PA molecule, and the results of the clinical trials that have demonstrated the safety and efficacy of TNK.

II. DESIGN AND CHARACTERIZATION OF TNK-t-PA

A. Protein Engineering of t-PA

1. Background and Rationale for t-PA Mutagenesis

From a clinical perspective, the therapeutic goals for a second-generation form of t-PA include more rapid lysis, a greater degree or frequency of reperfusion, a reduced incidence of hemorrhagic sequelae, as well as increased ease of administration. From a biochemical point of view, it was difficult to identify specific molecular changes in the t-PA protein itself that would result in a new thrombolytic agent with enhanced activity. In an effort to understand better the structural and functional characteristics of t-PA, numerous investigators have created and evaluated a wide variety of t-PA variants. When the t-PA gene was sequenced in 1984, it was apparent that some of the intron/exon splice junctions were in linking regions between domains or "modules" of the protein [8]. It was then suggested that the domain structures of t-PA could be correlated with individual functions [9]. Many t-PA variants were constructed by rearranging the gene sequence to alter the order or composition of its domains [10,11]. However, domain deletion or insertion variants of t-PA generally exhibit decreased fibrinolytic activities in specific functional assays [12]. A higher resolution functional analysis was required for the design of a second-generation form of t-PA.

Tissue plasminogen activator, a 65-kDa glycoprotein, is composed of 527 amino acids that are organized in five distinct modules: finger (F), growth factor (G), two kringle regions (K1, K2), and a serine protease domain (P) that are homologous with modules found in numerous plasma proteins (Fig. 1). Plasmin cleaves t-PA between Arg 275 and Ile 276: the resultant two-

TNK-tPA

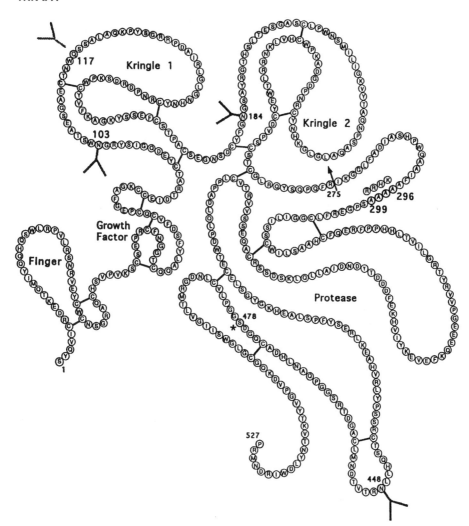

Figure 1   The molecular structure of TNKase.

chain t-PA (alteplase) is composed of an A-chain (amino acids 1 to 275, containing F, G, K1, and K2 domains) linked to the B-chain or protease domain (amino acids 276–527) by a disulfide-connecting Cys264 to Cys395. t-PA has 35 cysteines that form 17 disulfide bonds, with one unpaired cysteine at position 83 [13]. Most of the disulfides are intradomain linkages that have been assigned on the basis of homology with other well-characterized proteins, such as fibronectin, epidermal growth factor, and plasminogen [14,15].

Beginning in 1988, a systematic effort was undertaken to create and evaluate site-directed mutants of t-PA using a battery of in vitro and in vivo assays [16]. Efforts focused on three areas for potential improvement: (1) decreasing the plasma clearance rate of t-PA; (2) increasing the fibrin specificity; and (3) decreasing the inhibition of t-PA by plasma protease inhibitors. Approximately 80 mutants of t-PA were constructed using a strategy of clustered charged-to-alanine scanning mutagenesis in which a few charged amino acids (Arg, Lys, His, Asp, or Glu) were substituted with alanine [16]. This strategy allowed rapid screening of surface determinants on t-PA that mediate interactions with other protein cofactors, such as the hepatic receptors for t-PA, fibrin or fibrinogen, plasminogen, and plasminogen activator inhibitor (PAI). This work identified potentially interesting regions in the kringle 1 domain and in the protease region that mediated such functions as hepatic clearance, fibrin specificity, and resistance to PAI (see Fig. 1).

2. "T": Insertion of a Neoglycosylation Site

In the mutagenesis studies, some t-PA variants had sufficiently reduced plasma clearance to provide effective thrombolysis when the variant was administered as a bolus. It was an unexpected type of mutation, T103N (which has a novel glycosylation site on kringle 1), that produced a variant with the most suitable pharmacokinetic profile [17,18]. An eight-fold longer half-life was observed in vivo for the T103N variant of t-PA (abbreviated as the "T" mutation); however, this variant exhibited reduced fibrin binding and decreased in vitro or in vivo fibrinolytic activity when compared with wild-type t-PA [19].

3. "N": Deletion of a Glycosylation Site

The T103N mutation introduced an additional glycosylation site resulting in the kringle 1 domain having two carbohydrate moieties at positions 103 and 117 [20]. t-PA variants with two carbohydrate groups in kringle 1 exhibited decreased fibrinolytic activity. A key factor for achieving full fibrinolytic activity of t-PA appeared to be maintenance of high fibrin affinity, which was accomplished by addition of the N117Q mutation. This mutation resulted in deletion of a high mannose glycosylation site on kringle 1. The combination of T103N and N117Q mutations yielded a molecule (abbreviated "TN") with normal fibrin affinity and full plasma clot lysis activity as well as a longer circulating half-life, which resulted in significantly increased specific fibrinolytic activity [19].

4. "K": Charge Neutralization at the Active Site

The mutation of T103N, N117Q in t-PA yielded a variant with a long circulating plasma half-life and normal fibrinolytic activity, which was used to evaluate the efficacy of bolus administration. There is, however, a potential problem that must be addressed when considering bolus administration of a fully active t-PA. When t-PA is given as a bolus (or even as an infusion at high doses), the plasma levels of enzyme rapidly increase, and plasminogen becomes activated systemically as well as on the surface of the clot. Systemic plasmin generation leads to decreased levels of circulating plasminogen, fibrinogen, and α_2-antiplasmin. The undesirable consequence of systemic plasminogen activation is the potential for bleeding complications. Bleeding may be related to plasminemia, rather than fibrinogen depletion itself; both peripheral and intracranial hemorrhage are associated with systemic plasminogen activation [21]. One way to reduce systemic activation is to make t-PA even more fibrin-specific; that is, its reduced activity in the absence of a fibrin clot. Systematic mutagenesis was applied to t-PA with the hope of increasing its fibrin specificity. Fortunately, mutations in the protease domain were found that have this property [16]; the best-characterized example is a tetra-alanine substitution at positions 296–299 [22,23] Interestingly, this mutation KHRR(296–299)AAAA (abbreviated as the "K" mutation) results in a t-PA variant that is also substantially resistant to the plasminogen activator inhibitor, type-1 (PAI-1) [18,19,24].

Table 1 Characteristics of Mutations in TNK–t-PA

Substitution		Description
T	T103N	Adds a new glycosylation site on kringle-1, which decreases the rate of clearance; this extra glycosylation site decreases fibrin binding.
N	N117Q	Removes the existing glycosylation site on kringle-1, and in combination with glycosylation at the 103 position, the T103N, N117Q mutant has normal fibrin binding.
K	KHRR (296–299) AAAA	Increases the fibrin specificity, conserves fibrinogen, and increases resistance to the naturally occurring inhibitor, PAI-1

5. "TNK" Variant of t-PA

To create a variant of t-PA with reduced clearance, enhanced fibrin-specificity, and PAI-1 resistance, the mutations in three regions were combined in T103N, N117Q, KHRR(296–299)AAAA–t-PA. The resulting variant (TNK–t-PA) is substantially more potent than the wildtype parent. TNK–t-PA has substantially slower in vivo clearance (1.9 vs. 16.1 mL/min kg^{-1} for TNK–t-PA and t-PA, respectively, in rabbits), equivalent fibrin binding and plasma clot lysis activity, more than a tenfold increased fibrin specificity, and more than 80-fold increased resistance to PAI-1 [19]. In vivo models of fibrinolysis in rabbits indicate that TNK–t-PA (by bolus) achieves 50% lysis of a whole-blood clot in one-third the time required by an equivalent dose of t-PA (as an infusion). In the same model, the TNK variant is 8- and 13-fold more potent than t-PA toward whole blood clots and platelet-enriched clots, respectively. TNK–t-PA conserves fibrinogen and, because of its slower clearance and normal clot lysis activity, is effective as a bolus at a relatively low dose [19]. As a result of the modifications in the protein sequence at the three sites as just described, TNK–t-PA displays the characteristics summarized in Table 1.

A full description of the characterization and evaluation of TNK–t-PA in various animal models is described in detail elsewhere [25–32]. In addition, the preclinical experience, including pharmacokinetic, toxicokinetic, and metabolic analyses of TNK are described in these references. Finally, the preclinic pharmacodynamic and toxological studies of TNK have also been described elsewhere [30,31].

III. INITIAL CLINICAL EXPERIENCE

TNK–t-PA has been successfully tested in four completed clinical trials, and is now being studied in at least four phase IV combination trials. These studies and the planned phase IV trials will be described in this section.

A. Phase I: TIMI 10A

1. Study Design and Goals

The first clinical study of TNK [33], called "TIMI 10A," was designed to assess the pharmacokinetic characteristics of TNK in patients undergoing acute myocardial infarction. Patients presenting to the hospital with symptoms of an acute myocardial infarction of 12-h, or fewer, in duration were eligible. They were immediately given a bolus of TNK–t-PA as well as aspirin and intravenous heparin. Patients received one of eight ascending doses of TNK–t-PA from 5 to 50 mg as a single intravenous bolus. The 113 patients all underwent 90-min angiography to evaluate the status of the infarct-related coronary artery. The primary endpoint of this trial was pharmacokinetics and safety.

2. Study Results

As expected from preclinical data, the clearance of TNK–t-PA was slower than t-PA. Overall the clearance of TNK–t-PA was 151 ± 56 mL/min, which is significantly slower than the clearance of 572 ± 132 mL/min [31]. Even at the highest dose tested, TNK–t-PA does not appear to induce a "fibrinolytic state." There was no significant decrease in either fibrinogen or plasminogen concentrations as the dose of TNK–t-PA was increased from 5 to 50 mg. Similarly, the decreases in the α_2-antiplasmin levels to approximately 20% below baseline were much less than the 40–45% decrease found with t-PA. TNK–t-PA (at doses of 30–50 mg) also gave encouraging initial indications for angiographic efficacy, with rates of TIMI-2 and TIMI-3 flow comparable or superior to 90-min of t-PA.

3. Summary of Phase I

In conclusion, the preliminary results from the phase I trial are: (1) TNK–t-PA has a prolonged half-life, such that it can be administered as a single bolus; (2) TNK–t-PA appears to be more fibrin-specific than t-PA; (3) initial infarct-related coronary artery patency profile shows promising rates of TIMI grade 3 flow at 90 min at the 30- to 50-mg doses; and (4) the safety and tolerability in this initial cohort appears acceptable.

B. Phase II: TIMI-10B (Angiographic) and ASSENT-1 (Safety)

The phase II clinical trials of TNK–t-PA were designed to determine the angiographic efficacy of various doses of TNK—*TIMI-10B* [34], and to determine the safety (rates of death and intracerebral hemorrhage) of the various doses—*ASSENT-1* [35]. The trials enrolled concurrently and served as the basis for selecting a single dose for the phase III pivotal trial.

1. TIMI-10B Study Design and Goals

The TIMI 10B trial was designed to be conducted in parallel with the ASSENT-1 trial and to compare the angiographic efficacy of two doses (30 and 50 mg) of TNK with the standard dose of t-PA as a means of determining the appropriate dose of TNK to use in a large, pivotal phase III trial. Eligible patients were randomized to treatment with either bolus TNK and a dummy t-PA infusion or dummy TNK and standard t-PA infusion. Angiographic assessment of vessel patency was performed at 90 min after the initiation of thrombolytic treatment. Enrollment for the 50-mg dose was stopped and enrollment into a 40-mg cohort was substituted, after 3 of the 76 patients in the 50-mg study arm experienced an ICH. At the same time, the dose of heparin recommended in the study was decreased. A total of 886 patients were eventually randomized (837 were efficacy-evaluable), 311 to t-PA, 302 to 30-mg TNK, 148 to 40-mg TNK, and 76 to 50-mg TNK.

2. TIMI-10B Study Results

The primary endpoint of the trial was to determine the rate of TIMI-3 flow at 90 min in the treatment groups. Randomization resulted in groups that were well balanced in most respects. The rates of TIMI-3 flow for the groups are shown in the Table 2.

Table 2 TIMI-3 Flow at Different Doses

	30 mg TNK	40 mg TNK	50 mg TNK	t-PA
$N =$	302	148	76	311
% with TIMI-3 flow at 90 min	54.3	62.8	65.8	62.7

Analysis of patency using the TIMI frame count method gave similar results. When the results were analyzed based on a "weight-corrected" dose (dose administered per patient weight), there was a tendency toward better patency at doses in excess of 0.5 mg/kg. Similarly, when patients were stratified into dose/weight tertiles, significant differences were seen between the tertile groups, with higher dose/weight groups showing improved posttreatment flow.

Pharmacokinetic analysis corroborated the findings of the TIMI-10A trial and found that Tenecteplase exhibited biphasic elimination from the plasma with a mean initial half-life of 22 min and a mean terminal half-life of 115 min. The mean plasma clearance was 105 mL/min and did not depend on tenecteplase dose over the dose range studied. In comparison, rt-PA has a fourfold faster plasma clearance [34a]. Coagulation assays demonstrated that, compared with the standard dose of t-PA, TNK caused much less depletion of α_2-antiplasmin, fibrinogen, and plasminogen.

3. Summary of TIMI-10B

The conclusion of the TIMI-10B trial was that the 40-mg dose of TNK was comparable with that of the standard 90-min t-PA regimen. Weight-based dosing analysis suggested a benefit for using weight-based dosing in future trials.

4. ASSENT-1: Study Design and Goals

The ASSENT-1 trial was designed to be conducted in parallel with the TIMI-10B trial and to determine the safety of two doses (30 and 50 mg) of TNK. No t-PA comparator arm was included in the trial. Eligible patients were randomized to treatment with one of two doses of bolus TNK. No angiographic assessment was included in this trial. Although none of the 73 patients in the 50-mg study arm of ASSENT-1 experienced an ICH, the enrollment to the 50-mg dose was stopped owing to the three intracranial hemorrhages in the TIMI-10B study and enrollment into a 40-mg cohort was substituted. At the same time, the recommended dose of heparin was decreased. A total of 3235 patients were eventually randomized, 1701 to 30 mg TNK, 1457 to 40 mg TNK, and 73 to 50 mg TNK.

5. ASSENT-1 Study Results

The primary aim of the trial was to estimate the rate of ICH flow within 30 days in the treatment groups. Randomization resulted in groups that were well balanced. The rates of ICH for these groups are shown in the Table 3.

6. Summary of ASSENT-1

The conclusion of the ASSENT-1 trial was that a dose of TNK of approximately 0.5 mg/kg would likely be as safe and effective as the standard 90-min t-PA regimen for the treatment of acute MI.

Table 3 Rates of ICH at Different Dosages

	30 mg TNK	40 mg TNK	50 mg TNK
$N =$	1705	1457	73
Rate of ICH at 30 days	0.94	0.62	0
CI	0.5–1.5	1.3–1.2	0.0–4.9

Table 4 Additional Endpoints in the ASSENT-1 Study

	30 mg TNK	40 mg TNK	50 mg TNK
$N =$	1705	1457	73
Mortality at 30 days	6.9	6.0	4.1
Recurrent MI	8.2	5.9	5.5
Total Stroke	1.5	1.5	0

C. Phase III: ASSENT-2 (Pivotal)

ASSENT-2 Study Design and Goals

The ASSENT-2 trial [36] (Table 5) was designed to compare the covariate-adjusted 30-day mortality of a weight-adjusted dose of TNK with the standard 90-min t-PA regimen. Eligible patients were randomized to treatment with either weight-tiered TNK or to the standard 90-min t-PA regimen (see following). No angiographic assessment was included in this trial. A total of 16,949 patients were enrolled, 8461 to TNK and 8488 to t-PA.

2. ASSENT-2 Study Results

The primary aim of the trial was to determine the covariate-adjusted 30-day mortality in the treatment groups. Randomization resulted in groups that were well balanced. Thirty-day follow-up was available for 99.97% (16,943/16,949) of patients. The adjusted mortality rates for the groups are shown in Table 6.

The Kaplan–Meier survival curves for the two groups was superimposable and the prespecified analysis for equivalence was fulfilled. The efficacy and safety for TNK and t-PA were comparable across subgroups and for secondary endpoints.

Additional endpoints in the ASSENT-2 study are listed in Table 7. The rates of total bleeding and major bleeding were both less in the TNK-treated patients as compared with the

Table 5 Weight-Adjusted Dosing of TNK–t-PA

Patient weight (kg)	TNK–t-PA dose (mg)	Volume of TNK–t-PA (mL)
< 60	30	6
> 60 and < 70	35	7
> 70 and < 80	40	8
> 80 and < 90	45	9
> 90	50	10

Table 6 ASSENT-2 Study Results

	TNK	t-PA
$N =$	8461	8488
Adjusted 30-day mortality	6.189	6.15
Unadjusted 30-day mortality	6.16	6.18

Table 7 Additional Endpoints

	TNK	t-PA	p =
$N =$	8461	8488	
Total bleeding episodes	26.4	28.9	0.0003
Major bleeding episodes	4.6	5.9	0.0002
Transfusions	4.2	5.5	0.0013
ICH	0.9	0.9	1.0

t-PA-treated patients, suggesting that the enhanced fibrin specificity of TNK did result in an improved side effect profile.

3. Summary of ASSENT-2

The conclusion of the ASSENT-2 trial was that the mortality following treatment of acute myocardial infarction with TNK, administered as a bolus over 5 s, was equivalent to that after the standard 90-min t-PA dosage. The point estimates for ICH were nearly identical for the two treatment regimens. There was a statistically significant decrease in non-cerebral bleeding and transfusions in the TNK group. Because a single bolus administration of TNK could lead to a shorter time to treatment, the authors suggested that prehospital treatment should be tested.

IV. FUTURE STUDIES

Currently, there are several studies underway that are examining a reduced dose of TNK administered in conjunction with a glycoprotein IIb/IIIa inhibitor and the use of TNK with low molecular weight heparins. In the FASTER trial, TNK is used with tirofiban; in the ENTIRE trial, TNK is used in conjunction with abciximab and enoxaparin; in the INTEGRITI trial, TNK is used with eptifibatide, and in the ASSENT 3 trial, TNK is used with abciximab and enoxaparin. In addition, ASSENT 3 PLUS is examining whether administration of TNK in the prehospital setting (ambulance) is safe and potentially more effective than administration only in the hospital setting.

REFERENCES

1. Hoylaerts M, Rijken D, Lijnen H, Collen D. J Biol Chem 1982; 257:2912–2919.
2. Van de Werf F, Ludbrook P, Bergmann S, Tiefenbrunn A, Fox K, deGeest H, Verstraete M, Collen D, and Sobel B. Coronary thrombolysis with tissue-type plasminogen activator in patients with evolving myocardial infarction. N Engl Med 1984; 310:609–613.

3. Bergmann S, Fox K, Ter-Pogossian M, Sobel B, and Collen D. Clot-selective coronary thrombolysis with tissue-type plasminogen activator. Science 1983; 220:1181–1183.
4. NINDS rt-PA Stroke Study Group. Tissue plasminogen activator for acute ischemic stroke. The National Institute of Neurological Disorders and Stroke rt-PA Stroke Study Group [see comments]. N Engl J Med 1995; 333:1581–1587.
5. GUSTO Investigators. An international randomized trial comparing four thrombolytic strategies for acute myocardial infarction. The GUSTO investigators [see comments]. N Engl J Med 1993; 329:673–682.
6. GUSTO Investigators. The effects of tissue plasminogen activator, streptokinase, or both on coronary-artery patency, ventricular function, and survival after acute myocardial infarction. The GUSTO Angiographic Investigators [see comments] [published erratum appears in N Engl J Med 1994 Feb 17; 330:516]. N Engl J Med 1993; 329:1615–1622.
7. Stump D, Califf R, Topol E, Sigmon K, Thornton D, Masek R, Anderson L, Collen D. Pharmacodynamics of thrombolysis with recombinant tissue-type plasminogen activator. Correlation with characteristics of and clinical outcomes in patients with acute myocardial infarction. The TAMI Study Group. Circulation 1989; 80(5):1122–1230.
8. Ny T, Elgh F, Lund B. The structure of the human tissue-type plasminogen activator gene: correlation of intron and exon structures to functional and structural domains. Proc Natl Acad Sci USA 1984; 81:5355–5359.
9. van Zonneveld A, Veerman H, Pannekoek H. Autonomous functions of structural domains on human tissue-type plasminogen activator. Proc Natl Acad Sci USA 1986; 83:4670–4674.
10. Lijnen H, Collen D. Strategies for the improvement of thrombolytic agents. Thromb Haemost 1991; 66:88–110.
11. Higgins D, Bennett W. Tissue plasminogen activator: the biochemistry and pharmacology of variants produced by mutagenesis. Annu Rev Pharmacol Toxicol 1990; 30:91–121.
12. Keyt B, Paoni N, Bennett W. Site-directed mutagenesis of tissue-type plasminogen activator. In Cleland J, Craik, C, eds. Protein Engineering: Principles and Practices, New York: J. W. Wiley & Sons, 1996; 435–466.
13. Sehl LC, Nguyen HV, Berleau LT, Arcila P, Bennett WF, and Keyt BA. Locating the unpaired cysteine of tissue-type plasminogen activator. Protein Eng 1996; 9(2): 283–290.
14. Banyai L, Varadi A, and Patthy L. Common evolutionary origin of the fibrin-binding structures of fibronectin and tissue-type plasminogen activator. FEBS Lett 1983; 163:37–41.
15. Pennica D, Holmes W, Kohr W, Harkins R, Vehar G, Ward C, Bennett W, Yelverton E, Seeberg P, Heyneker H, Goeddel D, Collen D. Cloning and expression of human tissue-type plasminogen activator cDNA in E. coli. Nature 1983; 301:214–221.
16. Bennett W, Paoni N, Keyt B, Botstein D, Jones A, Presta L, Wurm F, Zoller M. High resolution analysis of functional determinants on human tissue-type plasminogen activator. J Biol Chem 1991; 266:5191–5201.
17. Refino CJ, Paoni NF, Keyt BA, Pater CS, Badillo JM, Wurm FM, Ogez J, Bennett WF. A variant of t-PA T103N, KHRR 296–299 AAAA; that, by bolus, has increased potency and decreased systemic activation of plasminogen. Thromb Haemost 1993; 70:313–319.
18. Paoni NF, Keyt BA, Refino CJ, Chow AM, Nguyen HV, Berleau LT, Badillo JM, Pena LC, Brady K, Wurm FM, Ogez J, Bennett WF. A slow clearing, fibrin-specific, PAI-1 resistant variant of t-PA T103N, KHRR 296–299 AAAA;. Thromb Haemost 1993; 70(2): 307–312.
19. Keyt BA, Paoni NF, Refino CJ, Berleau L, Nguyen H, Chow A, Lai J, Pena L, Pater C, Ogez J, Etcheverry T, Botstein D, Bennett WF. A faster-acting and more potent form of tissue plasminogen activator. Proc Natl Acad Sci USA 1994; 91:3670–3674.
20. Guzzetta AW, Basa LJ, Hancock WS, Keyt BA, Bennett WF. Identification of carbohydrate structures in glycoprotein peptide maps by the use of LC/MS with selected ion extraction with special reference to tissue plasminogen activator and a glycosylation variant produced by site directed mutagenesis. Anal Chem 1993; 65:2953–2962.
21. Bovill EG, Terrin ML, Stump DC, Berke AD, Frederick M, Collen D, Feit F, Gore JM, Hillis D, Lambrew CT, Leiboff, R Mann, KG Markis JE, Pratt CM, Sharkey SW, Sopko G, Tracy R, Chesebro

JH. Hemorrhagic events during therapy with recombinant tissue-type plasminogen activator, heparin, and aspirin for acute myocardial infarction. Results of the Thrombolysis in Myocardial Infarction (TIMI), Phase II Trial. Ann of Intern Med 1991; 115:256–265.

22. Paoni NF, Chow AM, Pena LC, Keyt BA, Zoller MJ, Bennett WF. Making tissue-type plasminogen activator more fibrin specific. Protein Eng 1993; 6:529–534.

23. Paoni NF, Refino CJ, Brady K, Pea LC, Nguyen HV, Kerr EM, van Reis R, Botstein D, Bennett WF. Protein Eng 1992; 5:259–266.

24. Madison EL, Goldsmith EJ, Gerard RD, Gething MJ, Sambrook JF. Nature 1989; 339:721–724.

25. Refino CJ, Keyt BA, Paoni NF, Badillo J, Pater CS, Van Peborgh J, Pena L, Berleau LT, Nguyen HV, Bennett, WF. Thromb. Haemost 1993; 69:841.

26. Berleau L, Refino C, Modi N, Bennett W, Keyt B. Interspecies scaling of WT-tPA and TNK-tPA: prediction of TNK-tPA clearance in humans [abstr]. Fibrinolysis 1994; 8(suppl) 1:26.

27. DeGuzman G, Richardson L, Berleau L, Keyt B, Baumgardner M, Zioncheck T. Hepatic uptake and processing of TNK-tPA. Pharm Res 1995; 123:332.

28. Benedict CR, Refino CJ, Keyt BA, Pakala R, Paoni NF, Thomas GR, Bennett WF. New variant of human tissue plasminogen activator TPA with enhanced efficacy and lower incidence of bleeding compared with recombinant human TPA. Circulation 1995; 92:3032–3040.

29. Gross M, Bussiere J, Prince B, Schultz J, Christian B. Pre-clinical toxicity assessment of TNK-tPA in dogs following IV bolus administration. Toxicologist 1996; 30(1 part 2):337–338.

30. Kadota T, Kondoh H, Chikazawa H, Kuroyanagi K, Ishikawa K, Kawano S. Cefepime (diHCl/L-arginine blend): intravenous continuous infusion and/or single dose subcutaneous toxicity study in rats and dogs [in Japanese]. Jpn J Antibiot 1992; 45:612–619.

31. Tanswell P, Tebbe U, Neuhaus KL, Glasle SL, Wojcik J, Seifried E. Pharmacokinetics and fibrin specificity of alteplase during accelerated infusions in acute myocardial infarction [see comments]. J Am Coll Cardiol 1992;19:1071–1075.

32. McCluskey ER, Keyt BA, Refino CJ, Modi NB, Zioncheck TF, Bussiere JL, Love, TW. The biochemistry, pharmacology and initial clinical experience with TNK-tPA In: Sasahara, AA, Loscalso, J. eds. New Therapeutic Agents in Thrombosis and Thrombolysis. NY: Marcel Dekker, 1997.

33. Cannon CP, McCabe CH, Gibson CM, Ghali M, Sequeira RF, McKendall GR, Breed J, Modi NB, Fox NL, Tracy RP, Love TW, Braunwald E, the TIMI 10A Investigators. TNK-tissue plasminogen activator in acute myocardial infarction. Results of the Thrombolysis in Myocardial Infarction (TIMI); 10A dose-ranging trial. Circulation 1997; 95:351–356.

34. Cannon CP, Gibson CM, McCabe CH, Adgey AAJ, Schweiger MJ, Sequeira RF, Grollier G, Giuliano RP, Frey M, Mueller HS, Steingart RM, Weaver WD, Van de Werf F, Braunwald E, for the Thrombolysis in Myocardial Infarction (TIMI); 10B Investigators. TNK-tissue plasminogen activator compared with front-loaded alteplase in acute myocardial infarction. Results of the TIMI 10B trial. Circulation 1998; 98:2805–2814.

34a. Modi NB, Fox NL, Clow FW, Tanswell P, Cannon CP, Van de Werf F, Brainwald E. Pharmacokinetics and pharmacodynamics of tenecteplase: results from a phase II study in patients with acute myocardial infarction. J Clin Pharma 2000; 40(5): 508–515.

35. Van de Werf F, Cannon CP, Luyten A, Houbracken K, McCabe CH, Berioli S, Bluhmki E, Sarelin H, Wang-Clow F, Fox NL, Braunwald E, the ASSENT-1 investigators. Safety assessment of single-bolus administration of TNK tissue-plasminogen activator in acute myocardial infarction: the ASSENT-1 trial. Am Heart J 1999; 137:786–791.

36. Assessment of the Safety and Efficacy of a New Thrombolytic (ASSENT-2); Investigators. Single-bolus tenecteplase compared with front-loaded alteplase in acute myocardial infarction: the ASSENT-2 double-blind randomised trial. Lancet 1999; 354:716–722.

32

Lanoteplase

Robert P. Giugliano
Harvard Medical School and Brigham and Women's Hospital, Boston, Massachusetts, U.S.A.

I. INTRODUCTION

In the era before the introduction of fibrinolytic therapy for the treatment of acute ST-elevation myocardial infarction, mortality in the first month following acute infarction was approximately 13% [1]. Shortly following the demonstration by deWood [2] that intracoronary thrombus resulting in total occlusion of the coronary artery was the predominant underlying patho-physiology of transmural infarction, drugs that dissolve intracoronary thrombus by activating the fibrinolytic system were developed and studied in large-scale clinical trials. These drugs, more accurately referred to as "fibrinolytic agents," activate plasminogen to the active enzyme plasmin which, in turn, digests fibrin to soluble degradation products. The benefit of fibrinolytic therapy in acute myocardial infarction is related to early achievement of infarct-related artery patency, whereby rapid coronary reperfusion limits infarct size, decreases left ventricular dysfunction, and improves survival [1,3–7].

First-generation fibrinolytic drugs (urokinase, streptokinase, anisoylated plasminogen–streptokinase activator complex), which are effective, but not fibrin-specific, are associated with anaphylaxis (urokinase, streptokinase), and are subject to a phenomenon known as "plasmino-gen steal" which reduces their ability to lyse thrombi because of gradual depletion of the plasminogen pool. Second-generation agents (tissue plasminogen activator [t-PA], single-chain urokinase-type plasminogen activator [scu-PA]) were developed as more fibrin-specific drugs in the hopes of improving efficacy while reducing the systemic lytic state and thus improving safety. Modest reductions in mortality were achieved, although safety, in particular the risk of intracranial hemorrhage, was not improved [5,8]. Third-generation fibrinolytic drugs (reteplase [r-PA], tenecteplase [TNK–t-PA], lanoteplase [n-PA]), with longer half-lives that permitted bolus administration, were subsequently developed. In this chapter, we will focus on one of these agents, lanoteplase, and review the relevant pharmacobiology and clinical trial results.

II. PHARMACOBIOLOGY

A. Molecular Structure

Lanoteplase (synonyms: ΔFE1X PA, n-PA, novel plasminogen activator, SUN9216) is a rationally designed mutant of t-PA with greater fibrinolytic potency and a prolonged plasma half-life suitable for single-bolus administration. Lanoteplase is derived from t-PA by deletion of the fibronectin finger-like and epidermal growth factor domains and mutation of Asn-117 to Gln-117 (designated Gln-39 in lanoteplase) in the kringle 1 domain (Fig. 1). Eighty-one amino acid residues (Cys-6 through Ile-86) are eliminated with deletion of the finger-like and epidermal growth factor domains, resulting in decreased clearance and some loss of fibrin specificity. An N-linked glycosylation site is removed with the mutation of Asn-117 to Gln-117 in an attempt to restore fibrin specificity, based on the prior observations that nonglycosylated wild-type t-PA binds to fibrin better than wild-type t-PA [9]. This point mutation at site 117 also prolongs the half-life by preventing clearance of lanoteplase by the mannose receptor.

Lanoteplase is produced by cell culture fermentation using an established ovarian cell line (CHO) from the Chinese hamster. The purified protein is primarily a single-chain molecule with the plasmin cleavage site intact. Of the two potential sites for N-linked glycosylation, one site is variably occupied (Asn-106), while the other (Asn-370) is fully occupied. The species with a single carbohydrate moiety at Asn-370 predominates. The molecular weight of lanoteplase is 53.6 kDa (including the carbohydrate moiety), compared with 70 kDa for alteplase.

B. Pharmacokinetic Properties

Lanoteplase was intentionally designed to be administered as a single bolus. This was achieved by reducing the plasma clearance and thereby prolonging the circulating plasma half-life. Pharmacokinetic parameters of lanoteplase have been assessed in both healthy male subjects and patients with acute myocardial infarction.

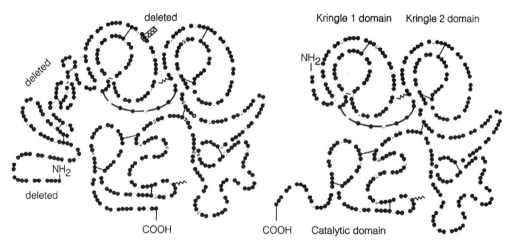

Figure 1 Schematic representation of the primary structure of tissue plasminogen activator (t-PA, left) and lanoteplase (n-PA, right): Lanoteplase has the fibronectin finger-like and epidermal growth factor domains removed and Asn-117 has been substituted for Gln-117 (designated Gln-39 in lanoteplase) in kringle 1.

In 30 healthy adult Japanese men who received lanoteplase in doses ranging from 0.05 to 2.0 mg, lanoteplase had a two-component (biphasic) mode of elimination [10]. The total body clearance (CL_{tot}) was 249–417 mL/min, volume of distribution at steady state (V_{dss}) 10–17 L, initial half-life ($t_{1/2\alpha}$) 8.2–12.6 min, and terminal half-life ($t_{1/2\beta}$) of 30–55 min. In comparison, the pharmacokinetic profile of t-PA in healthy volunteers revealed a CL_{tot} of 600–640 mL/min, V_d of 4.6–7.4 L, $t_{1/2\alpha}$ of 3–4 min, and $t_{1/2\beta}$ of 26–34 min, confirming the desired slower clearance and longer half-life of lanoteplase in healthy volunteers.

Similar pharmacokinetic data were obtained in patients with acute myocardial infarction [11] treated with one of four doses of lanoteplase (15, 30, 60, or 120 kU/kg) versus accelerated administration of alteplase. The plasma clearance of lanoteplase was approximately 10% of that of alteplase (lanoteplase: 40 ± 8 to 57 ± 19 mL/min; alteplase: 550–680 mL/min), thus resulting in a much longer initial half-life ($t_{1/2\alpha}$ lanoteplase: 31 ± 4 to 47 ± 13 min; $t_{1/2\beta}$ alteplase: 3.5 min) and terminal half-life ($t_{1/2\beta}$ lanoteplase: 444 ± 122 to 714 ± 301 min; $t_{1/2\beta}$ alteplase: 72 min). The volume of distribution at steady state for lanoteplase 15–120 kU/kg ranged from 12.1 ± 7.5 to 27.8 ± 15.7 L, which is 1.5–3 times greater than the V_{dss} of alteplase (8.4 L). The areas under the time–concentration curve (AUCs) of these four doses of lanoteplase were 955 ± 210, 1806 ± 221, 3579 ± 1018, and $10,266 \pm 919$ ng $\times$ h $\times$ mL^{-1}, respectively. Lanoteplase is metabolized mainly by the liver, and its metabolites are excreted in the urine. Lanoteplase has not been detected in urine, indicating that unchanged lanoteplase is not excreted in the urine.

C. Pharmacodynamic Properties

Measurable changes in coagulation and fibrinolytic system parameters are detectable as soon as 5 min following administration of lanoteplase in healthy volunteers [10]. After a dose of lanoteplase (in the absence of heparin), plasma levels of α_2-plasmin inhibitor (α_2-PI), plasminogen, fibrinogen, and plasminogen activator inhibitor-1 (PAI-1) were reduced, while fibrinogen degradation products (FDP), plasmin activity, α_2-plasmin inhibitor complex (PIC), and fibrinopepetide Bβ 15–42 were increased. Euglobulin lysis time was shortened, while the prothrombin time, activated partial thromboplastin time, α^2-macroglobulin data were minimally changed, and results for the thrombin time were inconclusive.

In patients with acute myocardial infarction, who also received aspirin and heparin, administration of four different doses of lanoteplase resulted in dose-related decreases in fibrinogen, plasminogen, and α_2-antiplasmin at 60 min that, for the three lower doses, returned to baseline by 24 h [11]. However, at the highest dose studied (120 kU/kg, the dose eventually selected for phase III testing), fibrinogen (−73%), plasminogen (−73%), and α_2-antiplasmin (−74%) were markedly decreased with nadir levels occurring 2 h postdose, and remained far below baseline at 24 h (−44% to −55%). In comparison (Table 1), following alteplase administration, α_2-antiplasmin (− 72%), fibrinogen (−50%), and plasminogen (−59%) were not quite as depressed, and were closer to baseline (−18% to −34%) at 24 h.

Following administration of 120 kU/kg of lanoteplase, maximum levels of D-dimer (36-fold), FDP (53-fold), and PAI-1 (2.8-fold) were noted at 2–4, 4–8, and 6 h respectively. PAI-1 returned to near baseline (1.5-fold) by 12 h, but D-dimer (4.5-fold) and FDP (36-fold) were still elevated at 24 h. In comparison (see Table 1) following alteplase, all three parameters (D-dimer [32-fold], FDP [51-fold], and PAI-1 [3.9-fold]) attained maximum concentration at an earlier timepoint (2 h), and two of the three (D-dimer [2.5-fold] and FDP [2.6-fold]) returned closer to baseline by 24 h compared with 120 kU/kg of lanoteplase.

Based on the foregoing results, we can conclude that the 120-kU/kg dose of lanoteplase is less fibrin-specific than t-PA. Less fibrin-specific plasminogen activators induce more extensive

Table 1 Pharmacological Characteristics of Alteplase and Lanoteplase

Characteristic	Alteplase (t-PA)	Lanoteplase (n-PA)
Plasma half-life $\pm$ SD (min)	3.5 ± 1.4	47 ± 13[b]
Plasma clearance $\pm$ SD (ml/min)	572 ± 132[a]	57 ± 19[b]
Excretion	Hepatic	Hepatic
Mode of administration	Bolus + infusion over 90 min[a]	Single bolus
Dose	≤ 100 mg[a]	120 kU/kg
Weight-adjusted	Yes, if weight < 67 kg	Yes
Fibrin specificity	++	+
$\downarrow$ Fibrinogen[c]	50%	75%[b]
$\downarrow$ Plasminogen[c]	59%	73%[b]
$\downarrow$ α_2-Antiplasmin[c]	72%	74%[b]
	Peak (h) 24 h	Peak[b] (h) 24 h
$\uparrow$ D-Dimer	$32 \times$ (2 h) $2.5 \times$	$36 \times$ (2–4 h) $4.5 \times$
$\uparrow$ FDP	$51 \times$ (2 h) $2.6 \times$	$53 \times$ (4–8 h) $36 \times$
$\uparrow$ PAI-1	$3.9 \times$ (2 h) $1.9 \times$	$2.8 \times$ (6 h) $1.5 \times$

[a]Alteplase: 15-mg bolus, 0.75 mg/kg, not exceeding 50 mg over 30 min, and 0.5 mg/kg, not exceeding 35 mg over the next hour.
[b]Lanoteplase 120 kU/kg.
[c]2 h postdose.

systemic plasminogen activation, and after saturation of α_2-antiplasmin, excess plasmin may degrade several proteins, including fibrinogen, factor V, and factor VIII [12,13]. The clinical implications are that administration of 120 kU/kg of lanoteplase compared with alteplase may cause a greater systemic coagulopathy, may require less adjunctive antithrombin, and may have the potential for more bleeding.

III. ANGIOGRAPHIC EVALUATION

Four studies [14–17] evaluated the angiographic efficacy of lanoteplase in patients with an acute myocardial infarction. Three of these studies [14–16] were performed in Japan in patients who had acute myocardial infarction with demonstrated total occlusion of the infarct artery by coronary angiography before administration of fibrinolytic therapy (Table 2). The fourth trial [17] was a randomised, double-blind, dose-ranging comparison of lanoteplase (15–120 kU/kg) versus alteplase (accelerated administration = 15-mg bolus, then 0.75 mg/kg [50 mg maximum] over 30 min, followed by 0.50 mg/kg [35 mg maximum] over 60 min) (Fig. 2).

In the first study [14], open-label lanoteplase in doses of 50, 100, or 150 kU/kg was administered in 139 Japanese patients younger than 75 years of age with acute myocardial infarction following angiographic documentation of complete coronary artery occlusion. Heparin was administered as a bolus of 5000 U at the time of angiography, with subsequent heparin administration at the physician's discretion. TIMI grade 3 flow at 60 min was achieved in 51, 39, and 51% of patients with coronary patency (TIMI 2 or 3 flow) in 72, 65, and 76%, respectively. The mean times to reperfusion among those with open arteries at 60 min were 24 ± 15, 29 ± 16, and 21 ± 14 min, and the mean ST resolution (all three doses pooled) was 36% at 60 min and 84% at discharge. Angiographic reocclusion (in patients with a patent infarct artery at 60 min) occurred in 16, 6, and 9%, respectively as determined by predischarge

Table 2 Angiographic Results in Early Phase II Studies

	Ref. 14 ($n = 129$)		Ref. 15 ($n = 171$)		Ref. 16 ($n = 187$)	
	Minutes to		Minutes to		Minutes to	
	TIMI 3	reperfusion	TIMI 3	reperfusion	TIMI 3	reperfusion
nPA (kU/kg)						
25	—	—	43%	28	—	—
50	51%	24	43%	29	—	—
75	—	—	47%	22	46%	22
100	39%	29	—	—	—	—
150	51%	21			—	—
t-PA (mg)						
65	—	—	—	—	49%	27

angiography. Major or minor hemorrhage occurred in 0, 9, and 17% of patients, respectively, including one intracranial hemorrhage in a patient receiving 150 kU/kg.

A second study [15] in 183 patients was nearly identical except that it was double-blinded and lower doses (25, 50, and 75 kU/kg) of lanoteplase were studied. TIMI grade 3 flow at 60 min was achieved in 43, 43, and 47% of patients with coronary patency (TIMI 2 or 3 flow) in 63, 74, and 75%, respectively. The mean times to reperfusion among those with open arteries at 60 min were 28 ± 15, 29 ± 16, and 22 ± 11 min, and the mean ST resolution (all three doses pooled) was 39% at 60 min and 83% at discharge. Angiographic reocclusion occurred in 13, 16, and 15% of patients, respectively. Major or minor hemorrhage occurred in 5, 5, and 3% of patients

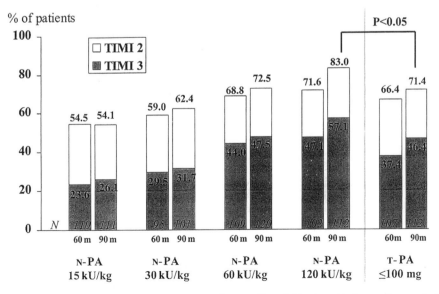

Figure 2 Rates of TIMI grades 2 and 3 flow at 60 and 90 min with lanoteplase and alteplase in the InTIME I trial.

respectively, with no intracranial hemorrhage at these reduced doses of lanoteplase in 183 patients.

The third angiographic trial [16] compared 75 kU/kg lanoteplase with alteplase 65 mg over 60 min among 205 patients in an otherwise similar fashion, as described in the two preceding studies [14–15]. TIMI 3 flow at 60 min was present in 46 versus 49%, and coronary patency in 74 versus 67% of patients receiving lanoteplase and alteplase, respectively (both p = NS). The mean time to reperfusion was shorter in patients receiving lanoteplase (22 vs. 29 min, p = 0.05). Bleeding was similar between the two groups (7 vs. 5%, p = NS), and no intracranial hemorrhages occurred.

Lastly, lanoteplase in doses ranging from 15 kU/kg to 120 kU/kg, was evaluated in 602 patients in a double-blind, randomized, double-placebo trial, InTIME (intravenous nPA for Treatment of Infarcting Myocardium Early) I [17]. Eligible patients included men or women aged 18–80 years, presenting within 6 h of suspected acute myocardial infarction, with ST-segment elevation or new left bundle-branch block, and the ability to undergo coronary angiography within 60 min. Aspirin (150–325 mg/day) and heparin (5000 U bolus then 1000 U/h infusion for at least 48 h titrated to achieve an aPTT of 60–85 s) were administered in all patients. Patients were randomized to receive 15, 30, 60, or 120 kU/kg of lanoteplase or ≤100 mg of alteplase (accelerated 90-min administration) in a 1 : 1 : 1 : 1 : 1 fashion.

The proportion of patients achieving TIMI grade 3 flow at 60 and 90 min demonstrated a dose-related increase with successively higher doses of lanoteplase (p < 0.001 logistic model for dose–response) (see Fig. 2). Higher rates of TIMI 3 flow were observed for 60 and 120 kU/kg lanoteplase compared to alteplase, although these differences did not achieve statistical significance. At 90 min, coronary patency with the 120-kU/kg dose was 83% compared with 71% for alteplase (p < 0.05).

Major and moderate bleeding did not differ between the various doses of lanoteplase (4.9–8.1%) and alteplase (10.5%). No intracranial hemorrhage occurred in the 124 patients who received 120 kU/kg of lanoteplase (upper bound of the 95% confidence interval = 2.4%), whereas 1 of the 124 patients (0.8%) who received alteplase suffered a hemorrhagic stroke. Rates of death (0.9–4.9%), reinfarction (0–3.3%), heart failure (4.6–6.6%), and composite outcome of any of the foregoing, or major bleeding (6.5–12.3%) were no different among the four doses of lanoteplase. The rates of each of these four clinical endpoints were numerically highest for alteplase (death 6.5%, reinfarction 6.5%, heart failure 8.9%, composite 21.8%). Given the excellent angiographic results and favorable initial clinical profile of lanoteplase 120 kU/kg, the large phase III trial, InTIME-II, was performed to compare the clinical outcomes of this dose of lanoteplase with alteplase.

IV. CLINICAL EFFICACY AND SAFETY

InTIME-II [18] was a randomized, double-blind, multicenter, equivalence trial designed to test whether 120-kU/kg single-bolus lanoteplase was at least as effective as 100 mg or less of accelerated alteplase in reducing mortality and major morbidity in patients with suspected myocardial infarction presenting within 6 h of symptom onset. A total of 15,078 patients were enrolled at 855 hospitals in 35 countries. Patients also received aspirin (150–325 mg p.o. or 150–500 mg i.v.) and intravenous heparin (bolus: 70 U/kg [maximum 4000 units], infusion: 15 U/kg h^{-1} [maximum 1000 units] for 24–48 h adjusted to achieve an aPTT of 50–70 s). The primary outcome was all-cause mortality through 30 days. Daily aspirin was continued at a dose of 100–325 mg.

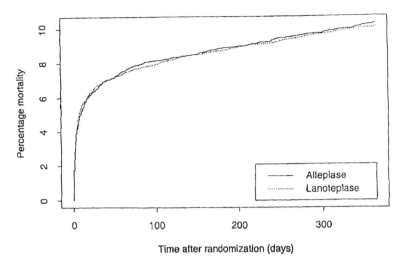

Figure 3 Mortality rates through 1 year in the InTIME II trial.

Results at 30 days indicated that lanoteplase was as effective as alteplase relative to mortality (30-day mortality: lanoteplase 6.77% vs. alteplase 6.60%, difference 0.17%; 95% CI 0.9–1.18; p = 0.048 for equivalence) [18]. The mortality curves were superimposable between the two treatment groups from 24 h through 1-year (Fig. 3) [18,19]. The secondary endpoint of death plus disabling stroke (Rankin score ≥ 3) was likewise similar between the two groups at 30 days (lanoteplase 7.2% vs. alteplase 7.0%; p = NS) and at 6 months (lanoteplase 8.9% vs. alteplase 9.0%). Trends toward a reduction in reinfarction, severe heart failure, the need for emergency or any revascularization, and severe recurrent ischemia were observed with inpatients randomized to lanoteplase (Table 3).

Table 3 Clinical Outcomes During Hospitalization and Through 30 Days in the InTIME II Trial Comparing Alteplase (t-PA) with Lanteplase (n-PA)

Event	Lanteplase (%)	Alteplase (%)	p
During index hospitalization			
Severe heart failure	2.1	2.4	0.30
Reinfarction	3.9	4.5	0.07
Need for emergency revascularization	5.4	6.2	0.04
Any revascularization	23.0	24.4	0.053
Severe recurrent ischemia	16.6	17.7	0.08
Through 30 days			
Severe heart failure	2.3	2.6	0.19
Reinfarction	5.0	5.5	0.14
Need for emergency revascularization	6.3	7.0	0.06
Any revascularization	25.8	26.9	0.15
Severe recurrent ischemia	19.8	20.9	0.17

Overall, the incidence of stroke was similar in the two treatment groups: lanoteplase 1.89% versus alteplase 1.52% (p = 0.10). However, the rate of intracranial hemorrhage (ICH) was significantly higher with lanoteplase (1.12% vs. 0.64%, p = 0.004). Excluding ICH, there were no differences between the treatment group in major bleeding (lanoteplase 0.5% vs. alteplase 0.6%) or moderate bleeding (lanoteplase 2.4% vs. alteplase 2.4%), however lanoteplase was associated with more minor bleeding than alteplase (19.7% vs. 14.8%, p < 0.0001).

Retrospective analyses of the aPTT values and ICH rates in InTIME-II revealed that lanoteplase was associated with a prolonged aPTT at 6 h that was on average 20 s greater than that observed with alteplase (Fig. 4) [20], perhaps owing to the lower fibrin specificity of lanoteplase. This, in turn, was hypothesized as a potential explanation for the higher rate of ICH with lanoteplase. The notion that higher doses of heparin are associated with increased ICH risk is consistent with observations from an experimental model of spontaneously hypertensive rats administered t-PA that revealed a potentiation of ICH by heparin [21]. The increased risk of ICH in this rat model was dependent on the heparin dose, and proportional to the prolongation of the aPTT. Such a mechanism may also explain the increased risk of ICH as aPTT levels increased beyond 70 s in GUSTO-I [22].

Thus, lanoteplase administered without a heparin bolus was subsequently studied in an open-label registry known as InTIME-IIb [20]. Heparin was administered as an initial infusion of 15 U/kg h^{-1} (maximum 1000 U/h), and patients who received a prior bolus of heparin were not eligible for participation. All patients received lanoteplase as the initial fibrinolytic agent. Otherwise, the study protocol was identical with InTIME-II.

Preliminary data reveal that by omitting the heparin bolus, the peak aPTT following lanoteplase plus heparin infusion was lowered by approximately 20 s, and the profile of the aPTT over time was nearly identical with that measured with alteplase and heparin bolus plus infusion in InTIME-II (see Fig. 4) [20]. Furthermore, the ICH rate with lanoteplase without a heparin bolus was markedly reduced to 0.50% in the per-protocol treatment group [23] in InTIME-IIb, less than half the rate that occurred with lanoteplase and heparin bolus plus infusion in InTIME-II (Fig. 5) [20]. Furthermore, unadjusted 30-day mortality rates were not statistically different (see Fig. 5) between patients receiving lanoteplase with (InTIME-II) versus without (InTIME-IIb) a heparin bolus, and after multivariate adjustment to account for the higher baseline risk in

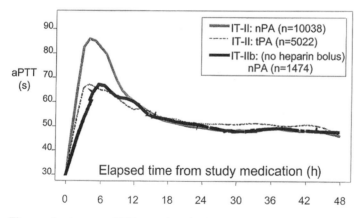

Figure 4 Average aPTT over time in InTIME-II and InTIME-IIb: In InTIME-II, lanoteplase (n-PA) was administered with adjunctive heparin bolus (70 U/kg, maximum 4000 U) and heparin infusion (15 U/kg h^{-1}, maximum initial infusion 1000 U/h) for 24–48 h adjusted to an aPTT of 50–70 s. In InTIME-IIb, the initial heparin bolus was omitted.

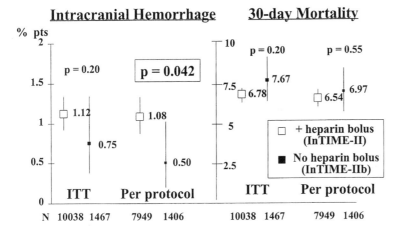

Figure 5 Intracranial hemorrhage and 30-day mortality rates in InTIME-II and InTIME-IIb with lanoteplase and different heparin regimens in intention-to-treat (ITT) and per protocol populations. See text and legend of Figure 4 for details of the treatment regimens.

patients enrolled in InTIME-IIb, the mortality rates were nearly identical (ITT cohort: OR = 1.04, p = 0.79; per protocol cohort: OR 0.99, p = 0.97) [20].

These observations emphasize the need for the evaluation of alternative lower-dose antithrombotic regimens in future trials of reperfusion regimens for myocardial infarction to reduce the risk of ICH [23]. Indeed, it remains controversial whether less fibrin-specific agents (e.g., streptokinase, possibly lanoteplase) require any heparin to be effective [24].

V.   CONCLUSIONS

Lanoteplase is a fibrinolytic derived from t-PA with a reduced plasma clearance and a prolonged half-life such that it can be administered as a single bolus. The efficacy and safety of lanoteplase have been investigated in several clinical studies, including angiographic and mortality trials. Dose-finding angiographic trials indicated that the 120-kU/kg dose achieved patency rates that were at least as good as front-loaded alteplase, whereas the phase-III InTIME II trial demonstrated that the 120-kU/kg dose lanoteplase was as effective as alteplase in mortality.

However, the rate of intracranial hemorrhage was significantly higher in patients receiving lanoteplase in InTIME-II, and further development of this compound has been halted. Subsequent analyses suggest that a higher early aPTT peak is associated with the less fibrin-specific drug lanoteplase compared with alteplase. This early peaking of the aPTT is obviated by omitting the initial heparin bolus, and in one pilot experience [20,23], resulted in a marked reduction in intracranial bleeding.

Although lanoteplase is unlikely to be marketed, important issues raised during its development include (1) confirmation that a single-bolus fibrinolytic is as effective as accelerated alteplase in reducing mortality in acute myocardial infarction; (2) question of how to balance safety and efficacy of new agents; (3) reaffirmation that heparin may be an important determinant of bleeding risk in patients treated with fibrinolytic therapy.

REFERENCES

1. Gruppo Italiano Per Lo Studio Della Streptochinasi Nell'Infarto Miocardico (GISSI). Effectiveness of intravenous thrombolytic treatment in acute myocardial infarction. Lancet 1986; 1:397–401.
2. DeWood MA, Spores J, Notske R, Mouser LT, Burroughs R, Golden MS, Lang HT. Prevalence of total coronary occlusion during the early hours of transmural myocardial infarction. N Engl J Med 1980; 303:897–902.
3. Braunwald E. The open-artery theory is alive and well-again. N Engl J Med 1993; 329:1650–1652.
4. Cannon CP. Optimizing the medical management of acute coronary syndromes. J Thromb Thrombolysis 1999; 7:171–189.
5. Global Utilization of Streptokinase, and Tissue Plasminogen Activator for Occluded Coronary Arteries (GUSTO); Investigators. An international randomized trial comparing four thrombolytic strategies for acute myocardial infarction. N Engl J Med 1993; 329:673–682.
6. The GUSTO Angiographic Investigators. The effects of tissue plasminogen activator, streptokinase, or both on coronary-artery patency, ventricular function, and survival after acute myocardial infarction. N Engl J Med 1993; 329:1615–1622.
7. Simes RJ, Topol EJ, Holmes DR Jr., White HD, Rutsch WR, Vahanian A, Simoons ML, Morris D, Betriu A, Califf RM. Link between the angiographic substudy and mortality outcomes in a large randomized trial of myocardial reperfusion: importance of early and complete infarct artery reperfusion. Circulation 1995; 91:1923–1928.
8. Tebbe U, Michels R, Adgey J, Boland J, Caspi A, Charbonnier B, Windeler J, Barth H, Groves R, Hopkins GR, Fennell W, Betriu A, Ruda M, Miczoch J. Randomized double-blind study comparing saruplase with streptokinase therapy in acute myocardial infarction: the COMPASS equivalence trial. J Am Coll Cardiol 1998; 31:487–493.
9. Hansen L, Blue Y, Barone K, Collen D, Larsen GR. Functional effects of asparagine-linked oligosaccharide on natural and variant human tissue-type plasminogen activator. J Biol Chem 1988; 263:15713–15719.
10. Phase I study of novel plasminogen activator, SUN9216 on the safety, pharmacological activity, and pharmacokinetics in healthy volunteers. Suntory Limited Protocol No. BA1101 Draft Report.
11. Liao W–C, Beierle FA, Stouffer BC, Dockens RC, Abbud ZA, Tay LK, Knaus DM, Raymond RH, Chew PH, Kostis JB. Single bolus regimen of lanoteplase (nPA); in acute myocardial infarction: pharmacokinetic evaluation from InTIME-I study. Circulation 1997; 96(suppl I);I-260–I-261.
12. Collen D. Fibrin-selective thrombolytic therapy for acute myocardial infarction. Circulation 1996; 93:857–865.
13. Collen D, Haber E. The fibrinolytic system and thrombolytic therapy. In: Chien EW, ed. Molecular Basis of Cardiovascular Disease. A Companion to Braunwald's Heart Disease. Philadelphia; W. B. Saunders 1999; 537–565.
14. Phase-II safety and efficacy of SUN9216 by i.v. bolus injection in patients with acute myocardial infarction: a multi-center study of clinical phase-II. Suntory Limited Protocol BA2201 Draft Report.
15. Yui Y, Saoky N, Iwade K, et al. A double-blind, dose-finding study for the i.v. bolus injection of SUN9216 (modified tissue plasminogen activator); in acute myocardial infarction: clinical late phase-II study. Jpn Pharmacol Ther 1997; 25:245–271.
16. Yui Y, Kawai T, Hosoda S, et al. Clinical efficacy of SUN9216 (modified tissue plasminogen activator); as compared to alteplase in patients with acute myocardial infarction: a multicenter randomized double-blind comparative study. Jpn Pharmacol Ther 1997; 25:269–302.
17. Den Heijer P, Vermeer F, Abrosioni E, Sadowski Z, Lopez-Sendon JL, von Essen R, Beaufils P, Thadani U, Adgey J, Pierard L, Brinker J, Davies RF, Smalling RW, Wallentin L, Caspi A, Pangerl A, Trickett L, Hauck C, Henry D, Chew P, for the INTIME Investigators. Evaluation of a weight-adjusted single-bolus plasminogen activator in patients with myocardial infarction. Circulation 1998; 98:2117–2125.
18. InTIME-II Investigators. Intravenous nPA for the treatment of infarcting myocardium early: InTIME-II, a double blind comparison of single bolus lanoteplase vs. accelerated alteplase for the treatment of patients with acute myocardial infarction. Eur Heart J; 2000; 21:2005–2013.

19. Antman EM, Wilcox RG, Giugliano RP, McCabe CH, Foxley A, Pangerl A, Chew PH, Skene AM, Neuhaus KL, Braunwald E, Investigators obot I-I. Long-term comparison of lanoteplase and alteplase in ST elevation myocardial infarction: 6 month followup in the InTIME-II trial. Circulation 1999; 100:I-498.
20. Giugliano RP, Antman EM, McCabe CH, Cutler SS, Chew P, Braunwald E. Omission of heparin bolus lowers rate of intracranial hemorrhage with lanoteplase. J Am Coll Cardiol 2000; 35 (suppl A):407A.
21. Paoni NF, Steinmetz HG, Gillett N, et al. An experimental model of intracranial hemorrhage during thrombolytic therapy with t-PA. Thromb Haemost 1996; 75:820–826
22. Granger CB, Hirsch J, Califf RM, Col J, White HD, Betriu A, Woodlief LH, Lee KL, Bovill EG, Simes RJ, Topol EJ. Activated partial thromboplastin time and outcome after thrombolytic therapy for acute myocardial infarction: results from the GUSTO-I trial. Circulation 1996; 93:870–878.
23. Giugliano RP, McCabe CH, Antman EM, Cannon CP, Van de Werf F, Wilcox RG, Braunwald E. Lower dose heparin with fibrinolysis is associated with lower rates of intracranial hemorrhage. Am Heart J 2001; 141:742–750.
24. GISSI-2: a factorial randomised trial of alteplase versus streptokinase and heparin versus no heparin among 12,490 patients with acute myocardial infarction. Gruppo Italiano per lo Studio della Sopravvivenza nell'Infarto Miocardico. Lancet 1990; 336:65–71.

33

Monteplase: Pharmacological and Clinical Experience

Chuichi Kawai
Takeda General Hospital and Kyoto University, Kyoto, Japan

Suguru Suzuki
Eisai Company Ltd., Tsukuba, Japan

SUMMARY

The most important characteristics to be improved for an ideal thrombolytic drug are simple and rapid administration, fibrin specificity, and an improved safety profile compared with tissue plasminogen activator (t-PA). We have developed a novel modified t-PA, monteplase (Cleactor) that was constructed by replacing a single amino acid, cysteine 84 with serine, in the epidermal growth factor domain. Monteplase has a decreased clearance and slightly less fibrin specificity than t-PA, allowing bolus intravenous administration and providing potent efficacy for thrombolysis without causing bleeding complications in in vitro and in vivo models. In canine coronary thrombolysis models, early complete reperfusion with a bolus intravenous injection of monteplase protected left ventricular function, 4 h or 1 week after treatment. Dose-finding, efficacy, and safety studies revealed that, due to its prolonged half-life, a single-bolus intravenous injection of monteplase resulted in a higher rate of early recanalization of infarct-related arteries than that of native t-PA in patients with acute myocardial infarction. There was no evidence for a higher incidence in bleeding complications in monteplase-treated patients than with native t-PA-treated patients. Thus, on the basis of preclinical and clinical investigations, monteplase is a safe and efficacious novel thrombolytic agent.

I. PRECLINICAL PROFILE OF MONTEPLASE

A. Mutagenesis and Biochemical Characterization

Tissue plasminogen activator (t-PA) is composed of 527 amino acids and consists of five structural domains (or modules): finger (F), epidermal growth factor (G), two kringles (K1, K2), and a protease domain (P). Three N-linked carbohydrate chains are attached to Asn-117 in K1 domain, Asn-184 in K2, and Asn-448 in P domain. In addition, threonine 61 in G domain is fucosylated [1]. Interestingly, t-PA contains 35 cysteine residues and 34 of them are involved in forming 17 disulfide bonds, thus leaving one cysteine residue free. Comparison of the amino acid sequence in G domains from various other plasma proteins showed that cysteine 83 is an unpaired cysteine residue [2]. We have mutated cysteine 83 or cysteine 84 to serine, expressed mutant proteins in BHK cells, and characterized their products. Initial findings demonstrated that cysteine 84 to serine (Cys-84-Ser) mutant cleared more slowly and lysed clots more efficiently than wild-type t-PA in vivo [3–5]. Systematic analysis involving cysteine-to-alanine mutations have located cysteine 83 as the unpaired residue and confirmed the altered properties of Cys-84-Ala mutant [6].

We have also investigated the immunogenic profiles of several mutant t-PAs, including Cys-84-Ser mutant in chimpanzees, to assess how structural modification of t-PA alters its immunogenic properties. This study demonstrated that neither wild-type t-PA nor Cys-84-Ser mutant elicited antibodies against those exogenous proteins and we concluded that Cys-84-Ser mutant was not immunogenic [7]. These characteristics of the Cys-84-Ser mutant, designated E6010 or monteplase, have led to further development of this mutant protein as an improved thrombolytic agent with potential clinical use. The primary structure of monteplase is shown in Figure 1. Extensive work in protein chemistry identified unexpected, but distinct, structural differences of monteplase when compared with t-PA. Different pairing of the disulfide bonds, loss of fucosylation at Thr-61 and an altered carbohydrate structure at Asn-117, were the major differences (Table 1). Single amino acid substitution of cysteine-84 to serine resulted in these complex and unexpected structural changes [8].

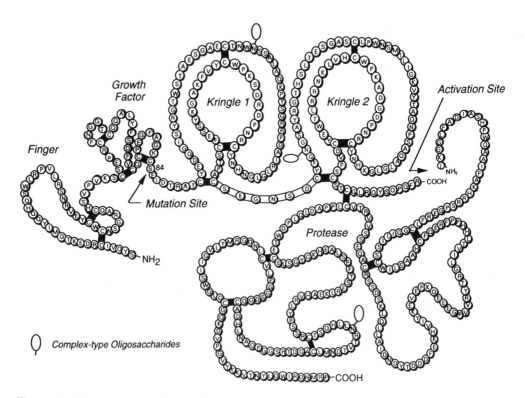

Figure 1   Primary structure of monteplase.

Table 1 Comparison of the Structure of Monteplase with t-PA

Structure	t-PA	Monteplase
Disulfide bonds in G domain	Cys-51–Cys62	Cys51–Cys73
	Cys56–Cys73	Cys56–Cys62
	Cys75–Cys84	Cys75–Cys83
	Cys83 unpaired	Ser84
Fucosylation of Ihr61	Yes	No
Carbohydrate on Asn117	High-mannose type	Complex type
Carbohydrate on Asn184	Complex type	Complex type
Carbohydrate on Asn448	Complex type	Complex type

Functional analysis in vitro revealed that fibrin binding by monteplase was decreased to about 30% of that of rt-PA (Fig. 2) [9]. The activator activity of monteplase was enhanced about 15-fold in the presence of fibrin fragments; this was one-eighth of the increase observed with rt-PA [10]. Fibrinogen consumption in various species (human, rat, dog, rabbit, and pig plasma) was examined [11]. Only at the highest dose, both monteplase and t-PA depleted blood coagulation and fibrinolysis parameters significantly. The lower efficiency in plasminogen activation and the lower fibrin affinity of monteplase might be attributed to the structural changes. Quantitative analyses of the interaction of rt-PA with PAI-1 indicated that the rate of complex formation of monteplase with PAI-1 was similar to that of rt-PA. The second-order rate constants of monteplase and single-chain form rt-PA to PAI-1 were 0.70 and 0.68 $M^{-1}s^{-1} \times 10^{7}$, respectively [12]. In summary, in experiments conducted in vitro, monteplase exhibited activities that were somewhat reduced from those of t-PA.

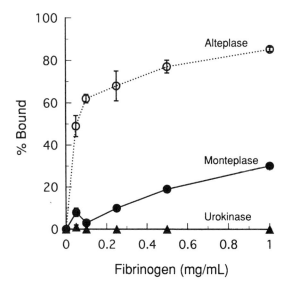

Figure 2 Binding of monteplase, alteplase, and urokinase to forming fibrin clots: Samples of 500 ng/mL (final concentration) of each activator were mixed with the indicated concentrations of fibrinogen. After clotting with thrombin the activator concentration in the supernatant was determined by enzyme-linked immunosorbent assay [ELISA]. Data are means ± the standard error ($n = 4$). (From Ref. 9.)

B. In Vivo Animal Model (Pharmacokinetics, Toxicology, and Pharmacology)

1. Pharmacokinetics of Monteplase

a. Pharmacokinetics of Monteplase in Rats.   Blood or plasma concentration, distribution, metabolism and excretion of monteplase were studied in male rats after a single intravenous administration of $[^{125}I]$-monteplase and compared with those of $[^{125}I]$-rt-PA [13].

After a single intravenous administration of $[^{125}I]$-monteplase, plasma clearances of TCA-precipitable radioactivity, immunoreactivity, fibrinolytic activity and unchanged monteplase were 10.3, 11.2, 3.1, and 5.5 times lower than those after dosing with $[^{125}I]$-rt-PA, respectively. In plasma, the complexes of $[^{125}I]$-monteplase with α_2-macroglobulin (molecular weight approximately 700 kDa) and with α_2-plasmin inhibitor (molecular weight approximately 180 kDa) were observed after dosing of $[^{125}I]$-monteplase, similar to $[^{125}I]$-rt-PA. After a single intravenous administration of $[^{125}I]$-monteplase, liver levels of TCA-precipitable radioactivity reached a maximum level at 15 min after administration, accounting for about 19% of administered radioactivity. For $[^{125}I]$-rt-PA, a maximum level was reached at 5 min after administration accounting for about 54% of administered dose. These results suggest that the differences in the distribution to the liver between monteplase and rt-PA resulted in the difference of plasma clearances.

Within 7 days after a single intravenous administration of $[^{125}I]$-monteplase, 96.05 and 5.32% of the administrated radioactivity were excreted into the urine and feces, respectively. Biliary excretion of radioactivity was 17.01% of the dose within 48 h after a single intravenous administration of $[^{125}I]$-monteplase. Both radioactivity excreted in the urine and in bile consisted mainly of small-molecular-weight metabolites or $[^{125}I]$.

b. Pharmacokinetics of Monteplase in Dogs.   The clearance of monteplase was evaluated in dogs following bolus intravenous injections [14]. The half-lives for α- and β-phases of plasma immunoreactive monteplase concentration were 4.76 and 50.8 min, and those of rt-PA were 3.56 and 36.0 min, respectively. The area under the curve (AUC) for immunoreactive monteplase was 2.4-fold greater than for rt-PA (63.52 $\mu g \cdot min\ mL^{-1}$ for monteplase, and 26. 43 $\mu g \cdot min\ mL^{-1}$ for rt-PA). Thus, the clearance of monteplase was slower than that of rt-PA.

c. Pharmacokinetics of Monteplase in Humans (Phase I Study).   The pharmacokinetics of monteplase were studied in four healthy volunteers following single intravenous administration of a dose of 6.0 mg/body [15]. The half-lives for α- and β-phases of plasma immunoreactive monteplase concentration were 23.66 min and 7.82 h, respectively. A one-compartment model was used for the analysis of the plasma fibrinolytic activity of monteplase concentration, since the β-phase for fibrinolytic activity of monteplase could not be defined owing to insufficient analytical sensitivity of this assay. The half-life of plasma fibrinolytic activity of monteplase concentration was 29.43 min. The AUCs for monteplase were 267.30 $\mu g \cdot min\ mL^{-1}$ (immunoreactivity), and 64.89 $\mu g \cdot min\ mL^{-1}$ (fibrinolytic activity).

2. Preclinical Toxicology of Monteplase

Acute toxicity studies were carried out using mice (dose levels: 80 and 160 mg/kg), rats (40, 80, and 160 mg/kg), and cynomolgus monkeys (40, 80, and 160 mg/kg) [16]. However, the lethal dosage level was more than 160 mg/kg in all animals. In rats a 4-week repeated intravenous-administration toxicity study of monteplase (dose levels: 1, 3, and 10 mg/kg day^{-1}) was conducted [17]. Increased mesangial matrix of glomeruli and plasma level of total cholesterol in the 3-mg/kg day^{-1} group were noted at the end of the treatment. Increased hemorrhage-related lesions thought to be secondary to the pharmacological action of the monteplase in the 3-mg/kg day^{-1} group were also seen. In the 10-mg/kg day^{-1} group, flushing and swelling of the nose and perinasal region, increased plasma level of triglyceride, and decreased plasma level of alkaline phosphatase were observed at the end of the treatment. Based on these results, the nontoxic dose was determined as $1\,mg/kg\,day^{-1}$. In cynomolgus monkeys, a 4-week repeated intravenous administration toxicity study of monteplase (dose levels: 1, 3, and $10\,mg/kg\,day^{-1}$) was performed [18]. A slight degree of hemorrhage-related lesions, and a decreased plasma level of hematological, coagulation and fibrinolysis parameters were observed in the 1-mg/kg or higher dose groups at the end of the treatment. In the 3-mg/kg dose group, pale visible mucosa, and swelling and induration at the injection site were observed. Two animals of the 10-mg/kg dose group became moribund. The morbidity was thought to be due to the anemia resulting from fibrinolysis-related hemorrhage (e.g., bloody stool). All findings noted in the 1-mg/kg group were thought to be secondary to the pharmacological action of monteplase and, therefore, the nontoxic dose was determined as $1\,mg/kg\,day^{-1}$.

3. Pharmacology of Monteplase

a. Thrombolytic Effect of Monteplase in a Canine Model with Copper Coil-Induced Coronary Artery Thrombi. The thrombolytic properties of monteplase were compared with a native human t-PA, tisokinase (Plasvata; Asahi Kasei Kogyo Co., Ltd., Tokyo, Japan) in a canine model with copper coil-induced coronary artery thrombi [19]. Tisokinase is a single-chain–form glycoprotein that is composed of 527 amino acids and is produced by diploid fibroblasts derived from human lungs [20]. The half-lives for α- and β-phases of plasma immunoreactive tisokinase concentration in healthy volunteers were 4 and 40 min, respectively [21]. These half-lives were almost equivalent to those of alteplase [22].

A model of copper coil-induced coronary artery thrombi 1, 3, and 6 h after thrombus formation was prepared using anesthetized dogs. The thrombolytic efficacy of bolus intravenous injection of monteplase (0.1, 0.2, and 0.4 mg/kg) and tisokinase (250 kIU/kg), or continuous intravenous infusion of tisokinase over 1 hr (125, 250, and 500 kIU/kg) were evaluated by three criteria: reperfusion rate, time to reperfusion, and reocclusion rate on coronary angiography.

The summary of the results is shown in Figure 3. The reperfusion rate was significantly higher, than that of the vehicle control group after bolus intravenous injection of monteplase at doses 0.1, 0.2, and 0.4 mg/kg for thrombi aged 3 and 6 h that had enriched fibrin with clear fibrin network and aggregated platelets. The reperfusion rate of bolus intravenous injection of monteplase was similar to that of continuous intravenous infusion of tisokinase. Monteplase significantly shortened the reperfusion time at doses of 0.2 and 0.4 mg/kg for thrombi aged 3 and 6 h, compared with the control group. There was a tendency to shorten the reperfusion time with the bolus intravenous injection of monteplase at doses of 0.2 and 0.4 mg/kg for thrombi aged 3 h, compared with the continuous intravenous infusion of tisokinase at all doses. Reocclusion was observed in only one or none of the animals (25% or less) in all drug-treated dose groups, either in monteplase or in tisokinase, 1 or 2 h after administration for thrombi aged 1, 3, or 6 h, except for in the 0.1-mg/kg monteplase group for thrombi aged 6 h in which reocclusion of three out of five animals (60%) was observed. Therefore, compared with continuous intravenous infusion of tisokinase, bolus intravenous injection of monteplase for thrombi aged 1, 3, and 6 h did not cause any significant difference in the reocclusion rate.

b. Effect of Monteplase on Recovery of Ventricular Function after Coronary Thrombolysis in a Canine Thrombosis Model. The purpose of thrombolytic therapy, after the onset of symptoms, is to achieve early initiation of coronary artery reperfusion to limit infarct size, to preserve left ventricular function, and to reduce mortality [23,24].

With the centerline method [25] in a canine copper coil-induced coronary thrombosis model, left ventricular function after coronary thrombolysis induced by monteplase was

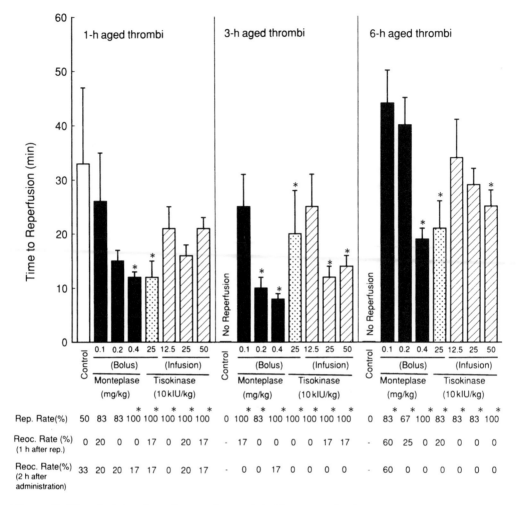

	Control	|	0.1	0.2	0.4	25	12.5	25	50
Rep. Rate(%)	50		83	83	100	100	100	100	100
Reoc. Rate (%) (1 h after rep.)	0		20	0	0	17	0	20	17
Reoc. Rate(%) (2 h after administration)	33		20	20	17	17	0	20	17

Control	0.1	0.2	0.4	25	12.5	25	50
0	100	83	100	100	100	100	100
-	17	0	0	0	0	17	17
-	0	0	17	0	0	0	0

Control	0.1	0.2	0.4	25	12.5	25	50
0	83	67	100	83	83	83	100
-	60	25	0	20	0	0	0
-	60	0	0	0	0	0	0

Figure 3 Thrombolytic effect of monteplase and tisokinase, a native human t-PA, on coronary artery thrombi of different durations: Data are the mean, and the vertical bars are the standard error of the time to reperfusion in a successful reperfusion. Closed bars show bolus intravenous injection of monteplase; and dotted and hatched bars show bolus intravenous injection and continuous intravenous infusion of tisokinase, respectively. Open bar shows control. The reperfusion rate (Rep. Rate, %) is expressed as {(the number of animals that showed recanalization 60 min after the drug administration)/ 6} $\times$ 100, and the reocclusion rate (Reoc. Rate, %) as {(the number of animals that showed reocclusion)/(the number of animals that showed recanalization)} $\times$ 100. (*: $p < 0.05$ vs. control). (From Ref. 19.)

compared with that induced by rt-PA or urokinase [26]. Thirty minutes after occlusion, monteplase (0.2 mg/kg), rt-PA (0.6 mg/kg for 1 h) or urokinase (60 kIU/kg for 1 h) was administered intravenously. Animals with sustained copper coil-occlusion served as the nonreperfused control. Left ventriculography (LVG) and coronary angiography (CAG) were obtained before and 30 min after coronary artery occlusion, immediately after coronary reperfusion, and at 1, 2, 3 and 4 h after coronary reperfusion. Left ventricular ejection fraction was obtained by analysis of the left ventriculogram at end diastole and end systole in LVGs.

Time to complete reperfusion was about 20 min in all drug-treated groups. Figure 4 shows the left ventricular ejection fraction in each group. In the monteplase group, the left ventricular

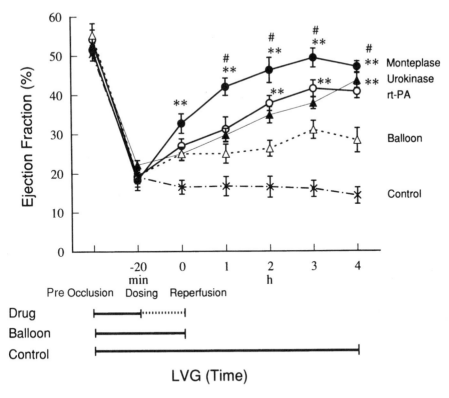

Figure 4 Changes in left ventricular contractility (left ventricular ejection fraction): Data are the mean, and the vertical bars are the standard error ($n = 6$, **: $p < 0.01$ vs. control, #: $p < 0.05$ vs. balloon). (From Ref. 26.)

ejection fraction recovered significantly, beginning immediately after reperfusion, compared with that in a nonreperfused control group. In the rt-PA group, left ventricular ejection fraction recovered significantly 2 h or more after reperfusion compared with that in a nonreperfused control group. In the urokinase group, left ventricular ejection fraction recovered significantly 4 h after reperfusion. In contrast, in the balloon reperfusion group, the recovery of left ventricular ejection fraction was not significant, even at 4 h after reperfusion. These results suggest that coronary reperfusion with monteplase induced earlier recovery of left ventricular function than that in the rt-PA or urokinase groups.

   c. Effect of Thrombolysis with Monteplase on the Protection against Deterioration of Left Ventricular Function during Coronary Occlusion in a Canine Model with Laser Ablation-Induced Acute Myocardial Infarction. The effects of a single intravenous bolus injection of monteplase on prognosis after 1 week using a canine thrombosis model were examined [27]. This model was produced by selective injection of an artificial autologous thrombus into the coronary artery stenosed by laser ablation under closed chest conditions. Animals were randomly assigned to receive either a placebo (control group), 0.22 mg/kg (group L, clinical dose) or 0.44 mg/kg (group H) bolus injection of monteplase. LVG and CAG were obtained before and after coronary artery occlusion, and at 30 and 60 min and 1 week after dosing with monteplase. Reperfusion rate at 1 h after treatment and patency rate 1 week after treatment in control, groups L and H were 10% (1/10), 50% (5/10), and 70% (7/9); and 0% (0/6), 33% (2/6), and 88% (7/8), respectively. Thus, a significantly higher reperfusion rate at 1 h

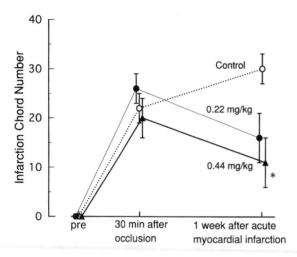

Figure 5 Changes in regional left ventricular wall motion expressed as infarction chord number: Data are the mean, and the vertical bars are the standard error ($n = 6$–10). Regional wall motion is expressed as the infarction chord number (i.e., the number of chords showing less than minus 2 standard deviations among chords located in regions dominated by the left anterior descending artery; (*: $p < 0.05$ vs. control). (From Ref. 27.)

after treatment and patency rate 1 week after treatment were seen in the H group compared with the control group. One week after treatment, the survival rates in control, groups L and H were 60% (6/10), 70% (7/10), and 80% (8/10), respectively.

The left ventricular function in each group is shown in Figure 5. The infarction chord number, as an index of regional ventricular wall motion, was significantly lower in the H group than that of control group, indicating that coronary thrombolysis with monteplase protected against loss of ventricular function after coronary occlusion. The results of this study suggest that the reperfusion of the occluded coronary artery and maintenance of the coronary patency with monteplase may improve the prognosis following acute myocardial infarction.

II. CLINICAL EXPERIENCE

A novel modified t-PA—monteplase—has been granted permission for clinical use as a single bolus injection in the treatment of acute myocardial infarction by the Japanese Government after serial clinical trials, including prospective, randomized, double-blind multicenter studies on dose-finding, efficacy and safety aspects.

A. Dose-Finding Study

1. Methods

A prospective, randomized, double-blind multicenter trial [28] of a single bolus injection was carried out to determine the optimal dose of monteplase in 177 patients with acute myocardial infarction of less than 6-h duration. All patients provided informed consent, and the protocol was approved by the institutional review committee of each of the 62 participating hospitals. The patients were divided into three groups receiving three different doses; namely, 0.12 mg/kg (low-dose group, Group L; $n = 59$) 0.22 mg/kg (medium-dose group, group M; $n = 51$), and

0.32 mg/kg (high dose group, group H; $n = 67$). The primary endpoint, a thrombolysis in myocardial infarction (TIMI) grade 2 or 3 recanalization rate of the infarct-related coronary artery 60 min after treatment, was initiated in each of the three groups. Secondary endpoints included recanalization of the infarct-related artery at 15, 30 and 45 min after treatment initiation, and therapy-related bleeding complications. Only patients with an angiographically confirmed 100% occlusion of the infarct-related artery despite the pretreatment of intravenous heparin and intracoronary nitroglycerin administration were enrolled in the study. Monteplase was administered intravenously within 2 min, according to the dose assigned to each patient.

2. Results

At 60 min after administration of monteplase, group M (0.22 mg/kg of monteplase) demonstrated the highest recanalization rate of TIMI grade 2 or 3, (78 or 69%, respectively). The recanalization rate of TIMI grade 2 or 3 in group M was significantly higher than that in group L (66 or 41%), respectively; however, the recanalization rate of TIMI grade 2 or 3 in group H was 72% or 61%, respectively, and showed no significant difference from those of group M (Fig. 6).

Bleeding complications including hemorrhage at the site of puncture requiring blood transfusion, gum bleeding, gastrointestinal bleeding requiring blood transfusion and cerebral hemorrhage increased in parallel with the doses (Table 2). As a result, it was decided that the optimal single-bolus dose of monteplase was 0.22 mg/kg.

The plasma concentration level of monteplase increased in parallel with the doses, reaching maximum at 60 min, and began to decrease at 120 min, becoming half the maximum value at 60 min. The plasma level of plasminogen, fibrinogen, and α_2-plasmin inhibitor (α_2-PI) significantly decreased at 60 and 120 min, respectively, and returned to near-baseline levels at 24 h. The rate of decrease was in parallel with the doses; and the values of plasminogen and

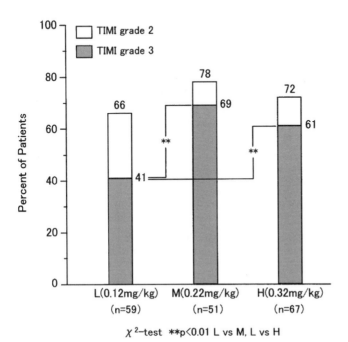

Figure 6 Recanalization rate of infarct-related arteries at 60 min after three doses (L: 0.12 mg/kg, M: 0.22 mg/kg, H: 0.32 mg/kg) of monteplase administration.

Table 2 Bleeding Events

	No. of patients		
Events	L $n = 64$	M $n = 58$	H $n = 68$
Puncture site (requiring blood transfusion)	0	0	2
Gingival bleeding	1	2	4
Gastrointestinal bleeding (requiring blood transfusion)	0	0	1
Cerebral hemorrhage	0	1	2
Total events	1 (2%)	3 (5%)	9 (13%)

fibrinogen at 60 min to 24 h after the treatment in groups M and H were significantly lower than those in group L. The plasma levels of α_2-PI plasmin complex (PIC) in groups M and H were significantly higher than those in group L at 60 and 120 min. The plasma D-dimer level increased significantly higher in group H than in groups M and L at 60 and 120 min (Fig. 7).

B. Efficacy and Safety Study

From data in the dose-finding study [28], a prospective, randomized, double-blind multicenter trial [29] was designed to examine the efficacy and safety of monteplase in comparison with native t-PA in patients with acute myocardial infarction.

1. Methods

The patients provided informed consent, and the protocol was approved by the institutional review board of each of the 84 participating hospitals. Patients were randomly assigned to receive either an intravenous bolus injection of 0.22 mg/kg of monteplase within 2 min, followed by a 1-hour infusion of placebo native t-PA, or intravenous-bolus injection of placebo monteplase within 2 min, followed an intravenous infusion of 28.8 mg (14.4 million IU) of native t-PA, tisokinase. One-tenth of the total native t-PA dose or its placebo was given as a bolus injection over a period of 1–2 min; the remainder was infused over 60 min.

The study was scheduled to be performed with 100 patients in each group. This sample size gave an 80% power to detect a 20% absolute difference in TIMI grades 2 or 3 recanalization at 60 min after treatment. The entry criteria were: (1) patients with acute myocardial infarction within 6 h of the onset; (2) angiographically confirmed total occlusion of the infarct-related coronary artery after intracoronary administration of nitrates; and (3) weight less than 100 kg and preferable age younger than 75 years. Patients were excluded from the enrollment according to the ordinary exclusion criteria for thrombolysis treatment.

The primary endpoint was to determine the TIMI grade 2 or 3 recanalization rate of the infarct-related coronary artery at 60 min after treatment in the two treatment groups. Secondary endpoints included the recanalization rate of the infarct-related coronary artery at 15, 30, and 45 min after treatment, and therapy-related bleeding complications. From 60 min after drug administration, percutaneous transluminal coronary angioplasty and other adjunct therapies were permitted at the discretion of the attending physician. Differences in the recanalization rate at

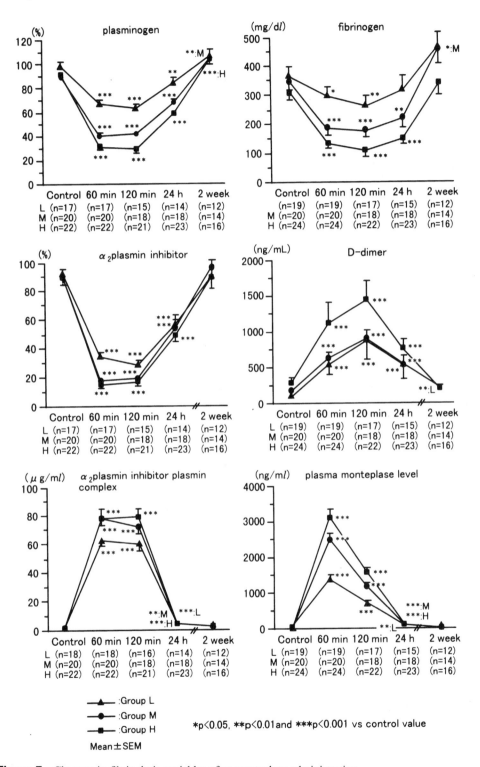

Figure 7 Changes in fibrinolytic variables after monteplase administration.

each assessment time were analyzed using the chi-square (χ^2) analysis with the Yates correction for continuity.

2. Results

A total of 97 patients in the monteplase group and 102 in the native t-PA group satisfied the entry criteria and provided angiograms of good quality that could be evaluated. The baseline characteristics of the patients showed no significant differences between the two groups for age, male predominance, body weight, or mean length of time from symptom onset to treatment initiation, and sites of the infarct-related coronary artery.

The recanalization rate of TIMI grade 2 or 3 at 60 min was 79% or 53%, respectively, in the monteplase group and 65 or 36%, respectively, in the native t-PA group; the differences in the recanalization rates between the two groups were significant (p < 0.05). The recanalization rate increased with time after treatment in both groups, but monteplase produced a significantly higher recanalization rate than native t-PA at each assessment time, particularly at 15 and 30 min (p < 0.001 for TIMI grade 2; p < 0.01 for TIMI grade 3) (Fig. 8). Using a single bolus injection of 0.22 mg/kg of monteplase, the rate of TIMI grade 2 or higher, recanalization was 78% at 60 min in the previous dose-finding study, which is similar to the 79% observed in the present efficacy and safety study.

Bleeding complications including bleeding at the puncture site requiring blood transfusion, gingival bleeding, hematemesis requiring blood transfusion, and cerebral hemorrhage occurring in eight monteplase-treated and six native t-PA-treated patients (Table 3). One fatal cerebral hemorrhage developed in the native t-PA group. However, there was no significant difference in the occurrence of bleeding complications between the two groups.

Among the patients who demonstrated recanalization of TIMI grade 2 or 3 at 60 min after treatment, reinfarction developed in 2 (3%) of 77 monteplase group patients and 4 (6%) of 66

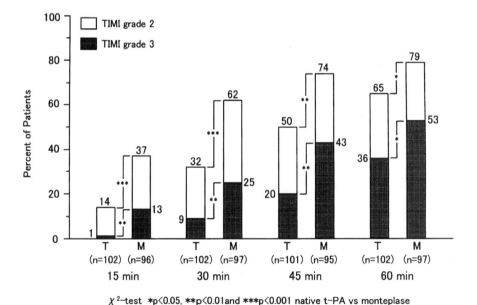

χ^2–test *p<0.05, **p<0.01and ***p<0.001 native t-PA vs monteplase

Figure 8 Recanalization rate of infarct-related arteries at each assessment time after administration of t-PA (tisokinase, T; and monteplase, M).

Table 3 Bleeding Events

Events	No. of patients	
	E6010 $n = 104$	Native t-PA $n = 107$
Puncture site (requiring blood transfusion)	1	1
Gingival bleeding	6	4
Hematemesis (requiring blood transfusion)	1	0
Cerebral hemorrhage	0	1
Total events	8 (8%)	6 (6%)

native t-PA group patients within 24 h, whereas 4 (5%) and 7 (11%) patients, respectively, showed evidence of reinfarction within 7 days. These differences were not significant.

Plasma fibrinolytic variables including plasminogen, fibrinogen, α_2-PI decreased whereas D-dimer increased after both monteplase and native t-PA treatment, and returned to near baseline levels 24 hour after drug administration.

3. Discussion

a. Pharmacokinetic Considerations. The total thrombolytic activity during the first 60 min after drug administration (i.e., AUCs derived from analyses of monteplase, and tisokinase, native t-PA, in plasma multiplied by the specific activity of each drug), revealed that a single-bolus intravenous injection within 2 min of 13.2 mg of monteplase (0.22 mg/kg, assuming the average body weight of Japanese patients to be 60 kg) (73,507 IU $\cdot$ min mL^{-1}) was comparable with a continuous intravenous injection over one of 28.8 mg of tisokinase (70,050 IU $\cdot$ min mL^{-1}) [15,30]. The percentage of binding to fibrin of tisokinase was 68%, whereas that of alteplase was 66%; these values are practically equivalent. Therefore, plasminogen-activating capacity of tisokinase is believed to be comparable with that of alteplase [31]. The dose of tisokinase adjusted for body weight (assuming an average body weight of 60 kg for Japanese patients) is 0.48 mg/kg, which appears low compared with studies of native t-PA performed in the United States and Europe. However, intravenous infusion of this regimen of tisokinase (28.8 mg) achieved a recanalization rate of TIMI 2 or higher in 72.6% at 60 min in the Japanese population [32]. As previously described, 0.22 mg/kg of monteplase was determined to be the optimal single-bolus injection dose for thrombolysis in the dose-finding study. These are the reasons for using the dose of 0.22 mg/kg for monteplase and 28.8 mg for tisokinase in the present comparative study for the treatment of acute myocardial infarction.

b. Bleeding Complications. A single-bolus injection of monteplase within 2 min caused no higher rate of bleeding complications than those in a continuous intravenous infusion of tisokinase over 60 min.

c. Reinfarction Rate. The study protocol specified no particular adjunctive therapy after drug administration for 60 min. However, the rates of reinfarction in patients treated with monteplase were less than these in patients treated with tisokinase both within 24 h and 7 days after treatment, although the differences were not significant.

d. Recanalization Rate. The percentage of recanalized patients with TIMI grade 2 or 3 at 60 min after the administration of the drug, and at each assessment time was significantly higher in patients treated with 2 min intravenous-bolus injection of monteplase than in those treated with 1-h–continuous intravenous-infusion of tisokinase (p < 0.05). The present findings clearly demonstrated that monteplase achieved the earlier and higher recanalization rate with an easier, therefore, more convenient, method of a single-bolus injection, than for tisokinase, a native t-PA, which requires a continuous-intravenous injection. This is very important in the treatment of acute myocardial infarction in which early recanalization of a culprit coronary artery within the "golden hours" is crucial in determining future fate of the patient.

III. CONCLUSIONS

Monteplase can be easily administered by a single-intravenous–bolus injection within 2 min and achieves a higher rate of early recanalization of a culprit coronary artery compared with native t-PA in patients with acute myocardial infarction. There were no higher rates of bleeding complications in monteplase-treated than in native t-PA–treated patients. As a result, monteplase may open a new era in the thrombolytic treatment of acute myocardial infarction.

REFERENCES

1. Kyte BA, Paoni NF, Bennett WF. Site-directed mutagenesis of tissue-type plasminogen activator. In: Cleland JL, Craik CS, eds. Protein Engineering: Principles and Practices. New York: Wiley, 1996; 435–466.
2. Banyai L, Varadi A, Patthy L. Common evolutionary origin of the fibrin-binding structures of fibronectin and tissue-type plasminogen activator. FEBS Lett 1983; 163:37–41.
3. Yoshitake S, Kato H, Hashimoto A, Ikeda Y, Kuwada M, Mulvihill E. Characterization of various forms of modified human tissue plasminogen activators in vitro [abstr]. Thromb Haemost 1989; 62:542.
4. Suzuki S, Nagaoka N, Suzuki N, Fujimori T, Yoshitake S. In vivo thrombolytic activities of modified human tissue plasminogen activators in rat arterio–venous shunt model [abstr]. Thromb Haemost 1989; 62:543.
5. Yuzuriha T, Mizuo H, Miyake Y. Novel modified human tissue plasminogen activators prolonged plasma clearance in vivo [abstr]. Thromb Haemost 1989; 62:543.
6. Sehl LC, Nguyen HV, Berleau LT, Arcilla P, Bennett WF, Kyte BA. Locating the unpaired cysteine of tissue-type plasminogen activator. Protein Eng 1996; 9:283–290.
7. Katsutani N, Yoshitake S, Takeuchi H, Kelliher JC, Couch RC, Shionoya H. Immunogenic properties of structurally modified human tissue plasminogen activators in chimpanzee and mice. Fundam Appl Toxcol 1992; 19:555–562.
8. Hayashi Y, Hamako J, Shikata Y, Kuwada M, Sato T, Titani K, Mizuochi T. Amino acid substitution by site-directed mutagenesis of human tissue plasminogen activators resulted in the altered processing of asparagine-linked oligosaccharide [abstr]. Glycoconjugate J 1991; 8:152.
9. Kasai S, Hashimoto A. [A comparative study of fibrin clot binding properties of E6010 with natural t-PA] [in Japanese]. Jpn Pharmacol Ther 1998; 26:989–992.
10. Suzuki S, Kasai S, Mizuo H, Mizui Y, Nagaoka N, Kikuchi K, Hashimoto A, Yuzuriha T, Yoshitake S. [A comparative study of clot affinity and fibrinolytic and fibrinogenolytic properties of E6010 with rt-PA (alteplase) and urokinase] [in Japanese]. Jpn Pharmacol Ther 1994; 22 (suppl 2):s-353–s-368.
11. Nagaoka N, Suzuki S, Suzuki N, Yoshitake S. [A comparative study of fibrinolytic properties of E6010, alteplase and urokinase in various animal species] [in Japanese]. Jpn Pharmacol Ther 1994; 22 (suppl 2):s-369–s-378.
12. Sakata Y, Kasai S, Suzuki S. [Characterization of a mutant tissue-type plasminogen activator (Cys 84 to Ser), E6010] [in Japanese]. Hematol Oncol 1994; 28:358–362.

13. Mizuo H, Seko T, Nose K, Ando T, Kagei Y, Kikuchi K, Mishima M, Ueda M, Nakata H, Horie T, Yuzuriha T. [Studies on the metabolic fate of modified recombinant tissue-type plasminogen activator (E6010) (1): Blood or plasma concentration, distribution, metabolism and excretion in rats after a single intravenous administration of ^{125}I-recombinant tissue-type plasminogen activator (rt-PA)]. [in Japanese]. Xenobiol Metab Dispos 1996; 11:556–584.

14. Suzuki S, Saito M, Suzuki N, Kato H, Nagaoka N, Yoshitake S, Mizuo H, Yuzuriha T, Yui Y, Kawai C. Thrombolytic properties of a novel modified human tissue-type plasminogen activator (E6010): a bolus injection of E6010 has equivalent potency of lysing young and aged canine coronary thrombi. J Cardiovasc Pharmacol 1991; 17:738–746.

15. Ohnishi A, Takazawa K, Fujita M, Shimomura M, Ishii M, Sanma H, Shimamura Y, Hasegawa J, Morishita N. [Phase I study of the modified tissue plasminogen activator E6010]. [in Japanese]. Jpn J Clin Pharmacol Ther 1994; 25:551–562.

16. Sumigama S, Shirakabe A, Chimoto T, Miyagawa H, Yamatsu K, Ohnishi M, Nakama K, Okazaki K, Nagata R. [Acute toxicity study of E6010 by intravenous administration in mice, rats and cynomolgus monkeys]. [in Japanese]. Jpn Pharmacol Ther 1994; 22 (suppl 2):s-193–s-199.

17. Sumigama S, Shirakabe A, Chimoto T, Miyagawa H, Aoki T, Katsutani N, Tagaya O, Miura K, Yamatsu K. [E6010 subacute toxicity study in rats on repeated intravenous administration for 4 weeks followed by a 2-week recovery period]. [in Japanese]. Jpn Pharmacol Ther 1994; 22 (suppl 2):s-201–s-232.

18. Okazaki K, Ohnishi M, Samejima H, Nagata R, Chimoto T, Tatsuo I, Shionoya H, Yamatsu K. [A 4-week repeated dose toxicity study of E6010 administered intravenously to cynomolgus monkeys followed by a 4-week recovery period]. [in Japanese]. Jpn Pharmacol Ther 1994; 22 (suppl 2):s-233–s-253.

19. Suzuki S, Takamura T, Ono H, Saito M, Ikeda Y, Kasai S, Kato H, Mizuo H, Goto M, Fujisawa M, Higashibara K, Tsukidate K, Yamanishi Y. [Thrombolytic properties of a novel modified t-PA, E6010 in a canine model with copper coil-induced coronary artery thrombi—comparison with tisokinase]. [in Japanese]. Jpn Pharmacol Ther 1996; 24:1287–1304.

20. Hasegawa A, Yamashita H, Kondo S, Kiyota T, Hayashi H, Yoshizaki H, Murakami A, Shiratsuchi M, Mori T. Proteose peptone enhances production of tissue-type plasminogen activator from human diploid fibroblasts. Biochem Biophys Res Commun 1988; 150:1230–1236.

21. Tanaka M. Tisokinase. Drugs Today 1992; 28:36–39.

22. Verstraete M, Bounameaux H, De Cock F, Van de Werf F, Collen D. Pharmacokinetics and Systematic fibrinogenolytic effects of recombinant human tissue-type plasminogen (rt-PA) in humans. J Pharmacol Exp Ther 1985; 235:506–512.

23. Linderer T, Schroder R, Arntz R, Heineking ML, Wunderlich W, Kohl K, Forycki F, Henzgen R, Wagner J. Prehospital thrombolysis: beneficial effects of very early treatment on infarct size and left ventricular function. J Am Coll Cardiol 1993; 22:1304–1310.

24. Califf RM, the GUSTO-I Investigators. One-year results from the global utilization of eptokinase and t-PA for occluded coronary arteries (GUSTO-I) trial. Circulation 1996; 94:1233–1238.

25. Sheehan FH, Braunwald E, Canner P, Dodge HT, Gore J, Natta PV, Passamani ER, Williams DO, Zaret B, Co-Investigators. The effect of intravenous thrombolytic therapy on left ventricular function: a report on tissue-type plasminogen activator and streptokinase from the thrombolysis in myocardial infarction (TIMI phase I) trial. Circulation 1987; 75:817–829.

26. Suzuki S, Saito M, Yui Y, Kawai C. A novel modified t-PA, E-6010, induces faster recovery of ventricular function after coronary thrombolysis than native t-PA in a canine model. Jpn Circ J 1995; 59:205–212.

27. Suzuki S, Saito M, Abe Y, Ono H, Takamura T, Yamanishi Y, Nakamura F, Tomaru T. [Effects of intravenous bolus injection of a novel thrombolytic drug, E-6010, on improved prognosis in a canine model with laser ablation-induced coronary artery thrombi]. [in Japanese]. Jpn Pharmacol Ther 1998; 26:993–1009.

28. Kawai C, Hosoda S, Kimata S, Kanmatsuse K, Suzuki S, Motomiya T, Yabe Y, Takatsu F, Yui Y, Kodama K, Minamino T, Sato H, Nobuyoshi M, Nakashima M. [Coronary thrombolysis in acute

myocardial infarction of E6010 (novel modified t-PA): a multicenter, double-blind, dose-finging study]. [in Japanese]. Jpn Pharmacol Ther 1994; 22:3925–3950.
29. Kawai C, Yui Y, Hosoda S, Nobuyoshi M, Suzuki S, Sato H, Takatsu F, Motomiya T, Kanmatsuse K, Kodama K, Yabe Y, Minamino T, Kimata S, Nakashima M. on behalf of the E6010 Study Group. A propective, randomized double-blind multicenter trial of a single bolus injection of the novel modified t-PA E6010 in the treatment of acute myocardial infarction: comparison with native t-PA. J Am Coll Cardiol 1997; 29:1447–1453.
30. Mori T, Nishino N, Shizume K, Sakakibara K, Ko T, Sugawara Y, Takada Y, Takada A. [Changes in various parameters of fibrinolysis in persons infused with tissue plasminogen activator—special reference to plasminogen activator inhibitor]. [in Japanese]. Jpn Pharmacol Ther 1988; Suppl. 6:1589–1596.
31. Murakami A, Yoshizaki H, Shirato S, Kondou S, Kiyota T, Hayashi H. [Characterization of tissue plasminogen activator (AK-124) in fibrinolysis]. [in Japanese]. Jpn Pharmacol Ther 1991; 19:59–64.
32. Hirosawa K, Suzuki S, Kawai C, Yui Y, Hosoda S, Kimata S, Abe H, Aoki N, Nakashima M, Kajiwara N, Kanmatsuse K, Takano T, Motomiya T, Minamino T, Kodama K, Sato H, Nobuyoshi M, Mitsudo K, Hayasaki K. [Intravenous coronary thrombolysis in acute myocardial infarction by AK-124 (tissue plasminogen activator): multicenter, double-blind study in comparison with urokinase]. [in Japanese]. Jpn Pharmacol Ther 1991; 19:1003–1032.

34

Pharmacological Action of and Clinical Experience with Pamiteplase, a Novel, Modified, Tissue-Type Plasminogen Activator

Tomihisa Kawasaki, Masanori Suzuki, Masao Katoh, and Kohki Hayamizu
Yamanouchi Pharmaceutical Company, Ltd., Ibaraki, Japan

SUMMARY

Tissue-type plasminogen activator (t-PA), a potent thrombolytic protein that, owing to its strict fibrin specificity, has greater safety and efficacy than urokinase and streptokinase. However, because of extremely short half-life, administration must be performed by high-dose infusion, which increases the possibility of systemic bleeding. Consequently, the medical community has sought a thrombolytic agent with the efficacy of t-PA, but with a prolonged plasma half-life that would allow administration by intravenous (i.v.) bolus injection. To this end, many genetically modified t-PA analogues were created and screened for thrombolytic activity by Yamanouchi Pharmaceutical, and the in vivo pharmacokinetics of each was assessed. Of these, pamiteplase, an engineered t-PA analogue that has a deleted K1 domain and a point mutation (^{275}Arg $\rightarrow$ Glu) at the site of the K2 domain linkage to the L-chain, exhibits reduced plasma clearance, but maintains both the specific activity and fibrin specificity of native t-PA. Experiments in several animal models of thrombosis confirmed pamiteplase dissolves thrombi without activating systemic fibrinolysis when an i.v. bolus is administered. In clinical trials on patients with acute myocardial infarction (AMI), pamiteplase was administered by i.v. bolus injection at doses of 0.05, 0.1, or 0.2 mg/kg. Coronary angiography showed that TIMI grade 2 or 3 reperfusion is achieved in 70–75% of patients given 0.1 or 0.2 mg/kg of pamiteplase. However, the incidence of hemorrhagic side effects caused by pamiteplase increases significantly at 0.2 mg/kg. As further indication of its safety, no antipamiteplase antibodies have been detected thus far in the blood of AMI patients given pamiteplase during either trials or clinical administration. These results show the great clinical advantage of pamiteplase administration for patients with AMI.

I. INTRODUCTION

Pamiteplase (Solinase; development code, YM866), developed by Yamanouchi Pharmaceutical Co., Ltd., is a novel thrombolytic agent obtained by modifying the gene that encodes tissue-type plasminogen activator (t-PA) [1]. It possesses a pronounced affinity for fibrin and retains essentially the same specific activity as native t-PA in vitro [2]. However, pamiteplase remains in plasma markedly longer than native t-PA in several animals [2,3] and in humans [4]. This review describes the limitations of thrombolytic agents that spurred the development of pamiteplase, outlines the biochemical and pharmacological properties of pamiteplase, summarizes clinical trial results, and reviews current and future status of the drug.

II. LIMITATIONS OF THROMBOLYTIC AGENTS

Thrombolytic therapy of acute myocardial infarction (AMI) is based on the premise that coronary artery thrombosis is its proximate cause [5]. In this scenario, the rupture of an atheromatous plaque produces a thrombus that occludes a coronary vessel, thus causing myocardial ischemia and cell necrosis. This occlusion leads to loss of ventricular function and possibly death. Consequently, one approach to treat the resulting AMI consists of pharmacological dissolution of the thrombus by intravenous (i.v.) infusion of plasminogen activators that activate the fibrinolytic system. The rationale for thrombolytic therapy in AMI is that early and sustained recanalization of blocked coronary vessels reduces cell death and infarct size; this preserves mycocardial function and improves early and late survival [6]. This hypothesis has been borne out by the demonstrated beneficial effects of thrombolytic therapy in AMI patients; consequently, thrombolysis has become a routine treatment [7].

Tissue-type plasminogen activator (t-PA) (Fig. 1, left) has a high affinity for fibrin, and its efficacy as a thrombolytic agent to treat AMI is well established [8]. Despite its widespread use, it has some significant limitations that limit its usefulness: resistance to recanalization within 90 min is observed in 15–40% of patients [9], whereas angiographically documented acute coronary reocclusion occurs in 5–25% of patients [10]. Time to reperfusion is sometimes slow, with restoration of anterograde coronary flow requiring on average 45 min or more from start of therapy. Additionally, because t-PA inhibits clot formation, substantial bleeding may take place elsewhere in the body; the incidence of intracerebral bleeding following t-PA infusion ranges from 0.3 to 0.7% [11]. Because of these drawbacks, the residual mortality in t-PA-treated patients is only 50% that of patients who did not receive thrombolytic treatment. Furthermore, all available thrombolytic agents, except anistreplase [12], are removed rapidly from the blood; their therapeutic use requires continuous i.v. infusion of large amounts of material that may contribute to therapeutic complications.

III. ORIGIN OF PAMITEPLASE

In patients with AMI, the benefit of thrombolysis is enhanced by early treatment to reestablish coronary patency. Consequently, a thrombolytic agent that can be given not by continuous infusion, but by bolus administration to speed treatment, has been urgently sought by physicians. Yamanouchi Pharmaceutical Company set out to design a thrombolytic agent with prolonged plasma half-life that preserved or enhanced the high specificity of t-PA for fibrin. The basic strategy to achieve this was to modify the t-PA molecule using genetic engineering. At that time (the mid-1980s), however, little formation was available concerning the relation of the structure of

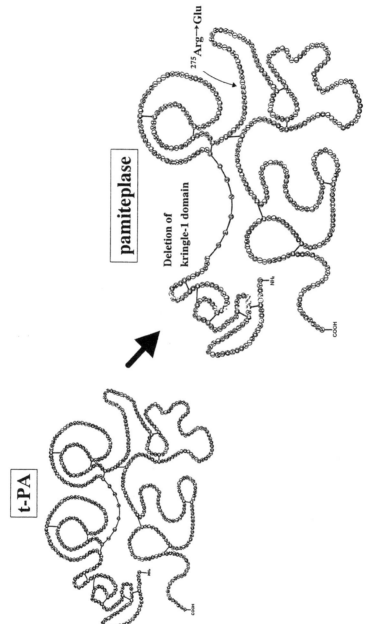

Figure 1 Structures of the native t-PA (left) and pamiteplase (right).

t-PA to its strong affinity for fibrin and its short plasma half-life. Consequently, structure–function mutagenesis studies were conducted to assign biological function to the protein domains.

Tissue-plasminogen activator consists of a heavy chain (H-chain) and a light chain (L-chain) that are connected to each other by one disulfide bond (see Fig. 1, left) [13]. The L-chain has serine protease activity. The H-chain is composed of four domains: finger, EGF-like (EGF), kringle-1 (K1), and kringle-2 (K2) in order from the N-terminal end [13]. To determine the function of each domain, modified t-PA genes were prepared to which one or two domains had been deleted. A Chinese hamster ovary (CHO) cell subline was also selected to express the proteins from these modified genes. Specific activity, fibrin affinity, and fibrin dependency (the ratio of plasminogen-activating activities in the presence or absence of fibrin) were examined, together with plasma half-life following i.v. bolus injection of each modified t-PA into rabbits [3]. The screening revealed that specific activity, fibrin affinity, and fibrin dependency decreased greatly after the deletion of each domain. However, removal of either the EGF domain or the K1 domain prolonged the plasma half-life to about 15–20 min (native t-PA: removed within 5 min), although no change in plasma half-life occurred when the K2 domain was deleted. Since a mutant protein with a deleted K1 domain (amino acids in positions 92–173 of the t-PA) had only a slightly decreased specific activity and fibrin activity compared with native t-PA, it was designated ΔK1–t-PA and was selected as the framework molecule for further development. The next step was to modify ΔK1–t-PA to increase its specificity for fibrin, its specific activity, or both.

The action of proteases such as plasmin splits one-chain t-PA between the arginine at position 275 and the isoleucine at position 276 into H- and L-chains, thereby forming a two-chain t-PA [14]. Studies indicated that mutant t-PA molecules with changes at this cleavage site, which prevent the formation of the two-chain form, have higher affinities for fibrin than native two-chain t-PA [15]. Therefore, a change was made in the ΔK1–t-PA gene that on amino acid substitution produced (^{275}Arg $\rightarrow$ Glu). This resulted in greatly improved affinity of the ΔK1–t-PA proteins for fibrin; affinity levels of this engineered protein were about the same level as native t-PA. Moreover, this mutant protein retained the markedly longer half-life of the ΔK1–t-PA framework molecule. This mutant t-PA was named pamiteplase (see Fig. 1, right); it was designated as a candidate for drug development and prepared in large quantities to proceed with pharmacological and toxicological evaluation.

Methods for manufacturing pamiteplase in large quantities were examined both before preclinical studies and thereafter [1]. These studies resulted in the following process: The modified gene is introduced into CHO cells, which are induced to secrete the pamiteplase protein into the supernatant culture medium. The protein is then purified by a four-stage procedure that uses a combination of ion-exchange and hydrophobic chromatographies [1]. Two types of glycosylation occur on native t-PA: first, three sugar chains are attached to the K1 domain, K2 domain, and L-chain, respectively; and second, two sugar chains are attached to the K1 domain and L-chain, respectively. Two types of glycosylation are also observed in the pamiteplase: two sugar chains are attached to the K2 domain and L-chain, and a sugar chain is attached to the L-chain. Of these two types, the latter alone is selected at the stage of purification. The pamiteplase obtained from this process shows almost the same specific activity as that of the native therapeutic t-PA alteplase (Activase) manufactured by Genentech, Inc., as determined by the fibrin clot lysis assay [2].

IV. BIOCHEMICAL PROPERTIES OF PAMITEPLASE

The in vitro biochemical properties of pamiteplase were compared with those of alteplase in humans and several animal species. The enzymatic activities of pamiteplase and alteplase were

Table 1 Kinetic Constants of Pamiteplase with Chromogenic Substrate

	K_m (mM)	K_{cat} (s^{-1})	K_{cat}/K_m (s^{-1} mM^{-1})
Pamiteplase	2.6 ± 0.2	15 ± 2.7	5.6 ± 1.1
Alteplase	1.2 ± 0.2	15 ± 2.3	13 ± 2.5
One-chain t-PA	1.9 ± 0.3	8.9 ± 0.8	4.8 ± 0.6
Two-chain t-PA	0.7 ± 0.2	27 ± 2.7	41 ± 5.9

(Mean $\pm$ SD, $n = 3$)

tested by both an assay of fibrin clot lysis time and an indirect chromogenic assay, calibrated to the international t-PA standard (83/517) [2]. The specific activity of pamiteplase was 570,000 IU/mg as determined by the clot-lysis assay, and 800,000 IU/mg as determined by the chromogenic assay. In comparison, the specific activity of alteplase was 600,000 IU/mg as determined by the clot-lysis assay, and 650,000 IU/mg as determined by the chromogenic assay; these results indicate that the specific activity of pamiteplase is comparable with that of alteplase. The kinetic constants of pamiteplase determined from conversion of the chromogenic substrate S-2288 were calculated from double-reciprocal plots, and the data were compared with data for alteplase, one-chain t-PA, and two-chain t-PA (Table 1). The K_m value of pamiteplase is 2.6 mM, the K_{cat} value is 15 s^{-1}, and the K_{cat}/K_m value is 5.6 s^{-1} mM^{-1}; these values are comparable with those of one-chain t-PA (1.9 mM, 8.9 s^{-1}, and 4.8 s^{-1} mM^{-1}, respectively) [2]. These results reflect that more than 98% of the pamiteplase protein consists of the one-chain form. Functionally, the binding of pamiteplase to fibrin clots in vitro was almost the same as that exhibited by alteplase, and was significantly greater than the binding exhibited by urokinase (Fig. 2). Similarly, the binding of pamiteplase to soluble fibrin (DESAFIB, American Diagnostica) and lysine sepharose was on the same order as the binding to fibrin clots [2]. Additionally, the fibrin

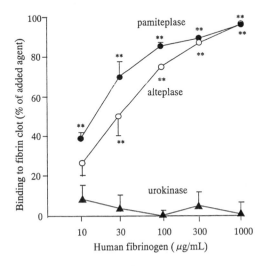

Figure 2 Binding of pamiteplase (closed circles), alteplase (open circles), and urokinase (closed triangles) to fibrin clots. Each agent (5 µg/mL) was incubated with one of several concentrations of fibrinogen and thrombin for 1 h. The amounts of each thrombolytic agent bound to fibrin clots were determined by enzyme-linked immunosorbent assay (ELISA). Each value represents the mean $\pm$ SEM ($n = 5$). **: p < 0.01 (compared with urokinase, Tukey's test).

dependency of pamiteplase was determined by the Glu–plasminogen activation rate induced by the t-PA analogues in the presence or absence of DESAFIB; interestingly, the fibrin dependency of pamiteplase was approximately ten times greater than that of alteplase (Fig. 3) [2]. Since the fibrin dependency of the ΔK1–t-PA framework molecule was comparable with that of alteplase, the high fibrin dependency of pamiteplase must be conferred by the point mutation that changes the amino acid residue in position 275 from arginine to glutamic acid. The in vitro clot lysis caused by pamiteplase in isolated plasma was compared with that of alteplase. The ED_{50} values of $[^{125}I]$-fibrin-labeled plasma clot lysis after 2 h of incubation with pamiteplase and alteplase were 0.28 and 0.07 μg/mL, respectively; these results indicate that the plasma clot lysis activity of pamiteplase is about four times less than that of alteplase [2]. However, no difference was

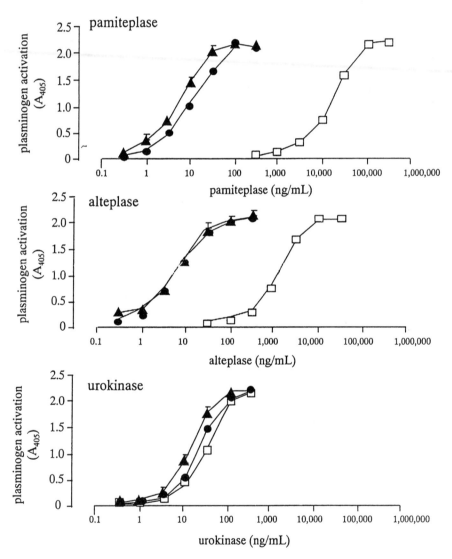

Figure 3 Fibrin dependency of plasminogen activation by pamiteplase, alteplase, and urokinase in the absence (open squares) or presence (closed circles) of fibrin clots, or the presence of soluble fibrin (DESAFIB, closed triangles). Each value represents the mean ± SEM ($n = 5$).

found between the lytic activities of pamiteplase and alteplase in plasma clot lysis assays conducted for short periods. Similar results were also observed in the clot-lysis assay using plasma clots from dogs as the substrate. Additionally, the inhibition of pamiteplase and alteplase activities by plasminogen activator inhibitor-1 (PAI-1) was comparable. These findings suggest that the thrombolytic activity of pamiteplase is influenced by other protease inhibitors present in the plasma.

V. PHARMACOLOGICAL PROPERTIES OF PAMITEPLASE

Pharmacological studies on pamiteplase were conducted using several thrombosis models. The thrombolytic activity of pamiteplase was compared with that of alteplase in dogs who had copper coil-induced coronary thromboses. Each coronary thrombus was allowed to set for 1, 3, or 6 h before either agent was administered. Pamiteplase was administered by i.v. bolus injection, but alteplase was administered either as a bolus or a 60-min i.v. infusion. In this experiment, pamiteplase was two- to four-times more effective in lysing thrombi than a bolus injection of alteplase; the difference in thrombolysis was apparent in 3- and 6 h-old thrombi (Fig. 4) [16]. Additionally, coronary reperfusion was achieved more rapidly with pamiteplase than with an i.v. infusion of alteplase [16]. Recanalization occurred in all animals injected with doses of more

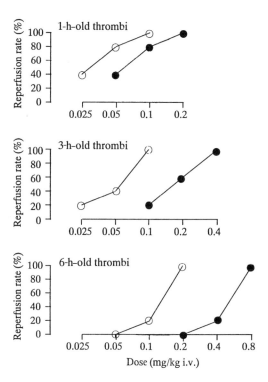

Figure 4 Thrombolytic effects of pamiteplase (open circles) and alteplase (closed circles) in dogs. Formation of thrombi was induced by a copper coil. The occlusive thrombi were allowed to set for 1, 3, or 6 h before either drug was administered. The drugs were administered by i.v. bolus injection, and coronary reperfusion was confirmed angiographically. The reperfusion rate is expressed as the percentage of individuals achieving reperfusion from a group of five animals.

than 0.1 mg/kg of pamiteplase, and no acute occlusion occurred [16]. Depletion of plasma fibrinogen to 70% of baseline levels was observed in animals given 0.2 mg/kg pamiteplase, 0.4 mg/kg alteplase by bolus, and 0.6 mg/kg alteplase by infusion [16]. These results suggest that pamiteplase, administered by i.v. bolus injection, exerts a thrombolytic effect superior to that of either a bolus injection or infusion of alteplase, without inducing excessive systemic fibrinolysis.

In the same thrombosis model, the effect of pamiteplase on left ventricular ejection fraction (LVEF) and myocardial infarct size after thrombolysis were compared with those of alteplase [17]. Pamiteplase administered by i.v. bolus injection at a dose of 0.05 mg/kg and alteplase by i.v. bolus followed by continuous infusion (0.038 mg/kg plus 0.342 mg/kg h^{-1} for 1 h) produced reperfusion in all animals, with a same median time to reperfusion. The LVEF significantly decreased 15 min after occlusion of the coronary artery induced by a copper coil. Pamiteplase improved LVEF within 3 h of administration, and alteplase improved LVEF within 4 h of administration. In contrast, LVEF did not improve in the vehicle group (Fig. 5). Only small areas of myocardial infarction were observed in the pamiteplase- and alteplase-treated groups. The areas of the left ventricular myocardium suffering from infarcts were $0.6 \pm 0.5\%$ in pamiteplase-treated animals, $0.8 \pm 0.5\%$ in alteplase-treated animals, and $18.2 \pm 4.2\%$ in vehicle-treated animals (Fig. 6). Additionally, the thrombolytic effect of pamiteplase was evaluated in a canine femoral arterial thrombosis model [18], a rat carotid artery thrombosis model [19], a guinea pig photochemically induced platelet-rich thrombosis model [20], and a rabbit jugular vein thrombosis model [21]. In all these experiments, pamiteplase, given by i.v. bolus administration, restored patency of occluded blood vessels and showed greater thrombolytic activity than alteplase. From these in vitro and in vivo studies, the clinically effective dose of pamiteplase in humans, to be administered by i.v. bolus, was set at 0.1–0.2 mg/kg.

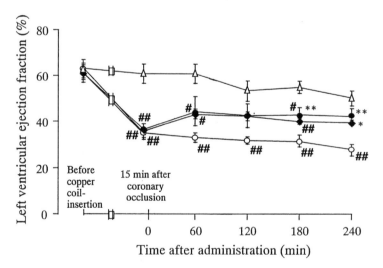

Figure 5 Effects of pamiteplase and alteplase on left ventricular ejection fraction in dogs with induced coronary thrombi. Administration of test drugs began 15 min after coronary occlusion was confirmed angiographically. Pamiteplase (0.05 mg/kg) and alteplase (0.038 mg/kg) were administered by i.v. bolus injection, followed by continuous infusion (0.342 mg/kg h^{-1} for 1 h). Symbols represent sham-operated animals (open triangles); and vehicle- (open circles), pamiteplase-treated (closed circles), or alteplase-treated animals (closed diamonds). Each value represents the mean $\pm$ SEM of five animals. #: $p < 0.05$; ##: $p < 0.01$: significantly different from the sham-operated group (Tukey's test). *: $p < 0.05$; **: $p < 0.01$; significantly different from the vehicle group (Tukey's test).

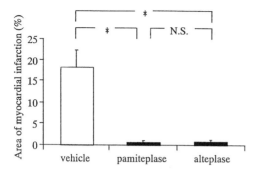

Figure 6 Effects of pamiteplase and alteplase on myocardial infarct area in dogs with induced coronary thrombi. Administration of test drugs began 15 min after coronary occlusion was confirmed angiographically. Pamiteplase (0.05 mg/kg) and alteplase (0.038 mg/kg) were administered by i.v. bolus injection, followed by continuous infusion (0.342 mg/kg h^{-1} for 1 h). The hearts were removed form sacrificed animals 4 h after start of test drug administration. The hearts were removed with 2,3,5-triphenyl tetrazolium chloride (TTC). Each value represents the mean ± SEM from five animals. **: p < 0.01; significantly different from the vehicle group (Tukey's test). N.S. indicates no significant difference between two groups (Tukey's test).

VI. CLINICAL TRIAL RESULTS

A phase I trial in healthy volunteers [4] was performed, and was followed by a trial in AMI patients; these trials were conducted to evaluate the efficacy and safety of pamiteplase. In the phase I trial [4], pamiteplase was given intravenously by bolus injection at doses ranging from 0.1 to 4 mg or by continuous infusion for 1 h to deliver a dose of 4 mg: no problematic findings were observed; no elevation in antibody titer against pamiteplase was noted; no significant change in fibrinogen level or bleeding time was observed. The total clearance of pamiteplase from the body (Cl$_{tot}$) calculated from the concentration of biologically active substance was 19–26% that of native t-PA. These results clearly show that there was no safety problem associated with pamiteplase administration, and that its residence time in blood was markedly longer than that of native t-PA. The efficacy and safety of pamiteplase were then evaluated in patients with AMI; the drug was delivered directly into the coronary artery [22]. One of three doses—4, 8, or 12 mg—was administered to each of 92 patients with an established complete occlusion of the coronary artery; patency, classified as grade 2 or 3 according to the TIMI classification [8], was restored in 82.8% (n = 29) of patients receiving 4 mg, in 78.6% (n = 28) of patients receiving 8 mg, and in 86.2% (n = 29) of patients receiving 12 mg [22]. These results demonstrate that pamiteplase dissolved coronary artery thrombi in humans.

An early phase II trial was conducted to investigate (1) the efficacy and safety of pamiteplase treatment delivered within 6 h of the onset of acute myocardial infarction, and (2) the preliminary optimal clinical doses of pamiteplase. This study used single i.v. bolus doses of 0.05, 0.1, 0.2, or 0.3 mg/kg [23]. Coronary angiography performed 60 min after pamiteplase administration showed that TIMI grade 2 or 3 patency was restored in 61.5% (n = 26) of patients receiving 0.05 mg/kg, in 71.4% (n = 28) of patients receiving 0.1 mg/kg, in 79.6% (n = 54) of patients receiving 0.2 mg/kg, and in 72.7% (n = 33) of patients receiving 0.3 mg/kg [23]. Of these doses, three—0.05, 0.1, and 0.2 mg/kg—were selected for a late-phase II trial [24], which was conducted in a double-blind manner, to find an optimal dose range. Patency was restored 60 min after administration in 52.2% (n = 46) of patients receiving 0.05 mg/kg, in 70.4% (n = 54) of patients receiving 0.1 mg/kg, and in 75.0% (n = 48) of patients receiving

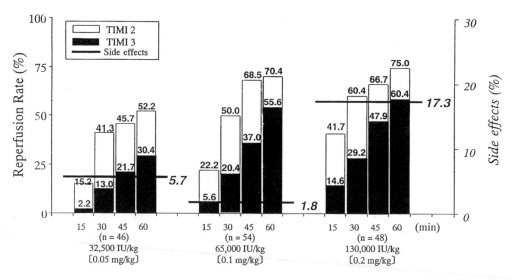

Figure 7 Reperfusion of coronary arteries of AMI patients, and rate of side effects, at 15, 30, 45, and 60 min after the administration of pamiteplase: Results from phase 2 clinical study.

0.2 mg/kg, suggesting that a sufficient effect was produced at a dose of 0.1 mg/kg or higher (Fig. 7). However, the incidence of side effects was 5.7, 1.8, and 17.3% for doses of 0.05, 0.1, and 0.2 mg/kg, respectively, and a significant increase in hemorrhagic side effects was noted at 0.2 mg/kg. Table 2 shows a list of the type and the incidence of hemorrhagic side effects reported during this study. Three hemorrhagic side effects occurred in three patients given 0.05 mg/kg, one event occurred in one patient given 0.1 mg/kg, and 12 events occurred in nine patients given 0.2 mg/kg. Consequently, 0.1 mg/kg was established as the optimal dose for a phase III study.

Table 2 Hemorrhagic Side Effects and Their Incidence During a Late-Phase 2 Trial of Pamiteplase

	Dose											
Patients	0.05 mg/kg 53				0.1 mg/kg 56				0.2 mg/kg 52			
No. of side effects	3				1				9			
Incidence of side effects	5.7%				1.8%				17.3%			
Causality of test drug[a]	S	R	U	T	S	R	U	T	S	R	U	T
No. of events	1	2	0	3	1	0	0	1	6	5	1	12
Details of the event												
Hemorrhage at the puncture site, hematoma	1		1				0		2	2		4
Gingival bleeding		1	1		1		1		1	2		3
Hematuria, intrabladder bleeding		1	1				0		1			1
Hemorrhagic shock			0				0		1			1
Cardiac tamponade			0				0			1	1	2
Postoperative bleeding			0				0		1			1

[a]S, suspected; R, related; U, undetermined; T, total.

A phase III double-blind intergroup comparative study using tisokinase [25], a native t-PA isolated from human diploid fibroblasts codeveloped by Asahi Chemical Industry Co. and Kowa Co. [26], was conducted. In this study, pamiteplase at a dose of 0.1 mg/kg delivered by i.v. bolus injection showed the same thrombolytic activity as that of tisokinase at a dose of 1.44×10^7 IU delivered by i.v. infusion over 60 min, with 10% given as an initial-bolus administration. This study also suggests the possibility that patency may be restored earlier in patients given pamiteplase by i.v. bolus injection than a native t-PA administered by i.v. bolus followed by continuous infusion. In addition, although most of the side effects from pamiteplase are hemorrhagic changes, such as hemorrhage at a puncture site, hematoma, gingival bleeding, and hematuria, the incidence of these changes was similar to corresponding values for tisokinase. The results of these studies taken together indicate pamiteplase is a useful coronary thrombolysis agent with excellent ease-of-use in emergency situations.

VII. DISCUSSION

In patients with AMI, the success rate of thrombolytic therapy diminishes as the time after the onset of the infarct increases [7], probably because of progressive cross-linking of the fibrin network [27]. Therefore, coronary artery recanalization must be accomplished as rapidly as possible to restore left ventricular function and thereby reduce mortality [28]. Although many techniques are available to accomplish this task, clinical trials have shown that t-PA removes thrombi more effectively than urokinase or streptokinase, the leading agents for non-invasive recanalization, because of its greater affinity for fibrin [7]. However, t-PA has a short biological half-life that requires complex techniques for its administration. To solve this problem, pamiteplase, a mutant t-PA protein, was engineered. This protein essentially retains the specific activity and fibrin affinity of native t-PA, but has a prolonged plasma biological half-life. Therefore, an i.v. bolus injection of pamiteplase would be expected to have greater thrombolytic efficacy than native t-PA. This is indeed what has been observed in pharmacological studies that used several different thrombosis models: an i.v. bolus injection of pamiteplase does exert a thrombolytic effect superior to either a bolus injection or infusion of native t-PA [16–21]. Consequently, this protein was quickly developed as a therapeutic agent.

Clinical studies have confirmed both the safety and the efficacy of pamiteplase. The phase I trial in healthy volunteers revealed no problem with its safety, and confirmed that its residence time in blood was longer than that of native t-PA [4]. These findings are important because they show pamiteplase may reduce or eliminate two primary problems associated with other thrombolytic agents: (1) an increased risk of bleeding complications, and (2) complicated administration methods of these drugs [10,29,30].

Concerning the efficacy of pamiteplase, an early phase II trial [23] indicated that 71.4–79.6% of patients receiving 0.1–0.3 mg/kg pamiteplase had the patency of the occluded artery restored to TIMI grade 2 or better within 60 min after an i.v. bolus injection. These results demonstrate that pamiteplase administered by i.v. bolus injection at these doses exhibits as effective thrombolysis as native t-PA delivered by continuous i.v. infusion, which has a reperfusion rate of 68.9–72.5% [29–31]. The incidence of hemorrhagic side effects in patients given 0.05, 0.1, or 0.2 mg/kg of pamiteplase was close to the incidence reported for native t-PA [29,30]. However, during these studies, hemorrhagic side effects occurred more frequently in patients given 0.3 mg/kg of pamiteplase than at other doses, suggesting that 0.3 mg/kg is less safe than the lower doses. Additionally, in a late-phase II trial conducted in a double-blind manner, 0.1 mg/kg was selected as the optimal dose for a double-blind phase III trial because of a significant increase in hemorrhagic side effects in patients given 0.2 mg/kg (see Table 2) [24].

Finally, results from a phase III double-blind intergroup comparison between pamiteplase and tisokinase revealed the thrombolytic efficacy of, and the incidence of hemorrhagic side effects associated with, 0.1 mg/kg pamiteplase administered by i.v. bolus injection were the same as those of a typical clinical dose of the native t-PA tisokinase administered by i.v. infusion over 60 min, following an initial bolus injection of 10% of the total dose [25]. Taken together, the results of these clinical studies demonstrate that 0.1 mg/kg of pamiteplase administered by i.v. bolus injection exerts a thrombolytic efficacy and elicits an incidence of hemorrhagic side effects almost equal to those of native t-PA infused intravenously over 60 min. Furthermore, the thrombolytic activity of pamiteplase is almost the same as that of E6010, another mutant t-PA developed by Eisai Co., Ltd. that can be administered by i.v. bolus injection [32].

Although these results indicate that pamiteplase is as effective as native t-PA, they do not show its true therapeutic potential. Because pamiteplase can be administered by i.v. bolus injection, earlier recanalization might be possible than for administration of native t-PA by i.v. continuous infusion. The coronary angiography findings from a phase III study [25] showed that the recanalization rate of pamiteplase 30 min after administration tended to show a significant increase compared with tisokinase. This is probably because a high plasma concentration of pamiteplase is achieved soon after i.v. bolus injection, and because its high plasma concentration lasts longer than native t-PAs. Because early recanalization of the occluded coronary blood flow is critical to the survival and recovery of patients with AMI, pamiteplase might lessen mortality and improves cardiac function more effectively than native t-PA. This hypothesis is the subject of future studies.

Although some safety information has been discussed, two points should be addressed. First, in clinical studies the incidence of hemorrhage side effects after an i.v. bolus injection of pamiteplase as almost the same as that of native t-PA administered by i.v. continuous infusion [29–31]. Therefore, since concomitant use of antithrombotic agents, such as heparin and aspirin, increases the risk of hemorrhage in patients receiving t-PA [33], pamiteplase administration should probably be conducted with the same level of caution exercised during the administration of native t-PAs. Additionally, special caution should be paid to the possibility of cerebral hemorrhage, as this is a complication observed after administration of native t-PA [11,34]. Second, because genetic engineering is used to manufacture pamiteplase, there are concerns that the synthetic protein itself or remnants of the manufacturing process might cause immune problems. As a final indication of its safety, no antipamiteplase antibody, antibody against a CHO-protein-derived foreign substance, or anti-BSA antibody was detected during clinical studies on pamiteplase [4,22–25], indicating that administration of pamiteplase does not affect the immune system and thus reducing possible physical concerns about anaphylaxis.

In conclusion, in both pharmacological and clinical studies pamitaplase administered by i.v. bolus injection is as safe and as efficacious as native t-PA administered by i.v. infusion over 60 min. These results demonstrate the usefulness of engineering proteins to enhance their favorable properties; for pamiteplase, this meant engineering t-PA to provide extended action by changing its structure to resist degradation and slow elimination. The success of this agent not only demonstrates the rewards awaiting those who boldly venture into this promising new field, but also the benefits awaiting those who cannot be helped today.

VIII. CURRENT STATUS AND FUTURE DIRECTIONS

Pamiteplase was launched in February 1999 in Japan as a drug to treat "coronary thrombolysis in AMI within 6 h of onset" with the instruction that a "single intravenous dose of 0.1 mg/kg (65,000 IU/kg) should be administered in about 1 min." Although this drug is now used in Japan to treat the acute stages of AMI, the mainstream of reperfusion therapy shifted from thrombolysis therapy to percutaneous transluminal coronary angioplasty (PTCA) and the indwelling stent method during the clinical development of the present drug. However, according to a 1998 report on PTCA, many patients underwent thrombolytic therapy that resulted in restored patency before PTCA. Analysis indicated that a statistically significant improvement in cardiac function (left ventricular ejection fraction and wall motion) occurred in these patients [35].

Many in the medical community have come to appreciate the efficacy of thrombolytic therapy, especially its ability to restore coronary patency quickly. Therefore, it is likely that modified t-PA for i.v. bolus injection will prove increasingly useful in treating not only cardiac ischemic disorders, but also the hyperacute stages of cerebral embolism. This method of treating some cerebral thromboses with thrombolytic agents within 3 h of onset has been accepted in the United States [36]. This method is also the subject of much discussion in Japan. Therefore, we hope that thrombolytic therapy, especially easy-to-administer agents such as pamiteplase, will continue to contribute to reduced mortality from improved prognosis of many occlusive vascular disorders.

ACKNOWLEDGMENTS

The authors thank Mr. S. E. Johnson for editing the manuscript.

REFERENCES

1. Kawauchi Y, Morinaga T, Yokota M, Kinoshita A, Kawamura K, Suzuki Y, Takayama M, Furuichi K, Gushima H. Gene construction and large scale production of a novel fibrinolytic agent (YM866) in CHO cells. Thromb Haemost 1991; 65:1193.
2. Katoh M, Suzuki Y, Miyamoto I, Watanabe T, Mori K, Arakawa H, Gushima H. Biochemical and pharmacokinetic properties of YM866, a novel fibrinolytic agent. Thromb Haemost 1991; 65:1193.
3. Katoh M, Shimizu Y, Kawauchi Y, Ishida J, Takayam M, Yokota M, Yano E, Kawasaki T, Katsuta K, Yano S, Morinaga T, Tsuju, Kinoshita A, Gomi Y, Takemoto T, Itoh K, Ezoe H, Gusima H. Comparison of clearance rate of various tissue plasminogen activator (t-PA) analogues. Thromb Haemost 1989; 62:542.
4. Hashimoto K, Oikawa K, Miyamoto I, Hayamizu K, Abe Y. Phase I study of novel modified tissue-type plasminogen activator. YM866. J Med Pharm Sci 1996; 36:623–646.
5. DeWood MA, Spores J, Notske R, Mousea LT, Burroughs R, Golden MS, Lang HT. Prevalence of total coronary occlusion during the early hours of transmural myocardial infarction. N Eng J Med 1980; 303–897–902.
6. Simoons ML, Serruys PW, van den Brand M, Res J, Verheugt FW, Krauss XH, Remme WJ, Bar F, Zwaan C, Laarse A, Vermeer F, Lubsen J. Early thrombolysis in acute myocardial infarction: limitation of infarct size and improved survival. J Am Coll Cardiol 1986; 7:717–728.
7. Topol EJ, Bates ER, Walton JA Jr, Baumann G, Wolfe S, Maino J, Bayer L, Gorman L, Kleine EM, O'Neill WW. Community hospital adminstration of intravenous tissue plasminogen activator in acute myocardial infarction: improved timing, thrombolytic efficacy and ventricular function. J Am Coll Cardiol 1987; 10:1173–1177.
8. Chesebro JH, Knatterud G, Roberts R, Borer J, Cohen LS, Daren J, Dodge HT, Francis CK, Hilis D, Ludbrook P, Markis JE, Mueller H, Passamani ER, Powers ER, Rao AK, Robertson T, Ross A, Ryan TJ, Sobel BE, Willerson J, Williams, SO, Zaret BL, Braunwald E. Thrombolysis in myocardial infarction (TIMI) trial, phase I: a comparison between intravenous tissue plasminogen activator and intravenous streptokinase. Clinical findings through hospital discharge. Circulation 1987; 76:142–154.

9. Mueller HS, Rao AK, Forman SA. Thrombolysis in myocardial infarction (TIMI): comparative studies of coronary reperfusion and systemic fibrinogenolysis with two forms of recombinant tissue-type plasminogen activator. J Am Coll Cardiol 1987; 10:479–490.

10. Gold HK, Leinbach RC, Garabedian HD, Yasuda T, Johns JA, Grossbard EB, Palacios I, Collen D. Acute coronary reocclusion after thrombolysis with recombinant human tissue-type plasminogen activator: prevention by a maintenance infusion. Circulation 1986; 73:347–352.

11. Sherry S. Tissue plasminogen activator (t-PA). Will it fulfil its promise? N Engl J Med 1985; 313:1014–1017.

12. Bell WR Jr. Evaluation of thrombolytic agents. Drugs 1997; 54 (suppl 3):11–16.

13. Pennica D, Holmes WE, Kohr WJ, Harkins RN, Vehar GA, Ward CA, Bennett WF, Yelverton E, Seeburg PH, Heyneker HL, Goeddell DV, Colleen D. Cloning and expression of human tissue-type plasminogen activator cDNA in E. coli. Nature 1983; 301:214–221.

14. Petersen LC, Johannessen M, Foster D, Kumar A, Mulvihill E. The effect of polymerized fibrin on the catalytic activities of one-chain tissue-type plasminogen activator as revealed by an analogue resistant to plasmin cleavage. Biochim Biophys Acta 1988; 952:245–254.

15. Tate KM, Higgins, DL, Holmes WF, Winkler ME, Heynecker HL, Vehar GA. Functional role of proteolytic cleavage at arginine-275 of human tissue plasminogen activator as assessed by site-directed mutagenesis. Biochemistry 1987; 26:338–343.

16. Kawasaki T, Katoh M, Kaku S, Gushima H, Takenaka T, Yui Y, Kawai C. Thrombolytic activity of a novel modified tissue-type plasminogen activator, YM866, in a canine model of coronary artery thrombosis. Jpn J Pharmacol 1993; 63:9–16.

17. Suzuki M, Funatsu T, Tanaka H, Usuda S. YM866, a novel modified tissue-type plasminogen activator, affects left ventricular function and myocardial infarct development in dogs with coronary artery thrombi. Jpn J Pharmacol 1998; 77:177–183.

18. Kawasaki T, Kaku S, Sakai Y, Takenata T. Comparative study of a mutant tissue-type plasminogen activator, YM866, with a tissue-type plasminogen activator in a canine model of femoral arterial thrombosis. J. Pharm Pharmacol 1996; 48:1041–1048.

19. Kawasaki T, Kawamura S, Katoh S, Takenaka T. Experimental model of carotid artery thrombosis in rats and the thrombolytic activity of YM866, a novel modified tissue-type plasminogen activator. Jpn J Pharmacol 1993; 63:135–142.

20. Kawasaki T, Kaku S, Takenaka T, Yanagi K, Ohshima N. Thrombolytic activity of YM866, a novel modified tissue-type plasminogen activator, in a photochemically induced platelet-rich thrombosis model. J Cardiovasc Pharmacol 1994; 23:884–889.

21. Kawasaki T, Kaku S, Sakai Y, Takenaka T. Thrombolytic activity of YM866, a novel modified tissue-type plasminogen activator, in a rabbit model of jugular vein thrombosis. Drug Dev Res 1994; 33:33–38.

22. Haze K, Kawai C, Hosoda S, Aoki N, Takano T, Kanmatsuse K, Motomiya T, Sumiyoshi T, Yui, Y, Minamino R, Kodama K, Sato H, Nobuyoshi M. Efficacy and safety of intracoronary administration of YM866 (modified tissue-type plasminogen activator) in patients with acute myocardial infarction. Jpn Pharmacol Ther 1996; 24:2467–2490.

23. Sumiyoshi T, Kawai C, Hosoda S, Aoki N, Takano T, Kanmatsuse K, Motomiya T, Yui Y, Minamino T, Kodama K, Haze K, Satoh H, Nobuyoshi M. Clinical evaluation of intravenous bolus injection of YM866 (modified tissue-type plasiminogen activator) in patients with acute myocardial infarction; multi-center early phase II study. Med Pharm 1996; 36:951–980.

24. Kodama K, Kawai C, Hosoda S, Aoki N, Takano T, Kanmatsuse K, Motomiya T, Sumiyoshi T, Yui Y, Minamino R, Haze K, Satoh H, Nobuyoshi M, Origasa H. Clinical evaluation of intravenous bolus injection of YM866 (modified tissue-type plasminogen activator) in patients with acute myocardial infarction—multicenter double blind dose-finding trial. J New Remedies Clin 1996; 45:2031–2063.

25. Yui, Y, Kawai C, Hosoda S, Aoki N, Takano T, Kanmatsuse K, Motomiya T, Sumiyoshi T, Minamino T, Kodama K, Haze K, Satoh H, Nobuyoshi M, Origasa H. Randomised, double-blind multicenter clinical trial of YM866 (modified t-PA) by intravenous bolus injection in patients with acute myocardial infarction in comparison with tisokinase (native t-PA). J New Remedies Clin 1996; 45:2175–2210.

26. Hasegawa A, Yamashita H, Kondo S, Kiyota T, Hayashi H, Yoshizaki H, Murakami A, Shiratsuchi M, Mori T. Protease peptone enhances production of tissue-type plasminogen activator from human diploid fibroblasts. Biochem Biophys Res Commun 1988; 150:1230–1236.

27. Loven M, Frade LJ, Torrado MC, Navarro JL. Thrombus age and tissue plasminogen activator-mediated thrombolysis in rats. Thromb Res 1989; 56:67–76.

28. Flameng W, Van de Werf F, Vanhaeckle J, Collen D. Coronary thrombolysis and infarct size reduction after intravenous infusion of tissue-type plasminogen activator in nonhuman primates. J Clin Invest 1985; 75:84–90.

29. Shintani H, Kawai C, Kanmatsuse K, Kimata S, Takano T, Takeyama Y, Yui Y, Nakashima M. Examination on clinical usefulness of continuous intravenous administration of GMK-527 (alteplase: rt-PA) in patients with acute myocardial infarction: multi-institutional double blind study with urokinase as control. Jpn J Clin Exp Med 1991; 156:429–451.

30. Hirosawa K, Suzuki S, Kawai C, Yui Y, Hosoda S, Kimata S, Abe Y, Aoki N, Nakashima M, Kajiwara N, Kanmatsuse K, Takano T, Motomiya T, Minamino R, Kodama K, Sato H, Nobuyoshi M, Mitsufuji K, Hayasaki K. Clinical evaluation of intravenous administration of AK-124 (tissue plasminogen activator) in patients with acute myocardial infarction: multi-institutional double blind study with urokinase as control. Jpn Pharmacol Ther 1991; 19:1003–1032.

31. Katoh K, Kawai C, Hosoda S, Nakashima M, Kanazawa T, Hiramori K, Kimata S, Aizawa T, Kajiwara N, Kanmatsuse K, Takano T, Tanaka K, Sugimoto T, Aoki N, Yabe Y, Mizuno Y, Matsuda T, Fujita M, Yui Y, Kodama K, Haze K, Nakamura M. Investigation of clinical usefulness of MMR701 (nateplase; t-PA) in patients with acute myocardial infarction—phase III study with urokinase as a control. J Clin Ther Med 1994; 10:633–668.

32. Kawai C, Yui Y, Hosoda S, Nobuyoshi M, Suzuki S, Sato H, Takatsu F. Motomiya T, Kanmatsuse K, Kodama K, Yabe Y, Minamino T, Kimata S, Nakashima M. A prospective, randomised, double-blind multicenter trial of a single bolus injection of the novel modified t-PA E6010 in the treatment of acute myocardial infarction: comparison with native t-PA. E6010 Study Group. J Am Coll Cardiol 1997; 29:1447–1453.

33. Bovill EG, Tracy RP, Knatterud GL, Stone PH, Nasmith J, Gore JM. Thompson BW, Tofler GH, Kleiman NS, Cannon C, Braunwald E. Hemorrhagic events during therapy with recombinant tissue plasminogen activator, heparin, and aspirin for unstable angina (Thrombolysis in Myocardial Ischemia, phase IIIB trial). Am J Cardiol 1997; 79:391–396.

34. Simoons ML, Maggioni AP, Knatterud G, Leimberger JD, de Jaegere P, van Domburg R, Boersma E, Franzosi MG, Califf R, Schroder R, Braunwald E. Individual risk assessment for intracranial haemorrhage during thrombolytic therapy. Lancet 1993; 342:1523–1528.

35. Ross A. Plasminogen activator and angioplasty compatibility trial (PACT). Am Heart J 1998; 135:1103–1104.

36. The NINDS rt-PA study group. Tissue plasminogen activator for acute ischemic stroke. N Engl J Med 1995; 333:1581–1587.

35

Recombinant, Glycosylated Prourokinase: Preclinical and Clinical Studies

Gregory A. Schulz, R. Bruce Credo, Debra A. Schuerr, Sandra E. Burke, Jack Henkin, and Bruce A. Wallin
Abbott Laboratories, Abbott Park, Illinois, U.S.A.

SUMMARY

Recombinant, glycosylated prourokinase (r-proUK; ABT-187, Prolyse®) is a single-chain urokinase-type plasminogen activator that is purified to homogeneity from the culture medium of hybridoma cells. Preclinical data from in vitro clot lysis experiments in human plasma and a canine femoral artery thrombosis model have demonstrated the efficacy of r-proUK as a potent thrombolytic agent. The lytic activity of r-proUK is significantly enhanced by the concomitant administration of heparin as adjunctive therapy. Fibrinogen, plasminogen, and α_2-antiplasmin levels are unaltered or only minimally so, in the femoral artery occlusion model. Thus, ABT-187 was characterized as a stable, potent, glycosylated r-proUK that can achieve rapid thrombolysis with only minimal perturbations of the clotting or fibrinolytic systems.

In the clinical experience to date, data from two pilot studies were obtained to evaluate the safety and efficacy of r-proUK in patients with acute myocardial infarction. The first was an open, multicenter study comparing two different doses of r-proUK, 60 and 80 mg; each dose was given as a bolus plus infusion over 60 or 90 min ($n = 46$). The second study was a double-blind, multicenter trial in which 85 patients received either a priming bolus dose of 250,000 IU of recombinant urokinase, followed immediately by 60 mg of r-proUK, or a placebo priming agent followed immediately by 80 mg r-proUK. In study 1, the 90-min patency rate was 66.7% in 21 patients receiving 60 mg over 60 min and 72.2% in 18 patients receiving 60 mg over 90 min. In study 2, the 90-min patency rates were 45.5% in the 60-mg–primed group, infused over 60 min (11 patients) and 80.8% in the primed group infused over 90 min (26 patients). In the 80-mg–nonprimed group, the 90-min patency rate was 100% in the 6 patients infused over 60 min and 69.2% in the 26 patients infused over 90 min. The rate of angiographic reocclusion in those who had no coronary intervention was 1.4% during the 18 h following the acute phase. Only 4.6% of patients experienced severe bleeding complications, with no patient developing brain hemorrhage.

Two trials have been conducted in acute ischemic stroke caused by thromboembolic occlusion of the middle cerebral artery (MCA) in which r-proUK was delivered through a superselective microcatheter directly into the clot in the MCA, beginning within 6 h of symptom onset. In a pilot study (PROACT I), recanalization, safety, and clinical outcomes were compared in 40 patients randomized to receive either 6 mg of r-proUK ($n = 26$) or a placebo ($n = 14$). Heparin was administered intravenously, either as a bolus of 100 U/kg followed by 1000 U/h (high-dose heparin group, $n = 16$), or a 2000-U bolus followed by an infusion of 500 U/h (lower-dose heparin group). The recanalization rate, assessed angiographically after the 2-h–study infusion, was 58% (r-proUK) versys 15% (placebo). At 2 h in the r-proUK group, 19% showed complete lysis and 39% partial lysis, whereas in the placebo group, only partial lysis occurred (20%). In the high-dose heparin group, recanalization was 82%, contrasted with 40% in the lower-dose heparin group. The frequency of brain hemorrhage with neurological deterioration was similar in the r-proUK and placebo groups (15.4 vs. 14.3%, respectively) although there appeared to be a higher rate of hemorrhage with deterioration in the high-dose heparin group. In the few patients assessed by the clinical outcome scales, the patients who recanalized under r-proUK treatment did better at 90 days (although not statistically significant), suggesting that improved outcome at 90 days and longer may be related to recanalization.

In a second study (PROACT II), 180 patients with angiographically confirmed MCA stroke were randomized to receive either 9 mg of r-proUK over 120 min in conjunction with the low-dose intravenous heparin regimen established in PROACT I ($n = 121$), or to a control group consisting of low-dose intravenous heparin alone ($n = 59$). The primary endpoint was the clinical outcome of functional independence at 90 days. Recanalization was also assessed at 120 min. At the 90-day clinical assessment, r-proUK had a 15% absolute benefit over control in the rate of patients achieving functional independence (40 vs. 25%, $p = 0.043$). This clinical benefit was achieved in spite of a higher rate of symptomatic intracranial hemorrhage in the r-proUK group at 36 h following initiation of therapy (10.2%) compared with control (1.8%), $p = 0.06$. The MCA recanalization rate at 2 h showed a highly significant increase for r-proUK (66%) versus control (18%), $p < 0.001$. Thus, PROACT II was the first ischemic stroke trial showing clinical benefit of thrombolysis initiated within 6 h of symptom onset, potentially widening the window of opportunity.

r-proUK has also been used in a phase 2 dose-ranging trial in the treatment of acute limb ischemia in the lower extremity caused by a thromboembolic arterial occlusion. This trial (PURPOSE) was a randomized, double-blind, parallel multicenter study designed to compare three doses of intra-arterial, catheter-directed r-proUK (2, 4, or 8 mg/h for 8 h, then 0.5 mg/h) with urokinase from a human tissue–culture-based source (4000 IU/min for 4 h, then 2000 IU/min), in the treatment of acute lower extremity occlusions in both native arteries and bypass grafts of 14-days duration or less. The primary outcome was complete ($> 95\%$) clot lysis of the occluding thrombus after 8 h of infusion.

In the 228 patients enrolled and treated in this trial, symptoms were present for an average of 4.5 days at the time of enrollment, and 68% of the patients had an occlusion in a bypass graft as opposed to a native arterial segment. The frequency of achieving complete clot lysis in 8 h increased from 39.3% in the 2-mg r-proUK group to 56.0% in the 8-mg r-proUK group, with 49.1% in the urokinase group. This apparent dose–response relation for r-proUK evident at 8 h was no longer apparent at 24 h. The risk of a major bleeding complication was low and appeared similar among all treatment groups.

In summary, r-proUK (ABT-187, Prolyse) is a glycosylated plasminogen activator expressed from a mouse hybridoma cell line that is exceedingly stable in vivo, maintaining clot-selectivity over a broad range of clinical dosing schedules, rapid acting, and with high efficacy for lysing clots, which can be achieved safely.

I. INTRODUCTION

Prourokinase (proUK) is the single-chain zymogen of the serine protease urokinase (UK, or urokinase-type plasminogen activator; u-PA). In a number of physiological systems and pathological conditions, the urokinase-mediated activation of plasminogen to plasmin is critically involved in the lytic mechanism of fibrinolysis and the maintenance of vascular patency. Both the proUK zymogen and urokinase, the active two-chain enzyme, have been employed as potent fibrinolytic agents for patients with thromboembolic diseases, including myocardial infarction [1], peripheral vascular occlusions [2,3], pulmonary embolism [4,5], and ischemic stroke [6,7].

II. BIOCHEMICAL CHARACTERIZATION OF RECOMBINANT PROUROKINASE

For the development of recombinant prourokinase (ABT-187) as a therapeutic agent, we have employed an expression system using mouse hybridoma SP2/0 cells [8]. From this genetic construct, r-proUK (ABT-187) is expressed as a mosaic single-chain glycoprotein of 411 amino acids. Figure 1 illustrates both the complete primary sequence of the molecule [9] and the structural domains of prourokinase, coded by discrete exons [10,11].

Conversion of ABT-187 to an active two-chain form (r-UK) occurs by the hydrolysis of the Lys^{158}–Ile^{159} amide bond [12]. Within the context of fibrinolysis, the enzymes plasmin [13] and kallikrein [14,15], which are known to activate prourokinase in vitro, are considered important catalysts in the physiological activation of the zymogen. In addition, cathepsin B [16],

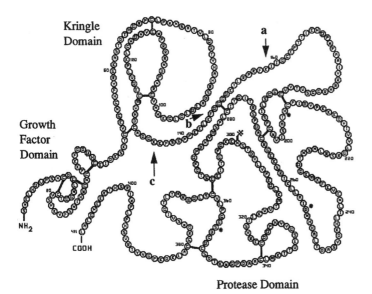

Figure 1 Primary structure of r-proUK (ABT-187): asterisks mark the locations of the amino acids involving the active site of UK (His-204, Asp-255, and Ser-356). Arrows mark the sites of cleavage by proteolytic enzymes. Cleavage at site a (Lys 158–Ile 159) produces active two-chain high-molecular-weight UK; cleavage at sites a and b, or a and c generate low-molecular-weight UK. Cleavage at sites b or c generate low-molecular-weight r-proUK molecules. The symbol at residue Asn-302 represents the site of N-linked glycosylation.

thermolysin [17], and a cellular protease of transformed fibroblasts [18] have also been catalytic here. The specific hydrolysis of prourokinase by thrombin at the Arg[156]–Phe[157] amide bond leads to inactivation of the zymogen [14].

ABT-187 shares many structural elements in common with the naturally occurring proUK product from kidney cells [19], including the presence of an N-linked oligosaccharide moiety at residue Asn[302]. ABT-187 contains neutral and amino sugars, as well as neuraminic acids. In addition, ABT-187 contains a single O-linked fucose residue at position Thr[18] [20]. In comparison, the proUK product harvested from a bacterial expression system (*Escherichia coli*) does not contain carbohydrate [21]. Lenich et al. claim that the presence of oligosaccharide at position Asn[302] influences the activity of proUK/UK and could be the major factor responsible for enhanced activity observed in one such *E. coli*-derived proUK [22].

III. IN VITRO CLOT LYSIS STUDIES WITH RECOMBINANT PROUROKINASE

We used an in vitro clot lysis system with human plasma [23] to characterize the lytic potential of ABT-187 and its high-molecular-weight two-chain form. ABT-187 is an efficient and potent thrombolytic agent that exhibits both a lag phase to the onset of lysis (Fig. 2) and a threshold effect (Fig. 3). The duration of the lag phase decreases with increasing concentrations of

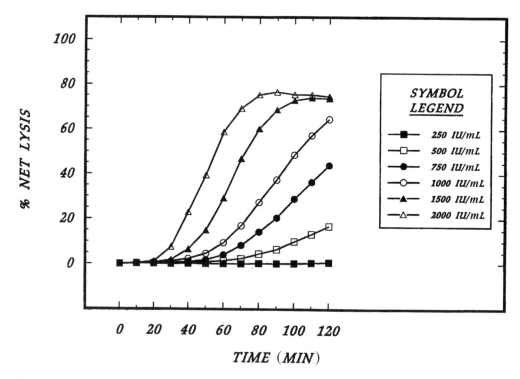

Figure 2 Dose–response curves for the in vitro lysis of clots prepared from fresh-frozen plasma. ^{125}I-labeled clots were prepared by adding radioactive fibrinogen, calcium, and thrombin to human plasma. After a 30-min incubation, the clots were washed, and then added to a volume of 2.5-mL plasma. Lysis was initiated by the addition of r-proUK (ABT-187). The mean values for net lysis were calculated by correcting for the levels of autolysis (< 11%) from replicate tubes to which no plasminogen activator was added.

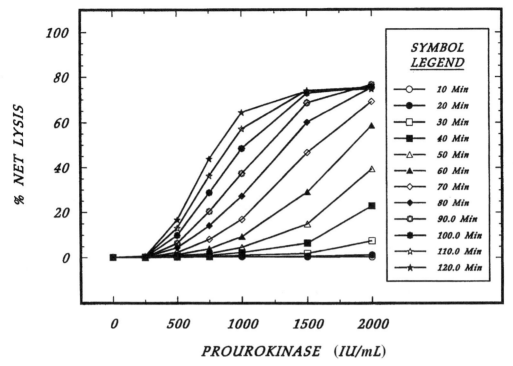

Figure 3 Concentration dependence for the in vitro lysis of human clots by r-proUK (ABT-187). The threshold effect of r-proUK in this assay system is apparent; at a concentration of ABT-187 less than 250 IU/mL, no net lysis was observed over the 120-min lysis period. The mean values for net lysis were calculated by correcting for the levels of autolysis (< 11%) from replicate tubes to which no plasminogen activator was added.

r-proUK, over a concentration range of 250–2000 IU/mL. The threshold effect is observed as an absence of lysis when the concentration of r-proUK was 250 IU/mL or less, even for rather lengthy observation periods (6 h). Clot lysis assays performed with two-chain urokinase, either high-molecular-weight (r-UK) or low-molecular-weight (Abbokinase), do not reveal the presence of the lag phase (data not shown). However, the threshold effect is present.

To study the lag phase, we performed a series of clot lysis reactions using r-proUK with various concentrations of its active two-chain counterpart (r-UK). The data presented in Figure 4 reveal that with a total concentration of r-proUK equal to 200 IU/mL, the addition of more than 4% r-UK significantly augments the lytic profiles, with a noticeable diminution of the time to the onset of lysis. In a similar lysis study utilizing r-proUK with 10% r-UK (total concentration of r-proUK equal to 500 IU/mL), we have observed nearly 50% lysis within 60 min, without an alteration in the fibrinogen level. These results are consistent with the findings of DeClerck et al. [24], which indicate that effective clot lysis with proUK does not require complete conversion of the zymogen to its two-chain counterpart and, moreover, lysis may precede the systematic degradation of plasma fibrinogen.

IV. PRECLINICAL PHARMACOLOGY OF RECOMBINANT PROUROKINASE

In our laboratories, studies to test the in vivo efficacy of r-proUK have been conducted in a well-characterized canine model of femoral artery thrombosis (Fig. 5). The model, which uses a

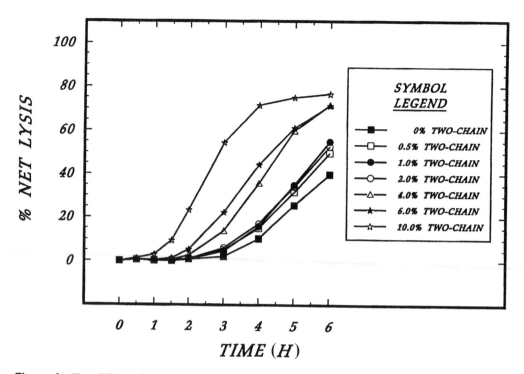

Figure 4 The addition of high-molecular-weight two-chain urokinase (r-UK) enhances the lytic profiles of r-proUK (ABT-187). The total concentration of potential urokinase activity from both r-proUK and r-UK was 200 IU/mL. The mean values for net lysis were calculated by correcting for the levels of autolysis (< 11%) from replicate tubes to which no plasminogen activator was added.

radiolabeled thrombus, measures the degree of clot lysis, as well as the simultaneous restoration of blood flow. In addition, hemostatic and fibrinolytic parameters including fibrinogen, plasminogen, and α_2-antiplasmin are also monitored throughout the protocol. We have used this experimental procedure to study the effects of several thrombolytic agents, in both the absence and presence of adjuncts to thrombolysis such as heparin. In the studies to be described, animals were prepared for clot formation by modification of the method of Badylak et al. [25], in which an isolated portion of the femoral artery is heat-damaged to expose underlying collagen, providing an area that can support a well-formed thrombus. Access to the main vessel is provided by cannulation of the profunda femoris branch of the femoral artery, which also allows instillation of ^{125}I-fibrinogen and thrombin into the vessel (Fig. 5). After a 45–90-min–aging period, the ligatures holding the thrombus in place are removed, and a gamma probe is placed over the radiolabeled clot to monitor the loss of radioactivity during the course of the protocol. After a suitable equilibration period, during which the thrombus is monitored for stability and a lytic baseline is established, the thrombolytic dose regimen is initiated.

We have demonstrated dose-related clot lysis using four doses of r-proUK in this model. Animals were randomized to receive either vehicle or 50,000, 100,000, 150,000, and 220,000 IU of r-proUK. Each dose was given as a 1-min intravenous-bolus injection, and the animals were monitored for 2 h after the initial treatment. The results are illustrated in Figure 6. In the vehicle control group, the decrease in radioactivity from the labeled clot was $11 \pm 3\%$ at the end of the observation period, not unlike the low-dose ABT-187 group, which showed $12 \pm 5\%$ at the same time point. Higher doses of 100,000, 150,000, and 220,000 IU of ABT-187 resulted in clot lysis

Method for Canine Femoral Artery Clot Lysis Model

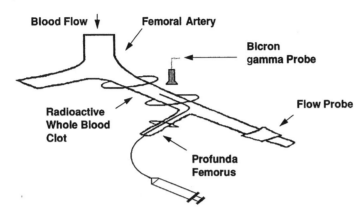

Figure 5 Schematic diagram showing the methodology for the preparation and monitoring of an experimental thrombus in the canine femoral artery.

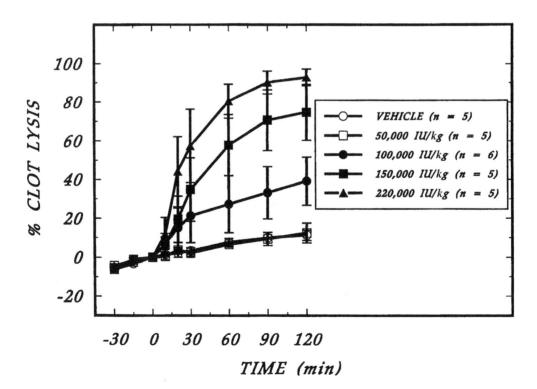

Figure 6 Dose–response curves (0–120 min) for the lytic effect of r-proUK in the canine femoral artery model. r-proUK (ABT-187) or vehicle was initiated at time 0, followed by a 30-min equilibration period.

Table 1 Treatment Regimens

Group	Treatment	Regimen	N
1	r-proUK	Bolus/bolus, 50%/50% at 0 and 15 min	7
2	r-proUK	Bolus/bolus, 50%/50% at 0 and 30 min	7
3	r-proUK	Bolus/infusion, 20%/80% infused to 30 min	7
4	r-proUK	Bolus/infusion, 20%/80% infused to 60 min	7
5	r-proUK	Bolus/infusion, 50%/50% infused to 30 min	7
6	Vehicle	Bolus/infusion, 50%/50% infused to 30 min	4

of 39 ± 12, 75 ± 14, and $93 \pm 4\%$, respectively. Blood samples drawn during the treatment protocol were assayed for fibrinogen, plasminogen, and α_2-antiplasmin levels; the results indicate that only α_2-antiplasmin was reduced in these animals, and that this finding was noted only at the two highest dose levels.

In another study, a variety of doses and dosing regimens were investigated. Thus, we examined a single dose of ABT-187 using different dosing regimens to compare the degree of clot lysis resulting from these treatments, with a detailed analysis of blood flow restoration. The experiments were carried out in our canine femoral artery thrombosis model. Thirty-nine male, beagle dogs were studied according to a randomization schedule. ABT-187 at one regimen per dog and the vehicle (2.9 mg/mL NaCl, 30 mg/mL mannitol, 3.8 mg/mL citric acid, pH = 5) were studied in six groups of animals. In all five drug treatment groups, r-proUK was administered at the same total dose of 80,000 U/kg, whereas the dosing regimens varied. The dose was typically divided into an initial loading bolus, followed by either another bolus or infusions of various lengths. The six treatment groups and regimens are shown in Table 1.

The lytic effect of r-proUK in this animal model is shown in Figure 7, in which clot lysis is expressed as the loss of counts from the radiolabeled thrombus over time. At the end of 2 h, clot lysis was 52 ± 7, 62 ± 7, 41 ± 8, 66 ± 5, and $73 \pm 4\%$ in groups 1, 2, 3, 4, and 5, respectively; a bolus/infusion regimen of the vehicle (group 6) produced a $12 \pm 6\%$ loss of counts at 120 min.

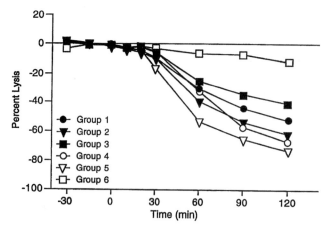

Figure 7 Clot lysis, expressed as a loss of counts from a radiolabeled thrombus over the 2-h period after drug or vehicle administration. See Table 8 for description of treatment groups. Data points are mean values. SEM for values at the end of 2 h are stated in the text, as are statistical differences.

Therefore, of the three regimens that demonstrated the greatest clot lysis (groups 2, 4, and 5), the regimen in which 50% of the total dose was given as a bolus and 50% as a 30-min infusion (group 5) appeared to result in the most optimal efficacy. Beginning at the 10-min time point in group 4 and the 30-min time point in groups 1, 2, 3, and 5, clot lysis was significantly different ($p < 0.05$) from the control values obtained before treatment in all the r-proUK-treated groups. Comparisons among groups revealed that, at 90 and 120 min, group 5 was significantly different from groups 3 and 6; however, no significant difference was observed between group 5 and groups 1, 2, or 4.

In addition to clot lysis, the restoration of blood flow is an important therapeutic endpoint in thrombolysis. The times to reflow and the total patency times for each of the groups were noted. Only one animal in the vehicle treatment group (group 6) exhibited restoration of flow during the observation period. The 50%/50% bolus/infusion regimen (group 5) produced the most rapid flow restoration (41 ± 12 min) and the greatest total patency time (60 ± 17 min) during the 120-min observation period. However, these differences in flow restoration and patency time for group 5 were not statistically significant when compared with the other treatment groups.

The results of this study indicate that, in our thrombosis model, optimal clot lysis and recovery of femoral artery blood flow is attained using a regimen in which 50% of the total dose (80,000 U/kg) is given as an intravenous bolus, followed immediately by the remaining 50% given as a 30-min infusion. However, clot lysis in this group is not significantly different from that attained in the animals that received only bolus dosing (50%/50% at 0 and 30 min; group 2), nor in group 4 that received a 20% bolus followed by 80% by a 60-min infusion. This may be attributed to relatively small groups of dogs which received each regimen and to the variability that can be observed when clot lysis alone is used as an endpoint in these experiments. Consequently, we conducted a detailed analysis of femoral artery blood flow to confirm our findings. After examination of the flow data, our conclusion on the regimen used in group 5 is somewhat strengthened by the fact that the time to reflow after this regimen is shorter, and the total patency time during the 2-h observation period is longer, when comparisons are made with the other treatment groups. However, it must also be stated that lack of statistical significance for groups 2 and 4 relative to group 5 indicates that use of a dosing regimen that provides a large bolus (group 2) followed by a prolonged infusion (group 4) might also afford a reasonable therapeutic approach.

In another study, the effects of ABT-187 were examined in the presence and absence of heparin, which was given immediately after clot formation. The heparin (bovine lung) dose was given as a bolus–infusion regimen that comprised a bolus of 500 U followed immediately by an infusion of 350 U/h until the end of the experiment. This dose of heparin was determined to maintain the activated partial thromboplastin time (APTT) at 1.5–2.0 times control. ABT-187 was given in a regimen in which 50% of the total dose (100,000 IU/kg) was given as a 30-min infusion. Four treatment groups (vehicle, vehicle + heparin, ABT-187 alone, and ABT-187 + heparin) were examined in this study. In each group, fibrinogen, plasminogen, and α_2-antiplasmin were monitored in plasma samples obtained at various time points throughout the 4-h protocol. The results of ABT-187 treatment in the presence and absence of heparin are illustrated in Figure 8. Vehicle infusion, as well as vehicle in the presence of heparin, resulted in a loss of radioactivity of $26 \pm 3\%$ and $28 \pm 5\%$, respectively. In contrast, animals that received ABT-187 alone showed clot lysis of $50 \pm 4\%$, whereas those treated with heparin and ABT-187 had significantly greater lysis of $85 \pm 5\%$ ($p < 0.05$).

Of equal importance is the data on restoration of blood flow, which was monitored throughout the experiment using an electromagnetic flow sensor placed distally to the thrombus. Dogs that received vehicle alone, vehicle plus heparin, or ABT-187 alone, showed virtually no

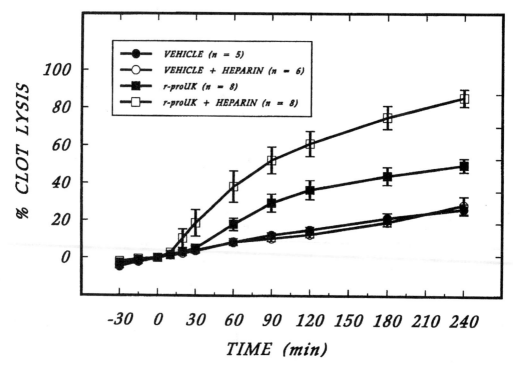

Figure 8 The effect of r-proUK and heparin on clot lysis in the canine femoral artery. Clot lysis is expressed as the percentage loss of radioactivity from the ^{125}I-labeled thrombus over a 4-h period, following administration of ABT-187 or vehicle, in the absence and presence of heparin. Treatment with heparin was initiated 45–90 min before administration of ABT-187 at $t = 0$. Clot lysis values are mean SEM.

restoration of blood flow, despite 50% clot lysis in the group that received ABT-187. However, when heparin was added to the treatment regimen, blood flow, expressed in Figure 9 as conductance (the reciprocal of femoral vascular resistance), was markedly increased. It is likely that the presence of heparin facilitates lysis and reflow by preventing the accretion of additional fresh fibrin on the existing radiolabeled thrombus. It is of particular interest that the restoration of blood flow was initiated within minutes of ABT-187 treatment in the animals receiving heparin and ABT-187.

The clot specificity of ABT-187 is clearly illustrated by the data shown in Table 2. Fibrinogen, plasminogen, and α_2-antiplasmin were virtually unchanged in plasma samples obtained at the end of the 30-min infusion period, as well as at the end of the 4-h observation. Therefore, these experiments indicate that treatment with r-proUK in the presence of heparin results in significant clot lysis and full restoration of blood flow in a vessel that was previously totally occluded by thrombus. Moreover, the concomitant administration of ABT-187 and heparin does not result in significant alteration of the fibrinolytic and hemostatic parameters in plasma. These experimental findings are consistent with the clot-specific fibrinolytic mechanism of ABT-187 and the absence of plasmin activity (fibrinogenolysis) in the systemic circulation.

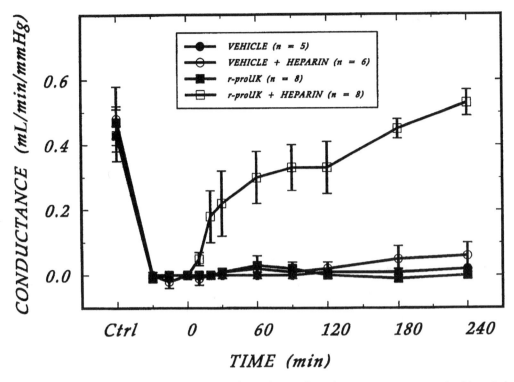

Figure 9 Vascular conductance in the canine femoral artery in each treatment group over the 4-h period following administration ($t = 0$) of ABT-187 or vehicle, in the absence and presence of heparin. Control values for conductance in each animal were obtained before the formation of the radioactive thrombus in the vessel. During the 30-min period before the start of drug treatment, no flow was observed in any animal, indicating the presence of a totally occlusive blood clot. Conductance values are mean SEM.

Table 2 The Effect of Prourokinase on the Plasma Levels of Coagulation Proteins in the Canine Femoral Artery Clot Lysis Model

		Fibrinogen (mg/dL)	Plasminogen (% of control)	Antiplasmin (% of control)
Vehicle	Control	276 ± 27	101 ± 5	105 ± 4
	30 min	235 ± 53	109 ± 5	115 ± 5
	240 min	299 ± 39	94 ± 2	112 ± 6
Pro-UK with Heparin	Control	277 ± 20	96 ± 6	111 ± 4
	30 min	263 ± 21	91 ± 6	98 ± 4
	240 min	288 ± 20	93 ± 5	104 ± 4

V. CLINICAL STUDIES WITH RECOMBINANT PROUROKINASE

A. Initial Studies in Myocardial Infarction

Two pilot studies were conducted to evaluate the safety and efficacy of r-proUK in the treatment of patients with acute myocardial infarction [26]. Both were dose-ranging studies, but the second study was designed to assess the efficacy of preactivating the thrombolytic system by administering recombinant urokinase before the administration of r-proUK.

1. Study Designs

The first study was an open, multicenter, dose-ranging study designed to evaluate two different doses of r-proUK; 60 and 80 mg. One-third of the total dose was administered as a bolus, with the remaining two-thirds as an infusion over a 60- or 90-min period.

The second study was a double-blind, multicenter trial that was conducted in two phases. In phase I, patients randomly received either a dose of 250,000 IU of recombinant urokinase (r-UK) as a priming agent immediately before the treatment dose of 60 mg of r-proUK, or a placebo priming agent followed immediately by the administration of 80 mg of r-proUK. The priming agent (r-UK or placebo) was administered as a bolus (over a 2-min period) followed immediately by a bolus of one-fourth of the total dose of r-proUK and an infusion of the remainder of the dose over a 90-min period. After the enrollment in phase I was completed, the protocol was amended to repeat the administration of 60 or 80 mg of r-proUK (primed and nonprimed), but with an infusion time of 60 min.

All patients received one aspirin tablet (325 mg) orally before the start of thrombolytic therapy and daily through hospital discharge. Heparin was administered intravenously throughout the study to maintain the activated partial thromboplastin time (aPTT) at two times the control value.

In the first study, coronary angiography was performed at the standard 90 min after initiation of study drug, but angiography of the infarct-related artery (IRA) was strongly encouraged at the 60-min mark, to assess early patency results for this new agent. Angiograms obtained 24 h after therapy were encouraged in the initial study and were required in patients in study 2 whose infarct-related arteries were open at the 90-min angiogram.

The primary endpoint for each study was the patency of the IRA at 90 min. Secondary endpoints included (1) patency of the IRA at 60 min, (2) reocclusion rate at the 24-h angiogram, and (3) the frequency of occurrence of negative clinical events related to the underlying coronary artery disease (e.g., recurrent ischemia, reinfarction, congestive heart failure, pulmonary edema, cardiogenic shock, emergency coronary artery bypass graft, stroke, or death). Side effects of therapy, particularly bleeding complications, were assessed during the first 3 days after the start of therapy.

During the course of the studies, each patient's AMI was to be treated as necessary. However, only mechanical intervention (PTCA) was allowed for treatment of an occluded IRA, after 48 h from the initiation of thrombolytic therapy had passed. The patient was to be followed for safety evaluations only for the 72 h following thrombolytic therapy.

Blood samples for determination of serum creatine kinase (CK) and the myocardial band fraction of CK (CK-MB) were obtained before r-proUK therapy and at 6-h intervals for 24 h following initiation of therapy. Blood samples for determination of plasma fibrinogen, fibrinogen degradation products (FDP), plasminogen, α_2-antiplasmin, fibrinopeptide A, and thrombin–antithrombin III complex (TAT-III) levels were obtained before treatment, and at various intervals following initiation of r-proUK therapy.

Throughout both clinical trials, every patient was observed for bleeding complications and other adverse reactions. It was not necessary to report bleeding manifestations associated with catheterization procedures. However, all of the following were considered to be bleeding complications: hematomas, ecchymoses, and oozing around the catheter site if they were of greater severity than would normally be expected; minor unexpected blood loss (< 250 mL) of no clinical significance, not requiring transfusion; moderate blood loss (250–500 mL); severe blood loss (> 500 mL), requiring transfusion replacement; life-threatening bleeding complications, such as intracranial hemorrhage, or other internal or external bleeding sufficient to cause hypotension.

2. Results

a. Patient Population.   Forty-six patients were enrolled in study I. A total of 85 patients were randomized in study II. Sixty-five patients were enrolled in the first phase of study II and 20 patients were enrolled in the second phase of the study. Only evaluable patients (i.e., patients who met specific criteria regarding disease presentation and treatment with study drug) were included in the analysis of efficacy presented here. Based on these criteria, three patients in study I and ten patients in study II were excluded from all "evaluable patient" efficacy analyses. Hence, 43 patients in I and 74 patients in II were evaluable patients. All patients who received any study drug were included in the safety analyses.

Comparison of the data from the two studies suggests that the patients enrolled in study I may have had more advanced vascular disease than those enrolled in study II, as evidenced by a higher rate of previous cardiovascular conditions or events.

The distribution of infarct locations showed that in study I, more than half of the patients had anterior infarctions. In contrast, fewer than half of the patients enrolled in study II had anterior infarctions.

b. Patency Evaluations.   In both studies the primary response variable for assessing the efficacy of r-proUK was the patency of the IRA at 90 min after the initiation of r-proUK administration. When possible, the IRA patency was also evaluated at 60 min. Only data obtained before any intervention were used in these patency analyses.

90-MINUTE PATENCY EVALUATION FOR EVALUABLE PATIENTS.   Thirty-nine (39) evaluable patients were included in the 90-min patency evaluation for study I. Patency rates were 66.7 and 72.2% for patients who received 60-min infusions and 90-min infusions, respectively, with a combined 90-min patency rate of 69.2%.

Thirty-seven (37) evaluable patients were included in the 90-min patency evaluation for patients who received 60 mg of r-proUK primed with r-UK in study II. The patency rate for the patients who received 60-min infusions was 45.5%, and the rate for patients who received 90-min infusions was 80.8%. The combined patency rate for the patients who received 60 mg of r-proUK after priming with 250,000 IU of r-UK was 70.3%.

Thirty-two (32) evaluable patients were included in the 90-min patency evaluation for patients who received 80 mg of r-proUK in study II. The patency rate for the six patients who received 60-min infusions was 100%, and the rate for patients who received 90-min infusions was 69.2%. The combined patency rate for the patients who received 80 mg of r-proUK was 75.0%. In study II, the 90-min patency following a 60-min infusion of 80 mg of r-proUK (nonprimed) was significantly greater than that following a 60-min infusion of 60 mg of r-proUK (primed), 100 versus 45.5% ($p = 0.043$).

The combined patency rate for all evaluable patients who received study drug over a 60-min infusion period in either study was 65.8%, and the combined rate for the patients who received study drug over a 90-min period was 74.3%. The overall 90-min patency across all treatment regimens in either study was 71.3%.

TIMI GRADE 3 PATENCY RESULTS AT THE 90-MIN ANGIOGRAM.   The number of evaluable patients exhibiting TIMI grade 3 patency at the 90-min angiogram was 42.1% in all the 60-min infusion group patients and 55.7% in the 90-min infusion group.

60-MINUTE PATENCY EVALUATION FOR EVALUABLE PATIENTS.   The IRA patency at 60 min was a secondary endpoint for study I only. Thirty-four (34) evaluable patients were included in the 60-min patency evaluation for study I. Patency rates were 83.3 and 56.3% for patients who received 60-min infusions and 90-min infusions, respectively, with a combined 60-min patency rate of 70.6%.

Nineteen (19) evaluable patients were included in the 60-min patency evaluation for patients who received 60 mg of r-proUK primed with r-UK. The patency rate for the patients who received 60-min infusions was 37.5%, and the rate for patients who received 90-min infusions was 45.5%.

Nineteen (19) evaluable patients were included in the 60-min patency evaluation for patients who received 80 mg of r-proUK in study II. The patency rate for the four patients who received 60-min infusions was 100%, and the rate for patients who received 90-min infusions was 60.0%. The combined patency rate for the patients who received 80 mg of r-proUK was 68.4%.

There was no statistically significant difference between the 60-min patency rates for the 60-mg (primed) and the 80-mg (nonprimed) treatment groups following either 60-min or 90-min infusions.

The combined patency rate for all evaluable patients who received study drug over a 60-min infusion period in either study was 73.3%, and the combined rate for the patients who received study drug over a 90-min period in either study was 54.8%.

REOCCLUSION.   The proportion of patients with angiographically documented reocclusion during the 24 h following treatment was a secondary endpoint for study II, but not for study I. However, angiographic evidence of reocclusion was obtained for a number of patients in Study I, and these data are included in the analysis. Of the patients who were patent at the 90-min angiogram, 70 had repeat angiography at approximately the 24-h mark. Of these 70 patients, only 1 patient who had no coronary intervention reoccluded [1.4%; 95% (CI; 0.1%–4.1%)]. The reason the remaining patients were not restudied was primarily related to physician discretion at particular sites and not to clinical event rates.

c. Clinical Endpoints.   The occurrences of any in-hospital clinical endpoints were similar between the two studies.

IN-HOSPITAL MORTALITY.   One patient died in the hospital during the course of these two studies. In study I, the patient, a 70-year-old white man, experienced ventricular tachycardia during administration of r-proUK, while en route to the study center by helicopter. He was defibrillated on arrival at the emergency room and was intubated. Angiography revealed occlusions of the LAD and circumflex arteries. Despite maximal cardiorespiratory support, including intra-aortic balloon and balloon angioplasty of both arteries, the patient died of irreversible ventricular failure.

BLEEDING COMPLICATIONS.   All bleeding complications were reported by the investigators as mild, moderate, severe, or life-threatening. The overall incidence of severe or life-threatening bleeding complications for both studies was 4.6%. There were no statistically significant differences between the 60-mg, primed, and the 80-mg, nonprimed, doses in the incidence of severe or life-threatening bleeding complications in study II. Because the two 60-mg–dose regimens in study I were administered sequentially, not in a randomized manner, no statistical tests were applied to the data.

d. Coagulation Studies.   Blood samples for measurement of plasma fibrinogen, plasminogen, α_2-antiplasmin, and fibrin(ogen) degradation products (FDP) were obtained before treatment and at specific times after initiation of thrombolytic therapy. The nadir values of fibrinogen, plasminogen, and α_2-antiplasmin were recorded as percentage change from baseline. Peak values of FDP were recorded as percentage of baseline.

Medians of the percentage decrease from baseline in plasma fibrinogen ranged from 22 to 74%. Priming with 250,000 IU of r-UK did not appear to affect the decrease in observed fibrinogen values. A slightly greater decrease was observed in the two groups treated with 90-min infusions, than for the 60-min infusions. However, these differences were not clinically significant. As might be expected, the 80-mg infusions produced greater decreases in fibrinogen than did the 60-mg doses.

As with plasminogen, the various dosage regimens had no consistent effect on the decreases in α_2-antiplasmin. These median decreases ranged from 49 to 83%, when compared with baseline.

One of the two regimens used in study I (60 mg infused over 60 min) produced the greatest increase in FDP, which might indicate that the clot load in this treatment group was greater than that in study II.

e. Fibrinopeptide A and TAT-III. In both studies, blood samples were obtained before treatment and at various times after treatment for determination of fibrinopeptide A and thrombin–antithrombin-III complex (TAT-III).

In 1988 Gulba et al. published data showing that an increase in TAT-III following thrombolysis of an occluded coronary artery was predictive of reocclusion. The data from these two studies do not appear to support Gulba's finding. In both studies, the patients whose IRAs did not reocclude experienced modest increases in TAT-III after thrombolysis, similar to that seen in the patients who reoccluded. The patients in study I who reoccluded did not experience an increase in TAT-III.

Similarly, the changes observed in fibrinopeptide A were not indicative of reocclusion. Medians of the percentage decrease from baseline in plasminogen values ranged from 36 to 61%. Neither the dose, duration of infusion, nor priming with r-UK had any observable effect on the decrease in plasminogen value.

On the basis of this experience, it was felt that r-proUK was a rapid-acting, effective fibrin-specific thrombolytic agent. Reocclusion was unusually low, in contrast with other thrombolytic agents and was considered an unique feature of prourokinase. Additionally, no strokes, thrombotic or hemorrhagic, were noted in either of the clinical studies. Subsequent to this early experience in patients with acute myocardial infarction, attention was directed toward stroke as the next area of clinical investigation with r-proUK.

B. Acute Ischemic Stroke

Two clinical trials in acute ischemic stroke have been conducted with recombinant prourokinase (r-proUK). These trials were conducted under the acronym PROACT (prolyse in acute cerebral thromboembolism) and involved an initial feasibility trial (PROACT I) and a larger phase 3 trial for registration (PROACT II). Both trials involved catheter-directed delivery of prourokinase directly into a thromboembolic occlusion in the middle cerebral artery (MCA) within 6 h of symptom onset. These two trials are summarized next.

1. PROACT I

PROACT I [27] was a multicenter, prospective, randomized, placebo-controlled, double-blind study conducted in the United States and Canada from January 1994 through February 1995. This study was an initial feasibility study of the effects of r-proUK delivered by intra-arterial (IA) infusion in subjects presenting with acute thromboembolic stroke of the MCA. Subjects who met all of the clinical, CT scan, and angiographic entrance criteria and, in those whom treatment could be initiated within 6 h of symptom onset were randomized to either 6-mg r-proUK or saline placebo administered over 2 h through a superselective microcatheter directly into the clot. Intravenous heparin was instituted at the time of angiography and was continued for 4 h. Three doses of heparin were used during this study. The initial heparin dosage regimen consisted of a bolus of 10,000 U (subsequently revised to a bolus of 100 U/kg after the first subject was enrolled), followed by a 1000-U/h infusion (high-dose heparin). The heparin dosage was later modified after 11 patients had been treated with r-proUK to a 2000-U bolus followed by a 500-U/h–infusion (low-dose heparin) to diminish the risk of hemorrhagic transformation. Subjects were monitored for safety and secondary clinical efficacy outcomes for 90 days.

The primary clinical endpoint for this study was MCA recanalization 120 min after the start of study drug administration. Angiography was performed at this time using a modification of the TIMI perfusion grade scale, to assess patency of the previously occluded vessel. Subjects were grouped as complete, partial, or no recanalization based on the TIMI perfusion scores of previously occluded vessel(s).

Forty-six (46) subjects were randomized and 40 subjects received treatment. A total of 26 subjects received r-proUK and 14 subjects received saline placebo. Of the 26 subjects who received r-proUK, 11 received the high-dose heparin regimen (> 2000-U–bolus dose), and 15 subjects received the low-dose heparin regimen (< 2000-U–bolus dose). Of the 14 subjects who received placebo, 5 received a high dose of heparin and 9 received a low dose of heparin. The results reported for PROACT I are for all treated subjects, unless otherwise specified. The recanalization results from PROACT I are presented by heparin dose in Table 3.

For all treated subjects, there was a statistically significantly higher rate of recanalization at 120 min following initiation of r-proUK versus saline placebo (p= 0.017). This difference was most pronounced for subjects receiving r-proUK and concurrent high-dose heparin (p < 0.001) vs. those receiving concurrent low-dose heparin (NS). The r-proUK recanalization rates were more than twofold higher with concurrent high-dose heparin (80%) versus concurrent low-dose heparin (41%).

The higher rate of recanalization with r-proUK and concurrent high-dose heparin was achieved at the cost of an increased rate of symptomatic intracranial hemorrhage. The rate of hemorrhagic transformation with clinical deterioration in the high-dose heparin group was 27.3% in the r-proUK group in contrast with an incidence of 20% in the placebo group, during the 10-day–observation period. In the low-dose heparin group, it was 6.7% in the r-proUK group and 11.1% in the placebo group.

Specific bleeding complications include injection site hematoma and hemorrhage, hematoma (nonspecific), hematuria, melena, mouth hemorrhage, epistaxis, hematocrit decrease and hemoglobin decrease.

Additional adverse events reported by one subject in the placebo treatment group (and no subjects in the r-proUK group) include generalized edema, sepsis, arrhythmia, atrial flutter, bradycardia, hypertension, hypotension, hypervolemia, convulsion, nervousness, atelectasis, cough increased, dry eyes, and oliguria.

Table 3   Recanalization by Heparin Dose in PROACT I

Heparin dose	Treatment group	N	Partial/complete recanalization at 120 min	p
High[a]	r-proUK	11	9 (81.8%)	< 0.001
	Placebo	5	0 (0.0%)	
Low[a]	r-proUK	15	6 (40.0%)	0.657
	Placebo	9	2 (22.2%)	
All	r-proUK	26	15 (57.7%)	0.017
	Placebo	14	2 (14.3%)	

[a] High dose: 100-U/kg bolus + 1000 U/h × 4 h; Low-dose: 2000-U bolus + 500 U/h × 4 h.

Subjects were also monitored for possible complications of the diagnostic and interventional angiographic procedures employed in this study. Adverse events noted as procedural complications in two treated r-proUK subjects and in one treated placebo subject were aspiration pneumonia, neurological deterioration, hematoma, and renal failure. Adverse events noted as procedural complications in subjects who were randomized, but did not receive an infusion of r-proUK or placebo, were vasospasm (cerebral ischemia) and neurological deterioration. Deaths reported in the 90-day follow-up period for subjects who had procedural complications (three subjects) were due to respiratory arrest, cardiorespiratory arrest, and cerebral infarction. Only the death owing to cerebral infarction was thought to be possibly procedurally related, per report.

Subjects who received only a diagnostic angiogram, and were not randomized, were also monitored for procedural-related complications. No procedural complications were noted.

2. PROACT II

PROACT II [28] was a multicenter, prospective, randomized, open-treatment, controlled study in subjects presenting with an acute stroke from thrombotic or thromboembolic occlusion of the middle cerebral artery (MCA). Subjects who presented with clinical evidence of acute ischemic stroke in the MCA territory within 6 h of the projected time of intervention were to be screened. Subjects who met all of the clinical, neurological, CT scan, and angiographic criteria were randomized in a 2 : 1 ratio to receive an intra-arterial infusion of 9 mg of r-proUK over 120 min, with concurrent low-dose heparin or an intravenous infusion of heparin alone (control). The intravenous heparin therapy consisted of a 2000-U bolus, followed by a 500-U/h infusion for 4 h in both groups. Randomized subjects were monitored for safety and clinical efficacy outcomes for 90 days.

One hundred eighty subjects were randomized, of which 162 (108 r-proUK and 54 control) were treated as randomized. The 13 subjects in the r-proUK group who were not treated as randomized did not receive any r-proUK, and the 5 subjects in the control group who were not treated as randomized received a thrombolytic agent on study days 1 or 2 (2 received intra-arterial r-proUK and 3 received intra-arterial urokinase).

The primary endpoint for this study was defined as the percentage of subjects achieving a modified Rankin disability score of ≤ 2 at 90 days following therapy (slight or no disability, able to function independently). Other efficacy endpoints consisted of the percentage of subjects having a Barthel Index of ≥ 60 (able to live at home with or without assistance) at 90 days, an NIHSS score of ≤ 1 (essentially normal neurological function) at 90 days following therapy, and recanalization with restoration of blood flow at 120 min after initiation of study drug infusion. All primary efficacy analyses were adjusted for baseline NIHSS strata (4–10, 11–20, and 21–30). The principal safety outcome was hemorrhagic transformation causing neurological deterioration within 36 h of treatment.

The results of the functional (modified Rankin and Barthel Index) and neurological (NIHSS) examinations performed on all randomized patients at the 90-day visit are presented in Table 4. Among randomized subjects, the NIHSS stratum-adjusted percentage of subjects with modified Rankin scores ≤ 2 at 90 days was statistically significantly higher among r-proUK subjects than among control subjects (40 vs. 25%, p = 0.043). Additionally, the stratum-adjusted proportions of r-proUK subjects attaining a Barthel Index ≥ 60 (able to live at home, but may require some assistance) and NIHSS ≤ 1 (normal or near normal neurological function) at 90 days were higher than those for control; however, statistical significance was not achieved for any of these secondary clinical comparisons.

The results of the 120-min recanalization assessments in PROACT II for all subjects treated as randomized are presented by treatment group in Table 5.

Table 4 90-Day Functional and Neurological Assessments Stratified by Baseline NIHSS Score For All Randomized Subjects in PROACT II

Endpoint baseline NIHSS	r-proUK		Control	
Modified Rankin ≤2	N		N	
≤10	16	10 (63%)	8	5 (63%)
11–20	75	34 (45%)	37	9 (24%)
> 20	30	4 (13%)	14	1 (7%)
Overall adjusted rate		40%[a]		25%
NIHSS ≤1	N		N	
≤10	16	7 (44%)	8	3 (38%)
11–20	75	13 (17%)	37	4 (11%)
> 20	30	1 (3%)	14	0 (0%)
Overall adjusted rate		18%		12%
Barthel Index ≥ 60	N		N	
≤10	16	11 (69%)	8	7 (88%)
11–20	75	44 (59%)	37	18 (49%)
> 20	30	10 (33%)	14	3 (21%)
Overall adjusted rate		54%		47%

[a] $p < 0.05$ compared with control for corresponding value. Using carry-forward methods and imputation for death for randomized subjects. Surviving subjects without a value to carry forward to the 90-day time point were considered failures for that time point.

At 120 min the rate of complete and partial recanalization for subjects treated as randomized was statistically significantly higher for the r-proUK group (66%) compared with the control group (18%), $p < 0.001$.

Mortality rates for PROACT II through the 90-day visit are presented by treatment group in Table 6.

Among randomized subjects, 25.6% (31/121) of the r-proUK subjects and 27.1% (16/59) of the control subjects died by their 90-day follow-up. Among subjects who were treated as randomized, 25.9% (28/108) of the r-proUK subjects and 24.1% (13/54) of the control subjects died by their 90-day follow-up. These differences between treatment groups were not statistically significant.

Deaths reported for subjects who were randomized to receive r-proUK (31) were due to progression of metastatic cancer, aspiration pneumonia, acute infarction of brain secondary to

Table 5 Recanalization Response in Subjects Treated as Randomized in PROACT II

Endpoint baseline NIHSS	r-proUK			Control			
	Complete	Partial	Nonrespond	Complete	Partial	Nonrespond	
120 min							
≤10	2/13	6/13	5/13	1/7	4/7	2/7	
11–20	16/70	29/70	25/70	0/31	4/31	27/31	
< 20	3/25	15/25	7/25	0/12	0/12	12/12	
Complete/partial overall stratum adjusted rate		66%			18%		< 0.001***

*** Statistically significant difference at the 0.001 level.

Table 6 Mortality Rates at 90-Day Follow-up in PROACT II

Data set	r-proUK	Control	p-Value
Randomized subjects	31/121 (25.6%)	16/59 (27.1%)	0.858
Subjects treated as randomized	28/108 (25.9%)	13/54 (24.1%)	0.850

embolized mural thrombus from inominate artery, cardiac failure, cerebral hemorrhage, transtentorial herniation of the brain, cerebral edema, cerebral herniation, respiratory arrest, pneumonia, stroke progression, sudden death, respiratory failure, acute renal failure and sepsis, cardiac arrhythmia and heart failure, ventricular fibrillation, cardiopulmonary, cerebrovascular accident, cerebral infarction, and cerebral emboli. Deaths reported for subjects who were randomized to receive control (16) were due to recurrent cerebral infarction, cerebral edema, cerebrovascular accident, respiratory failure, respiratory arrest, sepsis, cardiac arrest, myocardial infarction, congestive heart failure, progression of left MCA infarction, embolic stroke, stroke with respiratory arrest and cerebral herniation, and respiratory distress.

Table 7 summarizes all intracranial hemorrhages in PROACT II for subjects treated as randomized. Within 10 days of randomization, there was no statistically significant difference between treatment groups for the percentages of subjects (treated as randomized) experiencing any intracranial hemorrhage. Within 36 h of randomization, the percentages of r-proUK subjects treated as randomized experiencing any intracranial hemorrhage was significantly higher for the r-proUK group compared with the control group (p = 0.002). The percentage of subjects experiencing intracranial hemorrhage with neurological deterioration was greater among r-proUK subjects compared with control subjects at 36 h and 10 days, but those differences were not statistically significant.

Among subjects treated as randomized, nonhemorrhagic adverse events were reported for 75% of the r-proUK subjects and 64.8% of the control subjects, p = 0.198. Adverse events experienced by more than 10% of subjects in either treatment group included urinary tract infection (14.8% of r-proUK subjects vs. 9.3% of control subjects), brain edema (11.1% of r-proUK subjects vs. 3.7% of control subjects), cerebral infarct (10.2% of r-proUK subjects vs. 11.1% of control subjects), and aspiration pneumonia (7.4% of r-proUK subjects vs. 11.1% of control subjects).

Subjects were also monitored for possible complications of the diagnostic angiography and interventional procedures utilized in this study. Subjects were monitored for these procedural complications whether or not an infusion of r-proUK was administered. Among randomized subjects, 25 (20.7%) r-proUK and 14 (23.7%) control subjects experienced a procedural complication. Among subjects who underwent cerebral angiography and were not subsequently randomized (group III subjects) 19 (6.5%) subjects experienced procedural complications. The primary procedural complications reported were bleeding at the catheter entry site and hematuria

Table 7 Intracranial Hemorrhage (ICH) in Subjects Treated as Randomized in PROACT II

Event category	r-proUK ($n = 108$) N (%)	Control ($n = 54$) N (%)	p-Value
ICH (10 days)	57 (52.8%)	23 (42.6%)	0.246
ICH (36 h)	50 (46.3%)	11 (20.4%)	0.002**
ICH with deterioration (10 days)	13 (12.0%)	2 (3.7%)	0.148
ICH with deterioration (36 h)	11 (10.2%)	1 (1.9%)	0.063

** Statistically significant at $p < 0.01$.

secondary to the insertion of a urinary catheter before beginning cerebral angiography. This was seen in 7.4% of the r-proUK subjects, 16.9% of the control subjects, and 4.8% of the group III subjects. Two subjects, one in the r-proUK group, and one in the control group (who received intra-arterial urokinase), experienced intracranial hemorrhage with neurological deteriorations that were listed by the investigator as a procedural complication. Other complications were a worsening of neurological symptoms, anaphylaxis owing to contrast, and other.

C. Peripheral Arterial Occlusion

1. The PURPOSE Trial

The PURPOSE trial [29] was a phase II dose-ranging, parallel, randomized, double-blind, multicenter, comparative trial in the treatment of peripheral native artery and bypass graft thromboembolic occlusions. The objective was to evaluate and compare the safety and efficacy of three doses of r-proUK and one dose of tissue–culture-derived UK (ABT-790; Abbokinase, urokinase for injection). In addition, the study was to determine the optimum dose of r-proUK that is safe and effective in lysing blood clots in thrombosed peripheral native arteries or in bypass grafts.

The primary endpoint was the proportion of subjects who had complete clot lysis (> 95%) at the 8-h angiogram. Secondary endpoints included the proportion of subjects who had reestablishment of antegrade blood flow (TIMI perfusion grade 2 or 3) at 8 h or less after the start of study drug treatment as documented by angiography, the proportion of subjects without distally migrated clot in the target limb at any time during the study drug infusion as documented by angiography, the proportion of subjects with amputation-free survival at 30 days after treatment, and the proportion of subjects without adverse events or bleeding complications.

Eligible subjects were those presenting with clinical signs and symptoms of peripheral arterial occlusion (PAO) for ≤14 days in whom it was safe to administer thrombolytic therapy. Following angiographic confirmation of the completely occlusive clot, the subject was randomly assigned, in a blinded manner, to receive one of three doses of r-proUK or UK in a 1 : 1 : 1 : 1 ratio. Randomization was stratified based on whether the occlusion was in a native artery or in bypass graft. The study drug was to be administered directly into the clot by a multi-side-hole catheter (catheter of choice) until complete lysis (> 95% lysis) was achieved, or until a maximum of 24 h elapsed, or for 8 h if no clot lysis was observed at the 8-h angiogram. The study drug was to be administered as a bolus, using a lacing technique, over 5 min, followed by an infusion. The dosage and treatment groups used are presented in Table 8.

The target enrollment was to include 240 subjects enrolled at approximately 40 sites. A total of 241 subjects were randomized into the study and 227 subjects received study drug treatment. The results from this study for treated subjects are shown in Table 9.

Table 8 Dosage and Treatment Groups for PURPOSE Trial

Dose group	Maximum initial bolus administered over 5 min	Dosing for up to first 8 h	Dosing for maximum of additional 16 h	Total maximum drug exposure
1 (r-proUK)	2.0 mg	2 mg/h	0.5 mg/h	26 mg
2 (r-proUK)	4.0 mg	4 mg/h	0.5 mg/h	44 mg
3 (r-proUK)	8.0 mg	8 mg/h	0.5 mg/h	80 mg
4 (UK)	250,000 IU	4000 IU/min×4 h; 2000 IU/min×4 h	2000 IU/min×16 h	3,610,000 IU

Table 9 Results from PURPOSE Trial

	Group 1 r-proUK 2 mg $n = 61$	Group 2 r-proUK 4 mg $n = 55$	Group 3 r-proUK 8 mg $n = 52$	Group 4 UK 250,000 IU $n = 59$
Mean total dose (mg r-proUK or million IU UK) + SEM	21.6 ± 0.60	37.3 ± 0.73	67.2 ± 1.83	2.5 ± 0.12
Mean total infusion time (h) + SEM	16.7 ± 0.89	15.5 ± 0.94	12.7 ± 0.97	15.3 ± 0.91
No. of subjects with > 95% lysis at the 8-h angiogram	24/61 (39.3%)	24/54 (44.4%)[a]	28/50 (56.0%)[a]	28/57 (49.1%)[a]
No. of subjects with antegrade flow at 8 h angiogram	45/61 (73.8%)	40/54 (74.1%)[a]	36/50 (72.0%)[a]	39/56 (69.6%)[a]
No. of subjects without distal emboli	49/61 (80.3%)	44/55 (80.0%)	44/52 (84.6%)	53/59 (89.8%)
% of subjects with 30-day amputation-free survival + SE	93.4 ± 3.17	85.1 ± 4.86	86.1 ± 4.91	84.5 ± 4.76

[a] Subject(s) did not have an "8-h" angiogram and were excluded from the analysis.

Bleeding complications were reported from all four treatment groups and from each group, there were more subjects reporting entry-site bleeding complications than nonentry. A summary of the reported treatment–emergent-bleeding complications (entry and nonentry) for treated subjects, grouped by relation to study drug infusion, is provided in Table 10.

Specific nonentry-site–bleeding complications included anemia, ecchymosis, epistaxis, eye hemorrhage, gastrointestinal hemorrhage, gum hemorrhage, hematemesis, hematuria, hemoptysis, hemorrhage, hypochromic anemia, melena, petechia, rectal hemorrhage, and retroperitoneal hemorrhage.

Serious bleeding complications and nonhemorrhagic adverse events were reported for 48 subjects (4 subjects did not receive the therapy to which they were randomized) and there were 11 deaths (1 subject did not receive therapy to which he was randomized), of which 8 occurred during the initial hospitalization.

VI. DISCUSSION

Recombinant prourokinase (ABT-187; Prolyse) is a fully glycosylated recombinant product, obtained in large quantities from a mouse myeloma expression system. The presence of the N-

Table 10 Bleeding Complications for Treated Subjects in PURPOSE Trial

	Group 1 r-proUK 2 mg total $n = 61$	Group 2 r-proUK 4 mg total $n = 55$	Group 3 r-proUK 8 mg total $n = 52$	Group 4 UK 250,000 IU total $n = 59$
Relation	n (%)	n (%)	n (%)	n (%)
Probably	5 (8.2%)	7 (12.7%)	9 (17.3%)	6 (10.2%)
Possibly	7 (11.5%)	11 (20.0%)	17 (32.7%)	16 (27.1%)
Probably not	11 (18.0%)	9 (16.4%)	6 (11.5%)	8 (13.6%)
Not related	11 (18.0%)	7 (12.7%)	6 (11.5%)	4 (6.8%)
	34 (55.7%)	34 (61.8%)	38 (73.1%)	34 (57.6%)

linked oligosaccharide at position Asn[302], including the terminal neuraminic acid residues, has been implicated in the overall stability of this agent. The presence of the carbohydrate on ABT-187 increases its resistance to proteolytic degradation and influences its circulation time in plasma, and its catalytic potential.

The data we have obtained with our experimental models, using both an in vitro clot lysis system and a canine femoral artery thrombosis model, are consistent with the clot-specific mechanism that has been reported for the catalytic action of proUK. Moreover, the lytic potential of r-proUK is significantly enhanced by coadministration with heparin, and effective lysis can be achieved without systemic plasmin activation and perturbation of the normal coagulation and fibrinolytic parameters. This finding is of clinical importance in that nearly all of the patients receiving thrombolytic therapy, are treated in a parallel manner with anticoagulant, most notably heparin therapy. Although other antithrombin agents may be more potent in minimizing the additional generation of thrombin (and, hence, fibrin) within the clot network [30], it is apparent that the presence of heparin in the systemic circulation is of clinical importance.

Another aspect that may be of importance in the clinical arena is the ability of the various plasminogen activators to lyse thrombi of differing compositions. Several investigators have examined the lytic susceptibility (either in vitro or ex vivo) of arterial and venous clots [31], the influence of clot age [32], and the availability of plasminogen within the clots [33,34].

In a quantitative study, Brommer and Bockel have tried to correlate the fibrin and plasminogen content of human arterial thrombi with their ex vivo susceptibility to lysis with several of the available thrombolytic agents (t-PA, SK, UK, and proUK) [32]. They concluded that the plasminogen content of aged arterial thrombi is sufficient for rapid thrombolysis, and only after months, do fibrin and plasminogen become degraded to the extent that the clots become resistant to thrombolysis. It is intriguing to question at what point in the aging process in vivo clots do become resistant to lytic therapy; and whether the ability of r-proUK to maintain the integrity of such old or plasminogen-depleted clots may contribute to the excellent safety profile of this activator.

The clinical studies described represent use of Abbott's recombinant glycosylated prourokinase in humans. Acute myocardial infarction patients were chosen as the population for initial studies because they provide a better model than other patients for evaluating the systemic effects of the agent. The treatment regimen for this indication involves the systemic administration of substantial doses of r-proUK over a relatively short period. In contrast, most other indications in which thrombolytic therapy is used employ local, low-dose, catheter-directed administration of the thrombolytic agent directly into the clot over a period of several hours.

There was some evidence in the results of these studies to suggest that the patients enrolled in study I had more advanced coronary artery disease than those enrolled in study II. For example, the previous cardiovascular histories of the patients in study I indicated a considerably greater incidence of peripheral vascular disease, angina on exercise, previous myocardial infarction, and congestive heart failure, compared with the patients in study II. Furthermore, there was a greater incidence of recurrent ischemia in the patients in study I than in the patients in study II. However, this difference probably had no effect on the primary study endpoints, IRA patency.

Six different dose regimens were studied in the two trials. Sixty (60) and 80 mg of r-proUK were evaluated using 60- and 90-min infusions. In addition, because studies in animals had indicated that the onset of lytic action of r-proUK could be accelerated by pretreatment with a small dose of urokinase, two groups of patients were given 250,000 IU infusions of r-UK followed by 60 mg of r-proUK infused over 60 or 90 min.

Because of the small number of patients in each treatment group, it was not possible to select one dose regimen as being superior to the others. Moreover, the priming dose of r-UK

(250,000 IU) was apparently not large enough to accelerate the rate of clot lysis. However, the overall 90-min patency rate, combining all treatment regimens, was 71.3%.

A major finding of the study was the relatively low 24-h reocclusion rate of 1.4%, (95% CI; 0.1–4.1%), which compares very favorably with other agents. Specifically, the reocclusion rate for "front-loaded" alteplase with an aggressive intravenous heparin regimen has been reported to be 7.8% [35]. In earlier studies, reocclusion after alteplase treatment has been even higher, a finding consistent with the mounting evidence that the currently available drugs expose both injured endothelium and clot-bound thrombin, resulting in increased levels of thrombin activity after treatment which may lead to reocclusion [36–39]. The low rate observed in these patients is also remarkable when compared with the results of other prourokinase studies. Of the 191 patients given prourokinase and assessed for reocclusion in this and the PRIMI study [40], the reocclusion rate is 3.7%, (95%, CI; 1.0–6.4%). This low rate of reocclusion needs to be confirmed by studies of more patients, because this could be of significant clinical importance (e.g., the rate is very similar to that observed when alteplase is administered with hirudin, an antithrombin potentially improved over heparin [41,42]. The findings in this study also contrast to other prourokinase studies in which there was extensive secondary depletion of fibrinogen. This suggests that factors other than fibrinogen depletion may be related to the low rate of reocclusion seen with prourokinase. Prourokinase can bind to platelet and endothelial membranes and, perhaps, in some way this protects the artery from reocclusion [43]. In this study, the secondary markers of thrombin activation (i.e., antithrombin III and fibrinopeptide A levels were highest at the initiation of treatment and did not rise significantly following treatment). There was also no difference between the baseline levels in those patients and patients with occluded arteries at 90 min. Elevated thrombin antithrombin III and fibrinopeptide A levels occur following treatment with thrombolytic drugs and appear to be associated with thrombolysis drug failures and reocclusion [36–39]. The aggressive use of heparin as well as possible features of prourokinase itself may have contributed to the low rate of occlusion observed in this study.

The final high rate of patency and low rate of reocclusion were associated with few significant clinical events following treatment, including only one death and no strokes (hemorrhagic or thrombotic) were observed, although the number of patients studied is too small to define precisely these uncommon event rates. The incidence of reinfarction was also low (2%). Thus, these preliminary observations suggest a favorable, overall benefit and risk profile with r-proUK.

In the pilot stroke study, MCA recanalization frequency in patients receiving direct intra-arterial recombinant r-proUK within 6 h of stroke onset was significantly greater than placebo and cannot be ascribed to mechanical clot disruption. There was no difference in brain hemorrhage with clinical neurological deterioration between the r-proUK and placebo groups. Patients receiving r-proUK who recanalized, had better neurological outcomes at 90 days.

PROACT I was the first thrombolysis stroke trial to examine the role of concomitant heparin therapy. Animal data suggests that heparin doses sufficient to increase the activated partial thromboplastin time by 1.5 times control markedly increase the recanalization efficacy of r-proUK [44]. Unfortunately, although high-dose heparin doubled the recanalization rate in PROACT I it also resulted in four times the number of clinically significant brain hemorrhages. The lower-heparin–dose regimen represents a compromise between the positive recanalization and negative hemorrhage effects of heparin when combined with r-proUK. The role of antithrombotic therapy in preventing reocclusion was not addressed in this study.

A second study utilizing intra-arterial delivery of r-proUK to treat acute ischemic stroke caused by occlusion of the middle cerebral artery (PROACT II) resulted in significant clinical benefit at 3 months for the r-proUK group versus untreated controls. This study, utilizing a 50%

higher dose of r-proUK with concurrent subtherapeutic heparin, may potentially widen the treatment window for thrombolysis in the treatment of acute ischemic stroke from 3 to 6 h from symptom onset.

In summary, r-proUK (ABT-187) is a glycosylated single-chain recombinant proUK that is exceedingly stable, rapid-acting, and safe in the clinical doses used. The results from the two studies of acute myocardial infarction indicate that r-proUK (ABT-187, Prolyse) is an effective agent in opening and maintaining the patency of occluded coronary arteries. In addition, in middle cerebral artery thromboembolic stroke, r-proUK administered intra-arterially by catheter into the substance of the occluding clot results in a significantly greater frequency of recanalization and significant clinical benefit at 3 months compared with untreated controls. These positive results were achieved without significantly increasing hemorrhage complications, especially the occurrence of symptomatic brain hemorrhage. An additional clinical trial in patients with peripheral arterial occlusions was carried out in approximately 227 patients, and the three regimens of r-proUK were compared with the "standard" regimen of urokinase. The highest recanalization rate was achieved with the highest dose (8 mg/h) of r-proUK. However, this group also had the highest bleeding rate. The mean infusion time to achieve the high recanalization rate was almost 3 h less than the standard urokinase. There were, however, no differences among the different groups in the 30-day amputation rate.

Other trials will be needed to confirm the efficacy and safety of r-proUK.

REFERENCES

1. Weaver WD, Hartmann JR, Anderson JL, Reddy PS, Sobolski JC, Sasahara AA. New recombinant glycosylated prourokinase for treatment of patients with acute myocardial infarction. J Am Coll Cardiology 1994; 24:1242.
2. McNamara TO, Bomberger RA, Merchant RF. Intra-arterial urokinase as the initial therapy for acutely ischemic lower limbs. Circulation 1991; 83:106.
3. Ouriel K, Shortell CK, DeWeese JA, Green RM, Francis CW, Azodo MVU, Gutierrez OH, Manzione JV, Cox C, Marder VJ. A comparison of thrombolytic therapy with operative revascularization in the initial treatment of acute peripheral arterial ischemia. J Vasc Surg 1994; 19:1021.
4. Goldhaber SZ, Polak JF, Feldstein ML, Meyerovitz MF, Creager MA. Efficacy and safety of repeated boluses of urokinase in the treatment of deep venous thrombosis. Am J Cardiol 1994; 73:75.
5. Sasahara AA, McIntyre KM, Cella G, Palla A, Sharma GVRK. The clinical and hemodynamic features of acute pulmonary embolism. Curr Pulmonol 1988; 9:305.
6. del Zoppo GJ, Pessin MS, Mori E, Hacke W. Thrombolytic intervention in acute thrombotic and embolic stroke. Semin Neurol 1991; 11:368.
7. Higashida RT, Halbach VV, Tsai FY, Dowd CF, Hieshima GB. Interventional neurovascular techniques for cerebral revascularization in the treatment of stroke. Am J Roentgenol 1994; 163:793.
8. Lo K–M, Gilles SD. High level expression of human proteins in murine hybridoma cells: induction by methotrexate in the absence of gene amplification. Biochim Biophys Acta 1991; 445:215.
9. Kasai S, Arimura H, Nishida M, Suyama T. Primary structure of single-chain pro-urokinase. J Biol Chem 1985; 260:12382.
10. Riccio A, Grimaldi G, Verde P, Sebastio G, Boast S, Blasi F. The human urokinase–plasminogen activator gene and its promoter. Nucleic Acids Res 1985; 13:2759.
11. Patthy L. Evolutionary assembly of blood coagulation proteins. Sem Thromb Haemost 1990; 16:245.
12. Kasai S, Arimura H, Nishida M, Suyama T. Proteolytic cleavage of single chain pro-urokinase induces conformational change which follows activation of the zymogen and reduction of its high affinity for fibrin. J Biol Chem 1985; 260:12377.
13. Nolan C, Hall LS, Barlow GH, Tribby E II. Plasminogen activator from human embryonic kidney cell cultures—evidence for a proactivator. Biochim Biophys Acta 1977; 496:384.

14. Ichinose A, Fukikawa K, Suyama T. The activation of pro-urokinase by plasma kallikrein and its inactivation by thrombin. J Biol Chem 1985; 261:3486.

15. Loza J–P, Gurewich V, Johnstone M, Pannell R. Platelet-bound prekallikrein promotes pro-urokinase-induced clot lysis: a mechanism for targeting the factor XII dependent intrinsic pathway of fibrinolysis. Thromb Haemost 1994; 71:347.

16. Kobayshi H, Schmitt M, Goretzki L, Chucholowski N, Calvete J, Kramer M, GÜnzler WA, Jänicke F, Graeff H. Cathepsin B efficiently activates the soluble and the tumor cell receptor-bound form of the proenzyme urokinase-type plasminogen activator (pro-uPA). J Biol Chem 1991; 266:5147.

17. Marcotte P, Henkin J. Activation of pro-urokinase by thermolysin: characterization of the reaction and its utility. Fibrinolysis 1990; 4(suppl 3):28.

18. Berkenpas M, Quigley JP. Secretion of two-chain active plasminogen activator from *rsv*-transformed chicken embryo fibroblasts: evidence for a plasmin-independent converting activity. Fibrinolysis 1989; 3(suppl 1):3.

19. Novokhatny V, Medved L, Mazar A, Marcotte P, Henkin J, Ingham K. Domain structure and interactions of recombinant urokinase-type plasminogen activator. J Biol Chem 1992; 267:3878.

20. Kentzer EJ, Buko AM, Menon G, Sarin VK. Carbohydrate composition and presence of a fucose protein linkage in recombinant human pro-urokinase. BBRC 1990; 171:401.

21. Holmes WE, Pennica D, Blaber M, Rey M, Günzler WA, Steffans GJ, Heynecher, HL. Cloning and expression of the gene for pro-urokinase in *Escherichia coli*. Biotechnology 1985; 3:923.

22. Lenich C, Pannell R, Henkin J, Gurewich V. The influence of glycosylation on the catalytic and fibrinolytic properties of pro-urokinase. Thromb Haemost 1992; 68:539.

23. Zamarron C, Lijnen HR, Van Hoef B, Collen D. Biological and thrombolytic properties of proenzyme and active forms of human urokinase—I. Fibrinolytic and fibrinogenolytic properties in human plasma in vitro of urokinases obtained from human urine or by recombinant DNA technology. Thromb Haemost 1984; 52:19.

24. DeClerck PJ, Lijnen HR, Verstreken M, Moreau H, Collen D. A monoclonal antibody specific for two-chain urokinase-type plasminogen activator. Application to the study of the mechanism of clot lysis with single-chain urokinase-type plasminogen activator in plasma. Blood 1990; 75:1794.

25. Badylak SF, Poehlman ET, Williams C, Klabunde RE, Turek J, Schoenlein W. A simple canine model of arterial thrombosis with endothelial injury suitable for investigation of thrombolytic agents. J Pharmacol Methods 1988; 19:293.

26. Weaver WD, Hartmann JR, Anderson JL, Reddy PS, Sobolski JC, Sasahara AA. For the Prourokinase Study Group. New recombinant glycosylated prourokinase for treatment of patients with acute myocardial infarction. J Am Coll Cardiol 1994; 24:1242–1248.

27. del Zoppo GJ, Higashida RT, Furlan AJ, Pessin MS, Gent M, and the PROACT Investigators. PROACT: a phase II randomized trial of recombinant prourokinase by direct arterial delivery in acute middle cerebral artery stroke. Stroke 1998; 29:4–11.

28. Furlan A, Higashida R, Wechsler L, Gent M, Rowley H, Kase C, Pessin M, Ahuja A, Callahan F, Clark W, Silver F, Rivera F, for the PROACT Investigators. Intra-arterial prourokinase for acute ischemic stroke: the PROACT II study: a randomized controlled trial. JAMA 1999; 282:2003–2011.

29. Ouriel K, Kandarpa K, Schuerr D, Hultquist M, Hodkinson G, Wallin B. Prourokinase versus urokinase for recanalization of peripheral occlusions, safety and efficacy: the PURPOSE trial. JVIR 1999; 10:1083–1091.

30. Weitz JI, Hudoba M, Massei D, Maraganore J, Hirsh J. Clot-bound thrombin is protected from inhibition by heparin-antithrombin III but is susceptible to inactivation by antithrombin III-independent inhibitors. J Clin Invest 1990; 86:385.

31. van Loon BJP, Rijken DC, Brommer EJP, van der Maas APC. The amount of plasminogen, tissue-type plasminogen activator and plasminogen activator inhibitor type 1 in human thrombi and the relation to ex-vivi lysibility. Thromb Haemost 1992; 67:101.

32. Brommer EJP, van Bockel JH. Composition and susceptibility to thrombolysis of human arterial thrombi and the influence of their age. Blood Coagul Fibrinol 1992; 3:717.

33. Gottlob R. Plasminogen and plasmin inhibitors in arterial and venous thrombi of various ages. In: Davidson JF, Samama MM, Desnoyers PC, eds. Progress in Chemical Fibrinolysis and Thrombolysis. New York: Raven Press, 1975; 23.

34. Sabovic M, Lijnen HR, Keber D, Collen D. Correlation between progressive adsorption of plasminogen to blood clots and their sensitivity to lysis. Thromb Haemost 1990; 64:450.

35. The GUSTO Angiographic Investigators. An angiographic study within the global randomized trial of aggressive vs. standard thrombolytic strategies in patients with acute myocardial infarction. N Engl J Med 1993; 329:1615–1622.

36. Gash AK, Spann JF, Sherry S, Belber AD, Carabello BA, McDonough MT, Mann RH, McCann WD, Gault JH, Gentzler RD, Kent RL. Factors influencing reocclusion after coronary thrombolysis for acute myocardial infarction. Am J Cardiol 1986; 56:176–177.

37. Eidt JF, Allison P, Noble S, Ashton J, Golino P, McNatt J, Buja LM, Willerson JT. Thrombin is an important mediator of platelet aggregation in stenosed canine coronary arteries with endothelial injury. J Clin Invest 1992; 84:18–27.

38. Owen J, Friedman KD, Grossman BA, Wilkins C, Berke AD, Powers ER. Thrombolytic therapy with tissue plasminogen activator or streptokinase induces transient thrombin activity. Blood 1988; 72:616–620.

39. Fitzgerald DJ, Fitzgerald GA. Role of thrombin and thromboxane A_2 in reocclusion following coronary thrombolysis with tissue-type plasminogen activator. Proc Natl Acad Sci USA 1989; 86:7585–7589.

40. PRIMI Trial Study Group. Randomized double-blind trial of myocardial infarction. Lancet 1989; 1:863–868.

41. Weitz JL, Hudoba M, Massel D, Maraganore J, Hirsh J. Clot-bound thrombin is protected from inhibition by heparin–antithrombin but is susceptible to inactivation by antithrombin III independent inhibitors. J Clin Invest 1990; 86:385–391.

42. Rudd MA, George D, Johnstone MT, Moore RT, Collins L, Rabbani LE, Loscalzo J. Effect of thrombin inhibition on the dynamics of thrombolysis and on platelet function during thrombolytic therapy. Circ Res 1992; 70:829–834.

43. Gurewich V, Johnstone M, Loza JP, Pannell R. Pro-urokinase and prekallikrein are both associated with platelets: implications for the intrinsic pathway of fibrinolysis and for therapeutic thrombolysis. FEBS Lett 1993; 318:317.

44. Abbott Laboratories Scientific Report, PPRd/89/541. Evaluation of recombinant prourokinase (ABT-187) in the canine femoral artery clot lysis model (Dec. 27, 1989). IND 3472, Serial No. 000.

36

A Mutant Form of Prourokinase That Spares Hemostatic Fibrin

Victor Gurewich
Harvard Medical School and Beth Israel Deaconess Medical School, Boston, Massachusetts, U.S.A.

Jian-ning Liu
Nanjing University, Nanjing, China

SUMMARY

The u-PA paradigm of fibrinolysis is predicated on pro-uPA (pro-UK) remaining a zymogen in blood and being activated to two-chain u-PA (UK) selectively on the fibrin surface. Under these conditions, pro-UK-induced thrombolysis is fibrin-specific, and lysis is augmented by a hypercatalytic transitional state during the conversion of pro-UK to UK. Unfortunately, at the pharmacological doses used for therapeutic thrombolysis, pro-UK is unstable in blood and is activated to UK systemically. When this happens, the advantages of pro-UK over UK are lost. This instability of pro-UK is related to its relatively high intrinsic activity, which activates free plasminogen at pharmacological concentrations. Therefore, mutations were designed, produced, and characterized to reduce this intrinsic activity. A histidine[300] mutation (H-pro-UK) is described that is more than four times more stable in blood, and that induces effective, fibrin-specific clot lysis in vitro and in vivo, partly related to the fact that whereas its intrinsic activity is reduced, H-UK is almost twice as active as UK. An additional property of H-pro-UK is that in a study in dogs, it caused no increase in bleeding time at thrombolytic doses, in contrast to t-PA and pro-UK. A mechanism for the selective sparing of hemostatic fibrin is proposed.

I. INTRODUCTION

The design of the mutant prourokinase (pro-UK), which is described in this chapter, was based on certain problems and understandings that have emerged in the field of thrombolysis, which will be briefly reviewed. The first problem is that interest in this field is declining. Second, the t-PA paradigm of thrombolysis, which has formed most of our experience, appears to have reached its therapeutic limits. Third, u-PA, which represents a fundamentally different paradigm, has undergone only limited testing. And finally, the pharmacological exploitation of this zymogen–enzyme paradigm of thrombolysis is handicapped by the instability of the zymogen form of u-PA in plasma.

II. THROMBOLYSIS—QUO VADIS?

The leading two causes of death worldwide, according to the World Health Organization (WHO, 1998), are ischemic heart disease and cerebrovascular disease [1]. Because a thrombus triggers about 90% of heart attacks and 80% of strokes, thrombolytic therapy remains a potentially valuable therapeutic option. Moreover, as demographic changes have increased the number of older people, cardiovascular disease has become a leading cause of death, even in developing countries [2]. In addition, thrombolysis is of recognized importance in the treatment of venous thromboembolism and peripheral arterial occlusions.

Despite this large and growing need, there has been a striking diminution of interest in thrombolysis in recent years. This is evident from the decline in publications [3], and most notably, by the fact that primary angioplasty is rapidly replacing thrombolysis as the treatment of choice for acute myocardial infarction (AMI). As a result, the sale of thrombolytic agents has fallen significantly in recent years.

Percutaneous transluminal coronary angioplasty (PTCA; with or without a stent) has been compared with thrombolysis by tissue plasminogen activator (t-PA) or streptokinase (SK) in numerous clinical trials, and the over-all results are favorable for PTCA [4], despite its practical limitations. However, the trend to replace thrombolysis with PTCA for the primary treatment of AMI in most tertiary care centers has created a dilemma that has yet to be solved.

Thrombolysis and PTCA are competitive reperfusion techniques, rather than being complementary. This is because current thrombolytic agents, including SK, t-PA, and mutants of t-PA, are inimical to PTCA. Therefore, there is a problem of what to do for patients with AMI who are awaiting determination of what reperfusion method to use, or who are waiting for the catheterization room to be prepared and the necessary personnel to be assembled. The urgency of the problem was summarized in the journal Lancet [5]: *Right now we are doing nothing at all for our patients in a very crucial hour.* Indeed, the first hour is the time when the results of reperfusion, regardless of the method, are the best. In a study of this problem at three medical centers, substantial treatment delays were documented caused by confusion over which reperfusion treatment to use. It was concluded that this delay was largely responsible for many adverse outcomes [6].

Therefore, a thrombolytic agent that is complementary or synergistic with invasive reperfusion, such as PTCA, would fill a vital need.

III. THROMBOLYSIS: LESSONS FROM PAST EXPERIENCE

A. The t-PA Paradigm

The success of SK in the treatment of AMI refocused attention on the thrombus as being the trigger of most heart attacks, a fact that had been neglected for decades. Since that time, an occlusive thrombus has been the main target of the primary treatment of AMI. However, SK was a suboptimal thrombolytic for three reasons: Its efficacy is limited by an inevitable wholesale consumption of plasminogen; it induces a bleeding diathesis due to its nonspecific mode of action; and it is antigenic.

The development of t-PA, a natural plasminogen activator with strong fibrin-binding and resultant fibrin-specific mode of action, promised to herald a new and much improved era of therapeutic thrombolysis. In addition, because t-PA was thought to be responsible for physiological fibrinolysis, it was a rational choice for development as a therapeutic plasminogen activator. Surprisingly, early clinical experience in AMI with recombinant t-PA revealed limited efficacy at fibrin-specific doses. However, at higher doses, at which fibrin specificity was compromised, coronary artery patency rates with t-PA were almost twice as great as with SK. Therefore, when the first megatrial (GISSI-2) showed no clinical benefit in AMI, compared with SK, it was an inexplicable finding and an unanticipated setback.

All together, three megatrials with t-PA were completed, involving a total of more than 90,000 patients with AMI, who showed either no difference [7,8] or little difference [9] in mortality compared with SK. This discrepancy between the superior coronary patency rates associated with t-PA and the noncorresponding clinical outcome remains a puzzle, and has been referred to as the "t-PA paradox" [3]. This paradox cannot be explained by a higher rate of reocclusion compared with SK [10], and is presumably related to other secondary effects of t-PA [11]. Since the clinical results with t-PA mutants, reteplase, tenecteplase, and lanotaplase, are virtually identical with t-PA [12,13], despite their exceptionally high patency rates, similar adverse secondary effects also appear to accompany these forms of t-PA.

B. The u-PA Paradigm

By contrast to t-PA, u-PA does not bind to fibrin and its physiological role was believed not to be fibrinolysis, but rather to be extravascular plasminogen activation, promoted and targeted by a u-PA receptor found on many cell types. Nevertheless, pro-uPA or pro-UK was capable of clot lysis with a fibrin-specificity comparable with t-PA [14]. The mechanism for this was related to the fact that pro-UK is a zymogen in blood plasma that is activated to UK when it comes in contact with a clot. Its pharmacological properties have undergone relatively limited testing.

Most of the clinical experience has been with *rec.* pro-UK from *E. coli* (saruplase) produced by Grünenthal. The largest clinical trial involved 3089 patients with AMI, randomized to receive either saruplase or SK. The 30-day mortality was 5.7% for saruplase and 6.7% for SK, a difference that did not reach statistical significance. The hemorrhagic stroke rate was similar to that reported for t-PA, being 0.9% for saruplase, compared with 0.3% for SK [15].

All of the clinical trials with saruplase administered the activator at an infusion rate of 80 mg in 60 min. At this dose, most of the pro-UK is converted systemically to UK, and the benefits of the zymogen form are lost, as illustrated in Figure 1. Under these conditions, the clinical results are related more to the effects of high-dose UK, than to pro-UK. Therefore, the stability of the zymogen form of u-PA at pharmacological concentrations is a critical factor for its pharmacological exploitation.

Only two clinical studies involving at least 100 patients with AMI have been published in whom lower infusion rates of pro-UK were used [16,17]. The results were quite promising because exceptionally low mortality, reocclusion, and bleeding rates were found. The findings are in support of the concept that exploitation of the mechanism of action illustrated in Figure 1 (bottom) may give superior clinical results to those obtained when the mechanism illustrated in Figure 1 (top) is used. Nevertheless, there was an average of about 50% fibrinogen degradation in these trials with substantial individual differences, which were unpredictable. Finally, the long-standing belief that the u-PA paradigm of fibrinolysis is responsible mainly for extravascular plasminogen activation is belied by several animal studies. In gene-targeted mice, animals made deficient in u-PA developed some spontaneous intravascular fibrin deposits, whereas those made deficient in t-PA did not [18]. When both activators were absent, severe intravascular thrombosis occurred, indicating that u-PA and t-PA compensate for each other, implying that they are both required for physiological fibrinolysis, but that u-PA may have the dominant role. Similarly, in endotoxin-induced thrombosis in mice, fibrin dissolution correlated with u-PA, rather than t-PA, expression [19]. Spontaneous lysis of vena caval thrombosis in rats was also correlated more with u-PA than with t-PA activity [20], as was also true with the spontaneous lysis of pulmonary emboli in dogs [21].

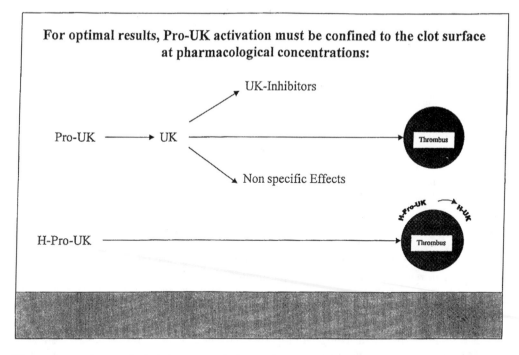

Figure 1 At pharmacological doses, pro-UK is unstable in blood plasma and is subject to activation to UK, which complexes with inhibitors and induces nonspecific plasminogen activation, as illustrated in the top schema. In the physiological mechanism of action, pro-UK activation is limited to the fibrin surface, as illustrated in the bottom schema. The mutant, H-pro-UK, remains stable at pharmacological concentrations, and thereby retains the advantages of efficacy and safety of the physiological mechanism of action of native pro-UK.

Therefore, the biological role of u-PA-mediated plasminogen activation seems to be important for intravascular fibrinolysis, encouraging its testing as a therapeutic agent. However, marshalling its physiological fibrin-targeted properties, which include a hypercatalytic transitional state during its conversion to UK on a fibrin clot [22], requires that it remain stable in blood at pharmacological concentrations.

IV. MUTANT PRO-UK

A. Design

Because limited plasma stability was the property of pro-UK that appeared to limit its pharmacological use, this property was investigated. It was previously found that above a certain concentration in vitro or in vivo, pro-UK is activated to UK in blood plasma. The concentration at which this occurs is quite variable among individuals both in vitro and in vivo. There are probably several plasma factors involved in the stability of pro-UK in this medium, but this subject remains largely unstudied. However, when spontaneous activation occurs, all of the advantages of pro-UK over UK are lost (see Fig. 1).

As previous studies suggested that pro-UK has an exceptionally high intrinsic activity, compared with other zymogens in the serine protease family [23,24], it was postulated that this activity initiated nonspecific plasminogen activation at pharmacological doses. The plasmin that is generated by this reaction then converts pro-UK to UK which, in turn, activates more plasminogen.

The structural basis of this high intrinsic activity was, therefore, investigated and was identified to be related to one charged residue (Lys[300]) [25]. This is situated in a flexible loop region of pro-UK [26]. When this residue is replaced by a neutral hydrophobic amino acid (Ala[300]), about 100-fold reduction in the intrinsic activity of pro-UK occurs. The Ala[300]-pro-UK is stable in plasma at high concentrations (> 50 μg/mL instead of ∼2 μg/mL) [25]. Unfortunately, this mutant has very little fibrinolytic activity in vitro in a plasma milieu.

A series of site-directed mutations at the Lys[300] position, and elsewhere within the flexible loop, were made and characterized [26,27]. Eventually, a Lys[300]→His mutation was found to have both an increased plasma stability and fibrinolytic efficacy in vitro and in vivo.

B. Characterization of His[300] pro-UK (H-pro-UK)

The intrinsic activity of H-pro-UK against amidolytic substrate was fourfold lower than native pro-UK, and the mutant was stable in plasma at a concentration more than fourfold greater than pro-UK. This is illustrated by the experiment shown in Figure 2, in which fibrinogen concentrations were measured after 6 h incubation (37°) of pro-UK or H-pro-UK in citrate or hirudin plasma. Incidentally noted from this experiment was the finding that both pro-UK and H-pro-UK are more stable in hirudin than citrate plasma. This phenomenon has not been explained.

The kinetics of activation of His[300]-pro-UK by plasmin or kallikrein were the same as those of pro-UK. However, the two-chain activity of H-pro-UK (H-UK) against amidolytic

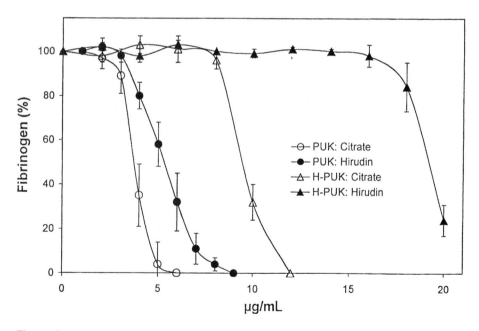

Figure 2 Experiment in which pro-UK (PUK) or H-pro-UK (H-PUK) were incubated (37°C) in citrate or hirudin plasma for 6 h. At the end of this time period, aprotinin was added and the fibrinogen concentration determined and compared with baseline (100%). As shown, in citrate plasma, PUK induced fibrinogen degradation (associated with conversion to UK) at a concentration above 2 μg/mL, and in hirudin plasma, above 3 μg/mL. By contrast, H-PUK remained stable up to 9 μg/mL in citrate and > 16 μg/mL in hirudin plasma. The explanation for the difference between citrate and hirudin plasmas is unknown.

substrate or plasminogen was almost twice that of UK. Consistent with this, the maximum rate of fibrin-specific clot lysis in a plasma milieu by H-pro-UK (calculated from the slope of the clot lysis curves) was 61%/h compared with 41% for pro-UK. Therefore, although the intrinsic activity of H-pro-UK was lower, providing it with significantly greater plasma stability, the two-chain activity of H-UK was significantly greater than UK, making it a more efficient plasminogen activator.

In vivo clot lysis experiments were performed in dogs, an animal for which response to human u-PA is similar to that of man [14]. Radiolabeled clots were made from dog blood and embolized to the lungs and blood samples obtained over time as previously described [14]. The lytic efficacy of H-pro-UK was compared with pro-UK, t-PA, and saline. The pro-UK ($20 \, \mu g/kg \, min^{-1}$) and t-PA ($10 \, \mu g/kg \, min^{-1}$) were administered at a maximum fibrin-specific infusion rate. The H-pro-UK was infused at 20, 40, and $60 \, \mu g/kg \, min^{-1}$ and remained fibrin-specific (no fibrinogen degradation) at the maximum dose. Fifty percent clot lysis occurred in 90 min with pro-UK, compared with 10 min for H-pro-UK at the highest infusion rate. At an infusion rate of $40 \, \mu g/kg \, min^{-1}$, clot lysis by H-pro-UK was comparable with that induced by $20 \, \mu g/kg \, min^{-1}$ of pro-UK [32].

Therefore, H-pro-UK induces far more rapid fibrin-specific clot lysis than is possible with pro-UK or t-PA, but higher infusion rates are required. This is made possible by H-pro-UK, without compromising fibrin specificity, because of its improved plasma stability and the higher catalytic activity of H-UK. Because clot lysis was much more rapid, the total dose of H-pro-UK to achieve 100% clot lysis in the dog was less than that required for pro-UK.

The bleeding time was measured in all of the animals given the maximum dose of H-pro-UK, and the standard dose of t-PA or pro-UK. Measurements were made at 0, 20, and 60 min after the start of the infusion using a standard filter-paper dabbing technique. The bleeding time was measured at the site of a 1-cm^2 skin incision over the abdomen from which the epidermis was peeled off, exposing several superficial vessels of comparable size. One of these was cut at each time point. The bleeding time was 1.2 ± 0.2 at baseline, and 1.2 ± 0.1 at 20 min for saline and H-pro-UK, compared with 2.2 ± 0.15 for t-PA and pro-UK. At 60 min, the bleeding times in the saline and H-pro-UK animals remained unchanged, whereas it went to more than 5 min for t-PA and 4 ± 0.2 min in the pro-UK animals.

Total bleeding was also measured from the number of standard gauze pads totally discolored by blood when placed sequentially on the wound. The number of pads was 1 for the saline animals, 1+ for the H-pro-UK, and 5.5 ± 1 for pro-UK, and 8.25 ± 0.5 for t-PA.

Therefore, in these animals, H-pro-UK induced highly effective clot lysis at a dose that had little apparent effect on hemostasis. This dissociation between thrombolysis and lysis of hemostatic fibrin requires some explanation. For this, the differences between the t-PA and u-PA paradigms of fibrinolysis, and some of the differences between a fibrin thrombus and hemostatic fibrin will be reviewed.

V. TWO PARADIGMS OF FIBRINOLYSIS AND TWO TYPES OF FIBRIN CLOTS

A. Fibrinolysis

The t-PA paradigm of fibrin-mediated plasminogen activation has been defined and well understood for almost 20 years [28]. Its basis is a ternary complex related to the binding of both t-PA and plasminogen to fibrin which substantially facilitates plasminogen activation. The fibrin fragment that promotes plasminogen activation by t-PA is fragment D. This is significant because it is present in intact fibrin. As a result, t-PA-induced clot lysis is not preceded by any lag phase and is little affected by either plasmin or carboxypeptidase pretreatment (to remove carboxy-terminal lysines) of clots [29]. That is to say, t-PA specifically activates the fibrin-bound plasminogen that is present before fibrin degradation commences and new plasminogen binding sites are created.

The u-PA paradigm is quite different and complementary to the foregoing pathway. Aside from the fact that pro-UK does not bind to fibrin and is a zymogen, its fibrinolytic [29] or plasminogen activating activity [30] is promoted by fibrin fragment E. This is generated only after fibrin degradation has been initiated and contains a new plasminogen-binding site consisting of carboxy-terminal lysines [31]. As a result of this mode of action, clot lysis by pro-UK is preceded by a lag phase [14] (the time required to generate fragment E), is promoted by pretreatment of a fibrin clot by plasmin and inhibited by pretreatment with carboxypeptidase [29]. Therefore, pro-UK is inactive against intact fibrin and requires some degradation of the fibrin with formation of new plasminogen binding sites for activity; in direct contrast to t-PA.

B. Hemostatic Fibrin versus a Fibrin Thrombus

Hemostatic fibrin serves the physiological function of sealing leaks in blood vessels and, therefore, has been referred to as "good" fibrin. Because the vasculature, especially in the elderly, is in a state of frequent repair, lysis of "good fibrin" is one of the risks that accompany therapeutic thrombolysis and is largely responsible for a stroke rate of about 1% and an incidence of serious hemorrhage of about 10%.

An important difference between hemostatic fibrin and a fibrin thrombus is that the latter occludes a vessel and induces stasis. This triggers the local release of t-PA from the vessel, and owing to the arrested flow, the t-PA is able to bind to the fibrin clot. As a result, lysis is initiated in the occluding thrombus and new plasminogen-binding sites are created. This concept is illustrated in Figure 3. Plasminogen bound to these new sites is activatable by pro-UK, whereas t-PA will preferentially activate plasminogen on intact fibrin, which also corresponds to hemostatic fibrin. This will not occur at physiological concentrations of t-PA owing to the presence of inhibitors and the protective effect of blood flow. The concept provides a possible explanation for why the intracranial bleeding rate with t-PA is greater than with SK, despite the relative fibrin specificity of the former.

The highly selective activity of pro-UK against partially degraded fibrin versus intact fibrin is dependent on it remaining in the zymogen form in the blood. As noted above, the instability in blood of native pro-UK at pharmacological doses undermines this objective and has limited its therapeutic exploitation. Once pro-UK is activated to UK, its selective mode of action is lost. The design of H-pro-UK was intended to keep this from happening and the results of the experimental animal studies indicate that when this objective is achieved, hemostatic fibrin is protected. A similar dissociation between the lysis of occlusive clots and hemostatic fibrin by H-pro-UK was also found in experiments with rhesus monkeys.

VI. CONCLUSION

Pro-UK induces fibrinolysis according to a paradigm that depends on it remaining in the zymogen form in blood. However, at pharmacological doses, pro-UK is relatively unstable and is converted to UK, a nonspecific plasminogen activator.

H-pro-UK is a site-directed mutant, which differs from pro-UK by 1 residue out of 411. This mutation reduces the intrinsic activity fourfold but increases the two-chain activity almost twofold. The reduced intrinsic activity substantially improves plasma stability and, thereby,

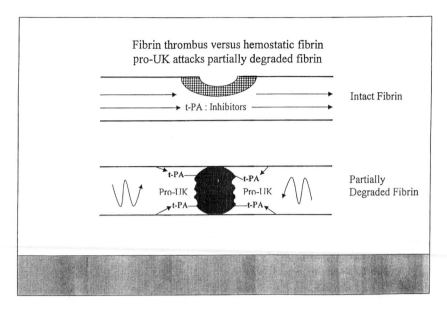

Figure 3 Two vessels are illustrated to provide a hypothesis to explain why H-pro-UK spared hemostatic fibrin at doses that induced effective clot lysis. The hypothesis is based on two principles: the difference between hemostatic fibrin and a fibrin thrombus, and the fact that pro-UK preferentially activates plasminogen bound to partially degraded, rather than to intact fibrin [29,30]. Hemostatic fibrin seals a vessel (top), remains intact because it is non-occlusive, and does not interrupt blood flow (straight arrows). By contrast, a fibrin thrombus (bottom) is occlusive, interrupts blood flow (wavy arrows), and induces the local release of t-PA from the vessel wall, which binds to the fibrin and initiates its degradation, as illustrated by the serrated edges. As a result, new plasminogen-binding sites are exposed. Plasminogen bound to these sites is selectively activated by pro-UK. Since H-pro-UK is a more stable form of pro-UK, it can exploit the natural selective activation of plasminogen on a thrombus over that on intact (hemostatic) fibrin of pro-UK at thrombolytic doses.

allows the physiological, fibrin-dependent properties of pro-UK to be better exploited at the pharmacological concentrations required for effective clot lysis.

One of these physiological properties is that pro-UK is relatively inactive against plasminogen bound to intact fibrin, and instead preferentially lyses partially degraded fibrin. Because hemostatic fibrin generally remains intact, it is resistant to degradation by low-dose pro-UK or pharmacological doses of H-pro-UK. At doses of H-pro-UK which induced highly effective clot lysis, hemostatic fibrin is not significantly affected. The bleeding time and blood loss from a standard wound were no different from that in the placebo animals, in contrast to those treated with pro-UK or t-PA.

REFERENCES

1. Balter M. AIDS now the world's fourth biggest killer [News of the Week] (article). Science 1999; 284:1101.
2. The hidden epidemic of cardiovascular disease [unsigned editorial]. Lancet 1998; 352:1795.
3. Gurewich V. Fibrinolysis: an unfinished agenda. Blood Coagul Fibrinol 2000; 11:401–407.
4. Weaver WD, Simes RJ, Betriu A, Grines CL, Zijlstra F, Garcia E, Grinfeld L, Gibbons RJ, Ribeiro EE, DeWood MA, Ribichini F. Comparison of primary coronary angioplasty and intravenous thrombolytic therapy for acute myocardial infarction. JAMA 1997; 278:2093–2098.

5. Lancet 1998; 351:421. [News].
6. Liu J, Gurewich V. A comparative study of the promotion of tissue plasminogen activator and pro-urokinase-induced plasminogen activation by fragments D and E-2 of fibrin. J Clin Invest 1991; 88:2012–2017.
7. Gruppo Italiano per lo studio della Sopravvivenza nell'Infarto miocardico. GISSI-2 a factorial randomised trial of alteplase versus no heparin among 12,490 patients with acute myocardial infarction. Lancet 1990; 336:65–71.
8. ISIS-3 (Third International Study of Infarct Survival Collaborative Group). ISIS-3; a randomised comparison of streptokinase versus anistreplase and of aspirin and heparin versus heparin alone among 41,299 cases of suspected acute myocardial infarction. Lancet 1992; 339:753–770.
9. Topol E, the GUSTO Investigators. An international randomized trial comparing four thrombolytic strategies for acute myocardial infarction. N Engl J Med 1993; 329:673–682.
10. Reiner JS, Lundergan CF, van den Brand M, the GUSTO Angiographic Investigators. Early angiography cannot predict postthrombolytic coronary reocclusion: observations from the GUSTO angiographic study. J Am Coll Cardiol 1994; 24:1439–1444.
11. Gurewich V, Muller J. Is coronary thrombolysis associated with side effects which significantly compromise clinical benefits? Am J Cardiol 1996; 77:756–758.
12. The Global Use of Strategies to Open Occluded Coronary Arteries (GUSTO III) Investigators. A comparison of reteplase with alteplase for acute myocardial infarction. N Engl J Med 1997; 337:1118–1123.
13. ASSENT-2 Investigators. Single-bolus tenecteplase compared with front-loaded alteplase in acute myocardial infarction: the ASSENT-2 double-blind randomised trial. Lancet 1999; 354: 716–722.
14. Gurewich V, Pannell R, Louie S, Kelley P, Suddith RL, Greenlee R. Effective and fibrin-specific clot lysis by a zymogen precursor form of urokinase (pro-urokinase). A study in vitro and in two animal species. J Clin Invest 1984; 73:1731–1739.
15. Tebbe U, Michels R, Adgey J, Boland J, Caspi A, Charbonnier B, Windeler J, Barth H, Groves R, Hopkins GR, Fennell W, Betriu A, Ruda M, Mlczoch J. Randomised, double-blind study comparing saruplase with streptokinase therapy in acute myocardial infarction: the COMPASS equivalence trial. J Am Coll Cardiol 1998; 31:487–493.
16. Zarich SW, Kowalchuk GJ, Weaver WD, Loscalzo J, Sassower M, Manzo K, Byrnes C, Muller JE, Gurewich V for the PATENT Study Group. Sequential combination thrombolytic therapy for acute myocardial infarction: results of the pro-urokinase and t-PA enhancement of thrombolysis (PATENT) trial. J Am Coll Cardiol 1995; 26:374–379.
17. Weaver WD, Hartmann JR, Anderson JL, Redd PS, Sobolski JC, Sasahara AA. New recombinant glycosylated pro-urokinase for treatment of patients with acute myocardial infarction. J Am Coll Cardiol 1994; 24:1242–1248.
18. Carmeliet P, Schoonjan L, Kiecken L, Ream B, Degen J, Bronson R, DeVos R, van den Oord JJ, Collen D, Mulligan RC. Physiological consequences of loss of plasminogen activator gene function in mice. Nature 1994; 368:419–424.
19. Yamamoto K, Loskutoff DJ. Fibrin deposition in tissue from endotoxin-treated mice correlates with decreases in the expression of urokinase-type but not tissue-type plasminogen activator. J Clin Invest 1996; 97:2440–2451.
20. Northeast ADR, Soo KS, Bobrow LG, Gaffney PH, Burnand KG. The tissue plasminogen activator and urokinase response in vivo during natural resolution of venous thrombus. J Vasc Surg 1995; 22:573–579.
21. Lang IM, Marsh JJ, Konopka RG, Olman MA, Binder BR, Moser KM, Schleef RR. Factors contributing to increased vascular fibrinolytic activity in mongrel dogs. Circulation 1993; 87:1990–2000.
22. Liu J, Pannell R, Gurewich V. A transitional state of pro-urokinase which has a higher catalytic efficiency against Glu-plasminogen than urokinase. J Biol Chem 1991; 267:15289–15292.
23. Pannell R, Gurewich V. The activation of plasminogen by single-chain urokinase or by two-chain urokinase—a demonstration that single chain urokinase has a low catalytic activity (pro-urokinase). Blood 1987; 69:22–26.

24. Gurewich V. Pannell R, Broeze RJ, Mao JI. Characterization of the intrinsic fibrinolytic properties of pro-urokinase through a study of plasmin resistant mutant forms produced by site specific mutagenesis of lysine 158. J Clin Invest 1988; 82:1956–1962.
25. Liu JN, Tang W, Sun ZY, Kung W, Pannell R, Sarmientos P, Gurewich V. A site-directed mutagenesis of pro-urokinase which substantially reduces its intrinsic activity. Biochemistry 1996; 35:14070–14076.
26. Sun Z, Jiang Y, Ma Z, Wu H, Liu BF, Xu Y, Tang W, Chen Y, Li C, Zhu D, Gurewich V, Liu J. Identification of flexible loop (297–313) of urokinase-type plasminogen activator, which helps determine its catalytic activity. J Biol Chem 1997; 272:2318–23823.
27. Sun Z, Lui BF, Chen Y, Gurewich V, Zhu D, Liu J. Analysis of the forces which stabilize the active conformation of urokinase-type plasminogen activator. Biochemistry 1998; 37:2935–2940.
28. Hoylaerts M, Rijken DC, Lijnen DC, Collen D. Kinetics of the activation of plasminogen by human tissue plasminogen activator. J Biol Chem 1982; 257:2912–2919.
29. Pannell R, Black J, Gurewich V. The complementary modes of action of tissue plasminogen activator (t-PA) and pro-urokinase (pro-UK) by which their synergistic effect on clot lysis may be explained. J Clin Invest 1988; 81:853–859.
30. Liu J, Gurewich V. A comparative study of the promotion of tissue plasminogen activator and pro-urokinase-induced plasminogen activation by fragments D and E-2 of fibrin. J Clin Invest 1991; 88:2012–2017.
31. Harpel PC, Chang TS, Verderber E. Tissue plasminogen activator and urokinase mediate the binding of *glu*-plasminogen to plasma fibrin I. Evidence for new binding sites in plasmin-degraded fibrin I. J Biol Chem 1985; 260:4432–4440.
32. Liu JN, Liu JX, Liu BF, Sun Z, Zuo JL, Zhang P, Zhang J, Chen Y, Gurewich V. Circ Res 2002; 90: 757–763.

37

Recombinant Staphylokinase for Thrombolytic Therapy

Peter Sinnaeve, H. Roger Lijnen, and Désiré Collen
Catholic University of Leuven, Leuven, Belgium

SUMMARY

Staphylokinase (Sak), a bacterial profibrinolytic agent, readily available by recombinant DNA technology, is a 136-amino–acid, single-chained polypeptide, with a unique structure and mechanism of action and of fibrin specificity. Preclinical investigations disclosed attractive characteristics, including high-thrombolytic potency, also toward platelet-rich thrombi and fibrin specificity in human plasma.

A randomized multicenter trial in 100 patients with acute myocardial infarction demonstrated that, relative to accelerated alteplase (recombinant–tissue-type plasminogen activator; rt-PA), Sak was significantly more fibrin-specific and at least as efficient: 20 mg Sak over 30 min, the dose tested in the second half of this trial, induced optimal coronary reperfusion (TIMI perfusion grade 3) in 74% of 23 patients (versus 58% of 52 patients treated with accelerated alteplase). Surprisingly, a survival advantage was found in favor of Sak in this small-scaled study.

In an open-label, angiographically controlled, dose-finding study, patients (≤ 80 years), with an acute myocardia insufficiency (AMI) within 6 h of symptom onset, received Sak (wild-type variant Sak42D) as a bolus, followed by an intravenous infusion over a 30-min period. Three incremental doses of Sak were studied: 15 mg ($n = 21$); 30 mg ($n = 31$); and 45 mg ($n = 30$). Surprisingly, there was no difference in TIMI 3 patency rates between the three doses given (62, 65, and 63%, respectively). Four patients had a major bleeding, nine had a minor bleeding, but there was no relation between dose of Sak and the extent of bleeding. Sak did not significantly affect plasma fibrinogen and plasminogen levels irrespective of the dose, confirming its fibrin-selectivity.

In patients with peripheral arterial occlusion (PAO), the recanalization rate and speed in 191 patients with angiographically documented PAO was studied following intra-arterial, catheter-directed Sak, given as a 2-mg bolus, followed by a 1-mg/h continuous infusion. Sak compared favorably with data reported for established thrombolytic agents: after 12 ± 1-mg Sak infused over 14 ± 0.7 h, recanalization was complete in 158 (83%) patients, partial in 24 (13%) patients, but failed completely in 7 (4%) patients.

Also, in six patients with severe clinical symptoms of acute deep venous thrombosis, confirmed by duplex ultrasound and extending at least into the common iliac vein, catheter-directed Sak (wild-type Sak42D) was administered directly into the thrombus as a 2-mg bolus followed by a 1-mg/h continuous infusion until patency was obtained. In four patients, subsequent 0.5 mg/h was given to clear any remaining clot. Complete lysis at the end of the treatment, as revealed by venography, was obtained in five patients.

A disadvantage of Sak is its antigenicity. Neutralizing antibody titers are low at baseline and during the first week after administration, but they increase steeply and remain elevated thereafter, precluding repeated use. Surprisingly, however, the antigenicity of Sak in laboratory animals and patients could be significantly attenuated, while preserving thrombolytic potential, by replacing selected clusters of charged amino acids by alanine.

In conclusion, presumably by virtue of a specificity for fibrin that exceeds by far that of any other approved plasminogen activator, Sak represents a potent thrombolytic agent in patients with arterial occlusive thrombosis or deep venous thrombosis. The initial clinical experience to date using single-bolus PEGylated Sak with prolonged half-life is encouraging, but still needs to be expanded to determine the optimal dose. Also, the optimal conjunctive antithrombotic therapy, the value in the treatment of other thromboembolic disorders and, ultimately, the merits in terms of safety and survival relative to both established and new thrombolytics remains to be established.

I. INTRODUCTION

Although thrombolytic therapy has markedly reduced mortality following acute myocardial infarction (MI) [1] and is gaining increasing acceptance for the treatment of various other thromboembolic disorders (including deep venous thrombosis, pulmonary embolism, and peripheral arterial occlusive disease) [2,3], the optimal thrombolytic strategy is yet to be realized [4]. Indeed, failed, suboptimal or delayed thrombus dissolution and reocclusion frequently prevent appreciable tissue preservation [5]. Because of an inherent bleeding risk, the therapeutic window of thrombolytics is relatively small and may be further narrowed by the conjunctive use of powerful antiplatelet and anticoagulant drugs. These general shortcomings and other disadvantages, particular to certain agents (including the high cost for recombinant tissue-type plasminogen activator [rt-PA], acute hypotension, and allergic reactions with streptokinase [SK] and derivatives, and lack of fibrin selectivity with SK and urokinase), inspire the search for newer and better fibrinolytic agents [6]. In this perspective a new light has been shed on an old (pro)fibrinolytic agent: staphylokinase (Sak).

II. HISTORICAL OVERVIEW

Already in 1908, H. Much reported that *Staphylococcus aureus* contained a clot-dissolving compound that he named staphylokinase (Sak) [7]. In their classic paper on SK, W. S. Tillett and R. L. Garner also mentioned the ability of staphylococcal strains to liquefy coagulated plasma [8]. In 1948, C. H. Lack disclosed that Sak does not lyse fibrin directly, but rather, it acts as a plasminogen activator [9].

Two observations may explain the delay in the development of Sak as a thrombolytic agent. First, in spite of its thrombolytic potency, the potential of Sak as a drug and notably the feasibility of standard dosing, were questioned in view of a wide range of inhibitor activity, presumed to be antibody-related, in the serum of a population sample [10]. Second, Sak administration to dogs induced massive bleeding with a high fatality rate [11]. In retrospect, the choice of the dog for these first animal experiments may have been unfortunate because Sak in this species, in contrast to most other species studied, lacks fibrin specificity [12].

The notion that thrombolytic strategies need to be optimized to attain their full therapeutic potential, on the one hand, and reappraisal of promising physicochemical characteristics of Sak and novel efficient production methods, on the other hand, have recently fueled renewed interest in this bacterial plasminogen activator.

III. STRUCTURE AND PRODUCTION OF STAPHYLOKINASE

Sak is a 136-amino–acid protein (comprising 45 charged amino acids) secreted by *S. aureus* strains after lysogenic conversion or transformation with bacteriophages. The primary structure of Sak shows no homology with that of other plasminogen activators (Fig. 1). Four natural variants that have been characterized (Sak42D, SakϕC, SakSTAR, and ATCC 29213 Sak), which differ at amino acid positions 33, 34, 36, and 43 of the mature protein only (Fig. 2) and have a very similar plasminogen-activating potential [13–16].

Staphylokinase folds into a compact ellipsoidal structure in which the core of the protein is composed exclusively of hydrophobic amino acids. It is folded into a mixed five-stranded, slightly twisted β-sheet that wraps around a central α-helix and has two additional short two-stranded β-sheets opposing the central sheet [17].

The purification of Sak from selected *S. aureus* strains for in vivo use has been disappointing because of low expression and concomitant secretion of potent exotoxins. Recently, large quantities of two variants of wild-type Sak (variants SakSTAR and Sak42D) have become available by introducing recombinant plasmids into *Escherichia coli* that subsequently produce intracellular Sak, up to 10–15% of total cell protein [18]. This material, after purification, allowed extended preclinical and early clinical evaluation.

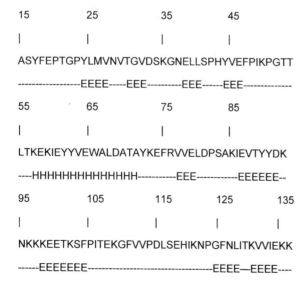

```
15          25          35          45

|           |           |           |

ASYFEPTGPYLMVNVTGVDSKGNELLSPHYVEFPIKPGTT

-----------------EEEE-----EEE----------EEE------EEE-------------

55          65          75          85

|           |           |           |

LTKEKIEYYVEWALDATAYKEFRVVELDPSAKIEVTYYDK

----HHHHHHHHHHHHHHH-----------EEE------------EEEEEE--

95          105         115         125         135

|           |           |           |           |

NKKKEETKSFPITEKGFVVPDLSEHIKNPGFNLITKVVIEKK

------EEEEEEE-----------------------------EEEE—EEEE----
```

Figure 1 Primary and secondary structure of staphylokinase: the amino acids are represented by their single-letter symbols: (E) indicates extended β-sheet; (H) indicates α-helix; (-) indicates random coil. For the 15-NH$_2$-terminal amino acids, no structural data are available.

NH2-Ser...	...33.....	..34.....	...36......	..43... ..Lys-COOH
Sak42D	Asp	Gly	Arg	Arg
SakΦC	Asp	Gly	Gly	His
SakSTAR	Asp	Ser	Gly	His
ATCC29213	Glu	Gly	Glu	His

Figure 2 Amino acid differences between four natural staphylokinase variants (Sak42D, SakφC, SakSTAR, and ATCC 29213Sak).

IV. MECHANISM OF FIBRIN SPECIFICITY

The mechanism of action and of fibrin specificity were elucidated to a large extent [see Refs. 19 and 20 for review]. Staphylokinase forms a 1 : 1 stoichiometric complex with plasmin(ogen). It is not an enzyme, and generation of an active site in its equimolar complex with plasminogen requires conversion of plasminogen to plasmin. In plasma, in the absence of fibrin, no significant amounts of plasmin–staphylokinase complex are generated because traces of plasmin are inhibited by α_2-antiplasmin. In the presence of fibrin, generation of the active complex is facilitated because traces of fibrin-bound plasmin are protected from α_2-antiplasmin, and inhibition of the complex by α_2-antiplasmin at the clot surface is delayed more than 100-fold. Furthermore, staphylokinase does not bind to a significant extent to plasminogen in circulating plasma, but binds with high affinity to plasmin and to plasminogen, which is bound to partially degraded fibrin. Recently, biochemical studies with highly purified recombinant Sak, initial experiments in animal models of thrombosis, and pilot studies in patients with acute myocardial infarction or peripheral arterial occlusion, have revealed that Sak is an efficient, highly fibrin-specific plasminogen activator [19,20].

V. CLINICALLY ATTRACTIVE CHARACTERISTICS SUGGESTED BY PRECLINICAL EXPERIMENTS

Extensive in vitro and laboratory animal experiments [reviewed in Refs. 19 and 20] demonstrated that in most species studied, Sak is a potent and rapidly acting plasminogen activator. As SK and Sak have functional similarities, yet also important differences, preclinical studies frequently compared these indirect plasminogen activators of bacterial origin. In human plasma, Sak, but not SK, proved to be extremely fibrin-specific. On a theoretical basis, fibrin specificity may improve efficacy and safety of thrombolytic therapy: the "plasminogen-steal" phenomenon and plasminemia-induced paradoxic prothrombotic effects are avoided, which may ameliorate efficacy; a "systemic plasminolytic state," and the resulting hemostatic perturbations are prevented, which may benefit safety. Also the ease of administration may improve: a high affinity for fibrin prolongs the biological half-life beyond the plasma half-life and thus may allow bolus administration even for fibrin-specific agents with a short circulatory half-life. These postulated advantages of fibrin specificity await thorough clinical validation.

In contrast with SK, Sak efficiently lysed not only platelet-poor but also platelet-rich plasma clots [21]. Retracted and mechanically compressed plasma clots were also sensitive to lysis with Sak but not with SK. This differential lysability may be explained by the expulsion of clot-associated plasminogen following retraction or compression. In contrast with non–fibrin-specific plasminogen activators, fibrin-specific agents, such as Sak, spare circulating plasmino-gen that can be recruited into the thrombus and subsequently be activated [21]. These properties may be clinically important because platelets contribute largely to reocclusion and because high platelet content of a clot, together with thrombus retraction and ageing, limits the thrombolytic efficacy of conventional agents. Clinically relevant doses of Sak did not affect platelet function [22]. In rabbits, Sak, in contrast with rt-PA, did not prolong surface-bleeding times unless aspirin and heparin were added [23]. In the cuticle-bleeding–time model, the lesser hemorrhagenic effect of Sak could be attributed to its fibrinogen-sparing potential.

Relative to SK, Sak appeared to be equally sensitive to inhibition with aprotinin, but considerably more sensitive to the antifibrinolytic effects of tranexamic acid in a hamster pulmonary embolism model [24]. The higher antifibrinolytic potency of tranexamic acid (which prevents binding of plasminogen to fibrin) toward Sak than toward SK is most likely related to the requirement of fibrin-bound plasminogen for efficient fibrinolysis with Sak.

The immunogenicity of SK and Sak (SakSTAR variant) was compared in a dog [25] and in a baboon [26] extracorporeal thrombosis model. Serial administration of SK induced rapidly increasing IgG-related SK-neutralizing activities in plasma and a progressive resistance to clot lysis in both species, and severe hypotensive reactions especially in baboons. With Sak, induction of Sak-neutralizing activities was less consistent and thrombolytic potency was relatively maintained while no acute hypotension occurred.

Recent improvements in thrombolytic treatment regimens include the development of fibrin-selective agents that can be administered as a single bolus [27]. Derivatization of proteins with polyethylene glycol (PEG) reduces plasma clearance and immunogenicity. Consequently, PEGylation of Sak might lead to variants with reduced half-life that are less immunogenic. Two Sak variant with reduced immunogenicity and conserved thrombolytic property (SakSTAR SY160 [K35A, E65Q, K74R, E80A, D82,A, T90A, E99D, T101S, E108A, K109A, K130T, K135R], or SakSTAR SY161 [K35A, E65Q, K74Q, E80A, D82,A, T90A, E99D, T101S, E108A, K109A, K130T, K135R]) have been derivatized with maleimide-polyethylene glycol (PEG) to reduce its clearance [27]. PEG side chains with an M_r of 5 (P5), 10 (P10), or 20 (P20) kDa were chemically linked to a thiol on cysteine, replacing a serine residue in position 3. Dose- and time-dependent lysis of ^{125}I-fibrin-labeled human plasma clots submerged in human plasma was equally effective compared with wild-type SakSTAR. The clearance of these PEGylated variants in hamsters and rabbits were inversely proportional to the molecular weights of the PEG side chains: a reduction of 2.5 times for P5, 5 times for P10, and 20 times for P20, respectively. In a hamster model of pulmonary embolism, PEGylated SakSTAR variants induced dose-related clot lysis with C_{50} values (causing 50% clot lysis in 2 h) inversely proportional to the size of the PEG molecules, without significant change in fibrinogen and α_2-antiplasmin levels.

Thus, promising properties of Sak, deduced from in vitro and laboratory animal experi-ments, included high thrombolytic efficacy, also toward platelet-rich and retracted thrombi, rapid onset of action, remarkable fibrin specificity, low bleeding risk, high sensitivity to inhibition by antifibrinolytic agents, and reduced antigenicity and allergenicity relative to SK. Furthermore, the prolonged plasma half-life of SakSTAR derivatized with maleimide polyethylene-glycol (MPG) promises new perspectives for single-bolus administration of SakSTAR variants in patients with acute myocardial infarction.

VI. CLINICAL EXPERIENCE WITH RECOMBINANT STAPHYLOKINASE

A. Acute Myocardial Infarction

In a first pilot recanalization study, ten patients with angiographically confirmed infarct-related artery occlusion (TIMI grade 0 flow) were treated with 10-mg-intravenous Sak (variant SakSTAR), given as a 1-mg bolus, followed by infusion of 9 mg over 30 min [28,29]. Angiography was repeated every 10 min for up to 40 min. Within 40 min all but one of the occluded coronary arteries were recanalized (TIMI grade 3 flow in eight and TIMI grade 2 flow in one patient). The mean (±SEM) time delay to reperfusion in recanalized arteries, 20 ± 4.0 min, compared favorably with the 45-min, or more, delays reported for rt-PA and SK [30]. Plasma levels of fibrinogen, plasminogen, and α_2-antiplasmin did not decrease. Sak antigen disappeared from plasma with a mean initial half-life of 6.3 min and a terminal half-life of 37 min [28]. Thus, Sak was able to induce rapid and sustained restoration of normal coronary artery flow at a dose that did not induce a systemic lytic state.

Subsequently, a multicenter randomized trial ("STAR trial") compared the effects of Sak versus the present standard regimen, accelerated and weight-adjusted rt-PA, on early coronary artery patency in 100 patients with acute MI [31]. Patients randomized to intravenous Sak were given 10 mg over 30 min, as in the pilot trial, and 20 mg, over 30 min, in the second half, always with an initial 10% bolus. The primary study endpoint, TIMI perfusion grade 3 at 90 min, was reached in 58% of patients treated with rt-PA ($n = 52$) and in 62% of patients treated with Sak ($n = 48$) (in 50% after 10 mg Sak ($n = 25$) and in 74% after 20 mg Sak ($n = 23$)). Although 20 mg of Sak produced the greatest recanalization benefit, the differences in 90-min coronary artery patency between groups (rt-PA, 10 and 20 mg Sak) were not statistically significant, probably because of the small numbers of patients. Again, Sak proved to be highly fibrin-specific, preserving plasma fibrinogen, plasminogen, and α_2-antiplasmin levels after infusions of 10, 20, and also of 40-mg Sak in five additional MI patients, whereas rt-PA caused a very significant drop of fibrinogen (mean decrease versus pretreatment of 30% at 90 min) and of plasminogen and α_2-antiplasmin (mean decreases of 60% at 90 min). The frequencies of hemorrhagic, thrombotic, electrical, mechanical, or allergic complications and of nonpharmacological reperfusion procedures following Sak and rt-PA were comparable. However, all five in-hospital deaths, all caused by early cardiogenic shock, appeared in the cohort randomized to rt-PA, resulting in an unexpected, and possibly coincidental, borderline significant mortality difference in favor of Sak ($0.25 < p < 0.05$). Thus, relative to accelerated rt-PA, Sak was significantly more fibrin-specific and induced early, stable, and complete patency of the infarct-related vessel at least as frequently, especially at a 20-mg dose without apparent excess acute toxicity.

To establish the optimal dose of Sak required to achieve TIMI-3 flow at 90 min within an acceptable safety profile, the CAPTORS trial (Collaborative Angiographic Patency Trial of Recombinant Staphylokinase) was initiated [32]. In this open-label angiographically controlled, dose-finding study, patients (80 years, or younger) with an AMI within 6 h of symptom onset received Sak (Sak42D) as a bolus (20% of total dose) followed by an intravenous infusion over a 30-min period. Three incremental doses of Sak were studied: 15 mg ($n = 21$), 30 mg ($n = 31$), and 45 mg ($n = 30$). Surprisingly, there was no difference in TIMI-3 patency rates between the three doses given (62, 65, and 63%, respectively). Four patients had a major bleeding, nine had a minor bleeding, but none had intracranial hemorrhage. There was no relation between the dose of Sak and the extent of bleeding. No patients experienced allergic reactions. Two patients died; one because of a cardiogenic shock in association with severe puncture site bleeding, and a second one because of a cardiogenic shock after the 90-min angiogram. Sak did not significantly affect plasma fibrinogen and plasminogen levels irrespective of the dose. α_2-Antiplasmin levels, however, showed a borderline significant reduction by dose ($p = 0.053$).

A second multicenter randomized trial compared the effects of double-bolus Sak administration versus the accelerated and weight-adjusted rt-PA, on early coronary artery patency in 102 patients with acute MI [33]. Patients randomized to double-bolus Sak ($n = 50$) were given 15 mg over 5 min, with a second bolus of 15 mg, 30 min later. Of the patients receiving double-bolus Sak, 68% had a TIMI-3 flow after 90 min, versus 57% after rt-PA administration (RR 1.3, 95% CI 0.8 to 2.0; $p = 0.3$). At 24 h, TIMI perfusion grade 3 rates were 100% in the Sak group, and 79% in the rTPA-treated group ($p = 0.005$). This difference at 24 h is possibly related to the low procoagulant and proaggregatory side effects of Sak [34]. The rates of hemorrhagic, mechanical, and electrical complications did not significantly differ between treatment groups. Double-bolus administration of Sak also preserved plasma fibrinogen and plasminogen levels, whereas α_2-antiplasmin levels had marginally, but significantly, decreased (91% of pretreatment) values. In contrast, rt-PA caused a significant drop of fibrinogen (mean decrease versus pretreatment of 30% at 90 min) and of plasminogen and α_2-antiplasmin (mean decreases of 54 and 56% at 90 min, respectively, $p < 0.0001$ vs. Sak).

Single-bolus administration has become a preferred regimen for treatment with thrombolytic agents. Two Sak variants with reduced immunogenicity and conserved thrombolytic potential (Sak SY160 and SY161) have been derivatized with maleimide-polyethylene glycol (PEG) to reduce the clearance [27]. The PEG side chain was chemically linked to a thiol on cysteine replacing a serine residue in position 3. These PEGylated variants detected only one-third of the antibodies generated by wild-type Sak in patients with acute myocardial infarction. Clearance of SakSTAR variants derivatized with PEG with an M_r of 5000 (P5), 10,000 (P10), or 20,000 (P20) after single-bolus administration in patients with evolving AMI was 2.5- to 5-fold, 5- to 20-fold, or 20-fold reduced compared with wild-type Sak [27]. Fourteen of the 18 patients who received an intravenous bolus of a reduced dose of 5 mg SakSTAR-P5 had TIMI grade 3 at 60 min (78, 95%; CI 55–91%). Of these 14 patients, 13 had a corrected TIMI frame count of ≤ 30 (20 ± 6). Eleven additional patients received a 2.5-mg bolus of SakSTAR-P5, resulting in TIMI grade 3 flow in seven patients at 60 min (63, 95%; CI 35–85%). Treatment-related complications included a Mallory–Weiss bleeding in a patient also receiving abciximab after PTCA at 60 min, and a large puncture-site hematoma requiring transfusion in a second patient. There were no allergic reactions or hemodynamic problems. Fibrinogen, plasminogen and α_2-antiplasmin remained unchanged at 60 min in patients receiving both 2.5 and 5 mg SakSTAR-P5, indicating a high-fibrin selectivity. These results show that single-bolus administration of low-dose PEGylated Sak is both safe and effective in the treatment of patients with AMI. Subsequently, an ongoing angiographic-controlled dose-finding trial (CAPTORS II) using single bolus PEGylated Sak will determine the optimal dose and safety profile.

From these studies it is concluded that Sak is a potent, rapidly acting and very fibrin-specific thrombolytic agent in MI patients. Its fibrin specificity, safety, and efficacy for coronary thrombolysis appear to compare well with these of the present gold standard: accelerated rt-PA. Initial studies on single-bolus PEGylated Sak administration have yielded encouraging results, and further studies to determine the optimal dose are currently being undertaken. However, the relative benefit of PEGylated Sak versus plasminogen activators in current clinical (or experimental) use in terms of reduction of MI-associated mortality and morbidity, awaits larger comparative clinical trials.

B. Peripheral Arterial Occlusion

Thirty patients (37–86 years of age) with limb ischemia or incapacitating claudication of less than 120 days duration and with angiographically documented thromboembolic peripheral arterial occlusion (PAO), mostly owing to in situ thrombosis of native femoropopliteal arteries, were treated in a pilot study [35]. Intra-arterial, catheter-directed Sak was given as a bolus of 1 mg, followed by a continuous infusion of 0.5 mg/h in 20 patients and as a bolus of 2 mg, followed by an infusion of 1 mg/h in 10 patients, together with heparin. After 7.0 ± 0.7 mg Sak, infused over 8.7 ± 1.0 h, recanalization was complete in 25 patients (83%), partial in 2, and absent in 3. Bad prognostic signs (including poor distal run-off, long duration, and distal localization of occlusion) characterized the three PAOs without macroscopic clot lysis.

These promising results prompted administration of Sak to 191 subsequent patients with angiographically documented PAO [36]. Intra-arterial, catheter-directed Sak was given as a bolus of 2 mg, followed by a continuous infusion of 1 mg/h, together with heparin at 1000 U/h. After 12 ± 1 mg Sak infused over 14 ± 0.7 h, recanalization was complete in 158 (83%), partial in 24 (13%), but failed completely in 7 (4%) patients. No difference in patency rates was observed between patients with symptom duration of 14 days or less or more than 14 days before enrollment. Complete lysis was achieved less frequently when acute occlusions (14 days or less) of native arteries occurred at popliteal level or lower (60%) as compared with more proximal occlusions (95%). Thrombolysis alone was sufficient in 61 (32%) patients, but other patients underwent either angioplasty and stenting (47%), bypass surgery (24%), or surgical thrombectomy (4%). Major hemorrhagic complications occurred in 23 (12%) patients, and included intracranial hemorrhage in 4 patients and severe puncture site hematoma requiring transfusion in 15 patients, and low gastrointestinal bleeding in 4 patients. Two patients developed an allergic reaction with severe hypotension within 15 min of onset of Sak infusion. Circulating fibrinogen remained unchanged during Sak therapy, but plasminogen and α_2-antiplasmin were marginally (10%), but significantly, lower after infusion. Ten patients died within the first year after treatment, and 16 amputations were performed in 162 patients who were followed for 1 year.

Thus, Sak appeared a valuable adjunct to endovascular and surgical revascularization techniques, with rapid and efficient restoration of vessel patency and of limb viability in the great majority of patients with acute to subacute PAO.

C. Deep-Venous Thrombosis

Six patients with severe clinical symptoms of acute deep-venous thrombosis, confirmed by duplex ultrasound and extending at least into the common iliac vein, received catheter-directed Sak [37]. Wild-type Sak42D was administered directly into the thrombus as a 2-mg bolus, followed by a 1-mg/h continuous infusion until patency was obtained. In four patients, subsequent 0.5 mg/h was given to clear any remaining clot. Concomitant heparin was given at 1000 U/h to achieve an aPTT prolongation of 1.5–2.5 times the control value. Complete lysis at the end of the treatment, as revealed by venography was obtained in five patients. In the sixth patient, patency was restored, and residual mural thrombus resistant to lysis with Sak was treated by stenting. Rethrombosis within 24 h in this patient was successfully treated with a rotating impeller followed by an infusion of r-tPA for 5 h. Again, treatment with Sak did not significantly alter fibrinogen, plasminogen or α_2-antiplasmin levels, despite prolonged infusion. Complications consisted of minor puncture site hematomas in four patients and a mild transient epistaxis in one of them. These results suggest that catheter-directed infusion of Sak is an effective and safe treatment in patients with extensive deep-venous thrombosis.

VII. ANTIGENICITY OF STAPHYLOKINASE AND ENGINEERED VARIANTS

The rather low-grade antigenicity of Sak, as suggested by early dog and baboon experiments, unfortunately could not be extended to patients: the vast majority of patients with either MI [31] or PAO [36] developed neutralizing antibodies to Sak, albeit after a long lag phase of 10–12 days, that remained elevated well above pretreatment levels for several months after administration [38]. However, the titers of preformed anti-Sak antibodies in the general population appeared to be lower than those of anti-SK antibodies and even systemic *S. aureus* infections failed to induce Sak-neutralizing antibodies in most patients, possibly reflecting the low proportion of *S. aureus* strains that produce Sak [39]. The current clinical experience suggest that major allergic reactions to Sak are rare. However, the boost of neutralizing antibody titers, on infusion of Sak, predicts therapeutic refractoriness on repeated administration. Therefore, the restriction to single-use applies probably to both SK and Sak. The absence of cross-reactivity to SK of antibodies elicited by Sak, and vice versa, suggests that the consecutive use of both plasminogen activators is not mutually exclusive.

Wild-type Sak contains three nonoverlapping immunodominant epitopes, at least two of which could be eliminated, albeit with partial inactivation of the molecule, by site-directed mutagenesis to alanine for selected clusters of two or three charged amino acids [40–42]. The recombinant combination mutants SakSTAR.M38 (with Lys35, Glu38, Lys74, Glu75, and Arg77, replaced by Ala) and SakSTAR.M89 (with Lys74, Glu75, Arg77, Glu80, and Asp82, replaced by Ala) had a reduced immunoreactivity toward a panel of murine monoclonal anti-SakSTAR antibodies and toward antibodies elicited in patients by treatment with SakSTAR. Relative to wild-type SakSTAR, SakSTAR.M38 and SakSTAR.M89 induced less circulating neutralizing activity and less resistance to thrombolysis on repeated infusion, following intensive immunization of rabbits [41] or baboons [43]. In a comparative study in 16 patients with PAO, intra-arterially SakSTAR.M38 and SakSTAR.M89 were equally fibrin-specific and thrombolytically effective, but significantly less antigenic than wild-type SakSTAR [35]. Subsequently, eight variants from a total of 350 "clustered-charge-to-alanine" variants of Sak, where shown to have intact or increased specific activity, maintained fibrinolytic potency and fibrin selectivity, and a markedly reduced reactivity with antiSak antibodies in pooled immunized patient plasma [42]. When given intra-arterially to patients with PAO, these agents induced significant Sak-neutralizing activity ($\geq 5\,\mu g/mL$) in only 28 out of 60 patients (47, 95% CI 35–59%) compared with 57 out of 70 patients (81, 95%: CI 72–91%, $p < 0.0001$) treated with wild-type Sak.

Following single bolus administration of reduced dose PEGylated Sak variants (SY160 and SY161), overt immunization ($\geq 5\,\mu g/mL$) at 3–4 weeks was seen in 10 of 15 patients treated with 5 mg, and in 2 of 7 patients treated with 2.5 mg [27]. SY160-P5- and SY161-P5-neutralizing activity increased to median values of $11\,\mu g$ of Sak variant neutralized per mL of plasma in patients treated with 5 mg, as compared with $21\,\mu g/mL$ in 10 patients treated with a 30-min infusion of 30-mg wild-type Sak ($p = 0.002$) (Fig. 3). After 2.5 mg of PEGylated variant, median neutralizing activity was only $3\,\mu g$ Sak neutralized per mL of plasma ($p = 0.0013$ vs. wild-type Sak). This decreased immunogenicity possibly relates to the combination of B-cell epitope elimination, PEGylation, and a reduced dose.

These studies prove the principle that Sak variants with reduced recognition of antibodies elicited with wild-type Sak and reduced antibody induction, but intact thrombolytic potency can be generated. Ongoing research intends to further unravel the mechanisms involved in the humoral and cellular immune response to Sak. Further reduction of the immunogenicity might also be better approached via additional elimination of T-cell epitopes.

VIII. CONCLUSION

Sak, a profibrinolytic agent produced by *S. aureus*, that is now readily available by recombinant DNA technology, induces efficient and rapid recanalization in patients with occlusive arterial

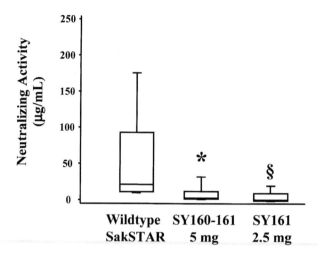

Figure 3 Antibody induction by PEG-SakSTAR: Neutralizing antibody activity 3–4 weeks after administration of wild-type Sak, Sak SY160-P5, and Sak SY161-P5 in patients with acute myocardial infarction. Neutralizing activity was significantly less in patients treated with a single bolus of 5 mg (* $p = 0.002$) and 2.5 mg (§ $p = 0.0013$) SY160 or 161, as compared with 10 patients treated with a 30-minute infusion of 30-mg wild-type Sak.

thrombosis and deep venous thrombosis (Table 1). Its fibrin specificity at clinically effective doses by far exceeds that of any commercially available plasminogen activator. Likewise, the speed and rate of clot lysis compare favorably with established agents, but definition of the relative benefits, especially in terms of reduction of mortality and morbidity, awaits larger comparative trials. Polyethylene glycol derivatization allows single-bolus administration of reduced-dose Sak. However, the optimal dose and safety profile of this promising agent remain to be determined. The antigenicity of wild-type Sak argues against repeated administration but the current, albeit limited, experience with selected recombinant mutants indicates that the immunoreactivity and antigenicity of this bacterial protein can at least be attenuated, while preserving fibrinolytic activity and fibrin specificity.

Table 1 Clinical Trials Using Staphylokinase

Indication	Study	Year	Variant	Number of patients receiving staphylokinase
Acute myocardial infarction	Pilot study	1993	SakSTAR	5
	STAR trial	1995	SakSTAR	48
	Bolus trial	1996	SakSTAR	12
	Double-bolus trial	1997	SakSTAR	50
	CAPTORS I	2000	Sak42D	82
	PEG-STAR	2000	PEG-STAR	18
	CAPTORS II	2001	PEG-STAR	Ongoing
Peripheral arterial occlusion		1995	SakSTAR	30
		2000	SakSTAR	191
Deep venous thrombosis		1998	Sak42D	6

REFERENCES

1. Anderson HV, Willerson JT. Thrombolysis in acute myocardial infarction. N EngI J Med 1993; 329:703–709.
2. Verstraete M. Use of thrombolytic drugs in non-coronary disorders. Drugs 1994; 38:801–821.
3. Verstraete M. Thrombolysis for arterial conditions other than myocardial infarction. Coronary Artery Dis 1994; 5:317–321.
4. Collen D, Lijnen HR. Basic and clinical aspects of fibrinolysis and thrombolysis. Blood 1991; 78:3114–3124.
5. Lincoff AM, Topol EJ. Illusion of reperfusion. Does anyone achieve optimal reperfusion during acute MI? Circulation 1993; 88:1361–1374.
6. Collen D. Is there an optimal thrombolytic regimen? Coronary Artery Dis 1994; 5:287–291.
7. Much H. Über eine Vorstufe des Fibrinfermentes in Kulturen von *Staphylokokkus aureus*. Biochemische Zeitschrift 1908; 14:143–155.
8. Tillett WS, Garner RL. The fibrinolytic activity of hemolytic streptococci. J Exp Med 1933; 58:485–502.
9. Lack CH. Staphylokinase: an activator of plasma protease. Nature 1948; 161:559–560.
10. Sweet B, McNicol GP, Douglas AS. In vitro studies of staphylokinase. Clin Sci 1965; 29:375–382.
11. Lewis JH, Keber CW, Wilson JH. Effects of fibrinolytic agents and heparin on intravascular clot lysis. Am J Physiol 1964; 207:1044–1048.
12. Collen D, Van Hoef B, Schlott B, Hartmann M, Gührs KH, Lijnen HR. Mechanisms of activation of mammalian plasma fibrinolytic systems with streptokinase and with recombinant staphylokinase. Eur J Biochem 1990; 21:307–314.
13. Sako T, Tsuchicla N. Nucleoticle sequence of the staphylokinase gene from *Staphylococcus aureus*. Nucleic Acids Res 1983; 11:7679–7693.
14. Behnke D, Gerlach D. Cloning and expression in *Escherichia coli, Bacillus subtilis* and *Streptococcus sanguis* of a gene for staphylokinase: a bacterial plasminogen activator. Mol Gen Genet 1987; 210:528–534.
15. Collen D, Zhao ZA, Holvoet P, Marynen P. Primary structure and gene structure of staphylokinase. Fibrinolysis 1992; 6:226–231.
16. Kim S–H, Chun H–S, Han MH, Park N–Y, Suk K. A novel variant of staphylokinase gene from *Staphylococcus aureus* ATCC 29213. Thromb Res 1997; 87:387–395.
17. Rabijns A, De Bondt HL, De Ranter C. Three-dimensional structure of staphylokinase, a plasminogen activator with therapeutic potential. Nat Struct Biol 1997; 4:357–360.
18. Schlott B, Hartmann M, Gührs KH, Birsch–Hirschfeld E, Pohl D, Vanderschueren S, Van de Werf F, Michoel A, Collen D, Behnke D. High yield production and purification of recombinant staphylokinase for thrombolytic therapy. Biotechnology 1994; 12:185–189.
19. Lijnen HR, Collen D. Staphylokinase, a fibrin-specific bacterial plasminogen activator. Fibrinolysis 1996; 10:119–126.
20. Collen D. Staphylokinase: a potent, uniquely fibrin-selective thrombolytic agent. Nat Med 1998; 4:279–284.
21. Lijnen HR, Van Hoef B, Vandenbossche L, Collen D. Biochemical properties of natural and recombinant staphylokinase. Fibrinolysis 1992; 6:214–225.
22. Lijnen HR, Van Hoef B, Collen D, Interactions of staphylokinase with human platelets. Thromb Haemost 1995; 73:472–477.
23. Vanderschueren S, Collen D. Comparative effects of staphylokinase and alteplase in rabbit bleeding time models. Thromb Haemost 1996; 75:816–819.
24. Lijnen HR, Stassen JM, Collen D. Differential inhibition with antifibrinolytic agents of staphylokinase and streptokinase induced clot lysis. Thromb Haemost 1995; 73:845–849.
25. Collen D, De Cock F, Van Linthout I, Declerck PJ, Lijnen HR, Stassen JM. Comparative thrombolytic and immunogenic properties of staphylokinase and streptokinase. Fibrinolysis 1992; 6:232–242.
26. Collen D, De Cock F, Stassen JM. Comparative immunogenicity and thrombolytic properties toward arterial and venous thrombi of streptokinase and recombinant staphylokinase in baboons. Circulation 1993; 87:996–1006.

27. Collen D, Sinnaeve P, Demarsin E, Moreau H, De Maeyer M, Jespers L, Laroche Y, Van de Werf F. Polyethylene glycol-derivatized cysteine-substitution variants of recombinant staphylokinase for single-bolus treatment of acute myocardial infarction. Circulation 2000; 102:1766–1772.
28. Collen D, Van de Werf F. Coronary thrombolysis with recombinant staphylokinase in patients with evolving myocardial infarction. Circulation 1993; 87:1850–1853.
29. Vanderschueren S, Collen D, Van de Werf F. Coronary reperfusion in patients with an acute myocardial infarction following intravenous administration of recombinant staphylokinase [abstr]. J Am Coll Cardiol 1994; 315A.
30. Collen DC, Gold HK. New developments in thrombolytic therapy. Thromb Res 1990; Suppl X:105–131.
31. Vanderschueren S, Barrios L, Kerdsinchai P, Van den Heuvel P, Hermans L, Vrolix M, De Man F, Benit E, Muyldermans L, Collen D, Van de Werf F. A randomized trial of recombinant staphylokinase versus alteplase for coronary artery patency in acute myocardial infarction. Circulation 1995; 92:2044–2049.
32. Armstrong P, Burton J, Palisaitis D, Thompson C, Van de Werf F, Rose B, Collen D, Teo K. Collaborative angiographic patency trial of recombinant staphylokinase (CAPTORS). Am Heart J 2000; 139:820–823.
33. Vanderschueren S, Collen D, Van de Werf F. A pilot study on bolus administration of recombinant staphylokinase for coronary artery thrombolysis. Thromb Haemost 1996; 76:541–544.
34. Okada K, Lijnen H, Moreau H, Vanderschueren S, Collen D. Procoagulant properties of intravenous staphylokinase versus tissue-type plasminogen activator. Thromb Haemost 1996; 76:857–859.
35. Vanderschueren S, Stockx L, Wilms G, Verhaeghe R, Lacroix H. Vermylen J, Collen D. Thrombolytic therapy of peripheral arterial occlusion with recombinant staphylokinase. Circulation 1995; 92:2050–2057.
36. Heymans S, Vanderschueren S, Verhaeghe R, Stockx L, Lacroix H, Nevelsteen A, Laroche Y, Collen D. Outcome and one year follow-up of intra-arterial staphylokinase in 191 patients with peripheral arterial occlusion. Thromb Haemost 2000; 83:666–671.
37. Heymans S, Verhaeghe R, Stockx L, Collen D. Feasibility study of catheter-directed thrombolysis with recombinant staphylokinase in deep venous thrombosis. Thromb Haemost 1998; 79:517–519.
38. Vanderschueren SMF, Stassen JM, Collen D. On the immunogenicity of recombinant staphylokinase in patients and in animal models. Thromb Haemost 1994; 72:297–301.
39. Declerck PJ, Vanderschueren S, Billiet J, Moreau H, Collen D. Prevalence and induction of circulating antibodies against recombinant staphylokinase. Thromb Haemost 1994; 71:129–133.
40. Collen D, Bernaerts R, Declerck P, De Cock F, Demarsin E, Jenné S, Laroche Y, Lijnen HR, Silence K, Verstreken M. Recombinant staphylokinase variants with altered immunoreactivity. I. Construction and characterization. Circulation 1996; 94:197–206.
41. Collen D, Moreau H, Stockx L, Vanderschueren S. Recombinant staphylokinase variants with altered immunoreactivity. II. Thrombolytic properties and antibody induction. Circulation 1996; 94:197–206.
42. Laroche Y, Heymans S, Capaert S, De Cock F, Demarsin E, Collen D. Recombinant staphylokinase variants with reduced antigenicity due to elimination of B-lymphocyte epitopes. Blood 2000; 96:1425–1432.
43. Vanderschueren S, Stassen JM, Collen D. Comparative antigenicity of wild-type staphylokinase (SakSTAR) and a selected mutant (SakSTAR.M38) in a baboon thrombolysis model. J Cardiovasc Pharm 1996; 27(6):809–815.

38

Desmodus rotundus (Vampire Bat) Plasminogen Activator DSPAα₁: A Superior Thrombolytic Created by Evolution

Wolf–Dieter Schleuning* and Peter Donner
Schering AG, Berlin, Germany

SUMMARY

Thrombolytic therapy with plasminogen activators (PAs) is now performed routinely for the treatment of acute myocardial infarction. However, thrombolytic agents such as streptokinase (SK), tissue-type plasminogen activator (t-PA), and urokinase-type plasminogen activators (u-PA) exhibit various shortcomings relative to their pharmacodynamic and pharmacokinetic characteristics and additionally may cause life-threatening side effects. With the aim of creating an improved fibrinolytic agent in mind, we have cloned and expressed the plasminogen activators from the saliva of the vampire bat *Desmodus rotundus*, originally described by Hawkey (1966). Four *Desmodus rotundus* salivary plasminogen activators (DSPAs) were identified which—like t-PA and u-PA—are composed of various conserved domains known from related proteins. DSPAα₁ and DSPAα₂ exhibit the structural formula finger (F), EGF (E), kringle (K), protease (P), DSPAβ, and the γ formulas EKP and KR, respectively. Subtle sequence differences and data from Southern blot hybridization analysis indicate that the four enzymes are coded by four different genes and are not generated by differential splicing of a single primary transcript. A preliminary biochemical and pharmacological analysis indicated that DSPAα₁ exhibited the most favorable profile and was, therefore, chosen for further study. A recombinant CHO-cell line for the production of DSPA and a purification protocol were established to obtain material that fulfilled the specifications for preclinical and clinical development.

The most important property that distinguishes DSPA from other plasminogen activators is its extraordinary fibrin specificity. In fact, the activity of DSPAα₁ is 105,000 times higher in the presence of fibrin than in its absence. The respective factor for t-PA is only 550. Likewise, fibrinogen, which is a fairly potent cofactor of plasminogen activation by t-PA, has hardly any effect on DSPAα₁. Therefore the factor of fibrin selectivity expressed as the quotient of activity in the presence of fibrin versus activity in the presence of fibrinogen is 12,900 for DSPA but only 72 for t-PA. Therefore, DSPAα₁ could fulfill the hopes originally linked to t-PA: plasminogen

---

**Current affiliation*: PAION GmbH Research Center, Berlin, Germany

activation restricted to the clot surface, without the systemic activation that inexorably leads to fibrinogen consumption, "plasminogen steal," and degradation of clotting factors VIII and V.

This fibrin specificity and selectivity of DSPAα$_1$ may translate into a more favorable side-effect profile. Pharmacological studies using a lung embolism model in rats demonstrated that recombinant DSPAα$_1$ is more potent and more clot-specific than t-PA. A higher-potency, clot specificity, and prolonged half-life of DSPAα$_1$ over t-PA were also verified in an arterial thrombosis model in rats. In a coronary thrombosis model of acute myocardial infarction in dogs, DSPAα$_1$ led to a faster recanalization and a lower incidence of reocclusion than did t-PA. On the other hand, a lower incidence of bleeding was observed in a rat mesenteric vein model. DSPAα$_1$ was characterized pharmacokinetically in rats and cynomolgus monkeys. In comparison with t-PA, a lower total clearance and a longer terminal half-life could be demonstrated. These data encourage the development of an intravenous bolus regimen in humans. A detailed toxicological study has been performed in rats and monkeys. No direct toxic effects could be observed, and effects appeared only at extremely high doses of DSPAα$_1$. A phase I clinical trial with healthy volunteers was performed in which subtherapeutic doses were applied by intravenous bolus administration. No relevant clinical changes nor negative effects on blood coagulation were observed. In addition, the pharmacokinetic predictions obtained from animal studies could be confirmed and the therapeutically effective dose of DSPAα$_1$ was predicted to be 0.5 mg/kg of body weight.

In summary, our data strongly support the notion that DSPAα$_1$ may be a safer thrombolytic than others currently in use.

I. INTRODUCTION

The treatment of acute myocardial infarction (AMI) by thrombolytic therapy was first attempted in the 1950s [1]. Moving from the experimental stage to mainstream clinical practice, however, took 25 years, a time during which a number of hurdles—conceptual as well as technical—had to be overcome [2,3]. First, elaborate studies were required, including the development of advanced-imaging techniques to create consensus among cardiologists that the main pathophysiological event underlying AMI is coronary thrombosis and not vasospasm. Second, it was feared—not without reason—that thrombolytic therapy could have serious risks and side effects.

Streptokinase, the first fibrinolytic agent to become available, is of streptococcal origin; therefore, it exhibits antigenicity. Most patients carry neutralizing antibodies and immunological memory against this agent, creating individual differences in dose response and the risk of allergic reactions. Furthermore, streptokinase does not discriminate between clot-bound and circulating plasminogen, thereby promoting systemic plasminogen activation with the consequences of plasminogen, α$_2$-antiplasmin, and fibrinogen consumption, and the degradation of clotting factors [4]. Urokinase (u-PA), a plasminogen activator originally purified from urine and later from cell culture supernatants of embryonic kidney cells, is superior to streptokinase because of its lack of antigenicity, but is likewise not specific for clot-bound plasminogen. Tissue-type plasminogen activator (t-PA), discovered in the late 1940s [5] and purified in the 1970s [6,7], could be made available in quantities sufficient for clinical trials only after the advent of recombinant DNA technology [8]. t-PA exhibits "fibrin specificity" (i.e., its activity is strongly enhanced in the presence of fibrin). This raised the hope that in a clinical setting the negative effects of systemic plasminogen activation could be avoided [9,10]. These expectations were only partially fulfilled. It took an extensive clinical trial (GUSTO: *G*lobal *U*tilization of *S*treptokinase and *t*-PA for *O*ccluded Coronary Arteries) to demonstrate that the fibrin specificity demonstrated *in vitro* translated into a better tolerance of the drug *in vivo*. The trial [11] unequivocally demonstrated the advantages of an accelerated t-PA regimen over streptokinase. Total mortality was significantly lower, and therapeutic benefit was clearly correlated with early onset of recanalization. t-PA, a fibrinolytic agent with a certain degree of fibrin specificity, has been superior to streptokinase, a non–fibrin-specific fibrinolytic. The demonstration of significant differences between the two agents however, required many patients, and even the optimized front-loading t-PA regimen achieved satisfactory patency at 90 min (TIMI grade 3) in only 53% of patients.

These shortcomings notwithstanding, GUSTO paved the way for ideas of how an earlier and more complete recanalization and, therefore, a further increase of total survival after AMI might be achieved, by a more aggressive bolus administration of a more fibrin-dependent thrombolytic. The well-known weaknesses of t-PA, such as its short half-life and limited fibrin specificity, set relatively narrow limits to any further improvement of the therapeutic regimen. The administration of high doses of t-PA to overcome its unfavorable pharmacokinetics was associated with the induction of plasminemia, coagulopathy, intracerebral hemorrhage, and stroke. Because of limited fibrin specificity, high plasma levels of t-PA deplete the levels of circulating plasminogen (an effect known as "plasminogen steal"), and thereby lower the amount of plasminogen available for activation at the clot surface. Therefore the superiority of fibrin-specific clot lysis demonstrated by GUSTO cannot be fully realized using currently available thrombolytic agents. As a consequence, considerable efforts have been directed at the improvement of fibrin specificity and the pharmacokinetic parameters of t-PA and other thrombolytic agents by mutagenesis, molecular chimerism or other forms of derivatization.

Many of these proteins, such as t-PA–deletion mutants, u-PA–t-PA hybrids, molecular chimeras between u-PA and antifibrin monoclonal antibodies, and hybrids between plasminogen and u-PA and t-PA, were investigated in vitro and in some cases *in vivo* [12]. So far none of these products has been proved to exhibit distinct advantages over t-PA. Clinical trials for a finger-EGF–deletion mutant of t-PA [13] and the so-called TNK mutant of t-PA [14] have been performed, but no decisive advantages over t-PA could be demonstrated.

Stimulated by earlier, mainly zoological work, we have chosen a different path to generate a novel thrombolytic. The digestive fluids of hematophageous animals such as leeches, ticks, hookworms, and mosquitos are a rich source of factors that interfere with the clotting system [15]. Building on observations from the 1930s [16], Christine Hawkey discovered in the 1960s a highly potent plasminogen activator in the saliva of the common vampire bat *Desmodus rotundus* [17], which was later partially purified and characterized by Cartwright [18]. Evolution has optimized this enzyme to support the feeding habit of the animal, (i.e., the digestion of relatively large, freshly formed clots). This target bears little resemblance to the physiological targets of other plasminogen activators, with their more subtle functions regulating cell function and matrix deposition during wound healing. Dissolution of freshly formed clots would, in fact, countervene the benefits of blood coagulation during the sealing of fresh wounds. It is a plausible hypothesis that the dissolution of an intravascular thrombus is more easily achieved by an agent optimized by evolution exclusively for fibrinolysis, rather then by u-PA or t-PA with their more complex multifunctional physiological roles.

Cartwright noticed the superior ability of partially purified DSPA (desmokinase in his nomenclature) to lyse preformed clots and suggested its use in medicine. However, in the days "before cloning," the dream of generating quantities of material sufficient for clinical testing could not be realized. At a time when cDNA cloning and heterologous expression have become routine laboratory practice, we and others [19,51] decided to build on this work and to lay down an experimental framework that enabled us to generate material in sufficient quality and quantity to allow preclinical and clinical investigations.

II. NATURAL HISTORY OF VAMPIRE BATS

Among the three known species of vampire bats, the white-winged *Diaemus youngi*, the hairy-legged *Diphylla ecaudata*, and the common *Desmodus rotundus*, only the latter one has become the object of scientific study. This is not only due to its wider distribution, but also because it presents a threat to livestock as a carrier of rabies virus. Vampire bats are unique among bats not only because of their diets but also because of a variety of fascinating morphological, physiological, and behavioral adaptations, which are related to their feeding habits. Foraging animals leave their caves at night and preferentially attack large farm or wild animals and, rarely, humans. They inflict a tiny, superficial, and apparently painless wound by removing a piece or skin with their razor-sharp incisors. The blood oozing from the wound is taken up by two channels on the undersite of the tongue while saliva flows down the groove on its dorsal surface. Back in the caves, unsuccessful kin profit from an unusual altruistic behavioral trait: they are fed by regurgitated blood. An excellent monograph on the natural history of vampire bats has been published by Greenhall and Schmidt [20].

III. BIOCHEMISTRY

A. Purification

The vampire bats used for our studies were collected from their resting places in natural caves in the Mexican state of Guerrero and maintained in captivity for several months. Saliva was collected by stimulating salivation by placing a small droplet of 1% pilocarpine nitrate in the buccal mucosa using a Pasteur pipette extended with a piece of silicone rubber tubing. Saliva was collected, using the same device, and placed in polystyrol tubes immersed in, melting ice. The saliva was subsequently frozen and shipped in dry ice for further processing. Saliva was fractionated by matrix-bound *Erythrina latissima* protease inhibitor [21]. Three isoenzymes with molecular weights of 52 kDa (DSPAα), 46 kDa (DSPAβ), and 42 kDa (DSPAγ) were identified [22]. All of these differed in their N-terminal amino acid sequences and could be further separated by hydrophobic interaction chromatography [23,24]. We did not follow the nomenclature "bat-PA" proposed by Gardell et al. [22], but chose DSPA (*D. rotundus* salivary plasminogen activator) for the following reasons:

1. There are several hundred species of bats, but only three species of vampire bats. We believe that the name of the enzyme should contain a scientifically sound reference to its origin in addition to an unequivocal description of its function.
2. DSPA represents an evolutionary adaptation to a specific feeding habit and as such is clearly distinct from other plasminogen activators, such as u-PA and t-PA, that have so far been found in all mammals investigated and are likely to occur also in bats. The designation Bat-PA does not take account of this distinctive characteristic and invites confusion with bat t-PA or u-PA.

B. Cloning and Expression

RNA was isolated from *Desmodus rotundus* salivary glands, used as a template for cDNA synthesis, and cloned into the λZAP vector according to standard procedures [25]. Candidate clones were isolated after screening the cDNA library using human t-PA cDNA as a probe. Hybridizing clones were partially sequenced and correspond to four distinct forms, which were described as DSPA α_1, α_2, β, and γ [51]. The cDNA sequences of the two largest forms (α_1 and

α_2) were closely related (80 differences for a total of 2245 nucleotides). DSPAα_2 cDNA exhibited six nucleotide differences with a sequence published previously [22]. DSPAβ cDNA was shortened by an internal 138-nucleotide deletion, but otherwise, displayed only one nucleotide difference when compared with DSPAα_2 cDNA. DSPAγ cDNA was even shorter (249-nucleotide-long deletion) and differed from DSPAα_1 and β-cDNA in 54 and 23 positions, respectively. When the sequences of DSPAs were aligned with t-PA. it became clear that they exhibited a modular structure characteristic of t-PA and u-PA, DSPAα_1 and DSPAα_2 consisted of an array of structural motifs: finger (F), epidermal growth factor (E), kringle (K), and protease (P). The formulas for DSPAβ and DSPAγ were EKP and KP, respectively (Fig. 1). Remarkably, the K motif more closely resembled kringle 1 than kringle 2 of t-PA. DSPAβ is closely related to DSPAα_2, whereas DSPAγ has diverged somewhat more, but still resembles α_2 more than α_1. All DSPA forms exhibited a potential N-glycosylation site in the protease domain. A further glycosylation site was found in the kringle of DSPAα_1 at the same position as in t-PA, whereas in α_2 and β it was located at a different position in the kringle. N-glycosylation is not a prerequisite for the fibrinolytic activity of any of the DSPA isoforms. No DSPAα_2 protein has been identified in *D. rotundus* saliva, indicating that this form is of low abundance in the specimens investigated. The structural features as well as the results of Southern blot experiments clearly indicated that the four forms of DSPA are products of different genes and are not generated by differential mRNA splicing as suggested by other authors [22].

C. DSPA Gene Expression in Heterologous Host Cells

For a preliminary characterization, expression plasmids coding for DSPAα_1, α_2, β, and γ were transiently transfected into COS-1 cells. Supernatants of the transfected cells were analyzed by radial lysis in plasminogen-containing casein and fibrin agar plates using a modification of Astrup's radial fibrinolysis assay [26]. All four forms of DSPA exhibited a ratio of fibrinolytic versus caseinolytic activity that was significantly higher than t-PA, as had already been observed with material purified from saliva. As DSPAα_1 exhibited the most favorable profile in these preliminary assays, it was decided to focus on this isoenzyme for further pharmacological and clinical studies. To this end a stable recombinant Chinese hamster ovarian (CHO)-cell line was established. The expression plasmid pSVPA 11 was transfected into dhfr$^-$CHO cells [27] using the calcium phosphate method and dhfr$^+$-positive cells were selected in MEM without nucleosides, supplemented with 2.5% dialyzed fetal calf serum. DSPAα_1 was isolated from the cell culture supernatants by affinity chromatography using *Erythrina latissima* trypsin inhibitor (ETI) immobilized on Sepharose [27].

D. Enzymology

"Fibrin specificity" is generally understood to be a property of plasminogen activators, which exhibit a higher catalytic efficiency in the presence of fibrin than in its absence. Indeed, whereas the catalytic efficiency of streptokinase or urokinase is unaffected by fibrin, t-PA-catalyzed generation of plasmin is considerably stimulated in its presence and to a lesser extent also by fibrinogen, fibrin degradation products, β-amyloid, and other less well-defined cofactors [10,28–30]. The underlying mechanism of this "cofactor dependence" has been intuitively attributed to "fibrin binding" by most authors, but as we will see later, its physicochemical basis is formed by more complex protein–protein interactions.

A detailed enzymological analysis was performed on the four DSPA forms and on a series of muteins to investigate the molecular basis of their striking fibrin dependence [31]. In the assay

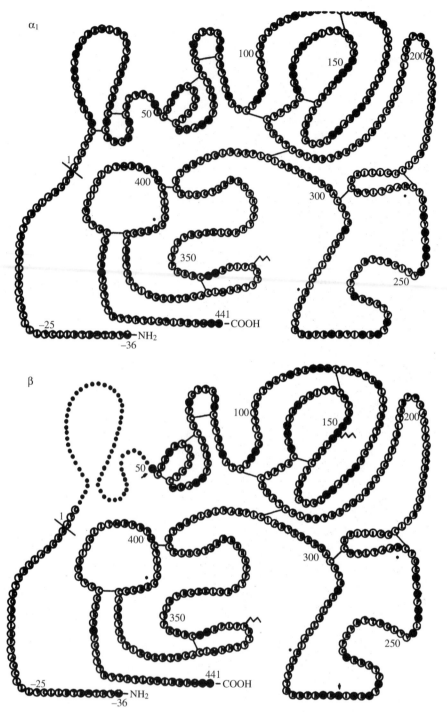

Figure 1 Schematic representation of DSPAα_1, $-\alpha_2$, $-\beta$, and $-\gamma$. Position 1 corresponds to the N terminus of the mature protein. Lines joining Cys residues were drawn in analogy to putative disulfide bridges in human t-Pa. The active site residues are shown with filled triangles. Short zigzag lines indicate potential N-linked glycosylation sites. Missing domains in DSPAβ and $-\gamma$ are indicated by a dotted outline. The amino acid differences between the different forms are shown in filled circles. Arrows point to positions mutated in DSPAβ or $-\gamma$ but not $-\alpha_2$, and crosses indicate positions conserved in DSPAγ, but not in DSPAα_2 or $-\beta$ when compared with DSPAα_1. (From Ref. 52.)

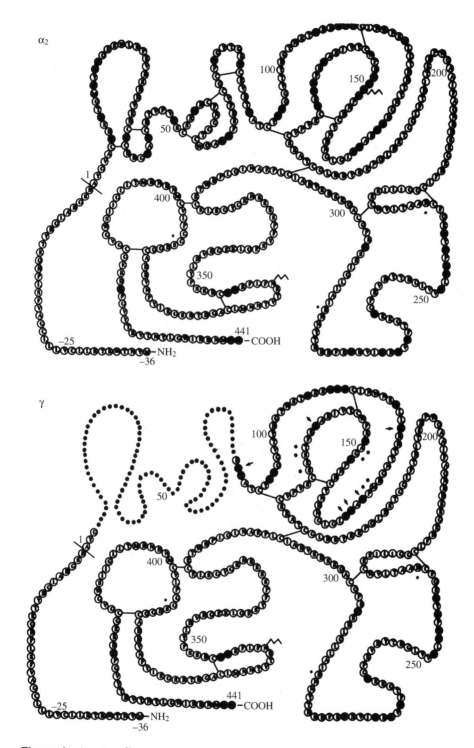

Figure 1 (*continued*)

system used, plasminogen activation is measured by the determination of the generated plasmin in real-time. Briefly, the results were as follows.

1. Fibrin binding of DSPAs is exclusively dependent on the presence of a finger region; consequently, DSPAα_1 and α_2, but not DSPAβ and γ, bind to fibrin.
2. None of the DSPAs contains a lysine-binding site.
3. All DSPAs are single-chain molecules displaying substantial amidolytic activity, but are almost inactive in a plasminogen activation assay in the absence of fibrin.
4. Upon addition of fibrin, the catalytic efficiency (k_{cat}/K_m) of plasminogen activation by DSPAα_1 increases 105,000-fold, whereas the corresponding value for t-PA is only 550.
5. The catalytic efficiency (k_{cat}/K_m) of DSPAα_1 and t-PA in the presence of fibrin is almost equal, but decreases dramatically with the loss of the finger and the kringle domain.
6. The ratio of the biomolecular rate constants of plasminogen activation in the presence of fibrin versus fibrinogen (fibrin selectivity) of DSPAα_1, α_2, β, γ was 13,000, 6500, 250, and 90, respectively. The corresponding value for t-PA is only 72 (Table 1).

Similar investigations with equivalent results have been performed by Bergum and Gardell [32], who additionally demonstrated that t-PA, in contrast to DSPAα_2, (bat-PA), is stimulated by the fragment X polymer, a fibrin degradation product that is generated during fibrinolysis.

These results establish a new paradigm for the molecular basis of "fibrin specificity." This term, commonly used as a measure of the degree to which a plasminogen activator is stimulated

Table 1 Kinetic Parameters of Glu-Plasminogen Activation by DSPAs and t-PA: Influence of Fibrinogen and Fibrin

Enzyme	Cofactor	k_{cat}/k_m [M^{-1} s^{-1}]	Stimulation factor	Ratio Fbn/Fbg
DSPAα_1	None	6.5 ± 3.9	1	
	Fbg	53 ± 28	8	
	Fbn	$684,000 \pm 198,000$	102,100	12,900
DSPAα_2	None	9.8 ± 8.0	1	
	Fbg	79 ± 34	8	
	Fbn	$517,000 \pm 187,000$	52,700	6,550
DSPAβ	None	6.0 ± 5.0	1	
	Fbg	42 ± 7	7	
	Fbn	$9,900 \pm 1,300$	1,650	235
DSPAγ	None	4.4 ± 2.8	1	
	Fbg	39.0 ± 7	9	
	Fbn	$3,510 \pm 850$	800	90
sct-PA	None	34 ± 14	1	
	Fbg	638 ± 92	19	
	Fbn	$525,000 \pm 61,000$	15,480	820
t-PA	None	$1,760 \pm 450$	1	
	Fbg	$13,600 \pm 2,230$	8	
	Fbn	$972,000 \pm 382,000$	550	72
Cleavable	None	135 ± 130	1	
DSPAα_1	Fbg	516 ± 126	4	
	Fbn	$565,000 \pm 215,000$	4,180	1,100

Source: Ref. 31.

by fibrin, is unfortunately ambiguous because it is mostly understood without reference to other cofactors. Ideally, the most "fibrin-specific" plasminogen activator would activate clot-bound plasminogen without affecting circulating plasminogen levels. That circulating fibrinogen is a relatively potent cofactor of t-PA-mediated plasminogen activation must be taken into account, however. A more meaningful quantitative parameter than "fibrin specificity," is therefore "fibrin selectivity," the quotient of the stimulatory effect of fibrin versus fibrinogen, which more accurately ascribes to a PA the preference for clot-bound versus circulating plasminogen. This factor is 13,000 for DSPAα₁ whereas it is only 72 for t-PA. What is the molecular basis of this striking difference? A plausible explanation was recently put forward by J. Weitz, Hamilton Civic Hospital Research Centre, Ontario (personal communication). Using light-scattering spectroscopy, this author characterized two fibrin-binding sites on t-PA, one high-affinity site associated with the finger and one low-affinity site associated with kringle 2. The kringle 2-binding site is also able to react with fibrinogen and fibrin fragments. As this site is missing in DSPA, it cannot react with fibrinogen or fibrin fragments; hence, the striking superiority of DSPA in fibrin selectivity. The absence of a plasmin-sensitive cleavage site in the peptide connecting the kingle and the protease domain is another distinguishing structural feature of all DSPA forms. If such a site is introduced, fibrin selectivity decreases by a factor of 10. Likewise, the fibrin selectivity of t-PA increases by a similar factor if this site is eliminated. DSPAβ and γ, which have no finger domain and therefore do not bind to fibrin, still exhibit fibrin selectivity. Therefore, fibrin binding is only one of several protein–protein interactions that determine fibrin selectivity. Other interactions are associated with the absence of a fibrinogen-binding site on the DSPA-kringle, the state of folding of the single-chain molecule, and other unknown structural elements of the protease domain [31]. DSPAα₂ (bat-PA) is also slightly less susceptible than t-PA to inactivation by plasminogen activator inhibitor 1 (PAI-1). The k_{ass} values for the interaction between PAI-1 and DSPAα₂ and two-chain t-PA (in the presence of fibrinogen) are 4.4×10^6 and 13.1×10^6 $M^{-1}s^{-1}$, respectively [33]. In a similar assay system in the presence of fibrin, Gruber [34] compared DSPAα₁ ($k_{ass} = 0.7 \times 10^6$ $M^{-1}s^{-1}$) and two–chain t-PA ($k_{ass} = 2.5 \times 10^6$ $M^{-1}s^{-1}$).

IV. PHARMACOLOGY

A. In Vitro Clot Lysis

Whole-blood clot lysis [35] is employed to determine the activity of a fibrinolytic agent in a "seminatural" environment (i.e., in the presence of all the cofactors and inhibitors known or unknown that are also likely to be present *in vivo*. Whole human blood clots were generated *in vitro*, aged for 1 h, and placed in autologous plasma in the presence of varying concentrations of either t-PA or DSPAα₁. The thrombolytic potential of both PAs, expressed as percentage change in clot wet weight and plasma fibrinogen content, were determined after a 6-h incubation. Both t-PA and DSPAα₁ exhibited a very similar thrombolytic profile (Fig. 2). In contrast to t-PA, however, only minimal fibrinogen degradation was observed in the DSPA-containing sample [23].

We have also compared the fibrin selectivity of t-PA and its mutant TNK-(t-PA) with that of DSPAα₁. Kinetic analysis of plasminogen activation revealed that TNK-(t-PA) is approximately eightfold more fibrin-selective than wild-type t-PA. However, the fibrin selectivity of DSPAα₁ is still 12-fold higher than that of TNK-(t-PA). DSPAα₁ clearly exhibits a higher efficacy than TNK-(t-PA) and t-PA in a whole human blood clot lysis assay at low concentrations (1–5 nM). At higher concentrations (≥10 nM), DSPAα₁ and TNK-(t-PA) are equally effective. Between 5 and 25 nM the efficacy of t-PA is very similar to that of DSPAα₁. The induction of

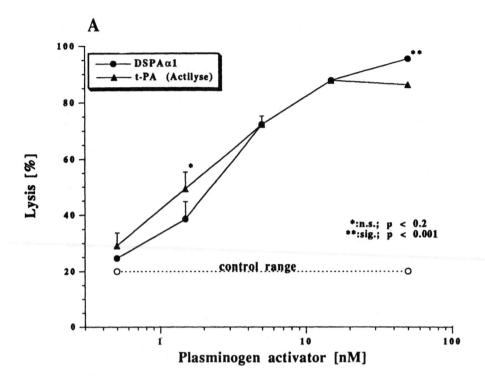

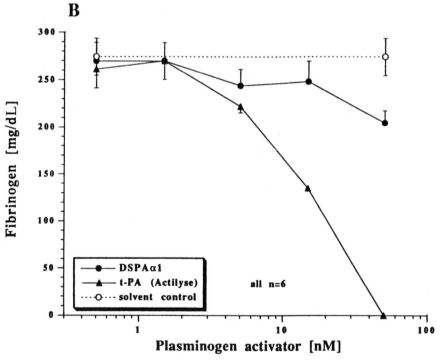

Figure 2 Human whole-blood clot lysis in vitro: (A) concentration response curves for tissue-type plasminogen activator (Actilyse) and DSPAα1; (B) fibrinogen concentrations after 6 h of incubation. (From Ref. 23.)

clot lysis by 50 nM t-PA is less efficacious, however, and at 100 nM t-PA, only incomplete clot lysis is achieved due to "plasminogen steal." The plasminogen steal effect is not observed at any concentration during DSPAα_1-mediated clot lysis, but is flagrant at concentrations above 100 nM TNK-(t-PA).

DSPAα_1-mediated clotlysis is not accompanied by fibrinogenolysis, even at the highest concentration. In contrast, complete clot lysis induced by t-PA, in particular at higher concentrations (25–100 nM), is compromised by severe fibrinogen degradation. Even at 10-nM t-PA, the level of functional fibrinogen is diminished by 70%. Whereas TNK-(t-PA) is clearly more fibrin-selective than t-PA, at elevated concentrations, complete clot lysis is achieved only at the expense of notable fibrinogenolysis, indicating that the fibrin selectivity of TNK-(t-PA) is still unsatisfactory. The consumption of α_2-antiplasmin corroborates our findings concerning fibrinogenolysis. α_2-Antiplasmin is virtually undetectable in plasma samples containing 10 nM and higher concentrations of t-PA and TNK-(t-PA), whereas DSPAα_1 samples still contain measurable amounts of α_2-antiplasmin even at 100 nM. Therefore, DSPAα_1 is the only plasminogen activator with strict fibrin cofactor requirements and is more potent than t-PA and TNK-(t-PA) at low doses [36].

Hare and Gardell [37] compared DSPAα_2 (bat-PA), t-PA, and streptokinase in a plasma clot lysis model using radiolabeled fibrinogen. Excessive fibrinogen degradation was observed only in the samples containing t-PA and streptokinase. In addition, the authors clearly demonstrated that the addition of a clot lysate did not stimulate DSPAα_2 activity, indicating that soluble fibrin degradation products do not influence DSPA activity.

B. Carotid and Femoral Artery Thrombosis in Rabbits

Thrombosis was induced by a copper coil inserted in the common carotid artery of groups of six anesthetized rabbits. Thrombolysis was initiated in the presence of heparin and aspirin. With this experimental approach, DSPAα_1 was at least as efficacious as t-PA and probably two to three times more potent [38]. In contrast to t-PA, no significant fibrinogenolysis or plasminogen depletion could be detected with DSPAα_1. α_2-Antiplasmin plasma levels decreased to a smaller extent than with t-PA. The plasma half-life of DSPAα_1 exceeded that of t-PA at all doses (Fig. 3).

In a rabbit model of femoral arterial thrombosis, DSPAα_2 (bat-PA) was evaluated and compared with t-PA [39]. A thrombus was formed by injecting autologous whole blood, Ca^{2+}, and thrombin into an isolated segment of the femoral artery. Following a 60-min–aging period, DSPAα_2 or t-PA was given by bolus intravenous injection, and blood flow restoration was measured with an electromagnetic flow probe. At 14 and 42 nmol/kg, t-PA reperfused 15 and 78% of the rabbits, respectively, whereas with 4.7, 8.1, 14, and 42 nmol/kg DSPAα_2 the reperfusion rates were 0, 50, 75, and 80%. The thrombolytic efficacy of DSPAα_2 at 14 nmol/kg was comparable with a threefold higher dose of t-PA (42 nmol/kg). Although the incidence of reperfusion by DSPAα_2 was not significantly different at 42 and 14 nmol/kg, other indices of efficacy, such as median time to reperfusion and residual thrombus mass, improved significantly when the threefold-higher dose was administered. Analysis of serial blood samples revealed that the administration of t-PA (42 nmol/kg), but not of DSPA, at the same dose elicited a marked decrease in the levels of plasma fibrinogen. This finding confirms the remarkable fibrin selectivity already noted using purified reagents as well as whole-blood clot lysis.

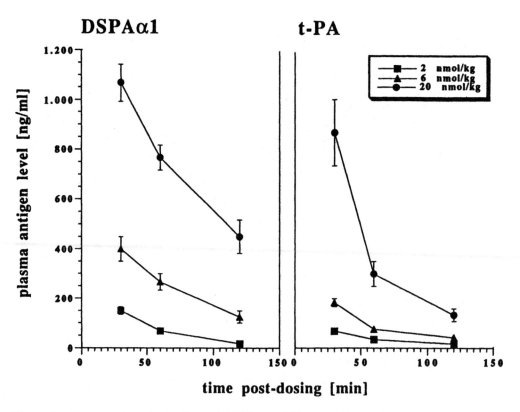

Figure 3 Plasma antigen levels (mean ± SEM, $n = 6$–7) of DSPAα_1 and tissue-type plasminogen activator (t-PA) following intravenous-bolus injection at 30, 60, and 120 min. (From Ref. 38.)

C. Myocardial Infarction in Dogs

Copper coil-induced myocardial infarction in dogs is widely considered as one of the best models of human myocardial infarction. The thrombolytic properties of t-PA and DSPAα_1, therefore, were tested in this way [40]. A copper coil was inserted into the coronary artery of an anesthetized animal, leading to the local formation of a thrombus. All dogs received heparin. Whereas control animals did not reperfuse within 180 min, intravenous bolus administration of DSPAα_1 at 25, 50, and 100 µg/kg resulted in a 100% incidence of recanalization within 37, 23, and 18 min, respectively. t-PA at 63 and 125 µg/kg reopened the coronary arteries in 33 and 50% of cases within 40 min. Eighty-three percent of the arteries were still patent 3 h after 50 and 100 µg/kg DSPAα_1, whereas only 20% (one in five) of all coronaries originally recanalized with either dose of t-PA were still open after 3 h (Fig. 4). The clearance of DSPAα_1 was lower than that of t-PA owing to a prolonged terminal half-life.

D. Experimental Pulmonary Embolism in Rats

The thrombolytic properties of DSPAα_1 and t-PA were compared in a rat model of pulmonary embolism [41]. Whole-blood clots, produced *in vitro* and labeled with [^{125}I]-fibrinogen, were embolized into the lungs of anesthetized rats. Thrombolysis was calculated from the difference between initial clot radioactivity and that remaining in the lungs after 60 min. When DSPAα_1 was

Table 2 Venipuncture Bleeding Time (BT) in Rats

Treatment	Dose (nmol/kg)	BT prolongation	Rebleeding
Control		0/8	0/8
t-PA	10	1/6	1/6
	30	6/6 [4][a]	3/6
	100	4/6 [4][a]	3/6
DSPAα₁	100	0/6	0/6
	300	1/6	5/6

[a]In brackets: number of animals showing severe bleeding, BT for longer than 10 min.

used, thrombolysis was achieved significantly faster than with t-PA. Moreover, t-PA significantly decreased fibrinogen, plasminogen and α_2-antiplasmin. Compared with t-PA, DSPAα₁ was clearly the more potent and more clot-selective ("fibrin-selective") thrombolytic agent.

E. Bleeding Models

The propensity for bleeding induction by DSPAα₁ as compared with t-PA and streptokinase was studied in a venipuncture model in rat mesenteric arcade veins [42]. Venipuncture bleeding time (5 min after thrombolysis induction) was prolonged >3 min in six of six animals given 30 nmol/kg t-PA, but in only one of six animals treated with 300 nmol/kg DSPAα₁. Sixty minutes after administration of the thrombolytic agents, venipuncture bleeding time with t-PA was still prolonged to 7.7 ± 3.5 min, but to only 2.5 ± 1.8 min after treatment with DSPα₁. Rebleeding occurred in three of six animals treated with 30-nmol/kg t-PA, in none of those treated with up to 100-nmol/kg DSPA, and in five of the six treated with 300-nmol/kg DSPAα₁ (Table 2).

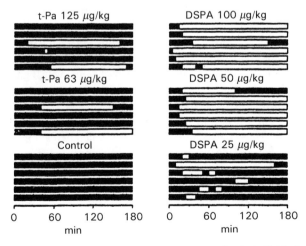

Figure 4 Patency profiles of coronary arteries in individual dogs after intravenous bolus administration of different amounts (as indicated) of DSPAα₁, tissue-type plasminogen activator (t-PA), or solvent (control). Each bar represents the angiographically defined patency status of a single dog coronary artery throughout the observation period of 180 min after dosing. Solid bars reflect periods of coronary occlusion; open bars depict periods of arterial reflow. (From Ref. 40.)

In aspirin-pretreated rabbits, the administration of 14 or 42 nmol/kg DSPAα$_2$ increased the template bleeding time to an extent similar to the administration of 42 nmol/kg of t-PA. The cuticle bleeding times in the same animals were prolonged only after the injection of t-PA. Even when the rabbits were pretreated with aspirin, only mild and transient bleeding was observed with DSPAα$_2$. Furthermore, the severity of bleeding from surgical sites was far more extensive in those rabbits that received t-PA rather than DSPAα$_2$ [39].

In another experiment, cuticle bleeding time was measured in anesthetized rabbits to assess the potential bleeding risks that may occur after bolus administration of DSPAα$_2$ (bat-PA) or t-PA [43]. Bleeding times were elevated only minimally with DSPAα$_2$, whereas t-PA exhibited a 6.2-fold increase. In contrast to DSPAα$_2$, t-PA induced a massive activation of systemic plasminogen and subsequent degradation of coagulation factors VIII and fibrinogen. The consumption of these factors may be the key event in t-PA-mediated coagulopathy.

With use of the same dosages, an equally severe degradation of factor VIII and fibrinogen by t-PA but not by DSPAα$_2$ was observed by another group using a rabbit ear puncture model of fibrinolytic bleeding [44]. However, the finding reported by these authors that bleeding occurs as frequently in animals treated with DSPAα$_2$ as in those treated with t-PA is surprising and puzzling in the light of the observed factor VIII and fibrinogen degradation by t-PA and in contrast to the results obtained by Mellott et al. [43].

It has been suggested that bleeding time is the best indicator of the risk of severe hemorrhage in patients treated with thrombolytic agents. If this assessment is correct, the results of the bleeding models suggest that thrombolysis with DSPAα$_1$ is superior in terms of therapeutic safety to other agents, currently approved for clinical use. There are, however, examples of cases in which bleeding was extended, despite an only moderately prolonged bleeding time, just as there are numerous examples of patients with massive prolongation of bleeding times who do not bleed. Thus, a definitive statement on improved safety associated with the therapeutic use of DSPAα$_1$ will have to await the results of clinical trials.

V. PHARMACOKINETICS

A sandwich enzyme-linked immunosorbent assay (ELISA) using affinity-purified and peroxidase-labeled DSPAα$_1$ antibodies raised in rabbits was developed. Its lower limit of detection was 3 ng/mL in undiluted, spiked plasma, and its accuracy was 98–108%, with a precision of 3–9.5%. No cross-reactivity with human t-PA or endogenous matrix constituents interfering with assay results was observed [45]. After intravenous administration of DSPAα$_1$ at 1 and 3 mg/kg to cynomolgus monkeys, antigen levels in plasma were dose dependent in both genders and exhibited a triphasic disposition profile with half-lives of 0.04–0.26, 0.6–3, and 4–8.5 h. The mean residence time of DSPAα$_1$ ranged from 3–9 h, and total clearance was approximately 2 mL/min kg^{-1} independent of sex and dose. These data showed a long systemic circulation of the antigen, linear pharmacokinetics, and no sex-specific pharmacokinetic differences in the dose range investigated.

In a second study, DSPAα$_1$ was characterized pharmacokinetically in rats and cynomolgus monkeys after intravenous-bolus administration of ^{125}I-labeled protein. Furthermore, several toxicokinetic studies with single or repeated administration of unlabeled DSPAα$_1$ were monitored by ELISA and fibrin clot lysis assay [FCLA) to measure antigen and activity levels. The dose range used in both species was 1–30 mg/kg. In both species, DSPAα$_1$ was characterized by long terminal half-lives of 1–2 h and 5–8 h with bi- or triphasically declining plasma levels. The terminal phase represented a partial AUC of 42–57% in monkeys. Total clearance accounted for 6–11 mL/min kg^{-1} and approximately 2 mL/min kg^{-1} in rats and monkeys, respectively. The volume of distribution in the central compartment was 0.5–

0.1 L/kg in both species. Pharmacokinetics were linear, and no sex-specific differences were observed. In both species, plasma antigen and activity levels and thus, the pharmacokinetics, exhibited a linear correlation, with a slope close to 1 over the dose range of 1–30 mg/kg. The use of ^{125}I-labeled protein provided only limited additional information for the early postdose phase, owing to rapid iodine exchange. In terms of distribution in rats, radiolabel indicative for DSPAα₁ (i.e., until 30 min postapplication) was found in the highly perfused organs and tissues. By means of allometric extrapolation, a total clearance of approximately $1\,\text{mL/min}\,\text{kg}^{-1}$ was predicted for humans (Hildebrand and Bhargava, unpublished).

DSPAα₁, therefore, displayed an advantageous pharmacokinetic and pharmacodynamic profile, especially for its low total clearance, its long terminal half-life, and the complete fibrinolytic activity of antigen present in the plasma, as compared to other established protein fibrinolytics including t-PA. Animal data are encouraging relative to the envisaged therapeutic dosage in humans (i.v. bolus) and indicate that DSPAα₁ treatment may have a reduced risk of reocclusion, compared with t-PA.

These data confirm previous observations made in dogs in the context of a coronary thrombolysis model [40]. The half-life of DSPAα₁ in dogs was greatly prolonged compared with t-PA [46], with the mean residence time being approximately 40–50 times longer. The clearance of DSPAα₁ was approximately five to nine times slower than that of t-PA, the t-PA mutant analogue TNK being cleared about half as fast as the wild-type. Again, the faster clearance of TNK–(t-PA) over t-PA [47] may translate into a minor advantage of TNK–(t-PA) over t-PA in both relative potency and total patency (including reocclusion). BM 06.022, another mutant consisting of the kringle 2 and protease domains of human t-PA, has a half-life of 13 min and a clearance of $5.1\,\text{mL} \times \text{min}^{-1} \times \text{kg}^{-1}$ in dogs [48]. It is being pursued in clinical trials as a less costly alternative to t-PA. The intention was to use BM 06.022 by single-intravenous–bolus injection. However, results obtained in a canine model of coronary thrombosis as well as first results in myocardial infarction patients indicate that the prolongation of half-life achieved with BM 06.022 may not be sufficient and that a second bolus application may be necessary to avoid early reocclusion and to achieve a satisfying degree of reperfusion [49,50]. DSPAα₁ may be the only fibrin-specific tbrombolytic agent available with a half-life long enough to allow single-bolus administration in myocardial infarction patients, because its pharmacokinetics are superior to all the afore-cited mutant forms of t-PA as well as DSPAα₂ (bat-PA).

The thrombolysis experiments performed with DSPAα₂ in a canine model of arterial thrombosis by Mellot et al. [46] are relevant to pharmacokinetics and are, therefore, also described here in detail. The reperfusion incidences after the administration of t-PA and DSPAα₂ at 14 nmol/kg were 50 and 88%, respectively. The mean times to reperfusion were not significantly different in the DSPAα₂ and t-PA treatment groups. All animals reoccluded during the 4-h trial; however, the mean time to reocclusion in the dogs treated with DSPAα₂, 144 min, was significantly delayed compared with that of t-PA-treated dogs; 37 min.

The approximately sixfold longer mean residence time of DSPAα₂ relative to t-PA was a likely contributor to the delayed reocclusion and superior thrombolytic efficacy in the DSPA treatment group. The clearance profile for t-PA was monoexponential, with a $t_{1/2}$ of 2.4 min. The clearance profile for DSPAα₂ was biexponential, with a $t_{1/2}$ of 0.9 min and a $t_{1/2}\beta$ of 20.2 min. Interestingly, the steady-state volume of distribution displayed by DSPAα₂ was 16-fold greater than that of t-PA. It was proposed that some DSPA was initially sequestered in an extraplasma compartment following administration and subsequently released back slowly into circulation; however, no experimental data were provided to support this suggestion.

The fibrinogen levels were essentially unaffected following the administration of DSPAα₂ or t-PA. Nevertheless, the absence of fibrinogenolysis in the DSPAα₂ treatment group is remarkable in the light of DSPA's prolonged mean residence time. It is also noteworthy that the mean residence time of DSPAα_2, albeit significantly longer than that of t-PA, is still six to eight times shorter than that of DSPAα_1. Indeed, this may be why a stronger tendency to reocclusion was apparent in experiments conducted with DSPAα_2 than in experiments with DSPAα_1.

VI. TOXICOLOGY

No direct toxic effects could be observed in systemic tolerance studies performed with DSPAα_1 in monkeys. Secondary effects such as bleeding, extended hematoma formation, haematological alterations, as well as organ changes, as a consequence of blood loss, were observed only at extremely high doses of DSPAα_1 up to 2×30-mg/kg intravenous bolus over 9 days or 30 mg/kg intravenous bolus over 15 days. In these studies the systemic burden of DSPAα_1 per single application represented approximately 70 times that described for the accelerated t-PA treatment scheme in humans [52].

With single intravenous-bolus applications of DSPAα_1 quantities of more than 10 mg/kg, we observed cardiac lesions (myonecrosis, myocarditis) in rats. These effects of treatment with plasminogen activators, such as streptokinase and eminase, have already been described [53,54] and are species-dependent. In monkeys no such effects were detected at any of the doses investigated. Such observations might be of limited relevance for the application of DSPAα_1 in humans.

The induction of an immunological memory, but no antibody formation, in monkeys was observed after single-bolus injections greater than 1 mg/kg body weight, whereas specific antibody formation with neutralizing capacity was observed at higher doses ($>$10 mg/kg).

In rats, antibody formation was observed only after repeated injections of DSPAα_1 in 40% of the treated animals. However, no effect on the endogenous fibrinolytic potential or any neutralization of rat t-PA activity or cross-reactivity with human t-PA was found in animals with substantial antibody titers [55]. In addition, antibodies raised in rabbits immunized with DSPAα_1 did not recognize any human t-PA in an ELISA-type assay (Fig. 5). These data indicate that antibody formation is not a major concern that might forbid a second therapeutic application, as persistence of DSPAα_1-specific antibodies did not result in any adverse effects in hemostatic or other parameters.

These detailed toxicological studies in rats and monkeys revealed no negative results that would preclude the use of DSPAα_1 in humans.

VII. PHASE I CLINICAL STUDIES

A phase I clinical trial with healthy volunteers was performed to determine the pharmacokinetics and the safety and tolerability of DSPAα_1. Subtherapeutic doses of 0.01, 0.03, and 0.05 mg/kg body weight DSPAα_1 were applied by intravenous-bolus administration. The study was designed as an open, uncontrolled interindividual group comparison. The pharmacokinetic parameters were determined by measuring DSPAα_1 antigen by ELISA from baseline up to 36 h after injection. Cardiovascular monitoring was extended over 1 h, and laboratory parameters such as DSPAα_1 activity (fibrin clot lysis assay) hemodynamics, and adverse events were monitored up to 24 h postinjection. The development of DSPAα_1 antibodies was checked for up to 3 months after the injection.

No clinically relevant changes or trends in hematology or clinical chemistry, and no negative clinical effects on blood coagulation, were observed. No formation of antibodies could

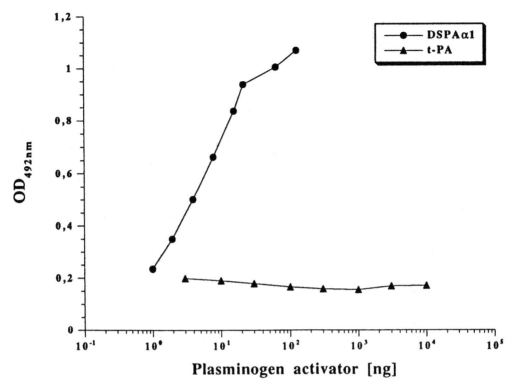

Figure 5 Cross-reactivity of human t-PA with DSPAα₁ antiserum raised in rabbits performed in an ELISA-type assay. (From Ref. 45.)

be detected. Therefore, there were no safety-related concerns in the dose range tested, and the pharmacokinetic prediction from animal studies was confirmed in humans. Based on the available pharmacokinetic data and in comparison with pharmacokinetic and clinical data of t-PA, the therapeutically effective dose of DSPAα₁ was predicted to be 0.5 mg/kg body weight (M. Mahler and W. Seifert, personal communication).

VIII. CLINICAL STUDIES WITH rDSPAα₁

A phase IIa study was conducted to evaluate the efficacy, safety, and tolerability of rDSPAα₁ as a thrombolytic agent in the treatment of patients with acute myocardial infarction. The study was designed as a non randomized, open-label, prospective dose-finding study in which patients received intravenous bolus of either 0.5 mg/kg or 0.75 mg/kg of rDSPAα₁, administered over 1–2 min, followed by intravenous heparin.

Efficacy was determined by measuring coronary angiography patency rates at 90 min after onset of thrombolysis while safety was assessed by recording the occurrence of bleedings, allergic, and other early or late complications. In addition the impact of rDSPAα₁ on the hemostatic system and the development of rDSPAα₁ antibodies after treatment were determined.

A total of 26 patients (19 men and 7 women) were enrolled into the study, with a mean age of 61 years (range 41–75) and a mean weight of 76 kg (range 62–92). The follow-up period of observation was 6 months. 18 patients received 0.5 mg/kg and 8 patients received 0.75 mg/kg of rDSPAα$_1$.

Early patency, as defined by a TIMI grade III score at the 90-min coronary angiogram, was achieved in 65% (17 of the 26 patients). Late patency (90 min to 24 h) was demonstrated in 21 patients. Out of the remaining five patients three died within 8 h after inclusion and two refused the 24 to 36 h angiogram.

The laboratory data from the study confirmed the high fibrin specificity of rDSPAα$_1$ as demonstrated by normal levels of fibrinogen. Other laboratory parameters—plasminogen, hematocrit, hemoglobin, activated partial thromboplastin time, creatine kinase, creatine kinase-MB, and α$_2$antiplasmin did not indicate any treatment-related safety issues.

The safety profile of rDSPAα$_1$ in this early study was typical for the administration of a thrombolytic in myocardial infarction. The serious adverse event reported was judged not to be rDSPAα$_1$ drug-related by the independent Safety Advisory Board. These events, rather, were indication-specific and typical for the natural course of disease.

This early study demonstrated that rDSPAα$_1$ acted as a typical plasminogen activator with comparable activity to other thrombolytics: the patency rate was 65%. Fibrin specificity was demonstrated by the fact that no fibrinogen depletion occurred. Almost all bleeding did not require any therapy. Bleeding also occurred more frequently in studies where angiography was performed and when patients were treated with high doses of heparin. Conclusions on efficacy and safety are hampered by the fact that patient number was small; however, proof of concept (thrombolysis) could be shown.

IX. CONCLUSIONS AND PERSPECTIVE

Following many years of controversy since the early 1980s, it has become generally accepted that the most significant pathophysiological event underlying AMI is the thrombotic occlusion of a coronary vessel and the subsequent myocardial damage caused by acute ischemia. It is therefore essential to reestablish coronary blood flow by surgical intervention or thrombolytic therapy as early as possible to keep myocardial necrosis at a minimum. It is well established that early mortality of AMI can be significantly reduced by either method and that the positive effects of early coronary recanalization also translate into a reduction of long-term mortality. Various thrombolytic agents are employed in various regimens, all of which are optimized to speed up the reopening of the coronary vessel while minimizing the associated risks; notably, hemorrhagic complications. In recent trials the most dangerous form of these—life-threatening intracranial bleeding—still exceeds 1% [56]. Nevertheless, even the most aggressive clinical regimens applied today do not achieve patency rates relevant for the prognosis of the patient (TIMI grade 3) [57] in more than 50% of the occluded vessels, and 20–30% of AMI patients do not respond to thrombolytic therapy at all. Moreover, acute reocclusion is seen in 25% of the patients who initially reperfuse, and the incidence of mortality is still intolerably high (approximately 10% in the Gruppo Italiano per lo studio della streptochinasi nell'infarto miocardia (GISSI-2)) [58] and in the ISIS-3 trial [59]. This limited efficacy and the fear of hemorrhagic side effects has encouraged the more widespread use of percutaneous transluminal coronary angioplasty (PTCA) which, however, excludes a large segment of the patient population for reasons of cost and the limited availability of the required facilities. Therefore, a further decrease of mortality from AMI can be achieved only by the development of more efficacious and safer thrombolytics. The introduction of a fibrinolytic agent that will not have hemorrhagic side effects would improve overall survival of AMI victims, most importantly, by increasing the number of patients eligible for therapy. Many patients today are excluded from the treatment because the risks of stroke or other complications outweigh possible benefits. DSPAα_1 is strictly fibrin-selective and not activated by fibrinogen, fibrin degradation products, or denatured protein, therefore does not lower the levels of plasminogen or coagulation factors during treatment. Unlike t-PA, DSPAα_1 is not activated by β-amyloid peptides, which frequently are deposited in the vasculature of older patients [30]. This is an important additional safety feature with a bearing on the risk of intracranial bleeding. In all relevant animal models, DSPAα_1 and DSPAα_2 were found to be more efficacious and less prone to side effects than any other thrombolytic agent currently in use.

The favorable pharmacokinetic profile of DSPAα_1 is likely to allow a single intravenous bolus regimen, which is much easier to apply than the combined front-loading and infusion regimens currently most widely used. Such a regimen will, for the first time, open the possibility of initiating thrombolytic therapy in the emergency vehicle or the home of the patient and therefore significantly broaden its current scope. It will thus establish a material underpinning for the vision that most patients who could benefit from thrombolytic therapy get a chance to receive it.

REFERENCES

1. Fletcher AP, Alkjaersig N, Sherry S. The clearance of heterologous protein from the circulation of normal and immunized man. J Clin Invest 1958; 37:1306–1315.
2. Laffel GL, Braunwald E. A new strategy for the treatment of acute myocardial infarction. N Engl J Med 1984; 311:710–717.
3. Altschule MD. The coronary occlusion story. Prolonged neglect of early clinicopathologic findings and of the experimental animal physiology they stimulated. Chest 1985; 87:81–84.
4. Collen D. On the regulation and control of fibrinolysis. Thromb Haemost 1980; 3:77–89.
5. Astrup, T, Permin PM. Fibrinolysis in animal organism. Nature 1947; 159:681–682.
6. Cole ER, Bachmann FW. Purification and properties of a plasminogen activator from pig heart. J Biol Chem 1977; 252:3729–3737.
7. Rijken DC, Collen D. Purification and characterization of the plasminogen activator secreted by human melanoma cells in culture. J Biol Chem 1981; 256:7035–7041.
8. Pennica D, Holmes WE, Kohr WJ. et al. Cloning and expression of human tissue-type plasminogen activator cDNA in E. coli. Nature 1983; 301:214–221.
9. Camiolo SM, Thorsen S, Astrup T. Fibrinogenolysis and fibrinolysis with tissue plasminogen activator, urokinase, streptokinase-activated human globulin, and plasmin. Proc Soc Exp Biol Med 1971; 138:277–280.
10. Hoylaerts M, Rijken DC, Lijnen HR, Collen D. Kinetics of the activation of plasminogen by human tissue plasminogen activator. J Biol Chem 1982; 257:2912–2919.
11. The GUSTO Investigators. An international randomized trial comparing four thrombolytic strategies for acute myocardial infarction. N Engl J Med 1993; 329:673–682.
12. Vertraete M, Ljinen HR, Collen D. Thrombolytic agents in development. Drugs 1995; 50:29–42.
13. Seifried E, Müller MM, Martin U, Künig R, Hombach U. Bolus application of a novel plasminogen activator in acute myocardial infarction patients: pharmacokinetics and effects on the hemostatic system. Ann NY Acad Sci 1992; 667:417–420.
14. Kety BA, Paoni NF, Refino CJ, et al. A faster-acting and more potent form of tissue plasminogen activator. Proc Natl Acad Sci USA 1994; 91:3670–3674.
15. Markwardt F. Coagulation inhibitors from blood-sucking animals. A new line of developing antithrombotic drugs. Pharmazie 1994; 49:313–316.
16. Bier O. Action anticoagulante et fibrinolytique de l'extrait des glances salivaires d'une chauve-souris hematophage Desmodus rufus. CR Soc Bio (Paris) 1932; 110:129.
17. Hawkey C. Plasminogen activator in the saliva of the vampire bat Desmodus rotundus. Nature 1966; 211:431–435.

18. Cartwright T. The plasminogen activator of vampire bat saliva. Blood 1974; 43:317–326.

19. Gardell SJ, Friedman PA. Vampire bat salivary plasminogen activator. In: Lorand L, Mann KG, eds. Methods in Enzymology: Proteolytic Enzymes in Coagulation, Fibrinolysis and Complement Activation, Vol. 223. San Diego, CA: Academic Press, 1993:233–249.

20. Greenhall AM, Schmidt U. Natural History of Vampire Bats. Boca Raton, FL: CRC Press, 1988.

21. Heussen G, Joubert F, Dowdle E. Purification of human tissue plasminogen activator with *Erythrina* trypsin inhibitor. J Biol Chem 1984; 259:11635–11638.

22. Gardell SL, Duong LT, Diehl RE, et al. Isolation, characterization and cDNA cloning of a vampire bat salivary plasminogen activator. J Biol Chem 1989: 264:17947–17952.

23. Schleuning W–D, Alagon A, Boidol W, et al. Plasminogen activators from the saliva of *Desmodus rotundus* (common vampire bat): unique fibrin specificity. Ann NY Acad Sci 1992; 667:395–403.

24. Petri T, Baldus B, Boidol W, et al. Novel plasminogen activators from the vampire bat *Desmodus rotundus*. In: Spier RE, Griffiths JB, MacDonald C, eds. Animal Technology: Developments, Processes and Products. Oxford: Butterworth-Heinemann, 1992; 599–604.

25. Maniatis T, Fritsch EF, Sambrook J. Molecular Cloning, A Laboratory Manual. Cold Spring Harbor NY: Cold Spring Habor Laboratory Press, 1989.

26. Astrup T, Müllertz S. The fibrin plate method for estimating fibrinolytic activity. Arch Biochem Biophys 1954; 40:346–351.

27. Petri T, Langer G, Bringmann P, et al. Production of vampire bat plasminogen activator DSPAα_1 in CHO and insect cells. J Biotechnol 1995; 39:75–83.

28. Weitz JI, Leslie B, Ginsberg I. Soluble fibrin degradation products potentiate tissue plasminogen activator-induced fibrinogen proteolysis. J Clin Invest 1991; 87:1082–1090.

29. Suenson E, Bjerrum P, Holm A, et al. The role of fragment X polymers in the fibrin enhancement of tissue plasminogen activator-catalyzed plasmin formation. J Biol Chem 1990; 265:22228–22237.

30. Kingston IB, Castro MJM, Anderson S. In vitro stimulation of tissue-type plasminogen activator by Alzheimer amyloid β-peptide analogues. Nat Med 1995; 1:138–142.

31. Bringmann P, Gruber D, Liese A, et al. Structural features mediating fibrin selectivity of vampire bat plasminogen activators. J Biol Chem 1995; 270:25596–25603.

32. Bergum PW, Gardell SJ. Vampire bat salivary plasminogen activator exhibits a strict and fastidious requirement for polymeric fibrin as its cofactor, unlike human tissue-type plasminogen activator. J Biol Chem 1992; 267:17726–17731.

33. Gardell SJ, Hare TR, Bergum PW, et al. Vampire bat plasminogen activator is quiescent in human plasma in the absence of fibrin unlike human tissue plasminogen activator. Blood 1990; 76:2560–2564.

34. Gruber D. Studien zum Wirkmechanismus neuer Plasminogen-Aktivatoren aus dem Speichel der Vampirfledermaus *Desmodus rotundus*. PhD dissertation, Freie Universität Berlin, Germany, 1995.

35. Beer JH, Kläy H–P, Herren T, Haeberli A, Straub PW. Whole blood clot lysis: enhanced by exposure to autologous but not to homologous plasma. Thromb Haemost 1994; 71:622–626.

36. Bringmann P, Liese A, Toschi L, Petri T, Schleuning W–D, Donner P. *Desmodus* salivary plasminogen activator α_1 is more potent and fibrin-selective in vitro than t-PA and TNK-(t-PA) [abstr 876]. Thromb Haemost 1995; 73:1129.

37. Hare TR, Gardell SJ. Vampire bat plasminogen activator promotes robust lysis of plasma clots in a plasma milieu without causing fluid phase plasminogen activation. Thromb Haemost 1992; 68:165–169.

38. Muschick P, Zeggert D, Dormer P, Witt W. Thrombolytic properties of *Desmodus* (vampire bat) salivary plasminogen activator DSPAα_1. Alteplase and streptokinase following intravenous bolus injection in a rabbit model of carotid artery. Fibrinolysis 1993: 7:284–290.

39. Gardell SJ, Ramjit DR, Stabilito II, et al. Effective thrombolysis without marked plasminemia after bolus intravenous administration of vampire bat salivary plasminogen activator in rabbits. Circulation 1991; 84:244–253.

40. Witt W, Maass B, Baldus B, Hildebrand M, Dormer P, Schleuning W–D. Coronary thrombolysis with *Desmodus* salivary plasminogen activator in dogs. Circulation 1994; 90:421–426.

41. Witt W, Baldus B, Bringmann P, Cashion L, Donner P, Schleuning W–D. Thrombolytic properties of *Desmodus rotundus* (vampire bat) salivary plasminogen activator in experimental pulmonary embolism in rats. Blood 1992: 79:1213–1217.

42. Gulba DC, Praus M, Witt W. DSPA alpha—properties of the plasminogen activators of the vampire bat *Desmondus rotundus*. Fibrinolysis 1995; 9:91–96.
43. Mellott MJ, Ramjit DR, Stabilito II, et al. Vampire bat salivary plasminogen activator evokes minimal bleeding relative to tissue-type plasminogen activator as assessed by a rabbit cubicle bleeding time model. Thromb Haemost 1995; 73:478–483.
44. Montoney M, Gardell SJ, Marder VJ. Comparison of the bleeding potential of vampire bat salivary plasminogen activator versus tissue plasminogen activator in an experimental rabbit model. Circulation 1995; 91:1540–1544.
45. Hildebrand M, Bunte T, Bringmann P, Schutt A. Development of an ELISA for the measurement of DSPAα₁ (*Desmodus rotundus* salivary plasminogen activator) in plasma and its application to investigate pharmacokinetics in monkeys. Fibrinolysis 1995; 9:107–111.
46. Mellott MJ, Stabilito II, Holohan MA, et al. Vampire bat salivary plasminogen activator promotes rapid and sustained reperfusion without concomitant systemic plasminogen activation in a canine model of arterial thrombosis. Arterioscler Thromb 1992; 12:212–221.
47. Collen D, Stassen JM, Refino CJ, et al. Comparative thrombolytic properties of recombinant tissue-type plasminogen activator (rt-PA) and of two plasminogen activator inhibitor-1 (PAI-1) resistant glycosylation variants in a combined arterial and venous thrombosis model in dogs [abstr]. Thromb Haemost 1993; 69:841.
48. Martin U, Fischer S, Kohnert U, et al. Properties of a novel plasminogen activator (BM 06.022) produced In *Escherichia coli*. Z Kardiol 1990; 79(suppl 3):167–170.
49. Martin U, Sponer G, König R, Smolarz A, Meyer–Sabellek W, Strein K. Double bolus administration of the novel recombinant plasminogen activator BM 06.022 improves coronary blood flow after reperfusion in a canine model of coronary thrombosis. Blood Coagul Fibrinol 1991; 3:139–147.
50. Neuhaus K–L, von Essen R, Vogt A. et al., GRECO Study Group. Dose-ranging study of a novel recombinant plasminogen activator in patients with acute myocardial infarction: results of the GRECO study [abstr]. Circulation 1991; 84(suppl II):II–573.
51. Krätzschmar J, Haendler B, Langer G, et al. The plasrninogen activator family from the salivary gland of the vampire bat *Desmodus rotundus*: cloning and expression. Gene 1991; 105:229–237.
52. Neuhaus K–L, Feuerer W, Jeep–Tebbe S, Niederer W, Vogt A, Tebbe U. Improved thrombolysis with a modified dose regimen of recombinant tissue-type plasminogen activator. J Am Coll Cardiol 1989; 14:1566–1569.
53. Waldmann G. Zur Pathogenese der Myocarditis rheumatica. In: Seidel K, ed. Beiräge zur Rheumatologie. Berlin: VEB Verlag Volk und Gesundheit, 1971:100–108.
54. Artus JA, Cockburn A, Fuller J, McMurdo AS, White DJ. The preclinical toxicology of anisoylated plasminogen streptokinase activator complex. Drugs 1987; 33:97–101.
55. Witt W, Kirchhoff D, Woy P, Zierz R, Bhargava AS. Antibody formation and effects on endogeneous fibrinolysis after repeated administration of DSPAα₁ in rats [abstr. 182]. Fibrinolysis 1994; 8:66.
56. De Jaegere PP, Arnold AA, Balk AH, Simoons ML. Intracranial hemorrhage in association with thrombolytic therapy: incidence and clinical predictive factors. J Am Coll Cardiol 1992; 1D:289–294.
57. Topol EJ. Validation of the early open infarct vessel hypothesis. Am J Cardiol 1993; 72:40G–45G.
58. Gruppo italiano per lo studio della streptochinasi nell'infarto miocardico. Effectiveness of intravenous thrombolytic treatment in acute myocardial infarction (GISSI). Lancet 1986; 1I:397–401.
59. ISIS 3 (Third International Study of Infarct Survival) Collaborative Study Group. ISIS 3: a randomized comparison of streptokinase vs tissue plasminogen activator vs anistreplase and of aspirin plus heparin vs aspirin alone among 41,299 cases of suspected acute myocardial infarction. Lancet 1992; 339:753–770.

39

Alfimeprase

Christopher F. Toombs

Amgen, Inc., Thousand Oaks, California, U.S.A.

SUMMARY

Alfimeprase is a recombinantly produced, truncated form of fibrolase, a known directly fibrinolytic zinc metalloprotease that was first isolated from the venom of the southern copperhead snake (*Agkistrodon contortrix contortrix*). Both fibrolase and alfimeprase have direct proteolytic activity against the fibrinogen Aα chain. In contrast, agents such as streptokinase or t-PA are not directly fibrinolytic; instead they promote thrombolysis through plasminogen activation. *In vivo* pharmacology studies have shown that thrombolysis with alfimeprase is up to six times more rapid than with plasminogen activators. Alfimeprase can be bound and neutralized by serum α_2-macroglobulin, a prevalent mammalian protease inhibitor, which is capable of forming a macromolecular complex with alfimeprase. As a result, systemic bleeding complications have been greatly reduced by the inhibitory effects of α_2-macroglobulin. However, when systemic dosages exceed the α_2-macroglobulin inhibitory capacity, toxicities appear, including hypotension and impaired hemostatis. The hypotensive effects have subsequently been found to be due to the generation of kinins and their effects evoked through the BK_2 receptor. However, these toxicities are not likely to be encountered in clinical testing as estimates of safe dosages have been calculated from more than 200 patients with peripheral vascular disease; clinically useful doses are likely to remain within these bounds. This chapter reviews the biochemical, in vitro, and in vivo characteristics of this novel-acting thrombolytic agent.

I. INTRODUCTION

Alfimeprase is a recombinantly produced truncated form of fibrolase, a known fibrinolytic zinc metalloprotease that was first isolated from the venom of *Agkistrodon contortrix contortrix*, the southern copperhead snake [1]. Fibrolase is a member of clan MB of metallopeptidases, family M12, subfamily B (the reprolysins), a grouping of proteolytic enzymes that comprise many enzymes originally characterized from snake venom.

The alfimeprase molecule differs slightly from fibrolase at the N terminus where alfimeprase contains 201 amino acids with an N terminal sequence of SFPQR···, in contrast

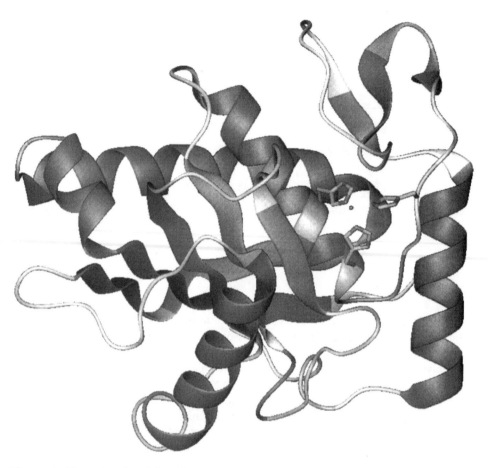

Figure 1 The active site of the alfimeprase molecule spans amino acids 139–159 and contains a zinc atom (sphere) which is complexed by three histidine residues (pentagons). This three-dimensional representation is positioned to see the active site. In three dimensions, the amino terminus is on the opposite side of the molecule and cannot be viewed in this projection.

to the N-terminal sequences of fibrolase, which begins with EQRFPQR··· and is 203 amino acids in length. The truncation was designed to prevent chemical reactions at amino acid residues that were capable of forming a variable quantity of cyclized glutamine (pyroglutamic acid), which is the basis for the two observed isoforms of fibrolase. Most of the studies described in this chapter were conducted with recombinant alfimeprase; however, in a few instances, where noted, a recombinant preparation of fibrolase was used.

Although alfimeprase is a modest two-amino acid truncation of fibrolase, the two enzymes are similar in enzymatic activity and the ability to be bound to and inhibited by α_2-macroglobulin. This is consistent with the data of Manning [2] indicating that the active site of the fibrolase spans amino acids 139–159, and its location, in three-dimensional space, is distant from the N-terminus where the truncation was made (see Fig. 1 for the predicted three-dimensional structure of fibrolase).

II. FIBRINOLYTIC ACTIVITY OF ALFIMEPRASE

Both fibrolase and alfimeprase are fibrinolytic, and fibrolase has been previously documented to have proteolytic activity against the fibrinogen Aα-chain, with reduced proteolytic cleavage of the Bβ-chain and no activity against the γ chain of fibrinogen [3]. In contrast, agents such as streptokinase, urokinase, and tissue-type plasminogen activator (t-PA) are plasminogen activators that promote thrombolysis by activation of the engogenous fibrinolytic system. Plasminogen activators catalyse the conversion of plasminogen into plasmin, a serine protease. It is through the generation of plasmin that the plasminogen activators ultimately effect fibrin degradation and, therefore, clot lysis. In contrast to the plasminogen activator class of thrombolytic drugs, fibrolase and alfimeprase do not rely on the endogeneous fibrinolytic system (conversion of plasminogen to plasmin). Hence, fibrolase and alfimeprase can be distinguished from the plasminogen activators by their unique mode of action and are defined as direct fibrinolytic agents.

The potential clinical advantages of such an agent are twofold: first, the demonstrated advantage in speed of lysis will be potentially advantageous as reperfusion may occur more quickly and salvage of ischemic tissues may be enhanced; second, the systemic inhibition of alfimeprase by α_2-macroglobulin may reduce the incidence of hemorrhagic complications.

III. SUBSTRATES OF ALFIMEPRASE AND FIBROLASE

Published literature on venom fibrolase has demonstrated the proteolytic activity against fibrinogen at the Lys[413]–Leu[414] site [4] and against the oxidized β-chain of insulin at the Ala[14]–Leu[15] site [5,6]. Alfimeprase also has proteolytic activity on these substrates. The degradation of the fibrinogen Aα chain can easily be demonstrated in a gel-based method, as first described with fibrolase by Ahmed [3] and replicated in Figure 2 using alfimeprase. To

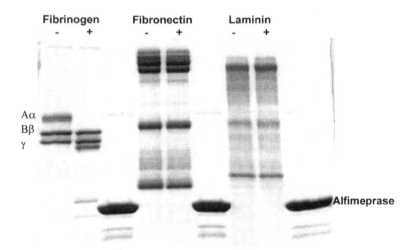

Figure 2 Samples of human fibrinogen, fibronectin, or laminin were incubated with alfimeprase (+ lanes) or buffer (− lanes) at 37°C for 30 minutes. Separation of the reaction mixture by SDS-PAGE and visualization of proteins with Coomassie staining reveals proteolytic degradation of the fibrinogen Aα chain in the presence of alfimeprase. In contrast, degradation of fibronectin or laminin was not observed. Purified alfimeprase, at an approximate molecular weight of 22.6 kD, appears in the lanes between each substrate protein.

explore other possible substrates for alfimeprase, a protein database search of amino acid sequences was conducted using the octapeptide sequences that surround the Lys^{413}–Leu^{414} (His-Thr-Glu-**Lys-Leu**-Val-Thr-Ser) and Ala^{14}–Leu^{15} (Leu-Val-Glu-**Ala-Leu**-Tyr-Leu-Val) cleavage sites in fibrinogen and oxidized β-chain of insulin, respectively. A search based on these sequences identified two proteins of potential interest, laminin β_3 precursor and fibronectin. Although these proteins contain potential cleavage sites, no cleavage of laminin or fibronectin by alfimeprase was observed in the gel-based assay that clearly shows proteolysis of fibrinogen A_{α} chain (Fig. 2). Hence, the presence of target peptide sequences within laminin and fibronectin does not correctly predict these proteins as alfimeprase substrates, suggesting that the target sequence must be properly oriented within the tertiary structure of a potential target protein such that it is accessible to proteolytic cleavage. Conversely, it is possible for other proteins, which were not identified by searches based on the octapeptide sequences containing Lys-Leu or Ala-Leu, to be substrates for alfimeprase owing to their tertiary structural motifs.

IV. α_2-MACROGLOBULIN

α_2-Macroglobulin is a prevalent protease inhibitor present in mammalian serum and is one of the largest of the serum proteins (725 kDa). The properties of α_2-macroglobulin that are relevant to alfimeprase are described in this section and for a more thorough review, see Barrett [7]. The specificity of α_2-macroglobulin for proteases is broad, encompassing serine, cysteine, aspartic, and metalloproteases classes. The α_2-macroglobulin molecule is a tetramer of identical subunits that are disulfide bonded in pairs with a noncovalent association of the half molecules. Thus, under reducing conditions, α_2-macroglobulin can be dissociated into its four monomeric subunits.

Each subunit of α_2-macroglobulin possesses a region that is very susceptible to proteolytic cleavage (the "bait" region). Proteolysis of the bait region induces a conformational change in α_2-macroglobulin, which entraps the protease within the α_2-macroglobulin molecule. This process is described in the literature as a "venus fly-trap" interaction. Once the protease is entrapped, the protease is sterically hindered and, therefore, cannot access macromolecular substrate.

In addition, a covalent bond can form between α_2-macroglobulin and many of the proteases that it entraps. As mentioned, entrapment of a protease induces a conformational change in the α_2-macroglobulin molecule. It is presumed that with this conformational change, a thioester bond on the interior of the α_2-macroglobulin molecule becomes reactive and can form a covalent bond with nucleophilic residues (such as lysine) of the entrapped protease. Thus, within the general circulation, α_2-macroglobulin can effectively neutralize a variety of proteases by entrapment of the protease which, in some instances, also becomes covalently bound to α_2-macroglobulin.

The conformational change in α_2-macroglobulin that is brought about by the entrapment of a protease results in a form that is recognized by the reticuloendothelial system. Clearance of α_2-macroglobulin–entrapped proteases is generally described with half-life values in minutes and is believed to occur through the low-density lipoprotein (LDL) receptor-related protein expressed on macrophages, hepatocytes, and fibroblasts.

A. Interaction of Alfimeprase with Purified Human α_2-Macroglobulin

α_2-Macroglobulin is a prevalent protease inhibitor, present in mammalian serum, that is capable of forming a macromolecular complex with alfimeprase. Unlike some proteases that can form a dissociable complex with α_2-macroglobulin, alfimeprase forms a complex and cannot be dissociated from α_2-macroglobulin under physiological conditions.

As shown in Figure 3, alfimeprase remains bound to α_2-macroglobulin even under the harsh laboratory conditions used to process samples for Western blotting (reducing agent, detergent, and boiling), confirming the nondissociable nature of the alfimeprase–α_2-macroglobulin complex.

Although α_2-macroglobulin is an effective protease inhibitor, its affinity for proteases varies. For example, plasmin can be inhibited by α_2-macroglobulin, but the interaction is slow. Therefore, we sought to describe the rate of inhibition of alfimeprase by α_2-macroglobulin.

As shown in Figure 3, when purified human α_2-macroglobulin and alfimeprase are incubated together, formation of the complex begins in seconds and is nearly complete within a few minutes. Although these data demonstrate that in vitro complex formation can be rapid, they only suggest the potential rapidity of complex formation in vivo.

B. Alfimeprase Binding to α_2-Macroglobulin Occurs in a 1 : 1 Molar Ratio

Trypsin is one example of protease that is bound and inhibited by α_2-macroglobulin, and it is possible for two trypsin molecules to become entrapped by α_2-macroglobulin; hence, the stoichiometry for trypsin–α_2-macroglobulin is 2 : 1. In contrast, venom fibrolase complexes

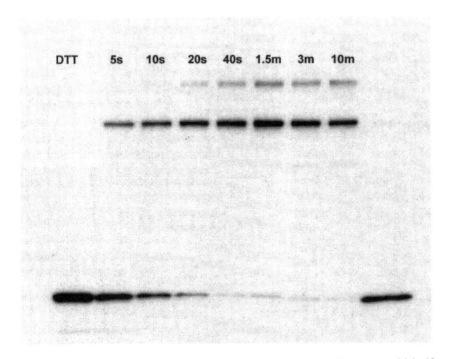

Figure 3 SDS-PAGE separation and Western blot visualization of the rate at which alfimeprase can form complex with purified human α_2-macroglobulin. Alfimeprase and purified human α_2- macroglobulin are incubated together and at various timepoints, the formation of complex is stopped by the addition of a buffer containing the reducing agent dithiothreotol (DTT). If α_2-macroglobulin is treated with DTT prior to the addition of alfimeprase (DTT lane), formation of the complex is completely prevented, indicating that DTT is an effective stopping agent. Upon the addition of alfimeprase, complex formation begins as early as 5 seconds (5s lane) and is nearly complete within 1.5 minutes (1.5m lane).

with α_2-macroglobulin in a 1 : 1 molar ratio; therefore, alfimeprase was also expected to bind in a 1 : 1 ratio. Even though the moderate truncation would not be expected to alter the 1 : 1 binding ratio, given that the molecular weight of alfimeprase (22.6 kDa) is similar to that of trypsin (23.8 kDa), we sought to determine empirically the stoichiometry of the interaction between alfimeprase and α_2-macroglobulin.

When alfimeprase and purified human α_2-macroglobulin are incubated together in equimolar ratios, virtually all of the alfimeprase is incorporated into a α_2-macroglobulin complex (Fig. 4). When alfimeprase is present in a twofold molar excess of α_2-macroglobulin, there is an ample amount of unbound alfimeprase remaining. This suggests that whereas α_2-macroglobulin can form complex with an equimolar quantity of alfimeprase, it cannot complex a twofold molar excess of alfimeprase, indicating that the stoichiometry of the interaction is 1 : 1.

C. α_2-Macroglobulin Binding in Human Plasma is Saturable

Although α_2-macroglobulin is one of the major plasma proteins, nonetheless, there is a finite quantity of α_2-macroglobulin available to bind and neutralize alfimeprase. The α_2-macroglobulin-binding capacity is, therefore, saturable. Figure 5 depicts a titration experiment in which a range of alfimeprase concentrations is added to a plasma sample from an individual human donor. When low concentrations of alfimeprase are added to plasma (< 30 µg of alfimeprase per milliliter of plasma), only the high-molecular-weight alfimeprase–α_2-macroglobulin complex

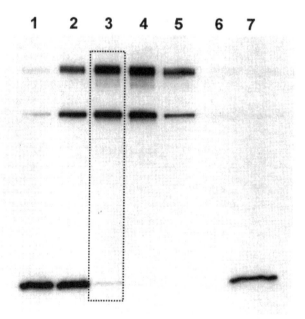

Figure 4 SDS-PAGE separation and Western blot visualization of alfimeprase combined with purified human α_2-macroglobulin, where alfimeprase and purified human α_2-macroglobulin were incubated at varying molar ratios. In lane 3 (dashed box), alfimeprase and α_2-macroglobulin are present in a 1:1 molar ratio and the immunoreactive bands are indicative of alfimeprase being present in the complexed form. When alfimeprase is present in molar excess of α_2-macroglobulin, unbound alfimeprase is present in the sample (lanes 1 and 2). Lane 1, a 10-fold molar excess; Lane 2, a 2-fold molar excess; Lane 3, an equimolar ratio; Lane 4, α_2-macroglobulin in 2-fold molar excess; Lane 5, α_2-macroglobulin in 10-fold molar excess; Lane 6, blank; Lane 7, purified alfimeprase.

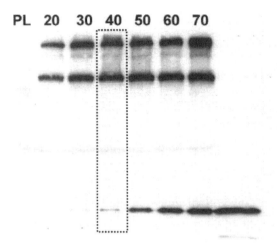

PL 20 30 40 50 60 70

Figure 5 SDS-PAGE separation and Western blot visualization of titration of plasma binding capacity with alfimeprase. In the lane loaded with plasma (PL) no immunoreactive bands are detected. At concentrations of $< 30\,\mu g/mL$ (20 and 30 lanes), alfimeprase is almost completely complexed with α_2-macroglobulin. At concentrations of $40\,\mu g/mL$ (40 lane) and higher (50, 60, and 70 lanes), the α_2-macroglobulin binding capacity in plasma has clearly been saturated and unbound alfimeprase can be detected in the sample. The last lane contains a purified alfimeprase standard, which migrates at approximately 22.6 kD.

form is detectable. At concentrations that approach and then slightly exceed the α_2-macroglobulin-binding capacity of this particular sample, the unbound alfimeprase begins to become detectable. Once the α_2-macroglobulin-binding capacity has been exceeded, the concentration of unbound alfimeprase rises proportionally as additional alfimeprase is added to the sample.

As these data demonstrate, the capacity for plasma to bind and neutralize alfimeprase is saturable and this is most likely a function of α_2-macroglobulin content. As α_2-macroglobulin is hypothesized to be the most important determinant of the alfimeprase safety profile, clinical dosing should be planned such that the total dose of alfimeprase administered remains within the plasma α_2-macroglobulin-binding capacity.

V. IN VITRO LYSIS OF CLOTTED HUMAN WHOLE BLOOD

The activity of alfimeprase has been demonstrated in an in vitro model of clot lysis. Human blood can be clotted by the addition of a high calcium concentration. Once formed, these clots can be solubilized with thrombolytic agents. The rate of clot lysis can be assessed by visual inspection of the clot mass.

As can be visually observed in the data of Figure 6, when a fixed amount of alfimeprase is used to degrade clots of varying sizes, the time required for clot dissolution increases proportionally with the mass of the clot.

A. In Vitro Lysis of Preformed Clots Mounted in PTFE Grafts

The activity of alfimeprase has been demonstrated in an in vitro model of clot lysis. Briefly, clots are formed from human whole blood to which thrombin and excessive calcium have been added.

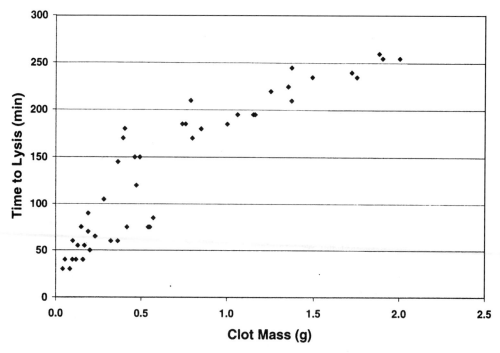

Figure 6 Scatter plot of individual clot lysis experiments. Retracted whole human blood clots were formed from citrated whole blood by the addition of excessive calcium and incubation for 90 minutes. The clotted blood was cut into various sizes, weighed and transferred to new tubes containing 2 mg of alfimeprase (0.4 mL of a 5 mg/mL solution). The tubes were inspected visually over a period of 5-hours and time to clot lysis was determined as the timepoint at which no visible clot mass remained.

The clots are incubated for 90 min. The clots are removed from the tubes and mounted in 5 cm sections of polytetrafluorethylene (PTFE) vascular graft material, which is then placed in a parallel branch of a closed-loop extracorporeal circuit, perfused with heparinized whole blood at 37°C. Flow through the circuit is initiated using a roller-pump and is adjusted so that perfusion remains at physiological pressure of approximately 60 mmHg.

An access port in the perfusion circuit is used to introduce a multiple sidehole drug delivery catheter. The catheter is advanced into the clot and positioned such that the sideholes are situated within the clot. Flow through the clotted graft segment is monitored with an ultrasonic Doppler flowprobe. At the initiation of the experiment, flow through the clotted graft segment is zero, and the time to clot lysis is determined as the time when flow through the graft segment has

Table 1 In Vitro Lysis of Human Clots in 5-cm PTFE Graft Segments

Drug	$n =$	Dose	Incidence of successful lysis	Time to lysis (min ± SD)
Alfimeprase	5	2 mg	40% (2 of 5)	52.3 ± 12.4
Alfimeprase	4	3 mg	100% (4 of 4)	38.9 ± 15.6[a]
Alfimeprase	5	5 mg	100% (5 of 5)	23.5 ± 4.7[a]
UK	9	30,000 U	100% (9 of 9)	56.7 ± 15.2

[a]Indicates $p < 0.05$ vs. urokinase group by ANOVA and Fishers PLSD testing.

Table 2 In Vitro Lysis of Human Clots in 14-cm PTFE Graft Segments

Drug	n =	Dose	Incidence of successful lysis	Time to lysis (min ± SD)
Alfimeprase	5	5 mg	40% (2 of 5)	41.2 ± 21.1
Alfimeprase	5	10 mg	100% (4 of 4)	38.3 ± 12.1
Alfimeprase	5	15 mg	100% (5 of 5)	31.8 ± 12.7

[a]Although time to lysis was shortest in the alfimeprase 15-mg group, the effect failed to reach statistical significance.

been restored. In most experiments, a precontracted clot was packed into a 5-cm length of PTFE, mounted in the perfusion circuit, and then treated with a variety of regimens. As shown in Table 1, a 2-mg dose of alfimeprase successfully dissolved the clot in only two of five cases. Doses of 3 mg and higher were uniformly effective in achieving clot lysis. Furthermore, lysis occurred more rapidly as the dose of alfimeprase was increased to 5 mg. The dose of urokinase that was used in the 5-cm segment was proportional to the urokinase dosage that was used to treat thrombotic occlusion in peripheral arteries. Treatment with 30,000 U of urokinase was also uniformly effective in achieving clot lysis. In a separate group of experiments, clotted blood was mounted in 14-cm segments of PTFE graft to determine alfimeprase's efficacy in larger clots. In the 5-cm segments, treatment with 5 mg of alfimeprase was consistently effective in achieving clot lysis. However, when 5 mg of alfimeprase was used in the 14-cm–graft segments, lysis was observed in only two of five experiments (40%). With 10 mg, alfimeprase was successful in four of four cases and, when the dose was raised further, clot lysis was observed in all cases and occurred more rapidly (Table 2).

Collectively, these data indicate that alfimeprase can effectively restore blood flow in this clotted graft model. Furthermore, these results show that for either the 5- or 14-cm–graft segment, an apparent dose–response relation is observed for both the incidence of and time to clot lysis.

VI. STUDIES THAT DEMONSTRATE BIOLOGICAL ACTIVITY IN ANIMALS

A. Thrombolysis in Acute Thrombosis of the Carotid Artery of Piglets and Rats

Pharmacology studies were conducted in carotid arteries that have been acutely thrombosed by locally injuring the vessel with anodal current. In these studies, an occlusive thrombus generally forms within 15 min. Once formed, the thrombosed carotid artery is observed for a period of 30 min to assure that the carotid occlusion is stable. Heparin and aspirin are then administered intravenously to prevent further propagation of the thrombus. In these studies, a small needle (30-g) was introduced into the artery in the vicinity of the occlusive thrombus and then cemented into place such that test agents could be administered locally.

Thrombolysis was attempted by intra-arterial (IA) infusion of test agents in a blinded fashion using numbered, coded syringes. While study drugs were being administered, flow through the carotid artery was monitored with a perivascular flow probe to determine the time at which reflow occurs. The time to lysis was recorded and group means were calculated for those experiments in which clot lysis was successful. Blood pressure and heart rate were observed during the study to monitor any untoward effects of the test agents. As a measure of the hemorrhagic potential of the test agents, any blood that was shed from the surgical site was collected with gauze swabs. The swabs were placed in a detergent solution to solubilize red blood cells and release hemoglobin, which was then quantified spectrophotometrically. Shed hemoglobin was mathematically converted into a volume of blood loss by using the hemoglobin concentration of whole blood (in grams per deciliter [g/dL]), which was measured for each animal.

The studies described in the following sections have been conducted using recombinant fibrolase or alfimeprase and have been compared with results obtained with either t-PA or urokinase (UK) as reference agents. In all studies, observations were continued for 90-min after initiation of the thrombolytic treatment regimen. Hemodynamic data are reported at baseline and after 15 min into the particular treatment regimen, a timepoint that coincides with the observation of hypotension following administration of alfimeprase in toxicology studies. Select data from these studies are presented as group means ± standard errors in the following sections.

1. Piglets: Comparison of Fibrolase and t-PA

Recombinant fibrolase was compared with t-PA in a piglet model of acute thrombosis and thrombolysis. Test agents were administered in a blinded fashion using numbered-coded pairs of syringes such that experiments were conducted and data collected without an awareness of the identity of treatment groups. Following administration of heparin (500-U/kg bolus + 500-U/kg h^{-1} infusion) and aspirin (5 mg/kg) in all animals, the first syringe was infused for 3 min and the second syringe was infused over the following 87 min for a total infusion time of 90 min. For fibrolase, the first syringe contained a fixed milligram dose of fibrolase and the second syringe contained saline. For t-PA, the first syringe contained one-third of the total milligram per kilogram dose and the second syringe contained the remaining two-thirds of the dose. In this way, the blind could be maintained while the dose of fibrolase was administered over 3 min and the dose of t-PA was administered as a 90-min "accelerated" infusion. The accelerated infusion of t-PA used in this study is qualitatively similar to the dosing recommendations for the clinical use of t-PA in the treatment of acute myocardial infarction.

As shown in Table 3, clot lysis in the 5- and 15-mg–fibrolase groups was more rapid than all other groups. In addition, t-PA (at 2 and 6 mg/kg) was associated with a significant amount of blood loss from the surgical site, whereas blood loss in the 2.5 and 5-mg–fibrolase treatment groups was not appreciably different from the negative-control group (saline). In the 15-mg–fibrolase group, blood loss was significantly different from the saline control group. Given the body weights of the piglets in the 15-mg group (5.3 ± 0.4 kg), this dosage was roughly equivalent to 3 mg/kg and likely to have exceeded the animal's capacity to systematically neutralize fibrolase. Whereas some changes in mean arterial pressure and heart rate reached statistical significance in saline and t-PA groups, no changes were noted in the fibrolase treatment groups.

2. Rats: Comparison of Alfimeprase and Urokinase

Alfimeprase has been compared with urokinase in a rat model of acute carotid thrombosis and thrombolysis. Test agents were administered in a blinded fashion using numbered-coded pairs of syringes such that experiments were conducted and data collected without an awareness of the identity of treatment groups. Following administration of heparin (100-U/kg bolus) and aspirin (5 mg/kg) in all animals, the first-coded syringe was infused for 6 min and the second-coded syringe was infused over the following 54 min for a total infusion time of 60 min. In the case of alfimeprase, the first syringe contained a fixed milligram dose of alfimeprase and the second syringe contained saline. In the case of UK, both the first and second syringes contained urokinase so that the delivery of urokinase would be by a 60-min infusion. In this way, the blind could be maintained while the dose of alfimeprase was administered over 6 min and the dose of

Table 3 Selected Parameters from a Comparison of r-Fibrolase and t-PA on Thrombolysis of Acutely Thrombosed Piglet Carotid Arteries

	Incidence of lysis (%)	Time to lysis (min)	Carotid flow (mL/min)		Blood volume loss (mL)	Mean arterial pressure (mmHg)		Heart Rate (min^{-1})	
			Base	90′Rx	90′Rx	Base	15′Rx	Base	15′Rx
Saline	0%	N/A	24.7	0.0	1.9	89.3	86.6	105	80*
($n = 8$)	(0 of 8)		±3.4	±0.0	±0.6	±4.8	±4.6	±11	±6
t-PA	30%	41.7	41.3	2.1	5.7	104.1	90.9	111	82*
1 mg/kg	(3 of 10)	±8.9	±4.7	±1.1	±1.2	±2.4	±4.7	±7	±3
($n = 10$)									
t-PA	70%	17.8	21.2	13.6	17.1*	96.0	90.2	111	90*
2 mg/kg	(7 of 10)	±5.7	±3.2	±3.0	±2.1	±4.3	±5.1	±15	±8
($n = 10$)									
t-PA	86%	51.5	30.6	6.1	9.8*	93.0	96.7	132	93*
6 mg/kg	(6 of 7)	±6.8	±4.9	±3.3	±1.9	±3.4	±5.7	±12	±8
($n = 7$)									
r-Fibrolase	64%	26.6	33.6	2.2	3.3	99.7	95.3	126	111
2.5 mg	(7 of 11)	±5.1	±4.1	±1.4	±1.5	±8.2	±7.2	±17	±12
($n = 11$)									
r-Fibrolase	100%	4.4*	26.0	8.1	1.7	88.2	89.2	107	109
5 mg	(11 of 11)	±0.9	±3.1	±2.1	±0.5	±5.3	±5.0	±9	±8
($n = 11$)									
r-Fibrolase	100%	6.1*	35.1	10.1	6.9*	87.0	88.7	98	88
15 mg	(7 of 7)	±2.0	±3.4	±2.4	±1.2	±6.6	±8.6	±12	±6
($n = 7$)									

Base: baseline timepoint following surgical instrumentation, but before the formation of thrombus. 15′Rx and 90′Rx; timepoints at 15 and 90 min following the administration of test agents.

Time to lysis: * indicates significant difference ($p < 0.05$) vs. all other groups by Kaplan Meier estimates.

Blood loss: * indicates significant differences ($p < 0.05$) from saline group by ANOVA.

Mean arterial pressure and Heart rate: *indicates significant difference ($p < 0.05$) from baseline timepoint by paired t-test. All data are presented as mean ± standard error.

urokinase was administered as a 60-min infusion. Although infusion of study medication was stopped at 60 min, animals were observed for an additional 30 min (90 min from initiation of treatment).

As shown in Table 4, clot lysis in the 2-mg–alfimeprase group was more rapid than all other groups. In addition, urokinase (at 250 U/min) was associated with a significant amount of blood loss from the surgical site, whereas blood loss in the urokinase 25-U/min or alfimeprase 2-mg groups was not statistically different from the negative-control group (saline). Although some changes in mean arterial pressure reached statistical significance in saline and urokinase 250-U/min groups, no changes were noted in the alfimeprase treatment group.

3. Thrombolysis of Acute Thrombosis in Exteriorized Thrombogenic Segments of Dacron Graft in Baboons

Studies have been conducted in baboons with permanently implanted, exteriorized arteriovenous shunts. In these studies, 5-cm × 3-mm segments of knitted Dacron graft were coated with

Table 4 Selected Parameters from a Comparison of Alfimeprase and Urokinase on Thrombolysis in Acutely Thrombosed Rat Carotid Arteries

	Incidence of lysis (%)	Time to lysis (min)	Carotid flow (mL/min)		Blood volume loss (mL)	Mean arterial pressure (mmHg)		Heart Rate (min^{-1})	
			Base	90'Rx	90'Rx	Base	15'Rx	Base	15'Rx
Saline (n = 6)	0% (0 of 6)	N/A	4.3 ±1.5	0.0 ±0.0	0.10 ±0.10	85.2 ±3.6	76.5* ±3.2	315 ±23	311 ±20
UK 25 U/min (n = 15)	47% (7 of 15)	55.3 ±4.3	3.2 ±0.4	0.7 ±0.3	1.06 ±0.41	87.7 ±3.6	87.1 ±3.4	306 ±9	313 ±8
UK 250 U/min (n = 15)	87% (13 of 15)	33.5 ±4.1	4.1 ±0.7	1.8 ±0.5	1.43* ±0.38	89.8 ±5.6	82.5* ±4.1	320 ±8	317 ±8
Alfimeprase 2 mg (n = 14)	71% (10 of 14)	6.3* ±1.6	3.8 ±0.5	2.1 ±0.7	0.97 ±0.21	87.1 ±4.6	84.5 ±3.6	305 ±9	310 ±9

Base: baseline timepoint following surgical instrumentation, but before the formation of thrombus. 15'Rx and 90'Rx; timepoints at 15 and 90 min following the administration of test agents.
Time to lysis: * indicates significant difference ($p < 0.05$) vs. all other groups by Kaplan Meier estimates.
Blood loss: * indicates significant differences ($p < 0.05$) from saline group by ANOVA.
Mean arterial pressure *indicates significant difference ($p < 0.05$) from baseline timepoint by paired t-test. All data are presented as mean ± standard error.

collagen and tissue factor. These coated grafts were then interposed between the arterial and venous arms of the shunt. Once the grafts had been positioned, flow through the circuit was monitored with a flow probe until the graft became completely occluded. Once the graft was occluded, a small (25-g) butterfly infusion set was used to puncture the tubing adjacent to the thrombosed graft and was then cemented in place. Thrombolytic agents were administered locally through the butterfly catheter, in the vicinity of the occluded segment (< 1 cm distance), and flow through the segment was continuously monitored with a flow probe to determine the time at which restoration of blood flow occurred.

As shown in Table 5, both alfimeprase and urokinase were effective in achieving thrombolysis in this model. As these exteriorized, occluded grafts were connected to the femoral artery/vein of a support animal, the systemic effects of these agents could be monitored as flow was restored and test articles enter the general circulation of the support animal. In the urokinase-treated grafts, there appeared to be a pronounced rise in circulating fibrin D-dimer in the support animal, coupled with a decrease in fibrinogen concentration. However, neither of these changes reached statistical significance. No change in D-dimer was noted in alfimeprase-treated animals and the change in fibrinogen appeared minimal. Collectively, these data suggest that in this model, local delivery of alfimeprase results in thrombolysis of the occluded shunt without production of a systemic lytic state in the support animal.

Table 5 Time to Lysis in Exteriorized Thrombosed Grafts and Changes in Systemic Hemostatic Parameters in Support Animal

Drug	Concentration	Total drug delivered (mg or U)	Time to lysis (min)	D-Dimer (ng/mL)			Fibrinogen (mg/dL)		
				Pre	Post	Δ%	Pre	Post	Δ%
Alfimeprase	1 mg/mL	0.3	15.5	228.7	224.6	−2%	4.3	4.2	−2%
n = 4		±0.1 mg	±6.7	±148.4	±134.3		±0.8	±0.8	
Alfimeprase	10 mg/mL	1.4	8.7*	96.3	108.0	+12%	2.8	2.6	−7%
(n = 3)		±0.8 mg	±4.7	±31.2	±5.5		±0.2	±0.1	
UK	5,000 U/mL	2,354	28.3	117.7	210.5	+79%	3.5	3.0	−14%
(n = 4)		±811 U	±9.7	±142.9	±183.1		±0.7	±0.8	
UK	50,000 U/mL	9,722	11.7	67.3	185.9	+176%	3.5	2.9	−17%
(n = 3)		7±4194 U	±5.0	±9.5	±71.6		±0.5	±0.3	

*p < 0.05 vs. UK 5000 U/mL group by ANOVA with Fishers PLSD test. Changes in fibrin D-dimer and fibrinogen were compared at baseline (Pre) and following delivery of test agent (Post). There were no significant changes in these parameters (baseline vs. posttreatment) in any group. All data are presented as mean ± standard deviation.

4. Thrombolysis in Subacute Thrombosis of Implanted Gore-Tex Grafts in Baboons

Additional baboon studies were conducted during which graft segments were implanted and allowed to thrombose. In these studies, an 8-cm–length of 4-mm-diameter Gore-Tex graft was used. Before implantation, the graft was coated with collagen and tissue factor, to increase its thrombogenicity. The baboons were anesthetized and an incision was made in the ventral surface of the neck to expose the carotid arteries bilaterally. The thrombogenic grafts were anastomosed into place in parallel to both the left and right common carotid arteries and observed until occlusion occurred. The surgical site was closed, and the animal recovered from anesthesia. After a period of 24 to 48-h, the animal was reanesthetized and a 4F multiple sidehole drug delivery catheter was introduced from a femoral site and advanced under fluoroscopic guidance to the carotids. The catheter was advanced into the clotted graft and positioned such that the sideholes were within the clot. Angiograms were performed using contrast medium infused by a separate catheter introduced through the brachial artery. An angiogram was performed before drug delivery to confirm that grafts remained occluded. Alfimeprase was delivered through the catheter as a 10-mg/mL solution at a delivery rate of 1 mL/h. Patency was checked every 15 min by performing additional angiograms.

Patency was restored in all of the thrombosed graft segments within 30–45 min following delivery of alfimeprase. Angiograms from an individual experiment (animal 6Q) are depicted in Figure 7, where flow through the occluded graft was restored using alfimeprase at a solution strength of 10 mg/mL, infused at 1 mL/h until patency was observed at 30 min (approximately 5 mg of alfimeprase infused).

5. Thrombolysis in Subacute Thrombosis of the Adult Pig Common Carotid Artery

Alfimeprase has been studied in a model of subacute thrombosis of the carotid artery in adult pigs (75–100 kg). The intent of these studies was to establish biological activity of alfimeprase in a thrombosis model that is relevant to the target clinical indication of peripheral arterial occlusion.

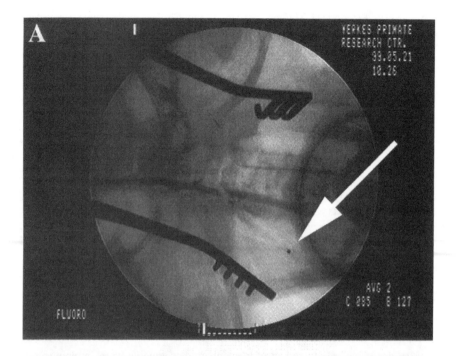

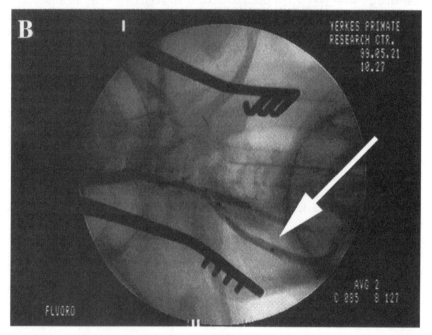

Figure 7 (A) Angiographic visualization of the left common carotid artery in a baboon and an occluded shunt, prior to the delivery of alfimeprase. The dark radiopaque marker tip of the drug delivery catheter can been seen within the graft (white arrow); however contrast media does not flow through the graft indicating that the graft is occluded. (B) Following delivery of 5 mg of alfimeprase (10 mg/mL at 1 mL/hr for 30 minutes), flow through the graft has been restored.

In this model the carotid artery is thrombosed along its entire length (~20 cm from origin at the aorta to the carotid bifurcation) by a combination of balloon injury, thrombin, and stasis. The size of the thrombus in this model approaches the size of thrombus encountered clinically in peripheral arterial occlusion. After successful thrombosis, the animal is allowed to recover for 4 days. A 4-day period was selected to allow extensive cross-linking of fibrin, remodeling of thrombus, and infiltration of cells.

On the fourth day, the animals are reanesthetized, the occlusion is reconfirmed and a multiple sidehole drug delivery catheter is advanced under fluoroscopic guidance and positioned such that the sideholes are located within the thrombus. Thrombolysis with alfimeprase has been angiographically observed using alfimeprase dosages that range from 10 to 30 mg (nonweight adjusted), as shown in Figure 8, demonstrating that alfimeprase is effective in restoring antegrade flow as assessed angiographically.

In conclusion, the results from these studies indicate that alfimeprase is efficacious in an animal model of thrombosis in which the thrombus is comparable in size and age with that frequently encountered in peripheral arterial occlusion. Whether the dose is expressed on a fixed basis (10–30 mg) or on a weight-adjusted basis (0.1–0.4 mg/kg), we have described dosages that appear to range from threshold or minimally active to fully efficacious. These dose ranges are recommended for use in clinical investigation in a peripheral thrombolysis application.

6. Summary Discussion of Animal Efficacy Data

Collectively, the efficacy of alfimeprase has been demonstrated in human clotted blood in vitro and in rat, piglet, adult pig, and baboon models of arterial thrombosis. The data presented in the preceding sections clearly establish the biological activity of alfimeprase across a broad range of species.

In all animals species tested, efficacious doses of alfimeprase have been established. In rats, local administration of alfimeprase (2 mg) successfully restored flow in 10 of 14 cases or 71%. In piglets, early experiments with local administration of fibrolase at 2.5, 5, or 15 mg led to successful restoration of flow in 64, 100, and 100% of cases, respectively. In baboon models, alfimeprase was administered locally as a continuous infusion until clot lysis occurred. As such, the incidence of clot lysis was 100% in baboon studies and total dosages in the range of 0.3–1.4 mg were required to achieve this effect. In the adult pig model, local inthrathrombus delivery of alfimeprase was effective in 100% of cases at a dose of 30 mg.

VII. SUMMARY OF MAJOR PHARMACOLOGICAL ACTIVITY

A. Speed of Clot Lysis

Where measured, time to clot lysis in the majority of studies with alfimeprase or fibrolase has been very rapid in comparison with the reference plasminogen activators used (t-PA and UK). In rats, time to lysis with alfimeprase was 6.3 min. In piglets, clot lysis with r-fibrolase was achieved within 10 min (except for the 2.5-mg r-fibrolase group, which required 26.6 min), whereas time to lysis with the plasminogen activators was in the range of 15–60 min. In the baboon exteriorized graft model, time to clot lysis with alfimeprase was 15 min or less, although the higher-dose regimen of urokinase used in this model was effective in 12 min. In the adult pig model, doses of 30 mg resulted in patency detected angiographically at 30 min, whereas patency with urokinase was not detected until 2 h or more.

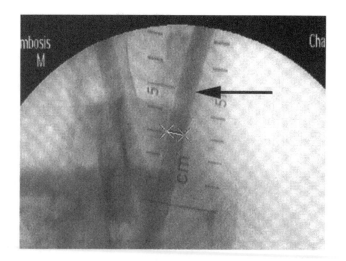

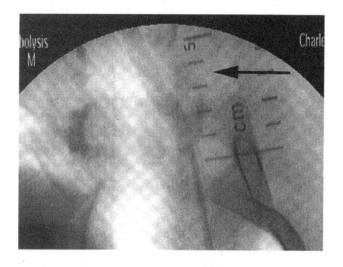

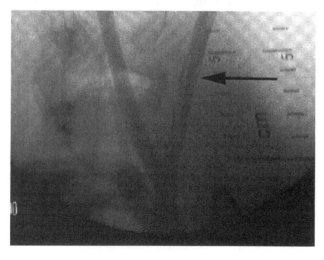

B. Hemorrhagic Potential

In several of the acute thrombosis experiments, the hemorrhagic potential of test agents was assessed by collecting and quantifying the blood shed from surgical sites. In rats, blood loss with alfimeprase was no different than the saline group, and blood loss with urokinase was significantly higher. In piglets, blood loss with r-fibrolase did not differ from the saline group at doses that were fully effective (> 80% incidence of clot lysis); however, when the dose of r-fibrolase was raised to that which amounted to more than 1 mg/kg on a weight-adjusted basis, hemorrhage was observed.

In the baboon exteriorized graft studies, hemostasis was assessed by measuring plasma fibrinogen and fibrin D-dimer in the support animal. In these studies, alfimeprase did not affect fibrinogen or D-dimer, whereas urokinase tended to increase circulating fibrin D-dimer and decrease fibrinogen, although these changes were not significant.

VIII. ADDITIONAL PHARMACOLOGY STUDIES

A. Effects of Alfimeprase on Fibrinogen and Platelet Aggregation In Vitro

Alfimeprase has been evaluated for potential effects on human plasma fibrinogen and platelet aggregation. Twenty healthy volunteers, who were self-reported to be aspirin-free for at least 10 days, served as donors for the collection of citrated whole blood and serum. The citrated whole blood was used for fibrinogen and platelet aggregation studies. The serum sample was frozen and shipped to a clinical laboratory for determination of serum α_2-macroglobulin concentration. The mean serum α_2-macroglobulin concentration for the group of 20 donors was 168 ± 9 mg/dL ($\pm$ standard error).

B. Fibrinogen

For fibrinogen studies, citrated plasma was prepared. The plasma samples were incubated with alfimeprase at concentrations of 0 (alfimeprase diluent), 10, 20, 40, and 100 μg/mL. Plasma fibrinogen was quantified at baseline (before the addition of any test agents) and at 30, 60, and 120 min after the addition of alfimeprase.

As the data in Table 6 indicate, plasma fibrinogen was not affected by incubation with alfimeprase at concentrations of 10 and 20 μg/mL. Presumably, the alfimeprase that was added to the sample was completely inhibited by the α_2-macroglobulin that was also present in the sample. In contrast, incubation of plasma with alfimeprase at 100 μg/mL resulted in complete degradation of fibrinogen in all plasma samples within the first 30 min of the incubation, suggesting that at an alfimeprase concentration of 100 μg/mL, the capacity for α_2-macroglobulin to bind and neutralize alfimeprase was exceeded.

Figure 8 (Top) Baseline angiogram in the adult porcine common carotid artery prior to balloon injury and the formation of an occlusive thrombus. The arrow indicates the position and the presence of contrast media in the left common carotid artery, indicating that the blood vessel is patent. (Center) Angiogram on day 4, prior to the administration of alfimeprase. The arrow indicates the position of the left common carotid artery, however, contrast media does not flow in the artery due to the presence of an occlusive thrombus. (Bottom) Angiogram at 2 hours following administration of 30 mg of alfimeprase through a multisideholded drug delivery catheter. The arrow indicates that flow has been restored in the left carotid artery. Minimal residual thrombus is visible in the lumen of the artery.

Table 6 Plasma Fibrinogen Following Incubation with Alfimeprase in Plasma of 20 Donors

Alfimeprase concentration (μg/mL)	Fibrinogen (mg/dL)			
	Baseline	30 min	60 min	120 min
0 (diluent)	204	187	185	177
	±9	±7	±7	±7
10	207	190	191	185
	±8	±7	±7	±7
20	208	200	201	198
	±8	±8	±8	±8
40	210	172	143	125*
	±8	±10	±17	±21
100	206	0	0	0*
	±9	±0	±0	±0

*Indicates significant differences ($p < 0.01$) of 120-min timepoint from baseline timepoint by paired t-test. Data are mean ± standard error.

In this in vitro study, at a concentration of 40 μg/mL, the group mean plasma fibrinogen dropped by about 40% ($p < 0.01$) during the 2-h incubation with alfimeprase. Donors with the highest α_2-macroglobulin concentration were resistant to the degradation of plasma fibrinogen when alfimeprase was added at a concentration of 40 μg/mL. In contrast, donors with a relatively low α_2-macroglobulin concentration were more vulnerable to alfimeprase (at 40 μg/mL), as assessed by the loss of plasma fibrinogen.

As shown in Figure 9, the results from the 20 donors were divided into two groups. In a group of 7 individuals in whom fibrinogen degradation was 50% or greater, the serum α_2-macroglobulin concentration averaged 135 mg/dL. In the remaining 13 individuals in whom fibrinogen was unaffected or there was less than a 50% loss in fibrinogen, the α_2-macroglobulin concentration averaged 186 mg/dL.

C. Platelet Aggregation

For platelet aggregation studies, citrated whole blood was used to prepare platelet-rich (PRP) and platelet-poor (PPP) plasmas. Citrated PRP was incubated with alfimeprase at concentrations of 0 (alfimeprase diluent), 10, 20, 40, and 100 μg/mL. Aggregation was induced by the addition of collagen (2 μg/mL). The platelet aggregation response was tested at baseline (before the addition of any test agents) and at 30, 60, and 120 min after the addition of alfimeprase.

In platelets, aggregation in the negative-control group declined slightly over time (2 h) consistent with the diminishing function of platelets ex vivo. Incubation of PRP with alfimeprase up to and including 40 μg/mL did not affect platelet aggregation.

When alfimeprase was incubated with PRP at 100 μg/mL (Table 7), a concentration which completely degraded plasma fibrinogen in all subjects studied (see previous section), a platelet aggregation response was still present, although it was 51%, compared with 78% in controls.

The retention of a platelet aggregation response when alfimeprase is incubated at 100 μg/mL appears to be consistent with the ability of platelets to release, on activation, the fibrinogen that is stored in platelet α-granules. This release of fibrinogen appears sufficient to support some, but not fully normal, platelet aggregation.

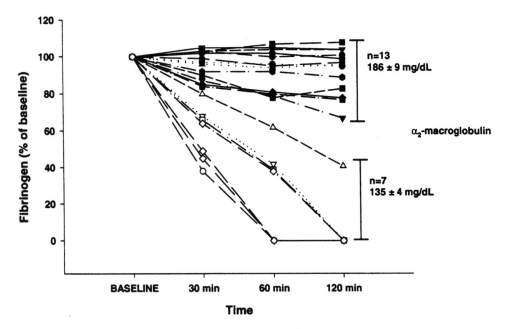

Figure 9 Individual plasma fibrinogen datapoints expressed as a percentage of baseline for plasma samples incubated with alfimeprase (40 μg/mL). Mean α_2-macroglobulin concentration (mean ± standard error) is shown for the group of 7 individuals (open symbols) where fibrinogen degradation was 50% or greater. In addition α_2-macroglobulin concentration is shown for the group 13 individuals (filled symbols) where fibrinogen was either unaffected by alfimeprase or where degradation was less than 50% of baseline.

Table 7 Platelet Aggregation Response to Collagen Following Incubation with Alfimeprase in Platelet-Rich Plasma

Alfimeprase concentration (μg/mL)	Platelet aggregation (%)			
	Baseline	30 min	60 min	120 min
0 (diluent)	89.7 ±1.8	90.1 ±1.7	88.2 ±2.1	78.2* ±3.3
10	92.5 ±1.6	88.4 ±1.9	87.8 ±2.0	83.9* ±2.6
20	91.7 ±1.7	87.9 ±1.7	87.1 ±2.0	81.4* ±3.2
40	90.2 ±1.6	85.8 ±1.8	85.4 ±2.4	79.2* ±3.0
100	89.4 ±1.6	82.5 ±2.0	77.2 ±2.0	51.2*† ±3.2

*$p < 0.01$ vs. baseline timepoint by paired t-test, indicating that in all groups there was a loss in platelet aggregation over time.
† $p < 0.01$ vs. all other groups at the 120-min timepoint by ANOVA indicating that the loss of platelet function was greatest in the alfimeprase 100-μg/mL group, as compared with all other groups.

D. Liberation of Fibrin D-Dimer from Preformed Human Whole Blood Clots: Effects of Alfimeprase and Urokinase

After the formation of a fibrin clot, the activity of factor XIII enhances the stability of a clot by mediating the cross-linking of fibrin monomers. Pharmacological dissolution of a fibrin clot with plasminogen activators is known to occur through the generation of plasmin, a serine protease. Plasmin proteolytically degrades fibrin in a way such as to solubilize and release a fragment of the cross-linked fibrin D peptides (the D-dimer). In clinical practice, the presence of D-dimer in the circulation is considered a marker of ongoing fibrinolysis.

Although it is known that plasmin-mediated dissolution of thrombus liberates the fibrin D-dimer, it is not known whether alfimeprase-mediated clot lysis would also do so. Given that the proteolytic specificity of alfimeprase differs from plasmin, it may be possible for alfimeprase to dissolve thrombus without liberating what would normally be detected as D-dimer in commercially available assays.

To determine whether alfimeprase-mediated clot lysis would liberate a measurable D-dimer, whole human blood was collected by venipuncture in three donors and clotted by the addition of excess calcium. The clots were washed, cut into approximate weights of 0.5 g (range 0.45–0.65 g) and transferred to new tubes. Alfimeprase (2 mg), urokinase (10,000–40,000 U), or an equivalent volume of saline was added to the reaction tubes and then allowed to incubate for 2 h. Aliquots were withdrawn from the tubes and were assayed for fibrin D-dimer in an ELISA assay specific for human D-dimer (TintElize Biopool International; Ventura, CA).

As is shown in Table 8, urokinase degrades clot and liberates fibrin D-dimer in a dose-dependent manner. Although in vitro clot lysis with alfimeprase was extensive ($> 95\%$ dissolution of clot mass), the quantity of D-dimer released was comparable with that observed with 10,000 U of urokinase, which degraded only approximately 30% of the thrombus mass.

These results indicate that degradation of human clot with urokinase releases D-dimer, in agreement with known biology. In addition, even though alfimeprase is clearly effective at

Table 8 Liberation of Fibrin D-Dimer During In Vitro Lysis of Clotted Whole Blood

Treatment	Fibrin D-dimer (μg/mL)		Dissolution of clot mass
	Baseline	120 min	
Saline 0.4 mL	0.0	1.1	None
$n = 5$	±0.0	±0.4	
Alfimeprase 2 mg	0.0	52.6	>95%
$n = 5$	±0.0	±8.7	
UK 10,000 U	0.1	47.8	∼30%
$n = 5$	±0.0	±16.7	
UK 20,000 U	1.3	230.0	∼40%
$n = 5$	±0.9	±82.1	
UK 40,000 U	1.2	307.0	∼50%
$n = 5$	±0.5	±147.9	

Aliquots were withdrawn from the tubes and were assayed for fibrin D-dimer in an ELISA assay specific for human D-dimer. Dissolution of clot mass was estimated visually for each group of five reaction tubes. Data are mean ± standard error.

degrading clot in this model, the release of D-dimer appeared lower than might be expected from the extent of clot lysis.

Although alfimeprase is an effective thrombolytic agent, it may not liberate soluble fragments of clot that are fully recognized as D-dimer in commercially available, immunoreactive assays for fibrin D-dimer. Given the differences in proteolytic specificity between alfimeprase and plasmin (formed by treatment with plasminogen activators), this result is plausible.

E. Hemodynamic Effects of Dosages of Alfimeprase That Are Predicted to Exceed α_2-Macroglobulin-Binding Capacity

In toxicology studies, dosages of alfimeprase that were expected to exceed the plasma α_2-macroglobulin binding capacity have been studied and observed to cause hypotension. In studies designed to assess the mechanism of alfimeprase-induced hypotension, guinea pigs were anesthetized, cannulated with arterial and venous catheters, and allowed to recover for at least 24 h. On the study day, the arterial cannula of the conscious guinea pig was connected to a pressure transducer. After an acclimation period of approximately 30 min, the guinea pigs received an intravenous-bolus dose of alfimeprase at 3 mg/kg, slightly exceeding a dose of 2.3 mg/kg, which was uniformly observed to exhibit clinical signs in guinea pig toxicological studies. Blood pressure responses were recorded for 60 min. Pretreatment of animals with varied pharmacological agents was used to identify the mechanism of the hypotensive response.

The hypotensive response to alfimeprase in toxic dosages is rapid and can correct spontaneously (Fig. 10). Pretreatment of animals with a bradykinin-2 (BK-2) receptor antagonist (HOE-140) was effective in preventing the hypotensive response. Pretreatment of animals with

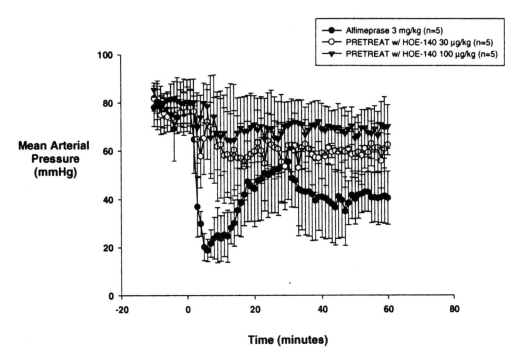

Figure 10 Mean arterial pressure in guinea pigs pretreated with HOE-140 prior to the administration of alfimeprase (3 mg/kg, iv)

L-NAME, indomethacin, or diphenydramine (to inhibit nitric oxide, prostanoids, or histamine, respectively) failed to have any effect on the hypotension that was observed. These data led us to conclude that alfimeprase is capable of generating a peptide that mimicked the effects of bradykinin at the BK-2 receptor. Further biochemical studies revealed that alfimeprase is actually capable of cleaving bradykinin from the low-molecular weight kininogen.

F. Potential Interaction of Alfimeprase and Plasminogen Activators

In clinical use it may be necessary to use plasminogen activators in patients who have previously received alfimeprase. Therefore, it was decided to determine whether there might be a deleterious drug interaction (e.g., exacerbation of bleeding) between alfimeprase and subsequently administered plasminogen activators.

   To evaluate a potential drug interaction, the hemorrhagic potential of the test articles was assessed in an experiment that is designed to quantify blood loss in an animal model. Guinea pigs were anesthetized and instrumented with arterial and venous catheters. During the course of the experiment, any blood that was shed from the surgical site was collected with gauze swabs. The swabs were placed in a detergent solution to solubilize red blood cells and release hemoglobin into solution. At specified timepoints, an aliquot of the detergent solution was removed and the hemoglobin content of the aliquot was determined in a spectrophotometer. Shed hemoglobin was mathematically converted into a volume of blood loss by using the hemoglobin concentration of whole blood (in g/dL), which was measured for each animal.

   Aspirin and heparin were administered to all animals. Administration of the test articles (alfimeprase, urokinase, or saline) was carried out using numbered, coded syringes so that the technicians were unaware of the particular treatment group.

   Guinea pigs first received an intravenous bolus of alfimeprase (0.5 mg/kg) or saline and the animal was monitored for 60-min. During this first 60-min observation, any blood shed from the surgical site was collected by cotton swabs and deposited into the detergent solution. After 60-min, animals were treated with one of two possible intravenous infusions of urokinase (low-dose: 2000-U bolus + 35-U/min infusion; or high-dose: 50,000-U bolus + 1,000-U/min infusion) or a volume-match bolus and infusion of saline. The animals were monitored for an additional 60-min observation period while the infusion of urokinase or saline continued. Any blood shed from the surgical site was collected by cotton swabs and deposited into the detergent solution.

   The results in Figure 11 indicate that following administration of alfimeprase (0.5 mg/kg) a hemorrhagic state did not develop during the first 60-min of the experiment, when compared with the saline control over the first 60-min. As alfimeprase alone did not produce a hemorrhagic state, we conclude that this dosage of alfimeprase (0.5 mg/kg) is nonhemorrhagic in guinea pigs.

   In contrast, in animals that received a saline infusion during the first 60-min of the experiment, a hemorrhagic state was clearly produced by the high-dose urokinase regimen within the first 15–30 min following the start of the infusion (SAL + UK high-dose group). As alfimeprase did not exacerbate the hemorrhage that was observed with high-dose urokinase infusion (alfimeprase + UK high dose group), we conclude a drug interaction (as measured by hemorrhagic potential) does not exist between alfimeprase and urokinase.

IX. CONCLUSIONS

The pharmacology of alfimeprase appears to demonstrate a high degree of novelty in relation to the plasminogen activator class of thrombolytic agents. Specifically, the animal data thus far

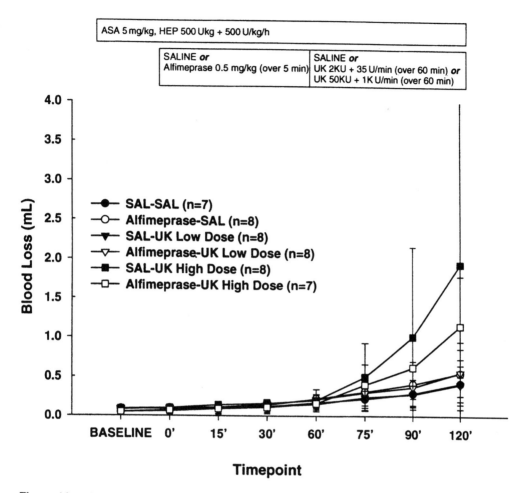

ASA 5 mg/kg, HEP 500 Ukg + 500 U/kg/h

SALINE *or*	SALINE *or*
Alfimeprase 0.5 mg/kg (over 5 min)	UK 2KU + 35 U/min (over 60 min) *or*
	UK 50KU + 1K U/min (over 60 min)

- ● SAL-SAL (n=7)
- ○ Alfimeprase-SAL (n=8)
- ▼ SAL-UK Low Dose (n=8)
- ▽ Alfimeprase-UK Low Dose (n=8)
- ■ SAL-UK High Dose (n=8)
- □ Alfimeprase-UK High Dose (n=7)

Figure 11 Blood shed from the surgical site was constantly collected and quantified. A hemorrhagic state was not observed following the administration of alfimeprase (0.5 mg/kg) and observation for one hour (0–60 minute timepoints). In contrast the high dose infusion regimen of urokinase clearly induces a hemorrhagic state. Results from the negative saline control (saline) group indicates that aspirin and heparin, as used, did not induce hemorrhage

indicate the speed of lysis appears greatly accelerated, and the potential risk of hemorrhagic complications appears greatly diminished. Despite the potential drawback in the requirement for local delivery of alfimeprase, the advantage gained in local delivery is more rapid thrombolysis combined with a reduced risk of bleeding. If these attributes are maintained as clinical safety and efficacy are assessed, alfimeprase will represent the first of a new therapeutic class (fibrinolytic metalloproteases) for use in thrombolysis.

REFERENCES

1. Randolph A, Chamberlain SH, Chu HL, Retzios AD, Markland FS Jr, Masiarz FR. Amino acid sequence of fibrolase, a direct-acting fibrinolytic enzyme from *Agkistrodon contortrix contortrix* venom. Protein Sci 1992; 1:590–600.

2. Manning MC. Sequence analysis of fibrolase, a fibrinolytic metalloproteinase from *Agkistrodon contortrix contortrix*. Toxicon 1995; 33:1189–1200.
3. Ahmed NK, Tennant KD, Markland FS, Lacz JP. Biochemical characteristics of fibrolase, a fibrinolytic protease from snake venom. Haemostasis 1990; 20:147–154.
4. Retzios AD, Markland FS. Fibrinolytic enzymes from the venoms of *Agkistrodon contortrix contortrix* and *Crotalus basiliscus basiliscus*; cleavage site specificity towards the alpha-chain of fibrin. Throm Res 1994; 74:355–367.
5. Pretzer D, Schulteis BS, Smith CD, Vander VD, Mitchell JW, Manning MC. Stability of the thrombolytic protein fibrolase: effect of temperature and pH on activity and conformation. Pharm Res 1991; 8:1103–1112.
6. Pretzer D. Schulteis B, Vander VD, Smith CD, Mitchell JW, Manning MC. Effect of zinc binding on the structure and stability of fibrolase, a fibrinolytic protein from snake venom. Pharm Res 1992; 9:870—877.
7. Barrett AJ. alpha-2 Macroglobulin. In: Barrett AJ, ed. Methods in Enzymology. Philadelphia; Academic Press, 1981; 737–754.

40

In Vitro and In Vivo Models to Investigate Clot Lysis and Thrombolysis

Jean Marie Stassen
Thromb-X N.V., Leuven, Belgium

SUMMARY

Thrombolytic therapy has become the standard of care for the treatment of numerous thrombotic diseases. The basic pharmacological work to identify effective agents relies heavily on preclinical experimental models. Treatment with thrombolytic agents induces an increased bleeding risk; therefore, the safety profile of new treatment strategies requires in-depth investigation in preclinical in vivo models. Many experimental models have been developed to investigate the mechanisms of thrombosis and to optimize antithrombotic and thrombolytic therapy.

Various models described in the literature, can be used to assess the safety and efficacy of fibrinolytic agents and thrombolytic regimens. However, with initiation of a test strategy, the following conceptual aspects are to be considered.

1. What are the effects of species differences?
2. What are the targets to be investigated: arterial versus venous thrombosis, whole-blood clots versus platelet-rich clots?
3. Are comparative data available that might reduce the number of animals needed?
4. Can different models (e.g., arterial, venous, and bleeding time models) be combined?

Frequently used experimental setups are summarized in this chapter. Furthermore, the order of description indicates a possible test strategy starting from in vitro experiments, followed by small-animal thrombosis model and ultimately by large-animal models.

However, simple experimental models are essential tools to investigate the efficacy and safety profiles of thrombolytic therapies.

I. INTRODUCTION

Thrombosis, a common disease clinically manifested by the accumulation of blood elements in blood vessels, is a major cause of mortality and morbidity in Western society. Multiple factors contribute to this pathology. It originates from a wide range of different underlying causes, depending on the occurrence in either the arterial or venous circulatory system.

651

The major cause of human arterial thrombosis is atherosclerosis. Thrombosis over atherosclerotic plaques is due to either superficial or to deep injury. In superficial injury endothelial denudation with thrombi adherent to the surface occurs. In deep injury major plaque rupture followed by exposure of the accumulated lipid core initiates rapid thrombus formation within the plaque. This thrombus may extend into the lumen, leading to occlusion [1,2]. In the last decades thrombolytic therapy has become the most effective therapeutic approach to treat acute thrombotic arterial occlusion [3–5].

Deep vein thrombosis (DVT), occurring after surgery, stroke, or myocardial infarction is the most common thromboembolic complication. Besides immobilization, the main risk factors are surgery, trauma, pregnancy, neoplasms, estrogen therapy, heart disease, and advanced age. Thrombolysis for the treatment of deep vein thrombosis can be an adjunct to anticoagulant therapy and new surgical techniques [6–8].

Pulmonary embolism (PE) a serious life-threatening complication of DVT is preferably treated with thrombolytic therapy, when extensive [9,10]. Despite numerous trials demonstrating the clinical benefits of thrombolytic therapy, it is not commonly used for the treatment of DVT and PE.

Ischemic strokes and transient ischemic attacks are major causes of serious physical disability and death. The eventual successful outcome depends highly on early restoration of blood flow. Thrombolytic therapy with recombinant tissue plasminogen activator (r-t-PA) to treat ischemic stroke according to the current AHA guidelines had a beneficial outcome [11–13].

The risk for anastomotic microvascular thrombosis in plastic and reconstructive surgery is especially prominent when vascular reconstruction is undertaken after a crushing injury or an avulsion [14]. The main risk factor in such cases may be areas of intimal/subintimal damage in macroscopically intact vessels, and thrombotic complications are, therefore, best avoided by extensive revision and generous use of interpositional vascular grafts [15]. Occasionally, however, surgical precautions alone are not sufficient to prevent thrombotic complications, and anatomical or other considerations may preclude more radical surgery. Preclinical and clinical results indicate that thrombolytic therapy in such cases might be a possible alternative [16–19].

The causes of the foregoing thrombotic diseases can all be summarized in alterations in the blood, the blood flow, or the vessel wall. To investigate underlying causes and to develop treatment strategies, many investigators have attempted to devise experimental methods that take into account all causes. Others have focused on some of the factors, as alteration of one factor might be severe enough to induce thrombosis [20–24].

To optimize existent therapy and to evaluate new thrombolytic strategies it is necessary to rely on animal models that mimic the thrombotic pathologies as just outlined. To study thrombosis experimentally, it is essential to produce thrombi in a consistent and reproducible manner. The reliability and reproducibility of each method is dependent on the procedure to monitor the thrombi produced. The use of a method for monitoring thrombi that allows their localization and quantification makes clear the deficiencies of producing experimental thrombi that involves rapid blood stasis and that reduce or eliminate cellular and metabolic activities and thereby reduce or eliminate stages of endogenous thrombogenesis or thrombolysis.

The aim of the present review is to describe in some animal models currently used in the experimental strategies to (1) increase the rate and extent of thrombolysis, (2) to overcome resistance to lysis, (3) to prevent thrombotic occlusion and reocclusion, and (4) to evaluate the effects of these procedures on bleeding tendency and hemostatic parameters. In contrast to the human pathology of thrombosis, animal models can only be seen as approaches to a certain disease state. To study treatment strategies, however, caution has to be taken in directly extrapolating the observations from animal experiments to the clinical situation. For it is evident

Table 1 Experimental Animal Models Used to Investigate Specific Problems Related to Efficacy and Safety of Thrombolytic Therapy of Arterial and Venous Thrombosis

Models and applications	Possible clot types	Ref.
Models to assess the thrombolytic efficacy		
In vitro clot lysis assays	All types	25
Extracorporeal clot lysis models	All types	28, 29, 31
Deep-vein thrombosis models	All types	30–32
Pulmonary embolism models	All types	33–36
Arterial thrombosis models	Microarterial	37
	Erythrocyte-rich clot	38, 39
	Platelet-rich clot	40–42
	Photo-induced thrombosis	43–46
	$FeCL_3$-induced thrombosis	47
Combined venous and arterial thrombosis models		31, 32, 48, 49
Acute myocardial infarction	Erythrocyte-rich-clot	53–55
	Platelet-rich clot	22, 57–59
Thrombotic stroke models	Platelet-rich-clot	66, 67
Embolic stroke models	All types	60, 62, 63, 68, 69
Models to assess the safety of thrombolytic therapy		
Template bleeding-time models	—	31, 78–83
Full-thickness ear puncture (rabbits only)	—	84, 85
Cuticle bleeding-time models	—	85, 86
Deep wound bleeding-time models	—	87
Hemorrhagic stroke model	—	88–91

[a]All types: Indicates that all possible manipulations with components of the blood can be performed before induction of clot formation.

that no one can master it fully or miss it completely, but each approach adds to our knowledge on this pathological mechanism and allows expansion of the methodology. The following survey concerning the production of experimental thrombosis might assist in the selection of which experimental system to use.

With the initiation and the outlining of a test strategy the following conceptual aspects have to be considered.

1. Do species differences influence the outcome?
2. Which are the targets to be investigated either arterial or venous thrombosis, or platelet-poor clots, erythrocyte-rich (whole-blood) clots or platelet-rich clots (Table 1)?
3. The existence of comparative data, which might reduce the number of animals needed?
4. Can different models (e.g., arterial and venous thrombosis models, and bleeding time models) be combined in the same animal?

II. EXPERIMENTAL MODELS TO ASSESS THE EFFICACY OF THROMBOLYTIC THERAPY

A. In Vitro Clot Lysis Assays

[125]I-Fibrin-labeled plasma clots are prepared from pooled plasma of different animal species. Following addition of $0.5\,\mu Ci$ of ^{125}I-labeled human fibrinogen (Amersham, UK) plasma is

clotted in a silicone tubing (internal diameter 4 mm) by addition of $CaCl_2$ (35-mM final concentration) and of 2 NIH U/mL human thrombin (Sigma, St. Louis, MO). After incubation at 37°C for 30 min the silicone tube containing the clot is cut in 5-mm pieces. The plasma clots (volume 60 µL) are extensively washed in saline for 1 h with changes every 15 min. The clots are immersed in 0.25 mL plasma of the same species. Lysis induced by different concentrations of plasminogen activators was quantified from the release of radioactivity from the clot. The concentration of plasminogen activator required to obtain 50% of clot lysis in 2 h (C_{50}), was determined [25].

B. Animal Models of Clot Lysis (see Table 1)

1. General Experimental Requirements

All studies with experimental animals should be approved by the local ethics committees and be carried out, conforming to the "Position of the American Heart Association on Research Animal Use," adopted November 11, 1984, Section 4 of the Animal Welfare Act, the guidelines of the International Committee on Thrombosis and Haemostasis, and the local ethics committees [26,27].

Commonly used anesthetics and their respective dosages in experimental animals used in the studies included in this review are summarized in Table 2. To allow accurate monitoring of the blood, radioactive thyroidal uptake of ^{125}I should be blocked by administration of NaI (≈ 100 µg/kg). The catheters used throughout this review were obtained from Portex, Hythe, UK. To monitor the blood flow an animal research Doppler flowmeter T106, with the corresponding perivascular flow probes of 1, 1.5, 2, or 3 mm, according to the size of the blood vessel, from Transonic Systems Inc., Ithaca, NY was used. In prolonged experiments the animals were given analgesic, antibiotic, and anti-inflammatory therapy.

2. Extracorporeal Clot Lysis Models

Extracorporeal loop thrombosis models allow repeated administration of thrombolytic substances to the same animal. For each experiment two clots of 0.3-mL normal plasma containing 0.5 µCi ^{125}I-labeled fibrinogen, 10 NIH U/mL of human thrombin, and 50 mmol/L $CaCl_2$ are prepared in tuberculin syringes into which a woollen thread was inserted to fix the clot (Fig. 1). The clot was aged for 30 min at 37°C and inserted into the extracorporeal arteriovenous loop [28,29]. A femoral or carotid artery was cannulated with a 4FG (Portex White) and connected through the tuberculin syringes to a punctured vein. The blood through the extracorporeal loop was maintained at 1 mL/min kg^{-1} body weight with a peristaltic pump. Thirty minutes before the start of the extracorporeal circulation the animals received an intravenous bolus of 1-mg/kg (dogs) or 7.5-mg/kg (rabbits) ridogrel (a combined thromboxane synthase inhibitor and prostaglandin endoperoxide receptor antagonist) (Janssen Pharmaceutics, Beerse, Belgium) to prevent platelet deposition in the loop. To prevent fibrin deposition, the animals were anticoagulated with heparin (100 U/kg followed by 50 U/kg h^{-1}) throughout the experiment. Thrombolysis was quantified 30 min after the end of the infusion by determination of the residual radioactivity in each two syringes.

3. Animal Models of Venous Thrombosis

b. Jugular Vein Thrombosis Models. The surgical procedure to produce the artificial thrombus is as follows: An external jugular vein is exposed through a 5- to 10-cm paramedial incision in the neck. The vein is cleared over a distance of 4–6 cm up to the main bifurcation of

Table 2 Commonly Used Premedication, Anesthesia of Some Experimental Animals: the Optimal Blood Sample Size Without Interfering with Hematological Parameters

Species	Premedication sedation	Anesthesia induction	Anesthesia maintenance	Blood sample number and size
Mouse	Atropine 12.5 µg/kg i.p.	Pentobarbital 60 mg/kg i.p.	Pentobarbital 10 mg/kg h^{-1} s.c. infusion	2×0.1 mL in 1 h
Hamster	Atropine 12.5 µg/kg i.p.	Pentobarbital 60 mg/kg i.p.	Pentobarbital 10 mg/kg h^{-1} i.p. infusion	3×0.2 mL in 1 h
Rat	Atropine 12.5 µg/kg i.p.	Pentobarbital 60 mg/kg i.p.	Pentobarbital 20 mg/kg h^{-1} i.p. infusion	4×0.5 mL in 1 h
Rabbit	Atropine 12.5 µg/kg i.m.	Rompun 13 mg/kg + ketamine 33 mg/kg i.m.	Rompun 6.6 mg/kg h^{-1} + ketamine 16 mg/kg h^{-1} i.v. infusion	10×2 mL in 1 h
Dog	Ketamine 10 mg/kg i.m.	Pentobarbital 30 mg/kg i.v.	Pentobarbital 8 mg/kg h^{-1} i.v. bolus	10×10 mL 1 h
Baboon	Ketamine 10 mg/kg i.m. + atropine 50 µg/kg	Pentobarbital 10 mg/kg i.v.	Pentobarbital 45 mg/kg i.v. bolus	8×10 mL 1 h

Route of administration: i.p., intraperitoneal; i.v., intravenous; i.m., intramuscular.
Rompun: Bayer, Leverkusen, Germany; Ketamin: Ketavet 100 mg/mL, Warner Lambert, Ann Harbor, MI; Pentobarbital: Nembutal, Abbott, North Chicago, IL.

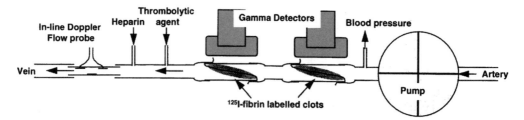

Figure 1 Schematic representation of the extracorporeal loop setup as it is used in baboons and in rabbits. (From Ref. 29.)

the external jugular vein and the facial vein. Small side branches are ligated and the facial vein is cannulated with a 3FG (Portex pink) catheter. A woollen thread is then introduced in the lumen of the jugular vein over a distance of 4 cm with the use of a straight 4-cm atraumatic needle. When bleeding has ceased, the vein is clamped both proximally and distally to isolate a vein segment, which is then emptied of all blood and the volume of the segment is measured by injection of saline [30,31].

Thrombus formation is induced by injecting 0.1 mL bovine thrombin (10 NIH U/mL) solution containing 10-mM $CaCl_2$, followed at once by the volume of fresh rabbit blood corresponding to the measured volume 1-µCi ^{125}I-labeled fibrinogen. Injection of air bubbles is avoided and mixing is ensured. Cotton swabs are placed over the vessel to absorb blood leaking from the vein segment. The clot is allowed to age for 30 min, before both vessel clamps are removed. A blood sample is drawn 1 min after removal of the vessel clamps to measure the baseline radioactivity in the blood. The cotton swabs are removed for radioisotope counting and the amount of radioactivity delivered to the clot is calculated by subtracting the swab losses, the radioactivity remaining in the syringe and the total blood radioactivity (assuming a blood volume of 60-mL/kg body weight) from the original amount of radioactivity in the syringe. The animals are anticoagulated with heparin (500 IU/kg as an intravenous bolus).

At the end of the experiment, the thrombosed segment of the jugular vein is removed after careful suturing of both ends, and the remaining radioactive material is measured. The extent of lysis is calculated as the difference between the radioactivity originally incorporated in the clot and the radioactivity in the vein segment and expressed as percentage of the original radio-activity.

b. Femoral Vein Thrombosis. The femoral vein is isolated between the inguinal ligament and the distal bifurcation, and all side branches are carefully ligated, except for a predominant musculocutaneous branch, which is cannulated. After introduction of a woollen thread in the lumen, a 4-cm–segment of the femoral vein is isolated between two vessel clamps, emptied, and flushed with saline through the side branch catheter. The segment is then filled with a mixture of a trace amount of ^{125}I-labeled human fibrinogen, 0.6–1.2 mL of fresh blood, and 2 U of thrombin. The venous vessel clamps are released and 60 min later the infusion protocol is started. The degree of clot lysis is determined as the residual radioactivity in the vein segment and expressed in percentage of the radioactivity at the end of the experiment (multiplied by 3 for extravascular distribution) and the radioactivity in the recovered thrombus with that originally present in the clot. This model was described in dogs and baboons [31,32].

4. Pulmonary Embolism Models

The use of pulmonary embolism models to study fibrinolysis and thrombolysis is described in several animal species including rabbits, hamsters, rats, ferrets, and mice [33–36]. The models are all based on the intravenous injection of an in vitro-formed radioactive thrombus, which is spontaneously embolized to the lungs.

The procedure for the production of a pulmonary embolus in hamsters is as follows [35]. A mixture of 600 µL of either fresh-frozen human plasma, fresh platelet-rich human plasma (platelet count 3×10^5/µL), or fresh platelet-enriched human plasma (platelet count 1.5×10^6/µL), 10 µL of human ^{125}I-labeled fibrinogen (≈ 1 µCi), and 100 µL of a mixture of human thrombin (10 NIH U/mL) and $CaCl_2$ (0.5 M) are aspirated into a 8FG catheter (Portex orange). The catheter is incubated for 30 min at 37°C, the plasma clot is then dislodged gently with positive pressure, cut in 1-cm segments (total volume approximately 50 µL), and the radioisotope content is measured. The clot is then aspirated into a 6FG catheter (Portex red) for injection. The jugular vein is exposed and the catheter containing the labeled plasma clot advanced into the brachiocephalic vein, where the clot is injected. The clot usually embolizes into one of the lungs but is occasionally trapped in the heart or fragmented into both lungs.

At the end of experiment, the animal is sacrificed, the heart and both lungs are removed, and their radioisotope content separately determined. The extent of clot lysis is determined as the difference between the radioactivity incorporated in the clot and the sum of the residual radioactivity in the lungs or the heart, and an isotope recovery balance is made.

5. Animal Models of Arterial Thrombosis

a. Peripheral Arterial Thrombosis

MICROARTERIAL THROMBOSIS IN RABBITS. Three-centimeter segments of the central arteries (diameters 0.8–1.2 mm) of both ears were prepared under a surgical microscope, moistened with Ringer's lactate, and placed between thin plastic foils in special vessel holders (S&T, Gestetten, Germany). To maximize blood flow, both animals and holders were maintained at temperatures of 39.5 ± 0.5°C and lidocaine (10 mg/mL Xylocaine; AB Astra, Sweden) was applied to the prepared vessels as required. Longitudinal arteriotomies (7 mm) were performed as follows. The lumen of the vessel was flattened between vascular clamps and denuded with a No. 15 scalpel blade, thereby exposing deep layers of the media. The arteriotomies were closed with running 10-0 monofilament sutures (Ethicon Inc., Sommerville, NJ). All vessel traumas are performed preferably by the same investigator. The patency is assessed at the end of the experiment by a standard empty/refill test distal from the injured side at regular intervals and the vessels are classified as patent or occluded [37].

ERYTHROCYTE-RICH ARTERIAL THROMBOSIS MODELS. The left femoral artery and the right femoral vein are exposed. The left deep femoral artery and the left superficial epigastric artery are cannulated. The blood flow in the left femoral artery is monitored throughout the experiment. A stenosis is produced proximal to the flow probe by stepwise constriction of the artery with two 3.0-vicryl sutures (Ethicon Inc., Sommerville, NJ) to reduce the flow to $\approx 40\%$ of baseline. A 1-cm segment of the femoral artery is clamped proximal and distal to the superficial epigastric artery, and the isolated segment is emptied by the side-branch catheter. The isolated segment is traumatized by external compression with a blunt forceps to provoke endothelial injury. Bovine thrombin (0.05 mL of 20 NIH U/mL) and freshly drawn blood (0.1 mL) are injected through the epigastric artery catheter; 10 min later, first the proximal and then the distal clamp is released. The absence of blood flow is monitored for 10 min to document stable occlusion. Immediately after confirming total occlusion, heparin is administered as an intravenous bolus of 200 U/kg followed by 70 U/kg every hour.

The recanalization is the time from administration of thrombolytic agent until reflow. Reocclusion is disappearance of the phasic pattern of blood flow. Partial reflow is defined as a blood flow between 15 and 50% of the poststenotic flow. Femoral arterial patency status is categorized as follows: (1) persistent occlusion: no significant blood flow; (2) reocclusion after reflow: reocclusion persisting until the end of the experiment, after initial reflow; (3) cyclic reflow: alternating reocclusion and recanalization following initial reflow; (4) persistent patency: persistent flow without reocclusion after initial reflow. At the end of the experiment, the segment was removed and fixed for pathological examination (see later under histologic examination) [38,39].

PLATELET-RICH ARTERIAL, THROMBOSIS MODELS.

Eversion Graft Thrombosis Models.   The models are derived from the model in rabbits developed by Kersh et al. [40]. The epigastric artery is cannulated with a 2FG catheter (Portex green) for intra-arterial administration of study drug. A 5-mm segment of the right femoral artery is excised between two ligations, stripped of excessive adventitial tissue, everted inside-out, and inserted in the left femoral artery under a surgical microscope (Wild M651, Heerbrugg, Switzerland) by end-to-end anastomosis using 10–12 interrupted sutures with 10-0–monofilament sutures (Ethicon Inc., Sommerville, NJ). The microvascular clamp, which clamps off the proximal and distal ends of the transected artery, is released [40–42].

Blood flow is continuously monitored with a 1.5-mm–Doppler flowprobe for at least 2 h. When the flow is decreased to ≤ 0.5 mL/min, the vessel is considered to be occluded and heparin is given through the cannulated femoral vein (bolus of 200 U/kg followed by 70 U/kg at hourly intervals). Occlusion occurs within 15 min in approximately 70% of the animals. In the rabbits with persistent patency at 15 min the everted segment is traumatized by external compression with blunt forceps for 1–2 s, once or twice at 5-min intervals, whereby occlusion is consistently obtained.

In dogs or baboons the everted segment from the left carotid artery is then inserted into the transsected femoral artery by end-to-end anastomosis using 12–16 interrupted sutures with 7-0–nylon monofilament sutures (Ethicon Inc., Sommerville, NJ). Intravenous heparin (4000-U bolus followed by 1000 U/h) is given 5 min before the microvascular clamps occluding the proximal and distal ends of the transsected artery are then released. Blood flow is restored to approximately 20% of baseline flow. This is followed by spontaneous occlusion of the everted segment graft, which persists for 60 min as determined by the flow measurements [31]. *Reperfusion* is defined as a blood flow of more than 25% of baseline flow. At the end of the experiment, the everted femoral arterial segment is fixed in 4% (w/v) formaldehyde for pathological examination.

Photo-Induced Arterial Thrombosis.   A photoinduced method to induce an arterial platelet-rich thrombosis (PIT) has been described in a wide range of animals and locations. All models are based on the same principle as described by Matsuno et al. [43,44].

The left femoral artery in rats is exposed over a length of 5-mm distal to the inguinal ligament and all adventitia was carefully removed. A 1-mm–Doppler flowprobe is positioned for the monitoring of the blood flow. An 3-mm–optic fiber connected to a xenon light source (Hamatsu Photonic, Hamamatsu, Japan) with a heat filter and a green filter (band with 54 nm centered at 540 nm) is positioned over the artery at a distance of 5 mm and proximal to the flowprobe. The light source is illuminated and the baseline blood flow is monitored for 10 min, after which an intravenous bolus injection of Rose Bengal (Sigma, St. Louis, MO) is administered. Within a very reproducible time range (350 ± 36 s) an occlusive platelet-rich thrombus was formed as observed from the decrease in blood flow and the histological observations. The light source is switch-off and the thrombus was aged for 30 min, after which thrombolytic therapy is initiated. Clot lysis is monitored by the reoccurrence of blood flow and by histological examination [43]. Use of this model was recently described in mice [45,46].

$FeCl_3$-Induced Thrombosis.   Thrombosis induced by ferric chloride is a widely used model to investigate the antithrombotic potential of antiplatelet agents and anticoagulants in

several animal species. Thrombosis is induced by impairment of the vessel by topical administration of ferric chloride. The occurrence and dissolution of a thrombus is monitored by perivascular blood flow measurement. This model was occasionally used to investigate the thrombolytic potency of t-PA [47].

6.   Combined Arterial and Venous Thrombosis Models

Experimental models such as platelet-rich carotid–femoral artery eversion graft and erythrocyte-rich femoral vein thrombosis models or combined platelet-rich femoral artery eversion graft and femoral vein thrombosis models were combined. The models combined venous and arterial techniques to induce thrombosis as described under the respective sections of venous and arterial thrombosis models. Such studies allowed direct comparisons of the thrombolytic efficacy toward arterial and venous thrombi of the investigated thrombolytic agents or regimens [31,32,48,49].

a. Acute Myocardial Infarction Models

LEFT ANTERIOR DESCENDING CORONARY ARTERY (LAD) COPPER COIL-INDUCED THROMBOSIS. The use of metal as a thrombogenic surface, to induce intravascular clot formation, was first described by Pearse in 1940. He placed metal tubes, tubular coiled springs, or flat springs in arteries of dogs to produce thrombosis and vascular occlusion [50]. Blair et al. applied the model to the coronary artery to induce acute myocardial infarction [51]. The thrombogenic coil was introduced through the coronary vessel wall in open chest preparations. Later this model was adapted by Kordenat et al. who inserted the thrombogenic coils through the left carotid artery under fluoroscopic guidance and demonstrated that it could be used for in situ clot lysis [52]. The model was used to evaluate the efficacy of thrombolytic agents in acute myocardial infarction in the dog [53–55].

The canine left carotid artery was exposed and a 3-mm–long copper coil (six turns of a 0.5-mm copper wire) with a diameter matching the LAD was inserted over an intracoronary guide wire (0.018-in. TSF wire; Cook, Bjearverskov, Denmark) into the LAD distal to the first main diagonal branch. An erythrocyte-rich thrombus forms within 15 min after introduction as evidenced, by electrocardiographic signs of transmural ischemia or by angiography of the left carotid artery (by 5F Lehman catheters, USCI Bard). The thrombus is aged for 60 min. An angiogram is performed to confirm total occlusion of the artery, after which intravenous thrombolytic therapy by the left brachial vein is initiated. Reperfusion and reocclusion are evaluated angiographically at 15-min intervals or whenever electrocardiographic signs suggestive of reperfusion or reocclusion occurred. Reflow is defined as Thrombolysis In Myocardial Infarction (TIMI) grade 2 or 3 flow, and occlusion as TIMI grade 0 or 1 perfusion [56].

ELECTRICALLY-INDUCED MYOCARDIAL INFARCTION IN DOGS.   A 2-cm segment of the artery is isolated proximal to the first obtuse marginal branch and instrumented with a Doppler flow probe, an intracoronary catheter electrode, and an adjustable mechanical occluder. The stimulation electrode is constructed from a 25-g stainless steel hypodermic needle tip attached to a 30-g Teflon-insulated, silver-coated copper wire. The vessel diameter is manipulated with a mechanical constrictor, constructed in a C-shape with a continuously adjustable D-shape Teflon occluder, which is complementary to the C-shape. The constrictor is adjusted to decrease the reactive hyperemic flow (resulting from a 10-s mechanical occlusion) by 30% without affecting mean resting coronary blood flow. Small coronary side branches over the exposed section of the LCX are ligated [22,57].

Thirty minutes after surgical preparation of the animal, a continuous anodal current is applied to the luminal surface of the artery by the intracoronary electrode. The anodal current is delivered by a 9-V nickel–cadmium battery with the anode connected in series with a 250-kΩ potentiometer to the intraluminal coronary artery electrode. The circuit is closed by placing the cathode in a cutaneous side. The anodal current is maintained until the blood flow in the artery stops and remains occlusive for 30 min. The resulting electrolytic lesion produces a thrombotic environment onto which an occlusive platelet-rich clot is formed [57–59]. Intravenous administration of investigational agents is started after complete stable occlusion for 30 min. Reperfusion and reocclusion criteria are as described earlier.

7. Animal Models of Stroke

Animal models of stroke permit a more detailed understanding of this complex disease. However, it has to be emphasized that the obtained results are largely dependent on species differences and the methods used. The effects of the thrombolytic agents in thrombotic and embolic stroke was investigated [60–65].

a. Middle Cerebral Artery Thrombosis. Matsuno et al. described a relatively simple model to induce a thrombotic middle cerebral artery (MCA) occlusion without craniotomy. As a result of this procedure an occlusive thrombus was induced in the MCA without opening the dura mater. To produce a stable MCA occlusion, as in the photoinduced thrombosis model, described earlier, the following procedure is used [66,67]. After injection of the photosensitive dye Rose Bengal (Sigma, St. Louis, MO) the MCA is irradiated with a high-intensity light with a wavelength of 540 nm for 8 min. A white platelet-rich thrombus, with an erythrocyte-rich end toward the boundaries of the irradiated area, is formed. Thirty minutes after thrombus formation, the lytic agents can be administered.

b. Embolic Stroke Models in Rats and Rabbits. Thrombolytic therapy in experimental embolic stroke was investigated in rats and rabbits [60,63,68]. The carotid arterial system is exposed and all accessible side branches of the internal and common carotid artery are ligated. The embolic stroke is induced by the directed injection of in vitro produced thrombi (single thrombus or a suspension of small blood clots) through a 2FG (Portex green) catheter, which is introduced in the external carotid artery and advanced to the carotid bifurcation. The preparatory work in this models is rather simple; however, the methods needed to quantify and monitor the type of experiments require highly sophisticated equipment [60,62,69].

C. Analytical Methods to Quantify Thrombolytic Efficacy

1. Blood Analysis

Before and during administration of the thrombolytic agents, and at the end of the experiments, blood samples are collected in 0.015-M citrate in the amounts indicated for each species in Table 2. The iodine 125 in blood is measured in a gamma counter. Platelet aggregation induced with approximately 10 µM ADP (Sigma, St. Louis, MO) or 0.1 mg/mL collagen (Sigma, St. Louis, MO) is individually titrated [70]. Fibrinogen is measured by a coagulation rate assay that is insensitive to therapeutic concentrations of heparin, α_2-antiplasmin is measured with a chromogenic substrate assay [30], and antigen levels with specific enzyme-linked immunosorbent assay (ELISA) assays [71–73].

2. Kinetics of Clot Lysis of Radioactive Clots

The time course of ^{125}I-fibrin-labeled venous clot lysis is monitored continuously by external gamma counting, using a 3×0.5-in. sodium iodide/thallium crystal (Bicron, Newbury, OH) positioned over the clot and connected to a dedicated Canberra-S100 system (Canberra-Packard, Meriden, CT) that allows direct data acquisition on a personal computer [35]. From the accumulated data, the rate of clot lysis can be obtained by fitting the obtained measurements with a single exponentially transformed function [74,75].

3. Analysis of Thrombolysis Data in Venous Clot Lysis Models

The relative thrombolytic potency and the specific thrombolytic activity can be derived by fitting the individual values of percentage lysis versus dose of thrombolytic agent administered, expressed in milligram per kilogram (mg/kg), or of percentage lysis versus steady-state plasminogen activator–related antigen level in plasma, expressed in micrograms per milliliter (μg/mL) with a double exponentially transformed sigmoidal function [74,75].

4. Histologic Examination

After fixation by superfusion and postfixation in formaldehyde, the segments of the blood vessels are embedded in paraffin blocks and sectioned longitudinally. Sections are stained with hematoxylin and eosin (Hd-E) and examined microscopically for the presence of intraluminal or mural thrombi. Alternatively, arteries are subjected to perfusion fixation with 0.1-M-cacodylate–buffered 2.5% glutaraldehyde for scanning electron microscopy [76].

The extent of thrombosis is semiquantitatively graded on a scale of 1–4 with 1 = no or minimal mural thrombus; 2 = mural thrombus occupying less than 50% of the luminal diameter throughout the length of the isolated arterial segment; 3 = thrombus occupying more than 50%, but less than 95% of the luminal diameter over a distance of at least the diameter of the vessel; 4 = complete occlusive or greater than 95% luminal thrombus. The composition of the thrombus is characterized as erythrocyte-rich (ER), platelet-rich (PR), or mixed with interlaced platelet-rich and erythrocyte-rich zones (MPE) [76].

5. Statistical Analysis

The values are expressed as mean ± SEM. The significance of differences between groups are determined with Student's t-test for paired or unpaired values. Fisher's exact test is used to compare the occurrence of reflow and reocclusion in the various groups. A Kruskal–Wallis nonparametric analysis of variance is performed on ranks of the ordered variable of arterial patency, which ranges from 0 = persistent occlusion, 1 = reocclusion after initial reflow and reocclusion, and 3 = persistent patency as determined with the blood flow meter. A similar analysis is performed on arterial patency, graded on pathological analysis, as described earlier. This form of analysis of variance is selected because of the nongaussian distribution of the patency-state variables [76].

IV. EXPERIMENTAL MODELS TO ASSESS THE SAFETY OF THROMBOLYTIC THERAPY

Bleeding constitutes the main side effect of thrombolytic therapy. Although it occurs most frequently in association with vascular puncture or other invasive procedures, it may occur unexpectedly, even in carefully selected patients. Spontaneous bleeding does not appear to correlate strongly with the extent of systemic fibrinolytic activation and fibrinogen breakdown, nor with any other demographic or clinical characteristic of the patient.

A. Bleeding Time Models

1. The Template Bleeding Time as an Index of Bleeding Tendency

In a study of 52 consecutive patients with acute myocardial infarction treated with TPA, in which spontaneous bleeding was observed in 13 patients, a transient prolongation of the template bleeding time predicted bleeding with a specificity and sensitivity of 69%. The template bleeding time constitutes a parameter that, to a limited extent, significantly correlates with spontaneous bleeding in association with thrombolytic therapy. Furthermore, this study revealed that aspirin intake is associated with an increased incidence of spontaneous bleeding in association with thrombolytic therapy [77].

2. Template Bleeding Time in Animals

Bleeding times are performed before, during intravenous administration of plasminogen activator, and toward the end of the experiment, with a spring-loaded blade device (Surgicutt International, Technidyne Corp, Edison, NJ; or Symplate, Organon Teknika, Turnhout, Belgium) applied to a carefully shaved foreleg of dogs and baboons [31,78–80] or sublingually in dogs [81]. In rabbits template bleeding times are either performed on the shaved hindleg or on the outside of the ear [82,83]. Alternatively a 3.5-mm full-thickness puncture with a number 11 scalpel blade is used to produce a standardized wound [84,85]. The accuracy of all these variations on the same method depends highly on the method used to quantify the bleeding time. The blood oozing from the wound is absorbed on a filter paper of any kind at 30-s intervals, carefully avoiding disruption of or trauma to the bleeding site. The bleeding time is the elapsed time from transsection until blood no longer stains the filter paper.

3. Cuticle Bleeding Time

This type of bleeding time measurement is described in dogs and rabbits and is performed only in acute experiments [85,86]. Before injury, all hair is shaved around the claws. A spring-loaded sliding blade guillotine nail clipper (Tecla Company Inc., Walled Lake, MI) is used to transsect the apex of the nail cuticle. Again, as for the template bleeding time, blood is blotted from the incision with a filter paper at 30-s intervals while care is taken to avoid contact with the incision. The bleeding time is the elapsed time from transsection until blood no longer stains the filter paper.

4. Deep Wound Bleeding Time

A deep surgical wound in the neck of the animal, isolating the carotid artery, is packed with gauze sponges to collect all blood loss into the wound. At 30-min intervals the gauze is replaced, and the sponges containing blood are immersed in Drabkin's reagent (Sigma, St. Louis, MO) which lyses the cells and forms a colored reaction product with hemoglobin. From this solution samples are read in a photometer at a wavelength of 550 nm. The amount of blood loss can be derived from a calibration curve containing known amounts of blood [87].

5. Hemorrhagic Stroke Models

The occurrence of hemorrhagic stroke after thrombolysis with TPA, and TNK–TPA to assess the safety of the respective agents was investigated in rabbits [88–91]. After thrombolytic therapy of embolic stroke in rabbits, as described under stroke models, the animals were allowed to recover for 24 h. The animals were sacrificed and the brains were removed and fixed in 10% formaldehyde for 2 weeks, checked for gross surface hemorrhage, and cut into 2.5-mm sections.

The sections were observed and scored (1 for a single hemisphere and 2 for hemorrhage on both hemispheres). The sum of the scores of all sections was thus assigned to each brain.

6. Strategies to Reverse and Prevent Bleeding Time Prolongation

The interactive effect of aspirin and TPA, TNK–TPA, BatPA, or staphylokinase on bleeding time prolongation and bleeding, be it to a different extent, was confirmed and observed in experimental animal studies in rabbits and dogs [83,85,86,92]. Injection of plasminogen activator inhibitor-1 in rabbits or of the plasmin inhibitor aprotinin in dogs on intravenous administration of TPA, immediately reverses the bleeding time prolongation and arrested the bleeding from incision sites [80]. Thus, although the mechanism of the prolongation of the bleeding time remains to be elucidated, the reversibility of this phenomenon argues against degradation of platelet membrane receptors. The phenomenon is suggestive of a plasmin-mediated disturbance of platelet function, which cannot be detected by ex vivo platelet aggregation. The combined results of both bleeding time methods in animals indicate that fibrinolytic bleeding time prolongation correlates with the fibrin specificity of thrombolytic agents in the nail cuticle bleeding time model and also with the use of conjunctive antithrombotic agents in the template bleeding time model. A possible explanation for the different sensitivities may relate to the size of the injured blood vessels (5–25 μm in template bleeding time and 50–250 μm in the cuticle bleeding time). In the first, the formed platelet plug may be sufficient to arrest bleeding, whereas the latter might require fibrin stabilization of the platelet plug. The precise mechanisms of hemostasis of both models remains unknown and the described differences need direct morphological confirmation. Nevertheless, the experimental data may provide a predictive index of the hemorrhagic diathesis occurring in some patients during thrombolytic therapy and may provide information on the mechanisms of spontaneous bleeding.

V. CONCLUSION

Although the remaining obstacles to consistent, rapid, persistent, and safe coronary recanalization remain complex, the conceptual framework is available for the development of improved thrombolytic therapy with plasminogen activators used in conjunction with specifically targeted antiplatelet and anticoagulant agents. Continued investigations along these new lines of research will probably provide new insights and progress toward the development of improved thrombolytic strategies, with minimized side effects. Although it is clear that compounds with antithrombin or antiplatelet properties may enhance and sustain the action of thrombolytic agents, their optimal use and potential hemorrhagic side effects remain to be further explored. Simple relevant animal models constitute essential experimental tools to investigate these problems. It is anticipated that optimized thrombolytic therapy will eventually consist of potent, specific plasminogen activators in combination with conjunctive (as opposed to adjunctive) anticoagulant or antiplatelet agents.

REFERENCES

1. Davies MJ, Thomas AC. Plaque fissuring—the cause of acute myocardial infarction, sudden ischaemic death, and crescendo angina. Br Heart J 1985; 53:363–373.
2. Davies MJ. Pathology of arterial thrombosis. Br Med Bull 1994; 50:789–802.
3. A comparison of reteplase with alteplase for acute myocardial infarction. The Global Use of Strategies to Open Occluded Coronary Arteries (GUSTO III) Investigators. N Engl J Med 1997; 337:1118–1123.

4. Single-bolus tenecteplase compared with front-loaded alteplase in acute myocardial infarction: the ASSENT-2 double-blind randomised trial. Assessment of the Safety and Efficacy of a New Thrombolytic, Investigators. Lancet 1999; 354:716–722.

5. Hampton JR. Thrombolytic therapy in acute myocardial infarction. Cardiovasc Drug Ther 1997; 11(suppl 1):241–246.

6. Haas S. Deep vein thrombosis: beyond the operating table. Orthopedics 2000; 23:s629–s632.

7. Schweizer J, Kirch W, Koch R, Elix H, Hellner G, Forkmann L, Graf A. Short- and long-term results after thrombolytic treatment of deep venous thrombosis. J Am Coll Cardiol 2000; 36:1336–1343.

8. Chang R, Cannon RO, 3rd, Chen CC, Doppman JL, Shawker TH, Mayo DJ, Wood B, Horne MK, 3rd. Daily catheter-directed single dosing of t-PA in treatment of acute deep venous thrombosis of the lower extremity. J Vasc Interven Radiol 2001; 12:247–252.

9. Goldhaber SZ. Pulmonary embolism thrombolysis: do we need another agent? Am Heart J 1999; 138:1–2.

10. Hamel E, Pacouret G, Vincentelli D, Forissier JF, Peycher P, Pottier JM, Charbonnier B. Thrombolysis or heparin therapy in massive pulmonary embolism with right ventricular dilation: Results from a 128-patient monocenter registry. Chest 2001; 120:120–125.

11. Kidwell CS, Liebeskind DS, Starkman S, Saver JL. Trends in acute ischemic stroke trials through the 20th century. Stroke 2001; 32:1349–1359.

12. Kaste M. Thrombolysis in ischaemic stroke—present and future: role of combined therapy. Cerebrovasc Dis 2001; 11:55–59.

13. Grotta IC, Welch KM, Fagan SC, Lu M, Frankel MR, Brott T, Levine SR, Lyden PD. Clinical deterioration following improvement in the NINDS rt-PA stroke trial stroke 2001; 32:661–668.

14. Pederson WC. Replantation. Plast Reconstr Surg 2001; 107:823–841.

15. Nystrom A, Backman C. Replantation of the completely avulsed thumb using long arterial and venous grafts. J Hand Surg [Br] 1991; 16:389–391.

16. Yii NW, Evans GR, Miller MJ, Reece GP, Langstein H, Chang D, Kroll SS, Wang B, Robb GL. Thrombolytic therapy: what is its role in free flap salvage? Ann Plast Surg 2001; 46:601–604.

17. Noguchi M, Matsusaki H, Yamamoto H. Intravenous bolus infusion of heparin for circulatory insufficiency after finger replantation. J Reconstr Microsurg 1999; 15:245–253.

18. Hashim HA, Atiyeh BS, Hamdan AM, Musharrafieh RS. Local intravenous thrombolysis with recombinant tissue plasminogen activatcr for salvage of forearm replantation. J Reconstr Microsurg 1996; 12:543–546.

19. Stassen JM, Lu G, Andreen O, Nystrom E, Nystrom A. Intraoperative thrombolytic treatment of microarterial occlusion by selective rt-PA infusion. Plast Reconstr Surg 1995; 96:1215–1217.

20. Dorffler-Melly J, Schwarte LA, Ince C, Levi M. Mouse models of focal arterial and venous thrombosis. Basic Res Cardiol 2000; 95:503–509.

21. Wessler S. The issue of animal models of thrombosis. Ann NY Acad Sci 1989; 556:366–370.

22. Bush LR, Shebuski RJ. In vivo models of arterial thrombosis and thrombolysis. FASEB J 1990; 4:3087–4098.

23. Stassen JM, Lijnen HR, Kieckens L, Cohen D. Small animal thrombosis models for the evaluation of thrombolytic agents. Circulation 1991; 83:1V65–72.

24. Henry R. Methods for inducing experimental thrombosis. Angiology 1962; 13:554–577.

25. Korninger C, Collen D. Studies on the specific fibrinolytic effect of human extrinsic (tissue-type) plasminogen activator in human blood and in various animal species in vitro. Thromb Haemost 1981; 46:561–565.

26. Giles AR. Guidelines for the use of animals in biomedical research. Thromb Haemost 1987; 58:1078–1084.

27. Wormuth HJ. Treatment of vertebrates according to Section 4 of the Animal Welfare Act. Dtsch Tierarztl Wochenschr 1992; 99:5–8.

28. Keyt BA, Paoni NP, Refino CJ, Berleau L, Nguyen H, Chow A, Lai J, Pena L, Pater C, Ogez J. A faster-acting and more potent form of tissue plasminogen activator. Proc Natl Acad Sci USA 1994; 91:3670–3674.

29. Refino CJ, Paoni NF, Keyt BA, Pater CS, Basillo JM, Wurm FM, Ogez J, Bennett WF. A variant of t-PA (TI03N, KHRR 296-299 AAAA) that, by bolus, has increased potency and decreased systemic activation of plasminogen. Thromb Haemost 1993; 70:313–319.

30. Collen D, Stassen TM, Verstraete M. Thrombolysis with human extrinsic (tissue-type) plasminogen activator in rabbits with experimental jugular vein thrombosis. Effect of molecular form and dose of activator, age of the thrombus, and route of administration. J Clin Invest 1983; 71:368–376.

31. Collen D, De Cock F, Stassen JM. Comparative immunogenicity and thrombolytic properties toward arterial and venous thrombi of streptokinase and recombinant staphylokinase in baboons. Circulation 1993; 87:996–1006.

32. Stassen TM, Rapold HT, Vanlinthout I, Collen D. Comparative effects of enoxaparin and heparin on arterial and venous clot lysis with alteplase in dogs. Thromb Haemost 1993; 69:454–459.

33. Butte AN, Houng AK, Jang IK, Reed GL. alpha 2-Antiplasmin causes thrombi to resist fibrinolysis induced by tissue plasminogen activator in experimental pulmonary embolism. Circulation 1997; 95:1886–1891.

34. Carmeliet P, Stassen TM, Schoonjans L, Ream B, van den Oord JJ, De Mol M, Mulligan RC, Collen D. Plasminogen activator inhibitor-1 gene-deficient mice. II. Effects on hemostasis, thrombosis, and thrombolysis. J Clin Invest 1993; 92:2756–2760.

35. Stassen TM, Vanlinthout I, Lijnen HR, Collen D. A hamster pulmonary embolism model for the evaluation of thrombolytic and pharmacokinetic properties of thrombolytic agents. Fibrinolysis 1990; 4(suppl):15–21.

36. Clozel JP, Holvoet P, Tschopp T. Experimental pulmonary embolus in the rat: a new in vivo model to test thrombolytic drugs. J Cardiovasc Pharmacol 1988; 12:520–525.

37. Arnljots B, Dougan P, Salemark L, Bergqvist D. Effects of streptokinase and urokinase on microarterial thrombosis and haemostasis. An experimental study in rabbits. Scand J Plast Recorstr Surg Hand Surg 1994; 28:9–13.

38. Gold HK, Yasuda T, Jang IK, Guerrero JL, Fallon JT, Leinbach RC, Collen D. Animal models for arterial thrombolysis and prevention of reocclusion. Erythrocyte-rich versus platelet-rich thrombus. Circulation 1991; 83(Suppl. IV):26–40.

39. Helft G, Bara L, Bloch MF, Samama MM. Comparative time course of thrombolysis induced by intravenous boluses and infusion of staphylokinase and tissue plasminogen activator in a rabbit arterial thrombosis model. Blood Coagul Fibrinol 1998; 9:411–417.

40. Kersh RA, Handren J, Hergrueter C, May JW Jr. Microvascular surgical experimental thrombosis model: rationale and design. Plast Reconstr Surg 1989; 83:866–872 [discussion 873–874].

41. Jang IK, Gold HK, Ziskind AA, Fallon JT, Holt RE, Leinbach RC, May JW, Collen D. Differential sensitivity of erythrocyte-rich and platelet-rich arterial thrombi to lysis with recombinant tissue-type plasminogen activator. A possible explanation for resistance to coronary thrombolysis. Circulation 1989; 79:920–928.

42. Hergrueter CA, Handren J, Kersh R, May JW Jr. Human recombinant tissue type plasminogen activator and its effect on microvascular thrombosis in the rabbit. Plast Reconstr Surg 1988; 81:418–424.

43. Matsuno H, Uematsu T, Nagashima S, Nakashima M. Photochemically induced thrombosis model in rat femoral artery and evaluation of effects of heparin and tissue-type plasminogen activator with use of this model. J Pharmacol Methods 1991; 25:303–317.

44. Fukuchi M, Uematsu T, Araki S, Nakashima M. Photochemically induced thrombosis of the rat coronary artery and functional evaluation of thrombus formation by occurrence of ventricular arrhythmias. Effects of acetylsalicylic acid and a thromboxane A_2 synthetase inhibitor of thrombus formation. Naunyn Schmiedebergs Arch Pharmacol 1992; 346:550–554.

45. Kawasaki T, Kaida I, Arnout J, Vermylen J, Hoylaerts MF. A new animal model of thrombophilia confirms that high plasma factor VIII levels are thrombogenic. Thromb Haemost 1999; 81:306–311.

46. Kawasaki T, Dewerchin M, Lijnen HR, Vermylen J, Hoylaerts MF. Vascular release of plasminogen activator inhibitor-1 impairs fibrinolysis during acute arterial thrombosis in mice. Blood 2000; 96:153–160.

47. Zhu Y, Carmeliet P, Fay WP. Plasminogen activator inhibitor-1 is a major determinant of arterial thrombolysis resistance. Circulation 1999; 99:3050–3055.

48. Baum PK, Martin D, Abendschein D. A preparation to study simultaneous arterial and venous thrombus formation in rabbits. J Invest Surg 2001; 14:153–160.
49. Collen D, Lu HR, Lijnen HR, Nelles L, Stassen JM. Thrombolytic and pharmacokinetic properties of chimeric tissue-type and urokinase-type plasminogen activators. Circulation 1991; 84:1216–1234.
50. Pearse HE. Experimental studies on gradual occlusion of large arteries. Ann Surgery 1940; 112:923–937.
51. Blair E, Nygren E, Cowley RA. A spriral wire technique for producing gradually coronary artery thrombosis. J Thorac Cardiovasc Surg 1964; 48:476–484.
52. Kordenat RK, Kezdi P, Powley D. Experimental intracoronary thrombosis and selective in situ lysis by catheter technique. Am J Cardiol 1972; 30:640–645.
53. Van de Werf F, Bergmann SR, Fox KA, et al. Coronary thrombolysis with intravenously administered human tissue-type plasminogen activator produced by recombinant DNA technology. Circulation 1984; 69:605–610.
54. Suzuki M, Funatsu T, Tanaka H, Usuda S. YM866, a novel modified tissue-type plasminogen activator, affects left ventricular function and myocardial infarct development in dogs with coronary artery thrombi. Jpn J Pharmacol 1998; 77:177–183.
55. Rapold HJ, Wu ZM, Stassen T, Van de Werf F, Collen D. Comparison of intravenous bolus injection or continuous infusion of recombinant single chain urokinase-type plasminogen activator (saruplase) for thrombolysis. A canine model of combined coronary arterial and femoral venous thrombosis. Blood 1990; 76:1558–1563.
56. TIMI Study Group. The Thrombolysis in Myocardial Infarction (TIMI) trial. Phase I findings. N Engl J Med 1985; 312:932–936.
57. Redlitz A, Nicolini FA, Malycky JL, Topol EJ, Plow EF. Inducible carboxypeptidase activity. A role in clot lysis in vivo. Circulation 1996; 93:1328–1330.
58. Tomoda H. Experimental study on the comparative thrombolytic effects of intracoronary and intravenous administration of urokinase. Jpn Heart J 1986; 27:259–265.
59. Roux SP, Tschopp TB, Kuhn H, Steiner B, Hadvary P. Effects of heparin, aspirin and a synthetic platelet glycoprotein IIb-IIIa receptor antagonist (Ro 43-5054) on coronary artery reperfusion and reocclusion after thrombolysis with tissue-type plasminogen activator in the dog. J Pharmacol Exp Ther 1993; 264:501–508.
60. Chapman DF, Lyden P, Lapchak PA, Nunez S, Thibodeaux H, Zivin J. Comparison of TNK with wild-type tissue plasminogen activator in a rabbit embolic stroke model. Stroke 2001; 32:748–752.
61. Small DL, Buchan AM. Animal models. Br Med Bull 2000; 56:307–317.
62. Vanderschueren S, Van Vlaenderen I, Collen D. Intravenous thrombolysis with recombinant staphylo-kinase versus tissue-type plasminogen activator in a rabbit embolic stroke model. Stroke 1997; 28: 1783–1788.
63. Overgaard K. Thrombolytic therapy in experimental embolic stroke. Cerebrovasc Brain Metab Rev 1994; 6:257–286.
64. del Zoppo GJ. Relevance of focal cerebral ischemia models. Experience with fibrinolytic agents. Stroke 1990; 21(Suppl. IV):155–160.
65. Futrell N, Millikan C, Watson BD, Dietrich WD, Ginsberg MD. Embolic stroke from a carotid arterial source in the rat: pathology and clinical implications. Neurology 1989; 39:1050–1056.
66. Umemura K, Toshima Y, Nakashima M. Thrombolytic efficacy of a modified tissue-type plasminogen activator, SUN9216, in the rat middle cerebral artery thrombosis model. Eur J Pharmacol 1994; 262:27–31.
67. Imura Y, Kiyota Y, Nagai Y, Nishikawa K, Terashita Z. Beneficial effect of CV-4151 (Isbogrel), a thromboxane A_2 synthase inhibitor, in a rat middle cerebral artery thrombosis model. Thromb Res 1995; 79:95–107.
68. Overgaard K, Sereghy T, Boysen G, Pedersen H, Hoyer S, Diemer NH. A rat model of reproducible cerebral infarction using thrombotic blood clot emboli. J Cereb Blood Flow Metab 1992; 12:484–490.
69. Zhang RL, Zhang L, Jiang Q, Zhang ZG, Goussev A, Chopp M. Postischemic intracarotid treatment with TNK–t-PA reduces infarct volume and improves neurological deficits in embolic stroke in the unanesthetized rat. Brain Res 2000; 878:64–71.

70. Kiss RG, Stassen JM, Deckmyn H, Roskams T, Gold HK, Plow EF, Collen D. Contribution of platelets and the vessel wall to the antithrombotic effects of a single bolus injection of Fab fragments of the antiplatelet GPIIb/IIIa antibody 7E3 in a canine arterial eversion graft preparation. Arterioscler Thromb 1994; 14:375–380.

71. Lijnen HR, Beelen V, Declerck PJ, Collen D. Bio-immunoassay for staphylokinase in blood. Thromb Haemost 1993; 70:491–494.

72. Darras V, Thienpont M, Stump DC, Collen D. Measurement of urokinase-type plasminogen activator (u-PA) with an enzyme-linked immunosorbent assay (ELISA) based on three murine monoclonal antibodies. Thromb Haemost 1986; 56:411–414.

73. Holvoet P. Cleemput H, Collen D. Assay of human tissue-type plasminogen activator (t-PA) with an enzyme-linked immunosorbent assay (ELISA) based on three murine monoclonal antibodies to t-PA. Thromb Haemost 1985; 54:684–687.

74. Holvoet P, Dewerchin M, Stassen JM, Lijnen HR, Tollenaere T, Gaffney PJ, Collen D. Thrombolytic profiles of clot-targeted plasminogen activators. Parameters determining potency and initial and maximal rates. Circulation 1993; 87:1007–1016.

75. Collen D, Lijnen HR, Vanlinthout I, Kieckens L, Nelles L, Stassen JM. Thrombolytic and pharmacokinetic properties of human tissue-type plasminogen activator variants, obtained by deletion and/or duplication of structural/functional domains, in a hamster pulmonary embolism model. Thromb Haemost 1991; 65:174–180.

76. Lu HR, Gold HK, Wu Z, et al. G4120, an Arg-Gly-Asp containing pentapeptide, enhances arterial eversion graft recanalization with recombinant tissue-type plasminogen activator in dogs. Thromb Haemost 1992; 67:686–691.

77. Gimple LW, Gold HK, Leinbach RC, Coller BS, Werner W, Yasuda T, Johns JA, Ziskind AA, Finkelstein D, Collen D. Correlation between template bleeding times and spontaneous bleeding during treatment of acute myocardial infarction with recombinant tissue-type plasminogen activator. Circulation 1989; 80:581–588.

78. Lu HR, Wu Z, Pauwels P, Lijnen HR, Collen D. Comparative thrombolytic properties of tissue-type plasminogen activator (t-PA), single-chain urokinase-type plasminogen activator (u-PA) and K1K2Pu (a t-PA/u-PA chimera) in a combined arterial and venous thrombosis model in the dog. J Am Coll Cardiol 1992; 19:1350–1359.

79. Imura Y, Stassen JM, Kurokawa T, Iwasa S, Lijnen HR, Collen D. Thrombolytic and pharmacokinetic properties of an immunoconjugate of single-chain urokinase-type plasminogen activator (u-PA) and a bispecific monoclonal antibody against fibrin and against u-PA in baboons. Blood 1992; 79:2322–2329.

80. Garabedian HD, Gold HK, Leinbach RC, Svizzero TA, Finkelstein DM, Guerrero JL, Collen D. Bleeding time prolongation and bleeding during infusion of recombinant tissue-type plasminogen activator in dogs: potentiation by aspirin and reversal with aprotinin. J Am Coil Cardiol 1991; 17:1213–1222.

81. Tschopp JF, Driscoll EM, Mu DX, Black SC, Pierschbacher MD, Lucchesi BR. Inhibition of coronary artery reocclusion after thrombolysis with an RGD-containing peptide with no significant effect on bleeding time. Coronary Artery Dis 1993; 4:809–817.

82. Mattson C, Wikstrom K, Sterky C, Pohl G. Synergism between tissue-type plasminogen activator and a genetically engineered variant lacking the finger domain, the growth factor domain and the first kringle domain. Thromb Haemost 1991; 65:286–290.

83. Vaughan DE, Declerck PJ, De Mol M, Collen D. Recombinant plasminogen activator inhibitor-1 reverses the bleeding tendency associated with the combined administration of tissue-type plasminogen activator and aspirin in rabbits. J Clin Invest 1989; 84:586–591.

84. Harpaz D, Chen X, Francis CW, Marder VJ, Meltzer RS. Ultrasound enhancement of thrombolysis and reperfusion in vitro. J Am Coll Cardiol 1993; 21:1507–1511.

85. Vanderschueren S. Collen D. Comparative effects of staphylokinase and alteplase in rabbit bleeding time models. Thromb Haemost 1996; 75:816–819.

86. Mellott MJ., Ramjit DR, Stabilito II, Hare TR, Senderak ET, Lynch JJ, Jr., Gardell SJ. Vampire bat salivary plasminogen activator evokes minimal bleeding relative to tissue-type plasminogen activator as assessed by a rabbit cuticle bleeding time model. Thromb Haemost 1995; 73:478–483.

87. Vlasuk GP, Dempsey EM, Oldeschulte GL, Bernardino VT, Richard BM, Rote WE. Evaluation of a novel small protein inhibitor of blood coagulation factor Xa (rNAP-5) in animal models of thrombosis. Circulation 1995; 95:abst. 3287.
88. Lapchak PA, Chapman DF, Zivin JA, Metalloproteinase inhibition reduces thrombolytic (tissue plasminogen activator)-induced hemorrhage after thromboembolic stroke. Stroke 2000; 31:3034–3040.
89. Hu B, Liu C, Zivin JA. Reduction of intracerebral hemorrhaging in a rabbit embolic stroke model. Neurology 1999; 53:2140–2145.
90. Thomas GR, Thibodeaux H, Errett CJ, Badillo JM, Wu DT, Refino CJ, Keyt BA, Bennett WF. Limiting systemic plasminogenolysis reduces the bleeding potential for tissue-type plasminogen activators but not for streptokinase. Thromb Haemost 1996; 75:915–920.
91. Lyden PD, Zivin JA, Clark WA, Madden K, Sasse KC, Mazzarella VA, Terry RD, Press GA. Tissue plasminogen activator-mediated thrombolysis of cerebral emboli and its effect on hemorrhagic infarction in rabbits. Neurology 1989; 39:703–708.
92. Thomas GR, Thibodeaux H, Errett CJ, Badillo JM, Keyt BA, Refino CJ, Zivin JA, Bennett WF. A long-half-life and fibrin-specific form of tissue plasminogen activator in rabbit models of embolic stroke and peripheral bleeding. Stroke 1994; 25:2072–2078[discussion 2078–2079].

41

Thrombolysis and Ultrasound

Charles W. Francis and Valentina Suchkova
University of Rochester Medical Center, Rochester, New York, U.S.A.

SUMMARY

Several small clinical studies have demonstrated that application of ultrasound using an endovascular catheter can recanalize occluded arterial vessels. The devices all use a wire operating between 19.5 and 45 kHz at high energy, resulting in direct mechanical or cavitational fragmentation of the thrombus. Careful catheter guidance is essential and vessel damage and perforation can occur. Studies are underway using lower intensity ultrasound delivered either by catheter or noninvasively in combination with fibrinolytic agents to accelerate thrombolysis. This approach will expose the vessel to lower intensities of ultrasonic energy, and the noninvasive transcutaneous application of ultrasound would simplify the approach.

I. INTRODUCTION

Vascular obstruction from thrombosis or thromboembolism results in common and serious clinical conditions including acute myocardial infarction, stroke, peripheral artery occlusion, deep-vein thrombosis, and pulmonary embolism. Remarkable improvements in management have resulted from the use of anticoagulants, antiplatelet agents, and risk modification to prevent initial or recurrent disease. Outcomes have also been improved by acute interventions to rapidly open occluded vessels using either mechanical approaches or thrombolysis. Thus, angioplasty has become accepted as a primary treatment for acute coronary thrombosis; other approaches to physically disrupt a clot or thrombus include mechanical atherectomy devices and the use of laser energy.

The use of thrombolytic therapy has also expanded as clinical trials have documented its ability to rapidly establish reperfusion and to improve outcomes in common thrombotic disorders. Large and convincing clinical trials have documented significant improvements in mortality and morbidity in acute myocardial infarction, improved outcomes in patients with peripheral arterial disease, and reduced disability in selected patients following stroke. Well-performed clinical trials have also focused attention on the limitations of thrombolytic therapy, including failure to establish reperfusion, bleeding complications, and delayed reperfusion with ischemic death of distal tissue before the blood supply is restored. Additionally, the underlying prothrombotic atherosclerotic lesion remains after thrombolysis, and therapy can fail because initial reperfusion is followed by prompt rethrombosis. In treatment of acute myocardial infarction, up to 20% of patients do not achieve reperfusion, and in those who do reperfuse the benefit decreases with longer periods of ischemia, emphasizing the need for rapidly acting therapy. This is even more critical for stroke, which must be treated very rapidly after onset of symptoms to achieve benefit, and the serious consequences of intracranial bleeding limit enthusiasm and widespread application. Problems with thrombolytic therapy of peripheral arterial disease include the requirement for proper catheter placement within the thrombus, the need for a longer duration of treatment, and the requirement for subsequent endovascular procedures or surgical reconstruction in the majority of patients. The limited use of thrombolysis in treatment of deep-vein thrombosis and pulmonary embolism reflects the high incidence of failure of thrombolysis and overall lower benefit/risk ratio.

These limitations of thrombolysis have spurred intense efforts to improve therapy, focusing on the development of new plasminogen activators, more effective and simpler dosing regimens, and the addition of adjunctive antiplatelet and anticoagulant therapies to increase reperfusion and reduce reocclusion. In this context, the use of ultrasound represents a completely different approach with new potential for opening occluded vessels. Depending on the intensity and frequency employed, ultrasound may accelerate enzymatic thrombolysis, or alternatively mechanical effects may predominate with physical disruption of thrombus. For both applications, there are important considerations related to tissue penetration and limiting adverse effects, including heating. A particular benefit of ultrasound is that the effects are limited to the insonified region so that its action is focused at the site of thrombosis, and systemic complications are limited. This chapter will review in vitro studies establishing the basis of using ultrasound, the biochemical and biophysical mechanisms of its action, animal studies, and initial clinical trials demonstrating the therapeutic potential.

II. IN VITRO STUDIES

The use of ultrasound for thrombolysis has evolved using two fundamentally different approaches to either disrupt the thrombus mechanically or to accelerate enzymatic fibrinolysis. The effect observed critically depends on ultrasound frequency and intensity. Several reports have established that a clot can be mechanically disrupted into small fragments using a wire vibrating at ultrasonic frequencies, in the absence of plasminogen activator [1–4]. The apparatus consists of an ultrasound transducer that is mechanically coupled to a wire ensheathed in a catheter, and ultrasound energy is transmitted to the tip, which vibrates with a high force, resulting in mechanical disruption of the clot. The catheter sizes have been typically 7F to 9F, although Steffen et al. [4] have investigated a 4.6F catheter with a length of 145 cm. When the device is activated, ultrasound energy is transmitted to the tip with a diameter of approximately 2 µm that vibrates with high force and displacement of up to 100 µm. Heating occurs routinely and is usually controlled with saline infusion through the catheter when it is activated.

Such devices can be used to mechanically disrupt either thrombus or atherosclerotic plaque. Siegel et al. [5] demonstrated that such a device could disrupt fibrous or calcified plaque in atherosclerotic arteries recovered at autopsy or surgery. Complete atherosclerotic occlusions of between 0.5 and 5 cm in length could be rapidly recanalized even if calcification was present. Effects on atherosclerotic and normal vessels differed, with less effect on the normal vessel wall, but thermal damage occurred in approximately one-third of trials, and perforation occurred in some. In a similar study, Ernst et al. [6] investigated the capacity of high intensity ultrasound to ablate atherosclerotic plaque and compared its effect with that on the normal vessel wall using samples obtained from autopsies. At high power, the ultrasound probe ablated atherosclerotic plaque effectively, but also perforated normal vessel wall. There was some selectivity depending on power levels, with greater effect on plaque and less normal vessel wall damage at power intensities of less than $68 \, \text{W/cm}^2$. With a different model, Dick et al. [7] showed that an intravascular 22.5-kHz–ultrasound device could disrupt thrombus trapped in a vena caval filter in vitro.

High-intensity ultrasound delivered using a transducer can also disrupt clots in vitro. Nishioka et al. [8] used a 24.9-kHz transducer at $2.9 \, \text{W/cm}^2$ to rapidly fragment thrombus, and this effect was increased by addition of cavitation nuclei in the form of dodecafluoropentane emulsion. Similarly, Porter et al. [9] investigated the effect of a 20-kHz transducer operating at $40 \, \text{W/cm}^2$, and demonstrated that it could disrupt clot in vitro, but that addition of microbubbles augmented the effect. Focused high-energy delivered as 1000 shocks at 24 kV was also able to ablate thrombi contained in arterial segments in vitro without damage to the vessel wall [10]. By using a somewhat different approach, Rosenschein et al. [11] tested a transducer with an acoustic lens to focus the energy and coupled this with an ultrasound-imaging system. This was used to treat clots inserted into bovine arterial segments at 500 kHz. Optimal parameters were a $1 : 15$ duty cycle and an intensity of over $35 \, \text{W/cm}^2$; these rapidly reduced a clot to small fragments. Arterial wall damage occurred at intensities over $45 \, \text{W/cm}^2$.

In general, ultrasound wires operating at approximately 20 kHz and high intensity can rapidly disrupt a clot into microscopic fragments and also have the potential to ablate atherosclerotic plaque. Disadvantages include the unknown effects of distal embolization of fragments, damage or perforation of the vessel wall, and heating. Technical problems include the limited flexibility of the ultrasound wire and breakage. In addition, the need for selective catheterization requires specialized facilities and highly trained personnel, which could result in treatment delays and limit wide clinical application. Clot disruption can also be achieved without catheterization by using an external transducer delivering high energy, and this effect is increased by addition of microbubbles.

The second approach to using ultrasound for thrombolysis is completely different conceptually and involves the use of lower-intensity ultrasound to accelerate enzymatic fibrinolysis with either minimal or no mechanical disruption of the clot. This approach is fundamentally a combination of a device delivering ultrasound energy and infusion of a plasminogen activator. The principal concept is that application of ultrasound will augment the effect of the plasminogen activator. This can be used to increase the frequency or speed of reperfusion or, alternatively, to decrease side effects by maintaining effectiveness of treatment at a lower dose of activator.

Critical issues in developing ultrasound to enhance enzymatic thrombolysis for therapeutic use have been identification of the optimum ultrasound frequency and defining the appropriate range of intensities. Several reports have demonstrated enhancement of thrombolysis with ultrasound at frequencies of 0.5 MHz and higher. Francis et al. [12] investigated the effect of ultrasound on fibrinolysis in vitro using plasma clots exposed to continuous-wave 1-MHz ultrasound at intensities up to $8 \, \text{W/cm}^2$. Significant acceleration of fibrinolysis induced by tissue-type plasminogen activator (t-PA) was observed at intensities of $1 \, \text{W/cm}^2$ and greater. There was no mechanical fragmentation of the clot, and fibrinolysis did not increase in the absence of plasminogen activator. Ultrasound exposure resulted in a marked reduction in the t-PA concentration required to achieve fibrinolysis. Acceleration of fibrinolysis was also observed with urokinase and streptokinase in addition to t-PA [13]. Ultrasound exposure, at the intensities used, resulted in a small increase in temperature that was insufficient to explain the enhancement of the fibrinolysis observed. The degree of ultrasound potentiation was dependent on intensity and also on activator concentration with greater acceleration of fibrinolysis at higher concentrations. The effect was greater at higher intensities and duty cycles, but was less at 3.4 MHz compared with 1 MHz. The results were similar to those observed by Lauer et al. [14] at 1.75 W/cm^2 and 50% duty cycle and, also, by Luo et al. [15] who observed acceleration of fibrinolysis with urokinase and streptokinase at 1 MHz and intensities of 1–2.2 W/cm^2. These results were confirmed by Harpaz et al. [16,17] who used a flow system to demonstrate increased in vitro reperfusion with application of 0.5-MHz ultrasound. Olsson et al. [18] and Nilsson et al. [19] also observed acceleration of in vitro fibrinolysis with streptokinase using ultrasound frequencies of 0.5–2.3 MHz in intensities up to 0.5 W/cm^2.

Ultrasound frequency is a critical parameter for effective thrombolysis because tissue penetration declines and heating increases at higher frequencies. Several reports indicate that enzymatic thrombolysis is enhanced at lower ultrasound frequencies. Tachibana et al. [20,21] demonstrated acceleration of urokinase-induced lysis of whole blood clots in the Chandler loop model with 48-kHz ultrasound, and Olsson et al. [18] demonstrated increased fibrinolysis in vitro with streptokinase using 170-kHz–pulsed ultrasound at 0.5 W/cm^2 and 1% duty cycle. Sehgal et al. [22] used ultrasound at 20 kHz and 1–2 W/cm^2 and showed enhancement of enzymatic fibrinolysis. Suchkova et al. [23] have investigated the potential of 40-kHz ultrasound and demonstrated significant acceleration of enzymatic fibrinolysis at intensities as low as 0.25 W/cm^2. The extent of fibrinolysis was dependent on intensity, and some mechanical disruption of the clot occurred at 40 kHz, which reached a maximum of 3.8% at 1.5 W/cm^2. The effects were strikingly greater than those observed previously at 1 MHz (Fig. 1). Samples of porcine rib cage were used to investigate tissue attenuation and heating at 40 kHz. The attenuation was only 1.7 ± 0.5 db through the intercostal space and 3.4 ± 0.9 db through porcine rib. Transmission through bone is challenging because of its relatively high absorption. However, temperature increments in rib at 40 kHz were less than 1°C/W cm^{-2}.

The capacity to enhance ultrasound at lower ultrasound frequencies is important for several reasons. First, at higher frequencies the attenuation of soft tissues reduces the intensity of the field to a degree that adequate treatment could be administered to clots in peripheral vessels, but

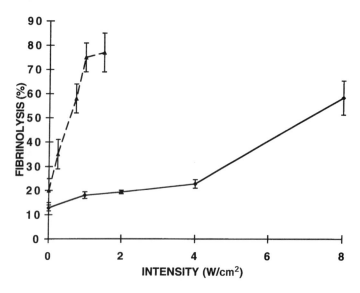

Figure 1   Comparison of the effects of ultrasound at 1 MHz and 40 kHz on fibrinolysis in vitro: The amount of fibrinolysis ($\pm$ SD) at 1 h was measured by solubilization of ^{125}I-fibrin labeled clots using identical systems except for ultrasound frequency. (From Ref. 23.)

heating would occur and could be limiting. The attenuation of bone is, however, an order of magnitude greater, and use of higher frequency ultrasound for noninvasive treatment of heart or brain would be precluded. In contrast, the depth of penetration at 40 kHz or lower frequencies in soft tissues is nearly infinite, and the rib cage transmits approximately one-half the intensity to the heart. Wavelengths of several centimeters mean that beam patterns are broad and relatively uniform even after passing through the chest wall. Also, there is a rather large-intensity window between the minimum values that are effective for enhancing thrombolysis and the values that would be thermally hazardous. At mid-kHz frequencies, even the brain may be accessible for noninvasive treatment with ultrasound. A review of published data [23] on attenuation of skull bone indicates that, even at 300 kHz, the intensity transmitted should be greater than one-third of incident level, and that attenuation is roughly proportional to the frequency, suggesting that at 40 kHz the ultrasound intensity reaching the brain with thermally acceptable levels should be great enough to enhance enzymatic thrombolysis.

This has recently been confirmed by Akiyama et al. [24], who found that 40% of ultrasound intensity could be transmitted through the temporal bone. Behrens et al. [25] investigated these effects within the range of 20–100 kHz and demonstrated a very low ultrasound attenuation through samples of different postmortem skulls by transtemporal and transoccipital insonation. Results showed an efficient homogeneous distribution of ultrasound intensity along the course of the middle cerebral artery main stem, indicating potential for insonation of this artery, and also suggesting that ultrasound exposure may be possible for basilar artery thrombosis.

Most studies examining enhanced fibrinolysis with ultrasound have focused on the potential use of external application, but miniaturized transducers have also been attached to catheters for endovascular use. This offers the potential to apply localized ultrasound at the site of thrombosis, while limiting insonation of normal tissue. Tachibana et al. [21] demonstrated enhanced clot lysis in vitro using a $2 \times 1 \times 5$-mm transducer operating at 225 kHz attached to a 2-mm–diameter catheter with a wire connecting it to an external power source. A similar enhancement of in vitro thrombolysis was found using a 170-kHz transducer at 0.5 W/cm^2 and 33% duty cycle with urokinase [26]. Shlansky–Goldberg et al. [27] also observed acceleration with a 64-kHz catheter-mounted transducer with a whole-blood clot in vitro using urokinase. Results with catheter-mounted transducers are qualitatively similar to those with larger transducers and offer the prospect of insonifying a much smaller area. They present technical challenges in fabricating high performance miniaturized transducers with satisfactory connection to an external power source and with appropriate cooling.

Taken together, the evidence is clear that ultrasound can accelerate thrombolysis in vitro with clots prepared from purified fibrin, plasma, or whole blood and with a variety of thrombolytic agents, including t-PA, streptokinase, and urokinase. The effect is large and intensity-dependent, and there is greater acceleration at lower that at higher frequencies. At lower intensities, the effects of ultrasound do not result primarily from mechanical disruption, but rather, are due to acceleration of enzymatic processes. The observed effect may be large with acceleration up to sevenfold in comparison with no ultrasound at 40 kHz. Ultrasound can also be used to mechanically fragment a clot using a wire placed in direct contact with the clot and activated at high power or by exposure to a sufficiently intense ultrasound field generated by a transducer.

III. MECHANISM OF EFFECT

Ultrasound can accelerate thrombolysis through multiple effects, and these differ for approaches that result in mechanical fragmentation as compared with those enhancing enzymatic fibrinolysis. Wires vibrating at ultrasonic frequencies and high intensity can mechanically fragment a clot through direct contact, but indirect effects through cavitation also play a role. In a study of the mechanism of ultrasound angioplasty, Rosenshein et al. [28] examined the effects of 20-kHz ultrasound at intensities up to $100 \, W/cm^2$. The cavitation threshold with this system was over 30 W, ultrasound ablation was evident only above the cavitation threshold, and its rate correlated with a level of ultrasound power. In hydroxyproline gelatin samples, the zone of ablation could be viewed with a telemicroscopy device, and this confirmed the role of cavitation and mechanical disruption of the gel. The cavitation-related bioeffect of ultrasound on blood elements was reported by Everbach et al. [29]. Human platelets with and without a microbubble echocontrast agent were exposed in vitro to $730 \, W/cm^2$ (I_{SSPA}) ultrasound pulses of duration 40–160 μs at 1 MHz and 20-Hz pulse repetition frequency. Inertial cavitation occurring within the samples accounted for up to 75% of the variation in the destruction of platelets and 83.5% of the release of bound radiolabel. When the echocontrast agent was absent, negligible cavitation occurred and the amount of platelet destruction was indistinguishable from sham (no-ultrasound) exposure. Therefore, microbubble echocontrast agents may interact with ultrasound to cause platelet lysis through the mechanism of inertial cavitation.

The mechanisms by which ultrasound enhances enzymatic thrombolysis are complex and multiple and relate primarily to enzyme transport, a rate-limiting step in therapeutic thrombolysis [30]. Mathematical modeling predicts and in vitro experiments demonstrate that effective delivery of thrombolytic agents into clots is the most important determinant of fibrinolytic rate [31]. Transport can occur by diffusion, but this is slow and limited by the need for a high concentration gradient. It can also occur by convection, which is more efficient but depends on the intrinsic resistance of the thrombus and the effective pressure gradient. Francis et al. [32] examined the effect of insonification on the distribution of plasminogen activator between clot and surrounding fluid in vitro. Plasma clots were overlaid with plasma containing ^{125}I-radiolabeled t-PA and then incubated in the presence of 1 MHz ultrasound at $4 \, W/cm^2$ or in the absence of ultrasound. The uptake of t-PA was significantly faster in the presence of ultrasound as compared with its absence. To determine the effect of ultrasound on the spatial distribution of enzyme, plasma clots were overlaid with plasma containing radiolabeled t-PA, incubated in the presence or absence of ultrasound, and then snap-frozen. The radioactivity in serial cryotome sections demonstrated that ultrasound altered the t-PA distribution, resulting in significantly deeper penetration of the enzyme into clots. Sakharov et al. [33] also showed ultrasound enhancement of fibrinolysis in vitro using several activators and concluded that it increased transport of plasminogen and activator to the clot surface. These results showed that exposure to ultrasound in the absence of fluid permeation through clots increases uptake and results in deeper penetration of enzyme, effects that would accelerate clot dissolution.

Since transport of fibrinolytic enzymes into clots by permeation is also an important determinant of the rate of fibrinolysis, Siddiqi et al. [34] examined the effect of ultrasound on fluid permeation through fibrin gels in vitro (Fig. 2). Exposure to 1-MHz ultrasound at $2 \, W/cm^2$ resulted in a significant increase in flow through the gel. The ultrasound-induced flow increase was intensity-dependent and reversible when ultrasound was discontinued. Degassing the fluid by autoclaving significantly reduced the ultrasound-induced increase in flow. These results indicated that exposure of fibrin gels to ultrasound increases pressure-mediated permeation and that the effect may be related to cavitation-induced changes in fibrin gel structure. The importance of cavitation is also supported by evidence demonstrating a reduction in ultrasound enhancement of fibrinolysis at high pressure that correlated with elimination of cavitation, as measured independently [35].

The state of fibrin polymerization is an important determinant of flow resistance in clots. Braaten et al. [36] examined the effects of ultrasound on the ultrastructure of fibrin gels using

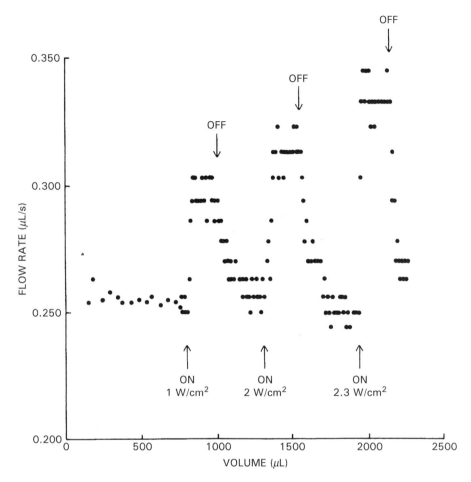

Figure 2 Effect of different ultrasound intensities on flow rate: Fibrin gels with a constant perfusion pressure were exposed to ultrasound at 1 W/cm^2 and 2.3 W/cm^2 using a duty cycle of 5 ms on, 5 ms off. In each case ultrasound was switched on as indicated and then switched off following achievement of a new steady-state flow rate (From Ref. 34.)

scanning electron microscopy. Gels exposed to ultrasound exhibited an increase in the number of fibrin fibers per unit volume accompanied by a concomitant decrease in mean fiber diameter. These effects were reversible, and there was no significant change in the structure of fibrin after ultrasound was discontinued. These results indicate that ultrasound exposure caused reversible disaggregation of fibrin fibers into smaller fibers, an effect that would alter flow resistance and create additional binding sites for fibrinolytic components, thereby improving fibrinolytic efficiency.

The binding of plasminogen activator and plasminogen to fibrin is important in the initiation of fibrinolysis. Because ultrasound caused an alteration in fibrin structure, Siddiqi et al. [37] characterized the effects of ultrasound on binding of t-PA to fibrin. Interaction of t-PA with fibrin involves two classes of binding sites, and ultrasound had little effect on the binding affinity of t-PA, but maximum binding was significantly increased. Ultrasound also affected the kinetics of t-PA binding to fibrin, significantly accelerating the rate of dissociation by approximately 70%. The findings indicated that ultrasound exposure may accelerate fibrinolysis by altering binding affinity, increasing maximum binding, and increasing access of t-PA to fibrin-binding sites.

Heating is another mechanism by which ultrasound can accelerate thrombolysis, as enzymatic reactions are temperature-dependent. Blinc et al. [13] examined the temperature-dependence of plasma clot lysis in vitro using t-PA at temperatures from 24 to 55°C. Up to 50°C there was a 1.1% increase in lysis per hour for every 1°C increase in temperature. In experiments using plasma clots in vitro, temperature increases caused by ultrasound were directly dependent on intensity, and were greater at higher frequencies. At 1 MHz, temperature increases of between 1° and 2° were observed at intensities shown to accelerate fibrinolysis. The temperature increments were sufficient to explain only a small portion of the acceleration of fibrinolysis.

IV. RESULTS IN ANIMAL MODELS

The favorable in vitro results demonstrating that ultrasound can mechanically disrupt clot formation or significantly accelerate fibrinolysis led to studies in several animal models (Table 1). The capacity of high-intensity ultrasound delivered by a catheter to disrupt arterial or venous thrombus with no administration of plasminogen activator was examined in several studies. In an early study, Trübestein et al. [38] formed thrombi in the iliac or femoral arteries or veins of dogs. They were then exposed to 26.5-kHz high-intensity ultrasound delivered through a catheter waveguide for intervals of 60 s on and 15 s off. Disrupted clot was aspirated using a suction device. Clots were recanalized within 2.5–5 min in both arteries and veins, and only minor endothelial cell damage was observed histologically, which resolved within 15 days. With use of a somewhat different approach, Rosenschein et al. [2] created femoral artery thrombi in dogs by damaging the endothelium with a catheter combined with external crush injury and temporary ligation. An ultrasound wire was then advanced to the site of thrombosis through a vascular sheath, and 20-kHz ultrasound was delivered at a power of 20 ± 10 W. As determined angiographically, ultrasound reduced obstruction from $93 \pm 11\%$ to $18 \pm 7\%$, recanalization occurred in all seven dogs tested. There was minimal evidence of vessel wall injury and no vessel perforation. In a canine coronary thrombosis model, Steffen et al. [4] achieved recanalization in 13 of 15 occluded coronary arteries in an average of 7 min using a 19.5-kHz ultrasound transducer. Although there was no vessel perforation or dissection, histological examination revealed focal mural thrombus remaining, and there was also evidence of vessel wall injury including transmural necrosis with hemorrhage in some cases. Ariani et al. [3] also examined effects of an ultrasound wire in a canine femoral artery thrombosis model. Ultrasound was delivered at 20 kHz with a catheter-ensheathed wire using angioscopic guidance to place the wire and probe in direct contact with the thrombus. Thrombi were successfully disrupted in 17 of 17 vessels with no evidence of distal embolization by angiography. The duration of treatment was 4 min or less, and power outputs of 15–20 W were used. There was little histological evidence of vessel damage with only nonocclusive mural thrombus remaining at the end of treatment. The effect of transcutaneous ultrasonic irradiation on the prevention of acute reocclusion was studied in dog femoral arteries by Yoshizawa et al. [39]. Continuous ultrasound of 200 kHz was delivered for 2 h, and patency was confirmed in seven of eight cases after ultrasound treatment.

An important part of the physical mechanism of ultrasound effect is cavitation, and this can be enhanced by increasing cavitation nuclei. This may be responsible for recent evidence indicating that stabilized microbubble echo contrast agents may be used to augment the effects of ultrasound on clot dissolution. Nishioka et al. [40] were able to reperfuse thrombosed rabbit femoral arteries with transcutaneous administration of 20-kHz ultrasound at 1.5 W/cm^2 in combination with the echo contrast agent, dodecafluoropentane, without administration of

Table 1 Thrombolysis with Ultrasound in Animal Models

Model	Thrombolytic agent	Ultrasound	Results	Ref.
Canine ileofemoral artery and vein (n = 20)	None	26.5 kHz catheter	Recanalization within 2.5–5 min	Trübestein, 1976 [38]
Rat femoral artery (n = 40)	Urokinase	48-kHz catheter	Reduced limb loss with US	Tachibana, 1985 [43]
Canine femoral artery (n = 7)	None	20-kHz; 20 ± 10-W catheter	Recanalization in 7/7	Rosenschein, 1990 [2]
Canine femoral artery (n = 17)	None	20-kHz; 15–20-W catheter	17/17 thrombi disrupted within 4 min	Ariani, 1991 [3]
Canine femoral artery (n = 10)	t-PA	200-kHz transcutaneous	Recanalizatioin in 7/8/10	Yoshizawa, 1992 [39]
Canine femoral artery (n = 10)	t-PA	200-kHz transcutaneous	Significant reduction in time to reflow with US plus t-PA	Hamano, 1992 [44]
Rabbit jugular vein (n = 6)	t-PA	1-MHz; 1.75-W/cm^2 catheter	US-enhanced t-PA-induced clot lysis	Lauer, 1992 [14]
Rabbit femoral artery (n = 27)	t-PA	1-MHz; 6.3-W/cm^2 catheter	Initial reflow faster with t-PA plus US, but also greater reduction	Kornowski, 1994 [45]
Rabbit small vessel (n = 18)	Streptokinase	1-MHz; 1-W/cm^2; 50% duty cycle	Accelerated clot lysis with SK plus US	Kashyap, 1994 [50]
Canine coronary artery (n = 18)	None	19.5-kHz; 2–5-W; 50% duty cycle	Recanalization of 15/18 arteries in mean of 7 min	Steffen, 1994 [4]
Rabbit ileofemoral artery (n = 19)	None	20-kHz; 1.5 W/cm^2; with DDFP; transcutaneous	82% recanalized	Nishioka 1997 [40]
Rabbit femoral artery (n = 32)	Streptokinase	1 MHz; 2 W/cm^2	Thrombolysis in 53% with US and 17% without	Riggs 1997 [47]

(continued)

Table 1 (*continued*)

Model	Thrombolytic agent	Ultrasound	Results	Ref.
Rabbit ileofemoral artery ($n = 15$)	Streptokinase	37 kHz; 160 W	Recanalization in 15/15	Luo 1997 [41]
Rabbit ileofemoral artery ($n = 10$)	None	37 kHz; 160 W ± PESDA pulse	All ileofemoral arteries treated with PESDA + US were recanalized	Birnbaum 1998 [42]
Rabbit retinal vein ($n = 27$)	Streptokinase	1 MHz; 1 W/cm^2; 10% duty cycle	64% of veins were recanalized after US + SK vs. 21% with SK alone	Larsson 1998 [49]
Canine coronary artery ($n = 24$)	t-PA	27 MHz; 0.9 W/cm^2	Transthoracic application of US augmented efficacy of t-PA-mediated thrombolysis	Siegel 2000 [51]
Rabbit femoral artery ($n = 29$)	Streptokinase	40 kHz; 0.75 W/cm^2	Increased thrombolysis with SK + US. Improvement of capillary perfusion and reversed muscle acidosis. Vasodilation of capillaries	Suchkova 2000 [52]

[a]All ultrasound is continuous wave unless indicated.

plasminogen activator. The high-intensity ultrasound, however, resulted in skin necrosis and severe histological changes owing to heating, but these could be minimized by using an appropriate cooling device [41]. The potential of microbubble echo contrast agents to enhance the effects of ultrasound in animal models is consistent with similar findings in vitro [26]. The study by Birnbaum et al. [42] evaluated a transcutaneous 37-kHz–pulsed ultrasound at a power range of 160 W with administration of PESDA microbubbles. All ten ileofemoral arteries treated with PESDA plus ultrasound were recanalized by angiography after ultrasound treatment.

Successful results have also been reported using ultrasound to accelerate enzymatic fibrinolysis in animal models. Tachibana et al. [43] injected an irritant into rat femoral arteries to produce distal thrombosis and ischemia. Treatment with intravenous urokinase alone was compared with urokinase in combination with 48-kHz ultrasound delivered with the leg in a waterbath. There was reduced limb loss with the combination compared with ultrasound alone or urokinase alone. In another report, the combination of t-PA and 200-kHz ultrasound delivered transcutaneously was used in a canine femoral artery thrombosis model [44]. The time to reflow was reduced from 58 ± 32 min with urokinase alone to 20 ± 20 min with the combination of urokinase and ultrasound. Kornowski et al. [45] used a rabbit femoral artery thrombosis model to compare treatment with t-PA alone or in combination with ultrasound at 1 MHz and 6.3 W/cm^2. Initial reflow occurred faster in animals treated with the combination of t-PA and ultrasound, but there was also greater reocclusion, so that arterial patency was overall lower with ultrasound than in its absence. These investigators observed a beneficial effect of aspirin in combination with ultrasound, suggesting that the higher rate of reocclusion with ultrasound was due to platelet activation, which had been observed earlier in in vitro studies [46].

Riggs et al. [47] also used a rabbit femoral artery thrombosis model, but treated with streptokinase in the presence or absence of ultrasound at 1 MHz and 2 W/cm^2. Thrombolysis occurred in 53% of animals receiving ultrasound as compared with 17% without. There was a maximum temperature increase of 4°C, and the endothelium showed only minimal histological changes. There was, however, evidence of increased platelet accumulation around the periphery of thrombi in ultrasound-treated animals, again consistent with the capacity of ultrasound to activate platelets. Luo et al. [48] used ultrasound at 26 kHz and a higher intensity of 18 W/cm^2 in a rabbit ileofemoral artery thrombosis model with streptokinase treatment. Recanalization occurred in 10 of 17 animals treated with both ultrasound and streptokinase, compared with only 1 of 12 treated with streptokinase and with 1 of 14 treated with ultrasound alone. Heating was a major problem in this experience with the occurrence of skin burns and tissue necrosis.

The effect of ultrasound on venous thrombolysis was investigated by Lauer et al. [14] in a rabbit model using ^{125}I-fibrin-labeled thrombi and external counting to monitor thrombolysis. Ultrasound was delivered at 1 MHz and 1.75 W/cm^2 through the skin in a waterbath with 2 s on and 2 s off. Animals that received the combination of t-PA and ultrasound showed a trend toward faster lysis that was not statistically significant. There was no histological evidence of vessel wall damage. Larsson et al. [49] used pulsed ultrasound of 1 MHz and 10% duty cycle in a rabbit retinal vein occlusion with low-dose streptokinase treatment. Adding pulsed low-energy ultrasound allowed use of a lower dose of streptokinase, while maintaining a good thrombolytic effect. With a different approach, Kashyap et al. [50] examined acceleration of fibrinolysis using ultrasound in a rabbit ear model of small-vessel injury. Full-thickness puncture wounds were made in rabbit ears, and the rabbits were rested for 2–3 h after cessation of bleeding for maturation of hemostatic plugs. Saline and streptokinase were then infused intravenously, and ultrasound was applied to some lesions at 1 MHz with a 50% duty cycle at 1 W/cm^2. Ear lesions in rabbits treated with saline alone showed no bleeding whether or not they were exposed to ultrasound. Streptokinase alone induced bleeding after 20 ± 6 min, whereas application of ultrasound significantly reduced the time to bleeding in streptokinase-treated rabbits to

8 ± 4 min (p < 0.002). Histological examination revealed that the application of ultrasound resulted in minor inflammatory changes. The findings indicated that the percutaneous application of ultrasound significantly accelerated streptokinase-induced fibrinolysis of hemostatic plugs in small vessels.

Siegel et al. [51] examined the effect of low-frequency ultrasound on coronary thrombolysis in a canine model. Thrombotic occlusion of the left anterior descending coronary artery was induced, and two groups of dogs were treated with either t-PA alone or in combination with 27-kHz ultrasound at $0.9 \, \mathrm{W/cm^2}$, delivered percutaneously through the chest to the artery. At 90 min there was significantly greater coronary flow in dogs receiving the combination of t-PA plus ultrasound than in those treated with t-PA alone.

Another recent study emphasizing the switch to lower-intensity ultrasound was reported by Suchkova et al. [52] using a rabbit femoral artery thrombosis model. Treatment was administered with either ultrasound alone at 40 kHz and $0.75 \, \mathrm{W/cm^2}$, streptokinase alone, or the combination of both ultrasound and streptokinase. Ultrasound or streptokinase alone resulted in minimal thrombolysis, but reperfusion was nearly complete with the combination after 120 min. The maximum temperature increase after 60 min of treatment was $1.6 \pm 1.3°C$ at the femoral artery and $1.1 \pm 0.7°C$ at the femur. A novel finding in these experiments was that ultrasound improved tissue perfusion independently of its effect on thrombolysis. In the absence of femoral artery flow, application of ultrasound caused capillary dilation, improved capillary perfusion, as measured with a laser–Doppler flowmeter, and also reversed muscle acidosis (Fig. 3). These effects were reversible and declined after ultrasound was removed. Histological examination showed that an ultrasound-exposed vessel had a tendency toward endothelial cell vacuolization with some cells lifted from the basement membrane.

In general, the results of animal experiments are consistent in demonstrating the potential of ultrasound for treating either arterial or venous thrombosis. In the absence of plasminogen

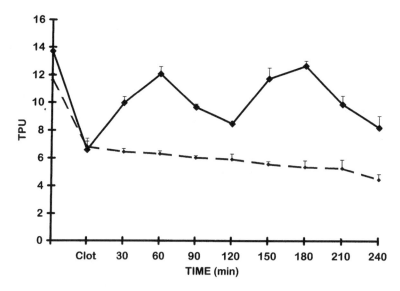

Figure 3 Effects of ultrasound on tissue perfusion: Perfusion was measured with a laser–Doppler probe placed over the gracilis muscle near the site of ligation of the rabbit femoral artery. In 9 control animals (dotted line) perfusion declined. The 9 animals receiving kHz ultrasound at $0.75 \, \mathrm{W/cm^2}$ (solid line) demonstrated increased perfusion until 60 min when the ultrasound was turned off. Ultrasound was applied again between 120 and 180 min and then turned off again. (From Ref. 52.)

activator, high-intensity ultrasound, delivered either through an endovascular catheter directly to the thrombus or externally, can result in mechanical fragmentation and vessel recanalization. Heating of endovascular devices and of insonified tissue is a problem The noninvasive transcutaneous delivery of lower-intensity ultrasound in combination with a plasminogen activator can accelerate thrombolysis with minimal evidence of vessel wall damage. This has been demonstrated in several animal models by independent groups of investigators, and the degree of enhancement appears to be large. Recent evidence indicates that ultrasound may have additional effects on vascular tone, resulting in vasodilation of capillary and improved collateral flow to ischemic tissue. This effect will also need to be considered in planning therapeutic application.

V. CLINICAL STUDIES

Initial clinical experience using catheter-delivered ultrasound has shown promise (Table 2). Siegel et al. [53] used an ultrasound wire, operating at 20 kHz and a power output of 20–35 W/cm^2, in a 7F catheter to treat eight patients with peripheral arterial obstruction. Recanalization occurred within 2 min in three of four patients with complete occlusions, and ultrasound administration reduced the degree of stenosis in others. Ultrasound energy with a frequency of 19.5 kHz, peak tip amplitude of 111 µm, and power output at the transducer at 25 W and 50% duty cycle, resolved vasospasm and induced arterial vasodilation [54]. In a subsequent larger study by the same group [55] percutaneous ultrasound angioplasty was performed on 50 peripheral arterial lesions in 45 patients using an ultrasound ablation system with a 2- or 3-mm tip operating at 19.5 kHz. Recanalization occurred in 30 of 35 totally occluded arteries, and stenosis was reduced in 13 of 15 patients. Arterial dissection occurred in 4 patients, and arterial perforation in an additional 4, but these were without serious clinical consequences. The application of ultrasonic angioplasty to recannalize totally occluded peripheral arteries in seven patients was reported by Rosenschein et al. [56]. A 1.6-mm–diameter flexible wire attached to an ultrasound-generating transducer operating at 20 kHz was advanced to the site of occlusion, and ultrasound was administered at energies between 5 and 35 W. This procedure achieved successful recanalization without perforation in all vessels with angiographic evidence of an average lumen patency of 82.5%. Preliminary experience using an ultrasound angioplasty device was also reported by Goyen et al. [57]. Nine patients with severe leg ischemia and subacute thrombotic arterial occlusions were treated with an ultrasound wire operating at 42 kHz and advanced to the site of occlusion. Successful recanalization was achieved in seven cases.

A number of studies have also investigated the potential of ultrasound to treat coronary artery thrombosis. Siegel et al. [58] performed a feasibility study of coronary ultrasound angioplasty in 19 patients. A 4.6F coronary catheter ultrasound-ablation device with a 1.7-mm–diameter ball tip was used operating at 19.5 kHz and a power of 16–20 W at the transducer in pulsed mode. In patients with unstable or exercise-induced myocardial ischemia, coronary artery stenosis was reduced by ultrasound and further by adjunctive balloon angioplasty. There were no ultrasound-related complications. In another preliminary study, ultrasonic coronary angioplasty was performed during coronary artery bypass grafting in 20 patients [59]. Several catheter systems were used to deliver ultrasound at 19.6 kHz in a pulsed mode (50% duly cycle of 30 ms) using a transducer with 16–20 W of output. Recanalization was achieved in 70% of attempts, but arterial perforation complicated the procedure in 10% of vessels. The three deaths that occurred in the study were thought to be unrelated to the ultrasound angioplasty procedure. Analysis of plaque debris revealed that 50% of the particles were less than 8 µm in diameter and over 95% were less than 25 µm in diameter. In a small study, 15 consecutive patients with

Table 2 Clinical Studies of Ultrasound and Thrombolysis

Location	Ultrasound	Result	Ref.
Peripheral artery ($n = 8$)	20 kHz; 20–35 W/cm^2	Perfusion and reduced arterial stenosis in 3/4	Siegel 1989 [53]
Peripheral artery ($n = 7$)	20 kHz; 5–35 W	Recanalization in 7/7	Rosenschein 1991 [56]
Peripheral artery ($n = 2$)	19.5 kHz; 25 W/cm^2; 50% duty cycle	Recanalization in 30/35 US-induced arterial vasodilation	Siegel 1992 [54]
Periphery artery ($n = 45$)	19.5 kHz; 25 W/cm^2	Stenosis decreased from 94 to 55% after US angioplasty	Siegel 1993 [55]
Periphery artery ($n = 9$)	42 kHz	Recanalization in 7/9	Goyen 2000 [57]
Coronary artery ($n = 19$)	9.5 kHz; 16–20 W; pulsed wave	Recanalization in 11/19	Siegel 1994 [58]
Coronary artery ($n = 20$)	19.6-kHz; 16–20 W; 50% duty cycle	70% of arteries were fully recanalized	Eccleston 1996 [59]
Coronary artery ($n = 14$)	19.5 kHz; 16–20 W; 50% duty cycle	Reperfusion in 13/14	Hamm 1997 [61]
Coronary artery ($n = 15$)	45 kHz; 18 W	US-induced reperfusion in 87%	Rosenschein 1997 [60]
Saphenous vein graft ($n = 20$)	41 kHz; 18 W	Reperfusion in 70%	Rosenschein 1999 [62]

[a]All ultrasound is continuous wave unless indicated.

anterior acute myocardial infarction and TIMI grade 0 or 1 flow in the left anterior descending artery underwent coronary ultrasound thrombolysis [60]. This device used a flexible wire in a 10F angioplasty guide catheter to direct the 1.6-mm tip to the site of thrombosis, and 45-kHz ultrasound at 18 W was delivered. Ultrasound induced successful reperfusion with TIMI grade 3 flow in 87% of the patients who were also treated with antiplatelet agents, anticoagulants, and adjunctive PTCA. There were no complications clearly related to the ultrasound procedure.

In a similar small study, Hamm et al. [61] used a 19.5-kHz–ultrasound wire directed through a 8F guiding catheter at power of 16–20 W using a 50% duty cycle. Intracoronary therapeutic ultrasound improved flow by at least 1 TIMI grade in 13 of 14 occluded arteries after a median of 85 s. All but one patient required adjunctive balloon angioplasty. Minor distal embolization was reported in two patients and non–flow-limiting dissection in five patients. Rosenschein et al. [62] have also reported successful recanalization of occluded saphaneous vein grafts using ultrasound. An ultrasound thrombolysis device with a 1.6-mm tip within a 7F guiding catheter operated at 41 kHz and 18W. Successful recanalization with the device was observed in 70% of patients with residual stenosis of $65 \pm 28\%$. Complications included one patient who had a non-Q–wave myocardial infarction, and distal embolization occurred in one additional patient. Adjunctive PTCA or stenting was required in all patients.

ACKNOWLEDGMENT

This work was supported by a Grant-in-Aid from the American Heart Association, New York State Affiliate.

REFERENCES

1. Hong AS, Chae J–S, Dublin SB, et al. Ultrasonic clot disruption: an in vitro study. Am Heart J 1990; 120:418–422.
2. Rosenschein U, Bernstein JJ, DiSegni E, et al. Experimental ultrasonic angioplasty: disruption of atherosclerotic plaque and thrombi in vitro and arterial recanalization in vivo. J Am Coll Cardiol 1990; 15:711–717.
3. Ariani M, Fishbein MC, Chae JS, et al. Dissolution of peripheral arterial thrombi by ultrasound. Circulation 1991; 84:1680–1688.
4. Steffen W, Fishbein MC, Luo H, et al. High intensity, low frequency catheter-delivered ultrasound dissolution of occlusive coronary artery thrombi: an in vitro and in vivo study. J Am Coll Cardiol 1994; 24:1571–1579.
5. Siegel RJ, Fishbein MC, Forrester J, et al. Ultrasonic plaque ablation. A new method for recanalization of partially or totally occluded arteries. Circulation 1988; 78:1443–1448.
6. Ernst A, Schenk EA, Cracewski SM, et al. Ability of high-intensity ultrasound to ablate human atherosclerotic plaques and minimize debris size. Am J Cardiol 1991; 68:242–246.
7. Dick A, Neuerburg J, Schmitz–Rode T, et al. Declotting of embolized temporary vena cava filter by ultrasound and the angiojet: comparative experimental in vitro studies. Invest Radiol 1998; 33:91–97.
8. Nishioka T, Luo H, Fishbein MC, et al. Dissolution of thrombotic arterial occlusion by high intensity, low frequency ultrasound and dodecafluoropentane emulsion: an in vitro and in vivo study. J Am Coll Cardiol 1997; 30:561–568.
9. Porter TR, LeVeen RF, Fox R, et al. Thrombolytic enhancement with perfluorocarbon-exposed sonicated dextrose albumin microbubbles. Am Heart J 1996; 132:964–968.
10. Rosenschein U, Yakubov SJ, Guberinich D, et al. Shock-wave thrombus ablation, a new method for noninvasive mechanical thrombolysis. Am J Cardiol 1992; 70:1358–1361.

11. Rosenschein U, Furman V, Kerner E, et al. Ultrasound imaging—guided noninvascular ultrasound tbrombolysis: preclinical results. Circulation 2000; 102:238–245.

12. Francis CW, Onundarson PT, Carstensen EL, et al. Characterization of ultrasound-potentiated fibrinolysis in vitro. J Clin Invest 1992; 90:2063–2068.

13. Blinc A, Francis CW, Trudnowski JL, Carstensen EL. Characterization of ultrasound-potentiated fibrinolysis in vitro. Blood 1993; 81:2636–2643.

14. Lauer CG, Burge R, Tang DB, et al. Effect of ultrasound on tissue-type plasminogen activator-induced thrombolysis. Circulation 1992; 86:1257–1264.

15. Luo H, Steffen W, Cercek B, et al. Enhancement of thrombolysis by external ultrasound. Am Heart J 1993; 125:1564–1569.

16. Harpaz D, Chen X, Francis CW, et al. Ultrasound enhancement of thrombolysis and reperfusion in vitro. J Am Coll Cardiol 1993; 21:1507–1511.

17. Harpaz D, Chen X, Francis CW, Meitzer RS. Ultrasound accelerates urokinase-induced thrombolysis and reperfusion. Am Heart J 1994; 127:1211–1219.

18. Olsson SB, Johnsson B, Hilsson A–M, Rouer A. Enhancement of thrombolysis by ultrasound. Ultrasound Med Biol 1994; 20:375–382.

19. Nilsson AM, Odselius R, Roijer A, Olsson SB. Pro- and antifibrinolytic effects of ultrasound on streptokinase-induced thrombolysis. Ultrasound Med Biol 1995; 21:833–840.

20. Tachibana S, Koga E. Ultrasonic vibration for boosting fibrinolytic effect of urokinase. Blood Vessel 1981; 12:450–453.

21. Tachibana K. Enhancement of fibrinolysis with ultrasound energy. J Vasc Intervent Radiol 1992; 3:299–303.

22. Seghal CM, Leveen RF, Shiansky–Goldberg RD. Ultrasound-assisted thrombolysis. Invest Radiol 1993; 28:939–943.

23. Suckhova V, Siddiqi FN. Carstensen EL, et al. Enhancement of fibrinolysis with 40 kHz ultrasound. Circulation 1998; 98:1030–1035.

24. Akiyama M, Ishibashi T, Amada T, Furuhata H. Low-frequency ultrasound penetrates the cranium and enhances thrombolysis in vitro. Neurosurgery 1998; 43:828–833.

25. Behrens S, Daffertshofer M, Spiegel D, Hennerici M. Low-frequency, low-intensity ultrasound accelerates thrombolysis through the skull. Ultrasound Med Biol 1999; 25:269–273.

26. Tachibana K, Tachibana S. Albumin microbubble echo-contrast material as an enhancer for ultrasound accelerated thrombolysis. Circulation 1995; 92:1148–1150.

27. Shlansky–Goldberg RD, Cines DB, Sehgal CM. Catheter-derived ultrasound potentiates in vitro thrombolysis. J Vasc Intervent Radiol 1996; 7:313–320.

28. Rosenschein U, Frimerman A, Laniado S, Miller HI. Study of the mechanism of ultrasound angioplasty from human thrombi and bovine aorta. Am J Cardiol 1994; 74:1263–1266.

29. Everbach EC, Makin IRS, Francis CW, Meltzer RS. Effect of acoustic cavitation on platelets in the presence of an echo-contrast agent. Ultrasound Med Biol 1998; 24:129–136.

30. Blinc A, Francis CW. Transport processes in fibrinolysis and fibrinolytic therapy. Thromb Haemost 1996; 76:481–491.

31. Diamond S, Anand S. Inner clot diffusion and permeation during fibrinolysis. Biophys J 1993; 65:2622–2643.

32. Francis CW, Blinc A, Lee S, Cox C. Ultrasound accelerates transport of recombinant tissue plasminogen activator into clots. Ultrasound Med Biol 1995; 21:419–424.

33. Sakharov DV, Barrett–Bergshoeff M, Hekkenberg RT, Rijken DC. Fibrin-specificity of a plasminogen activator affects the efficiency of fibrinolysis and responsiveness to ultrasound: comparison of nine plasminogen activators in vitro. Thromb Haemost 1999; 81:605–612.

34. Siddiqi F, Blinc A, Braaten J, Francis CW. Ultrasound increases flow through fibrin gels. Thromb Haemost 1995; 73:495–498.

35. Everbach EV, Francis CW. Cavitational mechanisms in ultrasound-accelerated thrombolysis. Ultrasound Med Biol 2000; 26:1153–1160.

36. Braaten JV, Goss RA, Francis CW. Ultrasound reversibly disaggregates fibrin fibers. Thromb Haemost 1997; 78:1063–1068.

37. Siddiqi F, Odrljin TM, Fay PJ, et al. Binding of tissue-plasminogen activator to fibrin: effects of ultrasound. Blood 1998; 91:2019–2025.

38. Trübestein G, Engel C, Etzerl F, et al. Thrombolysis by ultrasound. Clin Sci Mol Med 1976; 51:697s–698s.

39. Yoshizawa S. Ultrasonic irradiation method for prevention of acute reocclusion after thrombolysis. Tokyo Jikeikai Med J 1992; 107:265–274.

40. Nishioka T, Luo H, Fishbein MC, et al. Dissolution of thrombotic arterial occlusion by high intensity, low frequency ultrasound and dodecafluoropentane emulsion: an in vitro and in vivo study. J Am Coll Cardiol 1997; 30:561–568.

41. Luo H, Birnbaum Y, Fishbein MC, et al. Enhancement of thrombolysis in vivo without skin and soft tissue damage by transcutaneous ultrasound. Thromb Res 1997; 89:171–177.

42. Birnbaum, Y, Luo H, Nagai T, et al. Noninvasive in vivo clot dissolution without a thrombolytic drug. Recanalization of thrombosed ileofemoral arteries by transcutaneous ultrasound combined with intravenous infusion of microbubbles. Circulation 1998; 97:130–134.

43. Tachibana S. Application of ultrasonic vibration for boosting fibrinolytic effect of urokinase in rats. Blood Vessel 1985; 16:46–49.

44. Hamano K. Thrombolysis enhanced by transcutaneous ultrasonic irradiation. Tokyo Jikeikai Med J 1991; 106:533–542.

45. Kornowski R, Meltzer RS, Chernine A, et al. Does external ultrasound accelerate thrombolysis? Results from a rabbit model. Circulation 1994; 89:339–344.

46. Chater BV, Williams AR. Platelet aggregation induced in vitro by therapeutic ultrasound. Thromb Haemost 1977; 38:640–651.

47. Riggs PN, Francis CW, Bartos SR, Penney DP. Ultrasound enhancement of rabbit femoral artery thrombosis. Cardiovasc Surg 1997; 5:201–207.

48. Luo H, Nishioka T, Fishbein MC, et al. Transcutaneous ultrasound augments lysis of arterial thrombi in vivo. Circulation 1996; 94:775–778.

49. Larsson J, Carlson J, Olsson SB. Ultrasound enhanced thrombolysis in experimental retinal vein occlusion in the rabbit. Br J Ophthalmol 1998; 82:1438–1440.

50. Kashyap A, Blinc A, Marder VJ, et al. Acceleration of fibrinolysis by ultrasound in a rabbit ear model of small vessel injury. Thromb Res 1994; 76:475–485.

51. Siegel RJ, Atar S, Fishbein M, et al. Noninvasive, transthoracic, low-frequency ultrasound augments thrombolysis in a canine model of acute myocardial infarction. Circulation 2000; 101:2026–2029.

52. Suchkova VN, Baggs RB, Francis CW. Effect of 40 kHz ultrasound on acute thrombotic ischemia in a rabbit femoral artery thrombosis model: enhancement of thrombolysis and improvement in capillary muscle perfusion. Circulation 2000; 101:2296–2301.

53. Siegel RJ, Myler RK, Cumberland DC, DonMichael TA. Percutaneous ultrasonic angioplasty: initial clinical experience. Lancet 1989; 2:772.

54. Siegel RJ, Gaines P, Pocter A, et al. Clinical demonstration that catheter-delivered ultrasound energy reverses arterial vasoconstriction. J Am Coll Cardiol 1992; 20:732–735.

55. Siegel RJ, Gaines P, Crew JR, Cumberland DC. Clinical trial of percutaneous peripheral ultrasound angioplasty. J Am Coll Cardiol 1993; 22:480–488.

56. Rosenschein U, Rozenszajn LA, Kraus L, et al. Ultrasonic angioplasty in totally occluded peripheral arteries. Initial clinical, histological, and angiographic results. Circulation 1991; 83:1976–1986.

57. Goyen M, Kroger K, Buss C, Rudofsky G. Intravascular ultrasound angioplasty in peripheral arterial occlusion. Preliminary experience. Acta Radiol 2000; 41:122–124.

58. Siegel RM, Gunn J, Ahsan A, et al. Use of therapeutic ultrasound in percutaneous coronary angioplasty. Experimental in vitro studies and initial clinical experience. Circulation 1994; 89:1587–1592.

59. Eccleston DS, Cumpston GN, Hodge AJ, et al. Ultrasonic coronary angioplasty during coronary artery bypass grafting. Am J Cardiol 1996; 78:1172–1175.

60. Rosenschein U, Roth A, Rassin T, et al. Analysis of coronary ultrasound thrombolysis endpoints in acute myocardial infarction (ACUTE Trial): results of the feasibility phase. Circulation 1997; 95:1411–1416.
61. Hamm CW, Steffen W, Terres W, et al. Intravascular therapeutic ultrasound thrombolysis in acute myocardial infarctions. Am J Cardiol 1997; 80:200–204.
62. Rosenschein U, Gaul G, Erbel R, et al. Percutaneous transluminal therapy of occluded saphenous vein grafts. Can the challenge be met with ultrasound thrombolysis? Circulation 1999; 99:26–29.

Epilogue

The Management of Thrombotic and Cardiovascular Disorders in the 21st Century

Jawed Fareed and Debra A. Hoppensteadt
Loyola University Medical Center, Maywood, Illinois, U.S.A.

Over the past decade, interest in anticoagulant and thrombolytic drugs has grown dramatically as evidenced by a continual increase in the number of drugs introduced for both preclinical and clinical development. This book's second edition provides timely coverage of new therapeutic agents in thrombosis and thrombolysis and includes such topics as new heparins, synthetic heparinomimetic agents, antithrombin agents, anti-Xa agents, biotechnology-derived antithrombotic proteins, antiplatelet drugs, and novel thrombolytic agents. The developments are so rapid that an update on the additional information on these agents warrants inclusion and comments. The outstanding scientific research and development activities in the academic centers and pharmaceutical industry have resulted in a steady flow of new products. Third-party validation of developed products and extensive clinical trials have been carried out globally to validate the claims on the safety and efficacy of the newer drugs. The results of these studies constitute a significant portion of the progress reported at scientific forums. Through their fast-track developmental program and revised policies, the regulatory bodies, such as the European Medicine Evaluation Agency (EMEA), U. S. Food and Drug Administration (U. S. FDA), and other regional agencies, have continually contributed to the timely evaluation and approval of new drugs by providing input at various stages of drug development. Such close interactions have clarified various issues related to drug development and, in fact, have accelerated the approval process of many new drugs such as low-molecular-weight heparins (LMWHs), synthetic heparin pentasaccharide (Arixtra), newer antithrombin agents, and activated protein C (Xigris). Many new antiplatelet drugs and thrombolytic agents have also gained approval for multiple indications. The concept of polytherapy, including combinations of different drugs, has been introduced.

Owing to these rapid developments, several important issues related to current practices in anticoagulant therapy are recognized. These issues include the following:

1. The replacement of unfractionated heparin by LMWH in most indications.
2. The potential replacement of heparins by newly developed antithrombin and anti-Xa agents.

687

3. The feasibility of oral anti-Xa and anti-IIa agents as potential substitutes for oral anticoagulant drugs.
4. The development of synthetic heparinomimetics representing specific actions of heparins and their relative bioequivalence to heparin.
5. The development of recombinant antithrombotic agents, such as the activated protein C (APC), tissue factor pathway inhibitor, recombinant equivalent of serpins and thrombomodulin, with reference to their applications in specific disorders.
6. The development of newer antiplatelet drugs, such as the ADP receptor inhibitors, glycoprotein IIb/IIIa receptors, phosphodiesterase inhibitors, and specific cyclo-oxygenase (COX)-1 and COX-2 inhibitors and their relevance in the management of vascular disorders. The relevance of concomitant aspirin for the therapeutic index of each of these agents also requires additional investigations.
7. The design of newer thrombolytic agents, with specific reference to their endogenous interaction and pharmacodynamic differences, in terms of their relative clinical effects in stroke and myocardial infarction.
8. The recent recognition of the antithrombotic actions of statins, nitric oxide donors, and other nonanticoagulant drugs, and their effect on overall therapeutic approaches.

Despite several limitations, heparin is still the most widely used anticoagulant in the United States. Several oral formulations of heparin have been developed and tested in clinical trials. Although effective, the oral formulations of heparin failed to exhibit comparable efficacy to LMWHs in the management of deep venous thrombosis (DVT). In addition, several other chemically modified forms of heparin did not exhibit the expected pharmacological effects in either the preclinical or clinical settings. The LMWHs represent an optimal approach of using heparin components. It may be that the oral formulations exhibit efficacy in other indications.

Although heparin remains the sole anticoagulant used for surgical cardiovascular procedures, the continual expansion of the newer applications of LMWHs has added a new dimension to the overall management of thrombotic and cardiovascular disorders. Evidently, the LMWHs have achieved gold standard status in the management of thromboembolic disorders, and they now challenge other treatments, such as oral anticoagulants, for various indications. Several recent clinical trials have provided supportive data for the polytherapeutic use of LMWHs in the management of acute coronary syndromes, thrombotic stroke, and malignancy associated thrombotic events. LMWHs have also shown efficacy as surgical and interventional anti-coagulants. Unlike heparin, these drugs exhibit a better therapeutic index in these indications. LMWHs have also been evaluated recently in atrial fibrillation and cardiac transplantation. These drugs represent a refined use of heparins. LMWHs have multiple sites of action, which are limited not only to the inhibition of coagulation enzymes, but also profound actions on endothelial and blood cells. This observation has led to the development of the nonanticoagulant forms of LMWHs. Antithrombin agents such as hirudin and hirulog also have been compared with LMWHs for postsurgical prophylaxis of thromboembolism. Initial reports indicate favorable results with the use of recombinant hirudin for treatment of acute coronary syndromes; however, safety issues, such as bleeding, remain a concern. The understanding of the mechanisms of antithrombotic actions and the relevance of structural components of LMWHs have led to the development of synthetic analogues of heparin fragments. One remarkable approach, based on the elucidation of heparin's structure, has led to the synthesis of oligosaccharides with high affinity for antithrombin III (AT III). A synthetic pentasaccharide has undergone extensive clinical trials for both venous thromboembolic and coronary indications.

Although the development of the synthetic pentasaccharides represents a major advance in producing heparin-like drugs by using synthetic organic methods, this agent produces only a single pharmacological action of heparin. Furthermore, the pharmacological actions of these oligosaccharides are dependent on endogenous antithrombin. The U. S. FDA and EMEA have recently approved the use of synthetic heparin pentasaccharide, Arixtra, for the management of postorthopedic surgical thrombosis; however, bleeding risk was unexpectedly higher with this drug, and its use is not recommended in underweight patients. Pentasaccharide is likely to be equivalent to other modalities in the management of DVT prophylaxis; however, its use in other indications for which LMWHs are approved may not provide equivalence or superiority. Several additional clinical trials are being carried out with pentasaccharide in multiple indications, including treatment of thrombosis. Besides the lack of a clear clinical response, bleeding issues, lack of an antidote, drug interactions, product accumulation, and thrombocytopenia are some of the issues that will require clarifications. The current clinical trials may provide some of the answers on these issues.

There is much discussion of how LMWHs and related drugs mediate their effects. In addition to potentiation of AT III, several other mechanisms have been identified, including the release of tissue pathway inhibitor (TFPI), vascular effects, profibrinolytic effects, platelet selectin modulation, and growth factor modulation. Recently, published data suggest that LMWHs may also regulate thrombin-activatable fibrinolytic inhibitor (TAFI). Clinical trials in Europe have shown that subcutaneous LMWH, given once or twice daily, is at least as safe and effective as continuous intravenous heparin in the prevention of recurrent venous thrombo-embolism and is associated with reduced bleeding and lower mortality rates. In several recent studies, home administration of LMWH was as safe and effective as hospital administration of intravenous heparin in patients with proximal deep vein thrombosis. Initial evidence clearly suggests the LMWH may be a useful alternative to heparin in patients with pulmonary embolism. LMWHs also may be useful alternatives to heparin for arterial indications, such as treatment of unstable angina and stroke and the maintenance of peripheral arterial grafts. Recognizing the usefulness of LMWHs, the pharmaceutical industry has focused its attention on their use in the management of ischemic and thrombotic stroke. The success of early clinical trials also suggests that LMWH may be useful in the management of primary and secondary ischemic or thrombotic stroke. Although several clinical trials of the LMWHs did not show any improvement for the outcome in stroke, these drugs did show a clear reduction in the incidence of thrombotic complications in stroke patients. Thus, in the near future, the use of LMWH for prevention of thrombotic or ischemic stroke will be an important goal. LMWHs have also shown efficacy in the vascular dementia of the Alzheimer's type (SDAT). Thus, these drugs may become useful in neurological disorders. Their use as antithrombotic agents in the pregnant patient who requires long-term anticoagulation is, however, currently contraindicated owing to unexpected mortality.

Although LMWHs are proving to be as effective as, or safer than, heparin for various indications, it is important to realize that the differences in the manufacturing of various LMWHs lead to differences in the pharmacological profile. Although these differences have not been clinically validated, each of the LMWHs is expected to exhibit its own therapeutic index in a given clinical setting. Thus, the interchanging of LMWHs based on equivalent gravimetric or biological potency of standardized dosages may not be feasible. Optimized dosages of various LMWHs have been established for prophylaxis and treatment of DVT. Thus, each agent is given at a specified dosage. The optimized dosage of different LMWHs also differs for the management of acute coronary syndromes. The most notable differences are observed at higher dosages. When these agents are given intravenously for interventional cardiovascular procedures, each of the LMWHs produces a different anticoagulant response, regardless of the dosage equivalence at the gravimetric- or bioassay-adjusted potency. Therefore, the U. S. FDA, WHO, and professional organizations consider each drug distinct.

Because of the newer indications and length of therapy, some additional issues related to the optimal use of LMWHs remain to be addressed. Examples include monitoring, control of bleeding, and drug interactions. In addition, the use of high-dose subcutaneous LMWHs may require pharmacological antagonism. Several clinical trials have been designed to obtain information related to these issues. The differential clinical efficacy of various LMWHs was evident in the trials carried out with dalteparin (FRISC and FRIC), enoxaparin (ESSENCE), and nadroparin (FRAXIS).

The LMWHs have also shown remarkable clinical efficacy in the management of cancer-associated thrombosis. In addition, some of these clincial trials have shown that these drugs reduce the mortality in cancer patients. Thus, besides the anticoagulant effects, there may be additional actions of these agents that warrant further investigation.

Economic analyses of the treatment cost in various clinical settings show that although the cost of LMWH is marginally higher than the cost of heparin (40–150 dollars), the expected reduction in costs for all treatment-related clinical events is much higher for LMWHs (350–2700 dollars) than for heparin. Thus, LMWHs are an attractive alternative in an era of managed care health reform. Individual economic analysis for specific indications may provide additional information about reduced costs with the use of LMWHs for long-term outpatient treatment of such syndromes as unstable angina and ischemic cerebral events.

Additional depolymerization of LMWHs has resulted in the development of ultralow LMWHs. Several ultralow LMWHs have recently become available. Bemiparin represents such a product that is efficacious in the management of DVT in Europe. Several other agents are being clinically tested in some indications as vascular dementia, inflammatory bowel disease, and acute coronary syndromes.

Understanding the coagulation process has led to the identification of thrombin as a key enzyme in the thrombogenic processes. Several direct thrombin inhibitors have been developed over the past few years by different methods. Argatroban, hirulog, and hirudin have now become available for use. The recognition of heparin-induced thrombocytopenia (HIT) as the most catastrophic adverse effect of heparin, has led to the use of alternate anticoagulants. The antithrombin agents are most useful in this indication and have been specifically developed for this indication. Hirudin, the leech-derived protein, has been compared with heparin for various indications, including treatment and prophylaxis of venous and arterial thrombotic disorders. The use of hirudin has been reported to be associated with increased risk of bleeding, indicating that better monitoring and dose-adjustment protocols are needed, as well as antidotes. Clinical trials comparing hirudin and heparin as adjuncts in thrombolytic therapy for acute myocardial infarction (TIMI 9B) and acute coronary syndromes (GUSTO IIb) have now shown hirudin to be marginally (if at all) superior to heparin. Recently, several reports comparing the effects of heparin and hirudin have become available. A study comparing heparin and recombinant hirudin for the prophylaxis of DVT provided impressive data in favor of hirudin. In a second study, LMWHs was also compared with hirudin for postsurgical prophylaxis of DVT. The results favored hirudin.

Hirulog represents a designer antithrombin drug that combines the features of hirudin and other anticoagulant peptides. It is a reversible antithrombin agent and offers several advantages over hirudin. The FDA has approved this agent for anticoagulation during PTCA; hirulog is undergoing clinical trials for cardiovascular bypass surgery. Furthermore, antithrombin agents, such as argatroban and hirulog, may be useful in off-pump bypass surgery.

Argatroban, a small peptidomimetic thrombin inhibitor, is also approved by the U. S. FDA as an alternative anticoagulant for patients with HIT. It has been used successfully in Japan for over a decade in the treatment of thrombotic disorders. Several clinical trials in both Europe and the United States have been designed to investigate its use as an alternative to heparin in heparin-compromised patients and as a prophylactic agent to reduce late restenosis after PTCA and coronary directional atherectomy (CDA). As the half-life of argatroban is rather short, it has been administered by infusion protocols. For therapeutic anticoagulation, a level of 1–2 µg/mL is indicated, whereas for interventional cardiology procedures a level of 3–7 µg/mL is necessary. Argatroban also exhibits additional actions on blood vessels and may exert its clinical effects by multiple measures.

Owing to their weaker anticoagulant effects in global clotting tests, direct factor Xa inhibitors were not considered to be desirable anticoagulant and antithrombotic agents for developmental purposes. Given the favorable clinical results with pentasaccharide, however, strong interest in synthetic antifactor Xa drugs has reemerged. These agents may be useful in the prophylaxis of both arterial and venous thrombotic disorders and may offer a greater margin of safety than existing drugs. Additional advantages of direct thrombin and factor Xa inhibitors over heparin include subcutaneous and oral bioavailability. Although their biological half-life is usually less than 30 min, coupling them with larger agents, such as dextran or albumin, can prolong their half-life without affecting their pharmacological actions. Questions about monitoring and antagonism will have to be answered before thrombin and factor Xa inhibitors can be widely explored in clinical settings. Depending on their specificity for thrombin or factor Xa, they may be used as adjuncts with other classes of drugs, such as thrombolytic agents, for treatment of acute myocardial infarction. Low-molecular-weight thrombin and factor Xa inhibitors also may be used for localized delivery, stenting, and transdermal delivery.

Several anti-Xa drugs are now being developed for various indications. A major interest in the area is to develop oral anti-Xa drugs that can be used for the long-term management of both arterial and venous thrombosis. Owing to their better bioavailability, thrombin and factor Xa inhibitors combined may be more useful than the single agents. Optimal combinations for specific indications may be considered. As in the clinical development of LMWHs, thrombin and factor Xa inhibitors should be compared with heparin in terms of safety, efficacy, and cost.

In the search for antiplatelet agents to be used as antithrombotic drugs, it was recognized over 20 years ago that the platelet glycoprotein IIb/IIIa (GPIIb/IIIa) plays a key role in the final common pathway for platelet aggregation. Several reports that support the efficacy of impairing this pathway in arterial disorders have recently become available. In the EPILOG study, the combined effects of abciximab and heparin resulted in inhibition of restenosis. Many of the GPIIa/IIIb inhibitors, including abciximab, also inhibit the vitronectin receptor ($\alpha_v\beta_3$ integrin), which is implicated in endothelial and smooth-muscle cell migration. Thus, these agents exhibit multiple effects in addition to their antiplatelet functions. Another application of GPIIb/IIIa inhibitors is as alternative agents to aspirin in the management of unstable angina, non–Q-wave myocardial infarction, and ischemic or thrombotic stroke. The mechanism of the antiplatelet action of synthetic GPIIb/IIIa inhibitors and antibodies may be the same; however, major differences have been noted in their safety and efficacy. An emerging problem is therapeutic monitoring, which is being addressed with point-of-care systems. Thus, major clinical breakthroughs are expected with the use of these inhibitors in the management of cerebrovascular and cardiovascular disorders.

The introduction of novel antiplatelet drugs has added a new dimension to the management of arterial thrombosis, in particular thrombotic stroke. The availability of specific antagonists of the adenosine diphosphate (ADP) receptor (the thienopyridines, e.g., clopidogrel) have provided a new approach for several cardiovascular and cerebrovascular indications. Clopidogrel underwent extensive clinical trials to test its therapeutic efficacy in combined cardiovascular and cerebrovascular endpoints. The comparative results reported in several recent clinical trials have favored clopidogrel. However, in most of these studies, concomitant aspirin has been used. Clopidogrel has also been very important in preventing in-stent thrombosis.

Newer developments in thrombolytic therapy include recombinant tissue plasminogen activators (t-PAs). Bolus-injectable reteplase is a nonglycosylated plasminogen activator consisting of the Kringle 2 and protease domain of t-PA, and it exhibits a three- to four-fold longer half-life than t-PA. The INJECT trial demonstrated that reteplase is superior to streptokinase for management of acute myocardial infarction. Different variants of wild-type (wt) t-PA, recombinant staphylokinase, and DSPAα_1 and 2 (vampire bat PA) also have undergone clinical trials. Recombinant urokinase and prourokinase are now expressed in mammalian cell lines and are undergoing active clinical development. Molecular engineering of recombinant t-PA extends the biological half-life for bolus dosing, whereas staphylokinase and vampire bat plasminogen activator exhibit fibrin specificity. Additional clinical studies of such agents as tenectaplase, lanoteplase, monteplase, pamiteplase, and several other newly bioengineered agents have now become available. The thrombolytic agents have also found a place in the management of acute thrombotic stroke. The U. S. FDA has approved recombinant t-PA for these indications; however, caution should be exercised in the dosing of such agents. Optimal approaches to improve the safety/efficacy index are currently under investigation. The next few years will witness the emergence of longer-acting thrombolytics to facilitate bolus dosing and improved specificity for fibrin and other receptors to target thrombotic sites. New indications for thrombolytic therapy, such as stroke and microangiopathic syndromes, will be pursued. Thrombolytic agents have also been used with LMWHs and antiplatelet drugs to produce improved outcomes in specific indications.

Restenosis after cardiac interventions remains a major challenge. An optimal therapeutic approach is still unavailable, despite major scientific and financial undertakings. Even with the introduction of newer interventional cardiovascular and peripheral vascular procedures, late restenosis is commonly seen at a rate of 10–60%. Although the claimed efficacy of cardiovascular interventions exceeds that of medical and surgical approaches, restenosis is a major problem, resulting in angina and myocardial infarction. Several newer anticoagulant and antithrombotic drugs have been used to reduce restenosis. However, these approaches have met with limited success. Recent results with GPIIb/IIIa-targeting antibodies have been encouraging. With a better understanding of the pathophysiology of restenosis, improved drugs can be developed. Anticoagulant drugs, such as LMWHs and PEG hirudin, may prove useful. Mechanical devices such as stents and localized and programmed delivery of drugs may be expected to improve outcomes. Although monotherapy may be useful in the control of abrupt closure and subchronic occlusion, its role in late restenosis may be limited. Combined pharmacological and mechanical approaches, coupled with specialized delivery, have already provided favorable results. In this regard, heparin-coated stents and combination therapy that use clopidogrel have provided excellent results.

The coming years will witness dramatic developments in the management of thrombotic and cardiovascular disorders. Synthetic and recombinant approaches will provide cost-effective and clinically useful drugs. LMWHs and synthetic heparin analogues are expected to have significant effects on the overall management of thrombotic and cardiovascular disorders. Factors such as managed care, regulatory issues, polytherapy, and combined pharmacological and mechanical approaches will redirect the focus in management of venous and arterial thromboembolism, myocardial infarction, and thrombotic stroke. The direct antithrombin agents, such as hirudin and PEG hirudin, will be of great value for surgical anticoagulation and various acute indications. Postsurgical control of thrombotic processes may require a combination therapy and heparin-derived agents such as pentasaccharide and nonheparin glycosaminoglycans such as dermatan sulfate. Biotechnology-derived heparin analogues will also be developed.

Conventional drugs, such as heparin, oral anticoagulants, and aspirin, will remain the gold standards despite their known drawbacks. They require further optimization and can be used for various indications in a cost-effective manner. The newer drugs, however, provide alternatives that in the next few years may lead to improved, cost-compliant treatments. The actions of the nonanticoagulant drugs, such as the cholesterol-lowering agents (statins), specific inhibitors of cyclooxygenase, drugs capable of donating nitric oxide or upregulating its mediators, and drugs modulating endothelial function will also affect the combination therapy of thrombotic and cardiovascular diseases.

Index

695

About the Editors

ARTHUR A. SASAHARA is Professor of Medicine, Emeritus, Harvard Medical School, Boston, Massachusetts, and Senior Physician, Cardiovascular Division, Department of Medicine, Brigham and Women's Hospital, Boston, Massachusetts. He is the author, coauthor, editor, or coeditor of numerous journal articles, book chapters and books. He is a Fellow of the American College of Cardiology, the American Heart Association, the American College of Physicians, the American College of Chest Physicians, the International Society for Thrombosis and Hemostasis, and the International Society for Fibrinolysis and Thrombolysis, among others. In 1987, he became Venture Head, Thrombolysis Research, in 1993, Senior Venture Head, and in 1995, Senior Medical Consultant, Research and Development, Pharmaceutical Products Division, Abbott Laboratories, Abbott Park, Illinois. Dr. Sasahara received the A.B. degree (1951) from Oberlin College, Oberlin, Ohio, the M.D. degree (1955) from Case Western Reserve University School of Medicine, Cleveland, Ohio, and the A.M. (Hon.) degree (1974) from Harvard University, Cambridge, Massachusetts.

JOSEPH LOSCALZO is Wade Professor and Chairman, Department of Medicine, Professor of Biochemistry, and Director of the Whitaker Cardiovascular Institute, Boston University School of Medicine, Boston, Massachusetts. He is the author, coauthor, editor, or coeditor of numerous journal articles and book chapters and holds sixteen U.S. patents. He serves as Chair of the Board of Scientific Counselors of the National Heart, Lung, and Blood Institute of the National Institutes of Health and is Chair of the Research Committee of the American Heart Association. He is also an editorial board member for numerous journals, as well as Associate Editor of the New England Journal of Medicine. A Fellow of the American College of Cardiology, the American Heart Association Council on Clinical Cardiology, the American College of Physicians, and the Molecular Medicine Society, he is a member of the American Society for Clinical Investigations and the Association of American Physicians, among other organizations. Dr. Loscalzo received the A.B. degree (1972), the Ph.D. degree (1977) in biochemistry, and the M.D. degree (1977) from the University of Pennsylvania, Philadelphia.

ISBN 0-8247-0795-8

90000